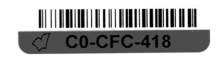

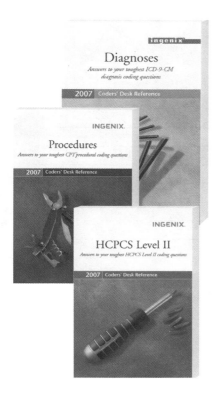

Get answers to your toughest coding questions from the experts.

2007 Coders' Desk Reference for Procedures

Item No.: 5700 $129.95
Available: December 2006   ISBN: 978-1-56337-848-5

2007 Coders' Desk Reference for Diagnoses

Item No.: 4995 $129.95
Available: September 2006   ISBN: 978-1-56337-921-5

2007 Coders' Desk Reference for HCPCS Level II

Item No.: 1083 $129.95
Available: December 2006   ISBN: 978-1-56337-849-2

With the nationwide shortage of coders continuing, new coders are expected to be proficient right away...while experienced coders are under pressure to be more productive than ever before. That's why Ingenix has created a comprehensive *Coders' Desk Reference* suite for all three code sets, creating an essential power suite for every health care professional.

- **Decrease coding time with comprehensive lay descriptions.** Clinical explanations clarify procedures in *Coders' Desk Reference for Procedures,* indicate the disease processes and causes of conditions in *Coders' Desk Reference for Diagnoses* and simplify HCPCS Level II codes by describing supplies and services in *Coders' Desk Reference for HCPCS Level II.*

- **Reduce costly claim delays and denials by always using the latest code sets.** All *Coders' Desk References* conform to standard code book organization and use updated codes for 2007.

- **New coders: Master the intricacies of coding, documentation and billing.** Veteran health care professionals:

Code faster and more efficiently. The suite offers advice to avoid common coding errors and includes anatomical charts, eponyms, acronyms and medical abbreviations.

INGENIX

Order Form

Information

Customer No. _____ Contact No. _____
Source Code _____
Contact Name _____
Title _____ Specialty _____
Company _____
Street Address _____
City (NO PO BOXES, PLEASE) _____ State _____ Zip _____
Telephone ( ) _____ Fax ( ) _____
IN CASE WE HAVE QUESTIONS ABOUT YOUR ORDER
E-mail _____ @ _____
REQUIRED FOR ORDER CONFIRMATION AND SELECT PRODUCT DELIVERY

Ingenix respects your right to privacy. We will not sell or rent your e-mail address or fax number to anyone outside Ingenix and its business partners. If you would like to remove your name from Ingenix promotion, please call 1.800.ingenix (464.3649), option 1.

Product

Item No.	Qty	Description	Price	Total

Subtotal _____
UT & VA residents, please add applicable Sales tax _____
(See chart on the left) Shipping & handling charges _____
All foreign orders, please call for shipping costs
Total _____

Payment

○Please bill my credit card ○MasterCard ○VISA ○Amex ○Discover
Card No. _____ Expires ___ (MONTH YEAR)
Signature _____
○Check enclosed, made payable to: Ingenix, Inc. ○Please bill my office
Purchase Order No. _____
ATTACH COPY OF PURCHASE ORDER

©2006 Ingenix, Inc. All prices subject to change without notice.

FOBA7

INGENIX®

CPT® Expert

2007

Notice

American Medical Association Notice

Our Commitment to Accuracy

Continuing Education Units for Certified Members of the American Academy of Professional Coders

Copyright

Acknowledgments

Brad Ericson, MPC, CPC, CPC-OS, *Product Manager*

Michael E. Desposito, *Director of Client Relations/Product Director*

Lynn Speirs, *Senior Director, Editorial/Desktop Publishing*

Karen Schmidt, BSN, *Technical Director*

Stacy Perry, *Manager, Desktop Publishing*

Lisa Singley, *Project Manager*

Wendy Gabbert, CPC, CPC-H, *Clinical/Technical Editor*

Karen H. Kachur, RN, CPC, *Clinical/Technical Editor*

Regina Magnani, RHIT, *Clinical/Technical Editor*

Sheri Poe Bernard, CPC, CPC-H, CPC-P, *Clinical/Technical Editor*

Kerrie Hornsby, *Desktop Publishing Specialist*

Kate Holden, *Editor*

About the Contributors

Wendy Gabbert, CPC, CPC-H
Clinical/Technical Editor

Ms. Gabbert has more than 20 years of experience in the health care field. She has extensive background in CPT/HCPCS and ICD-9-CM coding. She served several years as a coding consultant. Her areas of expertise include physician and hospital CPT coding assessments, chargemaster reviews, and the Outpatient Prospective Payment System (OPPS). She is a member of the American Academy of Professional Coders (AAPC).

Karen H. Kachur, RN, CPC
Clinical/Technical Editor

Ms. Kachur is a Clinical/Technical Editor for Ingenix with expertise in CPT/HCPCS and ICD-9-CM coding, in addition to physician billing, compliance, and fraud and abuse. Prior to joining Ingenix, she worked for many years as a staff RN in a variety of clinical settings including medicine, surgery, intensive care, psychiatry, and geriatrics. Ms Kachur has served as assistant director of a hospital utilization management and quality assurance department. She also has extensive experience as a nurse reviewer for Blue Cross/Blue Shield.

Regina Magnani, RHIT
Clinical/Technical Editor

Ms. Magnani has 25 years of experience in the health care industry in both health information management and patient financial services. Her areas of expertise include patient financial services, CPT/HCPCS and ICD-9-CM coding, the outpatient prospective payment system (OPPS), and chargemaster development and maintenance. She is an active member of the Healthcare Financial Management Association (HFMA), the American Health Information Management Association (AHIMA), and the American Association of Heathcare Administrative Management (AAHAM).

Sheri Poe Bernard, CPC, CPC-H, CPC-P
Clinical/Technical Editor

Ms. Bernard has been involved in product development at Ingenix for more than 14 years. She is currently secretary of the American Academy of Professional Coders' National Advisory Board, where she has served for six years. Prior to joining Ingenix, Ms. Bernard was a journalist specializing in medical reporting.

Contents

Introduction

Welcome to the Ingenix *CPT® Expert*, the definitive procedure coding source that combines the work of the American Medical Association (AMA) with the technical components you need for proper reimbursement and coding accuracy. *CPT Expert* not only provides you with the most recent version of the AMA's Physicians' Current Procedural Terminology (CPT®), but also with detailed coding instructions, clinical guidelines, lay definitions of complex procedures and medical terms, and summaries of the coverage policies used by federal and commercial payers.

CPT Expert includes the information needed to submit claims to commercial payers or federal intermediaries and carriers, and is correct at the time of printing. However, commercial payers and CMS may change payment rules at any time throughout the year. Commercial payers will announce changes through monthly news or information posted on their Web sites. CMS will post changes in policy on its website at *http://www.cms.hhs.gov/transmittals*. Local coverage determinations (LCDs) provide individual carrier guidelines for specific services. The existence of a procedure code does not imply coverage under any given insurance plan.

CPT Expert is based on the American Medical Association's Physicians' Current Procedural Terminology (CPT) coding system, which is copyrighted and owned by the physician organization. CPT is the nation's official, HIPAA compliant code set for procedures and services provided by physicians, ambulatory surgical centers, and hospital outpatient services, as well as laboratories, imaging centers, physical therapy clinics, urgent care centers, and others. **CPT Expert is not intended to be a replacement for the official AMA CPT manual.**

GETTING STARTED WITH *CPT EXPERT*

CPT Expert combines the most current material at publication time from the American Medical Association's CPT 2007, the Centers for Medicare and Medicaid Services online manual system, the Correct Coding Initiative, CMS fee schedules and rules, and Ingenix's own coding expertise.

Designed to be easy to use and full of information, this product is an excellent companion to your AMA CPT book, Medicare, Ingenix, or other resources. These are presented in black text or through use of an easy-to-spot color bar or icon. Coding guidelines, annotations and tips from Ingenix technical experts are designated in blue ink.

Icons derived from AMA guidelines or coding conventions are presented as circles. Icons derived from federal guidelines, data, or rules are square.

Blue Color Bar—Not Covered by Medicare
Services and procedures identified by this color bar are never a covered benefit under Medicare. Services and procedures that are not covered may be billed directly to the patient at the time of the service.

11975 Insertion, implantable contraceptive capsules ♀ Ⓔ

Yellow Color Bar—Unlisted Procedure
Unlisted CPT codes report procedures that have not been assigned a specific code number. An unlisted code delays payment due to the extra time necessary for review. When using an unlisted procedure code, include cover notes, documentation of medical necessity, and operative reports.

20999 Unlisted procedure, musculoskeletal system, general Ⓣ 80

Ⓣ Technical Component Only
Codes with this icon represent only the technical component (staff and equipment costs) of a procedure or service. Do not use either modifier 26 or TC with these codes.

77520 Proton treatment delivery; simple, without compensation Ⓢ Ⓣ

---

26 Professional Component
Only codes with this icon represent the physician's work or professional component of a procedure or service. Do not use either modifier 26 or TC with these codes.

77427 Radiation treatment management, five treatments Ⓔ 26 ▣

---

50 Bilateral Procedure
This icon identifies codes that can be reported bilaterally when the same surgeon provides the service for the same patient on the same date. Medicare allows payment for both procedures at 150 percent of the usual amount for one procedure. The modifier does not apply to bilateral procedures inclusive to one code.

27235 Percutaneous skeletal fixation of femoral fracture, proximal end, neck Ⓣ 50 ▣

---

80 Assist-at-Surgery Allowed

Services noted by this icon are allowed an assist at surgery with payment equal to 16 percent of the allowed amount for the global surgery for that procedure. No documentation is required.

80 Assist-at-Surgery Allowed with Documentation

Services noted by this icon are allowed an assistant at surgery with payment equal to 16 percent of the allowed amount for the global surgery for that procedure. Documentation is required.

+ Add-on Codes

This icon identifies procedures reported in addition to the primary procedure. The icon "+" denotes add-on codes. An add-on code is neither a stand-alone code nor subject to multiple procedure rules since it describes work in addition to the primary procedure.

⊘ Modifier 51 Exempt

Codes identified by this icon indicate that the procedure does not meet the definition of an add-on procedure and is not subject to multiple procedure rules.

⧉ Correct Coding Initiative (CCI)

CPT Expert identifies those codes with a corresponding CCI edit in Version 12.3, effective October 1, 2006. The CCI edits define correct coding practices that now serve as the basis of the national Medicare policy for paying claims. The code noted is the column 1 (comprehensive) code.

⊠ CLIA Waived Test

This icon identifies laboratory services that are not subject to the latest available Clinical Laboratory Improvement Amendments (CLIA) regulations.

⊚ Modifier 63 Exempt

This icon identifies procedures performed on infants that weigh less than 4 kg. Because of the complexity of performing procedures on infants less than 4 kg, this modifier may be added to the surgical codes to inform the payers of the special circumstance.

1–9 ASC Group

This icon identifies a service that is on the latest available list of Medicare covered ASC procedures, and identifies the ASC group, effective January 1, 2007.

⊙ Conscious Sedation

This icon identifies procedures that include conscious sedation. Conscious sedation codes should not be reported with these procedures.

A Age Edit

This icon denotes codes intended for use with a specific age group, such as neonate, newborn, pediatric, and adult. Carefully review the code description to assure the code you report most appropriately reflects the patient's age.

30460 Rhinoplasty for nasal deformity secondary to congenital cleft lip and/or palate, including columellar lengthening; tip only **7 62 80 ↵**

30400 Rhinoplasty, primary; lateral and alar cartilages and/or elevation of nasal tip **4 62 80 ↵**

+ 22216 each additional vertebral segment (List separately in addition to primary procedure) **62 ↵**

⊘ 50327 Backbench reconstruction of cadaver or living donor renal allograft prior to transplantation; venous anastomosis, each **62 80 ↵**

12051 Layer closure of wounds of face, ears, eyelids, nose, lips and/or mucous membranes; 2.5 cm or less **64 ⧉**

84830 Ovulation tests, by visual color comparison methods for human luteinizing hormone **♀ 80 ⊠**

44055 Correction of malrotation by lysis of duodenal bands and/or reduction of midgut volvulus (eg, Ladd procedure) **C 80 N1 ⊚**

50393 Introduction of ureteral catheter or stent into ureter through renal pelvis for drainage and/or injection, percutaneous **1 66 50 ↵**

⊙ 92986 Percutaneous balloon valvuloplasty; aortic valve **66 80 ↵**

49580 Repair umbilical hernia, younger than age 5 years; reducible **A 4 66 80 ↵**

M Maternity This icon identifies procedures that by definition should only be used for maternity patients generally between 12 and 55 years of age.	**59871** Removal of cerclage suture under anesthesia (other than local) Ⓜ ♀ 5 T 80 ⤴
♀ Female Only This icon identifies procedures that should only be reported for female patients.	**57220** Plastic operation on urethral sphincter, vaginal approach (eg, Kelly urethral plication) ♀ 3 T 80 ⤴
♂ Male Only This icon identifies procedures that should only be reported for male patients.	**52500** Transurethral resection of bladder neck (separate procedure) ♂ 3 T ⤴
MED: This notation precedes an instruction pertaining to this code in the Centers for Medicare and Medicaid Services' (CMS) Publication 100 (Pub 100) electronic manual or in a National Coverage Decision (NCD). These CMS sources present the rules for submitting these services to the federal government or its contractors and are included in the appendix of this book.	**46615** with ablation of tumor(s), polyp(s), or other lesion(s) not amenable to removal by hot biopsy forceps, bipolar cautery or snare technique 2 T 80 ⤴ **MED:** 100-2, 15, 260; 100-3, 100.2; 100-4, 12, 90.3; 100-4, 14, 10
AMA: This indicates discussion of the code in the American Medical Association's (AMA) *CPT Assistant* newsletter. Use the citation to find the correct issue.	**46083** Incision of thrombosed hemorrhoid, external 66 ⤴ **AMA:** 1997, Jun, 10
✔ Drug Not Approved by FDA The AMA CPT Editorial Panel is publishing new vaccine product codes prior to FDA approval. This symbol indicates which of these codes are pending FDA approval at press time. Check the Ingenix OnLine Web site (http://www.ingenixonline.com/content/pn/) or AMA Web site (http://www.ama-assn.org/ama/pub/category/3113.html) for updates to these codes as they pass through the FDA process.	Ø ✔ **90698** Diphtheria, tetanus toxoids, acellular pertussis vaccine, haemophilus influenza Type B, and poliovirus vaccine, inactivated (STaP - Hib - IPV), for intramuscular use

Ⓐ–Ⓨ OPPS OPSI Status Indicators

Status indicators identify how individual CPT codes are paid or not paid under the latest available hospital outpatient prospective payment system (OPPS). The same status indicator is assigned to all the codes within an Ambulatory Payment Classification (APC). Consult your payer or resource to learn which CPT codes fall within various APCs.

Ⓐ Indicates services that are paid under some other method such as the DMEPOS fee schedule or the physician fee schedule

Ⓑ Indicates codes that should not be used on an OPPS hospital outpatient bill (types 12X and 13X). Codes may be allowable on other types of bills.

Ⓒ Indicates inpatient procedures that are not paid under the OPPS

Ⓔ Indicates services for which payment is not allowed under the OPPS. In some instances, the service is not covered by Medicare. In other instances, Medicare does not use the code in question, but does use another code to describe the service

Ⓕ Corneal Tissue Acquisition; Certain CRNA Services; and Hepatitis B Vaccines which are paid at reasonable cost

Ⓖ Indicates a current drug or biological for which payment is made under the transitional pass-through payment methodology

Ⓗ Indicates a device for which payment is made under the transitional pass-through payment methodology

Ⓚ Indicates non-pass-through drugs and biologicals. radiopharmaceutical agents, brachytherapy sources, and blood and blood products

Ⓛ Indicates influenza or pneumonia vaccine paid as reasonable cost with no deductible or coinsurance

Ⓜ Services not billable to the fiscal intermediary and not payable under OPPS

Ⓝ Indicates services that are incidental, with payment packaged into another service or APC group

Ⓟ Indicates services paid only in partial hospitalization programs

Ⓠ Indicates packaged services subject to separate payment under OPPS payment methodology and paid when criteria is met

Ⓢ Indicates significant procedures for which payment is allowed under the hospital OPPS but to which the multiple procedure reduction does not apply

Ⓣ Indicates surgical services for which payment is allowed under the hospital OPPS. Services with this payment indicator are the only service to which the multiple procedure payment reduction applies

Ⓥ Indicates medical visits for which payment is allowed under the hospital OPPS

Ⓧ Indicates ancillary services for which payment is allowed under the hospital OPPS

Ⓨ Indicates nonimplantable durable medical equipment (DME) that is not paid under OPPS. True DME. Providers other than home health agencies bill to the DMERC.

Effective January 1, 2007

50393   **Introduction of ureteral catheter or stent into ureter through renal pelvis for drainage and/or injection, percutaneous** Ⓘ Ⓣ 50 ↵

For more information about ongoing development of the CPT coding system, consult the AMA Web site at URL http://www.ama-assn.org/

You may subscribe to an e-mail service to receive special reports when information in this book changes. Contact customer service at 1-800-INGENIX, option 1.

NOTE: All data current as of November 7, 2006.

Aorta — *continued*
Repair — *continued*
Thoracic Aneurysm with Graft, 33860-33877
Endovascular, 33880-33891, 75956-75959
Transposition of the Great Vessels, 33770-33781
Suspension, 33800
Suture, 33320-33322
Thoracic
Aneurysm, 33880-33889, 75956-75959
Ultrasound, 76770, 76775
Valve
Incision, 33415
Repair, 33400-33403
Left Ventricle, 33414
Supravalvular Stenosis, 33417
Replacement, 33405-33413
X-ray with Contrast, 75600-75630
Aorta–Pulmonary ART Transposition
See Transposition, Great Arteries
Aortic Sinus
See Sinus of Valsalva
Aortic Stenosis
Repair, 33415
Supravalvular, 33417
Aortic Valve
See Heart, Aortic Valve
Aortic Valve Replacement
See Replacement, Aortic Valve
Aortocoronary Bypass
See Coronary Artery Bypass Graft (CABG)
Aortocoronary Bypass for Heart Revascularization
See Artery, Coronary, Bypass
Aortography, 75600, 75605, 75630, 93544
with Ileofemoral Artery, 75630
See Angiography
Serial, 75625
Aortoiliac
Embolectomy, 34151, 34201
Thrombectomy, 34151, 34201
Aortopexy, 33800
Aortoplasty
Supravalvular Stenosis, 33417
AP, 51797
Apert–Gallais Syndrome
See Adrenogenital Syndrome
Apexcardiogram, 93799
Aphasia Testing, 96105
Apheresis
Therapeutic, 36511-36516
Apical–Aortic Conduit, 33404
Apicectomy
with Mastoidectomy, 69530, 69605
Petrous, 69530
Apicoectomy, 41899
Apoaminotransferase, Aspartate, 84550
Apolipoprotein
Blood or Urine, 82172
Appendectomy, 44950-44960
Laparoscopic, 44970
Appendiceal Abscess
See Abscess, Appendix
Appendico–Stomy, 44799
Appendico–Vesicostomy
Cutaneous, 50845
Appendix
Abscess
Incision and Drainage, 44900
Open, 44900
Percutaneous, 44901
Excision, 44950-44960
Application
Allergy Tests, 95044
Bone Fixation Device
Multiplane, 20692
Uniplane, 20690
Caliper, 20660
Cranial Tongs, 20660

Application — *continued*
Fixation Device
Shoulder, 23700
Halo
Cranial, 20661
Thin Skull Osteology, 20664
Femoral, 20663
Maxillofacial Fixation, 21100
Pelvic, 20662
Interdental Fixation Device, 21110
Neurostimulation, 64550
Radioelement, 77761-77778
with Ultrasound, 76965
Surface, 77789
Stereotactic Frame, 20660
Application of External Fixation Device
See Fixation (Device), Application, External
APPT
See Thromboplastin, Partial, Time
APPY, 44950-44960
APTT
See Thromboplastin, Partial, Time
Aquatic Therapy
with Exercises, 97113
Aqueous Shunt
to Extraocular Reservoir, 66180
Revision, 66185
Arch, Zygomatic
See Zygomatic Arch
Arm
See Radius; Ulna; Wrist
Excision
Bone, 25145
Excess Skin, 15836
Lipectomy, Suction Assisted, 15878
Removal
Foreign Body
Forearm or Wrist, 25248
Repair
Muscle, 24341
Tendon, 24341
Skin Graft
Delay of Flap, 15610
Full Thickness, 15220, 15221
Muscle, Myocutaneous, or Fasciocutaneous Flaps, 15736
Pedicle Flap, 15572
Split, 15100-15111
Tissue Transfer, Adjacent, 14020, 14021
Arm, Lower
Abscess, 25028
Excision, 25145
Incision and Drainage Bone, 25035
Amputation, 24900, 24920, 25900, 25905, 25915
Cineplasty, 24940
Revision, 25907, 25909
Angiography, 73206
Artery
Ligation, 37618
Biopsy, 25065, 25066
Bursa
Incision and Drainage, 25031
Bypass Graft, 35903
Cast, 29075
CT Scan, 73200-73206
Decompression, 25020-25025
Exploration
Blood Vessel, 35860
Fasciotomy, 24495, 25020-25025
Hematoma, 25028
Incision and Drainage, 23930
Lesion, Tendon Sheath
Excision, 25110
Magnetic Resonance Imaging (MRI), 73218-73220, 73223
Reconstruction
Ulna, 25337
Removal
Foreign Body, 25248

Arm, Lower — *continued*
Repair
Blood Vessel with Other Graft, 35266
Blood Vessel with Vein Graft, 35236
Decompression, 24495
Muscle, 25260, 25263, 25270
Secondary, 25265
Secondary
Muscle or Tendon, 25272, 25274
Tendon, 25260-25274, 25280-25295, 25310-25316
Secondary, 25265
Tendon Sheath, 25275
Replantation, 20805
Splint, 29125, 29126
Tenotomy, 25290
Tumor
Excision, 25075-25077
Ultrasound, 76880
Unlisted Services and Procedures, 25999
X-ray, 73090
with Upper Arm, 73092
Arm, Upper
Abscess
Incision and Drainage, 23930
See Elbow; Humerus
Amputation, 23900-23921, 24900, 24920
with Implant, 24931, 24935
Cineplasty, 24940
Revision, 24925, 24930
Angiography, 73206
Artery
Ligation, 37618
Biopsy, 24065, 24066
Bypass Graft, 35903
Cast, 29065
CT Scan, 73200-73206
Exploration
Blood Vessel, 35860
Hematoma
Incision and Drainage, 23930
Magnetic Resonance Imaging (MRI), 73218-73220, 73223
Muscle Revision, 24330, 24331
Removal
Cast, 29705
Foreign Body, 24200, 24201
Repair
Blood Vessel with Other Graft, 35266
Blood Vessel with Vein Graft, 35236
Muscle Revision, 24301, 24320
Muscle Transfer, 24301, 24320
Tendon, 24332
Tendon Lengthening, 24305
Tendon Revision, 24320
Tendon Transfer, 24301
Tenotomy, 24310
Replantation, 20802
Splint, 29105
Tumor
Excision, 24075-24077
Penetrating, 20103
Ultrasound, 76880
Unlisted Services and Procedures, 24999
Wound Exploration, 20103
X-ray, 73060
X-ray with Lower Arm
Infant, 73092
Arnold–Chiari Malformation Repair, 61343
AROM, 95851, 95852, 97110, 97530
Arrest, Epiphyseal
See Epiphyseal Arrest
Arrhythmias
Electrical Conversion Anesthesia, 00410
Induction, 93618

Arrhythmogenic Focus
Heart
Catheter Ablation, 93650-93652
Destruction, 33250, 33251
Arsenic, 82175
Heavy Metal Screen, 83015
ART, 86592, 86593
Arterial Catheterization
See Cannulation, Arterial
Arterial Dilatation, Transluminal
See Angioplasty, Transluminal
Arterial Grafting for Coronary Artery Bypass
See Bypass Graft, Coronary Artery, Arterial
Arterial Pressure
See Blood Pressure
Arterial Puncture, 36600
Arteriography, Aorta
See Aortography
Arteriosus, Ductus
See Ductus Arteriosus
Arteriosus, Truncus
See Truncus Arteriosus
Arteriotomy
See Incision, Artery; Transection, Artery
Arteriovenous Anastomosis, 36818-36820
Arteriovenous Fistula
Cannulization
Vein, 36815
Repair
Abdomen, 35182
Acquired or Traumatic, 35189
Head, 35180
Acquired or Traumatic, 35188
Lower Extremity, 35184
Acquired or Traumatic, 35190
Neck, 35180
Acquired or Traumatic, 35188
Thorax, 35182
Acquired or Traumatic, 35189
Upper Extremity, 35184
Acquired or Traumatic, 35190
Revision
Hemodialysis Graft or Fistula
with Thrombectomy, 36833
without Thrombectomy, 36832
Thrombectomy
Dialysis Graft
without Revision, 36831
Graft, 36870
Arteriovenous Malformation
Cranial
Repair, 61680-61692, 61705, 61708
Spinal
Excision, 63250-63252
Injection, 62294
Repair, 63250-63252
Arteriovenous Shunt
Angiography, 75790
Catheterization, 36145
Artery
Abdomen
Angiography, 75726
Catheterization, 36245-36248
Ligation, 37617
Adrenal
Angiography, 75731, 75733
Anastomosis
Cranial, 61711
Angiography, Visceral, 75726
Angioplasty, 75962-75968
Aorta
Angioplasty, 35452
Atherectomy, 35481, 35491
Aortoiliac
Embolectomy, 34151, 34201
Thrombectomy, 34151, 34201
Aortoiliofemoral, 35363
Arm
Angiography, 75710, 75716
Harvest of Artery for Coronary Artery Bypass Graft, 35600

Index

Artery — Arthrodesis

Index (side tab)

Biopsy — Blood (side tab)

Blood — *continued*
Nuclear Medicine
 Flow Imaging, 78445
 Plasma Iron
 Red Cell, 78140
 Red Cell Survival, 78130, 78135
Occult, 82270
Osmolality, 83930
Other Sources, 82271
Plasma
 Exchange, 36514-36516
Platelet
 Aggregation, 85576
 Automated Count, 85049
 Count, 85008
 Manual Count, 85032
Reticulocyte, 85046
Stem Cell
 Donor Search, 38204
 Harvesting, 38205-38206
 Transplantation, 38240-38242
  Cell Concentration, 38215
  Cryopreservation, 38207, 88240
  Plasma Depletion, 38214
  Platelet Depletion, 38213
  Red Blood Cell Depletion, 38212
  T–cell Depletion, 38210
  Thawing, 38208, 88241
  Tumor Cell Depletion, 38211
  Washing, 38209
Transfusion, 36430, 36440
 Exchange, 36455
 Newborn, 36450
 Fetal, 36460
 Push
  Infant, 36440
Unlisted Services and Procedures, 85999
Urine, 83491
Viscosity, 85810
Blood Banking
Frozen Blood Preparation, 86930-86932
Frozen Plasma Preparation, 86927
Physician Services, 86077-86079
Blood Cell
CD4 and CD8
 Including Ratio, 86360
Enzyme Activity, 82657
Exchange, 36511-36513
Sedimentation Rate
 Automated, 85652
 Manual, 85651
Blood Cell Count
Automated, 85049
B–Cells, 86355
Blood Smear, 85007, 85008
Differential WBC Count, 85004-85007, 85009
Hematocrit, 85014
Hemoglobin, 85018
Hemogram
 Added Indices, 85025-85027
 Automated, 85025-85027
 Manual, 85032
Microhematocrit, 85013
Natural Killer (NK) Cells, 86357
Red
 See Red Blood Cell (RBC), Count
Red Blood Cell, 85041
Reticulocyte, 85044, 85045
Stem Cells, 86367
T Cell, 86359-86361
White
 See White Blood Cell, Count
White Blood Cell, 85032, 85048, 89055
Blood Clot
Assay, 85396
Clot Lysis Time, 85175
Clot Retraction, 85170
Clotting Factor, 85250-85293
Clotting Factor Test, 85210-85244

Blood Clot — *continued*
Clotting Inhibitors, 85300-85302, 85305, 85307
Coagulation Time, 85345-85348
Factor Inhibitor Test, 85335
Blood Coagulation
Factor I, 85384, 85385
Factor II, 85210
Factor III, 85730, 85732
Factor IV, 82310
Factor IX, 85250
Factor V, 85220
Factor VII, 85230
Factor VIII, 85244, 85247
Factor X, 85260
Factor XI, 85270
Factor XIII, 85290, 85291
Blood Coagulation Defect
See Coagulopathy
Blood Coagulation Disorders
See Clot
Blood Coagulation Test
See Coagulation
Blood Component Removal
See Apheresis
Blood Count, Complete
See Complete Blood Count (CBC)
Blood Flow Check, Graft, 15860, 90940
Blood Gases
02, 82803-82810
by Pulse Oximetry, 94760
CO2, 82803
HCO3, 82803
Hemoglobin–Oxygen Affinity, 82820
O2 Saturation, 82805, 82810
p02, 82803
pCO2, 82803
pH, 82800, 82803
Blood Letting
See Phlebotomy
Blood Lipoprotein
See Lipoprotein
Blood, Occult
See Occult Blood
Blood Pool Imaging, 78472, 78473, 78481, 78483, 78494, 78496
Blood Pressure
Left Ventricular Filling, 0086T
Monitoring, 24 hour, 93784-93790
Venous, 93770
Blood Products
Irradiation, 86945
Pooling, 86965
Splitting, 86985
Blood Sample
Fetal, 59030
Blood Serum
See Serum
Blood Smear, 85060
Blood Syndrome
Chromosomal Analysis, 88245, 88248
Blood Test(s)
Nuclear Medicine
 Plasma Volume, 78110, 78111
 Platelet Survival, 78190, 78191
 Red Cell Volume, 78120, 78121
 Whole Blood Volume, 78122
Panels
 Electrolyte, 80051
 General Health Panel, 80050
 Hepatic Function, 80076
 Hepatitis, Acute, 80074
 Lipid Panel, 80061
 Metabolic
  Basic, 80048
  Comprehensive, 80053
 Obstetric Panel, 80055
 Renal Function, 80069
Volume Determination, 78122
Blood Transfusion, Autologous
See Autotransfusion
Blood Typing
ABO Only, 86900
Antigen Screen, 86903, 86904
Crossmatch, 86920-86922

Blood Typing — *continued*
Other RBC Antigens, 86905
Paternity Testing, 86910, 86911
Rh(D), 86901
Rh Phenotype, 86906
Blood Urea Nitrogen, 84520, 84525
Blood Vessel(s)
See Artery; Vein
Angioscopy
 Noncoronary, 35400
Endoscopy
 Surgical, 37500
Excision
 Arteriovenous
  Malformation, 63250-63252
Exploration
 Abdomen, 35840
 Chest, 35820
 Extremity, 35860
 Neck, 35800
Great
 Suture, 33320, 33321
Harvest
 Endoscopic, 33508
 Lower Extremity Vein, 35572
 Upper Extremity Artery, 35600
 Upper Extremity Vein, 35500
Kidney
 Repair, 50100
Repair
 Abdomen, 35221, 35251, 35281
  with Composite Graft, 35681-35683
  with Other Graft, 35281
  with Vein Graft, 35251
  See Aneurysm Repair; Fistula, Repair
 Aneurysm, 61705-61710
 Arteriovenous Malformation, 61680-61692, 61705-61710, 63250-63252
 Chest, 35211, 35216
  with Composite Graft, 35681-35683
  with Other Graft, 35271, 35276
  with Vein Graft, 35241, 35246
 Direct, 35201-35226
 Finger, 35207
 Graft Defect, 35870
 Hand, 35207
 Kidney, 50100
 Lower Extremity, 35226
  with Composite Graft, 35681-35683
  with Other Graft, 35271, 35276
  with Vein Graft, 35241, 35246
 Neck, 35201
  with Composite Graft, 35681-35683
  with Other Graft, 35261
  with Vein Graft, 35231
 Upper Extremity, 35206
  with Composite Graft, 35681-35683
  with Other Graft, 35266
  with Vein Graft, 35236
Shunt Creation
 with Bypass Graft, 35686
 with Graft, 36825, 36830
 Direct, 36821
 Thomas Shunt, 36835
Shunt Revision
 with Graft, 36832
Suture Repair, Great Vessels, 33320-33322
Bloom Syndrome
Chromosome Analysis, 88245
Blot Test, Ink
See Inkblot Test
Blotting, Western
See Western Blot
Blow–Out Fracture
Orbital Floor, 21385-21395

Blue, Dome Cyst
See Breast, Cyst
BMT, 38240, 38241, 38242
Boarding Home Care, 99324-99337
Bodies, Acetone
See Acetone Body
Bodies, Barr
See Barr Bodies
Bodies, Carotid
See Carotid Body
Bodies, Ciliary
See Ciliary Body
Bodies, Heinz
See Heinz Bodies
Bodies, Inclusion
See Inclusion Bodies
Bodies, Ketone
See Ketone Bodies
Body Cast
Halo, 29000
Removal, 29700, 29710, 29715
Repair, 29720
Risser Jacket, 29010, 29015
Turnbuckle Jacket, 29020, 29025
Upper Body and One Leg, 29044
Upper Body Only, 29035
Upper Body with Head, 29040
Upper Body with Legs, 29046
Body Composition
Dual Energy X–Ray Absorptiometry, 0028T
Body Fluid
Crystal Identification, 89060
Body of Vertebra
See Vertebral Body
Body Section
X-ray, 76100
 Motion, 76101, 76102
Body System, Neurologic
See Nervous System
BOH, 93600
Bohler Procedure, 28405
Bohler Splinting, 29515
Boil
See Furuncle
Boil, Vulva
See Abscess, Vulva
Bone
See Specific Bone
Ablation
 Tumor, 20982
Biopsy, 20220-20245
CT Scan
 Density Study, 77078-77079
Cyst
 Drainage, 20615
 Injection, 20615
Dual Energy X–ray
 Absorptiometry, 77080-77082
Excision
 Epiphyseal Bar, 20150
 Facial Bones, 21026
 Mandible, 21025
Fixation
 Caliper, 20660
 Cranial Tong, 20660
 External, 20690
 Halo, 20661-20663
 Interdental, 21110
 Multiplane, 20692
 Pin
  Wire, 20650
 Skeletal
  Humeral Epicondyle
   Percutaneous, 24566
  Stereotactic Frame, 20660
  Uniplane, 20690
Insertion
 Needle, 36680
 Osseointegrated Implant
  for External Speech Processor/Cochlear Stimulator, 69714-69718
Nuclear Medicine
 Density Study, 78350, 78351
 Imaging, 78300-78320

Index

Bone — Brain Ventriculography

Branchial Cleft
Cyst
Excision, 42810, 42815
Branchioma
See Branchial Cleft, Cyst
Breast
Abscess
Incision and Drainage, 19020
Augmentation, 19324, 19325
Bioimpedance, 0060T
Biopsy, 19100-19103
Cyst
Puncture Aspiration, 19000,
19001
Excision
Biopsy, 19100-19103
Capsules, 19371
Chest Wall Tumor, 19260-19272
Cyst, 19120
Lactiferous Duct Fistula, 19112
Lesion, 19120-19126
by Needle Localization, 19125,
19126
Mastectomy, 19300-19307
Nipple Exploration, 19110
Exploration, 19020
Implants
Insertion, 19340, 19342
Preparation of Moulage, 19396
Removal, 19328, 19330
Supply, 19396
Incision
Capsules, 19370
Injection
Radiologic, 19030
Magnetic Resonance Imaging (MRI),
77058-77059
Mammoplasty
Augmentation, 19324, 19325
Reduction, 19318
Mastopexy, 19316
Metallic Localization Clip Placement,
19295
Needle Biopsy, 19100
Needle Wire Placement, 19290,
19291
Periprosthetic Capsulectomy, 19371
Periprosthetic Capsulotomy, 19370
Reconstruction
with Free Flap, 19364
with Latissimus Dorsi Flap,
19361
with Other Techniques, 19366
with Tissue Expander, 19357
with Transverse Rectus Abdomi-
nis Myocutaneous (TRAM)
Flap, 19367-19369
Augmentation, 19324, 19325
Mammoplasty, 19318-19325
Nipple and Areola, 19350
Correction Inverted Nipples,
19355
Revision, 19380
Reduction, 19318
Removal
Capsules, 19371
Modified Radical, 19307
Partial, 19300
Radical, 19305-19307
Simple, Complete, 19303
Subcutaneous, 19304
Repair
Suspension, 19316
Stereotactic Localization, 77031
Ultrasound, 76645
Unlisted Services and Procedures,
19499
X-ray, 77055-77056, 77057
with Computer-aided Detection,
77051-77052
Mammography, 77051-77052
Localization Nodule, 77032
Breathing, Inspiratory Positive-Pres-
sure
See Intermittent Positive Pressure
Breathing (IPPB)

Breath Odor Alcohol
See Alcohol, Breath
Breath Test
Alcohol, Ethyl, 82075
Heart Transplant Rejection, 0085T
Helicobacter Pylori, 78267, 78268,
83013, 83014
Hydrogen, 91065
Bricker Operation
Intestines Anastomosis, 50820
Bristow Procedure, 23450-23462
Capsulorrhaphy, Anterior, 23450-
23462
Brock Operation, 33470-33475
Valvotomy, Pulmonary Valve, 33470-
33474
Broken, Nose
See Fracture, Nasal Bone
Bronchi
Aspiration
Catheter, 31720-31725
Endoscopic, 31645-31646
Biopsy
Endoscopic, 31625-31629,
31632, 31633
Brushing
Protected Brushing, 31623
Catheterization
with Bronchial Brush Biopsy,
31717
Insertion
with Intracavitary Radioele-
ment, 31643
Endoscopy
Aspiration, 31645, 31646
Biopsy, 31625, 31628, 31629,
31632, 31633
Destruction
Tumor, 31641
Dilation, 31630-31631, 31636-
31638
Excision
Lesion, 31640
Exploration, 31622
Foreign Body Removal, 31635
Fracture, 31630
Injection, 31656
Lesion, 31640, 31641
Stenosis, 31641
Tumor, 31640, 31641
Ultrasound, 31620
Exploration
Endoscopic, 31622
Fracture
Endoscopy, 31630
Injection
X-ray, 31656, 31715
Instillation
Contrast Material
Needle Biopsy, 31629, 31633
Reconstruction
Graft Repair, 31770
Stenosis, 31775
Removal
Foreign Body, 31635
Repair
Fistula, 32815
Stenosis
Endoscopic Treatment, 31641
Stent
Placement, 31636-31637
Revision, 31638
Tumor
Excision, 31640
Ultrasound, 31620
Unlisted Services and Procedures,
31899
X-ray
with Contrast, 71040, 71060
Bronchial Allergen Challenge
See Bronchial Challenge Test
Bronchial Alveolar Lavage, 31624
Bronchial Brush Biopsy
with Catheterization, 31717
Bronchial Brushings
Protected Brushing, 31623

Bronchial Challenge Test
with Antigens or Gases, 95071
with Chemicals, 95070
See also Allergy Tests
Bronchial Provocation Test
See Allergy Tests, Challenge Test,
Bronchial
Bronchoalveolar Lavage, 31624
Broncho-Bronchial Anastomosis,
32486
Bronchography, 71040, 71060
Catheterization
Injection
Transtracheal, 31715
Instillation
Contrast Material
Segmental
Injection, 31656
Bronchoplasty
Excision Stenosis and Anastomosis,
31775
Graft Repair, 31770
Reconstruction, Bronchi, 32501
Graft Repair, 31770
Stenosis, 31775
Bronchopneumonia, Hiberno-Vernal
See Q Fever
Bronchopulmonary Lavage, 31624
Bronchoscopy
Alveolar Lavage, 31624
Aspiration, 31645, 31646
Biopsy, 31625-31629, 31632, 31633
Brushing, Protected Brushing, 31623
Catheter Placement
Intracavity Radioelement, 31643
Diagnostic, 31622-31624, 31643
Dilation, 31630-31631, 31636-31638
Exploration, 31622
Fracture, 31630
Injection, 31656
Needle Biopsy, 31629, 31633
Removal
Foreign Body, 31635
Tumor, 31640, 31641
Stenosis, 31641
Stent Placement, 31631, 31636-
31637
Stent Revision, 31638
Ultrasound, 31620
X-ray Contrast, 31656
Bronchospasm Evaluation, 94060,
94070
Pulmonology, Diagnostic, Spirometry,
94010-94070
Bronkodyl
See Theophylline
Brow Ptosis
Repair, 67900
Brucella, 86000
Antibody, 86622
Bruise
See Hematoma
Brunschwig Operation, 58240
Pelvis, Exenteration, 58240
Brush Biopsy
Bronchi, 31717
Brush Border ab
See Antibody, Heterophile
BSO, 58720
Bucca
See Cheek
Buccal Mucosa
See Mouth, Mucosa
Bulbourethral Gland
Excision, 53250
Bulla
Incision and Drainage
Puncture Aspiration, 10160
Lung
Excision-Plication, 32141
Endoscopic, 32655
BUN, 84520-84545
Bunion Repair
with Implant, 28293
Bunionectomy, 28290-28299
Chevron Procedure, 28296

Bunion Repair — *continued*
Concentric Procedure, 28296
Joplin Procedure, 28294
Keller Procedure, 28292
Lapidus Procedure, 28297
Mayo Procedure, 28292
McBride Procedure, 28292
Mitchell Procedure, 28296
Silver Procedure, 28290
Burch Operation
Laparoscopic, 58152
Burgess Amputation
Disarticulation, Ankle, 27889
Burhenne Procedure, 43500
Bile Duct, Removal of Calculus,
43264, 47420, 47425, 47554
Percutaneous, 47630
Burkitt Herpesvirus
See Epstein-Barr Virus
Burns
Allograft, 15300-15321, 15330-
15336
Anesthesia, 01951-01953
Debridement, 15002-15003, 15004-
15005, 16020-16030
Dressing, 16020-16030
Escharotomy, 16035, 16036
Excision, 15002, 15004-15005
Initial Treatment, 16000
Tissue Culture Skin Grafts, 15100-
15157
Xenograft, 15400-15431
Burr Hole
Skull
with Injection, 61120
Biopsy, Brain, 61140
Catheterization, 61210
Drainage
Abscess, 61150, 61151
Cyst, 61150, 61151
Hematoma, 61154, 61156
Exploration
Infratentorial, 61253
Supratentorial, 61250
Implant
Cerebral Thermal Perfusion
Probe, 0077T
Neurostimulator Array,
61863-61868
Insertion
Catheter, 61210
Reservoir, 61210
Burrow's Operation, 14000-14350
Bursa
Ankle, 27604
Arm, Lower, 25031
Elbow
Excision, 24105
Incision and Drainage, 23931
Femur
Excision, 27062
Foot
Incision and Drainage, 28001
Hip
Incision and Drainage, 26991
Injection, 20600-20610
Ischial
Excision, 27060
Joint
Aspiration, 20600-20610
Drainage, 20600-20610
Injection, 20600-20610
Knee
Excision, 27340
Leg, Lower, 27604
Palm
Incision and Drainage, 26025,
26030
Pelvis
Incision and Drainage, 26991
Shoulder
Drainage, 23031
Wrist, 25031
Excision, 25115, 25116
Incision and Drainage, 25020
Infected Bursa, 25031

Cardiac Electroversion
See Cardioversion
Cardiac Event Recorder
Implantation, 33282
Removal, 33284
Cardiac Magnetic Resonance Imaging (CMRI)
Complete Study, 75554
Limited Study, 75555
Morphology, 75553
Velocity Flow Mapping, 75556
Cardiac Massage
Thoracotomy, 32160
Cardiac Output Measurement
by Indicator Dilution, 93561, 93562
Inert Gas Rebreathing
During Exercise, 0105T
During Rest, 0104T
Cardiac Pacemaker
See Heart, Pacemaker
Cardiac Rehabilitation, 93797, 93798
Cardiac Septal Defect
See Septal Defect
Cardiac Transplantation
See Heart, Transplantation
Cardiectomy
Donor, 33930, 33940
Cardioassist, 0049T, 92970, 92971
Cardiolipin Antibody, 86147
Cardiology
See Electrocardiography
Diagnostic
Acoustic Recording with Computer Analysis Heart Sounds, 0068T-0070T
Atrial Electrogram
Esophageal Recording, 93615, 93616
Cardioverter–Defibrillator
Evaluation and Testing, 93640-93642, 93741-93744
Echocardiography
Doppler, 93303-93321, 93662
Intracardiac, 93662
Transesophageal, 93318
Transthoracic, 93303-93317, 93350
Electrocardiogram
Evaluation, 93000, 93010, 93014
Microvolt T–wave, Alternans, 93025
Monitoring, 93224-93237
Patient–Demand, Single Event, 93268-93272
Rhythm, 93040-93042
Tracing, 93005
Transmission, 93012
Electrophysiologic
Follow–Up Study, 93624
Ergonovine Provocation Test, 93024
Evaluation
Heart Device, 93640
Heart
Stimulation and Pacing, 93623
Hemodynamic Monitoring
Non–invasive, 0086T
Implantable Loop Recorder System, 93727
Intracardiac Pacing and Mapping, 93631
3–D Mapping, 93613
Follow–up Study, 93624
Stimulation and Pacing, 93623
Intracardiac Pacing and Recording
Arrhythmia Induction, 93618-93620
Bundle of His, 93600
Comprehensive, 93619-93622
Intra–Atrial, 93602, 93610
Right Ventricle, 93603

Cardiology — continued
Diagnostic — continued
Intracardiac Pacing and Recording — continued
Tachycardia Sites, 93609
Ventricular, 93612
Intravascular Ultrasound, 92978, 92979
Left Ventricular Pressure Measurement, 0086T
M Mode and Real Time, 93307-93321
Pacemaker Testing, 93642
Antitachycardia System, 93724
Dual Chamber, 93731-93733
Leads, 93641
Single Chamber, 93734-93736
Perfusion Imaging, 78460, 78461
See Nuclear Medicine
Stress Tests
Cardiovascular, 93015-93018
Drug Induced, 93024
MUGA (Multiple Gated Acquisition), 78483
Tilt Table Evaluation, 93660
Vectorcardiogram
Evaluation, 93799
Tracing, 93799
Therapeutic
Angioplasty
Percutaneous, Transluminal, 92982, 92984
Cardioassist, 92970, 92971
Cardio Defibrillator Initial Set–up and Programming, 93745
Cardiopulmonary Resuscitation, 92950
Cardioversion, 92960, 92961
Intravascular Ultrasound, 92978, 92979
Pacing
Transcutaneous, Temporary, 92953
Thrombolysis
Coronary Vessel, 92975, 92977
Thrombolysis, Coronary, 92977
Valvuloplasty
Percutaneous, 92986, 92990
Cardiomyotomy
See Esophagomyotomy
Cardioplasty, 43320
Cardioplegia, 33999
Cardiopulmonary Bypass
with Prosthetic Valve Repair, 33496
Lung Transplant with
Double, 32854
Single, 32852
Cardiopulmonary Resuscitation, 92950
Cardiotomy, 33310, 33315
Cardiovascular Stress Test
See Exercise Stress Tests
Cardioversion, 92960, 92961
Care, Custodial
See Nursing Facility Services
Care, Intensive
See Intensive Care
Care, Neonatal Intensive
See Intensive Care, Neonatal
Care Plan Oversight Services
Home Health Agency Care, 99374, 99375
Hospice, 99377, 99378
Nursing Facility, 99379, 99380
Care, Self
See Self Care
Carneous Mole
See Abortion
Carnitine Total and Free, 82379
Carotene, 82380
Carotid Artery
Aneurysm Repair
Vascular Malformation or Carotid Cavernous Fistula, 61710

Carotid Artery — continued
Excision, 60605
Ligation, 37600-37606
Stent, Transcatheter Placement, 0075T-0076T
Transection
with Skull Base Surgery, 61609
Carotid Body
Lesion
Carotid Artery, 60605
Excision, 60600
Carotid, Common, 0126T
Carotid Pulse Tracing
with ECG Lead, 93799
Carpal Bone
See Wrist
Arthroplasty
with Implant, 25443
Cyst
Excision, 25130-25136
Dislocation
Closed Treatment, 25690
Open Treatment, 25695
Excision, 25210, 25215
Partial, 25145
Fracture, 25622-25628
with Manipulation, 25624, 25635
without Manipulation, 25622, 25630
Closed Treatment, 25622, 25630
Open Treatment, 25628, 25645
Incision and Drainage, 26034
Insertion
Vascular Pedicle, 25430
Osteoplasty, 25394
Repair, 25431-25440
Sequestrectomy, 25145
Tumor
Excision, 25130-25136
Carpals
Incision and Drainage, 25035
Carpal Tunnel
Injection
Therapeutic, 20526
Carpal Tunnel Syndrome
Decompression, 64721
Carpectomy, 25210, 25215
Carpometacarpal Joint
Arthrodesis
Hand, 26843, 26844
Thumb, 26841, 26842
Arthrotomy, 26070, 26100
Biopsy
Synovium, 26100
Dislocation
Closed Treatment, 26670
with Manipulation, 26675, 26676
Open Treatment, 26685, 26686
Exploration, 26070
Fusion
Hand, 26843, 26844
Thumb, 26841, 26842
Removal
Foreign Body, 26070
Repair, 25447
Synovectomy, 26130
Cartilage, Arytenoid
See Arytenoid
Cartilage, Ear
See Ear Cartilage
Cartilage Graft
Ear to Face, 21235
Harvesting, 20910, 20912
Rib to Face, 21230
Cartilaginous Exostosis
See Exostosis
Case Management Services
Team Conferences, 99361-99362
Telephone Calls, 99371-99373
Cast
See Brace; Splint
Body
Halo, 29000
Risser Jacket, 29010, 29015
Turnbuckle Jacket, 29020, 29025
Upper Body and Head, 29040

Cast — continued
Body — continued
Upper Body and Legs, 29046
Upper Body and One Leg, 29044
Upper Body Only, 29035
Clubfoot, 29450
Cylinder, 29365
Finger, 29086
Hand, 29085
Hip, 29305, 29325
Leg
Rigid Total Contact, 29445
Long Arm, 29065
Long Leg, 29345, 29355, 29365, 29450
Long Leg Brace, 29358
Patellar Tendon Bearing (PTB), 29435
Removal, 29700-29715
Repair, 29720
Short Arm, 29075
Short Leg, 29405-29435, 29450
Shoulder, 29049-29058
Unlisted Services and Procedures, 29799
Walking, 29355, 29425
Revision, 29440
Wedging, 29740, 29750
Windowing, 29730
Wrist, 29085
Casting
Unlisted Services and Procedures, 29799
Castration
See Orchiectomy
Castration, Female
See Oophorectomy
Cataract
Excision, 66830
Incision, 66820, 66821
Laser, 66821
Stab Incision, 66820
Removal
Extraction
Extracapsular, 66982, 66984
Intracapsular, 66983
Catecholamines, 80424, 82382-82384
Blood, 82383
Urine, 82382
Cathepsin–D, 82387
Catheter
See Cannulization; Venipuncture
Aspiration
Nasotracheal, 31720
Tracheobronchial, 31725
Bladder, 51701-51703
Irrigation, 51700
Breast
Cytology, 0046T, 0047T
for Interstitial Radioelement Application, 19296-19298
Bronchus for Intracavitary Radioelement Application, 31643
Central Venous
Repair, 36575
Replacement, 36580, 36581, 36584
Repositioning, 36597
Coronary Artery without Concomitant Left Heart Catheterization, 93508
Venous Coronary Bypass Graft without Concomitant Left Heart Catheterization, 93508
Declotting, 36550
Exchange
Drainage, 49423
Intravascular, 37209, 75900
Intracatheter
Irrigation, 99507
Obstruction Clearance, 36596
Pericatheter
Obstruction Clearance, 36595

Index

Colon — Computer–aided Detection

Colon — *continued*
  Incision
    Creation
      Stoma, 44320, 44322
    Exploration, 44025
    Revision
      Stoma, 44340-44346
  Lavage
    Intraoperative, 44701
  Lesion
    Destruction, 45383
    Excision, 44110, 44111
  Lysis
    Adhesions, 44005
  Obstruction, 44025, 44050
  Reconstruction
    Bladder from, 50810
  Removal
    Foreign Body, 44025, 44390,
      45379
    Polyp, 44392
  Repair
    Diverticula, 44605
    Fistula, 44650-44661
    Hernia, 44050
    Malrotation, 44055
    Obstruction, 44050
    Ulcer, 44605
    Volvulus, 44050
    Wound, 44605
  Stoma Closure, 44620, 44625
  Suture
    Diverticula, 44605
    Fistula, 44650-44661
    Plication, 44680
    Stoma, 44620, 44625
    Ulcer, 44605
    Wound, 44605
  Tumor
    Ablation, 45339
    Destruction, 45383
  Ultrasound
    Endoscopic, 45391-45392
    via Colotomy, 45355
    via Stoma, 44388-44397
    Virtual, 0066T-0067T
  Unlisted Services and Procedures,
    44799
  X–ray with Contrast
    Barium Enema, 74270, 74280
Colonna Procedure, 27120
  Acetabulum, Reconstruction, 27120
    with Resection, Femoral Head,
      27122
Colonography
  CT Scan, 0086T-0088T
Colonoscopy
  Biopsy, 45380
  Collection of Specimen, 45380
    via Colotomy, 45355
  Destruction
    Lesion, 45383
    Tumor, 45383
  Dilation, 45386
  Hemorrhage Control, 45382
  Injection, Submucosal, 45381
  Placement
    Stent, 45387
  Removal
    Foreign Body, 45379
    Polyp, 45384, 45385
  Ultrasound, 45391-45392
    Tumor, 45384, 45385
  via Stoma, 44388-44390
    Biopsy, 44393
    Destruction
      of Lesion, 44393
      of Tumor, 44393
    Exploration, 44388
    Hemorrhage, 44391
    Placement
      Stent, 44397
    Removal
      Foreign Body, 44390
      Polyp, 44392, 44394
      Tumor, 44392, 44394

Colonoscopy — *continued*
  Virtual, 0066T-0067T
Colon–Sigmoid
  See Colon
  Biopsy
    Endoscopy, 45331
  Endoscopy
    Ablation
      Polyp, 45339
      Tumor, 45339
    Biopsy, 45331
    Dilation, 45340
    Exploration, 45330, 45335
    Hemorrhage, 45334
    Needle Biopsy, 45342
    Placement
      Stent, 45327, 45345
    Removal
      Foreign Body, 45332
      Polyp, 45333, 45338
      Tumor, 45333, 45338
    Ultrasound, 45341, 45342
    Volvulus, 45337
  Exploration
    Endoscopy, 45330, 45335
  Hemorrhage
    Endoscopy, 45334
  Needle Biopsy
    Endoscopy, 45342
  Removal
    Foreign Body, 45332
  Repair
    Volvulus
      Endoscopy, 45337
  Ultrasound
    Endoscopy, 45341, 45342
Colorrhaphy, 44604
Color Vision Examination, 92283
Colostomy, 44320, 45563
  Abdominal
    Establishment, 50810
  Delayed Opening, 44799
  Home Visit, 99505
  Intestine, Large
    with Suture, 44605
  Perineal
    Establishment, 50810
  Revision, 44340
    Paracolostomy Hernia, 44345,
      44346
Colotomy, 44025
Colpectomy
  with Hysterectomy, 58275
    with Repair of Enterocele, 58280
  Partial, 57106
  Total, 57110
Colpoceliocentesis
  See Colpocentesis
Colpocentesis, 57020
Colpocleisis, 57120
Colpocleisis Complete
  See Vagina, Closure
Colpohysterectomies
  See Excision, Uterus, Vaginal
Colpoperineorrhaphy, 57210
Colpopexy, 57280
  Extra–peritoneal, 57282
  Intraperitoneal, 57283
  Laparoscopic, 57425
Colpoplasty
  See Repair, Vagina
Colporrhaphy
  Anterior, 57240, 57289
    with Insertion of Mesh, 57267
    with Insertion of Prosthesis,
      57267
  Anteroposterior, 57260, 57265
    with Enterocele Repair, 57265
    with Insertion of Mesh, 57267
    with Insertion of Prosthesis,
      57267
  Nonobstetrical, 57200
  Posterior, 57250
Colposcopy
  Biopsy, 56821, 57421, 57454-57455,
    57460

Colposcopy — *continued*
  Biopsy — *continued*
    Endometrial, 58110
    Cervix, 57421, 57452-57461
    Exploration, 57452
    Loop Electrode Biopsy, 57460
    Loop Electrode Conization, 57461
    Perineum, 99170
    Vagina, 57420-57421
    Vulva, 56820
      Biopsy, 56821
Colpotomy
  Drainage
    Abscess, 57010
  Exploration, 57000
Colpo–Urethrocystopexy, 58152,
  58267, 58293
  Marshall–Marchetti–Krantz proce-
    dure, 58152, 58267, 58293
  Pereyra Procedure, 58267, 58293
Colprosterone
  See Progesterone
Columna Vertebralis
  See Spine
**Column Chromatography/Mass Spec-
  trometry**, 82541-82544
**Combined Heart–Lung Transplanta-
  tion**
  See Transplantation, Heart–Lung
**Combined Right and Left Heart Car-
  diac Catheterization**
  See Cardiac Catheterization, Com-
    bined Left and Right Heart
Combined Vaccine, 90710
Comedones
  Opening or Removal of (Incision and
    Drainage)
    Acne Surgery, 10040
Commando–Type Procedure, 41155
Commissurotomy
  Right Ventricular, 33476, 33478
Common Sensory Nerve
  Repair, Suture, 64834
Common Truncus
  See Truncus, Arteriosus
Communication Device
  Non–speech–generating, 92605-
    92606
  Speech–generating, 92607-92609
Community/Work Reintegration
  See Physical Medicine/Therapy/ Oc-
    cupational Therapy
  Training, 97537
Compatibility Test
  Blood, 86920
  Electronic, 86923
Complement
  Antigen, 86160
  Fixation Test, 86171
  Functional Activity, 86161
  Hemolytic
    Total, 86162
  Total, 86162
Complete Blood Count, 85025-85027
Complete Colectomy
  See Colectomy, Total
Complete Pneumonectomy
  See Pneumonectomy, Completion
**Complete Transposition of Great
  Vessels**
  See Transposition, Great Arteries
Complex, Factor IX
  See Christmas Factor
Complex, Vitamin B
  See B Complex Vitamins
Component Removal, Blood
  See Apheresis
Composite Graft, 15760, 15770
  Vein, 35681-35683
    Autogenous
      Three or More Segments
        Two Locations, 35683
      Two Segments
        Two Locations, 35682
Compound B
  See Corticosterone

Compound F
  See Cortisol
Compression, Nerve, Median
  See Carpal Tunnel Syndrome
Computed Tomographic Scintigraphy
  See Emission Computerized Tomog-
    raphy
Computed Tomography (CT Scan)
  with Contrast
    Abdomen, 74160
    Arm, 73201
    Brain, 70460
    Ear, 70481
    Face, 70487
    Head, 70460
    Leg, 73701
    Maxilla, 70487
    Neck, 70491
    Orbit, 70481
    Pelvis, 72193
    Sella Turcica, 70481
    Spine
      Cervical, 72126
      Lumbar, 72132
      Thoracic, 72129
    Thorax, 71260
  without Contrast
    Abdomen, 74150
    Arm, 73200
    Brain, 70450
    Cardiac Structures, 0148T-0150T
    Coronary Arteries, 0146T-0147T
    Ear, 70480
    Face, 70486
    Head, 70450
    Heart, 0144T-0145T
    Leg, 73700
    Maxilla, 70486
    Neck, 70490
    Orbit, 70480
    Pelvis, 72192
    Sella Turcica, 70480
    Spine, Cervical, 72125
    Spine, Lumbar, 72131
    Spine, Thoracic, 72128
    Thorax, 71250
  without Contrast, followed by Con-
    trast
    Abdomen, 74170
    Arm, 73202
    Brain, 70470
    Ear, 70482
    Face, 70488
    Head, 70470
    Heart, 0151T
    Leg, 73702
    Maxilla, 70488
    Neck, 70492
    Orbit, 70482
    Pelvis, 72194
    Sella Turcica, 70482
    Spine
      Cervical, 72127
      Lumbar, 72133
      Thoracic, 72130
    Thorax, 71270
  Bone
    Density Study, 77078-77083
  Colon
    Colonography, 0066T-0070T
    Diagnostic, 0067T
    Screening, 0066T
    Virtual Colonoscopy, 0068T-
      0070T
  Drainage, 75898
  Follow–up Study, 76380
  Guidance
    3D Rendering, 76376-76377
    Cyst Aspiration, 77012
    Localization, 77011
    Needle Biopsy, 77012
    Radiation Therapy, 77014
Computer–aided Detection
  Chest Radiograph
  Mammography, 77051, 77052

CRIT, 85013
Critical Care Services, 99289-99292
    See Emergency Department Services;
        Prolonged Attendance
    Evaluation and Management, 99291-
        99292
        NULL
    Gastric Intubation, 91105
    Interfacility Transport, 99289, 99290
    Ipecac Administration for Poison,
        99175
    Neonatal
        Initial, 99295
        Low Birth Weight Infant, 99298-
            99299
        Subsequent, 99296
    Pediatric
        Initial, 99293
        Interfacility Transport, 99289,
            99290
        Subsequent, 99294, 99299
Cross Finger Flap, 15574
Crossmatch, 86920-86922
Crossmatching, Tissue
    See Tissue Typing
CRP, 86140
Cruciate Ligament
    Arthroscopic Repair, 29888, 29889
    Repair, 27407, 27409
        Knee with Collateral Ligament,
            27409
Cryoablation
    See Cryosurgery
Cryofibrinogen, 82585
Cryoglobulin, 82595
Cryopreservation
    Cells, 38207-38208, 88240, 88241
    Embryo, 89258
    Freezing and Storage, 38207, 88240
    Oocyte, 0059T
    Ovarian Tissue, 0058T
    Sperm, 89259
    Testes, 89335
        Embryo, 89352
        Oocytes, 89353
        Reproductive Tissue, 89354
        Sperm, 89356
        Thawing
Cryosurgery, 17000-17286, 47371,
    47381
    See Destruction
    Cervix, 57511
    Labyrinthotomy, 69801
    Lesion
        Anus, 46916, 46924
        Mouth, 40820
        Penis, 54056, 54065
        Skin
            Benign, 17000-17004
            Malignant, 17260-17286
            Pre Malignant, 17000-17004
        Vagina, 57061-57065
        Vulva, 56501-56515
        Warts, flat, 17110, 17111
Cryotherapy
    Acne, 17340
    Destruction
        Ciliary body, 66720
    Lesion
        Cornea, 65450
        Retina, 67208, 67227
    Retinal Detachment
        Prophylaxis, 67141
        Repair, 67101
    Trichiasis
        Correction, 67825
Cryptectomy, 46210, 46211
Cryptococcus
    Antibody, 86641
    Antigen Detection
        Enzyme Immunoassay, 87327
Cryptococcus Neoformans
    Antigen Detection
        Enzyme Immunoassay, 87327
Cryptorchism
    See Testis, Undescended

Cryptosporidium
    Antigen Detection
        Direct Fluorescent Antibody,
            87272
        Enzyme Immunoassay, 87328
Crystal Identification
    Any Body Fluid, 89060
CS, 99143-99150
C–Section, 59510-59515, 59618-59622
    See also Cesarean Delivery
CSF, 86325, 89050, 89051
CST, 59020
CTS, 29848, 64721
CT Scan
    with Contrast
        Abdomen, 74160
        Arm, 73201
        Brain, 70460
        Ear, 70481
        Face, 70487
        Head, 70460
        Leg, 73701
        Maxilla, 70487
        Neck, 70491
        Orbit, 70481
        Pelvis, 72193
        Sella Turcica, 70481
        Spine
            Cervical, 72126
            Lumbar, 72132
            Thoracic, 72129
        Thorax, 71260
    without Contrast
        Abdomen, 74150
        Arm, 73200
        Brain, 70450
        Ear, 70480
        Face, 70486
        Head, 70450
        Leg, 73700
        Maxilla, 70486
        Neck, 70490
        Orbit, 70480
        Pelvis, 72192
        Sella Turcica, 70480
        Spine
            Cervical, 72125
            Lumbar, 72131
            Thoracic, 72128
        Thorax, 71250
    without Contrast, followed by Con-
        trast
        Abdomen, 74170, 74175, 75635
        Arm, 73202, 73206, 73220,
            73223
        Brain, 70470, 70496
        Chest, 71275
        Ear, 70482
        Face, 70488
        Head, 70470, 70496
        Leg, 73702, 73706, 75635
        Maxilla, 70488
        Neck, 70492, 70498
        Orbit, 70482
        Pelvis, 72191, 72194
        Sella Turcica, 70482
        Spine
            Cervical, 72127
            Lumbar, 72133
            Thoracic, 72130
        Thorax, 71270, 71275
    3D Rendering, 76376-76377
    Bone
        Density Study, 77078-77083
    Colon
        Diagnostic, 0067T
        Screening, 0066T
    Drainage, 75989
    Follow-up Study, 76380
    Guidance
        Localization, 77011
        Needle Biopsy, 77012
        Radiation Therapy, 77014
        Tissue Ablation, 77013
        Vertebroplasty, 72292

CT Scan, Radionuclide
    See Emission Computerized Tomog-
        raphy
Cuff, Rotator
    See Rotator Cuff
Culdocentesis, 57020
Culdoscopy, 57452
Culdotomy, 57000
Culture
    Acid Fast Bacilli, 87116
    Amniotic Fluid
        Chromosome Analysis, 88235
    Bacteria
        Additional Methods, 87077
        Aerobic, 87040-87070
        Anaerobic, 87073-87076
        Blood, 87040
        Feces, 87045, 87046
        Other, 87070-87073
        Screening, 87081
        Urine, 87086, 87088
    Bone Marrow
        Chromosome Analysis, 88237
    Chlamydia, 87110
    Chorionic Villus
        Chromosome Analysis, 88235
    Fertilized Oocyte
        for In Vitro Fertilization, 89250
            with Co–Culture of Embryo,
                89251
            Assisted Microtechnique,
                89280, 89281
    Fungus
        Blood, 87103
        Hair, 87101
        Identification, 87106
        Nail, 87101
        Other, 87102
        Skin, 87101
    Lymphocyte
        Chromosome Analysis, 88230
    Mold, 87107
    Mycobacteria, 87116-87118
    Mycoplasma, 87109
    Oocyte/Embryo
        Extended Culture, 89272
        for In Vitro Fertilization, 89250
            with Co–Culture of Embryo,
                89251
    Pathogen
        by Kit, 87084
    Skin
        Chromosome Analysis, 88233
    Tissue
        Toxin
            Antitoxin, 87230
            Toxin Virus, 87252, 87253
    Tubercle Bacilli, 87116
    Typing, 87140-87158
    Unlisted Services and Procedures,
        87999
    Yeast, 87106
Curettage
    See Dilation and Curettage
    Cervix
        Endocervical, 57454, 57456,
            57505
    Cornea, 65435, 65436
        Chelating Agent, 65436
    Hydatidiform Mole, 59870
    Postpartum, 59160
Curettage, Uterus
    See Uterus, Curettage
Curettement
    Skin Lesion, 11055-11057, 17004,
        17110, 17270, 17280
Curietherapy
    See Brachytherapy
Custodial Care
    See Domicilary Services; Nursing
        Facility Services
Cutaneolipectomy
    See Lipectomy
**Cutaneous Electrostimulation, Anal-
    gesic**
    See Application, Neurostimulation

Cutaneous Tag
    See Skin, Tags
Cutaneous Tissue
    See Integumentary System
Cutaneous–Vesicostomy
    See Vesicostomy, Cutaneous
CVS, 59015
CXR, 71010-71035, 71090
Cyanide
    Blood, 82600
    Tissue, 82600
Cyanocobalamin, 82607, 82608
Cyclic AMP, 82030
**Cyclic Citrullinated Peptide (CCP),
    Antibody**, 86200
Cyclic GMP, 83008
Cyclic Somatostatin
    See Somatostatin
Cyclocryotherapy
    See Cryotherapy, Destruction, Ciliary
        Body
Cyclodialysis
    Destruction
        Ciliary Body, 66740
Cyclophotocoagulation
    Destruction
        Ciliary Body, 66710, 66711
Cyclosporine
    Assay, 80158
Cyst
    Abdomen
        Destruction
            Excision, 49200, 49201
    Ankle
        Capsule, 27630
        Tendon Sheath, 27630
    Bartholin's Gland
        Excision, 56740
        Repair, 56440
    Bile Duct
        Excision, 47715, 47719
    Bladder
        Excision, 51500
    Bone
        Drainage, 20615
        Injection, 20615
    Brain
        Drainage, 61150, 61151, 61156,
            62161, 62162
        Excision, 61516, 61524, 62162
    Branchial Cleft
        Excision, 42810, 42815
    Breast
        Incision and Drainage, 19020
        Puncture Aspiration, 19000,
            19001
    Calcaneus, 28100-28103
    Carpal, 25130-25136
    Choledochal
        Excision, 47715, 47719
    Ciliary Body
        Destruction, 66770
    Clavicle
        Excision, 23140-23146
    Conjunctiva, 68020
    Dermoid
        Nose
            Excision, 30124, 30125
    Drainage
        Contrast Injection, 49424
        with X–ray, 76080
    Excision
        Cheekbone, 21030
        Clavicle, 23140
            with Allograft, 23146
            with Autograft, 23145
        Femur, 27355, 27357, 27358
        Ganglion
            See Ganglion
        Humerus
            with Allograft, 23156
            with Autograft, 23155
        Hydatid
            See Echinococcosis
        Lymphatic
            See Lymphocele

Index

Cyst — Daily Living Activities

Dilation — *continued*
Trachea
Endoscopic, 31630, 31631, 31636-31638
Ureter, 50395, 52341, 52342, 52344, 52345
Endoscopic, 50553, 50572, 50953, 50972
Urethra, 52260, 52265
General, 53665
Suppository and/or Instillation, 53660, 53661
Urethral
Stenosis, 52281
Stricture, 52281, 53600-53621
Vagina, 57400
Dilation and Curettage
See Curettage; Dilation
Cervical Stump, 57558
Cervix, 57558, 57800
Corpus Uteri, 58120
Hysteroscopy, 58558
Induced Abortion, 59840
with Amniotic Injections, 59851
with Vaginal Suppositories, 59856
Postpartum, 59160
Dilation and Evacuation, 59841
with Amniotic Injections, 59851
Dimethadione, 82654
Dioxide, Carbon
See Carbon Dioxide
Dioxide Silicon
See Silica
Dipeptidyl Peptidase A
See Angiotensin Converting Enzyme (ACE)
Diphenylhydantoin
See Phenytoin
Diphosphate, Adenosine
See Adenosine Diphosphate
Diphtheria
Antibody, 86648
Immunization, 90698, 90700-90702, 90714-90715, 90718-90723
Dipropylacetic Acid
Assay, 80164
Direct Pedicle Flap
Formation, 15570-15576
Disability Evaluation Services
Basic Life and/or Disability Evaluation, 99450
Work–Related or Medical Disability Evaluation, 99455, 99456
Disarticulation
Ankle, 27889
Elbow, 20999
Hip, 27295
Knee, 27598
Shoulder, 23920, 23921
Wrist, 25920, 25924
Revision, 25922
Disarticulation of Shoulder
See Shoulder, Disarticulation
Disc Chemolyses, Intervertebral
See Chemonucleolysis
Discectomies
See Discectomy
Discectomies, Percutaneous
See Discectomy, Percutaneous
Discectomy
Anterior with Decompression
Cervical Interspace, 63075
Each Additional, 63076
Thoracic Interspace, 63077
Each Additional, 63078
Arthrodesis
Additional Interspace, 22534, 22585
Lumbar, 22533, 22558, 22630
Thoracic, 22532, 22556
Vertebra
Cervical, 22554
Cervical, 22220
Diskectomy
See Discectomy

Discectomy — *continued*
Lumbar, 22224, 22630
Percutaneous, 62287
Thoracic, 22222
Additional Segment, 22226
Discharge, Body Substance
See Drainage
Discharge Instructions
Heart Failure, 4014F
Discharge Services
See Hospital Services
Hospital, 99238, 99239
Nursing Facility, 99315, 99316
Observation Care, 99234-99236
Disc, Intervertebral
See Intervertebral Disc
Discission
Cataract
Laser Surgery, 66821
Stab Incision, 66820
Vitreous Strands, 67030
Discography
Cervical Disc, 72285
Injection, 62290, 62291
Lumbar Disc, 72295
Thoracic, 72285
Discolysis
See Chemonucleolysis
Disease
Durand–Nicolas–Favre
See Lymphogranuloma Venereum
Erb–Goldflam
See Myasthenia Gravis
Heine–Medin
See Polio
Hydatid
See Echinococcosis
Lyme
See Lyme Disease
Ormond
See Retroperitoneal Fibrosis
Peyronie
See Peyronie Disease
Posada–Wernicke
See Coccidioidomycosis
Disease/Organ Panel
See Organ/Disease Panel
Diskography
Dislocated Elbow
See Dislocation, Elbow
Dislocated Hip
See Dislocation, Hip Joint
Dislocated Jaw
See Dislocation, Temporomandibular Joint
Dislocated Joint
See Dislocation
Dislocated Shoulder
See Dislocation, Shoulder
Dislocation
Acromioclavicular Joint
Open Treatment, 23550, 23552
Ankle Joint
Closed Treatment, 27840, 27842
Open Treatment, 27846, 27848
Carpal, 25690
Closed Treatment, 25690
Open Treatment, 25695
Carpometacarpal Joint
Closed Treatment, 26641, 26645, 26670
with Anesthesia, 26675
Open Treatment, 26665, 26685, 26686
Percutaneous Fixation, 26676
Clavicle
with Manipulation, 23545
without Manipulation, 23540
Closed Treatment, 23540, 23545
Open Treatment, 23550, 23552
Elbow
with Manipulation, 24620, 24640
Closed Treatment, 24600, 24605, 24640
Open Treatment, 24586, 24615

Dislocation — *continued*
Hip Joint
without Trauma, 27265, 27266
Closed Treatment, 27250, 27252, 27265, 27266
Congenital, 27256-27259
Open Treatment, 27253, 27254, 27258, 27259
Interphalangeal Joint
Finger(s)/Hand
Closed Treatment, 26770, 26775
Open Treatment, 26785
Percutaneous Fixation, 26776
Toe(s)/Foot, 28660-28675
Closed Treatment, 28660, 28665
Open Treatment, 28675
Percutaneous Fixation, 28666
Knee
Closed Treatment, 27550, 27552
Open Treatment, 27556-27558, 27566, 27730
Recurrent, 27420-27424
Lunate, 25690-25695
with Manipulation, 25690, 26670-26676, 26700-26706
Closed Treatment, 25690
Open Treatment, 25695
Metacarpophalangeal Joint
Closed Treatment, 26700-26706
Open Treatment, 26715
Metatarsophalangeal Joint
Closed Treatment, 28630, 28635
Open Treatment, 28645
Percutaneous Fixation, 28636
Patella
Closed Treatment, 27560, 27562
Open Treatment, 27566
Recurrent, 27420-27424
Pelvic Ring
Closed Treatment, 27193, 27194
Open Treatment, 27217, 27218
Percutaneous Fixation, 27216
Percutaneous Fixation
Metacarpophalangeal, 26705
Peroneal Tendons, 27675, 27676
Radioulnar Joint
Closed Treatment, 25675
with Radial Fracture, 25520
Open Treatment, 25676
with Radial Fracture, 25525, 25526
Radius
with Fracture, 24620, 24635
Closed Treatment, 24620
Open Treatment, 24635
Closed Treatment, 24640
Shoulder
Closed Treatment
with Manipulation, 23650, 23655
with Fracture of Greater Humeral Tuberosity, 23665
Open Treatment, 23670
with Surgical or Anatomical Neck Fracture, 23675
Open Treatment, 23660
Recurrent, 23450-23466
Sternoclavicular Joint
Closed Treatment
with Manipulation, 23525
without Manipulation, 23520
Open Treatment, 23530, 23532
Talotarsal Joint
Closed Treatment, 28570, 28575
Open Treatment, 28546
Percutaneous Fixation, 28576
Tarsal
Closed Treatment, 28540, 28545
Open Treatment, 28555

Dislocation — *continued*
Tarsal — *continued*
Percutaneous Fixation, 28545, 28546
Tarsometatarsal Joint
Closed Treatment, 28600, 28605
Open Treatment, 28615
Percutaneous Fixation, 28606
Temporomandibular Joint
Closed Treatment, 21480, 21485
Open Treatment, 21490
Thumb
with Fracture, 26645
Open Treatment, 26665
Percutaneous Fixation, 26650, 26665
with Manipulation, 26641-26650
Closed Treatment, 26641, 26645
Open Treatment, 26665
Percutaneous Fixation, 26650
Tibiofibular Joint
Closed Treatment, 27830, 27831
Open Treatment, 27832
Vertebrae
Additional Segment, Any Level
Open Treatment, 22328
Cervical
Open Treatment, 22326
Closed Treatment
with Manipulation, Casting and/or Bracing, 22315
without Manipulation, 22310
Lumbar
Open Treatment, 22325
Thoracic
Open Treatment, 22327
Wrist
with Fracture
Closed Treatment, 25680
Open Treatment, 25685
Intercarpal
Closed Treatment, 25660
Open Treatment, 25670
Percutaneous, 25671
Radiocarpal
Closed Treatment, 25660
Open Treatment, 25670
Radioulnar
Closed Treatment, 25675
Open Treatment, 25676
Percutaneous Fixation, 25671
Dislocation, Radiocarpal Joint
See Radiocarpal Joint, Dislocation
Disorder
Blood Coagulation
See Coagulopathy
Penis
See Penis
Retinal
See Retina
Displacement Therapy
Nose, 30210
Dissection
Hygroma, Cystic
Axillary, 38550, 38555
Cervical, 38550, 38555
Lymph Nodes, 38542
Dissection, Neck, Radical
See Radical Neck Dissection
Distention
See Dilation
Diverticulectomy, 44800
Esophagus, 43130, 43135
Diverticulectomy, Meckel's
See Meckel's Diverticulum, Excision
Diverticulopexy
Esophagus, 43499
Pharynx, 43499
Diverticulum
Bladder
See Bladder, Diverticulum
Meckel's
Excision, 44800
Repair
Urethra, 53400, 53405

Index

Drainage — Ear, Nose, and Throat

Finger — *continued*
Unlisted Services and Proce-
dures/Hands or Fingers,
26989
X–ray, 73140
Finger Flap
Tissue Transfer, 14350
Finger Joint
See Intercarpal Joint
Finney Operation, 43850
FISH, 88365
Fishberg Concentration Test
Water Load Test, 89235
Fissurectomy, 46200
Fissure in Ano
See Anus, Fissure
Fistula
Anal
Repair, 46288, 46706
Arteriovenous, 36831-36833
Revision
with Thrombectomy, 36831
without Thrombectomy, 36832
Thrombectomy without revision,
36831
Autogenous Graft, 36825
Bronchi
Repair, 32815
Carotid–Cavernous Repair, 61710
Chest Wall
Repair, 32906
Conjunctiva
with Tube or Stent, 68750
without Tube, 68745
Enterovesical
Closure, 44660, 44661
Kidney, 50520-50526
Lacrimal Gland
Closure, 68770
Dacryocystorhinostomy, 68720
Nose
Repair, 30580, 30600
Window, 69666
Oval Window, 69666
Postauricular, 69700
Rectovaginal
with Concomitant Colostomy,
57307
Abdominal Approach, 57305
Transperineal Approach, 57308
Round Window, 69667
Sclera
Iridencleisis or Iridotasis, 66165
Sclerectomy with Punch or Scis-
sors with Iridectomy, 66160
Thermocauterization with Iridec-
tomy, 66155
Trabeculectomy ab Externo in
Absence Previous Surgery,
66170
Trabeculectomy ab Externo with
Scarring, 66172
Trephination with Iridectomy,
66150
Suture
Kidney, 50520-50526
Ureter, 50920, 50930
Trachea, 31755
Tracheoesophageal
Repair, 43305, 43312, 43314
Speech Prothesis, 31611
Transperineal Approach, 57308
Ureter, 50920, 50930
Urethra, 53400, 53405
Urethrovaginal, 57310
with Bulbocavernosus Trans-
plant, 57311
Vesicouterine
Closure, 51920, 51925
Vesicovaginal
Closure, 51900
Transvesical and Vaginal Ap-
proach, 57330
Vaginal Approach, 57320
X–ray, 76080

Fistula Arteriovenous
See Arteriovenous Fistula
Fistulectomy
See Hemorrhoids
Anal, 46060, 46270-46285
Fistulization
Conjunction to Nasal Cavity, 68745
Esophagus, 43350-43352
Intestines, 44300-44346
Lacrimal Sac to Nasal Cavity, 68720
Penis, 54435
Pharynx, 42955
Sclera, 0123T
Tracheopharyngeal, 31755
Fistulization, Interatrial
See Septostomy, Atrial
Fistulotomy
Anal, 46270, 46280
Fitting
Cervical Cap, 57170
Contact Lens, 92070, 92310-92313
See Contact Lens Services
Diaphragm, 57170
Low Vision Aid, 92354, 92355
See Spectacle Services
Spectacle Prosthesis, 92352, 92353
Spectacles, 92340-92342
Fitzgerald Factor, 85293
Fixation (Device)
See Application; Bone; Fixation;
Spinal Instrumentation
Application, External, 20690, 20692
Insertion, 22841-22844
Prosthetic, 22851
Reinsertion, 22849
Interdental without Fracture, 21497
Pelvic
Insertion, 22848
Removal
External, 20694
Internal, 20670, 20680
Sacrospinous Ligament
Vaginal Prolapse, 57282
Shoulder, 23700
Skeletal
Humeral Epicondyle
Percutaneous, 24566
Spinal
Insertion, 22841-22847
Prosthetic, 22851
Reinsertion, 22849
Fixation, External
See External Fixation
Fixation, Kidney
See Nephropexy
Fixation, Rectum
See Proctopexy
Fixation Test Complement
See Complement, Fixation Test
Fixation, Tongue
See Tongue, Fixation
Flank
See Back/Flank
Flap
See Skin Graft and Flap
Delay of Flap at Trunk, 15600
at Eyelids, Nose Ears, or Lips,
15630
at Forehead, Cheeks, Chin, Neck,
Axillae, Genitalia, Hands,
Feet, 15620
at Scalp, Arms, or Legs, 15610
Section Pedicle of Cross Finger,
15620
Free
Breast Reconstruction, 19364
Microvascular Transfer,
15756-15758
Grafts, 15574-15650, 15842
Composite, 15760
Derma–Fat–Fascia, 15770
Cross Finger Flap, 15574
Punch for Hair Transplant
Less than 15, 15775
More than 15, 15776
Island Pedicle, 15740

Flap — *continued*
Island Pedicle — *continued*
Neurovascular Pedicle, 15750
Latissimus Dorsi
Breast Reconstruction, 19361
Omentum
Free
with Microvascular Anastomo-
sis, 49906
Transfer
Intermediate of Any Pedicle,
15650
Transverse Rectus Abdominis Myocu-
taneous
Breast Reconstruction, 19367-
19369
Flatfoot Correction, 28735
Flea Typhus
See Murine Typhus
Fletcher Factor, 85292
Flow Cytometry, 88182-88189
Flow Volume Loop/Pulmonary, 94375
See Pulmonology, Diagnostic
Fluid, Amniotic
See Amniotic Fluid
Fluid, Body
See Body Fluid
Fluid, Cerebrospinal
See Cerebrospinal Fluid
Fluid Collection
Incision and Drainage
Skin, 10140
Fluid Drainage
Abdomen, 49080, 49081
Fluorescein
Angiography, Ocular, 92287
Intravenous Injection
Vascular Flow Check, Graft,
15860
Fluorescein, Angiography
See Angiography, Fluorescein
Fluorescent Antibody, 86255, 86256
Fluorescent In Situ Hybridization,
88365
Fluoride
Blood, 82735
Urine, 82735
Fluoroscopy
Bile Duct
Calculus Removal, 74327
Guide for Catheter, 74328, 74330
Chest
Bronchoscopy, 31622-31646
Complete (four views), 71034
Partial (two views), 71023
Drain Abscess, 75989
GI Tract
Guidance Intubation, 74340
Hourly, 76000, 76001
Introduction
GI Tube, 74340
Larynx, 70370
Nasogastric, 43752
Needle Biopsy, 77002
Pancreatic Duct
Catheter, 74329, 74330
Pharynx, 70370
Renal
Guide Catheter, 74475
Spine/Paraspinous
Guide Catheter
Needle, 77003
Unlisted Procedure, 76496
Ureter
Guidance Catheter, 74480
Vertebra
Osteoplasty, 72291-72292
X–ray with Contrast
Guidance Catheter, 74475
Flurazepam
Blood or Urine, 82742
Flush Aortogram, 75722, 75724
Flu Vaccines, 90645-90660
FNA
See Fine Needle Aspiration
Foam Stability Test, 83662

Fold, Vocal
See Vocal Cords
Foley Operation Pyeloplasty
See Pyeloplasty
Foley Y–Pyeloplasty, 50400, 50405
Folic Acid, 82747
RBC, 82746
Follicle Stimulating Hormone (FSH),
80418, 80426, 83001
Folliculin
See Estrone
Follitropin
See Follicle Stimulating Hormone
(FSH)
Follow–Up Services
See Hospital Services; Office and/or
Other Outpatient Services
Post–Op, 99024
Fontan Procedure, 33615, 33617
Food Allergy Test, 95075
See Allergy Tests
Foot
See Metatarsal; Tarsal
Amputation, 28800, 28805
Bursa
Incision and Drainage, 28001
Capsulotomy, 28260-28264
Cast, 29450
Cock Up Fifth Toe, 28286
Fasciectomy, 28060
Radical, 28060, 28062
Fasciotomy, 28008
Endoscopic, 29893
Hammertoe Operation, 28285
Incision, 28002-28005
Joint
See Talotarsal Joint; Tar-
sometatarsal Joint
Magnetic Resonance Imaging
(MRI), 73721-73723
Lesion
Excision, 28080, 28090
Magnetic Resonance Imaging (MRI),
73718-73720
Nerve
Excision, 28055
Incision, 28035
Neuroma
Excision, 28080
Ostectomy, Metatarsal Head, 28288
Reconstruction
Cleft Foot, 28360
Removal
Foreign Body, 28190-28193
Repair
Muscle, 28250
Tendon
Advancement Posterior Tibial,
28238
Capsulotomy; Metatarsopha-
langeal, 28270
Interphalangeal, 28272
Capsulotomy, Midfoot; Medial
Release, 28270
Capsulotomy, Midtarsal (Hey-
man Type), 28264
Extensor, Single, 28208
Secondary with Free Graft,
28210
Flexor, Single, with Free Graft,
28200
Secondary with Free Graft,
28202
Tenolysis, Extensor
Multiple through Same In-
cision, 28226
Tenolysis, Flexor
Multiple through Same In-
cision, 28222
Single, 28220
Tenotomy, Open, Extensor
Foot or Toe, 28234
Tenotomy, Open, Flexor,
28230
Toe, Single Procedure,
28232

Foot — *continued*
Replantation, 20838
Sesamoid
Excision, 28315
Skin Graft
Delay of Flap, 15620
Full Thickness, 15240, 15241
Pedicle Flap, 15574
Split, 15100, 15101
Splint, 29590
Strapping, 29540, 29590
Suture
Tendon, 28200-28210
Tendon Sheath
Excision, 28086, 28088
Tenolysis, 28220-28226
Tenotomy, 28230-28234
Tissue Transfer, Adjacent, 14040, 14041
Tumor
Excision, 28043-28046
Unlisted Services and Procedures, 28899
X–ray, 73620, 73630
Foot Abscess
See Abscess, Foot
Foot Navicular Bone
See Navicular
Forearm
See Arm, Lower
Forehead
Reconstruction, 21179-21180, 21182-21184
Midface, 21159, 21160
Reduction, 21137-21139
Rhytidectomy, 15824, 15826
Skin Graft
Delay of Flap, 15620
Full Thickness, 15240, 15241
Pedicle Flap, 15574
Tissue Transfer, Adjacent, 14040, 14041
Forehead and Orbital Rim
Reconstruction, 21172-21180
Foreign Body
Removal
Adenoid, 42999
Anal, 46608
Ankle Joint, 27610, 27620
Arm
Lower, 25248
Upper, 24200, 24201
Auditory Canal, External, 69200
with Anesthesia, 69205
Bile Duct, 43269
Bladder, 52310, 52315
Brain, 61570
Bronchi, 31635
Colon, 44025, 44390, 45379
Colon–Sigmoid, 45332
Conjunctival Embedded, 65210
Cornea
with Slip Lamp, 65222
without Slit Lamp, 65220
Duodenum, 44010
Elbow, 24000, 24101, 24200, 24201
Esophagus, 43020, 43045, 43215, 74235
External Eye, 65205
Eyelid, 67938
Finger, 26075, 26080
Foot, 28190-28193
Gastrointestinal, Upper, 43247
Gum, 41805
Hand, 26070
Hip, 27033, 27086, 27087
Hysteroscopy, 58562
Interphalangeal Joint
Toe, 28024
Intertarsal Joint, 28020
Intestines, Small, 44020, 44363
Intraocular, 65235
Kidney, 50561, 50580
Knee Joint, 27310, 27331, 27372
Lacrimal Duct, 68530

Foreign Body — *continued*
Removal — *continued*
Lacrimal Gland, 68530
Larynx, 31511, 31530, 31531, 31577
Leg, Upper, 27372
Lung, 32151
Mandible, 41806
Maxillary Sinus, 31299
Mediastinum, 39000, 39010
Metatarsophalangeal Joint, 28022
Mouth, 40804, 40805
Muscle, 20520, 20525
Stimulator
Skeletal, 20999
Nose, 30300
Anesthesia, under, 30310
Lateral Rhinotomy, 30320
Orbit, 61334, 67413, 67430
with Bone Flap, 67430
without Bone Flap, 67413
Pancreatic Duct, 43269
Pelvis, 27086, 27087
Penile Tissue, 54115
Penis, 54115
Pericardium, 33020
Endoscopic, 32658
Peritoneum, 49402
Pharynx, 42809
Pleura, 32150, 32151
Endoscopic, 32653
Posterior Segment
Magnetic Extraction, 65260
Nonmagnetic Extraction, 65265
Rectum, 45307, 45915
Scrotum, 55120
Shoulder, 23040, 23044
Complicated, 23332
Deep, 23331
Subcutaneous, 23330
Skin
with Debridement, 11010-11012
Stomach, 43500
Subcutaneous, 10120, 10121
with Debridement, 11010-11012
Tarsometatarsal Joint, 28020
Tendon Sheath, 20520, 20525
Toe, 28022
Ureter, 50961, 50980
Urethra, 52310, 52315
Uterus, 58562
Vagina, 57415
Wrist, 25040, 25101, 25248
Forensic Exam, 88040
Cytopathology, 88125
Phosphatase, Acid, 84061
Foreskin of Penis
See Penis, Prepuce
Formycin Diphosphate
See Fibrin Degradation Products
Fournier's Gangrene
See Debridement, Skin, Subcutaneous Tissue, Infected
Fowler Procedure
Osteotomy, 28305
Fowler–Stephens Orchiopexy, 54650
Fox Operation, 67921
Fraction, Factor IX
See Christmas Factor
Fracture
Femur
Neck
Closed Treatment, 27230
with Manipulation, 27232
Open Treatment, 27236
Percutaneous Fixation, 27235
Fracture, Treatment
Acetabulum
with Manipulation, 27222
without Manipulation, 27220
Closed Treatment, 27220, 27222
Open Treatment, 27226-27228

Fracture, Treatment — *continued*
Alveola
Closed Treatment, 21421
Open Treatment, 21422, 21423
Alveolar Ridge
Closed Treatment, 21440
Open Treatment, 21445
Ankle
with Manipulation, 27818
without Manipulation, 27816
Closed Treatment, 27816, 27818
Lateral, 27786, 27792, 27822
Closed Treatment, 27786
with Manipulation, 27788
Open Treatment, 27792
Malleolus
Bimalleolar
Closed Treatment, 27808
with Manipulation, 27810
Open Treatment, 27814
Medial, 27760-27766, 27808-27814
Closed Treatment, 27760
with Manipulation, 27762
Open Treatment, 27766
Open Treatment, 27822, 27823
Trimalleolar, 27816-27823
Closed Treatment, 27816
with Manipulation, 27818
Open Treatment, 27822
with Fixation, 27823
Ankle Bone
Medial, 27760, 27762
Bennett's
See Thumb, Fracture
Bronchi
Endoscopy, 31630
Calcaneus
with Manipulation, 28405, 28406
without Manipulation, 28400
Closed Treatment, 28400, 28405
Open Treatment, 28415, 28420
Percutaneous Fixation, 28436
Carpal, 25622-25628
Closed Treatment
with Manipulation, 25624, 25635
without Manipulation, 25622, 25630
Open Treatment, 25628, 25645
Carpal Scaphoid
Closed Treatment, 25622
Carpometacarpal
Closed Treatment, 26645
Open Treatment, 26665
Percutaneous Fixation, 26650
Cheekbone
with Manipulation, 21355
Open Treatment, 21360-21366
Clavicle
Closed Treatment, 23500, 23505
with Manipulation, 23505
without Manipulation, 23500
Open Treatment, 23515
Coccyx
Closed Treatment, 27200
Open Treatment, 27202
Colles–Reversed
See Smith Fracture
Craniofacial
Closed Treatment, 21431
Open Treatment, 21432-21435
Debridement
with Open Fracture, 11040-11044
Elbow
Closed Treatment, 24620, 24640
Open Treatment, 24586, 24587, 24635
Femur
with Manipulation, 27232, 27502, 27503, 27510
without Manipulation, 27230, 27238, 27246, 27500, 27501, 27508, 27516, 27517, 27520

Fracture, Treatment — *continued*
Femur — *continued*
Closed Treatment, 27230, 27238, 27240, 27246, 27500-27503, 27510, 27516, 27517
Distal, 27508, 27510, 27514
Epiphysis, 27516-27519
Intertrochanteric
Closed Treatment, 27238
with Manipulation, 27240
Intramedullary Implant, Shaft, 27245
Open Treatment, 27244
with Implant, 27245
Neck
Closed Treatment, 27230
with Manipulation, 27232
Open Treatment, 27236
Percutaneous Fixation, 27235
Open Treatment, 27244, 27245, 27248, 27506, 27507, 27511-27514, 27519
Percutaneous Fixation, 27235, 27509
Pertrochanteric
Closed Treatment, 27238
with Manipulation, 27240
Intermedullary Implant Shaft, 27245, 27500, 27502, 27506-27507
Open Treatment, 27244, 27245
Shaft, 27500, 27502, 27506, 27507
Subtrochanteric
Closed Treatment, 27238
with Manipulation, 27240
Intramedullary Implant, 27245
Open Treatment, 27244, 27245
Supracondylar, 27501-27503, 27509, 27511, 27513
Transcondylar, 27501-27503, 27509, 27511, 27513
Trochanteric
Closed Treatment, 27246
Open Treatment, 27248
Fibula
with Manipulation, 27781, 27788, 27810
without Manipulation, 27780, 27786, 27808
Closed Treatment, 27780, 27781, 27786, 27788, 27808, 27810
Malleolus, 27786-27814
Open Treatment, 27784, 27792, 27814
Shaft, 27780-27786, 27808
Frontal Sinus
Open Treatment, 21343, 21344
Great Toe
Closed Treatment, 28490
with Manipulation, 28490
Heel
Closed Treatment
with Manipulation, 28405, 28406
without Manipulation, 28400
Open Treatment, 28415, 28420
Humerus
with Dislocation
Closed Treatment, 23665
Open Treatment, 23670
with Shoulder Dislocation
Closed Treatment, 23675
Open Treatment, 23680
Closed Treatment, 24500, 24505
with Manipulation, 23605
without Manipulation, 23600
Condyle, 24582
Closed Treatment, 24576, 24577
Open Treatment, 24579

© 2006 Ingenix

Hand — *continued*
Implantation
Removal, 26320
Tube/Rod, 26392, 26416
Tube/Rod, 26390
Insertion
Tendon Graft, 26392
Magnetic Resonance Imaging (MRI), 73218-73223
Reconstruction
Tendon Pulley, 26500-26502
Repair
Blood Vessel, 35207
Cleft Hand, 26580
Muscle, 26591, 26593
Release, 26593
Tendon
Extensor, 26410-26416, 26426, 26428, 26433-26437
Flexor, 26350-26358, 26440
Profundus, 26370-26373
Replantation, 20808
Skin Graft
Delay of Flap, 15620
Full Thickness, 15240, 15241
Pedicle Flap, 15574
Split, 15100, 15101
Strapping, 29280
Tendon
Excision, 26390
Extensor, 26415
Tenotomy, 26450, 26460
Tissue Transfer, Adjacent, 14040, 14041
Tumor
Excision, 26115-26117
Unlisted Services and Procedures, 26989
X-ray, 73120, 73130
Hand Abscess
See Abscess, Hand
Hand(s) Dupuytren's Contracture(s)
See Dupuytren's Contracture
Handling
Device, 99002
Radioelement, 77790
Specimen, 99000, 99001
Hand Phalange
See Finger, Bone
Hanganutziu Deicher Antibodies
See Antibody, Heterophile
Haptoglobin, 83010, 83012
Hard Palate
See Palate
Harelip Operation
See Cleft Lip, Repair
Harii Procedure (Carpal Bone), 25430
Harrington Rod
Insertion, 22840
Removal, 22850
Hartmann Procedure, 44143
Laparoscopy
Partial Colectomy with Colostomy, 44206
Open, 44143
Harvesting
Bone Graft, 20900, 20902
Bone Marrow, 38230
Cartilage, 20910, 20912
Conjunctival Graft, 68371
Eggs for In Vitro Fertilization, 58970
Endoscopic
Vein for Bypass Graft, 33508
Fascia Lata Graft, 20920, 20922
Intestines, 44132, 44133
Kidney, 50300, 50320, 50547
Liver, 47133, 47140-47142
Lower Extremity Vein for Vascular Reconstruction, 35572
Skin, 15040
Stem Cell, 38205, 38206
Tendon Graft, 20924
Tissue Grafts, 20926

Harvesting — *continued*
Upper Extremity Artery
for Coronary Artery Bypass Graft, 35600
Upper Extremity Vein
for Bypass Graft, 35500
Hauser Procedure
Reconstruction, Patella, for Instability, 27420
Hayem's Elementary Corpuscle
See Blood, Platelet
Haygroves Procedure, 27120, 27122
HBcAb, 86704, 86705
HBeAb, 86707
HBeAg, 87350
HBsAb, 86706
HBsAg (Hepatitis B Surface Antigen), 87340
HCG, 84702, 84703
HCO3
See Bicarbonate
Hct, 85013, 85014
HCV Antibodies
See Antibody, Hepatitis C
HD, 27295
HDL (High Density Lipoprotein), 83718
Head
Angiography, 70496, 70544-70546
CT Scan, 70450-70470, 70496
Excision, 21015-21070
Fracture and/or Dislocation, 21310-21497
Incision, 21010, 61316, 62148
Introduction, 21076-21116
Lipectomy, Suction Assisted, 15876
Magnetic Resonance Angiography (MRA), 70544-70546
Nerve
Graft, 64885, 64886
Other Procedures, 21299, 21499
Repair
Revision and/or Reconstruction, 21120-21296
Ultrasound Examination, 76506, 76536
Unlisted Services and Procedures, 21499
X-ray, 70350
Headbrace
Application, 21100
Removal, 20661
Head Rings, Stereotactic
See Stereotactic Frame
Heaf Test
TB Test, 86580
Health Behavior
See Evaluation and Management, Health Behavior
Health Risk Assessment Instrument, 99420
Hearing Aid
Bone Conduction
Implant, 69710
Removal, 69711
Repair, 69711
Replace, 69710
Check, 92592, 92593
Hearing Aid Services
Electroacoustic Test, 92594, 92595
Examination, 92590, 92591
Hearing Evaluation, 92506
Hearing Tests
See Audiologic Function Tests; Hearing Evaluation
Hearing Therapy, 92507, 92601-92604
Heart
Ablation
Ventricular Septum
Non-surgical, 0024T
Accoustic Sound Recording, 0068T, 0069T, 0070T
Allograft Preparation, 33933, 33944
Angiocardiography, 93555
Angiography
Injection, 93542, 93543

Heart — *continued*
Angiography — *continued*
Injection — *continued*
See Cardiac Catheterization; Injection
Aortic Arch
with Cardiopulmonary Bypass, 33853
without Cardiopulmonary Bypass, 33852
Aortic Valve
Repair, Left Ventricle, 33414
Replacement, 33405-33413
Arrhythmogenic Focus
Catheter Ablation, 93650-93652
Destruction, 33250, 33251, 33261
Atria
See Atria
Biopsy, 93505
Radiologic Guidance, 76932
Blood Vessel
Repair, 33320-33322
Cardiac Output Measurements, 93561, 93562
Cardiac Rehabilitation, 93797, 93798
Cardioassist, 92970, 92971
Ventricular Assist Device Extra-corporeal, 0049T
Cardiopulmonary Bypass
with Lung Transplant, 32852, 32854
Cardioverter-Defibrillator
Evaluation and Testing, 93640, 93641, 93642
Catheterization, 93501, 93510-93533
Combined Right and Retrograde Left for Congenital Cardiac Anomalies, 93531
Combined Right and Transseptal Left for Congenital Cardiac Anomalies, 93532, 93533
Flow-Directed, 93503
Right for Congenital Cardiac Anomalies, 93530
See Catheterization, Cardiac
Closure
Septal Defect, 33615
Valve
Atrioventricular, 33600
Semilunar, 33602
Commissurotomy, Right Ventricle, 33476, 33478
Defibrillator
Insertion, 33240
Pads
Removal, 33243, 33244
Pulse Generator Only, 33241
Repair, 33218, 33220
Replacement, Leads, 33216, 33217, 33249
Destruction
Arrhythmogenic Focus, 33250, 33261
Electrical Recording
3-D Mapping, 93613
Acoustic Heart Sound, 0068T-0070T
Atria, 93602
Atrial Electrogram, Esophageal (or Trans-esophageal), 93615, 93616
Bundle of His, 93600
Comprehensive, 93619, 93620
Right Ventricle, 93603
Tachycardia Sites, 93609
Electroconversion, 92960, 92961
Electrophysiologic Follow-Up Study, 93624
Evaluation of Device, 93640
Excision
Donor, 33930, 33940
Tricuspid Valve, 33460, 33465
Exploration, 33310, 33315
Fibrillation
Atrial, 33254, 33255-33256

Heart — *continued*
Great Vessels
See Great Vessels
Heart-Lung Bypass
See Cardiopulmonary Bypass
Heart-Lung Transplantation
See Tranplantation, Heart-Lung
Hemodynamic Monitoring
Non-invasive, 0086T
Implantation
Artificial Heart, Intracorporeal, 0051T
Total Replacement Heart System, Intracorporeal, 0051T
Ventricular Assist Device, 33976
Extracorporeal, 0048T
Incision
Atrial, 33254, 33255-33256
Exploration, 33310, 33315
Injection
Radiologic, 93542, 93543
See Cardiac Catheterization, Injection
Insertion
Balloon Device, 33973
Defibrillator, 33212-33213
Electrode, 33210, 33211, 33214-33217, 33224-33225
Pacemaker, 33206-33208, 33212, 33213
Catheter, 33210
Pulse Generator, 33212-33214
Ventricular Assist Device, 33975
Intraoperative Pacing and Mapping, 93631
Ligation
Fistula, 37607
Magnetic Resonance Imaging (MRI)/with Contrast Material, 75553
without Contrast Material, 75552
Mitral Valve
See Mitral Valve
Muscle
See Myocardium
Myocardium
Imaging, Nuclear, 78466-78469
Perfusion Study, 78460-78465
Nuclear Medicine
Blood Flow Study, 78414
Blood Pool Imaging, 78472, 78473, 78481, 78483, 78494, 78496
Myocardial Imaging, 78466-78469
Myocardial Perfusion, 78460-78465, 78491, 78492
Shunt Detection (Test), 78428
Unlisted Services and Procedures, 78499
Open Chest Massage, 32160
Output
See Cardiac Output
Pacemaker
Conversion, 33214
Insertion, 33206-33208
Pulse Generator, 33212, 33213
Removal, 33233-33237
Replacement, 33206-33208
Catheter, 33210
Upgrade, 33214
Pacing
Arrhythmia Induction, 93618
Atria, 93610
Transcutaneous
Temporary, 92953
Ventricular, 93612
Pacing Cardioverter-Defibrillator
Evaluation and Testing, 93640-93642, 93740-93744
Insertion Single/Dual Chamber Electrodes, 33216, 33217, 33224-33225, 33249
Pulse Generator, 33240

Hemorrhoidectomy — *continued*
External Complete, 46250
Ligature, 46221
Simple, 46255
with Fissurectomy, 46257, 46258
Hemorrhoidopexy, 46947
Hemorrhoids
Destruction, 46934-46936
Incision
External, 46083
Injection
Sclerosing Solution, 46500
Ligation, 46945, 46946
Stapling, 46947
Suture, 46945, 46946
Hemosiderin, 83070, 83071
Hemothorax
Thoracostomy, 32020
Heparin, 85520
Clotting Inhibitors, 85300-85305
Neutralization, 85525
Protamine Tolerance Test, 85530
Heparin Cofactor I
See Antithrombin III
Hepatectomy
Extensive, 47122
Left Lobe, 47125
Partial
Donor, 47140-47142
Lobe, 47120
Right Lobe, 47130
Total
Donor, 47133
Hepatic Abscess
See Abscess, Liver
Hepatic Arteries
See Artery, Hepatic
Hepatic Artery Aneurysm
See Artery, Hepatic, Aneurysm
Hepatic Duct
Anastomosis
with Intestines, 47765, 47802
Exploration, 47400
Incision and Drainage, 47400
Nuclear Medicine
Imaging, 78223
Removal
Calculi (Stone), 47400
Repair
with Intestines, 47765, 47802
Unlisted Services and Procedures, 47999
Hepatic Haemorrhage
See Hemorrhage, Liver
Hepaticodochotomy
See Hepaticostomy
Hepaticoenterostomy, 47802
Hepaticostomy, 47400
Hepaticotomy, 47400
Hepatic Portal Vein
See Vein, Hepatic Portal
Hepatic Portoenterostomies
See Hepaticoenterostomy
Hepatic Transplantation
See Liver, Transplantation
Hepatitis A and Hepatitis B, 90636
Hepatitis Antibody
A, 86708, 86709
B core, 86704, 86705
Be, 86707
B Surface, 86706
C, 86803, 86804
Delta Agent, 86692
IgG, 86704, 86708
IgM, 86704, 86705, 86708, 86709
Hepatitis Antigen
B, 87515-87517
Be, 87350
B Surface, 87340, 87341
C, 87520-87522
Delta Agent, 87380
G, 87525-87527
Hepatitis A Vaccine
Adolescent
Pediatric
Three Dose Schedule, 90634

Hepatitis A Vaccine — *continued*
Adolescent — *continued*
Pediatric — *continued*
Two Dose Schedule, 90633
Adult Dosage, 90632
Hepatitis B and Hib, 90748
Hepatitis B Immunization, 90740-90747
Hepatitis B Vaccine
Dosage
Adolescent, 90743
Adult, 90746
Immunosuppressed, 90740, 90747
Pediatric, 90744
Adolescent, 90743-90744
Hepatitis B Virus E Antibody
See Antibody, Hepatitis
Hepatitis B Virus Surface ab
See Antibody, Hepatitis B, Surface
Hepatorrhaphy
See Liver, Repair
Hepatotomy
Abscess, 47010, 47011
Percutaneous, 47011
Cyst, 47010, 47011
Percutaneous, 47011
Hernia
Repair
with Spermatic Cord, 55540
Abdominal, 49560, 49565, 49590
Incisional, 49560
Recurrent, 49565
Diaphragmatic, 39502-39541
Chronic, 39541
Esophageal Hiatal, 39520
Neonatal, 39503
Epigastric, 49570
Incarcerated, 49572
Femoral, 49550
Incarcerated, 49553
Recurrent, 49555
Recurrent Incarcerated, 49557
Reducible, 49550
Incisional, 49561, 49566
Incarcerated, 49561
Inguinal, 49491, 49495-49500, 49505
Incarcerated, 49492, 49496, 49501, 49507, 49521
Infant, Incarcerated
Strangulated, 49496, 49501
Infant, Reducible, 49495, 49500
Laparoscopic, 49650, 49651
Pediatric, Reducible, 49500, 49505
Recurrent, Incarcerated
Strangulated, 49521
Recurrent, Reducible, 49520
Sliding, 49525
Strangulated, 49492
Lumbar, 49540
Lung, 32800
Orchiopexy, 54640
Recurrent Incisional
Incarcerated, 49566
Umbilicus, 49580, 49585
Incarcerated, 49582, 49587
Spigelian, 49590
Hernia, Cerebral
See Encephalocele
Hernia, Rectovaginal
See Rectocele
Hernia, Umbilical
See Omphalocele
Heroin, Alkaloid Screening, 82101
Heroin Screen, 82486
Herpes Simplex Virus
Antibody, 86696
Antigen Detection
Immunofluorescence, 87273, 87274
Nucleic Acid, 87528-87530

Herpes Simplex Virus — *continued*
Identification
Smear and Stain, 87207
Herpes Smear, 87207
Herpesvirus 4 (Gamma), Human
See Epstein–Barr Virus
Herpes Virus–6 Detection, 87531-87533
Herpetic Vesicle
Destruction, 54050, 54065
Heteroantibodies
See Antibody, Heterophile
Heterograft
Skin, 15400
Heterologous Tranplantations
See Heterograft
Heterologous Transplant
See Xenograft
Heterophile Antibody, 86308-86310
Heterotropia
See Strabismus
Hexadecadrol
See Dexamethasone
Hex B
See b–Hexosaminidase
Hexosephosphate Isomerase
See Phosphohexose Isomerase
Heyman Procedure, 27179, 28264
H Flu
See Hemophilus Influenza
Hgb, 85018
HGB, 83036, 83051, 83065, 83068
Hg Factor
See Glucagon
HGH (Human Growth Hormone), 80418, 80428, 80430, 83003, 86277
HHV–4
See Epstein–Barr Virus
HIAA (Hydroxyindolacetic Acid, Urine), 83497
Hibb Operation, 22841
Hib Vaccine
Four Dose Schedule
HbOC, 90645
PRP–T, 90648
PRP–D/Booster, 90646
PRP–OMP
Three Dose Schedule, 90647
Hickmann Catheterization
See Cannulization; Catheterization; Venous, Central Line; Venipuncture
Hicks–Pitney Test
Thromboplastin, Partial Time, 85730, 85732
Hidradenitis
See Sweat Gland
Excision, 11450-11471
Suppurative
Incision and Drainage, 10060, 10061
High Altitude Simulation Test, 94452-94453
High Density Lipoprotein, 83718
Highly Selective Vagotomy
See Vagotomy, Highly Selective
High Molecular Weight Kininogen
See Fitzgerald Factor
Highmore Antrum
See Sinus, Maxillary
Hill Procedure, 43324
Laparoscopic, 43280
Hinton Positive
See RPR
Hip
See Femur; Pelvis
Abscess
Incision and Drainage, 26990
Arthrocentesis, 20610
Arthrodesis, 27284, 27286
Arthrography, 73525
Arthroplasty, 27130, 27132
Arthroscopy, 29860-29863
Arthrotomy, 27030, 27033
Biopsy, 27040, 27041

Hip — *continued*
Bone
Drainage, 26992
Bursa
Incision and Drainage, 26991
Capsulectomy
with Release, Flexor Muscles, 27036
Cast, 29305, 29325
Craterization, 27070, 27071
Cyst
Excision, 27065-27067
Denervation, 27035
Echography
Infant, 76885, 76886
Endoprothesis
See Prosthesis, Hip
Excision, 27070
Excess Skin, 15834
Exploration, 27033
Fasciotomy, 27025
Fusion, 27284, 27286
Hematoma
Incision and Drainage, 26990
Injection
Radiologic, 27093, 27095, 27096
Manipulation, 27275
Reconstruction
Total Replacement, 27130
Removal
Cast, 29710
Foreign Body, 27033, 27086, 27087
Arthroscopic, 29861
Loose Body
Arthroscopic, 29861
Prosthesis, 27090, 27091
Repair
Muscle Transfer, 27100-27105, 27111
Osteotomy, 27146-27156
Tendon, 27097
Saucerization, 27070
Stem Prostheses
See Arthroplasty, Hip
Strapping, 29520
Tenotomy
Abductor Tendon, 27006
Adductor Tendon, 27000-27003
Iliopsoas Tendon, 27005
Total Replacement, 27130, 27132
Tumor
Excision, 27047-27049, 27065-27067
Radical, 27075, 27076
Ultrasound
Infant, 76885, 76886
X-ray, 73500-73520, 73540
with Contrast, 73525
Intraoperative, 73530
Hip Joint
Arthroplasty, 27132
Revision, 27134-27138
Arthrotomy, 27502
Biopsy, 27502
Capsulotomy
with Release, Flexor Muscles, 27036
Dislocation, 27250, 27252
without Trauma, 27265, 27266
Congenital, 27256-27259
Open Treatment, 27253, 27254
Manipulation, 27275
Reconstruction
Revision, 27134-27138
Synovium
Excision, 27054
Arthroscopic, 29863
Total Replacement, 27132
Hippocampus
Excision, 61566
Hip Stem Prosthesis
See Arthroplasty, Hip
Histalog Test
Gastric Analysis Test, 91052
Histamine, 83088

Incision and Drainage — Infusion Pump

Infusion Pump — *continued*
  Intraarterial
    Removal, 36262
    Revision, 36261
  Intravenous
    Insertion, 36563
    Removal, 36590
    Revision, 36576, 36578
  Maintenance, 95990, 96521, 96522
    Chemotherapy, Pump Services, 96521, 96522
  Spinal Cord, 62361, 62362
  Ventricular Catheter, 61215
Infusion Therapy, 62350, 62351, 62360-62362
  See Injection, Chemotherapy
  Arterial Catheterization, 36640
  Chemotherapy, 96401-96542
  Home Infusion Procedures, 99601-99602
  Intravenous, 90760-90761, 90765-90768
  Pain, 62360-62362, 62367-62368
  Transcatheter Therapy, 75896
Ingestion Challenge Test, 95075
  See Allergy Tests
Inguinal Hernia Repair
  See Hernia, Repair, Inguinal
INH
  See Drug Assay
Inhalation
  Pentamidine, 94642
Inhalation Provocation Tests
  See Bronchial Challenge Test
Inhalation Treatment, 94640, 94664, 99503
  See Pulmonology, Therapeutic
Inhibin A, 86336
Inhibition, Fertilization
  See Contraception
Inhibition Test, Hemagglutination
  See Hemagglutination Inhibition Test
Inhibitor, Alpha 1-Protease
  See Alpha-1 Antitrypsin
Inhibitor, Alpha 2-Plasmin
  See Alpha-2 Antiplasmin
Inhibitory Concentration, Minimum
  See Minimum Inhibitory Concentration
Initial Inpatient Consultations
  See Consultation, Initial Inpatient
Injection
  See Allergen Immunotherapy, Infusion
  Abdomen
    Air, 49400
    Contrast Material, 49400
  Angiography
    Coronary, 93556
    Pulmonary, 75746
  Ankle
    Radial, 27648
  Antibiotic Administration, 90772
  Antigen (Allergen), 95115-95125, 95145-95170
  Aorta (Aortography)
    Radiologic, 93544
  Aponeurosis, 20550
  Bladder
    Radiologic, 51600-51610
  Bone Marrow, into, 38999
  Brain Canal, 61070
  Breast
    Radiologic, 19030
  Bronchography
    Segmental, 31656
  Bursa, 20600-20610
  Cardiac Catheterization, 93539-93545
  Carpal Tunnel
    Therapeutic, 20526
  Chemotherapy, 96401-96402, 96450, 96542
  Cistern
    Medication or Other, 61055

Injection — *continued*
  Contrast
    Central Venous Access Device, 36598
    via Peritoneal Catheter, 49424
  Corpora Cavernosa, 54235
  Cyst
    Bone, 20615
    Kidney, 50390
    Pelvis, 50390
    Thyroid, 60001
  Elbow
    Arthrography, Radiologic, 24220
  Epidural
    See Epidural, Injection
  Esophageal Varices
    Endoscopy, 43243
  Esophagus
    Sclerosing Agent, 43204
    Sphincter, 0133T
    Submucosal, 43201
  Extremity
    Pseudoaneurysm, 36002
  Eye
    Air, 66020
    Medication, 66030
  Eyelid
    Subconjunctival, 68200
  Ganglion
    Anesthetic, 64505, 64510
  Ganglion Cyst, 20612
  Gastric Secretion Stimulant, 91052
  Gastric Varices
    Endoscopy, 43243
  Heart
    Therapeutic Substance into Pericardium, 33999
  Heart Vessels
    Cardiac Catheterization, 93539-93545
      See Catheterization, Cardiac
    Radiologic, 93545
  Hemorrhoids
    Sclerosing Solution, 46500
  Hip
    Radiologic, 27093, 27095
  Insect Venom, 95130-95134
  Intervertebral Disc
    Chemonucleolysis Agent, 62292
    Radiological, 62290, 62291
  Intra-amniotic, 59850-59852
  Intraarterial
    Diagnostic, 90773
    Therapeutic, 90773
  Intradermal, Tattooing, 11920-11922
  Intralesional, Skin, 11900, 11901
  Intramuscular, 90772
    Diagnostic, 90772
    Therapeutic, 90772, 99506
  Intravenous
    Diagnostic, 90774
    Therapeutic, 90774
    Vascular Flow Check, Graft, 15860
  Joint, 20600-20610
  Kidney
    Drugs, 50391
    Radiologic, 50394
  Knee
    Radiologic, 27370
  Lacrimal Gland
    Radiologic, 68850
  Left Heart
    Radiologic, 93543
  Lesion, Skin, 11900, 11901
  Ligament, 20550
  Liver, 47015
    Radiologic, 47500, 47505
  Lungs
    Radiologic, 93541
  Lymphangiography, 38790
  Mammary Ductogram
    Galactogram, 19030
  Muscle Endplate
    Cervical Spinal, 64613
    Extremity, 64614

Injection — *continued*
  Muscle Endplate — *continued*
    Facial, 64612
    Trunk, 64614
  Nerve
    Anesthetic, 64400-64530
    Neurolytic Agent, 64600-64680
  Orbit
    Retrobulbar
      Alcohol, 67505
      Medication, 67500
    Tenon's Capsule, 67515
  Pancreatography, 48400
  Paravertebral Facet Joint
    Nerve, 64470-64476
  Penis
    for Erection, 54235
    Peyronie Disease, 54200
      with Surgical Exposure of Plaque, 54205
    Radiology, 54230
    Vasoactive Drugs, 54231
  Pericardium
    Injection of Therapeutic Substance, 33999
  Peritoneal Cavity Air
    See Pneumoperitoneum
  Radiologic
    Breast, 19030
  Rectum
    Sclerosing Solution, 45520
  Right Heart
    See Cardiac Catheterization, Injection
    Injection of Radiologic Substance, 93542
  Sacroiliac Joint
    for Arthrography, 27096
  Salivary Duct, 42660
  Salivary Gland
    Radiologic, 42550
  Sclerosing Agent
    Esophagus, 43204
    Intravenous, 36470, 36471
  Sentinel Node Identification, 38792
  Shoulder
    Arthrography, Radiologic, 23350
  Shunt
    Peritoneal
      Venous, 49427
  Sinus Tract, 20500
    Diagnostic, 20501
  Spider Veins
    Telangiectasia, 36468, 36469
  Spinal Artery, 62294
  Spinal Cord
    Anesthetic, 62310-62319
    Blood, 62273
    Neurolytic Agent, 62280-62282
    Other, 62310, 62311
    Radiologic, 62284
  Spleen
    Radiologic, 38200
  Steroids for Urethral Stricture, 52283
  Subcutaneous
    Diagnostic, 90772
    Silicone, 11950-11954
    Therapeutic, 90772
  Temporomandibular Joint
    Arthrography, 21116
  Tendon Origin, Insertion, 20551
  Tendon Sheath, 20550
  Therapeutic
    Extremity Pseudoaneurysm, 36002
    Lung, 32960
    Thyroid, 60001
    Turbinate, 30200
  Thoracic Cavity
    See Pleurodesis, Chemical
  Trachea
    Puncture, 31612
  Transtracheal
    Bronchography, 31715

Injection — *continued*
  Trigger Point(s)
    One or Two Muscle Groups, 20552
    Three or More Muscle Groups, 20553
  Turbinate, 30200
  Unlisted, 90779
  Unlisted Services and Procedures, 90779
  Ureter
    Drugs, 50391
    Radiologic, 50684
  Ureteropyelography, 50690
  Venography, 36005
  Ventricular
    Dye, 61120
    Medication or Other, 61026
  Vitreous, 67028
    Fluid Substitute, 67025
  Vocal Cords
    Therapeutic, 31513, 31570, 31571
  Wrist
    Carpal Tunnel
      Therapeutic, 20526
    Radiologic, 25246
Inkblot Test, 96101-96103
Inner Ear
  See Ear, Inner
Innominate
  Tumor
    Excision, 27077
Innominate Arteries
  See Artery, Brachiocephalic
Inorganic Sulfates
  See Sulfate
Insemination
  Artificial, 58321, 58322, 89268
Insertion
  See Implantation; Intubation; Transplantation
  Balloon
    Intra-Aortic, 33967, 33973
  Breast
    Implants, 19340, 19342
  Cannula
    Arteriovenous, 36810, 36815
    ECMO, 36822
    Extra Corporeal Circulation for Regional Chemotherapy of Extremity, 36823
    Thoracic Duct, 38794
    Vein to Vein, 36800
  Catheter
    Abdomen, 49420, 49421
    Abdominal Artery, 36245-36248
    Aorta, 36200
    Bile Duct, 47525, 47530, 75982
      Percutaneous, 47510
    Bladder, 51045, 51701-51703
    Brachiocephalic Artery, 36215-36218
    Brain, 61210, 61770
    Breast
      for Interstitial Radioelement Application, 19296-19298
    Bronchi, 31717
    Bronchus
      for Intracavity Radioelement Application, 31643
    Cardiac
      See Catheterization, Cardiac
      Flow Directed, 93503
    Ear, Middle, 69405
    Eustachian Tube, 69405
    Flow Directed, 93503
    Gastrointestinal, Upper, 43241
    Jejunum, 44015
    Kidney, 50392
    Lower Extremity Artery, 36245-36248
    Nasotracheal, 31720
    Pelvic Artery, 36245-36248
    Pleural Cavity, 32019

Intracranial Neoplasm, Acoustic Neuroma
　See Brain, Tumor, Excision
Intracranial Neoplasm, Craniopharyngioma
　See Craniopharyngioma
Intracranial Neoplasm, Meningioma
　See Meningioma
Intracranial Nerve
　Electrocoagulation
　　Anesthesia, 00222
Intracranial Procedures
　Anesthesia, 00190, 00210-00222
Intrafallopian Transfer, Gamete
　See GIFT
Intraluminal Angioplasty
　See Angioplasty
Intramuscular Injection
　See Injection, Intramuscular
Intraocular Lens
　Exchange, 66986
　Insertion, 66983
　　Manual or Mechanical Technique, 66982, 66984
　　not Associated with Concurrent Cataract Removal, 66985
Intraoperative Manipulation of Stomach, 43659, 43999
Intraoral
　Skin Graft
　　Pedicle Flap, 15576
Intra–Osseous Infusion
　See Infusion, Intraosseous
Intrathoracic Esophagoesophagostomy, 43499
Intrathoracic System
　Anesthesia, 00500-00580
Intratracheal Intubation
　See Insertion, Endotracheal Tube
Intrauterine Contraceptive Device
　See Intrauterine Device (IUD)
Intrauterine Device (IUD)
　Insertion, 58300
　Removal, 58301
Intrauterine Synechiae
　See Adhesions, Intrauterine
Intravascular Stent
　See Transcatheter, Placement, Intravascular Stents
　X-ray, 75960
Intravascular Ultrasound
　Intraoperative, 37250, 37251
Intravenous Injection
　See Injection, Intravenous
Intravenous Pyelogram
　See Urography, Intravenous
Intravenous Therapy, 90760-90761, 90765-90768, 90774-90775
　See Injection, Chemotherapy
Intravesical Instillation
　See Bladder, Instillation
Intravitreal Injection
　Pharmacologic Agent, 67028
Intrinsic Factor, 83528
　Antibodies, 86340
Introduction
　Breast
　　Metallic Localization Clip Placement, 19295
　　Preoperative Placement, Needle, 19290-19291
　Contraceptive Capsules
　　Implantable, 11975-11977
　Drug Delivery Implant, 11981, 11983
　Gastrointestinal Tube, 44500
　　with Fluoroscopic Guidance, 74340
　Injections
　　Intradermal, 11920-11922
　　Intralesional, 11900, 11901
　　Subcutaneous, 11950-11954
　Tissue Expanders, Skin, 11960-11971
Intubation
　See Insertion
　Endotracheal Tube, 31500

Intubation — *continued*
　Eustachian Tube
　　See Catheterization, Eustachian Tube
　for Specimen Collection
　　Esophagus, 91000
　　Stomach, 91055
　　Gastric, 89130-89141, 91105
Intubation Tube
　See Endotracheal Tube
Intussusception
　Barium Enema, 74283
　Reduction
　　Laparotomy, 44050
Invagination, Intestinal
　See Intussesception
Inversion, Nipple
　See Nipples, Inverted
Investigation
　FDA Approved Chronic Care Drugs, 0130T
In Vitro Fertilization
　Biopsy Oocyte, 89290, 89291
　Culture Oocyte, 89250, 89251
　　Extended, 89272
　Embryo Hatching, 89253
　Fertilize Oocyte, 89250
　　Microtechnique, 89280, 89281
　Identify Oocyte, 89254
　Insemination of Oocyte, 89268
　Prepare Embryo, 89255, 89352
　Retrieve Oocyte, 58970
　Transfer Embryo, 58974, 58976
　Transfer Gamete, 58976
In Vivo NMR Spectroscopy
　See Magnetic Resonance Spectroscopy
Iodide Test
　Nuclear Medicine, Thyroid Uptake, 78000-78003
　Starch Granules, Feces
Iodine Test
　See Starch Granules, Feces
IOL, 66825, 66983-66986
Ionization, Medical
　See Iontophoresis
Iontophoresis, 97033
　Sweat Collection, 89230
IP
　See Allergen Immunotherapy
Ipecac Administration, 99175
IPPB (Intermittent Positive Pressure Breathing)
Iridectomy
　with Corneoscleral or Corneal Section, 66600
　with Sclerectomy with Punch or Scissors, 66160
　with Thermocauterizaton, 66155
　with Transfixion as for Iris Bombe, 66605
　with Trephination, 66150
　by Laser Surgery, 66761
　Peripheral for Glaucoma, 66625
Iridencleisis, 66165
Iridocapsulectomy, 66830
Iridocapsulotomy, 66830
Iridodialysis, 66680
Iridoplasty, 66762
Iridotasis, 66165
Iridotomy
　by Laser Surgery, 66761
　by Stab Incision, 66500
　Excision
　　with Corneoscleral or Corneal Section, 66600
　　with Cyclectomy, 66605
　　Optical, 66635
　　Peripheral, 66625
　Incision
　　with Transfixion as for Iris Bombe, 66505
　　Stab, 66500
　Optical, 66635
　Peripheral, 66625
　Sector, 66630

Iris
　Cyst
　　Destruction, 66770
　Excision
　　Iridectomy
　　　with Corneoscleral or Corneal Section, 66600
　　　with Cyclectomy, 66605
　　　Optical, 66635
　　　Peripheral, 66625
　　　Sector, 66630
　Incision
　　Iridotomy
　　　with Transfixion as for Iris Bombe, 66505
　　　Stab, 66500
　Lesion
　　Destruction, 66770
　Repair, 66680
　　Suture, 66682
　Revision
　　Laser Surgery, 66761
　　Photocoagulation, 66762
　Suture
　　with Ciliary Body, 66682
Iron, 83540
Iron Binding Capacity, 83550
Iron Hematoxylin Stain, 88312
Iron Stain, 85536, 88313
Irradiation
　Blood Products, 86945
Irrigation
　Bladder, 51700
　Caloric Vestibular Test, 92533, 92543
　Catheter
　　Brain, 62194, 62225
　Corpora Cavernosa
　　Priapism, 54220
　Penis
　　Priapism, 54220
　Peritoneal
　　See Peritoneal Lavage
　Rectum
　　for Fecal Impaction, 91123
　Shunt
　　Spinal Cord, 63744
　Sinus
　　Maxillary, 31000
　　Sphenoid, 31002
　Vagina, 57150
　Venous Access Device
Irving Sterilization
　Ligation, Fallopian Tube, Oviduct, 58600-58611, 58670
Ischial
　Excision
　　Bursa, 27060
　　Tumor, 27078, 27079
Ischiectomy, 15941
Ischium
　Pressure Ulcer, 15940-15946
ISG Immunization, 90281, 90283
Island Pedicle Flaps, 15740
Islands of Langerhans
　See Islet Cell
Islet Cell
　Antibody, 86341
Isocitrate Dehydrogenase
　See Isocitric Dehydrogenase
Isocitric Dehydrogenase
　Blood, 83570
Isolation
　Sperm, 89260, 89261
Isomerase, Glucose 6 Phophate
　See Phosphohexose Isomerase
Isopropanol
　See Isopropyl Alcohol
Isopropyl Alcohol, 84600
Isthmusectomy
　Thyroid Gland, 60210-60225
IUD, 58300, 58301
　Insertion, 58300
　Removal, 58301
IV, 90760-90761, 90765-90768, 90774-90775

IVC Filter
　Placement, 75940
IV, Coagulation Factor
　See Calcium
IVF (In Vitro Fertilization), 58970-58976, 89250-89255
IV Infusion Therapy
　See Allergen Immunotherapy; Chemotherapy; Infusion Injection, Chemotherapy, 96409, 96411, 96413-96417, 96542
IV Injection
　Injection, Intravenous, 90774-90775
Ivor Lewis, 43117
IVP, 50394, 74400
Ivy Bleeding Time, 85002
IX Complex, Factor
　See Christmas Factor

J

Jaboulay Operation
　Gastroduodenostomy, 43810, 43850, 43855
Jannetta Procedure
　Decompression, Cranial Nerves, 61458
Japanese, River Fever
　See Scrub Typhus
Jatene Procedure
　Repair, Great Arteries, 33770-33781
Jaw Joint
　See Facial Bones; Mandible; Maxilla
Jaws
　Muscle Reduction, 21295, 21296
　X–ray
　　for Orthodontics, 70355
Jejunostomy
　with Pancreatic Drain, 48001
　Catheterization, 44015
　Insertion
　　Catheter, 44015
　　Laparoscopic, 44186
　　Non–Tube, 44310
Jejunum
　Transfer with Microvascular Anastomosis, Free, 43496
Johannsen Procedure, 53400
Johanson Operation
　See Reconstruction, Urethra
Joint
　See Specific Joint
　Acromioclavicular
　　See Acromioclavicular Joint
　Arthrocentesis, 20600-20610
　Aspiration, 20600-20610
　Dislocation
　　See Dislocation
　Drainage, 20600-20610
　Finger
　　See Intercarpal Joint
　Fixation (Surgical)
　　See Arthrodesis
　Foot
　　See Foot, Joint
　Hip
　　See Hip, Joint
　Injection, 20600-20610
　Intertarsal
　　See Intertarsal Joint
　Knee
　　See Knee Joint
　Ligament
　　See Ligament
　Metacarpophalangeal
　　See Metacarpophalangeal Joint
　Metatarsophalangeal
　　See Metatarsophalangeal Joint
　Mobilization, 97140
　Nuclear Medicine
　　Imaging, 78300-78315
　Radiology
　　Stress Views, 77071
　Sacroiliac
　　See Sacroiliac Joint
　Shoulder
　　See Glenohumeral Joint

Lacrimal Duct — *continued*
　Insertion
　　Stent, 68815
　Removal
　　Dacryolith, 68530
　　Foreign Body, 68530
　　X–ray with Contrast, 70170
Lacrimal Gland
　Biopsy, 68510
　Close Fistula, 68770
　Excision
　　Partial, 68505
　　Total, 68500
　Fistulization, 68720
　Incision and Drainage, 68400
　Injection
　　X–ray, 68850
　Nuclear Medicine
　　Tear Flow, 78660
　Removal
　　Dacryolith, 68530
　　Foreign Body, 68530
　Repair
　　Fistula, 68770
　Tumor
　　Excision
　　　with Osteotomy, 68550
　　　without Closure, 68540
Lacrimal Punctum
　Closure
　　by Plug, 68761
　　by Thermocauterization, Ligation
　　　or Laser Surgery, 68760
　Dilation, 68801
　Incision, 68440
　Repair, 68705
Lacrimal Sac
　Biopsy, 68525
　Excision, 68520
　Incision and Drainage, 68420
Lacrimal System
　Unlisted Services and Procedures,
　　68899
Lacryoaptography
　Nuclear, 78660
Lactase Deficiency Breath Test, 91065
Lactate, 83605
Lactic Acid, 83605
Lactic Acid Measurement
　See Lactate
Lactic Cytochrome Reductase
　See Lactic Dehydrogenase
Lactic Dehydrogenase, 83615, 83625
Lactiferous Duct
　Excision, 19112
　Exploration, 19110
Lactoferrin
　Fecal, 83630-83631
Lactogen, Human Placental, 83632
Lactogenic Hormone
　See Prolactin
Lactose
　Urine, 83633, 83634
Ladd Procedure, 44055
Laki Lorand Factor
　See Fibrin Stabilizing Factor
L–Alanine
　See Aminolevulinic Acid (ALA)
Lamblia Intestinalis
　See Giardia Lamblia
Lambrinudi Operation
　Arthrodesis, Foot Joints, 28730,
　　28735, 28740
Lamellar Keratoplasties
　See Keratoplasty, Lamellar
Laminaria
　Insertion, 59200
Laminectomy, 63600
　Decompression
　　Cervical, 63001, 63015
　　　with Facetectomy and
　　　　Foraminotomy, 63045,
　　　　63048
　　Laminotomy
　　　Initial
　　　　Cervical, 63020

Laminectomy — *continued*
　Decompression — *continued*
　　Laminotomy — *continued*
　　　Initial — *continued*
　　　　Each Additional Space,
　　　　　63035
　　　　Lumbar, 63030
　　　Reexploration
　　　　Cervical, 63040
　　　　　Each Additional Inter-
　　　　　　space, 63043
　　　　Lumbar, 63042
　　　　　Each Additional Inter-
　　　　　　space, 63044
　　　Lumbar, 63005, 63017
　　　　with Facetectomy and
　　　　　Foraminotomy, 63046,
　　　　　63048
　　　Sacral, 63011
　　　Thoracic, 63003, 63016
　　　　with Facetectomy and
　　　　　Foraminotomy, 63047,
　　　　　63048
　Excision
　　Lesion, 63250-63273
　　Neoplasm, 63275-63290
　　Surgical, 63170-63200
Laminoplasty
　Cervical, 63050-63051
Laminotomy
　Cervical, One Interspace, 63020
　Lumbar, 63042
　　One Interspace, 63030
　　　Each Additional, 63035
　Re–exploration, Cervical, 63040
Langerhans Islands
　See Islet Cell
Language Evaluation, 92506
Language Therapy, 92507, 92508
LAP, 83670
Laparoscopic Appendectomy
　See Appendectomy, Laparoscopic
Laparoscopic Biopsy of Ovary
　See Biopsy, Ovary, Laparoscopic
Laparoscopy
　with X–ray, 47560
　Abdominal, 49320-49329
　Adrenalectomy, 50545
　Adrenal Gland
　　Biopsy, 60650
　　Excision, 60650
　Appendectomy, 44970
　Aspiration, 49322
　Biopsy, 47561, 49321
　　Lymph Nodes, 38570
　Cecostomy, 44188
　Cholangiography, 47560, 47561
　Cholecystectomy, 47562-47564
　Cholecystoenterostomy, 47570
　Closure
　　Enterostomy, 44227
　Colectomy
　　Partial, 44204-44208, 44213
　　Total, 44210-44212
　Colostomy, 44188
　Destruction
　　Lesion, 58662
　Diagnostic, 49320
　Drainage
　　Extraperitoneal Lymphocele,
　　　49323
　Ectopic Pregnancy, 59150
　　with Salpingectomy and/or
　　　Oophorectomy, 59151
　Enterolysis, 44180
　Esophagogastric Fundoplasty, 43280
　Fimbrioplasty, 58672
　Gastric Restrictive Procedures,
　　43644-43645, 43770-43774
　Gastrostomy
　　Temporary, 43653
　Hernia Repair
　　Initial, 49650
　　Recurrent, 49651
　Ileostomy, 44187
　Incontinence Repair, 51990, 51992

Laparoscopy — *continued*
　In Vitro Fertilization, 58976
　　Retrieve Oocyte, 58970
　　Transfer Embryo, 58974
　　Transfer Gamete, 58976
　Jejunostomy, 44186
　Kidney
　　Ablation, 50541-50542
　Ligation
　　Veins, Spermatic, 55500
　Liver
　　Ablation
　　　Tumor, 47370, 47371
　Lymphadenectomy, 38571-38572
　Lymphatic, 38570-38589
　Lysis of Adhesions, 58660
　Lysis of Intestinal Adhesions, 44180
　Mobilization
　　Splenic Flexure, 44213
　Nephrectomy, 50545-50548
　　Partial, 50543
　Orchiectomy, 54690
　Orchiopexy, 54692
　Ovary
　　Reimplantation, 59898
　　Suture, 59898
　Oviduct Surgery, 58670, 58671,
　　58679
　Pancreatic Islet Cell Transplantation,
　　0143T
　Pelvis, 49320
　Proctectomy, 45395, 45397
　Proctopexy, 45400, 45402
　Prostatectomy, 55866
　Pyloplasty, 50544
　Removal
　　Fallopian Tubes, 58661
　　Leiomyomata, 58545-58546
　　Ovaries, 58661
　　Spleen, 38120
　　Testis, 54690
　Resection
　　Intestines
　　　with Anastomosis, 44202,
　　　　44203
　Salpingostomy, 58673
　Splenectomy, 38120, 38129
　Stomach, 43651-43659
　　Gastric Bypass, 43644-43645
　　Gastroenterostomy, 43644-43645
　　Roux–en–Y, 43644
　Surgical, 38570-38572, 43651-
　　43653, 44180-44188, 44212,
　　44213, 44227, 44970, 45395-
　　45402, 47370, 47371, 49321-
　　49323, 49650, 49651, 50541,
　　50543, 50545, 50945-50948,
　　51992, 54690, 54692, 55550,
　　55866, 57425, 58545, 58546,
　　58552, 58554
　　with Guided Transhepatic
　　　Cholangiography, 47560-
　　　47561
　Unlisted Services and Procedures,
　　38129, 38589, 43289, 43659,
　　44238-45499, 47379, 47579,
　　49329, 49659, 50549, 50949,
　　51999, 54699, 55559, 58578,
　　58579, 58679, 59898
　Ureterolithotomy, 50945
　Ureteroneocystostomy, 50947-50948
　Urethral Suspension, 51990
　Vaginal Hysterectomy, 58550-58554
　Vaginal Suspension, 57425
　Vagus Nerves Transection, 43651,
　　43652
Laparotomy
　with Biopsy, 49000
　Exploration, 47015, 49000, 49002,
　　58960
　for Staging, 49220
　Hemorrhage Control, 49002
　Second Look, 58960
　Staging, 58960
　Surgical, 44050

Laparotomy, Exploratory
　See Abdomen, Exploration
Lapidus Procedure, 28297
Large Bowel
　See Anus; Cecum; Rectum
Laroyenne Operation
　Vagina, Abscess, Incision and
　　Drainage, 57010
Laryngeal Function Study, 92520
Laryngectomy
　Partial, 31367-31382
　Subtotal, 31367, 31368
　Total, 31360, 31365
Laryngocele
　Removal, 31300
Laryngofissure, 31300
Laryngography, 70373
　Instillation
　　Contrast Material
Laryngopharyngectomy
　See Excision, Larynx, with Pharynx
　Excision, Larynx, with Pharynx,
　　31390, 31395
Laryngopharynx
　See Hypopharynx
Laryngoplasty
　Burns, 31588
　Cricoid Split, 31587
　Laryngeal Stenosis, 31582
　Laryngeal Web, 31580
　Open Reduction of Fracture, 31584
Laryngoscopy
　Diagnostic, 31505
　Direct, 31515-31571
　Exploration, 31505, 31520-31526,
　　31575
　Fiberoptic, 31575-31579
　　with Stroboscopy, 31579
　Indirect, 31505-31513
　Newborn, 31520
　Operative, 31530-31561
Laryngotomy
　Diagnostic, 31320
　Partial, 31370-31382
　Removal
　　Tumor, 31300
　Total, 31360-31368
Larynx
　Aspiration
　　Endoscopy, 31515
　Biopsy
　　Endoscopy, 31510, 31535,
　　　31536, 31576
　Dilation
　　Endoscopic, 31528, 31529
　Endoscopy
　　Direct, 31515-31571
　　Excision, 31545-31546
　　Exploration, 31505, 31520-
　　　31526, 31575
　　Fiberoptic, 31575-31579
　　　with Stroboscopy, 31579
　　Indirect, 31505-31513
　　Operative, 31530-31561
　Excision
　　with Pharynx, 31390, 31395
　　Lesion, 31512, 31578
　　　Endoscopic, 31545-31546
　　Partial, 31367-31382
　　Total, 31360, 31365
　Exploration
　　Endoscopic, 31505, 31520-
　　　31526, 31575
　Fracture
　　Open Treatment, 31584
　Insertion
　　Obturator, 31527
　Nerve
　　Destruction, 31595
　Pharynx
　　with Pharynx, 31390
　Reconstruction
　　with Pharynx, 31395
　　Burns, 31588
　　Cricoid Split, 31587
　　Other, 31588

Lesion — *continued*
Intestines
Excision, 44110
Intestines, Small
Destruction, 44369
Excision, 44111
Iris
Destruction, 66770
Larynx
Excision, 31545-31546
Leg, Lower
Tendon Sheath, 27630
Lymph Node
Incision and Drainage, 38300, 38305
Mesentery
Excision, 44820
Mouth
Destruction, 40820
Excision, 40810-40816, 41116
Vestibule
Destruction, 40820
Repair, 40830
Nasopharynx
Excision, 61586, 61600
Nerve
Excision, 64774-64792
Nose
Intranasal
External Approach, 30118
Internal Approach, 30117
Orbit
Excision, 61333, 67412
Palate
Destruction, 42160
Excision, 42104-42120
Pancreas
Excision, 48120
Pelvis
Destruction, 58662
Penis
Destruction
Any Method, 54065
Cryosurgery, 54056
Electrodesiccation, 54055
Extensive, 54065
Laser Surgery, 54057
Simple, 54050-54060
Surgical Excision, 54060
Excision, 54060
Penile Plaque, 54110-54112
Pharynx
Destruction, 42808
Excision, 42808
Rectum
Excision, 45108
Removal
Larynx, 31512, 31578
Resection, 52354
Retina
Destruction
Extensive, 67227, 67228
Localized, 0017T, 67208, 67210
Radiation by Implantation of Source, 67218
Sclera
Excision, 66130
Skin
Abrasion, 15786, 15787
Biopsy, 11100, 11101
Destruction
Benign, 17000-17250
Malignant, 17260-17286
by Photodynamic Therapy, 96567
Excision
Benign, 11400-11471
Malignant, 11600-11646
Injection, 11900, 11901
Paring or Curettement, 11055-11057
Benign Hyperkeratotic, 11055-11057
Shaving, 11300-11313

Lesion — *continued*
Skin Tags
Removal, 11200, 11201
Skull
Excision, 61500, 61600-61608, 61615, 61616
Spermatic Cord
Excision, 55520
Spinal Cord
Destruction, 62280-62282
Excision, 63265-63273
Stomach
Excision, 43611
Testis
Excision, 54512
Toe
Excision, 28092
Tongue
Excision, 41110-41114
Uvula
Destruction, 42145
Excision, 42104-42107
Vagina
Destruction, 57061, 57065
Vulva
Destruction
Extensive, 56515
Simple, 56501
Wrist Tendon
Excision, 25110
Lesion of Sciatic Nerve
See Sciatic Nerve, Lesion
Leu 2 Antigens
See CD8
Leucine Aminopeptidase, 83670
Leukemia Lymphoma Virus I, Adult T Cell
See HTLV-I
Leukemia Lymphoma Virus I Antibodies, Human T Cell
See Antibody, HTLV-I
Leukemia Lymphoma Virus II Antibodies, Human T Cell
See Antibody, HTLV-II
Leukemia Virus II, Hairy Cell Associated, Human T Cell
See HTLV-II
Leukoagglutinins, 86021
Leukocyte
See White Blood Cell
Alkaline Phosphatase, 85540
Antibody, 86021
Histamine Release Test, 86343
Phagocytosis, 86344
Transfusion, 86950
Leukocyte Count
See White Blood Cell, Count
Leukocyte Histamine Release Test, 86343
Levarterenol
See Noradrenalin
Levator Muscle Rep
Blepharoptosis, Repair, 67901-67909
LeVeen Shunt
Insertion, 49425
Patency Test, 78291
Revision, 49426
Levulose
See Fructose
L Glutamine
See Glutamine
LH (Luteinizing Hormone), 80418, 80426, 83002
LHR (Leukocyte Histamine Release Test), 86343
Lidocaine
Assay, 80176
Lid Suture
Blepharoptosis, Repair, 67901-67909
Life Support
Organ Donor, 01990
Lift, Face
See Face Lift
Ligament
See Specific Site

Ligament — *continued*
Collateral
Repair, Knee with Cruciate Ligament, 27409
Dentate
Incision, 63180, 63182
Section, 63180, 63182
Injection, 20550
Release
Coracoacromial, 23415
Transverse Carpal, 29848
Repair
Elbow, 24343-24346
Knee Joint, 27405-27409
Ligation
Appendage
Dermal, 11200
Artery
Abdomen, 37617
Carotid, 37600-37606
Chest, 37616
Coronary, 33502
Coronary Artery, 33502
Ethmoidal, 30915
Extremity, 37618
Fistula, 37607
Maxillary, 30920
Neck, 37615
Temporal, 37609
Bronchus, 31899
Esophageal Varices, 43204, 43400
Fallopian Tube
Oviduct, 58600-58611, 58670
Gastroesophageal, 43405
Hemorrhoids, 46945, 46946
Oviducts, 59100
Salivary Duct, 42665
Shunt
Aorta
Pulmonary, 33924
Peritoneal
Venous, 49428
Thoracic Duct, 38380
Abdominal Approach, 38382
Thoracic Approach, 38381
Thyroid Vessels, 37615
Ureter, 53899
Vas Deferens, 55450
Vein
Clusters, 37785
Esophagus, 43205, 43244, 43400
Femoral, 37650
Gastric, 43244
Iliac, 37660
Jugular, Internal, 37565
Perforate, 37760
Saphenous, 37700-37735, 37780
Vena Cava, 37620
Ligature Strangulation
Skin Tags, 11200, 11201
Light Coagulation
See Photocoagulation
Light Scattering Measurement
See Nephelometry
Light Therapy, UV
See Actinotherapy
Limb
See Extremity
Limited Lymphadenectomy for Staging
See Lymphadenectomy, Limited, for Staging
Limited Neck Dissection
with Thyroidectomy, 60252
Limited Resection Mastectomies
See Breast, Excision, Lesion
Lindholm Operation
See Tenoplasty
Lingual Bone
See Hyoid Bone
Lingual Frenectomy
See Excision, Tongue, Frenum
Lingual Nerve
Avulsion, 64740
Incision, 64740
Transection, 64740

Lingual Tonsil
See Tonsils, Lingual
Linton Procedure, 37760
Lip
Biopsy, 40490
Excision, 40500-40530
Frenum, 40819
Incision
Frenum, 40806
Reconstruction, 40525, 40527
Repair, 40650-40654
Cleft Lip, 40700-40761
Fistula, 42260
Unlisted Services and Procedures, 40799
Lipase, 83690
Lip, Cleft
See Cleft Lip
Lipectomies, Aspiration
See Liposuction
Lipectomy, 15830-15839
Suction Assisted, 15876-15879
Lipids
Feces, 82705, 82710
Lipo–Lutin
See Progesterone
Lipolysis, Aspiration
See Liposuction
Lipophosphodiesterase I
See Tissue Typing
Lipoprotein, 83695
Blood, 0026T, 83700-83701, 83704, 83718-83719
LDL, 83700-83701, 83721
Lipoprotein, Alpha
See Lipoprotein
Lipoprotein, Pre–Beta
See Lipoprotein, Blood
Liposuction, 15876-15879
Lips
Skin Graft
Delay of Flap, 15630
Full Thickness, 15260, 15261
Pedicle Flap, 15576
Tissue Transfer, Adjacent, 14060, 14061
Lisfranc Operation
Amputation, Foot, 28800, 28805
Listeria Monocytogenes
Antibody, 86723
Lithium
Assay, 80178
Litholapaxy, 52317, 52318
Lithotripsy
with Cystourethroscopy, 52353
See Extracorporeal Shock Wave Therapy
Bile Duct Calculi (Stone)
Endoscopy, 43265
Bladder, 52353
Kidney, 50590
Pancreatic Duct Calculi (Stone)
Endoscopy, 43265
Ureter, 52353
Urethra, 52353
Lithotrity
See Litholapaxy
Liver
See Hepatic Duct
Ablation
Tumor, 47380-47382
Laparoscopic, 47370, 47371
Abscess
Aspiration, 47015
Incision and Drainage
Closed, 47011
Open, 47010
Percutaneous, 47011
Injection, 47015
Aspiration, 47015
Biopsy, 47100
Anesthesia, 00702
Cyst
Aspiration, 47015
Incision and Drainage
Open, 47010

Manipulation — *continued*
Dislocation and/or Fracture
Acetabulum, 27222
Acromioclavicular, 23545
Ankle, 27810, 27818, 27860
Carpometacarpal, 26670-26676
Chest Wall, 94667, 94668
Clavicle, 23505
Elbow, 24300, 24640
Epicondyle, 24565
Femoral, 27232, 27502, 27510, 27517
Petrochanteric, 27240
Fibula, 27781, 27788
Finger, 26725, 26727, 26742, 26755
Greater Tuberosity
Humeral, 23625
Hand, 26670-26676
Heel, 28405, 28406
Hip, 27257
Hip Socket, 27222
Humeral, 23605, 24505, 24535, 24577
Epicondyle, 24565
Intercarpal, 25660
Interphalangeal Joint, 26340, 26770-26776
Lunate, 25690
Malar Area, 21355
Mandibular, 21451
Metacarpal, 26605, 26607
Metacarpophalangeal, 26700-26706, 26742
Metacarpophalangeal Joint, 26340
Metatarsal Fracture, 28475, 28476
Nasal Bone, 21315, 21320
Orbit, 21401
Phalangeal Shaft, 26727
Distal, Finger or Thumb, 26755
Phalanges, Finger/Thumb, 26725
Phalanges
Finger, 26742, 26755, 26770-26776
Finger/Thumb, 26727
Great Toe, 28495, 28496
Toes, 28515
Radial, 24655, 25565
Radial Shaft, 25505
Radiocarpal, 25660
Radioulnar, 25675
Scapula, 23575
Shoulder, 23650, 23655
with Greater Tuberosity, 23665
with Surgical or Anatomical Neck, 23675
Sternoclavicular, 23525
with Surgical or Anatomical Neck, 23675
Talus, 28435, 28436
Tarsal, 28455, 28456
Thumb, 26641-26650
Tibial, 27532, 27752
Trans–Scaphoperilunar, 25680
Ulnar, 24675, 25535, 25565
Vertebral, 22315
Wrist, 25259, 25624, 25635, 25660, 25675, 25680, 25690
Foreskin, 54450
Globe, 92018, 92019
Hip, 27275
Interphalangeal Joint, Proximal, 26742
Knee, 27570
Osteopathic, 98925-98929
Physical Therapy, 97140
Shoulder
Application of Fixation Apparatus, 23700

Manipulation — *continued*
Spine
Anesthesia, 22505
Stoma, 44799
Tibial, Distal, 27762
Manometric Studies
Kidney
Pressure, 50396
Rectum
Anus, 91122
Ureter
Pressure, 50686
Ureterostomy, 50686
Manometry
Esophageal, 43499
Esophagogastric, 91020
Rectum
Anus, 90911
Mantoux Test
Skin Test, 86580
Manual Therapy, 97140
Maquet Procedure, 27418
Marcellation Operation
Hysterectomy, Vaginal, 58260-58270, 58550
Marshall–Marchetti–Krantz Procedure, 51840, 51841, 58152, 58267, 58293
Marsupialization
Cyst
Acne, 10040
Bartholin's Gland, 56440
Laryngeal, 31599
Splenic, 38999
Sublingual Salivary, 42409
Lesion
Kidney, 53899
Liver
Cyst or Abscess, 47300
Pancreatic Cyst, 48500
Urethral Diverticulum, 53240
Mass
Ablation
Kidney, 50542
Massage
Cardiac, 32160
Therapy, 97124
See Physical Medicine/Therapy/ Occupational Therapy
Masseter Muscle/Bone
Reduction, 21295, 21296
Mass Spectrometry and Tandem Mass Spectrometry
Analyte
Qualitative, 83788
Quantitative, 83789
Mastectomy
Gynecomastia, 19300
Modified Radical, 19307
Partial, 19301-19302
Radical, 19305-19306
Simple, Complete, 19303
Subcutaneous, 19304
Mastectomy, Halsted
See Mastectomy, Radical
Masters' 2–Step Stress Test, 93799
Mastoid
Excision
Complete, 69502
Radical, 69511
Modified, 69505
Petrous Apicectomy, 69530
Simple, 69501
Total, 69502
Obliteration, 69670
Repair
with Apicectomy, 69605
with Tympanoplasty, 69604
by Excision, 69601-69603
Fistula, 69700
Mastoid Cavity
Debridement, 69220, 69222
Mastoidectomy
with Apicectomy, 69605
with Labyrinthectomy, 69910
with Labyrinthotomy, 69802

Mastoidectomy — *continued*
with Petrous Apicectomy, 69530
with Skull Base Surgery, 61590, 61597
Decompression, 61595
Facial Nerve, 61595
with Tympanoplasty, 69604, 69641-69646
Ossicular Chain Reconstruction, 69636
and Synthetic Prosthesis, 69636
Cochlear Device Implantation, 69930
Complete, 69502
Revision, 69601-69605
Osseointegrated Implant
for External Speech Processor/Cochlear Stimulator, 69715, 69718
Ossicular Chain Reconstruction, 69605
Radical, 69511
Modified, 69505
Revision, 69602, 69603
Simple, 69501
Mastoidotomy, 69635-69637
with Tympanoplasty, 69635
Ossicular Chain Reconstruction, 69636
and Synthetic Prosthesis, 69637
Mastoids
Polytomography, 76101, 76102
X-ray, 70120, 70130
Mastopexy, 19316
Mastotomy, 19020
Maternity Care and Delivery, 0500F-0502F, 0503F, 59400-59898
See also Abortion, Cesarean Delivery, Ectopic Pregnancy, Vaginal Delivery
Maxilla
See Facial Bones; Mandible
Bone Graft, 21210
CT Scan, 70486-70488
Cyst, Excision, 21048, 21049
Excision, 21030, 21032-21034
Fracture
with Fixation, 21345-21347
Closed Treatment, 21345, 21421
Open Treatment, 21346-21348, 21422, 21423
Osteotomy, 21206
Reconstruction
with Implant, 21245, 21246, 21248, 21249
Tumor
Excision, 21048-21049
Maxillary Arteries
See Artery, Maxillary
Maxillary Sinus
See Sinus, Maxillary
Maxillary Torus Palatinus
Tumor Excision, 21032
Maxillectomy, 31225, 31230
Maxillofacial Fixation
Application
Halo Type Appliance, 21100
Maxillofacial Impressions
Auricular Prosthesis, 21086
Definitive Obturator Prosthesis, 21080
Facial Prosthesis, 21088
Interim Obturator Prosthesis, 21079
Mandibular Resection Prosthesis, 21081
Nasal Prosthesis, 21087
Oral Surgical Splint, 21085
Orbital Prosthesis, 21077
Palatal Augmentation Prosthesis, 21082
Palatal Lift Prosthesis, 21083
Speech Aid Prosthesis, 21084
Surgical Obturator Prosthesis, 21076

Maxillofacial Procedures
Unlisted Services and Procedures, 21299
Maxillofacial Prosthetics, 21076-21088
Unlisted Services and Procedures, 21089
Maydl Operation, 45563, 50810
Mayo Hernia Repair, 49580-49587
Mayo Operation
Varicose Vein Removal, 37700-37735, 37780, 37785
Mayo Procedure, 28292
Maze Procedure, 33254, 33255-33256
MBC, 87181-87190
McBride Procedure, 28292
McBurney Operation
Hernia Repair, Inguinal, 49495-49500, 49505
Incarcerated, 49496, 49501, 49507, 49521
Recurrent, 49520
Sliding, 49525
McCannel Procedure, 66682
McCauley Procedure, 28240
McDonald Operation, 57700
McKissock Surgery, 19318
McIndoe Procedure, 57291
McVay Operation
Hernia Repair, Inguinal, 49495-49500, 49505
Incarcerated, 49496, 49501, 49507, 49521
Laparoscopic, 49650, 49651
Recurrent, 49520
Sliding, 49525
Measles, German
See Rubella
Measles Immunization, 90705, 90707-90708, 90710
Measles Uncomplicated
Measurement
See Rubeola
Left Ventricular Filling Pressure, 0086T
Meat Fibers
Feces, 89160
Meatoplasty, 69310
Meatotomy, 53020, 53025
Contact Laser Vaporization
with/without Transurethral Resection of Prostate, 52648
with Cystourethroscopy, 52281
Infant, 53025
Non–Contact Laser Coagulation
Prostate, 52647
Transurethral Electrosurgical Resection
Prostate, 52601
Ureter, 52290
Urethral
Cystourethroscopy, 52290-52305
Meckel's Diverticulum
Excision, 44800
Unlisted Services and Procedures, 44899
Median Nerve
Decompression, 64721
Neuroplasty, 64721
Release, 64721
Repair
Suture
Motor, 64835
Transposition, 64721
Median Nerve Compression
See Carpal Tunnel Syndrome
Mediastinal Cyst
See Cyst, Mediastinal
Mediastinoscopy, 39400
Mediastinotomy
Cervical Approach, 39000
Transthoracic Approach, 39010
Mediastinum
See Chest; Thorax
Cyst
Excision, 32662, 39200

© 2006 Ingenix

Phalanx, Finger
　Craterization, 26235, 26236
　Cyst
　　Excision, 26210, 26215
　Diaphysectomy, 26235, 26236
　Excision, 26235, 26236
　　Radical
　　　for Tumor, 26260-26262
　Fracture
　　Articular
　　　with Manipulation, 26742
　　　Closed Treatment, 26740
　　　Open Treatment, 26746
　　Distal, 26755, 26756
　　　Closed Treatment, 26750
　　　Open Treatment, 26765
　　　Percutaneous, 26756
　　Open Treatment, 26735
　　Distal, 26765
　　　Percutaneous Fixation, 26756
　　Shaft, 26720-26727
　　　Open Treatment, 26735
　Incision and Drainage, 26034
　Ostectomy
　　Radical
　　　for Tumor, 26260-26262
　Repair
　　Lengthening, 26568
　　Nonunion, 26546
　　Osteotomy, 26567
　Saucerization, 26235, 26236
　Thumb
　　Fracture
　　　Shaft, 26720-26727
　Tumor
　　Excision, 26210, 26215
Phalanx, Great Toe
　See Phalanx, Toe
　Fracture
　　Closed Treatment, 28490
　　　with Manipulation, 28495, 28496
　　　Percutaneous Fixation, 28496
　　Open Treatment, 28505
Phalanx, Toe
　Condyle
　　Excision, 28126
　Craterization, 28124
　Cyst
　　Excision, 28108
　Diaphysectomy, 28124
　Excision, 28124, 28150-28160
　Fracture
　　with Manipulation, 28515
　　without Manipulation, 28510
　　Open Treatment, 28525
　Repair
　　Osteotomy, 28310, 28312
　Saucerization, 28124
　Tumor
　　Excision, 28108, 28175
Pharmaceutic Preparations
　See Drug
Pharmacotherapies
　See Chemotherapy
Pharyngeal Tonsil
　See Adenoids
Pharyngectomy
　Partial, 42890
Pharyngolaryngectomy, 31390, 31395
Pharyngoplasty, 42950
Pharyngorrhaphy
　See Suture, Pharynx
Pharyngostomy, 42955
Pharyngotomy
　See Incision, Pharynx
Pharyngotympanic Tube
　See Eustachian Tube
Pharynx
　See Nasopharynx; Throat
　Biopsy, 42800-42806
　Cineradiography, 70371, 74230
　Creation
　　Stoma, 42955
　Excision, 42145
　　with Larynx, 31390, 31395

Pharynx — *continued*
　Excision — *continued*
　　Partial, 42890
　　Resection, 42892, 42894
　Hemorrhage, 42960-42962
　Lesion
　　Destruction, 42808
　　Excision, 42808
　Reconstruction, 42950
　Removal, Foreign Body, 42809
　Repair
　　with Esophagus, 42953
　Unlisted Services and Procedures, 42999
　Video, 70371, 74230
　X-ray, 70370, 74210
Phencyclidine, 83992
Phenobarbital, 82205
　Assay, 80184
Phenothiazine, 84022
Phenotype Analysis
　by Nucleic Acid
　　Infectious Agent
　　　HIV-1 Drug Resistance, 87903, 87904
Phenotype Prediction
　by Generic Database
　　HIV-1
　　　Drug Susceptibility, 87900
　　Using Regularly Updated Genotypic Bioinformatics, 87900
Phenylalanine, 84030
Phenylalanine–Tyrosine Ratio, 84030
Phenylketones, 84035
Phenylketonuria
　See Phenylalanine
Phenytoin
　Assay, 80185, 80186
Pheochromocytoma, 80424
Pheresis
　See Apheresis
Phlebectasia
　See Varicose Vein
Phlebectomy
　Varicose Veins, 37765, 37766
Phlebographies
　See Venography
Phlebography, 76499
Phleborheography, 93965
Phleborrhaphy
　See Suture, Vein
Phlebotomy
　Therapeutic, 99195
Phonocardiogram
　Evaluation, 93799
　Intracardiac, 93799
　Tracing, 93799
Phoria
　See Strabismus
Phosphatase
　Alkaline, 84075, 84080
　　Blood, 84078
　Forensic Examination, 84061
Phosphatase, Acid, 84060
　Blood, 84066
Phosphate, Pyridoxal
　See Pyridoxal Phosphate
Phosphatidylcholine Cholinephosphohydrolase
　See Tissue Typing
Phosphatidyl Glycerol
Phosphatidylglycerol, 84081
　See Phosphatidylglycerol
Phosphocreatine Phosphotransferase, ADP
　See CPK
Phosphogluconate–6
　Dehydrogenase, 84085
Phosphoglycerides, Glycerol
　See Phosphatidylglycerol
Phosphohexose Isomerase, 84087
Phosphohydrolases
　See Phosphatase
Phosphokinase, Creatine
　See CPK

Phospholipase C
　See Tissue Typing
Phospholipid Antibody, 86147, 86148
Phospholipid Cofactor Antibody, 0030T
Phosphomonoesterase
　See Phosphatase
Phosphoric Monoester Hydrolases
　See Phosphatase
Phosphorous, 84100
　Urine, 84105
Phosphotransferase, ADP Phosphocreatine
　See CPK
Photochemotherapies, Extracorporeal
　See Photopheresis
Photochemotherapy, 96910-96913
　See Dermatology
　Endoscopic Light, 96570, 96571
Photocoagulation
　Endolaser Panretinal
　　Vitrectomy, 67040
　Focal Endolaser
　　Vitrectomy, 67040
　Iridoplasty, 66762
　Lesion
　　Cornea, 65450
　　Retina, 0017T, 67210, 67227, 67228
　Retinal Detachment
　　Prophylaxis, 67145
　　Repair, 67105
Photodensity
　Radiographic Absorptiometry, 77083
Photodynamic Therapy
　External, 96567
Photography
　Ocular
　　External, 92285
　　Internal, 92286, 92287
　Skin, Diagnostic, 96904
Photo Patch
　Allergy Test, 95052
　See Allergy Tests
Photopheresis
　Extracorporeal, 36522
Photophoresis
　See Actinotherapy; Photochemotherapy
Photoradiation Therapies
　See Actinotherapy
Photoscreen
　Ocular, 0065T
Photosensitivity Testing, 95056
　See Allergy Tests
Phototherapies
　See Actinotherapy
Phototherapy, Ultraviolet
　See Actinotherapy
Phrenic Nerve
　Anastomosis
　　to Facial Nerve, 64870
　Avulsion, 64746
　Incision, 64746
　Injection
　　Anesthetic, 64410
　Transection, 64746
Physical Examination
　Office and/or Other Outpatient Services, 99201-99205
Physical Medicine/Therapy/Occupational Therapy
　See Neurology, Diagnostic
　Activities of Daily Living, 97535, 99509
　Aquatic Therapy
　　with Exercises, 97113
　Athletic Training
　　Evaluation, 97005
　　Re-evaluation, 97006
　Check–Out
　　Orthotics/Prosthetics
　　　ADL, 97762
　Cognitive Skills Development, 97532
　Community/Work Reintegration, 97537

Physical Medicine/Therapy/Occupational Therapy — *continued*
　Evaluation, 97001, 97002
　Hydrotherapy
　　Hubbard Tank, 97036
　　Pool with Exercises, 97036, 97113
　Joint Mobilization, 97140
　Kinetic Therapy, 97530
　Manipulation, 97140
　Modalities
　　Contrast Baths, 97034
　　Diathermy Treatment, 97024
　　Electric Stimulation
　　　Attended, Manual, 97032
　　　Unattended, 97014
　　Hot or Cold Pack, 97010
　　Hydrotherapy (Hubbard Tank), 97036
　　Infrared Light Treatment, 97026
　　Iontophoresis, 97033
　　Microwave Therapy, 97024
　　Paraffin Bath, 97018
　　Traction, 97012
　　Ultrasound, 97035
　　Ultraviolet Light, 97028
　　Unlisted Services and Procedures, 97039
　　Vasopneumatic Device, 97016
　　Whirlpool Therapy, 97022
　Orthotics Training, 97760
　Osteopathic Manipulation, 98925-98929
　Procedures
　　Aquatic Therapy, 97113
　　Gait Training, 97116
　　Group Therapeutic, 97150
　　Massage Therapy, 97124
　　Neuromuscular Reeducation, 97112
　　Physical Performance Test, 97750
　　Therapeutic Exercises, 4018F, 97110
　　Traction Therapy, 97140
　　Work Hardening, 97545, 97546
　Prosthetic Training, 97761
　Sensory Integration, 97533
　Therapeutic Activities, 97530
　Unlisted Services and Procedures, 97139, 97799
　Wheelchair Management, 97542
　Work Reintegration, 97537
Physical Therapy
　See Physical Medicine/Therapy/Occupational Therapy
Physician Services
　Care Plan Oversight Services, 99374-99380
　　Home Health Agency Care, 99374
　　Hospice, 99377, 99378
　　Nursing Facility, 99379, 99380
　Direction, Advanced Life Support, 99288
　Prolonged
　　with Direct Patient Contact, 99354-99357
　　　Outpatient Office, 99354, 99355
　　with Direct Patient Services Inpatient, 99356, 99357
　　without Direct Patient Contact, 99358, 99359
　Standby, 99360
　Supervision, Care Plan Oversight Services, 99374-99380
Pierce Ears, 69090
Piercing of Ear Lobe, 69090
Piles
　See Hemorrhoids
Pilon Fracture Treatment, 27824
Pilonidal Cyst
　Excision, 11770-11772
　Incision and Drainage, 10080, 10081
Pin
　See Wire

© 2006 Ingenix

Index

© 2006 Ingenix

Repair — *continued*
  Body Cast, 29720
  Brain
    Wound, 61571
  Breast
    Suspension, 19316
  Bronchi
    Fistula, 32815
  Brow Ptosis, 67900
  Bunion, 28290-28299
  Bypass Graft, 35901-35907
    Fistula, 35870
  Calcaneus
    Osteotomy, 28300
  Cannula, 36860, 36861
  Carpal, 25440
  Carpal Bone, 25431
  Cervix
    Cerclage, 57700
      Abdominal, 59320, 59325
    Suture, 57720
  Chest Wall, 32905
    Closure, 32810
    Fistula, 32906
    Pectus Excavatum, 21740
  Chin
    Augmentation, 21120, 21123
    Osteotomy, 21121-21123
  Clavicle
    Osteotomy, 23480, 23485
  Cleft Hand, 26580
  Cleft Lip, 40525, 40527, 40700-
      40761
    Nasal Deformity, 40700, 40701,
      40720, 40761
  Cleft Palate
    See Cleft Palate Repair
  Colon
    Fistula, 44650-44661
    Hernia, 44050
    Malrotation, 44055
    Obstruction, 44050
  Cornea
    See Cornea, Repair
  Coronary Chamber Fistula, 33500,
      33501
  Cyst
    Bartholin's Gland, 56440
    Choledochal, 47719
    Liver, 47300
  Defibrillator, Heart, 33218, 33220
  Diaphragm
    for Eventration, 39545
    Hernia, 39502-39541
    Lacerations, 39501
  Ductus Arteriosus, 33820-33824
  Ear, Middle
    Oval Window Fistula, 69666
    Round Window Fistula, 69667
  Elbow
    Fasciotomy, 24350-24356
    Hemiepiphyseal Arrest, 24470
    Ligament, 24343-24346
    Muscle, 24341
    Muscle Transfer, 24301
    Tendon, 24340-24342
      Each, 24341
    Tendon Lengthening, 24305
    Tendon Transfer, 24301
    Tennis Elbow, 24350-24356
  Encephalocele, 62121
  Enterocele
    Hysterectomy, 58270, 58294
  Epididymis, 54900, 54901
  Epispadias, 54380-54390
  Esophagus, 43300, 43310, 43313
    Esophagogastrostomy, 43320
    Esophagojejunostomy, 43340,
      43341
    Fistula, 43305, 43312, 43314,
      43420, 43425
    Fundoplasty, 43324, 43325
    Muscle, 43330, 43331
    Preexisting Perforation, 43405
    Varices, 43401
    Wound, 43410, 43415

Repair — *continued*
  Eye
    Ciliary Body, 66680
      Suture, 66682
    Conjunctiva, 65270-65273
      Wound, 65270-65273
    Cornea, 65275
      with Glue, 65286
      Astigmatism, 65772, 65775
      Wound, 65275-65285
        Dehiscence, 66250
    Fistula
      Lacrimal Gland, 68770
    Iris
      with Ciliary Body, 66680
      Suture, 66682
    Lacrimal Duct
      Canaliculi, 68700
    Lacrimal Punctum, 68705
    Retina
      Detachment, 67101-67112
    Sclera
      with Glue, 65286
      with Graft, 66225
      Reinforcement, 67250, 67255
      Staphyloma, 66220, 66225
      Wound, 65286, 66250
    Strabismus
      Chemodenervation, 67345
    Symblepharon
      with Graft, 68335
      without Graft, 68330
      Division, 68340
    Trabeculae, 65855
  Eyebrow
    Ptosis, 67900
  Eyelashes
    Epilation
      by Forceps, 67820
      by Other than Forceps, 67825
    Incision of Lid Margin, 67830
      with Free Mucous Membrane
        Graft, 67835
  Eyelid, 21280, 21282
    Ectropion
      Blepharoplasty, 67916, 67917
      Suture, 67914
      Thermocauterization, 67915
    Entropion
      Blepharoplasty, 67923, 67924
      Suture, 67921-67924
      Thermocauterization, 67922
    Excisional, 67961, 67966
    Lagophthalmos, 67912
    Ptosis
      Conjunctivo–Tarso–Muller's
        Muscle–Levator Resec-
        tion, 67908
      Frontalis Muscle Technique,
        67901, 67902
      Levator Resection, 67903,
        67904
      Reduction of Overcorrection,
        67909
      Superior Rectus Technique,
        67906
    Retraction, 67911
    Wound
      Suture, 67930, 67935
  Eye Muscles
    Strabismus
      Adjustable Sutures, 67335
      One Horizontal Muscle, 67311
      One Vertical Muscle, 67314
      Posterior Fixation Suture
        Technique, 67334,
        67335
      Previous Surgery not Involving
        Extraocular Muscles,
        67331
      Release Extensive Scar Tissue,
        67343
      Superior Oblique Muscle,
        67318
      Two Horizontal Muscles,
        67312

Repair — *continued*
  Eye Muscles — *continued*
    Strabismus — *continued*
      Two or More Vertical Muscles,
        67316
    Wound
      Extraocular Muscle, 65290
  Facial Bones, 21208, 21209
  Facial Nerve
    Paralysis, 15840-15845
    Suture
      Intratemporal, Lateral to
        Geniculate Ganglion,
        69740
      Intratemporal, Medial to
        Geniculate Ganglion,
        69745
  Fallopian Tube, 58752
    Anastomosis, 58750
    Create Stoma, 58770
  Fascial Defect, 50728
  Femur, 27470, 27472
    with Graft, 27170
    Epiphysis, 27475-27485, 27742
      Arrest, 27185
      by Pinning, 27176
      by Traction, 27175
      Open Treatment, 27177,
        27178
    Osteoplasty, 27179
    Osteotomy, 27181
    Muscle Transfer, 27110
    Osteotomy, 27140, 27151, 27450,
        27454
      with Fixation, 27165
      with Open Reduction, 27156
    Femoral Neck, 27161
  Fibula
    Epiphysis, 27477-27485, 27730-
        27742
    Osteotomy, 27707-27712
  Finger
    Claw Finger, 26499
    Macrodactyly, 26590
    Polydactylous, 26587
    Syndactyly, 26560-26562
    Tendon
      Extensor, 26415-26434,
        26445, 26449, 26455
      Flexor, 26356-26358, 26440,
        26442
      Joint Stabilization, 26474
      PIP Joint, 26471
    Toe Transfer, 26551-26556
    Trigger, 26055
    Volar Plate, 26548
    Web Finger, 26560
  Fistula
    Carotid–Cavernous, 61710
    Ileoanal Pouch, 46710, 46712
    Mastoid, 69700
    Rectovaginal, 57308
  Foot
    Fascia, 28250
    Muscles, 28250
    Tendon, 28200-28226, 28238
  Gallbladder
    with Gastroenterostomy, 47741
    with Intestines, 47720-47740
    Laceration, 47999
  Great Arteries, 33770-33781
  Great Vessel, 33320-33322
  Hallux Valgus, 28290-28299
  Hamstring, 27097
  Hand
    Cleft Hand, 26580
    Muscles, 26591, 26593
    Tendon
      Extensor, 26410-26416,
        26426, 26428, 26433-
        26437
      Flexor, 26350-26358, 26440
      Profundus, 26370-26373
  Hearing Aid
    Bone Conduction, 69711

Repair — *continued*
  Heart
    Anomaly, 33600-33617
    Aortic Sinus, 33702-33722
    Artificial Heart
      Intracorporeal, 0052T, 0053T
    Atrial, 33254, 33255-33256
    Atrioventricular Canal, 33660,
        33665
      Complete, 33670
    Atrioventricular Valve, 33660,
        33665
    Blood Vessel, 33320-33322
    Cor Triatriatum, 33732
    Fibrillation, 33254, 33255-33256
    Infundibular, 33476, 33478
    Mitral Valve, 33420-33427
    Myocardium, 33542
    Outflow Tract, 33476, 33478
    Post–Infarction, 33542, 33545
    Prosthetic Valve, 33670, 33852,
        33853
    Prosthetic Valve Dysfunction,
        33496
    Pulmonary Artery Shunt, 33924
    Pulmonary Valve, 33470-33474
    Septal Defect, 33545, 33608,
        33610, 33681-33688,
        33692-33697
      Atrial and Ventricular, 33647
      Atrium, 33641
    Sinus of Valsalva, 33702-33722
    Sinus Venosus, 33645
    Tetralogy of Fallot, 33692
    Total Replacement Heart System
      Intracorporeal, 0052T, 0053T
    Tricuspid Valve, 33465
    Ventricle, 33611, 33612
      Obstruction, 33619
    Ventricular Tunnel, 33722
    Wound, 33300, 33305
  Hepatic Duct
    with Intestines, 47765, 47802
  Hernia, 50728
    with Spermatic Cord, 54640
    Abdomen, 49565, 49590
      Incisional or Ventral, 49560
    Epigastric, 49570
      Incarcerated, 49572
    Femoral, 49550
      Incarcerated, 49553
      Recurrent, 49555
      Recurrent Incarcerated, 49557
      Reducible Recurrent, 49555
    Incisional
      Incarcerated, 49561
      Recurrent Incarcerated, 49566
    Inguinal, 49491-49521
      Initial
        by Laparoscopy, 49650
        Incarcerated, 49496,
          49501, 49507
        Reducible, 49495, 49500,
          49505
        Strangulated, 49496,
          49501, 49507
      Recurrent
        by Laparoscopy, 49651
        Incarcerated, 49521
        Reducible, 49520
        Strangulated, 49521
      Sliding, 49525
    Intestinal, 44025, 44050
    Lumbar, 49540
    Lung, 32800
    Orchiopexy, 54640
    Parasternal, 49999
    Reducible
      Initial
        Epigastric, 49570
        Femoral, 49550
        Incisional, 49560
        Inguinal, 49495, 49500,
          49505
        Umbilical, 49580, 49585
        Ventral, 49560

© 2006 Ingenix

Replacement — *continued*
  Knee
    Total, 27447
  Mitral Valve, 33430
  Nerve, 64726
  Neurostimulator
    Pulse Generator/Receiver
      Intracranial, 61885
      Peripheral Nerve, 64590
      Spinal, 63685
  Ossicles
    with Prosthesis, 69633, 69637
  Ossicular Replacement
    See TORP (Total Ossicular Re-
      placement Prosthesis)
  Pacemaker, 33206-33208
    Catheter, 33210
    Electrode, 33210, 33211, 33216,
      33217
  Pacing Cardioverter–Defibrillator
    Leads, 33243, 33244
    Pulse Generator Only, 33241
  Penile
    Prosthesis, 54410, 54411, 54416,
      54417
  Prosthesis
    Skull, 62143
    Urethral Sphincter, 53448
  Pulmonary Valve, 33475
  Pulse Generator
    Brain, 61885
    Peripheral Nerve, 64590
    Spinal Cord, 63685
  Receiver
    Brain, 61885
    Peripheral Nerve, 64590
    Spinal Cord, 63685
  Skull Plate, 62143
  Spinal Cord
    Reservoir, 62360
  Stent
    Ureteral, 50382, 50387
  Tissue Expanders
    Skin, 11970
  Total Replacement
    See Hip, Total Replacement
  Total Replacement Heart System
    Intracorporeal, 0052T-0053T
  Tricuspid Valve, 33465
  Ureter
    with Intestines, 50840
    Electronic Stimulator, 53899
  Uterus
    Inverted, 59899
  Venous Access Device, 36582,
    36583, 36585
    Catheter, 36578
  Venous Catheter
    Central, 36580, 36581, 36584
Replantation, Reimplantation
  Adrenal Tissue, 60699
  Arm, Upper, 20802
  Digit, 20816, 20822
  Foot, 20838
  Forearm, 20805
  Hand, 20808
  Scalp, 17999
  Thumb, 20824, 20827
Report Preparation
  Extended, Medical, 99080
  Psychiatric, 90889
Reposition
  Toe to Hand, 26551-26556
Repositioning
  Central Venous Catheter, Previously
    Placed, 36597
  Electrode
    Heart, 33215, 33216, 33217,
      33226
  Gastrostomy Tube, 43761
  Heart
    Defibrillator
      Leads, 33215, 33216, 33226,
        33249
  Intraocular Lens, 66825
  Tricuspid Valve, 33468

Reproductive Tissue
  Cryopreserved
  Preparation
    Thawing, 89354
  Storage, 89344
Reprogramming
  Shunt
    Brain, 62252
Reptilase Test, 85635
  Time, 85635
Reptilase Time
  See Thrombin Time
Resection
  Abdomen, 51597
  Aortic Valve Stenosis, 33415
  Bladder Diverticulum, 52305
  Bladder Neck
    Transurethral, 52500
  Brain Lobe
    See Lobectomy, Brain
  Chest Wall, 19260-19272
  Diaphragm, 39560, 39561
  Humeral Head, 23195
  Intestines, Small
    Laparoscopic, 44202, 44203
  Mouth
    with Tongue Excision, 41153
  Myocardium
    Aneurysm, 33542
    Septal Defect, 33545
  Nasal Septum Submucous
    See Nasal Septum, Submucous
      Resection
  Nose
    Septum, 30520
  Ovary, Wedge
    See Ovary, Wedge Resection
  Palate, 42120
  Pancoast Tumor, 32503-32504
  Phalangeal Head
    Toe, 28153
  Prostate Transurethral
    See Prostatectomy, Transurethral
  Radical
    Abdomen, 51597
    Arm, Upper, 24077
    Elbow, 24077
      with Contracture Release,
        24149
    Foot, 28046
    Humerus, 24150, 24151
    Radius, 24152, 24153
    Tumor
      Ankle, 27615
      Calcaneus or Talus, 27647
      Clavicle, 23200
      Femur, 27365
      Fibula, 27646
      Humerus, 23220
      Humerus with Autograft,
        23221
      Humerus with Prosthetic Re-
        placement, 23222
      Knee, 27329, 27365
      Leg, Lower, 27615
      Leg, Upper, 27329
      Metatarsal, 28173
      Phalanx, Toe, 28175
      Scapula, 23210
      Tarsal, 28171
      Tibia, 27645
  Rhinectomy
    Partial, 30150
    Total, 30160
  Ribs, 19260-19272, 32900
  Synovial Membrane
    See Synovectomy
  Temporal Bone, 69535
  Tumor
    Lung, 32503-32504
  Ulna
    Arthrodesis
      Radioulnar Joint, 25830
  Ureterocele
    Ectopic, 52301
    Orthotopic, 52300

Resection — *continued*
  Vena Cava
    with Reconstruction, 37799
Resonance Spectroscopy, Magnetic
  See Magnetic Resonance Spec-
    troscopy
Respiration, Positive–Pressure
  See Pressure Breathing, Positive
Respiratory Pattern Recording
  Preventive
    Infant, 94772
Respiratory Syncytial Virus
  Antibody, 86756
  Antigen Detection
    Direct Fluorescent Antibody,
      87280
    Direct Optical Observation, 87807
    Enzyme Immunoassay, 87420
  Immuneglobulin, 90378, 90379
Response, Auditory Evoked
  See Auditory Evoked Potentials
Rest Home Visit
  See Domiciliary Services
Restoration
  Ventricular, 33548
Resuscitation
  See Cardiac Massage
  Cardiopulmonary (CPR), 92950
  Newborn, 99440
Reticulocyte
  Count, 85044, 85045
Retina
  Incision
    Encircling Material, 67115
  Lesion
    Extensive
      Destruction, 67227, 67228
    Localized
      Destruction, 0017T, 67208-
        67218
  Repair
    Detachment
      with Vitrectomy, 67108,
        67112
      by Scleral Buckling, 67112
      Cryotherapy or Diathermy,
        67101
      Injection of Air, 67110
      Photocoagulation, 67105
      Scleral Dissection, 67107
    Prophylaxis
      Detachment, 67141, 67145
    Retinopathy
      Destruction
        Cryotherapy, Diathermy,
          67227
        Photocoagulation, 67228
Retinacular
  Knee
    Release, 27425
Retinopathy
  Destruction
    Cryotherapy, Diathermy, 67227
    Photocoagulation, 67228
Retinopexy, Pneumatic, 67110
Retraction, Clot
  See Clot Retraction
Retrieval
  Transcatheter Foreign Body, 37203
Retrocaval Ureter
  Ureterolysis, 50725
**Retrograde Cholangiopancreatogra-
  phies, Endoscopic**
  See Cholangiopancreatography
Retrograde Cystourethrogram
  See Urethrocystography, Retrograde
Retrograde Pyelogram
  See Urography, Retrograde
Retroperitoneal Area
  Abscess
    Incision and Drainage
      Open, 49060
      Percutaneous, 49061
  Biopsy, 49010

Retroperitoneal Area — *continued*
  Cyst
    Destruction/Excision, 49200,
      49201
  Endometriomas
    Destruction/Excision, 49200,
      49201
  Exploration, 49010
  Needle Biopsy
    Mass, 49180
  Tumor
    Destruction
      Excision, 49200, 49201
Retroperitoneal Fibrosis
  Ureterolysis, 50715
Retropubic Prostatectomies
  See Prostatectomy, Retropubic
Revascularization
  Distal Upper Extremity
    with Interval Ligation, 36838
  Heart
    Arterial Implant, 33999
    Myocardial Resection, 33542
    Other Tissue Grafts, 20926
  Interval Ligation
    Distal Upper Extremity, 36838
  Penis, 37788
  Transmyocardial, 33140, 33141
Reversal, Vasectomy
  See Vasovasorrhaphy
Reverse T3, 84482
Reverse Triiodothyronine, 84482
Revision
  See Reconstruction
  Abdomen, Venous Shunt, 49429
  Aorta, 33404
  Atrial, 33254-33256
  Blepharoplasty, 15820-15823
  Breast
    Implant, 19380
  Bronchial Stent, 31638
  Bronchus, 32501
  Bypass Graft
    Vein Patch, 35685
  Cervicoplasty, 15819
  Cornea
    Prosthesis, 65770
    Reshaping
      Epikeratoplasty, 65767
      Keratomileusis, 65760
      Keratophakia, 65765
  Defibrillator Site
    Chest, 33223
  Ear, Middle, 69662
  External Fixation System, 20693
  Eye
    Aqueous Shunt, 66185
  Gastrostomy Tube, 44373
  Hip Replacement
    See Replacement, Hip, Revision
  Hymenal Ring, 56700
  Infusion Pump
    Intra–Arterial, 36261
    Intravenous, 36576, 36578,
      36582, 36583
  Iris
    Iridoplasty, 66762
    Iridotomy, 66761
  Jejunostomy Tube, 44373
  Lower Extremity Arterial Bypass,
    35879, 35881
  Pacemaker Site
    Chest, 33222
  Rhytidectomy, 15824-15829
  Semicircular Canal
    Fenestration, 69840
  Shunt
    Intrahepatic Portosystemic,
      37183
  Skin Pocket, Chest
    for Implantable Cardioverter–De-
      fibrillator, 33223
    for Pacemaker, 33222
  Sling, 53442
  Stapedectomy
    See Stapedectomy, Revision

Revision — *continued*
Stomach
for Obesity, 43848
Tracheostomy
Scar, 31830
Urinary–Cutaneous Anastomosis,
50727, 50728
Vagina
Graft, 57295
Sling
Stress Incontinence, 57287
Venous Access Device, 36576,
36578, 36582, 36583, 36585
Ventricle
Ventriculomyectomy, 33416
Ventriculomyotomy, 33416
Vesicostomy, 51880
Rh (D)
See Blood Typing
Rheumatoid Factor, 86430, 86431
Rh Immune Globulin
See Immune Globulins, Rho (D)
Rhinectomy
Partial, 30150
Total, 30160
Rhinomanometry, 92512
Rhinopharynx
See Nasopharynx
Rhinophyma
Repair, 30120
Rhinoplasty
Cleft Lip
Cleft Palate, 30460, 30462
Primary, 30400-30420
Secondary, 30430-30450
Rhinoscopy
See Endoscopy, Nose
Rhinotomy
Lateral, 30118, 30320
Rhizotomy, 63185, 63190
Rho(D) Vaccine, 90384-90386
Rho Variant Du, 86905
Rh Type, 86901
Rhytidectomy, 15824-15829
Cheek, 15828
Chin, 15828
Forehead, 15824
Glabellar Frown Lines, 15826
Neck, 15825, 15828
Superficial Musculoaponeurotic
System, 15829
Rhytidoplasties
See Face Lift
Rib
Antibody, 86756
Antigen Detection by Immunoassay
with Direct Optical Observation
Direct Fluorescense, 87280
Enzyme Immunoassay, 87420
Bone Graft
with Microvascular Anastomosis,
20962
Excision, 21600-21616, 32900
Fracture
Closed Treatment, 21800
External Fixation, 21810
Open Treatment, 21805
Free Osteocutaneous Flap with Mi-
crovascular Anastomosis,
20969
Graft
to Face, 21230
Resection, 19260-19272, 32900
X–ray, 71100-71111
Riboflavin, 84252
Richardson Operation Hysterectomy
See Hysterectomy, Abdominal, Total
Richardson Procedure, 53460
Rickettsia
Antibody, 86757
Ridell Operation
Sinusotomy, Frontal, 31075-31087
Ridge, Alveolar
See Alveolar Ridge
Right Atrioventricular Valve
See Tricuspid Valve

Right Heart Cardiac Catheterization
See Cardiac Catheterization, Right
Heart
Ripstein Operation
See Proctopexy
Risk Factor Reduction Intervention
Group Counseling, 99411, 99412
Individual Counseling, 99401-99404
Risser Jacket, 29010, 29015
Removal, 29710
RK, 65771
Rocky Mountain Spotted Fever, 86000
Roentgenographic
See X–Ray
Roentgenography
See Radiology, Diagnostic
Roentgen Rays
See X–Ray
ROM, 95851, 95852, 97110, 97530
Ropes Test, 83872
Rorschach Test, 96101-96103
Ross Procedure, 33413
Rotation Flap
See Skin, Adjacent Tissue Transfer
Rotator Cuff
Repair, 23410-23420
Rotavirus
Antibody, 86759
Antigen Detection
Enzyme Immunoassay, 87425
Rotavirus Vaccine, 90680
Round Window
Repair Fistula, 69667
Round Window Fistula
See Fistula, Round Window
Roux–en-Y Procedure, 43621, 43633,
43634, 43644, 43846, 47740,
47741, 47780, 47785, 48540
RPR, 86592, 86593
RSV
Antibody, 86756
Antigen Detection
Direct Fluorescent Antibody,
87280
Enzyme Immunoassay, 87420
Immuneglobulin, 90378, 90379
RT3, 84482
Rubbing Alcohol
See Isopropyl Alcohol
Rubella
Antibody, 86762
Vaccine, 90706-90710
Rubella HI Test
Hemagglutination Inhibition Test,
86280
Rubella Immunization, 90706-90710
Rubeola
Antibody, 86765
Antigen Detection
Immunofluorescence, 87283
Ruiz–Mora Procedure, 28286
Russel Viper Venom Time, 85612,
85613

S

Saccomanno Technique, 88108
Sac, Endolymphatic
See Endolymphatic Sac
Sacral Nerve
Implantation
Electrode, 64561, 64581
Insertion
Electrode, 64561, 64581
Sacroiliac Joint
Arthrodesis, 27280
Arthrotomy, 27050
Biopsy, 27050
Dislocation
Open Treatment, 27218
Fusion, 27280
Injection for Arthrography, 27096
X-ray, 72200, 72202, 73542
Sacrum
Pressure Ulcer, 15931-15937
Tumor
Excision, 49215

Sacrum — *continued*
X–ray, 72220
SAECG, 93278
Sahli Test
Stomach, Intubation with Specimen
Prep., 91055
Salicylate
Assay, 80196
Saline Load Test
Saline–Solution Abortion
See Abortion, Induced, by Saline
Salivary Duct
Catheterization, 42660
Dilation, 42650, 42660
Ligation, 42665
Repair, 42500, 42505
Fistula, 42600
Salivary Glands
Abscess
Incision and Drainage, 42310,
42320
Biopsy, 42405
Calculi
Excision, 42330-42340
Cyst
Drainage, 42409
Excision, 42408
Injection
X–ray, 42550
Needle Biopsy, 42400
Nuclear Medicine
Function Study, 78232
Imaging, 78230, 78231
Parotid
Abscess, 42300, 42305
Unlisted Services and Procedures,
42699
X–ray, 70380, 70390
with Contrast, 70390
Salivary Gland Virus
See Cytomegalovirus
Salmonella
Antibody, 86768
Salpingectomy, 58262, 58263, 58291,
58292, 58552, 58554, 58661,
58700
Ectopic Pregnancy
Laparoscopic Treatment, 59151
Surgical Treatment, 59120
Oophorectomy, 58943
Salpingohysterostomy
See Implantation, Tubouterine
Salpingolysis, 58740
Salpingoneostomy, 58673, 58770
Salpingo–Oophorectomy, 58720
Resection Ovarian Malignancy,
58950-58956
Resection Peritoneal Malignancy,
58950-58956
Resection Tubal Malignancy, 58950-
58956
Salpingostomy, 58673, 58770
Laparoscopic, 58673
SALT, 84460
Salter Osteotomy of the Pelvis
See Osteotomy, Pelvis
Sampling
See Biopsy; Brush Biopsy; Needle
Biopsy
Sang–Park Procedure
Septectomy, Atrial, 33735-33737
Balloon (Rashkind Type), 92992
Blade Method (Park), 92993
Sao Paulo Typhus
See Rocky Mountain Spotted Fever
SAST, 84450
Saucerization
Calcaneus, 28120
Clavicle, 23180
Femur, 27070, 27360
Fibula, 27360, 27641
Hip, 27070
Humerus, 23184, 24140
Ileum, 27070
Metacarpal, 26230
Metatarsal, 28122

Saucerization — *continued*
Olecranon Process, 24147
Phalanges
Finger, 26235, 26236
Toe, 28124
Pubis, 27070
Radius, 24145, 25151
Scapula, 23182
Talus, 28120
Tarsal, 28122
Tibia, 27360, 27640
Ulna, 24147, 25150
Sauve–Kapandji Procedure
Arthrodesis, Distal Radioulnar Joint,
25830
SBFT, 74249
Scabies
See Tissue, Examination for Ectopar-
asites
Scalenotomy
See Muscle Division, Scalenus Anti-
cus
Scalenus Anticus
Division, 21700, 21705
Scaling
See Exfoliation
Scalp
Skin Graft
Delay of Flap, 15610
Full thickness, 15220, 15221
Pedicle Flap, 15572
Split, 15100, 15101
Tissue Transfer, Adjacent, 14020,
14021
Tumor Resection
Radical, 21015
Scalp Blood Sampling, 59030
Scan
See Specific Site; Nuclear Medicine
Abdomen
See Abdomen, CT Scan
CT
See CT Scan
MRI
See Magnetic Resonance Imaging
PET
See Positron Emission Tomogra-
phy
Radionuclide
See Emission Computerized To-
mography
Scanning Radioisotope
See Nuclear Medicine
Scanogram, 77073
Scaphoid
Fracture
with Manipulation, 25624
Closed Treatment, 25622
Open Treatment, 25628
Scapula
Craterization, 23182
Cyst
Excision, 23140
with Allograft, 23146
with Autograft, 23145
Diaphysectomy, 23182
Excision, 23172, 23190
Partial, 23182
Fracture
Closed Treatment
with Manipulation, 23575
without Manipulation, 23570
Open Treatment, 23585
Ostectomy, 23190
Repair
Fixation, 23400
Scapulopexy, 23400
Saucerization, 23182
Sequestrectomy, 23172
Tumor
Excision, 23140, 23210
with Allograft, 23146
with Autograft, 23145
Radical Resection, 23210
X–ray, 73010
Scapulopexy, 23400

Scarification
Pleural, 32215
Scarification of Pleura
See Pleurodesis
Schauta Operation, 58285
Schede Procedure, 32905, 32906
Schilling Test, 78270, 78271
See Vitamin B–12 Absorption Study
Schlatter Operation Total Gastrectomy
See Excision, Stomach, Total
Schlicter Test, 87197
Schocket Procedure, 66180
See Aqueous Shunt
Schuchard Procedure
Osteotomy
Maxilla, 21206
Schwannoma, Acoustic
See Brain, Tumor, Excision
Sciatic Nerve
Decompression, 64712
Injection
Anesthetic, 64445, 64446
Lesion
Excision, 64786
Neuroma
Excision, 64786
Neuroplasty, 64712
Release, 64712
Repair
Suture, 64858
Scintigraphy
See Computed Tomographic Scintigraphy
See Emission Computerized Tomography
See Nuclear Medicine
Scissoring
Skin Tags, 11200, 11201
Sclera
Excision, 66130
Sclerectomy with Punch or Scissors, 66160
Fistulization
Iridencleisis or Iridotasis, 66165
Sclerectomy with Punch or Scissors with Iridectomy, 66160
Thermocauterization with Iridectomy, 66155
Trabeculectomy ab Externo in Absence of Previous Surgery, 66170
Trephination with Iridectomy, 66150
Incision
Iridencleisis or Iridotasis, 66165
Sclerectomy with Punch or Scissors with Iridectomy, 66160
Thermocauterization with Iridectomy, 66155
Trabeculectomy ab Externo in Absence of Previous Surgery, 66170
Trephination with Iridectomy, 66150
Lesion
Excision, 66130
Repair
with Glue, 65286
Reinforcement
with Graft, 67255
without Graft, 67250
Staphyloma
with Graft, 66225
without Graft, 66220
Wound (Operative), 66250
Tissue Glue, 65286
Scleral Buckling Operation
Retina, Repair, Detachment, 67107-67112
Scleral Ectasia
See Staphyloma, Sclera
Sclerectomy, 66160
Sclerotherapy
Venous, 36468-36471

Sclerotomy
See Incision, Sclera
Screening, Drug
See Drug, Screen
Scribner Cannulization, 36810
Scrotal Varices
See Varicocele
Scrotoplasty, 55175, 55180
Scrotum
Abscess
Incision and Drainage, 54700, 55100
Excision, 55150
Exploration, 55110
Hematoma
Incision and Drainage, 54700
Removal
Foreign Body, 55120
Repair, 55175, 55180
Ultrasound, 76870
Unlisted Services and Procedures, 55899
Scrub Typhus, 86000
Second Look Surgery
See Reoperation
Section
See Decompression
Cesarean
See Cesarean Delivery
Cranial Nerve, 61460
Spinal Access, 63191
Dentate Ligament, 63180, 63182
Gasserian Ganglion
Sensory Root, 61450
Medullary Tract, 61470
Mesencephalic Tract, 61480
Nerve Root, 63185, 63190
Spinal Accessory Nerve, 63191
Spinal Cord Tract, 63194-63199
Tentorium Cerebelli, 61440
Vestibular Nerve
Transcranial Approach, 69950
Translabyrinthine Approach, 69915
Sedation
Conscious (Moderate), 99143-99150
Seddon–Brookes Procedure, 24320
Sedimentation Rate
Blood Cell
Automated, 85652
Manual, 85651
Segmentectomy
Breast, 19301-19302
Lung, 32484
Selenium, 84255
Self Care
See Physical Medicine / Therapy / Occupational Therapy
Training, 97535, 99509
Sella Turcica
CT Scan, 70480-70482
X–ray, 70240
Semen Analysis, 89300-89321
with Sperm Isolation, 89260-89261
Sperm Analysis
Antibodies, 89325
Hyaluronan Binding Assay, 0087T
Semenogelase
See Antigen, Prostate Specific
Semicircular Canal
Incision
Fenestration, 69820
Revised, 69840
Semilunar
Bone
See Lunate
Ganglion
See Gasserian Ganglion
Seminal Vesicle
Cyst
Excision, 55680
Excision, 55650
Incision, 55600, 55605
Mullerian Duct
Excision, 55680

Seminal Vesicle — *continued*
Unlisted Services and Procedures, 55899
Seminal Vesicles
Vesiculography, 74440
X-ray with Contrast, 74440
Seminin
See Antigen, Prostate Specific
Semiquantitative, 81005
Sengstaaken Tamponade
Esophagus, 43460
Senning Procedure
See Repair, Great Arteries; Revision
Repair, Great Arteries, 33774-33777
Senning Type, 33774-33777
Sensitivity Study
Antibiotic
Agar, 87181
Disc, 87184
Enzyme Detection, 87185
Macrobroth, 87188
MIC, 87186
Microtiter, 87186
MLC, 87187
Mycobacteria, 87190
Antiviral Drugs
HIV–1
Tissue Culture, 87904
Sensor, Fetal Oximetry
Insertion
Cervix
Vagina
Sensorimotor Exam, 92060
Sensory Nerve
Common
Repair / Suture, 64834
Sensory Testing
Quantitative (QST), Per Extremity
Cooling Stimuli, 0108T
Heat–Pain Stimuli, 0109T
Touch Pressure Stimuli, 0106T
Using Other Stimuli, 0110T
Vibration Stimuli, 0107T
Sentinel Node
Injection Procedure, 38792
Separation
Craniofacial
Closed Treatment, 21431
Open Treatment, 21432-21436
Septal Defect
Repair, 33813, 33814
Septectomy
Atrial, 33735-33737
Balloon Type, 92992
Blade Method, 92993
Closed
See Septostomy, Atrial
Submuccous Nasal
See Nasal Septum, Submuccous Resection
Septic Abortion
See Abortion, Septic
Septoplasty, 30520
Septostomy
Atrial, 33735-33737
Balloon Type, 92992
Blade Method, 92993
Septum, Nasal
See Nasal Septum
Sequestrectomy
with Alveolectomy, 41830
Calcaneus, 28120
Carpal, 25145
Clavicle, 23170
Forearm, 25145
Humeral Head, 23174
Humerus, 24134
Olecranon Process, 24138
Radius, 24136, 25145
Scapula, 23172
Skull, 61501
Talus, 28120
Ulna, 24138, 25145
Wrist, 25145
Serialography
Aorta, 75625

Serodiagnosis, Syphilis
See Serologic Test for Syphilis
Serologic Test for Syphilis, 86592, 86593
Seroma, 10140
Incision and Drainage
Skin, 10140
Serotonin, 84260
Serum
Albumin
See Albumin, Serum
Antibody Identification
Pretreatment, 86975-86978
CPK
See Creatine Kinase, Total
Serum Immune Globulin, 90281-90283
Serum Globulin Immunization, 90281, 90283
Sesamoid Bone
Excision, 28315
Finger
Excision, 26185
Foot
Fracture, 28530, 28531
Thumb
Excision, 26185
Sesamoidectomy
Toe, 28315
Severing of Blepharorrhaphy
See Tarsorrhaphy, Severing
Sever Procedure, 23020
Sex Change Operation
Female to Male, 55980
Male to Female, 55970
Sex Chromatin
See Barr Bodies
Sex Chromatin Identification, 88130, 88140
Sex Hormone Binding Globulin, 84270
Sex–Linked Ichthyoses
See Syphilis Test
SG, 84315, 93503
SGOT, 84450
SGPT, 84460
Shaving
Skin Lesion, 11300-11313
SHBG, 84270
Shelf Procedure
Osteotomy, Hip, 27146-27151
Femoral with Open Reduction, 27156
Shiga–like Toxin
Enzyme Immunoassay, 87427
Shigella
Antibody, 86771
Shirodkar Operation, 57700
Shock Wave Lithotripsy, 50590
Shock Wave (Extracorporeal) Therapy, 0019T, 28890
Shock Wave, Ultrasonic
See Ultrasound
Shop Typhus of Malaya
See Murine Typhus
Shoulder
See Clavicle; Scapula
Abscess
Drainage, 23030
Amputation, 23900-23921
Arthrocentesis, 20610
Arthrodesis, 23800
with Autogenous Graft, 23802
Arthrography
Injection
Radiologic, 23350
Arthroplasty
with Implant, 23470, 23472
Arthroscopy
Diagnostic, 29805
Surgical, 29806-29826
Arthrotomy
with Removal Loose or Foreign Body, 23107
Biopsy
Deep, 23066
Soft Tissue, 23065

Spinal Cord — *continued*
Implantation
Electrode, 63650, 63655
Pulse Generator, 63685
Receiver, 63685
Incision, 63200
Dentate Ligament, 63180, 63182
Tract, 63170, 63194-63199
Injection
Anesthesia, 62310, 62311, 62319
Blood, 62273
CT Scan, 62284
Neurolytic Agent, 62280-62282
Other, 62310, 62311
X-ray, 62284
Insertion
Electrode, 63650, 63655
Pulse Generator, 63685
Receiver, 63685
Lesion
Destruction, 62280-62282
Excision, 63265-63273, 63300-63308
Needle Biopsy, 62269
Neoplasm
Excision, 63275-63290
Puncture (Tap)
Diagnostic, 62270
Drainage of Fluid, 62272
Lumbar, 62270
Reconstruction
Dorsal Spine Elements, 63295
Release, 63200
Removal
Catheter, 62355
Electrode, 63660
Pulse Generator, 63688
Pump, 62365
Receiver, 63688
Reservoir, 62365
Repair
Cerebrospinal Fluid Leak, 63707, 63709
Meningocele, 63700, 63702
Myelomenigocele, 63704, 63706
Section
Dentate Ligament, 63180, 63182
Tract, 63194-63199
Shunt
Create, 63740, 63741
Irrigation, 63744
Removal, 63746
Replacement, 63744
Stereotaxis
Aspiration, 63615
Biopsy, 63615
Creation Lesion, 63600
Excision Lesion, 63615
Stimulation, 63610
Syrinx
Aspiration, 62268
Tumor
Excision, 63275-63290
Spinal Cord Neoplasms
See Spinal Cord
Tumor
See Spinal Cord, Tumor; Tumor Excision
See Spinal Cord, Tumor; Tumor, Spinal Cord
Spinal Fluid
See Cerebrospinal Fluid
Spinal Fracture
See Fracture, Vertebra
Spinal Instrumentation
Anterior, 22845-22847
Removal, 22855
Internal Fixation, 22841
Pelvic Fixation, 22848
Posterior Nonsegmental
Harrington Rod Technique, 22840
Harrington Rod Technique Removal, 22850
Posterior Segmental, 22842, 22844
Posterior Segmental Removal, 22852
Prosthetic Device, 22851

Spinal Instrumentation — *continued*
Reinsertion of Spinal Fixation Device, 22849
Spinal Manipulation
See Manipulation, Chiropractic
Spinal Nerve
Avulsion, 64772
Transection, 64772
Spinal Tap
See Cervical Puncture; Cisternal Puncture; Subdural Tap; Ventricular Puncture
Cervical Puncture, 61050, 61055
Cisternal Puncture, 61050, 61055
Drainage of Fluid, 62272
Lumbar, 62270
Subdural Tap, 61000, 61001
Ventricular Puncture, 61020, 61026, 61105-61120
Spine
See Spinal Cord; Vertebra; Vertebral Body;
Allograft
Morselized, 20930
Structural, 20931
Autograft
Local, 20936
Morselized, 20937
Structural, 20938
Biopsy, 20250, 20251
CT Scan
Cervical, 72125-72127
Lumbar, 72131-72133
Thoracic, 72128-72130
Fixation, 22842
Fusion
Anterior, 22808-22812
Anterior Approach, 22548-22585, 22812
Exploration, 22830
Lateral Extracavitary, 22532-22534
Posterior Approach, 22590-22802
Insertion
Instrumentation, 22840-22848, 22851
Kyphectomy, 22818, 22819
Magnetic Resonance Angiography, 72159
Magnetic Resonance Imaging
Cervical, 72141, 72142, 72156-72158
Lumbar, 72148-72158
Thoracic, 72146, 72147, 72156-72158
Manipulation
Anesthesia, 22505
Myelography
Cervical, 72240
Lumbosacral, 72265
Thoracic, 72255
Total, 72270
Reconstruction
Dorsal Spine Elements, 63295
Reinsertion Instrumentation, 22849
Removal Instrumentation, 22850, 22852, 22855
Repair, Osteotomy
Anterior, 22220-22226
Posterior, 22210-22214
Cervical Laminoplasty, 63050-63051
Posterolateral, 22216
Standing X-ray, 72069
Ultrasound, 76800
Unlisted Services and Procedures, 22899
X-ray, 72020, 72090
with Contrast
Cervical, 72240
Lumbosacral, 72265
Thoracic, 72255
Total, 72270
Absorptiometry, 77080, 77081, 77083

Spine — *continued*
X-ray — *continued*
Cervical, 72040-72052
Lumbosacral, 72100-72120
Standing, 72069
Thoracic, 72070-72074
Thoracolumbar, 72080
Total, 72010
Spine Chemotherapy
Administration, 96450
See Chemotherapy
Spirometry, 94010-94070
See Pulmonology, Diagnostic
Patient Initiated, 94014-94016
Splanchnicectomy
See Nerves, Sympathectomy, Excision
Spleen
Excision, 38100-38102
Laparoscopic, 38120
Injection
Radiologic, 38200
Nuclear Medicine
Imaging, 78185, 78215, 78216
Repair, 38115
Splenectomy
Laparoscopic, 38120
Partial, 38101
Partial with Repair, Ruptured Spleen, 38115
Total, 38100
En Bloc, 38102
Splenoplasty
See Repair, Spleen
Splenoportography, 75810
Injection Procedures, 38200
Splenorrhaphy, 38115
Splenotomy, 38999
Splint
See Casting; Strapping
Arm
Long, 29105
Short, 29125, 29126
Finger, 29130, 29131
Foot, 29590
Leg
Long, 29505
Short, 29515
Oral Surgical, 21085
Ureteral
See Ureteral Splinting
Split Grafts, 15100-15121
Split Renal Function Test
See Cystourethroscopy, Catheterization, Ureteral
Splitting
Blood Products, 86985
Sprengel's Deformity, 23400
Spring Water Cyst
See Cyst, Pericardial
Spur, Bone
See Exostosis
Calcaneal
See Heel Spur
Sputum Analysis
SQ, 90772
SRH
See Somatostatin
Ssabanejew–Frank Operation
Incision, Stomach, Creation of Stoma, 43830-43832
Stabilizing Factor, Fibrin
See Fibrin Stabilizing Factor
Stable Factor, 85230
Stallard Procedure
See Conjunctivorhinostomy
Stamey Procedure, 51845
Standby Services, 99360
Standing X-ray, 72069, 73564, 73565
Stanftan
See Binet Test
Stapedectomy
with Footplate Drill Out, 69661
without Foreign Material, 69660
Revision, 69662

Stapedotomy
with Footplate Drill Out, 69661
without Foreign Material, 69660
Revision, 69662
Stapes
Excision
with Footplate Drill Out, 69661
without Foreign Material, 69660
Mobilization
See Mobilization, Stapes
Release, 69650
Revision, 69662
Staphyloma
Sclera
Repair
with Graft, 66225
without Graft, 66220
Starch Granules
Feces
State Operation
Proctectomy
Partial, 45111, 45113-45116, 45123
Total, 45110, 45112, 45120
with Colon, 45121
Statin Therapy, 4002F
Statistics/Biometry
See Biometry
Steindler Stripping, 28250
Steindler Type Advancement, 24330
Stellate Ganglion
Injection
Anesthetic, 64510
Stem, Brain
See Brainstem
Stem Cell
Cell Concentration, 38215
Count, 86367
Total Count, 86367
Cryopreservation, 38207, 88240
Donor Search, 38204
Harvesting, 38205-38206
Limbal
Allograft, 65781
Plasma Depletion, 38214
Platelet Depletion, 38213
Red Blood Cell Depletion, 38212
T–cell Depletion, 38210
Thawing, 38208, 38209, 88241
Transplantation, 38240-38242
Tumor Cell Depletion, 38211
Washing, 38209
Stenger Test, 92565, 92577
See Audiologic Function Test; Ear, Nose and Throat
Stenosis
Aortic
See Aortic Stenosis
Bronchi, 31641
Reconstruction, 31775
Excision
Trachea, 31780, 31781
Laryngoplasty, 31582
Reconstruction
Auditory Canal, External, 69310
Repair
Trachea, 31780, 31781
Tracheal
See Trachea Stenosis
Urethral Stenosis
See Urethral Stenosis
Stenson Duct
See Parotid Duct
Stent
Indwelling
Insertion
Ureter, 50605
Placement
Bronchoscopy, 31631, 31636-31637
Colonoscopy, 45387
via Stoma, 44397
Endoscopy
Gastrointestinal, Upper, 43256
Enteroscopy, 44370

Sympathectomy
with Rib Excision, 21616
Artery
Digital, 64820
Radial, 64821
Superficial Palmar Arch, 64823
Ulnar, 64822
Cervical, 64802
Cervicothoracic, 64804
Digital Artery with Magnification, 64820
Lumbar, 64818
Presacral, 58410
Thoracic, 32664
Thoracolumbar, 64809
Sympathetic Nerve
Excision, 64802-64818
Injection
Anesthetic, 64508, 64520, 64530
Sympathins
See Catecholamines
Symphysiotomy
Horseshoe Kidney, 50540
Symphysis, Pubic
See Pubic Symphysis
Syncytial Virus, Respiratory
See Respiratory Syncytial Virus
Syndactylism, Toes
See Webbed, Toe
Syndactyly
Repair, 26560-26562
Syndesmotomy
See Ligament, Release
Syndrome
Adrenogenital
See Adrenogenital Syndrome
Ataxia–Telangiectasia
See Ataxia Telangiectasia
Bloom
See Bloom Syndrome
Carpal Tunnel
See Carpal Tunnel Syndrome
Costen's
See Temporomandibular Joint (TMJ)
Erb–Goldflam
See Myasthenia Gravis
Ovarian Vein
See Ovarian Vein Syndrome
Synechiae, Intrauterine
See Adhesions, Intrauterine
Treacher Collins
See Treacher–Collins Syndrome
Urethral
See Urethral Syndrome
Syngesterone
See Progesterone
Synostosis (Cranial)
See Craniosynostosis
Synovectomy
Arthrotomy with
Glenohumeral Joint, 23105
Sternoclavicular Joint, 23106
Elbow, 24102
Excision
Carpometacarpal Joint, 26130
Finger Joint, 26135, 26140
Hip Joint, 27054
Interphalangeal Joint, 26140
Knee Joint, 27334-27335
Metacarpophalangeal Joint, 26135
Palm, 26145
Wrist, 25105, 25115-25119
Radical, 25115, 25116
Synovial
Bursa
See Bursa
Cyst
See Ganglion
Membrane
See Synovium
Popliteal Space
See Baker's Cyst

Synovium
Biopsy
Carpometacarpal Joint, 26100
Interphalangeal Joint, 26110
Knee Joint, 27330
Metacarpophalangeal Joint
with Synovial Biopsy, 26105
Excision
Carpometacarpal Joint, 26130
Finger Joint, 26135-26140
Hip Joint, 27054
Interphalangeal Joint, 26140
Knee Joint, 27334-27335
Syphilis ab
See Antibody, Treponema Pallidum
Syphilis Test, 86592, 86593
Syrinx
Spinal Cord
Aspiration, 62268
System
Endocrine
See Endocrine System
Hemic
See Hemic System
Lymphatic
See Lymphatic System
Nervous
See Nervous System

T

T–3, 84480
T3 Free
See Triiodothyronine, Free
T–4
T Cells, 86360, 86361
Thyroxine, 84436-84439
T4 Molecule
See CD4
T4 Total
See Thyroxine, Total
T–7 Index
Thyroxine, Total, 84436
Triiodothyronine, 84480-84482
T–8, 86360
Taarnhoj Procedure
Decompression, Gasserian Ganglion, Sensory Root, 61450
Tachycardia
Heart
Recording, 93609
Tacrolimus
Drug Assay, 80197
Tag, Skin
See Skin, Tags
TAH, 51925, 58150, 58152, 58200-58240, 58951, 59525
TAHBSO, 58150, 58152, 58200-58240, 58951
Tail Bone
Excision, 27080
Fracture, 27200, 27202
Takeuchi Procedure, 33505
Talectomy
See Astragalectomy
Talotarsal Joint
Dislocation, 28570, 28575, 28585
Percutaneous Fixation, 28576
Talus
Arthrodesis
Pantalar, 28705
Subtalar, 28725
Triple, 28715
Arthroscopy
Surgical, 29891, 29892
Craterization, 28120
Cyst
Excision, 28100-28103
Diaphysectomy, 28120
Excision, 28120, 28130
Fracture
with Manipulation, 28435, 28436
without Manipulation, 28430
Open Treatment, 28445
Percutaneous Fixation, 28436
Repair
Osteochondritis Dissecans, 29892

Talus — *continued*
Repair — *continued*
Osteotomy, 28302
Saucerization, 28120
Tumor
Excision, 27647, 28100-28103
Tap
Cisternal
See Cisternal Puncture
Lumbar Diagnostic
See Spinal Tap
Tarsal
Fracture
Percutaneous Fixation, 28456
Tarsal Bone
See Ankle Bone
Tarsal Joint
See Foot
Arthrodesis, 28730, 28735, 28740
with Advancement, 28737
with Lengthening, 28737
Craterization, 28122
Cyst
Excision, 28104-28107
Diaphysectomy, 28122
Dislocation, 28540, 28545, 28555
Percutaneous Fixation, 28545, 28546
Excision, 28116, 28122
Fracture
with Manipulation, 28455, 28456
without Manipulation, 28450
Open Treatment, 28465
Fusion, 28730, 28735, 28740
with Advancement, 28737
with Lengthening, 28737
Repair, 28320
Osteotomy, 28304, 28305
Saucerization, 28122
Tumor
Excision, 28104-28107, 28171
Tarsal Strip Procedure, 67917, 67924
Tarsal Tunnel Release, 28035
Tarsal Wedge Procedure, 67916, 67923
Tarsometatarsal Joint
Arthrodesis, 28730, 28735, 28740
Arthrotomy, 28020, 28050
Biopsy
Synovial, 28050, 28052
Dislocation, 28600, 28605, 28615
Percutaneous Fixation, 28606
Exploration, 28020
Fusion, 28730, 28735, 28740
Removal
Foreign Body, 28020
Loose Body, 28020
Synovial
Biopsy, 28050
Excision, 28070
Tarsorrhaphy, 67875
Median, 67880
Severing, 67710
with Transposition of Tarsal Plate, 67882
Tattoo
Cornea, 65600
Skin, 11920-11922
TB, 87015, 87116, 87190
TBG, 84442
TBS, 88164, 88166
TB Test
Antigen Response, 86480
Cell Mediated Immunity Measurement, 86480
Skin Test, 86580
T Cell Leukemia Virus I Antibodies, Adult
See Antibody, HTLV–I
T Cell Leukemia Virus I, Human
See HTLV I
T Cell Leukemia Virus II Antibodies, Human
See Antibody, HTLV–II
T Cell Leukemia Virus II, Human
See HTLV II

T–Cells
CD4
Absolute, 86361
Count, 86359
Depletion
Ratio, 86360
T Lymphotropic Virus Type III Antibodies, Human
See Antibody, HIV
T–Cell T8 Antigens
See CD8
TCT
See Thrombin Time
Td, 90718
Team Conference
Case Management Services, 99361-99373
Tear Duct
See Lacrimal Gland
Tear Gland
See Lacrimal Gland
Technique
Pericardial Window
See Pericardiostomy
TEE, 93312-93318
Teeth
X–ray, 70300-70320
Telangiectasia
Chromosome Analysis, 88248
Injection, 36468
Telangiectasia, Cerebello–Oculocutaneous
See Ataxia Telangiectasia
Telephone
Case Management Services, 99361-99373
Pacemaker Analysis, 93733, 93736
Transmission of ECG, 93012
Teletherapy
Dose Plan, 77305-77321
Temperature Gradient Studies, 93740
Temporal Arteries
See Artery, Temporal
Temporal, Bone
Electromagnetic Bone Conduction Hearing Device
Implantation/Replacement, 69710
Removal/Repair, 69711
Excision, 69535
Resection, 69535
Tumor
Removal, 69970
Unlisted Services and Procedures, 69979
Temporal, Petrous
Excision
Apex, 69530
Temporomandibular Joint (TMJ)
Arthrocentesis, 20605
Arthrography, 70328-70332
Injection, 21116
Arthroplasty, 21240-21243
Arthroscopy
Diagnostic, 29800
Surgical, 29804
Arthrotomy, 21010
Cartilage
Excision, 21060
Condylectomy, 21050
Coronoidectomy, 21070
Dislocation
Closed Treatment, 21480, 21485
Open Treatment, 21490
Injection
Radiologic, 21116
Magnetic Resonance Imaging, 70336
Meniscectomy, 21060
Prostheses
See Prosthesis, Temporomandibular
Reconstruction
See Reconstruction, Temporomandibular Joint
X–ray with Contrast, 70328-70332
Tenago Procedure, 53431

Tendinosuture
  See Suture, Tendon
Tendon
  Achilles
    See Achilles Tendon
  Arm, Upper
    Revision, 24320
  Finger
    Excision, 26180
  Forearm
    Repair, 25260-25274
  Graft
    Harvesting, 20924
  Insertion
    Biceps Tendon, 24342
  Lengthening
    Ankle, 27685, 27686
    Arm, Lower, 25280
    Arm, Upper, 24305
    Elbow, 24305
    Finger, 26476, 26478
    Forearm, 25280
    Hand, 26476, 26478
    Leg, Lower, 27685, 27686
    Leg, Upper, 27393-27395
    Toe, 28240
    Wrist, 25280
  Palm
    Excision, 26170
  Release
    Arm, Lower, 25295
    Arm, Upper, 24332
    Wrist, 25295
  Shortening
    Ankle, 27685, 27686
    Finger, 26477, 26479
    Hand, 26477, 26479
    Leg, Lower, 27685, 27686
  Transfer
    Arm, Lower, 25310, 25312, 25316
    Arm, Upper, 24301
    Elbow, 24301
    Finger, 26497, 26498
    Hand, 26480-26489
    Leg, Lower, 27690-27692
    Leg, Upper, 27400
    Pelvis, 27098
    Thumb, 26490, 26492, 26510
    Wrist, 25310, 25312, 25316, 25320
  Transplant
    Leg, Upper, 27396, 27397
  Wrist
    Repair, 25260-25274
Tendon Origin
  Insertion
    Injection, 20551
Tendon Pulley Reconstruction of Hand
  See Hand, Reconstruction, Tendon Pulley
Tendon Sheath
  Arm
    Lower
      Repair, 25275
  Finger
    Incision, 26055
    Incision and Drainage, 26020
    Lesion, 26160
  Foot
    Excision, 28086, 28088
  Hand
    Lesion, 26160
    Injection, 20550
  Palm
    Incision and Drainage, 26020
  Removal
    Foreign Body, 20520, 20525
  Wrist
    Excision, 25115, 25116
    Incision, 25000, 25001
    Repair, 25275
Tendon Shortening
  Ankle, 27685, 27686
  Leg, Lower, 27685, 27686

Tenectomy, Tendon Sheath
  See Excision, Lesion, Tendon Sheath
Tennis Elbow
  Repair, 24350-24356
Tenodesis
  Biceps Tendon
    at Elbow, 24340
    at Shoulder, 23430
  Finger, 26471, 26474
  Wrist, 25300, 25301
Tenolysis
  Ankle, 27680, 27681
  Arm, Lower, 25295
  Arm, Upper, 24332
  Finger
    Extensor, 26445, 26449
    Flexor, 26440, 26442
  Foot, 28220-28226
  Hand
    Extensor, 26445, 26449
    Flexor, 26440, 26442
  Leg, Lower, 27680, 27681
  Wrist, 25295
Tenomyotomy, 23405, 23406
Tenon's Capsule
  Injection, 67515
Tenoplasty
  Anesthesia, 01714
Tenorrhaphy
  See Suture, Tendon
Tenosuspension
  See Tenodesis
Tenosuture
  See Suture, Tendon
Tenosynovectomy, 26145, 27626
Tenotomy
  Achilles Tendon, 27605, 27606
  Anesthesia, 01712
  Ankle, 27605, 27606
  Arm, Lower, 25290
  Arm, Upper, 24310
  Finger, 26060, 26455, 26460
  Foot, 28230, 28234
  Hand, 26450, 26460
  Hip
    Abductor, 27006
    Adductor, 27000-27003
    Iliopsoas Tendon, 27005
  Leg, Upper, 27306, 27307, 27390-27392
  Toe, 28010, 28011, 28232, 28234, 28240
  Wrist, 25290
TENS, 64550, 97014, 97032
Tension Test, 95857
Tentorium Cerebelli
  Section, 61440
Terman–Merrill Test, 96101-96103
Termination, Pregnancy
  See Abortion
Tester, Color Vision
  See Color Vision Examination
Testes
  Cryopreservation, 89335
  Nuclear Medicine
    Imaging, 78761
  Undescended
    See Testis, Undescended
Testicular Vein
  See Spermatic Veins
Testimony, Medical, 99075
Testing
  Actigraphy, 0089T
  Neurobehavioral, 96116
  Neuropsychological, 96118-96120
    Intraoperative, 95920
  Psychological, 96101-96103
  Range of Motion
    Extremities, 95851
    Eye, 92018-92019
    Hand, 95852
    Rectum
      Biofeedback, 90911
    Trunk, 97530

Testing — *continued*
  Rectum
Testing, Histocompatibility
  See Tissue Typing
Testis
  Abscess
    Incision and Drainage, 54700
  Biopsy, 54500, 54505
  Cryopreservation, 89335
  Excision
    Laparoscopic, 54690
    Partial, 54522
    Radical, 54530, 54535
    Simple, 54520
  Hematoma
    Incision and Drainage, 54700
  Insertion
    Prosthesis, 54660
  Lesion
    Excision, 54512
  Needle Biopsy, 54500
  Nuclear Medicine
    Imaging, 78761
  Repair
    Injury, 54670
    Suspension, 54620, 54640
    Torsion, 54600
  Suture
    Injury, 54670
    Suspension, 54620, 54640
  Transplantation
    to Thigh, 54680
  Tumor
    Excision, 54530, 54535
  Undescended
    Exploration, 54550, 54560
  Unlisted Services and Procedures, 54699, 55899
Testosterone, 84402
  Response, 80414
    Stimulation, 80414, 80415
  Total, 84403
Testosterone Estradiol Binding Globulin
  See Globulin, Sex Hormone Binding
Test Tube Fertilization
  See In Vitro Fertilization
Tetanus, 86280
  Antibody, 86774
  Immunoglobulin, 90389
  Vaccine, 90703
Tetanus Immunization, 90698-90703, 90715, 90718, 90720-90723
Tetrachloride, Carbon
  See Carbon Tetrachloride
Tetralogy of Fallot, 33692-33697, 33924
THA, 27130-27134
Thal–Nissen Procedure, 43325
Thawing
  Cryopreserved
    Embryo, 89352
    Oocytes, 89356
    Reproductive Tissue, 89354
    Sperm, 89353
  Previously Frozen Cells, 38208, 38209
Thawing and Expansion
  of Frozen Cell, 88241
THBR, 84479
Theleplasty
  See Nipples, Reconstruction
Theophylline
  Assay, 80198
Therapeutic
  Abortion
    See Abortion, Therapeutic
  Apheresis
    See Apheresis, Therapeutic
  Drug Assay
    See Drug Assay
  Mobilization
    See Mobilization
  Photopheresis
    See Photopheresis

Therapeutic — *continued*
  Radiology
    See Radiology, Therapeutic
Therapeutic Activities
  Music
    Per 15 Minutes, 97530
Therapies
  Cold
    See Cryotherapy
  Exercise
    See Exercise Therapy
  Family
    See Psychotherapy, Family
  Language
    See Language Therapy
  Milieu
    See Environmental Intervention
  Occupational
    See Occupational Therapy
  Photodynamic
    See Photochemotherapy
  Photoradiation
    See Actinotherapy
  Physical
    See Physical Medicine/ Therapy/Occupational Therapy
  Speech
    See Speech Therapy
  Tocolytic
    See Tocolysis
  Ultraviolet
    See Actinotherapy
Therapy
  ACE Inhibitor Therapy
    See Performance Measures
  Beta Blocker Therapy
    See Performance Measures
  Desensitization
    See Allergen Immunotherapy
  Hemodialysis
    See Hemodialysis
  Hot Pack
    See Hot Pack Treatment
  Pharmacologic, for Cessation of Tobacco Use
    See Performance Measures
  Radiation
    See Irradiation
  Speech
    See Speech Therapy
  Statin Therapy, Prescribed
    See Performance Measures
  Warfarin, 4012F
Thermocauterization
  Ectropion
    Repair, 67922
  Lesion
    Cornea, 65450
Thermocoagulation
  See Electrocautery
Thermogram
  Cephalic, 93760
  Peripheral, 93762
Thermographies
  See Thermogram
Thermography, Cerebral
  See Thermogram, Cephalic
Thermotherapy
  Prostate, 53850-53853
    Microwave, 53850
    Radiofrequency, 53852
Thiamine, 84425
Thiersch Operation
  Pinch Graft, 15050
Thiersch Procedure, 46753
Thigh
  Excision
    Excess Skin, 15832
  Fasciotomy, 27025
    See Femur; Leg, Upper
Thin Layer Chromatographies
  See Chromatography, Thin–Layer
Thiocyanate, 84430
Thompson Procedure, 27430
Thompson Test
  Smear and Stain, Routine, 87205

Thyroid Hormone Uptake, 84479
Thyroid Isthmus
   Transection, 60200
Thyroid Simulator, Long Acting
   See Thyrotropin Releasing Hormone
     (TRH)
Thyroid Stimulating Hormone (TSH),
   80418, 80438-80440, 84443
Thyroid Stimulating Hormone Receptor ab
   See Thyrotropin Releasing Hormone
     (TRH)
Thyroid Stimulating Immune Globulins (TSI), 84445
Thyroid Suppression Test
   Nuclear Medicine, Thyroid Uptake,
     78000-78003
Thyrolingual Cyst
   See Cyst, Thyroglossal Duct
Thyrotomy, 31300
Thyrotropin Receptor ab
   See Thyrotropin Releasing Hormone
     (TRH)
**Thyrotropin Releasing Hormone
(TRH)**, 80438, 80439
Thyrotropin Stimulating Immunoglobulins, 84445
Thyroxine
   Free, 84439
   Neonatal, 84437
   Total, 84436
   True, 84436
Thyroxine Binding Globulin, 84442
TIBC, 83550
Tibia
   See Ankle
   Arthroscopy Surgical, 29891, 29892
   Craterization, 27360, 27640
   Cyst
     Excision, 27635-27638
   Diaphysectomy, 27360, 27640
   Excision, 27360, 27640
     Epiphyseal Bar, 20150
   Fracture
     with Manipulation, 27825
     without Manipulation, 27824
       Incision, 27607
     Arthroscopic Treatment, 29855,
       29856
       Plafond, 29892
     Closed Treatment, 27824, 27825
       with Manipulation, 27825
       without Manipulation, 27824
     Distal, 27824-27828
     Intercondylar, 27538, 27540
     Malleolus, 27760-27766, 27808-
       27814
     Open Treatment, 27535, 27536,
       27758, 27759, 27826-
       27828
     Plateau, 29855, 29856
       Closed Treatment, 27530,
        27532
     Shaft, 27752-27759
   Osteoplasty
     Lengthening, 27715
   Prophylactic Treatment, 27745
   Reconstruction, 27418
     at Knee, 27440-27443, 27446
   Repair, 27720-27725
     Epiphysis, 27477-27485, 27730-
       27742
     Osteochondritis Dissecans
       Arthroscopy, 29892
     Osteotomy, 27455, 27457, 27705,
       27709, 27712
     Pseudoarthrosis, 27727
   Saucerization, 27360, 27640
   Tumor
     Excision, 27635-27638, 27645
   X–ray, 73590
Tibial
   Arteries
     See Artery, Tibial

Tibial — *continued*
   Nerve
     Repair/Suture
       Posterior, 64840
Tibiofibular Joint
   Arthrodesis, 27871
   Dislocation, 27830-27832
   Disruption
     Open Treatment, 27829
   Fusion, 27871
TIG
   See Immune Globulins, Tetanus
Time
   Bleeding
     See Bleeding Time
   Prothrombin
     See Prothrombin Time
   Reptilase
     See Thrombin Time
Tinnitus
   Assessment, 92625
Tissue
   Culture
     Chromosome Analysis, 88230-
       88239
     Homogenization, 87176
     Non–neoplastic Disorder, 88230,
       88237
     Skin Grafts, 15040-15157
     Solid tumor, 88239
     Toxin/Antitoxin, 87230
     Virus, 87252, 87253
   Enzyme Activity, 82657
   Examination for Ectoparasites,
     87220
   Examination for Fungi, 87220
   Expander
     Breast Reconstruction with,
       19357
     Insertion
       Skin, 11960
     Removal
       Skin, 11971
     Replacement
       Skin, 11970
   Grafts
     Harvesting, 20926
   Granulation
     See Granulation Tissue
   Homogenization, 87176
   Hybridization In Situ, 88365-88368
   Mucosal
     See Mucosa
   Preparation
     Drug Analysis, 80103
   Soft
     Abscess, 20000, 20005
   Transfer
     Adjacent
       Eyelids, 67961
       Skin, 14000-14350
     Facial Muscles, 15845
     Finger Flap, 14350
     Toe Flap, 14350
   Typing
     HLA Antibodies, 86812-86817
     Lymphocyte Culture, 86821,
       86822
Tissue Adhesives
   Closure, Skin with
     Abdomen
       Complex, 13100-13102
       Intermediate, 12031-12037
       Intermediate Layered, 12031-
         12037
       Simple, 12001-12007
       Superficial, 12001-12007
     Arm, Arms
       Complex, 13120-13122
       Intermediate, 12031-12037
       Layered, 12031-12037
       Simple, 12001-12007
       Superficial, 12001-12007
     Axilla, Axillae
       Complex, 13131-13133
       Intermediate, 12031-12037

Tissue Adhesives — *continued*
   Closure, Skin with — *continued*
     Axilla, Axillae — *continued*
       Layered, 12031-12037
       Simple, 12001-12007
       Superficial, 12001-12007
     Back
       Complex, 13100-13102
       Intermediate, 12031-12037
       Layered, 12031-12037
       Simple, 12001-12007
       Superficial, 12001-12007
     Breast
       Complex, 13100-13102
       Intermediate, 12031-12037
       Layered, 12031-12037
       Simple, 12001-12007
       Superficial, 12001-12007
     Buttock
       Complex, 13100-13102
       Intermediate, 12031-12037
       Layered, 12031-12037
       Simple, 12001-12007
       Superficial, 12001-12007
     Cheek, Cheeks
       Complex, 13131-13133
       Intermediate, 12051-12057
       Layered, 12051-12057
       Simple, 12011-12018
       Superficial, 12011-12018
     Chest
       Complex, 13100-13102
       Intermediate, 12031-12037
       Layered, 12031-12037
       Simple, 12001-12007
       Superficial, 12001-12007
     Chin
       Complex, 13131-13133
       Intermediate, 12051-12057
       Layered, 12051-12057
       Simple, 12011-12018
       Superficial, 12011-12018
     Ear, Ears
       Complex, 13150-13153
       Intermediate, 12051-12057
       Layered, 12051-12057
         2.5 cm or less, 12051
       Simple, 12011-12018
       Superficial, 12011-12018
     External
       Genitalia
         Complex/Intermediate,
           12041-12047
         Layered, 12041-12047
         Simple, 12001-12007
         Superficial, 12041-12047
     Extremity, Extremities
       Complex/Intermediate,
         12031-12037
       Layered, 12031-12037
       Simple, 12001-12007
       Superficial, 12001-12007
     Face
       Complex/Intermediate,
         12051-12057
       Layered, 12051-12057
       Simple, 12011-12018
       Superficial, 12011-12018
     Feet
       Complex, 13131-13133
       Intermediate, 12041-12047
       Layered, 12041-12047
       Simple, 12001-12007
       Superficial, 12001-12007
     Finger, Fingers
       Complex, 13131-13133
       Intermediate, 12041-12047
       Layered, 12041-12047
       Simple, 12001-12007
       Superficial, 12001-12007
     Foot
       Complex, 13131-13133
       Intermediate, 12041-12047
       Layered, 12041-12047
       Simple, 12001-12007
       Superficial, 12001-12007

Tissue Adhesives — *continued*
   Closure, Skin with — *continued*
     Forearm, Forearms
       Complex, 13120-13122
       Intermediate, 12031-12037
       Layered, 12031-12037
       Simple, 12001-12007
       Superficial, 12001-12007
     Forehead
       Complex, 13131-13133
       Intermediate, 12051-12057
       Layered, 12051-12057
       Simple, 12011-12018
       Superficial, 12011-12018
     Genitalia
       Complex, 13131-13133
       External
         Complex/Intermediate,
           12041-12047
         Layered, 12041-12047
         Simple, 12001-12007
         Superficial, 12001-12007
     Hand, Hands
       Complex, 13131-13133
       Intermediate, 12041-12047
       Layered, 12041-12047
       Simple, 12001-12007
       Superficial, 12001-12007
     Leg, Legs
       Complex, 13120-13122
       Intermediate, 12031-12037
       Layered, 12031-12037
       Simple, 12001-12007
       Superficial, 12001-12007
     Lip, Lips
       Complex, 13150-13153
       Intermediate, 12051-12057
       Layered, 12051-12057
       Simple, 12011-12018
       Superficial, 12011-12018
     Lower
       Arm, Arms
         Complex, 13120-13122
         Intermediate, 12031-12037
         Layered, 12031-12037
         Simple, 12001-12007
         Superficial, 12001-12007
       Extremity, Extremities
         Complex, 13120-13122
         Intermediate, 12031-12037
         Layered, 12031-12037
         Simple, 12001-12007
         Superficial, 12001-12007
       Leg, Legs
         Complex, 13120-13122
         Intermediate, 12031-12037
         Layered, 12031-12037
         Simple, 12001-12007
         Superficial, 12001-12007
     Mouth
       Complex, 13131-13133
     Mucous Membrane
       Complex/Intermediate,
         12051-12057
       Layered, 12051-12057
       Simple, 12011-12018
       Superficial, 12011-12018
     Neck
       Complex, 13131-13133
       Intermediate, 12041-12047
       Layered, 12041-12047
       Simple, 12001-12007
       Superficial, 12001-12007
     Nose
       Complex, 13150-13153
       Intermediate, 12051-12057
       Layered, 12051-12057
       Simple, 12011-12018
       Superficial, 12011-12018
     Palm, Palms
       Complex, 13131-13133
       Intermediate, 12041-12047
       Layered, 12041-12047
       Simple, 12001-12007
       Superficial, 12001-12007

Vagotomy
With Gastroduodenostomy Revision/Reconstruction, 43855
With Gastrojejunostomy Revision/Reconstruction, 43865
With Partial Distal Gastrectomy, 43635
Abdominal, 64760
Highly Selective, 43641
Parietal Cell, 43641, 64755
Reconstruction, 43855
  with Gastroduodenostomy Revision, 43855
  with Gastrojejunostomy Revision, Reconstruction, 43865
Selective, 43640
Transthoracic, 64752
Truncal, 43640
Vagus Nerve
Avulsion
  Abdominal, 64760
  Selective, 64755
  Thoracic, 64752
Incision, 43640, 43641
  Abdominal, 64760
  Selective, 64755
  Thoracic, 64752
Injection
  Anesthetic, 64408
Transection, 43640, 43641
  Abdominal, 64760
  Selective, 43652, 64755
  Thoracic, 64752
  Truncal, 43651
Valentine's Test
Urinalysis, Glass Test, 81020
Valproic Acid
See Dipropylacetic Acid
Valproic Acid Measurement
See Dipropylacetic Acid
Valsalva Sinus
See Sinus of Valsalva
Valva Atrioventricularis Sinistra (Valva Mitralis)
See Mitral Valve
Valve
Aortic
  See Heart, Aortic Valve
Bicuspid
  See Mitral Valve
Mitral
  See Mitral Valve
Pulmonary
  See Pulmonary Valve
Tricuspid
  See Tricuspid Valve
Valvectomy
Tricuspid Valve, 33460
Valve Stenoses, Aortic
See Aortic Stenosis
Valvotomy
Mitral Valve, 33420, 33422
Pulmonary Valve, 33470-33474
Reoperation, 33530
Valvuloplasty
Aortic Valve, 33400-33403
Femoral Vein, 34501
Mitral Valve, 33425-33427
Percutaneous Balloon
  Aortic Valve, 92986
  Mitral Valve, 92987
  Pulmonary Valve, 92990
Prosthetic Valve, 33496
Reoperation, 33530
Tricuspid Valve, 33460-33465
Vancomycin
Assay, 80202
Van Den Bergh Test, 82247, 82248
Vanillymandelic Acid
Urine, 84585
Vanilmandelic Acid
See Vanillylmandelic Acid
Varicella (Chicken Pox)
Immunization, 90710, 90716
Varicella–Zoster
Antibody, 86787

Varicella–Zoster — *continued*
Antigen Detection
  Direct Fluorescent Antibody, 87290
Varices Esophageal
See Esophageal Varices
Varicocele
Spermatic Cord
  Excision, 55530-55540
Varicose Vein
with Tissue Excision, 37735, 37760
Ablation, 36475-36479
Removal, 37718, 37722, 37735, 37765-37785
Secondary Varicosity, 37785
Vascular Flow Check, Graft, 15860
Vascular Injection
Unlisted Services and Procedures, 36299
Vascular Lesion
Cranial
  Excision, 61600-61608, 61615, 61616
Cutaneous
  Destruction, 17106-17108
Vascular Malformation
Cerebral
  Repair, 61710
Finger
  Excision, 26115
Hand
  Excision, 26115
Vascular Procedure
Brachytherapy
  Intracoronary Artery, 92974
Intravascular Ultrasound
  Coronary Vessels, 92978, 92979
Stent
  Intracoronary, 92980, 92981
Vascular Procedures
Angioscopy
  Noncoronary Vessels, 35400
Endoscopy
  Surgical, 37500
Harvest
  Lower Extremity Vein, 35572
Intravascular Ultrasound
  Non–Coronary Vessels, 75945, 75946
Thrombolysis
  Coronary Vessels, 92975, 92977
  Cranial Vessels, 37195
Vascular Rehabilitation
See Peripheral Artery Disease Rehabilitation (PAD)
Vascular Studies
See Doppler Scan, Duplex, Plethysmography
Angioscopy
  Aorta, 93978, 93979
  Noncoronary Vessels, 35400
Artery Studies
  Extracranial, 93875-93882
  Extremities, 93922-93924
  Intracranial, 93886, 93888
  Lower Extremity, 93922-93926
  Middle Cerebral Artery, Fetal, 76821
  Umbilical Artery, Fetal, 76820
  Upper Extremity, 93930, 93931
Blood Pressure Monitoring, 24 Hour, 93784-93790
Cardiac Catheterization
  Imaging, 93555, 93556
Hemodialysis Access, 93990
Kidney
  Multiple Study with Pharmacological Intervention, 78709
  Single Study with Pharmacological Intervention, 78708
Penile Vessels, 93980, 93981
Plethysmography
  Total Body, 93720-93722
  Temperature Gradient, 93740
Thermogram
  Cephalic, 93760

Vascular Studies — *continued*
Thermogram — *continued*
  Peripheral, 93762
Unlisted Services and Procedures, 93799
Venous Studies
  Extremities, 93965-93971
  Venous Pressure, 93770
  Visceral Studies, 93975-93979
Vascular Surgery
Endoscopy, 37500
Unlisted Services and Procedures, 37799
Vas Deferens
Anastomosis
  to Epididymis, 54900, 54901
Excision, 55250
Incision, 55200
  for X–Ray, 55300
Ligation, 55450
Repair
  Suture, 55400
Unlisted Services and Procedures, 55899
Vasography, 74440
X–Ray with Contrast, 74440
Vasectomy, 55250
Laser Coagulation of Prostate, 52647
Laser Vaporization of Prostate, 52648
Reversal
  See Vasovasorrhaphy
Transurethral
  Cystourethroscopic, 52402
  Transurethral Electrosurgical Resection of Prostate, 52601
  Transurethral Resection of Prostate, 52648
Vasoactive Drugs
Injection
  Penis, 54231
Vasoactive Intestinal Peptide, 84586
Vasogram
See Vasography
Vasography, 74440
Vasointestinal Peptide
See Vasoactive Intestinal Peptide
Vasopneumatic Device Therapy, 97016
See Physical Medicine/Therapy/Occupational Therapy
Vasopressin, 84588
Vasotomy, 55200, 55300
Transurethral
  Cystourethroscopic, 52402
Vasovasorrhaphy, 55400
Vasovasostomy, 55400
VBAC, 59610-59614
V, Cranial Nerve
See Trigeminal Nerve
VDRL, 86592, 86593
Vectorcardiogram
Evaluation, 93799
Tracing, 93799
Vein
Ablation
  Endovenous, 36475-36479
Adrenal
  Venography, 75840, 75842
Anastomosis
  Caval to Mesenteric, 37160
  Intrahepatic Portosystemic, 37182-37183
  Portocaval, 37140
  Reniportal, 37145
  Saphenopopliteal, 34530
  Splenorenal, 37180, 37181
  Vein, 34530, 37180, 37181
    to Vein, 37140-37160, 37182-37183
Angioplasty
  Transluminal, 35460
Arm
  Harvest of Vein for Bypass Graft, 35500
  Venography, 75820, 75822

Vein — *continued*
Axillary
  Thrombectomy, 34490
Biopsy
  Transcatheter, 75970
Cannulization
  to Artery, 36810, 36815
  to Vein, 36800
Catheterization
  Central Insertion, 36555-36558
  Organ Blood, 36500
  Peripheral Insertion, 36568, 36569
  Removal, 36589
  Repair, 36575
  Replacement, 36578-36581, 36584
  Umbilical, 36510
Endoscopic Harvest
  for Bypass Graft, 33508
External Cannula Declotting, 36860, 36861
Extremity
  Non–Invasive Studies, 93965-93971
Femoral
  Repair, 34501
Femoropopliteal
  Thrombectomy, 34421, 34451
Guidance
  Fluoroscopic, 77001
  Ultrasound, 76937
Hepatic Portal
  Splenoportography, 75810
  Venography, 75885, 75887
Iliac
  Thrombectomy, 34401, 34421, 34451
Injection
  Sclerosing Agent, 36468-36471
Insertion
  IVC Filter, 75940
Interrupt
  Femoral Vein, 37650
  Iliac, 37660
  Vena Cava, 37620
Jugular
  Venography, 75860
Leg
  Harvest for Vascular Reconstruction, 35572
  Venography, 75820, 75822
Ligation
  Clusters, 37785
  Esophagus, 43205
  Jugular, 37565
  Perforation, 37760
  Saphenous, 37700-37735, 37780
  Secondary, 37785
Liver
  Venography, 75860, 75889, 75891
Neck
  Venography, 75860
Nuclear Medicine
  Thrombosis Imaging, 78456-78458
Orbit
  Venography, 75880
Placement
  IVC Filter, 75940
Portal
  Catheterization, 36481
Pulmonary
  Repair, 33730
Removal
  Clusters, 37785
  Saphenous, 37700-37735, 37780
  Varicose, 37765, 37766
Renal
  Venography, 75831, 75833
Repair
  Aneurysm, 36834
  Angioplasty, 75978
  Graft, 34520

X–ray — *continued*
Ribs, 71100-71111
Sacroiliac Joint, 72200, 72202, 73542
Sacrum, 72220
Salivary Gland, 70380
Scapula, 73010
Sella Turcica, 70240
Shoulder, 73020, 73030, 73050
Sinuses, 70210, 70220
Sinus Tract, 76080
Skull, 70250, 70260
Specimen
Surgical, 76098
Spine, 72020, 72090
Cervical, 72040-72052
Lumbosacral, 72100-72120

X–ray — *continued*
Spine — *continued*
Thoracic, 72070-72074
Thoracolumbar, 72080
Total, 72010
Standing
Spine, 72069
Sternum, 71120, 71130
Teeth, 70300-70320
Tibia, 73590
Toe, 73660
Total Body
Foreign Body, 76010
Unlisted Services and Procedures, 76120, 76125
Wrist, 73100, 73110

X–Ray Tomography, Computed
See CT Scan
Xylose Absorption Test
Blood, 84620
Urine, 84620

Y

YAG, 66821
Yeast
Culture, 87106
Yellow Fever Vaccine, 90717
Yersinia
Antibody, 86793
Y–Plasty, 51800

Z

Ziegler Procedure
Discission Secondary Membranous Cataract, 66820
ZIFT, 58976
Zinc, 84630
Zinc Manganese Leucine Aminopeptidase
See Leucine Aminopeptidase
Z–Plasty, 26121-26125, 41520
Zygoma
See Cheekbone
Zygomatic Arch
Fracture
with Manipulation, 21355
Open Treatment, 21356-21366
Reconstruction, 21255

Evaluation and Management

The following information is taken directly from the AMA's *Physicians' Current Procedural Terminology*.

CLASSIFICATION OF EVALUATION AND MANAGEMENT (E/M) SERVICES

The E/M section is divided into broad categories such as office visits, hospital visits, and consultations. Most of the categories are further divided into two or more subcategories of E/M services. For example, there are two subcategories of office visits (new patient and established patient) and there are two subcategories of hospital visits (initial and subsequent). The subcategories of E/M services are further classified into levels of E/M services that are identified by specific codes. This classification is important because the nature of physician work varies by type of service, place of service, and the patient's status.

The basic format of the levels of E/M services is the same for most categories. First, a unique code number is listed. Second, the place and/or type of service are specified (e.g., office consultation). Third, the content of the service is defined (e.g., comprehensive history and comprehensive examination). (See "Levels of E/M Services," for details on the content of E/M services.) Fourth, the nature of the presenting problem(s) usually associated with a given level is described. Fifth, the time typically required to provide the service is specified. (A detailed discussion of time begins on page 2.)

DEFINITIONS OF COMMONLY USED TERMS

Certain key words and phrases are used throughout the E/M section. The following definitions are intended to reduce the potential for differing interpretations and to increase the consistency of reporting by physicians in differing specialties.

NEW AND ESTABLISHED PATIENT

Solely for the purposes of distinguishing between new and established patients, professional services are those face-to-face services rendered by a physician and reported by a specific CPT code(s). A new patient is one who has not received any professional services from the physician, or another physician of the same specialty who belongs to the same group practice, within the past three years.

An established patient is one who has received professional services from the physician, or another physician of the same specialty who belongs to the same group practice, within the past three years.

In the instance where a physician is on call for or covering for another physician, the patient's encounter will be classified as it would have been by the physician who is not available.

No distinction is made between new and established patients in the emergency department. E/M services in the emergency department category may be reported for any new or established patient who presents for treatment in the emergency department.

Review the decision tree to help determine if an E/M service should be reported as a new or established patient.

CHIEF COMPLAINT

A concise statement describing the symptom, problem, condition, diagnosis or other factor that is the reason for the encounter, usually stated in the patient's words.

CONCURRENT CARE

Concurrent care is the provision of similar services, e.g., hospital visits, to the same patient by more than one physician on the same day. When concurrent care is provided, no special reporting is required.

COUNSELING

Counseling is a discussion with a patient and/or family concerning one or more of the following areas:

- Diagnostic results, impressions, and/or recommended diagnostic studies
- Prognosis
- Risks and benefits of management (treatment) options
- Instructions for management (treatment) and/or follow-up
- Importance of compliance with chosen management (treatment) options
- Risk factor reduction
- Patient and family education

(For psychotherapy, see 90804–90857.)

FAMILY HISTORY

A review of medical events in the patient's family that includes significant information about:

- The health status or cause of death of parents, siblings, and children
- Specific diseases related to problems identified in the Chief Complaint or History of the Present Illness, and/or System Review
- Diseases of family members which may be hereditary or place the patient at risk

HISTORY OF PRESENT ILLNESS

The history of present illness is a chronological description of the development of the patient's present illness from the first sign and/or symptom to the present. This includes a description of location, quality, severity, timing, context, modifying factors and associated signs and symptoms significantly related to the presenting problem(s).

LEVELS OF E/M SERVICES

Within each category or subcategory of E/M service, there are three to five levels of E/M services available for reporting purposes. Levels of E/M services are not interchangeable among the different categories or subcategories of service. For example, the first level of E/M services in the subcategory of office visit, new patient, does not have the same definition as the first level of E/M services in the subcategory of office visit, established patient.

The levels of E/M services include examinations, evaluations, treatments, conferences with or concerning patients, preventive pediatric and adult health supervision, and similar medical services, such as the determination of the need and/or location for appropriate care. Medical screening includes the history, examination, and medical decision-making required to determine the need and/or location for appropriate care and treatment of the patient (e.g., office and other outpatient setting, emergency department, nursing facility, etc.). The levels of E/M services encompass the wide variations in skill, effort, time, responsibility and medical knowledge required for the prevention or diagnosis and treatment of illness or injury and the promotion of optimal health. All physicians may use each level of E/M services.

The descriptors for the levels of E/M services recognize seven components, six of which are used in defining the levels of E/M services. These components are:

- History
- Examination
- Medical decision making
- Counseling
- Coordination of care
- Nature of presenting problem
- Time

The first three of these components (history, examination, and medical decision making) are considered the key components in selecting a level of E/M services. (See "Determine the Extent of History Obtained.")

The next three components (counseling, coordination of care, and the nature of the presenting problem) are considered contributory factors in the majority of encounters. Although the first two of these contributory factors are important E/M services, it is not required that these services be provided at every patient encounter.

Coordination of care with other providers or agencies without a patient encounter on that day is reported using the case management codes.

Evaluation and Management

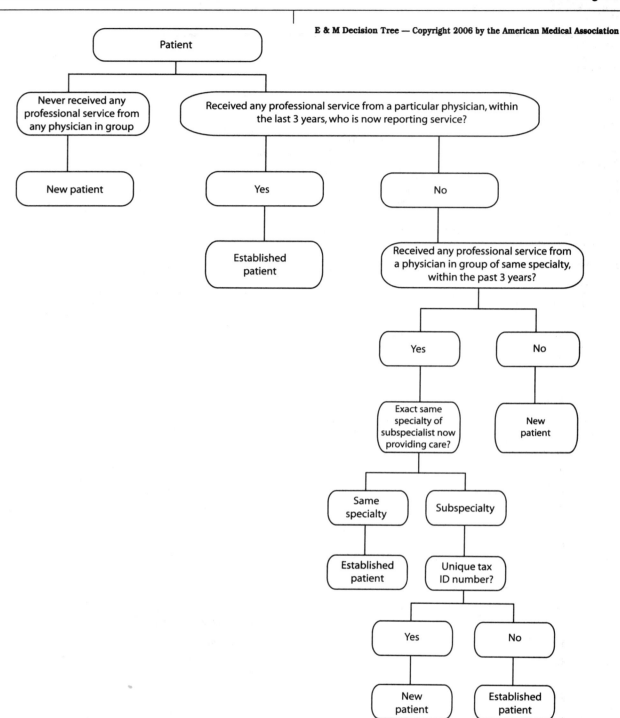

E & M Decision Tree — Copyright 2006 by the American Medical Association

The final component, time, is discussed in detail below.

Any specifically identifiable procedure (i.e., identified with a specific CPT code) performed on or subsequent to the date of initial or subsequent E/M services should be reported separately.

The actual performance and/or interpretation of diagnostic tests/studies ordered during a patient encounter are not included in the levels of E/M services. Physician performance of diagnostic tests/studies for which specific CPT codes are available may be reported separately, in addition to the appropriate E/M code. The physician's interpretation of the results of diagnostic tests/studies (i.e., professional component) with preparation of a separate distinctly identifiable signed written report may also be reported separately, using the appropriate CPT code with the modifier 26 appended.

The physician may need to indicate that on the day a procedure or service identified by a CPT code was performed, the patient's condition required a

significant separately identifiable E/M service above and beyond other services provided or beyond the usual preservice and postservice care associated with the procedure that was performed. The E/M service may be caused or prompted by the symptoms or condition for which the procedure and/or service was provided. This circumstance may be reported by adding the modifier 25 to the appropriate level of E/M service. As such, different diagnoses are not required for reporting of the procedure and the E/M services on the same date.

NATURE OF PRESENTING PROBLEM

A presenting problem is a disease, condition, illness, injury, symptom, sign, finding, complaint, or other reason for encounter, with or without a diagnosis being established at the time of the encounter. The E/M codes recognize five types of presenting problems that are defined as follows:

Minimal: A problem that may not require the presence of the physician, but service is provided under the physician's supervision.

Self-limited or minor: A problem that runs a definite and prescribed course, is transient in nature, and is not likely to permanently alter health status OR has a good prognosis with management/compliance.

Low severity: A problem where the risk of morbidity without treatment is low; there is little to no risk of mortality without treatment; full recovery without functional impairment is expected.

Moderate severity: A problem where the risk of morbidity without treatment is moderate; there is moderate risk of mortality without treatment; uncertain prognosis OR increased probability of prolonged functional impairment.

High severity: A problem where the risk of morbidity without treatment is high to extreme; there is a moderate to high risk of mortality without treatment OR high probability of severe, prolonged functional impairment.

PAST HISTORY

A review of the patient's past experiences with illnesses, injuries, and treatments that includes significant information about:

- Prior major illnesses and injuries
- Prior operations
- Prior hospitalizations
- Current medications
- Allergies (e.g., drug, food)
- Age appropriate immunization status
- Age appropriate feeding/dietary status

SOCIAL HISTORY

An age appropriate review of past and current activities that includes significant information about:

- Marital status and/or living arrangements
- Current employment
- Occupational history
- Use of drugs, alcohol, and tobacco
- Level of education
- Sexual history
- Other relevant social factors

SYSTEM REVIEW (REVIEW OF SYSTEMS)

An inventory of body systems obtained through a series of questions seeking to identify signs and/or symptoms which the patient may be experiencing or has experienced. For the purposes of the CPT coding system, the following elements of a system review have been identified:

- Constitutional symptoms (fever, weight loss, etc.)
- Eyes
- Ears, nose, mouth, throat
- Cardiovascular
- Respiratory
- Gastrointestinal
- Genitourinary
- Musculoskeletal
- Integumentary (skin and/or breast)
- Neurological
- Psychiatric
- Endocrine
- Hematologic/lymphatic
- Allergic/immunologic

The review of systems helps define the problem, clarify the differential diagnosis, identify needed testing, or serves as baseline data on other systems that might be affected by any possible management options.

TIME

The inclusion of time in the definitions of levels of E/M services has been implicit in prior editions of the CPT book. The inclusion of time as an explicit factor beginning in *CPT 1992* is done to assist physicians in selecting the most appropriate level of E/M services. It should be recognized that the specific times expressed in the visit code descriptors are averages, and therefore represent a range of times which may be higher or lower depending on actual clinical circumstances.

Time is not a descriptive component for the emergency department levels of E/M services because emergency department services are typically provided on a variable intensity basis, often involving multiple encounters with several patients over an extended period of time. Therefore, it is often difficult for physicians to provide accurate estimates of the time spent face-to-face with the patient.

Studies to establish levels of E/M services employed surveys of practicing physicians to obtain data on the amount of time and work associated with typical E/M services. Since "work" is not easily quantifiable, the codes must rely on other objective, verifiable measures that correlate with physicians' estimates of their "work". It has been demonstrated that physicians' estimations of intraservice time (as explained on the next page), both within and across specialties, is a variable that is predictive of the "work" of E/M services. This same research has shown there is a strong relationship between intra-service time and total time for E/M services. Intra-service time, rather than total time, was chosen for inclusion with the codes because of its relative ease of measurement and because of its direct correlation with measurements of the total amount of time and work associated with typical E/M services. Intra-service times are defined as face-to-face time for office and other outpatient visits and as unit/floor time for hospital and other inpatient visits. This distinction is necessary because most of the work of typical office visits takes place during the face-to-face time with the patient, while most of the work of typical hospital visits takes place during the time spent on the patient's floor or unit.

Face-to-face time (office and other outpatient visits and office consultations): For coding purposes, face-to-face time for these services is defined as only that time that the physician spends face-to-face with the patient and/or family. This includes the time in which the physician performs such tasks as obtaining a history, performing an examination, and counseling the patient.

Physicians also spend time doing work before or after the face-to-face time with the patient, performing such tasks as reviewing records and tests, arranging for further services, and communicating further with other professionals and the patient through written reports and telephone contact.

This non-face-to-face time for office services—also called pre- and post-encounter time—is not included in the time component described in the E/M codes. However, the pre- and post-face-to-face work associated with an encounter was included in calculating the total work of typical services in physician surveys.

Thus, the face-to-face time associated with the services described by any E/M code is a valid proxy for the total work done before, during, and after the visit.

Unit/floor time (hospital observation services, inpatient hospital care, and nursing facility): For reporting purposes, intra-service time for these services is defined as unit/floor time, which includes the time that the physician is present on the patient's hospital unit and at the bedside rendering services for that patient. This includes the time in which the physician establishes and/or reviews the patient's chart, examines the patient, writes notes and communicates with other professionals and the patient's family.

In the hospital, pre- and post-time includes time spent off the patient's floor performing such tasks as reviewing pathology and radiology findings in another part of the hospital.

This pre- and post-visit time is not included in the time component described in these codes. However, the pre- and post-work performed during the time spent off the floor or unit was included in calculating the total work of typical services in physician surveys.

Thus, the unit/floor time associated with the services described by any code is a valid proxy for the total work done before, during, and after the visit.

UNLISTED SERVICE

An E/M service may be provided that is not listed in this section of the CPT book. When reporting such a service, the appropriate "Unlisted" code may be used to indicate the service, identifying it by "Special Report," as discussed in the following paragraph. The "unlisted services" and accompanying codes for the E/M section are as follows:

99429	**Unlisted preventive medicine service**
99499	**Unlisted evaluation and management service**

RESULTS/TESTING/REPORTS

Results indicate the technical component of a procedure or service. Testing is the service that leads to the report and interpretation. Reports provide interpretation of the tests.

SPECIAL REPORT

An unlisted service or one that is unusual, variable, or new may require a special report demonstrating the medical appropriateness of the service. Pertinent information should include an adequate definition or description of the nature, extent, and need for the procedure; and the time, effort, and equipment necessary to provide the service. Additional items which may be included are complexity of symptoms, final diagnosis, pertinent physical findings, diagnostic and therapeutic procedures, concurrent problems, and follow-up care.

INSTRUCTIONS FOR SELECTING A LEVEL OF E/M SERVICE

IDENTIFY THE CATEGORY AND SUBCATEGORY OF SERVICE

The categories and subcategories of codes available for reporting E/M services are shown in table 1.

REVIEW THE REPORTING INSTRUCTIONS FOR THE SELECTED CATEGORY OR SUBCATEGORY

Most of the categories and many of the subcategories of service have special guidelines or instructions unique to that category or subcategory. Where these are indicated, e.g., "Inpatient Hospital Care," special instructions will be presented preceding the levels of E/M services.

REVIEW THE LEVEL OF E/M SERVICE DESCRIPTORS AND EXAMPLES IN THE SELECTED CATEGORY OR SUBCATEGORY

The descriptors for the levels of E/M services recognize seven components, six of which are used in defining the levels of E/M services. These components are:

- History
- Examination
- Medical decision making
- Counseling
- Coordination of care
- Nature of presenting problem
- Time

The first three of these components (i.e., history, examination, and medical decision making) should be considered the key components in selecting the level of E/M services. An exception to this rule is in the case of visits which consist predominantly of counseling or coordination of care. (See numbered paragraph 3, page 5.)

The nature of the presenting problem and time are provided in some levels to assist the physician in determining the appropriate level of E/M service.

DETERMINE THE EXTENT OF HISTORY OBTAINED

The extent of the history is dependent upon clinical judgment and on the nature of the presenting problem(s). The levels of E/M services recognize four types of history that are defined as follows:

Problem focused: Chief complaint; brief history of present illness or problem.

Expanded problem focused: Chief complaint; brief history of present illness; problem pertinent system review.

Detailed: Chief complaint; extended history of present illness; problem pertinent system review extended to include a review of a limited number of additional systems; pertinent past, family, and/or social history directly related to the patient's problems.

Comprehensive: Chief complaint; extended history of present illness; review of systems which is directly related to the problem(s) identified in the history of the present illness plus a review of all additional body systems; complete past, family, and social history.

The comprehensive history obtained as part of the preventive medicine evaluation and management service is not problem-oriented and does not involve a chief complaint or present illness. It does, however, include a comprehensive system review and comprehensive or interval past, family, and social history as well as a comprehensive assessment/history of pertinent risk factors.

TABLE 1

Categories and Subcategories of Service

Category/Subcategory	Code Numbers
Office or Other Outpatient Services	
New Patient	99201–99205
Established Patient	99211–99215
Hospital Observation Services	
Hospital Observation Discharge Services	99217
Initial Hospital Observation Services	99218–99220
Hospital Observation or Inpatient Care Services (Including Admission and Discharge Services)	99234–99236
Hospital Inpatient Services	
Initial Hospital Care	99221–99223
Subsequent Hospital Care	99231–99233
Hospital Discharge Services	99238–99239
Consultations	
Office Consultations	99241–99245
Initial Inpatient Consultations	99251–99255
Emergency Department Services	99281–99288
Pediatric Patient Transport	99289–99290
Critical Care Services	
Adult (over 24 months of age)	99291–99292
Pediatric	99293–99294
Neonatal	99295–99296
Continuing Intensive Care Services	99298–99300
Nursing Facility Services	
Initial Nursing Facility Care	99304–99306
Subsequent Nursing Facility Care	99307–99310
Nursing Facility Discharge Services	99315–99316
Other Nursing Facility Services	99318
Domiciliary, Rest Home or Custodial Care Services	
New Patient	99324-99328
Established Patient	99334–33337
Domiciliary, Rest Home (e.g., Assisted Living Facility), or Home Care Plan Oversight Services	99339–99340
Home Services	
New Patient	99341–99345
Established Patient	99347–99350
Prolonged Services	
With Direct Patient Contact	99354–99357
Without Direct Patient Contact	99358–99359
Standby Services	99360
Case Management Services	
Team Conferences	99361–99362
Telephone Calls	99371–99373
Care Plan Oversight Services	99374–99380
Preventive Medicine Services	
New Patient	99381–99387
Established Patient	99391–99397
Individual Counseling	99401–99404
Group Counseling	99411–99412
Other	99420–99429
Newborn Care	99431–99440
Special E/M Services	99450–99456
Other E/M Services	99499

DETERMINE THE EXTENT OF EXAMINATION PERFORMED

The extent of the examination performed is dependent on clinical judgment and on the nature of the presenting problem(s). The levels of E/M services recognize four types of examination that are defined as follows:

Problem focused: A limited examination of the affected body area or organ system.

Expanded problem focused: A limited examination of the affected body area or organ system and other symptomatic or related organ system(s).

Detailed: An extended examination of the affected body area(s) and other symptomatic or related organ system(s).

Comprehensive: A general multisystem examination or a complete examination of a single organ system. Note: The comprehensive examination performed as part of the preventive medicine evaluation and management service is multisystem, but its extent is based on age and risk factors identified.

For the purposes of these CPT definitions, the following body areas are recognized:

- Head, including the face
- Neck
- Chest, including breasts and axilla
- Abdomen
- Genitalia, groin, buttocks
- Back
- Each extremity

For the purposes of these CPT definitions, the following organ systems are recognized:

- Eyes
- Ears, nose, mouth, and throat
- Cardiovascular
- Respiratory
- Gastrointestinal
- Genitourinary
- Musculoskeletal
- Skin
- Neurologic
- Psychiatric
- Hematologic/lymphatic/immunologic

DETERMINE THE COMPLEXITY OF MEDICAL DECISION MAKING

Medical decision making refers to the complexity of establishing a diagnosis and/or selecting a management option as measured by:

- The number of possible diagnoses and/or the number of management options that must be considered
- The amount and/or complexity of medical records, diagnostic tests, and/or other information that must be obtained, reviewed, and analyzed
- The risk of significant complications, morbidity, and/or mortality, as well as comorbidities, associated with the patient's presenting problem(s), the diagnostic procedure(s) and/or the possible management options

Four types of medical decision making are recognized: straightforward; low complexity; moderate complexity; and high complexity. To qualify for a given type of decision making, two of the three elements in Table 2 must be met or exceeded.

Comorbidities/underlying diseases, in and of themselves, are not considered in selecting a level of E/M services unless their presence significantly increases the complexity of the medical decision making.

SELECT THE APPROPRIATE LEVEL OF E/M SERVICES BASED ON THE FOLLOWING

1. For the following categories/subcategories, all of the key components, i.e., history, examination, and medical decision making, must meet or exceed the stated requirements to qualify for a particular level of E/M service: office, new patient; hospital observation services; initial hospital care; office consultations; initial inpatient consultations; emergency department services; initial nursing facility care; domiciliary care, new patient; and home, new patient.

2. For the following categories/subcategories, two of the three key components (i.e., history, examination, and medical decision making) must meet or exceed the stated requirements to qualify for a particular level of E/M services: office, established patient; subsequent hospital care; subsequent nursing facility care; domiciliary care, established patient; and home, established patient.

3. When counseling and/or coordination of care dominates (more than 50%) the physician/patient and/or family encounter (face-to-face time in the office or other outpatient setting or floor/unit time in the hospital or nursing facility), then time may be considered the key or controlling factor to qualify for a particular level of E/M services. This includes time spent with parties who have assumed responsibility for the care of the patient or decision making whether or not they are family members (e.g., foster parents, person acting in locum parentis, legal guardian). The extent of counseling and/or coordination of care must be documented in the medical record.

DOCUMENTATION GUIDELINES

Originally jointly developed by the American Medical Association (AMA) and the Health Care Financing Administration (HCFA) in 1995, the documentation guidelines for E/M services experienced substantial revision in 1997. These documentation guidelines are not included in CPT guidelines and AMA policy does not endorse them. For the time being, physicians may use either the 1995 or 1997 guidelines for Medicare purposes. These can be found on the Internet at http://www.cms.hhs.gov/medlearn/emdoc.asp. A comparison of the two systems can be found at http://www.cms.hhs.gov/medlearn/appndix1.pdf.

COMPONENTS

HISTORY COMPONENT GUIDELINES

- The chief complaint, review of systems, and the past, family, and/or social history may be included as separate elements of the history. Or, this information may be included in the description of the history of the present illness.

- A review of systems and/or a past, family, and/or social history obtained during an earlier encounter does not need to be re-recorded if there is evidence that the physician reviewed and updated the previous information. This may occur when a physician updates his or her own record, or in an institutional setting or group practice where many physicians use a common record. The review and update may be documented by describing any new review of systems and/or past, family, and/or social history information or noting there has been no change in the information and indicating the date and location of the earlier review of systems and/or past, family, and/or social history.

- The review of systems and/or past, family, and/or social history may be recorded by ancillary staff or on a form completed by the patient. To document that the physician reviewed the information, there must be a notation supplementing or confirming the information recorded by others.

- If the physician cannot obtain a history from the patient or other source, the record should describe the patient's condition or other circumstance that precludes obtaining this information.

- The medical record should clearly reflect the chief complaint.

- To qualify for brief history of present illness, the medical record should describe one to three elements of the present illness.

- To qualify for extended history of present illness, the medical record should describe four or more elements of the present illness or associated comorbidities.

- To qualify for problem pertinent review of systems, the patient's positive responses and pertinent negatives for the system related to the problem should be documented.

- To qualify for extended review of systems, the patient's positive responses and pertinent negatives for two to nine systems should be documented.

- To qualify for complete review of systems, at least 10 organ systems must be reviewed. Those systems with positive or pertinent negative responses must be individually documented. For the remaining systems, a notation indicating all other systems are negative is permissible.

- At least one specific item from any of the three history areas must be documented for a pertinent past, family, and/or social history.

- At least one specific item from two of the three history areas must be documented for a complete past, family, and/or social history for the following categories of E/M services: office or other outpatient services, established patient; emergency department; subsequent nursing facility care; domiciliary care, established patient; and home care, established patient.

- At least one specific item from each of the three history areas must be documented for a complete past, family, and/or social history for the following categories of E/M services: office or other outpatient services, new patient; hospital observation services; hospital inpatient services, initial care; consultations; comprehensive nursing facility assessments; domiciliary care, new patient; and home care, new patient.

EXAMINATION COMPONENT GUIDELINES
- Specific abnormal findings and relevant negative findings of the examination of the affected or symptomatic body area(s) or organ system(s) should be documented. A notation of "abnormal" without elaboration is insufficient.

- Abnormal or unexpected findings of the examination of the unaffected or asymptomatic body area(s) or organ system(s) should be described.

- A brief statement or notation indicated "negative" or "normal" is sufficient to document normal findings related to unaffected area(s) or asymptomatic organ system(s).

- Examinations are divided into two different types, general multi-system examinations or single organ system examinations. Any physician can perform either type of examination in any specialty. The type is based upon clinical judgment, the patient's history, and the nature of presenting problems.

- Specific elements have been identified for each type of examination and for each specialty. The elements for each are not included in this book as the tables are too lengthy to be reproduced here. Obtain a copy of the complete documentation guidelines for specific details about each type of examination.

TABLE 2

Complexity of Medical Decision Making

Number of Diagnoses or Management Options	Amount and/or Complexity of Data to be Reviewed	Risk of Complications and/or Morbidity or Mortality	Type of Decision Making
minimal	minimal or none	minimal	straightforward
limited	limited	low	low complexity
multiple	moderate	moderate	moderate complexity
extensive	extensive	high	high complexity

MEDICAL DECISION MAKING COMPONENT GUIDELINES
Make sure the following components are documented:

- Number of diagnoses or management options

- An assessment, clinical impression, or diagnosis for each encounter. This information may be explicitly stated or implied in documented decisions regarding management plans and/or further evaluation.

- The initiation of, or changes in, treatment. Treatment includes a wide range of management options including patient instructions, nursing instructions, therapies, and medications.

- Amount/complexity of data reviewed

- In cases of referrals or consultations, who requests the advice, and to which provider the referral or consultation is made.

- If a diagnostic service is ordered, planned, scheduled, or performed at the time of the E/M encounter, the type of service (e.g., lab or x-ray).

- The review of lab, radiology, and/or other diagnostic tests. An entry in a progress note such as "WBC elevated" or "chest x-ray unremarkable" is acceptable.

- A decision to obtain old records or a decision to obtain additional history from the family, caretaker, or other source to supplement that obtained from the patient.

- Relevant findings from the review of old records, and/or the receipt of additional history from the family, caretaker, or other source. If there is no relevant information beyond that already obtained, that fact should be documented. A notation of "old records reviewed" or "additional history obtained from family" without elaboration is insufficient.

- The results of discussion of laboratory, radiology, or other diagnostic test with the physician who performed or interpreted the study.

- The direct visualization and independent interpretation of an image, tracing, or specimen previously or subsequently interpreted by another physician.

- Risks of complications, morbidity, mortality

- Comorbidities, underlying diseases, or other factors that increase the complexity of medical decision making by increasing the risk of complications, morbidity, and/or mortality.

- If a surgical or invasive diagnostic procedure is ordered, planned, or scheduled at the time of the E/M encounter, the type of procedure (e.g., laparoscopy).

- The specific procedure if performed at the time of the E/M encounter

- The referral for, or decision to perform, a surgical or invasive diagnostic procedure on an urgent basis.

CONTRIBUTING FACTORS
If the physician elects to report the level of service based on counseling and/or coordination of care, the total length of time of the encounter (face-to-face or floor time, as appropriate) as well as the time spent counseling should be documented. The record should describe the counseling and/or activities to coordinate care.

SUMMARY
- Clarify that a code may be selected and documented based on counseling/coordination of care, without reference needed to any other dimension of code selection (i.e., history, exam, and medical decision making).

- Emphasize that for established patients, only two of the three key components need be performed (i.e., history, examination, complexity of medical decision making).

- Simplify history selection by allowing documentation of two of the three history areas (HPI, ROS, and PFSH) instead of requiring all three to be documented.

- Add a note that, when a history cannot be obtained due to the patient's condition (e.g., inability to communicate, urgent, emergent situation), the history is deemed "comprehensive" for coding and documentation purposes.

- Simplify examination criteria by eliminating confusing instructions, while enhancing clinical flexibility by eliminating rigid distinctions between general multi-system vs. single system examinations.

- Simplify the medical decision making component by eliminating one level of complexity (straightforward)—the proposed levels are: low, moderate, and high complexity.

- Simplify the medical decision making component by allowing the highest complexity element (i.e., the number of diagnoses/risk of complications, diagnostic procedures/tests and or data to be reviewed, or management options) to drive the level of medical decision making selection. In addition to the noted changes in the glossary, clarifications in the proposed guidelines also include the following:

  — These documentation guidelines are not applicable to the preventive medicine services, critical care, or neonatal intensive care codes.

  — Any record format for documenting history (including preprinted history forms completed by the patient and reviewed by the physician) is acceptable.

— The chief complaint and reason for the encounter requirements are not applicable to subsequent inpatient hospital services.

— Definitions of chief complaint, reason for encounter, and brief/extended history of present illness have been added.

PLACE-OF-SERVICE DISTINCTIONS

The E/M code section is divided into subsections by type and place of service. Keep the following in mind when coding each service setting:

• A patient is considered an outpatient at a health care facility until formal inpatient admission occurs.

• Physicians, regardless of specialty, may use 99281–99285 for reporting emergency department services within hospital-based emergency facilities. Other Emergency Services (99288) is reserved for physician directed emergency care provided by the physician in a hospital emergency or critical care department in two-way communication with ambulance or rescue personnel outside the hospital.

• Consultation codes are linked to location.

• Initial hospital inpatient and hospital observation codes as well as initial nursing facility visit codes include evaluation and management services provided elsewhere (office visit codes or emergency department) by the admitting physician on the same day.

DOCUMENTING THE PATIENT RECORD

Physicians and staff members have developed numerous methods to document professional services, and there is no single "right" way as long as all pertinent components of the codes are documented. Some physicians check off a CPT code on an encounter form, while others make clinical notations in the patient's chart for the coding personnel to translate into codes.

E/M SUBCATEGORIES

E/M codes are intended to standardize the way physicians, coders, and claims processors code patient visits. The varied choices presented by E/M codes result in more consistent billing patterns.

OFFICE OR OTHER OUTPATIENT SERVICES

Use codes (99201–99215) to report the services for office or outpatient visits. The CPT book does not provide instructions for reporting multiple office or outpatient visits provided by the same physician on the same calendar date. The most common practice is to report a single visit code per day, evaluating all services provided during that day to arrive at the correct level of service. Prolonged service codes may be used to report services beyond the usual.

HOSPITAL OBSERVATION SERVICES

Codes 99217–99220 report E/M services provided to patients designated or admitted as "observation status" in a hospital. It is not necessary that the patient be located in an observation area designated by the hospital to use these codes; however, whenever a patient is placed in a separately designated observation area of the hospital or emergency department, these codes should be used.

INITIAL OBSERVATION CARE

When a patient is admitted to observation status in the course of an encounter in another site of service (e.g., hospital emergency department, physician's office, nursing facility). All related E/M services provided by that physician on the same day are included in the admission for hospital observation. Only one physician can report initial observation services. Do not use these observation codes for post-recovery of a procedure that is considered a global surgical service.

OBSERVATION CARE DISCHARGE SERVICES

Use 99217 only if discharge from observation status occurs on a date other than the initial date of observation status. The code includes final examination of the patient, discussion of the hospital stay, instructions for continuing care, and preparation of discharge records. If a patient is admitted to and subsequently discharged from observation status on the same date, report the service observation/inpatient hospital care codes 99234–99236.

HOSPITAL INPATIENT SERVICES

The codes for hospital inpatient services report admission to a hospital setting, follow-up care provided in a hospital setting, observation or inpatient care for same day admission and discharge, and hospital discharge day management. For inpatient care, the time component includes not only face-to-face time with the patient, but also any unit/floor time related to the patient's care. This time may include family counseling or discussing the patient's condition with the family, establishing and reviewing the patient's record, documenting within the chart, and communicating with other health care professionals, such as other physicians, nursing staff, and respiratory therapists.

Initial hospital care codes (99221–99223) are used by the admitting physician to report the first hospital inpatient encounter. All evaluation and management services provided by the admitting physician in conjunction with the admission regardless of the site of the encounter are included in the initial hospital care service. Services provided in the emergency room, observation room, physician's office, or nursing facility specifically related to the admission cannot be reported separately. Physicians, other than the admitting physician, should not use initial hospital care codes, but should report their services with the appropriate consultation or subsequent hospital care codes.

Codes 99238 and 99239 report hospital discharge day management, but exclude discharge of a patient from observation status. Discharge services for newborns or neonates may be reported with 99238 or 99239 for lengths of stay of more than one day. When a physician other than the attending physician provides concurrent care on discharge day, report these services using subsequent hospital care codes.

Observation or inpatient care services, which include admission and discharge services for the same date of service, are reported with 99234–99236. These codes are reported once and include all care provided by the admitting physician whether initiated at another site, within the observation unit, or on an inpatient basis.

CONSULTATIONS

Consultations are provided at the request of another physician or other appropriate source for the purpose of rendering an opinion or advice regarding the evaluation and management of a specific problem. Consultations in the CPT book fall under two subcategories: office or other outpatient consultations and inpatient consultations. If counseling dominates the encounter, time determines the correct code.

The general rules and requirements of a consultation are as follows:

• Requests for consultation must come from an attending physician or other appropriate source, and the necessity for this service must be documented in the patient's record.

• The consulting physician should provide communication regarding his/her findings to the requesting physician.

• The consultant may initiate diagnostic and/or therapeutic services, such as writing orders or prescriptions and initiating treatment plans.

• The opinion rendered and services ordered or performed and the physician ID number must be documented in the patient's medical record and a report of this information communicated to the requesting provider.

• Report separately any identifiable procedure or service performed on, or subsequent to, the date of the initial consultation. When the consultant assumes responsibility for the management of any or all of the patient's care subsequent to the consultation encounter, consult codes are no longer appropriate. Depending on the location, identify the correct subsequent or established patient codes.

• A consultation initiated by the patient or family rather than by a physician is reported with the appropriate office visit code.

• A consultation mandated by a third-party payer should be appended with modifier 32.

OFFICE OR OTHER OUTPATIENT SERVICES

NEW PATIENT

99201 Office or other outpatient visit for the evaluation and management of a new patient, which requires these three key components: a problem focused history; a problem focused examination; straightforward medical decision making. Counseling and/or coordination of care with other providers or agencies are provided consistent with the nature of the problem(s) and the patient's and/or family's needs. Usually, the presenting problem(s) are self limited or minor. Physicians typically spend 10 minutes face-to-face with the patient and/or family. Ⓥ 80 ☐

MED: 100-3,10.4; 100-3,40.5; 100-3,70.1; 100-3,70.2; 100-3,130.2; 100-3,130.3; 100-3,130.4; 100-3,130.5; 100-3,130.6; 100-3,130.7; 100-3,160.2; 100-3,160.7.1; 100-3,230.1; 100-3,250.1; 100-3,250.4; 100-3,270.4; 100-4,4,160; 100-4,12,30.6.7; 100-4,32,12.1

AMA: 2000,Feb,3, 9, 11; 1999,Jun,8; 1998,Jul,9; 1995,Summer,4; 1995,Spring,1; 1995,Fall,9; 1993,Summer,2; 1993,Spring,34; 1993,Fall,9; 1992,Summer,1, 24; 1992,Spring,9, 24; 1991,Winter,11

99202 Office or other outpatient visit for the evaluation and management of a new patient, which requires these three key components: an expanded problem focused history; an expanded problem focused examination; straightforward medical decision making. Counseling and/or coordination of care with other providers or agencies are provided consistent with the nature of the problem(s) and the patient's and/or family's needs. Usually, the presenting problem(s) are of low to moderate severity. Physicians typically spend 20 minutes face-to-face with the patient and/or family. Ⓥ 80 ☐

MED: 100-3,10.4; 100-3,40.5; 100-3,70.1; 100-3,70.2; 100-3,130.2; 100-3,130.3; 100-3,130.4; 100-3,130.5; 100-3,130.6; 100-3,130.7; 100-3,160.2; 100-3,160.7.1; 100-3,230.1; 100-3,250.1; 100-3,250.4; 100-3,270.4; 100-4,4,160; 100-4,12,30.6.7; 100-4,32,12.1

AMA: 2000,Feb,11; 1998,Jul,9; 1995,Summer,4; 1995,Spring,1; 1995,Fall,9; 1993,Summer,2; 1993,Spring,34; 1993,Fall,9; 1992,Spring,9, 24; 1992,Summer,1, 24; 1991,Winter,11

99203 Office or other outpatient visit for the evaluation and management of a new patient, which requires these three key components: a detailed history; a detailed examination; medical decision making of low complexity. Counseling and/or coordination of care with other providers or agencies are provided consistent with the nature of the problem(s) and the patient's and/or family's needs. Usually, the presenting problem(s) are of moderate severity. Physicians typically spend 30 minutes face-to-face with the patient and/or family. Ⓥ 80 ☐

MED: 100-3,10.4; 100-3,40.5; 100-3,70.1; 100-3,70.2; 100-3,130.2; 100-3,130.3; 100-3,130.4; 100-3,130.5; 100-3,130.6; 100-3,130.7; 100-3,160.2; 100-3,160.7.1; 100-3,230.1; 100-3,250.1; 100-3,250.4; 100-3,270.4; 100-4,4,160; 100-4,12,30.6.7; 100-4,32,12.1

AMA: 2000,Feb,11; 1998,Jul,9; 1995,Summer,4; 1995,Spring,1; 1995,Fall,9; 1993,Summer,2; 1993,Spring,34; 1993,Fall,9; 1992,Spring,9, 24; 1992,Summer,1, 24; 1991,Winter,11

99204 Office or other outpatient visit for the evaluation and management of a new patient, which requires these three key components: a comprehensive history; a comprehensive examination; medical decision making of moderate complexity. Counseling and/or coordination of care with other providers or agencies are provided consistent with the nature of the problem(s) and the patient's and/or family's needs. Usually, the presenting problem(s) are of moderate to high severity. Physicians typically spend 45 minutes face-to-face with the patient and/or family. Ⓥ 80 ☐

MED: 100-3,10.4; 100-3,70.1; 100-3,70.2; 100-3,130.2; 100-3,130.3; 100-3,130.4; 100-3,130.5; 100-3,130.6; 100-3,130.7; 100-3,160.2; 100-3,160.7.1; 100-3,230.1; 100-3,250.1; 100-3,250.4; 100-3,270.4; 100-4,4,160; 100-4,12,30.6.7; 100-4,32,12.1

AMA: 2000,Feb,11; 1998,Jul,9; 1995,Summer,4; 1995,Spring,1; 1995,Fall,9; 1993,Summer,2; 1993,Spring,34; 1993,Fall,9; 1992,Spring,9, 24; 1992,Summer,1, 24; 1991,Winter,11

99205 Office or other outpatient visit for the evaluation and management of a new patient, which requires these three key components: a comprehensive history; a comprehensive examination; medical decision making of high complexity. Counseling and/or coordination of care with other providers or agencies are provided consistent with the nature of the problem(s) and the patient's and/or family's needs. Usually, the presenting problem(s) are of moderate to high severity. Physicians typically spend 60 minutes face-to-face with the patient and/or family. Ⓥ 80 ☐

MED: 100-3,10.4; 100-3,40.5; 100-3,70.1; 100-3,70.2; 100-3,130.2; 100-3,130.3; 100-3,130.4; 100-3,130.5; 100-3,130.6; 100-3,130.7; 100-3,160.2; 100-3,160.7.1; 100-3,230.1; 100-3,250.1; 100-3,250.4; 100-3,270.4; 100-4,4,160; 100-4,12,30.6.7; 100-4,32,12.1

AMA: 2000,Feb,11; 1998,Jul,9; 1995,Summer,4; 1995,Spring,1; 1995,Fall,9; 1993,Summer,2; 1993,Spring,34; 1993,Fall,9; 1992,Spring,9, 24; 1992,Summer,1, 24; 1991,Winter,11

ESTABLISHED PATIENT

99211 Office or other outpatient visit for the evaluation and management of an established patient, that may not require the presence of a physician. Usually, the presenting problem(s) are minimal. Typically, 5 minutes are spent performing or supervising these services. Ⓥ 80 ☐

MED: 100-3,10.4; 100-3,40.5; 100-3,70.1; 100-3,70.2; 100-3,130.2; 100-3,130.3; 100-3,130.4; 100-3,130.5; 100-3,130.6; 100-3,130.7; 100-3,160.2; 100-3,160.7.1; 100-3,230.1; 100-3,250.1; 100-3,250.4; 100-3,270.4; 100-4,4,160; 100-4,12,30.6.7; 100-4,32,12.1

AMA: 2000,Feb,11; 1999,Oct,9; 1998,Jul,9; 1997,Feb,9; 1996,Oct,10; 1995,Summer,4; 1995,Spring,1; 1995,Fall,9; 1993,Spring,34; 1993,Summer,2; 1993,Fall,9; 1992,Summer,1, 24; 1992,Spring,9, 24; 1991,Winter,11

99212 Office or other outpatient visit for the evaluation and management of an established patient, which requires at least two of these three key components: a problem focused history; a problem focused examination; straightforward medical decision making. Counseling and/or coordination of care with other providers or agencies are provided consistent with the nature of the problem(s) and the patient's and/or family's needs. Usually, the presenting problem(s) are self limited or minor. Physicians typically spend 10 minutes face-to-face with the patient and/or family. Ⓥ 80 ☐

MED: 100-3,10.4; 100-3,40.5; 100-3,70.1; 100-3,70.2; 100-3,130.2; 100-3,130.3; 100-3,130.4; 100-3,130.5; 100-3,130.6; 100-3,130.7; 100-3,160.2; 100-3,160.7.1; 100-3,230.1; 100-3,250.1; 100-3,250.4; 100-3,270.4; 100-4,4,160; 100-4,12,30.6.7; 100-4,32,12.1

AMA: 2002,May,17; 2000,Jun,11; 2000,Feb,11; 1998,Jul,9; 1995,Summer,4; 1995,Spring,1; 1995,Fall,9; 1993,Fall,9; 1993,Summer,2; 1993,Spring,34; 1992,Summer,1, 24; 1992,Spring,9, 24; 1991,Winter,11

Evaluation and Management

99213 — 99220

99213   Office or other outpatient visit for the evaluation and management of an established patient, which requires at least two of these three key components: an expanded problem focused history; an expanded problem focused examination; medical decision making of low complexity. Counseling and coordination of care with other providers or agencies are provided consistent with the nature of the problem(s) and the patient's and/or family's needs. Usually, the presenting problem(s) are of low to moderate severity. Physicians typically spend 15 minutes face-to-face with the patient and/or family.   [V] [80] [⏸]

MED: 100-3,10.4; 100-3,40.5; 100-3,70.1; 100-3,70.2; 100-3,130.2; 100-3,130.3; 100-3,130.4; 100-3,130.5; 100-3,130.6; 100-3,130.7; 100-3,160.2; 100-3,160.7.1; 100-3,230.1; 100-3,250.1; 100-3,250.4; 100-3,270.4; 100-4,4,160; 100-4,12,30.6.7; 100-4,32,12.1

AMA: 1998,Jul,9; 1997,Jan,10; 1995,Summer,4; 1995,Spring,1; 1995,Fall,9; 1993,Summer,2; 1993,Spring,34; 1993,Fall,9; 1992,Spring,9, 24; 1992,Summer,1, 24; 1991,Winter,11

99214   Office or other outpatient visit for the evaluation and management of an established patient, which requires at least two of these three key components: a detailed history; a detailed examination; medical decision making of moderate complexity. Counseling and/or coordination of care with other providers or agencies are provided consistent with the nature of the problem(s) and the patient's and/or family's needs. Usually, the presenting problem(s) are of moderate to high severity. Physicians typically spend 25 minutes face-to-face with the patient and/or family.   [V] [80] [⏸]

MED: 100-3,10.4; 100-3,40.5; 100-3,70.1; 100-3,70.2; 100-3,130.2; 100-3,130.3; 100-3,130.4; 100-3,130.5; 100-3,130.6; 100-3,130.7; 100-3,160.2; 100-3,160.7.1; 100-3,230.1; 100-3,250.1; 100-3,250.4; 100-3,270.4; 100-4,4,160; 100-4,12,30.6.7; 100-4,32,12.1

AMA: 1998,Jul,9; 1995,Summer,4; 1995,Spring,1; 1995,Fall,9; 1993,Summer,2; 1993,Fall,9; 1993,Spring,34; 1992,Spring,9, 24; 1992,Summer,1, 24; 1991,Winter,11

99215   Office or other outpatient visit for the evaluation and management of an established patient, which requires at least two of these three key components: a comprehensive history; a comprehensive examination; medical decision making of high complexity. Counseling and/or coordination of care with other providers or agencies are provided consistent with the nature of the problem(s) and the patient's and/or family's needs. Usually, the presenting problem(s) are of moderate to high severity. Physicians typically spend 40 minutes face-to-face with the patient and/or family.   [V] [80] [⏸]

MED: 100-3,10.4; 100-3,40.5; 100-3,70.1; 100-3,70.2; 100-3,130.2; 100-3,130.3; 100-3,130.4; 100-3,130.5; 100-3,130.6; 100-3,130.7; 100-3,160.2; 100-3,160.7.1; 100-3,230.1; 100-3,250.1; 100-3,250.4; 100-3,270.4; 100-4,4,160; 100-4,12,30.6.7; 100-4,32,12.1

AMA: 1998,Jul,9; 1997,Jan,10; 1995,Summer,4; 1995,Spring,1; 1995,Fall,9; 1993,Summer,2; 1993,Spring,34; 1993,Fall,9; 1992,Spring,9, 24; 1992,Summer,1, 24; 1991,Winter,11

HOSPITAL OBSERVATION SERVICES

OBSERVATION CARE DISCHARGE SERVICES

If the patient is admitted to the hospital on the same day as admission to the observation area, consult CPT codes for Hospital Admission (99221-99223).

Consult CPT codes 99234-99236 for admission and discharge to observation area on same date.

99217   Observation care discharge day management (This code is to be utilized by the physician to report all services provided to a patient on discharge from "observation status" if the discharge is on other than the initial date of "observation status." To report services to a patient designated as "observation status" or "inpatient status" and discharged on the same date, use the codes for Observation or Inpatient Care Services [including Admission and Discharge Services, 99234-99236 as appropriate.])   [B] [80] [⏸]

MED: 100-1,5,70; 100-2,15,30; 100-4,11,40.1.3; 100-4,12,10; 100-4,12,30.6; 100-4,12,30.6.8; 100-4,12,100; 100-4,12,100.1.7; 100-4,12,100.1.8

AMA: 1998,May,1; 1998,Mar,1; 1997,Nov,2

INITIAL OBSERVATION CARE

NEW OR ESTABLISHED PATIENT

▲ **99218**   Initial observation care, per day, for the evaluation and management of a patient which requires these three key components: a detailed or comprehensive history; a detailed or comprehensive examination; and medical decision making that is straightforward or of low complexity. Counseling and/or coordination of care with other providers or agencies are provided consistent with the nature of the problem(s) and the patient's and/or family's needs. Usually, the problem(s) requiring admission to "observation status" are of low severity.   [B] [80] [⏸]

MED: 100-1,5,70; 100-2,15,30; 100-4,11,40.1.3; 100-4,12,10; 100-4,12,30.6; 100-4,12,30.6.8; 100-4,12,100; 100-4,12,100.1.7; 100-4,12,100.1.8

AMA: 1998,Mar,1; 1995,Fall,9; 1993,Spring,34

99219   Initial observation care, per day, for the evaluation and management of a patient, which requires these three key components: a comprehensive history; a comprehensive examination; and medical decision making of moderate complexity. Counseling and/or coordination of care with other providers or agencies are provided consistent with the nature of the problem(s) and the patient's and/or family's needs. Usually, the problem(s) requiring admission to "observation status" are of moderate severity.   [B] [80] [⏸]

MED: 100-1,5,70; 100-2,15,30; 100-4,11,40.1.3; 100-4,12,10; 100-4,12,30.6; 100-4,12,30.6.8; 100-4,12,100; 100-4,12,100.1.7; 100-4,12,100.1.8

AMA: 1998,Mar,1; 1995,Fall,16; 1993,Spring,34

99220   Initial observation care, per day, for the evaluation and management of a patient, which requires these three key components: a comprehensive history; a comprehensive examination; and medical decision making of high complexity. Counseling and/or coordination of care with other providers or agencies are provided consistent with the nature of the problem(s) and the patient's and/or family's needs. Usually, the problem(s) requiring admission to "observation status" are of high severity.   [B] [80] [⏸]

MED: 100-1,5,70; 100-2,15,30; 100-4,11,40.1.3; 100-4,12,10; 100-4,12,30.6; 100-4,12,30.6.8; 100-4,12,100; 100-4,12,100.1.7; 100-4,12,100.1.8

AMA: 1998,Mar,1; 1995,Fall,16; 1993,Spring,34

---

[26] Professional Component Only   [80]/[80] Assist-at-Surgery Allowed/With Documentation   Unlisted   Not Covered

[TC] Technical Component Only   **MED:** Pub 100/NCD References   **AMA:** CPT Assistant References   [1]-[9] ASC Group   ♂ Male Only   ♀ Female Only

10 — CPT Expert   CPT only © 2006 American Medical Association. All Rights Reserved. *(Black Ink)*   © 2006 Ingenix *(Blue Ink)*

HOSPITAL INPATIENT SERVICES

INITIAL HOSPITAL CARE

99221   Initial hospital care, per day, for the evaluation and management of a patient, which requires these three key components: a detailed or comprehensive history; a detailed or comprehensive examination; and medical decision making that is straightforward or of low complexity. Counseling and/or coordination of care with other providers or agencies are provided consistent with the nature of the problem(s) and the patient's and/or family's needs. Usually, the problem(s) requiring admission are of low severity. Physicians typically spend 30 minutes at the bedside and on the patient's hospital floor or unit.   Ⓑ 80 ⬚

MED: 100-2,6,10; 100-3,10.3; 100-3,70.1; 100-3,70.2; 100-3,130.1; 100-3,130.7; 100-4,12,30.6; 100-4,12,30.6.9; 100-4,12,100; 100-4,12,100.1.7; 100-4,12,100.1.8

AMA: 1998,Mar,1; 1996,Sep,10; 1996,Jul,11; 1995,Spring,1; 1995,Fall,9; 1993,Spring,34; 1992,Summer,1, 24; 1992,Spring,13, 24; 1992,Fall,1; 1991,Winter,11

99222   Initial hospital care, per day, for the evaluation and management of a patient, which requires these three key components: a comprehensive history; a comprehensive examination; and medical decision making of moderate complexity. Counseling and/or coordination of care with other providers or agencies are provided consistent with the nature of the problem(s) and the patient's and/or family's needs. Usually, the problem(s) requiring admission are of moderate severity. Physicians typically spend 50 minutes at the bedside and on the patient's hospital floor or unit.   Ⓑ 80 ⬚

MED: 100-2,6,10; 100-3,10.3; 100-3,70.1; 100-3,70.2; 100-3,130.1; 100-3,130.7; 100-4,12,30.6; 100-4,12,30.6.9; 100-4,12,100; 100-4,12,100.1.7; 100-4,12,100.1.8

AMA: 1998,Mar,1; 1996,Sep,10; 1996,Jul,11; 1995,Spring,1; 1995,Fall,9; 1993,Spring,34; 1992,Summer,1, 24; 1992,Spring,13, 24; 1992,Fall,1; 1991,Winter,11

99223   Initial hospital care, per day, for the evaluation and management of a patient, which requires these three key components: a comprehensive history; a comprehensive examination; and medical decision making of high complexity. Counseling and/or coordination of care with other providers or agencies are provided consistent with the nature of the problem(s) and the patient's and/or family's needs. Usually, the problem(s) requiring admission are of high severity. Physicians typically spend 70 minutes at the bedside and on the patient's hospital floor or unit.   Ⓑ 80 ⬚

MED: 100-2,6,10; 100-3,10.3; 100-3,70.1; 100-3,70.2; 100-3,130.1; 100-3,130.7; 100-4,12,30.6; 100-4,12,30.6.9; 100-4,12,100; 100-4,12,100.1.7; 100-4,12,100.1.8

AMA: 1998,Mar,1; 1996,Sep,10; 1996,Jul,11; 1995,Spring,1; 1995,Fall,9; 1993,Spring,34; 1992,Summer,1, 24; 1992,Spring,13, 24; 1992,Fall,1; 1991,Winter,11

SUBSEQUENT HOSPITAL CARE

99231   Subsequent hospital care, per day, for the evaluation and management of a patient, which requires at least two of these three key components: a problem focused interval history; a problem focused examination; medical decision making that is straightforward or of low complexity. Counseling and/or coordination of care with other providers or agencies are provided consistent with the nature of the problem(s) and the patient's and/or family's needs. Usually, the patient is stable, recovering or improving. Physicians typically spend 15 minutes at the bedside and on the patient's hospital floor or unit.   Ⓑ 80 ⬚

MED: 100-2,6,10; 100-3,10.3; 100-3,130.1; 100-3,130.7; 100-4,12,30.6; 100-4,12,30.6.9; 100-4,12,30.6.15; 100-4,12,100; 100-4,12,100.1.7; 100-4,12,100.1.8; 100-4,12,190

AMA: 1995,Spring,1; 1995,Fall,16; 1993,Spring,34; 1992,Summer,1, 24; 1992,Fall,1; 1992,Spring,13, 24; 1991,Winter,11

99232   Subsequent hospital care, per day, for the evaluation and management of a patient, which requires at least two of these three key components: an expanded problem focused interval history; an expanded problem focused examination; medical decision making of moderate complexity. Counseling and/or coordination of care with other providers or agencies are provided consistent with the nature of the problem(s) and the patient's and/or family's needs. Usually, the patient is responding inadequately to therapy or has developed a minor complication. Physicians typically spend 25 minutes at the bedside and on the patient's hospital floor or unit.   Ⓑ 80 ⬚

MED: 100-2,6,10; 100-3,10.3; 100-3,130.1; 100-3,130.7; 100-4,12,30.6; 100-4,12,30.6.9; 100-4,12,30.6.15; 100-4,12,100; 100-4,12,100.1.7; 100-4,12,100.1.8; 100-4,12,190

AMA: 2000,Jan,11; 1995,Spring,1; 1995,Fall,16; 1993,Spring,34; 1992,Summer,1, 24; 1992,Spring,13, 24; 1992,Fall,1; 1991,Winter,11

99233   Subsequent hospital care, per day, for the evaluation and management of a patient, which requires at least two of these three key components: a detailed interval history; a detailed examination; medical decision making of high complexity. Counseling and/or coordination of care with other providers or agencies are provided consistent with the nature of the problem(s) and the patient's and/or family's needs. Usually, the patient is unstable or has developed a significant complication or a significant new problem. Physicians typically spend 35 minutes at the bedside and on the patient's hospital floor or unit.   Ⓑ 80 ⬚

MED: 100-2,6,10; 100-3,10.3; 100-3,130.1; 100-3,130.7; 100-4,12,30.6; 100-4,12,30.6.9; 100-4,12,30.6.15; 100-4,12,100; 100-4,12,100.1.7; 100-4,12,100.1.8; 100-4,12,190

AMA: 1995,Spring,1; 1995,Fall,16; 1993,Spring,34; 1992,Summer,1, 24; 1992,Fall,1; 1992,Spring,13, 24; 1991,Winter,11

OBSERVATION OR INPATIENT CARE SERVICES (INCLUDING ADMISSION AND DISCHARGE SERVICES)

Consult CPT codes 99217-99220 for patients that are admitted and discharged from observation on different dates. Consult CPT codes 99221-99223 and 99238-99239 for patients admitted for inpatient care and discharged on different dates.

99234 Observation or inpatient hospital care, for the evaluation and management of a patient including admission and discharge on the same date which requires these three key components: a detailed or comprehensive history; a detailed or comprehensive examination; and medical decision making that is straightforward or of low complexity. Counseling and/or coordination of care with other providers or agencies are provided consistent with the nature of the problem(s) and the patient's and/or family's needs. Usually the presenting problem(s) requiring admission are of low severity. ⒷⒽⓀⓁ

> MED: 100-1,5,70; 100-2,6,10; 100-2,15,30; 100-3,10.3; 100-3,130.1; 100-3,130.7; 100-4,11,40.1.3; 100-4,12,10; 100-4,12,30.6; 100-4,12,30.6.9; 100-4,12,100; 100-4,12,100.1.7; 100-4,12,100.1.8
> AMA: 2002,Jun,10; 2000,Jan,11; 1998,May,1; 1998,Mar,1

99235 Observation or inpatient hospital care, for the evaluation and management of a patient including admission and discharge on the same date which requires these three key components: a comprehensive history; a comprehensive examination; and medical decision making of moderate complexity. Counseling and/or coordination of care with other providers or agencies are provided consistent with the nature of the problem(s) and the patient's and/or family's needs. Usually the presenting problem(s) requiring admission are of moderate severity. ⒷⒽⓀⓁ

> MED: 100-1,5,70; 100-2,6,10; 100-2,15,30; 100-3,10.3; 100-3,130.1; 100-3,130.7; 100-4,11,40.1.3; 100-4,12,10; 100-4,12,30.6; 100-4,12,30.6.9; 100-4,12,100; 100-4,12,100.1.7; 100-4,12,100.1.8
> AMA: 2002,Jun,10; 2000,Jan,11; 1998,May,1; 1998,Mar,1

99236 Observation or inpatient hospital care, for the evaluation and management of a patient including admission and discharge on the same date which requires these three key components: a comprehensive history; a comprehensive examination; and medical decision making of high complexity. Counseling and/or coordination of care with other providers or agencies are provided consistent with the nature of the problem(s) and the patient's and/or family's needs. Usually the presenting problem(s) requiring admission are of high severity. ⒷⒽⓀⓁ

> MED: 100-1,5,70; 100-2,6,10; 100-2,15,30; 100-3,10.3; 100-3,130.1; 100-3,130.7; 100-4,11,40.1.3; 100-4,12,10; 100-4,12,30.6; 100-4,12,30.6.9; 100-4,12,100; 100-4,12,100.1.7; 100-4,12,100.1.8
> AMA: 2002,Jun,10; 2000,Jan,11; 1998,May,1; 1998,Mar,1

HOSPITAL DISCHARGE SERVICES

99238 Hospital discharge day management; 30 minutes or less ⒷⒽⓀⓁ

> MED: 100-2,6,10; 100-3,10.3; 100-3,130.1; 100-3,130.7; 100-4,12,30.6; 100-4,12,30.6.9; 100-4,12,70; 100-4,12,100; 100-4,12,100.1.7; 100-4,12,100.1.8; 100-4,13,20; 100-4,13,90
> AMA: 1999,Jan,10; 1998,May,1; 1998,Mar,1, 11; 1997,Nov,4; 1993,Spring,4; 1992,Fall,1

These codes are to be utilized by the physician to report all services provided to a patient on the date of discharge, if other than the initial date of inpatient status. To report concurrent care services provided by a physician(s) other than the attending physician, use subsequent hospital care codes (99231-99233) on the day of discharge. For Observation Care Discharge, consult CPT code 99217. For observation or inpatient hospital care including the admission and discharge of the patient on the same date, consult CPT codes 99234-99236. For Nursing Facility Care Discharge, consult CPT codes 99315 and 99316. If discharge services are provided to newborns admitted and discharged on the same date, consult CPT code 99435.

99239 more than 30 minutes ⒷⒽⓀⓁ

> MED: 100-1,5,70; 100-2,6,10; 100-2,15,30; 100-3,10.3; 100-3,130.1; 100-3,130.7; 100-4,11,40.1.3; 100-4,12,10; 100-4,12,30.6; 100-4,12,30.6.9; 100-4,12,100; 100-4,12,100.1.7; 100-4,12,100.1.8
> AMA: 1999,Jan,10; 1998,May,1; 1998,Mar,1, 11; 1997,Nov,4

CONSULTATIONS

A consultation is an evaluation of a patient provided by a physician at the request of another physician or appropriate source. The consulting physician may order tests or therapeutic services at the time of the visit, and these would be reported separately. The request for the consultation as well as the consultant's opinion must be documented in the patient's chart. A written report must be sent back to the physician requesting the consult.

A consultation requested by the patient or family member and not by a physician or appropriate source should not be reported with consultation codes. Report the appropriate evaluation and management (E/M) code for this service.

Append modifier 32 if the request is made by a third-party payer.

If the consulting physician assumes care for all or a part of the patient's treatment, report the appropriate E/M code for this service. If there is a distinction between new or established patient in the E/M code set, the patient is considered an established patient.

OFFICE OR OTHER OUTPATIENT CONSULTATIONS

NEW OR ESTABLISHED PATIENT

Report the following codes for consultations performed in the physician's office or as an outpatient, including hospital observation, home services, domiciliary, rest home, or emergency department. Any follow-up visits in the office or facility at the request of the consultant or patient should be submitted with the appropriate evaluation and management code. If another request is made for a consultation by a physician or appropriate source, the consultation codes can be used again.

99241 Office consultation for a new or established patient, which requires these three key components: a problem focused history; a problem focused examination; and straightforward medical decision making. Counseling and/or coordination of care with other providers or agencies are provided consistent with the nature of the problem(s) and the patient's and/or family's needs. Usually, the presenting problem(s) are self limited or minor. Physicians typically spend 15 minutes face-to-face with the patient and/or family. ⓋⒽⓁ

> MED: 100-1,5,70; 100-2,15,30; 100-4,4,160; 100-4,11,40.1.3; 100-4,12,10; 100-4,12,30.6; 100-4,12,30.6.10; 100-4,12,30.6.15; 100-4,12,100; 100-4,12,100.1.7; 100-4,12,100.1.8
> AMA: 2002,Sep,11; 2002,Jul,2; 2001,Aug,1; 2000,Apr,10; 1999,Jun,10; 1997,Oct,1; 1995,Spring,1; 1993,Spring,1, 34; 1992,Spring,1, 13, 24; 1992,Summer,1; 1991,Winter,11

99242 Office consultation for a new or established patient, which requires these three key components: an expanded problem focused history; an expanded problem focused examination; and straightforward medical decision making. Counseling and/or coordination of care with other providers or agencies are provided consistent with the nature of the problem(s) and the patient's and/or family's needs. Usually, the presenting problem(s) are of low severity. Physicians typically spend 30 minutes face-to-face with the patient and/or family. ⓋⒽⓁ

> MED: 100-1,5,70; 100-2,15,30; 100-4,4,160; 100-4,11,40.1.3; 100-4,12,10; 100-4,12,30.6; 100-4,12,30.6.10; 100-4,12,30.6.15; 100-4,12,100; 100-4,12,100.1.7; 100-4,12,100.1.8
> AMA: 2002,Sep,11; 2002,Jul,2; 2001,Aug,1; 1995,Spring,1; 1993,Spring,1, 34; 1992,Summer,1; 1992,Spring,1, 13, 24; 1991,Winter,11

26 Professional Component Only   80/80 Assist-at-Surgery Allowed/With Documentation   Unlisted   Not Covered

TC Technical Component Only   MED: Pub 100/NCD References   AMA: CPT Assistant References   1-9 ASC Group   ♂ Male Only   ♀ Female Only

12 — CPT Expert   CPT only © 2006 American Medical Association. All Rights Reserved. (Black Ink)   © 2006 Ingenix (Blue Ink)

99243   Office consultation for a new or established patient, which requires these three key components: a detailed history; a detailed examination; and medical decision making of low complexity. Counseling and/or coordination of care with other providers or agencies are provided consistent with the nature of the problem(s) and the patient's and/or family's needs. Usually, the presenting problem(s) are of moderate severity. Physicians typically spend 40 minutes face-to-face with the patient and/or family. Ⓥ 80 ◪

MED: 100-1,5,70; 100-2,15,30; 100-4,4,160; 100-4,11,40.1.3; 100-4,12,10; 100-4,12,30.6; 100-4,12,30.6.10; 100-4,12,30.6.15; 100-4,12,100; 100-4,12,100.1.7; 100-4,12,100.1.8

AMA: 2002,Sep,11; 2002,Jul,2; 2001,Aug,1; 1995,Spring,1; 1993,Spring,1, 34; 1992,Summer,1; 1992,Spring,1, 13, 24; 1991,Winter,11

99244   Office consultation for a new or established patient, which requires these three key components: a comprehensive history; a comprehensive examination; and medical decision making of moderate complexity. Counseling and/or coordination of care with other providers or agencies are provided consistent with the nature of the problem(s) and the patient's and/or family's needs. Usually, the presenting problem(s) are of moderate to high severity. Physicians typically spend 60 minutes face-to-face with the patient and/or family. Ⓥ 80 ◪

MED: 100-1,5,70; 100-2,15,30; 100-4,4,160; 100-4,11,40.1.3; 100-4,12,10; 100-4,12,30.6; 100-4,12,30.6.10; 100-4,12,30.6.15; 100-4,12,100; 100-4,12,100.1.7; 100-4,12,100.1.8

AMA: 2002,Sep,11; 2002,Jul,2; 2001,Aug,1; 1995,Spring,1; 1993,Spring,1, 34; 1992,Summer,1; 1992,Spring,1, 13, 24; 1991,Winter,11

99245   Office consultation for a new or established patient, which requires these three key components: a comprehensive history; a comprehensive examination; and medical decision making of high complexity. Counseling and/or coordination of care with other providers or agencies are provided consistent with the nature of the problem(s) and the patient's and/or family's needs. Usually, the presenting problem(s) are of moderate to high severity. Physicians typically spend 80 minutes face-to-face with the patient and/or family. Ⓥ 80 ◪

MED: 100-1,5,70; 100-2,15,30; 100-4,4,160; 100-4,11,40.1.3; 100-4,12,10; 100-4,12,30.6; 100-4,12,100.1.7; 100-4,12,30.6.15; 100-4,12,100; 100-4,12,100.1.8

AMA: 2002,Sep,11; 2002,Jul,2; 2001,Aug,1; 1997,Oct,1; 1995,Spring,1; 1993,Spring,1, 34; 1992,Summer,1; 1992,Spring,1, 13, 24; 1991,Winter,11

INPATIENT CONSULTATIONS

NEW OR ESTABLISHED PATIENT

Report the following codes for consultations provided to inpatients, nursing home residents, or patients in a partial hospital setting. The consultant should only report one consultation code per admission. Additional visits during the admission should be reported with the appropriate evaluation and management code for subsequent hospital care or subsequent nursing facility care. This includes any services necessary for the consultant to complete his or her assessment, monitor progress, revise recommendations, or examine a new problem.

▲ 99251   Inpatient consultation for a new or established patient, which requires these three key components: a problem focused history; a problem focused examination; and straightforward medical decision making. Counseling and/or coordination of care with other providers or agencies are provided consistent with the nature of the problem(s) and the patient's and/or family's needs. Usually, the presenting problem(s) are self limited or minor. Physicians typically spend 20 minutes at the bedside and on the patient's hospital floor or unit. Ⓒ 80 ◪

MED: 100-2,6,10; 100-3,10.3; 100-3,70.1; 100-3,70.2; 100-3,130.1; 100-3,130.7; 100-3,160.7.1; 100-4,12,30.6; 100-4,12,30.6.10; 100-4,12,100; 100-4,12,100.1.7; 100-4,12,100.1.8; 100-4,12,190

AMA: 2002,Sep,11; 2001,Aug,1; 1997,Oct,1; 1995,Spring,1; 1993,Spring,34; 1992,Summer,1; 1992,Spring,1, 13, 24; 1991,Winter,11

▲ 99252   Inpatient consultation for a new or established patient, which requires these three key components: an expanded problem focused history; an expanded problem focused examination; and straightforward medical decision making. Counseling and/or coordination of care with other providers or agencies are provided consistent with the nature of the problem(s) and the patient's and/or family's needs. Usually, the presenting problem(s) are of low severity. Physicians typically spend 40 minutes at the bedside and on the patient's hospital floor or unit. Ⓒ 80 ◪

MED: 100-2,6,10; 100-3,70.1; 100-3,70.2; 100-3,130.1; 100-3,130.7; 100-3,160.7.1; 100-4,12,190

AMA: 2002,Sep,11; 2001,Aug,1; 1995,Spring,1; 1993,Summer,34; 1992,Summer,1; 1992,Spring,1, 13, 24; 1991,Winter,11

▲ 99253   Inpatient consultation for a new or established patient, which requires these three key components: a detailed history; a detailed examination; and medical decision making of low complexity. Counseling and/or coordination of care with other providers or agencies are provided consistent with the nature of the problem(s) and the patient's and/or family's needs. Usually, the presenting problem(s) are of moderate severity. Physicians typically spend 55 minutes at the bedside and on the patient's hospital floor or unit. Ⓒ 80 ◪

MED: 100-2,6,10; 100-3,10.3; 100-3,70.1; 100-3,70.2; 100-3,130.1; 100-3,130.7; 100-3,160.7.1; 100-4,12,30.6; 100-4,12,30.6.10; 100-4,12,100; 100-4,12,100.1.7; 100-4,12,100.1.8; 100-4,12,190

AMA: 2002,Sep,11; 2001,Aug,1; 1995,Spring,1; 1993,Summer,34; 1992,Summer,1; 1992,Spring,1, 13, 24; 1991,Winter,11

▲ 99254   Inpatient consultation for a new or established patient, which requires these three key components: a comprehensive history; a comprehensive examination; and medical decision making of moderate complexity. Counseling and/or coordination of care with other providers or agencies are provided consistent with the nature of the problem(s) and the patient's and/or family's needs. Usually, the presenting problem(s) are of moderate to high severity. Physicians typically spend 80 minutes at the bedside and on the patient's hospital floor or unit. Ⓒ 80 ◪

MED: 100-2,6,10; 100-3,10.3; 100-3,70.1; 100-3,70.2; 100-3,130.1; 100-3,130.7; 100-3,160.7.1; 100-4,12,30.6; 100-4,12,30.6.10; 100-4,12,100; 100-4,12,100.1.7; 100-4,12,100.1.8; 100-4,12,190

AMA: 2002,Sep,11; 2001,Aug,1; 1995,Spring,1; 1993,Summer,34; 1992,Summer,1; 1992,Spring,1, 13, 24; 1991,Winter,11

Evaluation and Management

99255 — 99284

▲ 99255   Inpatient consultation for a new or established patient, which requires these three key components: a comprehensive history; a comprehensive examination; and medical decision making of high complexity. Counseling and/or coordination of care with other providers or agencies are provided consistent with the nature of the problem(s) and the patient's and/or family's needs. Usually, the presenting problem(s) are of moderate to high severity. Physicians typically spend 110 minutes at the bedside and on the patient's hospital floor or unit.   [C] [80] ▣

MED: 100-2,6,10; 100-3,10.3; 100-3,70.1; 100-3,70.2; 100-3,130.1; 100-3,130.7; 100-3,160.7.1; 100-4,12,30.6; 100-4,12,30.6.10; 100-4,12,100; 100-4,12,100.1.7; 100-4,12,100.1.8; 100-4,12,190

AMA: 2002,Sep,11; 2001,Aug,1; 1995,Spring,1; 1993,Summer,34; 1992,Summer,1; 1992,Spring,1, 13, 24; 1991,Winter,11

EMERGENCY DEPARTMENT SERVICES

Emergency department (ED) service codes do not differentiate between new and established patients and are used by hospital-based and nonhospital-based physicians.

Time is not a descriptive component for the emergency department levels of E/M services since services are on a variable basis and usually involve multiple encounters with several patients over extended periods of time.

Use 99217-99220 to report evaluation and management services provided in the observation area of a hospital. Use 99291 and 99292 to report critical care provided in the emergency department.

An E/M service can be billed by a physician in addition to a surgical procedure when a separately identifiable E/M service is rendered. For example, if a physician sutures a scalp wound and performs a full neurological exam for a patient with head trauma, it would be proper to bill the surgery and the E/M service. This circumstance would be reported by adding modifier 25 to the appropriate E/M code. It would not be correct, however, if the evaluation only required identifying the need for sutures and confirming immunization status.

Associated with ED services is 99288 Physician direction of emergency medical systems (EMS) emergency care, advanced life support. The physician must be located in the ED or critical care department; be in two-way voice communication with the ambulance or rescue personnel outside the hospital; and direct the performance of necessary medical procedures.

NEW OR ESTABLISHED PATIENT

99281   Emergency department visit for the evaluation and management of a patient, which requires these three key components: a problem focused history; a problem focused examination; and straightforward medical decision making. Counseling and/or coordination of care with other providers or agencies are provided consistent with the nature of the problem(s) and the patient's and/or family's needs. Usually, the presenting problem(s) are self limited or minor.   [V] [80] ▣

MED: 100-1,5,70; 100-2,15,30; 100-3,70.1; 100-4,4,20.5; 100-4,4,160; 100-4,11,40.1.3; 100-4,12,10; 100-4,12,30.6; 100-4,12,30.6.11; 100-4,12,70; 100-4,12,100; 100-4,12,100.1.7; 100-4,12,100.1.8; 100-4,13,20; 100-4,13,90

AMA: 2002,Jul,2; 2000,Jan,11; 2000,Feb,11; 1995,Spring,1; 1993,Spring,34; 1992,Summer,1; 1992,Spring,24; 1991,Winter,11

99282   Emergency department visit for the evaluation and management of a patient, which requires these three key components: an expanded problem focused history; an expanded problem focused examination; and medical decision making of low complexity. Counseling and/or coordination of care with other providers or agencies are provided consistent with the nature of the problem(s) and the patient's and/or family's needs. Usually, the presenting problem(s) are of low to moderate severity.   [V] [80] ▣

MED: 100-1,5,70; 100-2,15,30; 100-3,70.1; 100-4,4,20.5; 100-4,4,160; 100-4,11,40.1.3; 100-4,12,10; 100-4,12,30.6; 100-4,12,30.6.11; 100-4,12,70; 100-4,12,100; 100-4,12,100.1.7; 100-4,12,100.1.8; 100-4,13,20; 100-4,13,90

AMA: 2002,Jul,2; 2000,Jan,11; 2000,Feb,11; 1995,Summer,1; 1995,Spring,1; 1993,Spring,34; 1992,Summer,1, 18; 1992,Spring,24; 1991,Winter,11

99283   Emergency department visit for the evaluation and management of a patient, which requires these three key components: an expanded problem focused history; an expanded problem focused examination; and medical decision making of moderate complexity. Counseling and/or coordination of care with other providers or agencies are provided consistent with the nature of the problem(s) and the patient's and/or family's needs. Usually, the presenting problem(s) are of moderate severity.   [V] [80] ▣

MED: 100-1,5,70; 100-2,15,30; 100-3,70.1; 100-4,4,20.5; 100-4,4,160; 100-4,11,40.1.3; 100-4,12,10; 100-4,12,30.6; 100-4,12,30.6.11; 100-4,12,70; 100-4,12,100; 100-4,12,100.1.7; 100-4,12,100.1.8; 100-4,13,20; 100-4,13,90

AMA: 2002,Jul,2; 2000,Jan,11; 2000,Feb,11; 1995,Summer,1; 1995,Spring,1; 1993,Spring,34; 1992,Summer,1, 18; 1992,Spring,24; 1991,Winter,11

99284   Emergency department visit for the evaluation and management of a patient, which requires these three key components: a detailed history; a detailed examination; and medical decision making of moderate complexity. Counseling and/or coordination of care with other providers or agencies are provided consistent with the nature of the problem(s) and the patient's and/or family's needs. Usually, the presenting problem(s) are of high severity, and require urgent evaluation by the physician but do not pose an immediate significant threat to life or physiologic function.   [V] [80] ▣

MED: 100-1,5,70; 100-2,15,30; 100-3,70.1; 100-4,4,20.5; 100-4,4,160; 100-4,11,40.1.3; 100-4,12,10; 100-4,12,30.6; 100-4,12,30.6.11; 100-4,12,70; 100-4,12,100; 100-4,12,100.1.7; 100-4,12,100.1.8; 100-4,13,20; 100-4,13,90

AMA: 2002,Jul,2; 2000,Jan,11; 2000,Feb,11; 1995,Summer,1; 1995,Spring,1; 1993,Spring,34; 1992,Summer,1, 18; 1992,Spring,24; 1991,Winter,11

[26] Professional Component Only   [80]/[80] Assist-at-Surgery Allowed/With Documentation   Unlisted   Not Covered

[TC] Technical Component Only   MED: Pub 100/NCD References   AMA: CPT Assistant References   [1]-[9] ASC Group   ♂ Male Only   ♀ Female Only

14 — CPT Expert   CPT only © 2006 American Medical Association. All Rights Reserved. (Black Ink)   © 2006 Ingenix (Blue Ink)

99285 Emergency department visit for the evaluation and management of a patient, which requires these three key components within the constraints imposed by the urgency of the patient's clinical condition and/or mental status: a comprehensive history; a comprehensive examination; and medical decision making of high complexity. Counseling and/or coordination of care with other providers or agencies are provided consistent with the nature of the problem(s) and the patient's and/or family's needs. Usually, the presenting problem(s) are of high severity and pose an immediate significant threat to life or physiologic function. [V] [80] [C]

MED: 100-1,5,70; 100-2,15,30; 100-3,70.1; 100-4,4,20.5; 100-4,4,160; 100-4,11,40.1.3; 100-4,12,10; 100-4,12,30.6; 100-4,12,30.6.11; 100-4,12,70; 100-4,12,100; 100-4,12,100.1.7; 100-4,12,100.1.8; 100-4,13,20; 100-4,13,90

AMA: 2002,Sep,11; 2002,Jul,2; 2000,Jan,11; 2000,Feb,11; 1999,Nov,2-3; 1995,Summer,1; 1995,Spring,1; 1993,Spring,34; 1992,Spring,24; 1992,Summer,1, 18; 1991,Winter,11

OTHER EMERGENCY SERVICES

99288 Physician direction of emergency medical systems (EMS) emergency care, advanced life support [B]

MED: 100-1,5,70; 100-2,15,30; 100-4,11,40.1.3; 100-4,12,10; 100-4,12,30.6; 100-4,12,30.6.11; 100-4,12,100; 100-4,12,100.1.7; 100-4,12,100.1.8

AMA: 1992,Summer,18

PEDIATRIC CRITICAL CARE PATIENT TRANSPORT

CPT codes 99289 and 99290 are reported for face-to-face physical attendance and direct face-to-face care provided by a physician during a transport of a critically ill or critically injured pediatric patient. from one facility to another. Time begins when the physician assumes primary responsiblity for the patient. Services requiring less than 30 minutes of face-to-face time, should not be reported with 99289 or 99290. The physician should not report procedures preformed by additional transport team members. Patient must be 24 months of age or younger.

The following procedures are included in CPT codes 99289 and 99290: routine monitoring, the interpretation of cardiac output measurements (93561, 93562), chest x-rays (71010, 71015, 71020), pulse oximetry (94760, 94761, 94762), blood gases, computer stored information (99090), gastric intubation (43752, 91105), temporary transcutaneous pacing (92953), ventilation management (94002-94004, 94660, 94662), and vascular access procedures (36000, 36400, 36405, 36406, 36410, 36415, 36540, 36600). The physician should separately report any additional procedures not listed above.

CRITICAL CARE SERVICES GUIDELINES

- Critical care codes include evaluation and management of the critically ill or injured patient, requiring direct delivery of medical care.
- Care provided to a patient who is not critically ill but happens to be in a critical care unit should be identified using subsequent hospital care codes or inpatient consultation codes as appropriate.
- Critical care of less than 30 minutes should be reported using an appropriate E/M code.
- Critical care codes identify the duration of time spent by a physician on a given date, even if the time is not continuous. Code 99291 reports the first hour and is used only once per date. Code 99292 reports each additional 30 minutes of critical care per date.
- Critical care of less than 15 minutes beyond the first hour or less than 15 minutes beyond the final 30 minutes should not be reported.

99289 Critical care services delivered by a physician, face-to-face, during an interfacility transport of critically ill or critically injured pediatric patient, 24 months of age or less; first 30-74 minutes of hands on care during transport [A] [N] [80] [C]

MED: 100-1,5,70; 100-2,15,30; 100-4,11,40.1.3; 100-4,12,10; 100-4,12,30.6; 100-4,12,30.6.12; 100-4,12,100; 100-4,12,100.1.7; 100-4,12,100.1.8

+ **99290** Critical care services delivered by a physician, face-to-face, during an interfacility transport of critically ill or critically injured pediatric patient, 24 months of age or less; each additional 30 minutes (List separately in addition to code for primary service) [A] [N] [80] [C]

MED: 100-1,5,70; 100-2,15,30; 100-4,11,40.1.3; 100-4,12,10; 100-4,12,30.6; 100-4,12,30.6.12; 100-4,12,100; 100-4,12,100.1.7; 100-4,12,100.1.8

Note that 99290 is an add-on code and must be used in conjuction with 99289.

Do not report these codes for pediatric critical care transport services of less than 30 minutes duration, in these instances, report the appropriate E/M code.

CRITICAL CARE SERVICES

Critical care is not specific to a location such as an ICU or CCU. Rather it is determined by the patient's critical condition requiring this type of physician care. Therefore, routine visits to a stabilized patient in an ICU are not necessarily critical care.

Services such as endotracheal intubation (31500) and the insertion and placement of a flow directed catheter (e.g., Swan-Ganz, 93503) may be reported separately. Append modifier 25 to the critical care code to indicate a separate service was performed.

The following CPT codes are considered part of critical care services and should not be separately reported: theinterpretation of cardiac output measurements (93561, 93562), interpretation of chest x-rays (71010, 71015, 71020), pulse oximetry (94760-94762), blood gases and other information stored in computers (e.g., blood pressures, hematologic date, ECGs (99090), gastric intubation (43752 and 91105), ventilation management (94002-94004, 94660, 94662), temporary transcutaneous pacing (92953), and vascular procedures (36000, 36410, 36415, 36540, and 36600). The physicians should separately report any procedures performed that are not listed above.

99291 Critical care, evaluation and management of the critically ill or critically injured patient; first 30-74 minutes [S] [80] [C]

MED: 100-1,5,70; 100-2,15,30; 100-4,4,20.5; 100-4,4,160; 100-4,11,40.1.3; 100-4,12,10; 100-4,12,30.6; 100-4,12,30.6.12; 100-4,12,100; 100-4,12,100.1.7; 100-4,12,100.1.8

AMA: 2003,Feb,15; 2002,Jul,2; 2000,Apr,6; 1999,Nov,3-5; 1998,Dec,6; 1996,Jan,7; 1995,Summer,1; 1993,Summer,1; 1992,Summer,18

+ **99292** each additional 30 minutes (List separately in addition to code for primary service) [N] [80] [C]

MED: 100-1,5,70; 100-2,15,30; 100-4,4,20.5; 100-4,11,40.1.3; 100-4,12,10; 100-4,12,30.6; 100-4,12,30.6.12; 100-4,12,100; 100-4,12,100.1.7; 100-4,12,100.1.8

AMA: 2003,Feb,15; 2000,Dec,15; 2000,Apr,6; 1998,Dec,6; 1996,Jan,7; 1995,Summer,1; 1993,Summer,1; 1992,Summer,18

Note that 99292 is an add-on code and must be used in conjunction with 99291.

INPATIENT NEONATAL AND PEDIATRIC CRITICAL CARE SERVICES

CPT codes 99295, 99296 are used to report services provided by a physician for a critically ill baby through the first 28 days of life. Code 99295 is for the date of admission and 99296 should be reported for subsequent days. Each code may only be reported once per day per patient.

Evaluation and Management

99293 — 99305

CPT codes 99293, 99294 are used to report services provided by a physician for a critically ill infant or child from 29 days through 24 months of age. Code 99293 is for the date of admission and 99294 should be reported for subsequent days. Each code may only be reported once per day per patient. Services for critically ill or injured patients older than 24 months would be reported with codes 99291, 99292.

Report critical care services provided in the outpatient setting (e.g., emergency department or office) for neonates and pediatric patients up through 24 months of age with the Critical Care codes 99291, 99292. If the same physician provides critical care on both an inpatient and outpatient basis, report only the appropriate Neonatal or Pediatric Critical Care code 99295-99296 for all critical care services provided on that day.

The pediatric and neonatal critical care codes include all the procedures listed in the hourly critical care codes (99291, 99292) plus these procedures: umbilical venous (36510) and umbilical arterial catheters (36660), other arterial catheters (36140, 36620), central (36555) or peripheral vessel catheterization (36000), vascular access procedures (36400, 36405, 36406), vascular punctures (36420, 36600), oral or nasogastric tube placement (43752), endotracheal intubation (31500), lumbar puncture (62270), suprapubic bladder aspiration (51000), bladder catheterization (51701, 51702), management of mechanical ventilation (94002-94004) or continuous positive airway pressure (CPAP) (94660), surfactant administration (94610), intravascular fluid administration (90760-90761), transfusion of blood components (36430, 36440), invasive or non-invasive electronic monitoring of vital signs, bedside pulmonary function testing (94375), and/or monitoring or interpretation of blood gases or oxygen saturation (94760-94762). Any services not contained in this list should be reported separately.

Initial NICU critical care does not include physician standby services (99360), attendance at delivery and initial stabilization (99436), or newborn resuscitation (99440) when the physician's presence for the delivery and resuscitation is required prior to transfer of the infant to the NICU. In addition, codes for prolonged physician services (99356 and 99357) may be used if prolonged, face-to-face services are required, prior to admission to NICU.

INPATIENT PEDIATRIC CRITICAL CARE

99293   **Initial inpatient pediatric critical care, per day, for the evaluation and management of a critically ill infant or young child, 29 days through 24 months of age**   Ⓐ Ⓒ 80 ◪

   MED: 100-4,12,30.6.12; 100-4,12,100; 100-4,12,100.1.7; 100-4,12,100.1.8
   AMA: 2003,Feb,15

99294   **Subsequent inpatient pediatric critical care, per day, for the evaluation and management of a critically ill infant or young child, 29 days through 24 months of age**   Ⓐ Ⓒ 80 ◪

   MED: 100-4,12,30.6.12; 100-4,12,100; 100-4,12,100.1.7; 100-4,12,100.1.8
   AMA: 2003,Feb,15

INPATIENT NEONATAL CRITICAL CARE

99295   **Initial inpatient neonatal critical care, per day, for the evaluation and management of a critically ill neonate, 28 days of age or less**   Ⓐ Ⓒ 80 ◪

   MED: 100-1,5,70; 100-2,15,30; 100-4,11,40.1.3; 100-4,12,10; 100-4,12,30.6; 100-4,12,30.6.12; 100-4,12,100; 100-4,12,100.1.7; 100-4,12,100.1.8
   AMA: 2003,Feb,15; 2000,Dec,14; 1999,Nov,5-6; 1998,Mar,11; 1997,Nov,4-5; 1993,Summer,1

99296   **Subsequent inpatient neonatal critical care, per day, for the evaluation and management of a critically ill neonate, 28 days of age or less**   Ⓐ Ⓒ 80 ◪

   MED: 100-1,5,70; 100-2,15,30; 100-4,11,40.1.3; 100-4,12,10; 100-4,12,30.6; 100-4,12,30.6.12; 100-4,12,100; 100-4,12,100.1.7; 100-4,12,100.1.8
   AMA: 2003,Feb,15; 2000,Dec,14; 1999,Nov,5-6; 1998,Mar,11; 1997,Nov,4-5; 1993,Summer,1

CONTINUING INTENSIVE CARE SERVICES

Codes 99298-9300 are used by the physician responsible for the ongoing intensive care for low birth weight (LBW, 1500-2500 grams present body weight) newborns, very low birth weight (VLBW, less than 1500 grams present body weight) newborns or normal weight (2501-5000 grams present body weight) infants that do not meet the criteria for critical care but require intensive observation, numerous interventions, and other intensive services. The codes are reported for subsequent day(s) of care. They are reported once per calendar day, per infant and are global codes. They include the same services that would be included in codes 99293-99296.

99298   **Subsequent intensive care, per day, for the evaluation and management of the recovering very low birth weight infant (present body weight less than 1500 g)**   Ⓐ Ⓒ 80 ◪

   MED: 100-1,5,70; 100-2,15,30; 100-4,11,40.1.3; 100-4,12,10; 100-4,12,30.6; 100-4,12,30.6.12; 100-4,12,100; 100-4,12,100.1.7; 100-4,12,100.1.8
   AMA: 2000,Dec,15; 1998,Nov,2-3

99299   **Subsequent intensive care, per day, for the evaluation and management of the recovering low birth weight infant (present body weight of 1500-2500 g)**   Ⓐ Ⓒ 80 ◪

   MED: 100-4,12,30.6; 100-4,12,30.6.12; 100-4,12,100; 100-4,12,100.1.7; 100-4,12,100.1.8

99300   **Subsequent intensive care, per day, for the evaluation and management of the recovering infant (present body weight of 2501-5000 g)**   Ⓝ 80

NURSING FACILITY SERVICES

INITIAL NURSING FACILITY CARE

Two main subcategories for these codes are Initial Facility Care and Subsequent Nursing Facility Care. Both apply to either new or established patients.

Physicians are responsible for ensuring that patients receive a multi-disciplinary plan of care, provide input in to the Resident Assessment Instrument (RAI) which includes the Minimum Data Set (MDS), Resident Assessment Protocols (RAPs) and utilization guidelines.

NEW OR ESTABLISHED PATIENT

Typical times have not been established for 99304-99306.

99304   **Initial nursing facility care, per day, for the evaluation and management of a patient which requires these three key components: a detailed or comprehensive history; a detailed or comprehensive examination; and medical decision making that is straightforward or of low complexity. Counseling and/or coordination of care with other providers or agencies are provided consistent with the nature of the problem(s) and the patient's and/or family's needs. Usually, the problem(s) requiring admission are of low severity.**   Ⓑ 80

99305   **Initial nursing facility care, per day, for the evaluation and management of a patient which requires these three key components: a comprehensive history; a comprehensive examination; and medical decision making of moderate complexity. Counseling and/or coordination of care with other providers or agencies are provided consistent with the nature of the problem(s) and the patient's and/or family's needs. Usually, the problem(s) requiring admission are of moderate severity.**   Ⓑ 80

---

26 Professional Component Only   80/80 Assist-at-Surgery Allowed/With Documentation   Unlisted   Not Covered

TC Technical Component Only   MED: Pub 100/NCD References   AMA: CPT Assistant References   1-9 ASC Group   ♂ Male Only   ♀ Female Only

16 — CPT Expert   CPT only © 2006 American Medical Association. All Rights Reserved. (Black Ink)   © 2006 Ingenix (Blue Ink)

99306   Initial nursing facility care, per day, for the evaluation and management of a patient, which requires these three key components: a comprehensive history; a comprehensive examination; and medical decision making of high complexity. Counseling and/or coordination of care with other providers or agencies are provided consistent with the nature of the problem(s) and the patient's and/or family's needs. Usually, the problem(s) requiring admission are of high severity.   B 80

SUBSEQUENT NURSING FACILITY CARE

Subsequent nursing facility care codes include reviewing medical records, tests, patient condition, response to treatment and any changes in the patient's staus since the patient's last assessment.

99307   Subsequent nursing facility care, per day, for the evaluation and management of a patient, which requires at least two of these three key components: a problem focused interval history; a problem focused examination; straightforward medical decision making. Counseling and/or coordination of care with other providers or agencies are provided consistent with the nature of the problem(s) and the patient's and/or family's needs. Usually, the patient is stable, recovering, or improving.   B 80

99308   Subsequent nursing facility care, per day, for the evaluation and management of a patient, which requires at least two of these three key components: an expanded problem focused interval history; an expanded problem focused examination; medical decision making of low complexity. Counseling and/or coordination of care with other providers or agencies are provided consistent with the nature of the problem(s) and the patient's and/or family's needs. Usually, the patient is responding inadequately to therapy or has developed a minor complication.   B 80

99309   Subsequent nursing facility care, per day, for the evaluation and management of a patient, which requires at least two of these three key components: a detailed interval history; a detailed examination; medical decision making of moderate complexity. Counseling and/or coordination of care with other providers or agencies are provided consistent with the nature of the problem(s) and the patient's and/or family's needs. Usually, the patient has developed a significant complication or a significant new problem.   B 80

99310   Subsequent nursing facility care, per day, for the evaluation and management of a patient, which requires at least two of these three key components: a comprehensive interval history; a comprehensive examination; medical decision making of high complexity. Counseling and/or coordination of care with other providers or agencies are provided consistent with the nature of the problem(s) and the patient's and/or family's needs. The patient may be unstable or may have developed a significant new problem requiring immediate physician attention.   B 80

NURSING FACILITY DISCHARGE SERVICES

99315   Nursing facility discharge day management; 30 minutes or less   B 80 □

MED: 100-1,5,70; 100-2,15,30; 100-4,11,40.1.3; 100-4,12,10; 100-4,12,30.6; 100-4,12,30.6.13; 100-4,12,100; 100-4,12,100.1.7; 100-4,12,100.1.8

AMA: 2002,Nov,11; 2002,May,19; 1998,May,1; 1997,Nov,5-6

99316   more than 30 minutes   B 80 □

MED: 100-1,5,70; 100-2,15,30; 100-4,11,40.1.3; 100-4,12,10; 100-4,12,30.6; 100-4,12,30.6.13; 100-4,12,100; 100-4,12,100.1.7; 100-4,12,100.1.8

AMA: 2002,Nov,11; 2002,May,19; 1998,May,1; 1997,Nov,5-6

OTHER NURSING FACILITY SERVICES

99318   Evaluation and management of a patient involving an annual nursing facility assessment, which requires these three key components: A detailed interval history; A comprehensive examination; and Medical decision making that is of low to moderate complexity. Counseling and/or coordination of care with other providers or agencies are provided consistent with the nature of the problem(s) and the patient's and/or family's needs. Usually, the patient is stable, recovering, or improving.   B 80

DOMICILIARY, REST HOME (EG, BOARDING HOME), OR CUSTODIAL CARE SERVICES

Domiciliary, Rest Home, or Custodial Care Service codes are used to report services provided for the evaluation and management of patients in a facility that provides room and board and long-term personal assistance such as an assisted living facility. Medical services are not part of the facility's services.

NEW PATIENT

99324   Domiciliary or rest home visit for the evaluation and management of a new patient, which requires these three key components: A problem focused history; A problem focused examination; and Straightforward medical decision making. Counseling and/or coordination of care with other providers or agencies are provided consistent with the nature of the problem(s) and the patient's and/or family's needs. Usually, the presenting problem(s) are of low severity. Physicians typically spend 20 minutes with the patient and/or family or caregiver.   B 80

99325   Domiciliary or rest home visit for the evaluation and management of a new patient, which requires these three key components: An expanded problem focused history; An expanded problem focused examination; and Medical decision making of low complexity. Counseling and/or coordination of care with other providers or agencies are provided consistent with the nature of the problem(s) and the patient's and/or family's needs. Usually, the presenting problem(s) are of moderate severity. Physicians typically spend 30 minutes with the patient and/or family or caregiver.   B 80

99326   Domiciliary or rest home visit for the evaluation and management of a new patient, which requires these three key components: A detailed history; A detailed examination; and Medical decision making of moderate complexity. Counseling and/or coordination of care with other providers or agencies are provided consistent with the nature of the problem(s) and the patient's and/or family's needs. Usually, the presenting problem(s) are of moderate to high severity. Physicians typically spend 45 minutes with the patient and/or family or caregiver.   B 80

99327   Domiciliary or rest home visit for the evaluation and management of a new patient, which requires these three key components: A comprehensive history; A comprehensive examination; and Medical decision making of moderate complexity. Counseling and/or coordination of care with other providers or agencies are provided consistent with the nature of the problem(s) and the patient's and/or family's needs. Usually, the presenting problem(s) are of high severity. Physicians typically spend 60 minutes with the patient and/or family or caregiver.   B 80

99328   Domiciliary or rest home visit for the evaluation and management of a new patient, which requires these three key components: A comprehensive history; A comprehensive examination; and Medical decision making of high complexity. Counseling and/or coordination of care with other providers or agencies are provided consistent with the nature of the problem(s) and the patient's and/or family's needs. Usually, the patient is unstable or has developed a significant new problem requiring immediate physician attention. Physicians typically spend 75 minutes with the patient and/or family or caregiver.   B 80

ESTABLISHED PATIENT

99334   Domiciliary or rest home visit for the evaluation and management of an established patient, which requires at least two of these three key components: A problem focused interval history; A problem focused examination; Straightforward medical decision making. Counseling and/or coordination of care with other providers or agencies are provided consistent with the nature of the problem(s) and the patient's and/or family's needs. Usually, the presenting problem(s) are self-limited or minor. Physicians typically spend 15 minutes with the patient and/or family or caregiver.   B 80

99335   Domiciliary or rest home visit for the evaluation and management of an established patient, which requires at least two of these three key components: An expanded problem focused interval history; An expanded problem focused examination; Medical decision making of low complexity. Counseling and/or coordination of care with other providers or agencies are provided consistent with the nature of the problem(s) and the patient's and/or family's needs. Usually, the presenting problem(s) are of low to moderate severity. Physicians typically spend 25 minutes with the patient and/or family or caregiver.   B 80

99336   Domiciliary or rest home visit for the evaluation and management of an established patient, which requires at least two of these three key components: A detailed interval history; A detailed examination; Medical decision making of moderate complexity. Counseling and/or coordination of care with other providers or agencies are provided consistent with the nature of the problem(s) and the patient's and/or family's needs. Usually, the presenting problem(s) are of moderate to high severity. Physicians typically spend 40 minutes with the patient and/or family or caregiver.   B 80

99337   Domiciliary or rest home visit for the evaluation and management of an established patient, which requires at least two of these three key components: A comprehensive interval history; A comprehensive examination; Medical decision making of moderate to high complexity. Counseling and/or coordination of care with other providers or agencies are provided consistent with the nature of the problem(s) and the patient's and/or family's needs. Usually, the presenting problem(s) are of moderate to high severity. The patient may be unstable or may have developed a significant new problem requiring immediate physician attention. Physicians typically spend 60 minutes with the patient and/or family or caregiver.   B 80

DOMICILIARY, REST HOME, (E.G., ASSISTED LIVING FACILITY) OR HOME CARE PLAN OVERSIGHT SERVICES

These codes are to report care plan oversight services provided under the individual supervision of a physician to a patient in a rest home, (e.g., assisted living facility), home, or in domiciliary care.

99339   Individual physician supervision of a patient (patient not present) in home, domiciliary or rest home (eg, assisted living facility) requiring complex and multidisciplinary care modalities involving regular physician development and/or revision of care plans, review of subsequent reports of patient status, review of related laboratory and other studies, communication (including telephone calls) for purposes of assessment or care decisions with health care professional(s), family member(s), surrogate decision maker(s) (eg, legal guardian) and/or key caregiver(s) involved in patient's care, integration of new information into the medical treatment plan and/or adjustment of medical therapy, within a calendar month; 15-29 minutes   B

99340   Individual physician supervision of a patient (patient not present) in home, domiciliary or rest home (eg, assisted living facility) requiring complex and multidisciplinary care modalities involving regular physician development and/or revision of care plans, review of subsequent reports of patient status, review of related laboratory and other studies, communication (including telephone calls) for purposes of assessment or care decisions with health care professional(s), family member(s), surrogate decision maker(s) (eg, legal guardian) and/or key caregiver(s) involved in patient's care, integration of new information into the medical treatment plan and/or adjustment of medical therapy, within a calendar month; 30 minutes or more   B

HOME SERVICES

Services and care provided at the patient's home or other private residence are reported from this subcategory. While not all payers will reimburse for physician home services, it is important to document home visits and submit a claim.

26 Professional Component Only   80/80 Assist-at-Surgery Allowed/With Documentation   Unlisted   Not Covered

TC Technical Component Only   MED: Pub 100/NCD References   AMA: CPT Assistant References   1-9 ASC Group   ♂ Male Only   ♀ Female Only

18 — CPT Expert   CPT only © 2006 American Medical Association. All Rights Reserved. (Black Ink)   © 2006 Ingenix (Blue Ink)

NEW PATIENT

99341   Home visit for the evaluation and management of a new patient, which requires these three key components: A problem focused history; A problem focused examination; and Straightforward medical decision making. Counseling and/or coordination of care with other providers or agencies are provided consistent with the nature of the problem(s) and the patient's and/or family's needs. Usually, the presenting problem(s) are of low severity. Physicians typically spend 20 minutes face-to-face with the patient and/or family.   B 80

> MED: 100-1,5,70; 100-2,15,30; 100-4,11,40.1.3; 100-4,12,10; 100-4,12,30.6; 100-4,12,30.6.14; 100-4,12,30.6.15
>
> AMA: 1998,Oct,6; 1997,Nov,6-8; 1997,Jun,6; 1995,Spring,1; 1993,Spring,34; 1992,Summer,1; 1992,Spring,24; 1991,Winter,11

99342   Home visit for the evaluation and management of a new patient, which requires these three key components: An expanded problem focused history; An expanded problem focused examination; and Medical decision making of low complexity. Counseling and/or coordination of care with other providers or agencies are provided consistent with the nature of the problem(s) and the patient's and/or family's needs. Usually, the presenting problem(s) are of moderate severity. Physicians typically spend 30 minutes face-to-face with the patient and/or family.   B 80

> MED: 100-1,5,70; 100-2,15,30; 100-4,11,40.1.3; 100-4,12,10; 100-4,12,30.6; 100-4,12,30.6.14; 100-4,12,30.6.15
>
> AMA: 1998,Oct,6; 1997,Nov,6-8; 1997,Jun,6; 1995,Spring,1; 1993,Spring,34; 1992,Summer,1; 1992,Spring,24; 1991,Winter,11

99343   Home visit for the evaluation and management of a new patient, which requires these three key components: A detailed history; A detailed examination; and Medical decision making of moderate complexity. Counseling and/or coordination of care with other providers or agencies are provided consistent with the nature of the problem(s) and the patient's and/or family's needs. Usually, the presenting problem(s) are of moderate to high severity. Physicians typically spend 45 minutes face-to-face with the patient and/or family.   B 80

> MED: 100-1,5,70; 100-2,15,30; 100-4,11,40.1.3; 100-4,12,10; 100-4,12,30.6; 100-4,12,30.6.14; 100-4,12,30.6.15
>
> AMA: 1998,Oct,6; 1997,Nov,6-8; 1997,Jun,6; 1995,Spring,1; 1993,Spring,34; 1992,Summer,1; 1992,Spring,24; 1991,Winter,11

99344   Home visit for the evaluation and management of a new patient, which requires these three components: A comprehensive history; A comprehensive examination; and Medical decision making of moderate complexity. Counseling and/or coordination of care with other providers or agencies are provided consistent with the nature of the problem(s) and the patient's and/or family's needs. Usually, the presenting problem(s) are of high severity. Physicians typically spend 60 minutes face-to-face with the patient and/or family.   B 80

> MED: 100-1,5,70; 100-2,15,30; 100-4,11,40.1.3; 100-4,12,10; 100-4,12,30.6; 100-4,12,30.6.14; 100-4,12,30.6.15
>
> AMA: 1998,Oct,6; 1997,Nov,6-8

99345   Home visit for the evaluation and management of a new patient, which requires these three key components: A comprehensive history; A comprehensive examination; and Medical decision making of high complexity. Counseling and/or coordination of care with other providers or agencies are provided consistent with the nature of the problem(s) and the patient's and/or family's needs. Usually, the patient is unstable or has developed a significant new problem requiring immediate physician attention. Physicians typically spend 75 minutes face-to-face with the patient and/or family.   B 80

> MED: 100-1,5,70; 100-2,15,30; 100-4,11,40.1.3; 100-4,12,10; 100-4,12,30.6; 100-4,12,30.6.14; 100-4,12,30.6.15
>
> AMA: 1998,Oct,6; 1997,Nov,6-8

ESTABLISHED PATIENT

99347   Home visit for the evaluation and management of an established patient, which requires at least two of these three key components: A problem focused interval history; A problem focused examination; Straightforward medical decision making. Counseling and/or coordination of care with other providers or agencies are provided consistent with the nature of the problem(s) and the patient's and/or family's needs. Usually, the presenting problem(s) are self limited or minor. Physicians typically spend 15 minutes face-to-face with the patient and/or family.   B 80

> MED: 100-1,5,70; 100-2,15,30; 100-4,11,40.1.3; 100-4,12,10; 100-4,12,30.6; 100-4,12,30.6.14; 100-4,12,30.6.15
>
> AMA: 1998,Oct,6; 1997,Nov,6-8

99348   Home visit for the evaluation and management of an established patient, which requires at least two of these three key components: An expanded problem focused interval history; An expanded problem focused examination; Medical decision making of low complexity. Counseling and/or coordination of care with other providers or agencies are provided consistent with the nature of the problem(s) and the patient's and/or family's needs. Usually, the presenting problem(s) are of low to moderate severity. Physicians typically spend 25 minutes face-to-face with the patient and/or family.   B 80

> MED: 100-1,5,70; 100-2,15,30; 100-4,11,40.1.3; 100-4,12,10; 100-4,12,30.6; 100-4,12,30.6.14; 100-4,12,30.6.15
>
> AMA: 1998,Oct,6; 1997,Nov,6-8

99349   Home visit for the evaluation and management of an established patient, which requires at least two of these three key components: A detailed interval history; A detailed examination; Medical decision making of moderate complexity. Counseling and/or coordination of care with other providers or agencies are provided consistent with the nature of the problem(s) and the patient's and/or family's needs. Usually, the presenting problem(s) are moderate to high severity. Physicians typically spend 40 minutes face-to-face with the patient and/or family.   B 80

> MED: 100-1,5,70; 100-2,15,30; 100-4,11,40.1.3; 100-4,12,10; 100-4,12,30.6; 100-4,12,30.6.14; 100-4,12,30.6.15
>
> AMA: 1998,Oct,6; 1997,Nov,6-8

99350　　Home visit for the evaluation and management of an established patient, which requires at least two of these three key components: A comprehensive interval history; A comprehensive examination; Medical decision making of moderate to high complexity. Counseling and/or coordination of care with other providers or agencies are provided consistent with the nature of the problem(s) and the patient's and/or family's needs. Usually, the presenting problem(s) are of moderate to high severity. The patient may be unstable or may have developed a significant new problem requiring immediate physician attention. Physicians typically spend 60 minutes face-to-face with the patient and/or family.　　B 80 ◻

MED: 100-1,5,70; 100-2,15,30; 100-4,11,40.1.3; 100-4,12,10; 100-4,12,30.6; 100-4,12,30.6.14; 100-4,12,30.6.15

AMA: 1998,Oct,6; 1997,Nov,6-8

PROLONGED SERVICES

PROLONGED PHYSICIAN SERVICE WITH DIRECT (FACE-TO-FACE) PATIENT CONTACT

These codes report services involving direct patient contact beyond the usual service, with separate codes for office or outpatient encounters (99354 and 99355) and for inpatient encounters (99356 and 99357). Prolonged physician services are add-on services and should be listed separately in addition to the E/M service. The codes report the total duration of face-to-face time spent by the physician on a given date, even if the time is not continuous.

Code 99354 or 99356 reports the first hour of prolonged service on a given date, depending on the place of service, with 99355 or 99357 used to report each additional 30 minutes for that date. Services lasting less than 30 minutes are not reportable in this category, and the services must extend 15 minutes or more into the next time period to be reportable. For example, services lasting one hour and 12 minutes are reported by 99354 or 99356 alone. Services lasting one hour and 17 minutes are reported by the code for the first hour plus the code for an additional 30 minutes.

+　**99354**　　Prolonged physician service in the office or other outpatient setting requiring direct (face-to-face) patient contact beyond the usual service (eg, prolonged care and treatment of an acute asthmatic patient in an outpatient setting); first hour (List separately in addition to code for office or other outpatient Evaluation and Management service)　　N 80 ◻

MED: 100-1,5,70; 100-2,15,30; 100-4,11,40.1.3; 100-4,12,10; 100-4,12,30.6; 100-4,12,30.6.15; 100-4,12,100; 100-4,12,100.1.7; 100-4,12,100.1.8

AMA: 2000,Sep,1; 1994,Spring,30, 32

Note that 99354 is an add-on code and must be used in conjunction with 99201-99215, 99241-99245, and 99301-99350.

+　**99355**　　each additional 30 minutes (List separately in addition to code for prolonged physician service)　　N 80 ◻

MED: 100-1,5,70; 100-2,15,30; 100-4,11,40.1.3; 100-4,12,10; 100-4,12,30.6; 100-4,12,30.6.15; 100-4,12,100; 100-4,12,100.1.7; 100-4,12,100.1.8

AMA: 2000,Sep,1; 1994,Spring,30, 32

Note that 99355 is an add-on code and must be used in conjunction with 99354.

+　**99356**　　Prolonged physician service in the inpatient setting, requiring direct (face-to-face) patient contact beyond the usual service (eg, maternal fetal monitoring for high risk delivery or other physiological monitoring, prolonged care of an acutely ill inpatient); first hour (List separately in addition to code for inpatient Evaluation and Management service)　　C 80 ◻

MED: 100-1,5,70; 100-2,15,30; 100-4,11,40.1.3; 100-4,12,10; 100-4,12,30.6; 100-4,12,30.6.15; 100-4,12,100; 100-4,12,100.1.7; 100-4,12,100.1.8

AMA: 1994,Spring,30, 32

Note that 99356 is an add-on code and must be used in conjunction with 99221-99233, 99251-99255.

+　**99357**　　each additional 30 minutes (List separately in addition to code for prolonged physician service)　　C 80 ◻

MED: 100-1,5,70; 100-2,15,30; 100-4,11,40.1.3; 100-4,12,10; 100-4,12,30.6; 100-4,12,30.6.15; 100-4,12,100; 100-4,12,100.1.7; 100-4,12,100.1.8

Note that 99357 is an add-on code and must be used in conjunction with 99356.

PROLONGED PHYSICIAN SERVICE WITHOUT DIRECT (FACE-TO-FACE) PATIENT CONTACT

These prolonged physician services without direct patient contact are used before and/or after face-to-face patient care and may include review of extensive records and tests, and communication (other than telephone calls, 99371-99373) with other professionals and/or the patient and family. These are beyond the usual services and include both inpatient and outpatient settings. Report these services in addition to other services provided, including any level of E/M service.

Use 99358 to report the first hour and 99359 for each additional 30 minutes. All aspects of time reporting are the same as explained above for direct patient contact services.

+　**99358**　　Prolonged evaluation and management service before and/or after direct (face-to-face) patient care (eg, review of extensive records and tests, communication with other professionals and/or the patient/family); first hour (List separately in addition to code(s) for other physician service(s) and/or inpatient or outpatient Evaluation and Management service)　　N

MED: 100-1,5,70; 100-2,15,30; 100-4,11,40.1.3; 100-4,12,10; 100-4,12,30.6; 100-4,12,30.6.15; 100-4,12,100; 100-4,12,100.1.7; 100-4,12,100.1.8

AMA: 1998,Nov,3; 1994,Spring,32

Note that 99358 is an add-on code and must be used in conjunction with other physician services, including E/M services at any level.

If telephone calls need to be reported, consult CPT codes 99371-99373.

+　**99359**　　each additional 30 minutes (List separately in addition to code for prolonged physician service)　　N

MED: 100-1,5,70; 100-2,15,30; 100-4,11,40.1.3; 100-4,12,10; 100-4,12,30.6; 100-4,12,30.6.15; 100-4,12,100; 100-4,12,100.1.7; 100-4,12,100.1.8

Note that 99359 is an add-on code and must be used in conjunction with 99358.

PHYSICIAN STANDBY SERVICES

Report code 99360 for physician standby services requested by another physician. The standby physician has no direct patient contact. The standby physician may not provide services to other patients or be proctoring another physician for the time to be reportable. Also, if the standby physician ultimately provides services subject to a surgical package, the standby is not separately reportable.

This code reports cumulative standby time by date of service. Less than 30 minutes is not reportable and a full 30 minutes must be spent for each unit of service

26 Professional Component Only　　　　80/80 Assist-at-Surgery Allowed/With Documentation　　Unlisted　　Not Covered

TC Technical Component Only　　MED: Pub 100/NCD References　　AMA: CPT Assistant References　　1-9 ASC Group　　♂ Male Only　　♀ Female Only

20 — CPT Expert　　　　CPT only © 2006 American Medical Association. All Rights Reserved. (Black Ink)　　　　© 2006 Ingenix (Blue Ink)

reported. For example, 25 minutes is not reportable and 50 minutes is reported as one unit (99360 x 1).

99360   **Physician standby service, requiring prolonged physician attendance, each 30 minutes (eg, operative standby, standby for frozen section, for cesarean/high risk delivery, for monitoring EEG)** B ⬚

> MED: 100-1,5,70; 100-1,5,90.2; 100-2,15,30; 100-2,15,80; 100-2,15,80.1; 100-4,11,40.1.3; 100-4,12,10; 100-4,12,30.6; 100-4,12,30.6.15; 100-4,16,10; 100-4,16,10.1; 100-4,16,110.4
> AMA: 1997,Nov,8; 1997,Aug,18; 1997,Apr,10; 1994,Spring,32
> To report hospital mandated on-call services, consult CPT codes 99026-99027.
>
> Note that 99360 may be reported in addition to 99431 or 99440 as appropriate. However, 99360 cannot be reported in addition to 99436.

CASE MANAGEMENT SERVICES

Physician case management is a process of involving direct patient care as well as coordinating and controlling access to the patient or initiating and/or supervising other necessary health care services. Case management services include team conferences (99361-99362) and telephone calls (99371-99373).

TEAM CONFERENCES

99361   **Medical conference by a physician with interdisciplinary team of health professionals or representatives of community agencies to coordinate activities of patient care (patient not present); approximately 30 minutes** N

> MED: 100-1,5,70; 100-2,15,30; 100-4,11,40.1.3; 100-4,12,10; 100-4,12,30.6; 100-4,12,30.6.16

99362   **approximately 60 minutes** N

> MED: 100-1,5,70; 100-2,15,30; 100-4,11,40.1.3; 100-4,12,10; 100-4,12,30.6; 100-4,12,30.6.16

ANTICOAGULANT MANAGEMENT

The services in this category are used to report the management of warfarin therapy. This includes the ordering, review, and interpretation of International Normalized Ratio (INR) testing, providing feedback to the patient, and adjusting the medication if necessary. Do not include the services described by these codes when determining the evaluation and management (E/M) code or care plan oversight code. The codes should not be reported in addition to 99371-99373, 0074T when the services are provided online or on the phone. Append modifier 25 to the appropriate E/M service. This service is provided as an outpatient only. If the service is initiated or continued in the inpatient or observation setting, a new period begins after discharge and should be reported with 99364. Codes 99363-99364 cannot be reported with 99217-99239, 99291-99300, 99304-99318 or other code(s) for physician management of INR testing for a patient with a mechanical heart valve. Do not report these codes for less than 60 continuous days of services. Do not report 99363 or 99364 if the specified minmum number of services are not performed.

● 99363   **Anticoagulant management for an outpatient taking warfarin, physician review and interpretation of International Normalized Ratio (INR) testing, patient instructions, dosage adjustment (as needed), and ordering of additional tests; initial 90 days of therapy (must include a minimum of 8 INR measurements)** E

● 99364   **each subsequent 90 days of therapy (must include a minimum of 3 INR measurements)** E

TELEPHONE CALLS

99371   **Telephone call by a physician to patient or for consultation or medical management or for coordinating medical management with other health care professionals (eg, nurses, therapists, social workers, nutritionists, physicians, pharmacists); simple or brief (eg, to report on tests and/or laboratory results, to clarify or alter previous instructions, to integrate new information from other health professionals into the medical treatment plan, or to adjust therapy)** B

> MED: 100-1,5,70; 100-2,15,30; 100-4,11,40.1.3; 100-4,12,10; 100-4,12,30.6; 100-4,12,30.6.16; 100-4,12,70; 100-4,13,20; 100-4,13,90
> AMA: 2000,May,11

99372   **intermediate (eg, to provide advice to an established patient on a new problem, to initiate therapy that can be handled by telephone, to discuss test results in detail, to coordinate medical management of a new problem in an established patient, to discuss and evaluate new information and details, or to initiate new plan of care)** B

> MED: 100-1,5,70; 100-2,15,30; 100-4,11,40.1.3; 100-4,12,10; 100-4,12,30.6; 100-4,12,30.6.16; 100-4,12,70; 100-4,13,20; 100-4,13,90
> AMA: 2000,May,11

99373   **complex or lengthy (eg, lengthy counseling session with anxious or distraught patient, detailed or prolonged discussion with family members regarding seriously ill patient, lengthy communication necessary to coordinate complex services of several different health professionals working on different aspects of the total patient care plan)** B

> MED: 100-1,5,70; 100-2,15,30; 100-4,11,40.1.3; 100-4,12,10; 100-4,12,30.6; 100-4,12,30.6.16; 100-4,12,70; 100-4,13,20; 100-4,13,90
> AMA: 2000,May,11

CARE PLAN OVERSIGHT SERVICES

Codes 99374-99380 report the services of a physician providing ongoing review and revision of a patient's care plan involving complex or multidisciplinary care modalities. Care plan oversight services are reported separately from any necessary office/outpatient, hospital, home, nursing facility, or domiciliary services. Only one physician may report these codes per patient per 30-day period. Also, low intensity and infrequent supervision services are not reported separately.

99374   **Physician supervision of a patient under care of home health agency (patient not present) in home, domiciliary or equivalent environment (eg, Alzheimer's facility) requiring complex and multidisciplinary care modalities involving regular physician development and/or revision of care plans, review of subsequent reports of patient status, review of related laboratory and other studies, communication (including telephone calls) for purposes of assessment or care decisions with health care professional(s), family member(s), surrogate decision maker(s) (eg, legal guardian) and/or key caregiver(s) involved in patient's care, integration of new information into the medical treatment plan and/or adjustment of medical therapy, within a calendar month; 15-29 minutes** B

> MED: 100-1,5,70; 100-2,15,30; 100-4,11,40.1.3; 100-4,12,10; 100-4,12,30.6
> AMA: 1997,Nov,8-9; 1994,Summer,9

99375   **30 minutes or more**   E

MED: 100-1,5,70; 100-2,15,30; 100-4,11,40.1.3; 100-4,12,10; 100-4,12,30.6

AMA: 1997,Nov,8-9; 1994,Summer,9

99377   **Physician supervision of a hospice patient (patient not present) requiring complex and multidisciplinary care modalities involving regular physician development and/or revision of care plans, review of subsequent reports of patient status, review of related laboratory and other studies, communication (including telephone calls) for purposes of assessment or care decisions with health care professional(s), family member(s), surrogate decision maker(s) (eg, legal guardian) and/or key caregiver(s) involved in patient's care, integration of new information into the medical treatment plan and/or adjustment of medical therapy, within a calendar month; 15-29 minutes**   B

MED: 100-1,5,70; 100-2,15,30; 100-4,11,10; 100-4,11,40.1.3; 100-4,12,10; 100-4,12,30.6

AMA: 1997,Nov,8-9

99378   **30 minutes or more**   E

MED: 100-1,5,70; 100-2,15,30; 100-4,11,10; 100-4,11,40.1.3; 100-4,12,10; 100-4,12,30.6

AMA: 1997,Nov,8-9

99379   **Physician supervision of a nursing facility patient (patient not present) requiring complex and multidisciplinary care modalities involving regular physician development and/or revision of care plans, review of subsequent reports of patient status, review of related laboratory and other studies, communication (including telephone calls) for purposes of assessment or care decisions with health care professional(s), family member(s), surrogate decision maker(s) (eg, legal guardian) and/or key caregiver(s) involved in patient's care, integration of new information into the medical treatment plan and/or adjustment of medical therapy, within a calendar month; 15-29 minutes**   B

MED: 100-1,5,70; 100-2,15,30; 100-4,11,40.1.3; 100-4,12,10; 100-4,12,30.6

99380   **30 minutes or more**   B

MED: 100-1,5,70; 100-2,15,30; 100-4,11,40.1.3; 100-4,12,10; 100-4,12,30.6

AMA: 1997,Nov,8-9

PREVENTIVE MEDICINE SERVICES

Preventive medicine codes are used to report periodic preventive medicine evaluation and management of infants, children, adolescents, and adults. Examples of services reported with these codes include well-child exams, annual gynecologic exams, and other annual or periodic exams specifically focused on promoting health and preventing illness.

Preventive medicine evaluation and management services can be reported with problem-oriented evaluation and management services (99201-99215) if the abnormality encountered or the pre-existing condition addressed during the preventive medicine exam requires significant additional work. Report with modifier 25 to indicate that a separately identifiable evaluation and management service was provided.

Codes 99381-99397 include counseling, anticipatory guidance, and risk factor reduction provided at the time of the preventive medicine service. Use 99401-99429

only when reporting counseling and risk factor reduction provided at a separate encounter. Report all ancillary lab, x-ray, and other procedures additionally.

NEW PATIENT

99381   **Initial comprehensive preventive medicine evaluation and management of an individual including an age and gender appropriate history, examination, counseling/anticipatory guidance/risk factor reduction interventions, and the ordering of appropriate immunization(s), laboratory/diagnostic procedures, new patient; infant (age younger than 1 year)**   A E

MED: 100-1,5,70; 100-2,15,30; 100-2,16,90; 100-4,11,40.1.3; 100-4,12,10; 100-4,12,30.6; 100-4,12,30.6.2

AMA: 2002,May,1; 1998,Nov,3-4; 1998,Jul,9; 1997,Aug,1; 1995,Spring,1; 1993,Spring,14, 34; 1992,Summer,1; 1992,Spring,24; 1991,Winter,11

If counseling/anticipatory guidance/risk factor reduction interventions are provided at an encounter separate from the preventive medicine examination, consult CPT codes 99401-99412.

99382   **early childhood (age 1 through 4 years)**   A E

MED: 100-1,5,70; 100-2,15,30; 100-2,16,90; 100-4,11,40.1.3; 100-4,12,10; 100-4,12,30.6; 100-4,12,30.6.2

AMA: 2002,May,1; 1998,Nov,3-4; 1998,Jul,9; 1997,Aug,1; 1995,Spring,1; 1993,Spring,14, 34; 1992,Summer,1; 1992,Spring,24; 1991,Winter,11

99383   **late childhood (age 5 through 11 years)**   A E

MED: 100-1,5,70; 100-2,15,30; 100-2,16,90; 100-4,11,40.1.3; 100-4,12,10; 100-4,12,30.6; 100-4,12,30.6.2

AMA: 2002,May,1; 1998,Nov,3-4; 1998,Jul,9; 1997,Aug,1; 1995,Spring,1; 1993,Spring,14, 34; 1992,Summer,1; 1992,Spring,24; 1991,Winter,11

99384   **adolescent (age 12 through 17 years)**   A E

MED: 100-1,5,70; 100-2,15,30; 100-2,16,90; 100-4,11,40.1.3; 100-4,12,10; 100-4,12,30.6; 100-4,12,30.6.2

AMA: 2002,May,1; 1998,Nov,3-4; 1998,Jul,9; 1997,Aug,1; 1995,Spring,1; 1993,Spring,14, 34; 1992,Summer,1; 1992,Spring,24; 1991,Winter,11

99385   **18-39 years**   A E

MED: 100-1,5,70; 100-2,15,30; 100-2,16,90; 100-4,11,40.1.3; 100-4,12,10; 100-4,12,30.6; 100-4,12,30.6.2

AMA: 2002,May,1; 1998,Nov,3-4; 1998,Jul,9; 1997,Aug,1; 1995,Spring,1; 1993,Spring,14, 34; 1992,Summer,1; 1992,Spring,24; 1991,Winter,11

99386   **40-64 years**   A E

MED: 100-1,5,70; 100-2,15,30; 100-2,16,90; 100-4,11,40.1.3; 100-4,12,10; 100-4,12,30.6; 100-4,12,30.6.2

AMA: 2002,May,1; 1998,Nov,3-4; 1998,Jul,9; 1997,Aug,1; 1995,Spring,1; 1993,Spring,14, 34; 1992,Summer,1; 1992,Spring,24; 1991,Winter,11

99387   **65 years and over**   A E

MED: 100-1,5,70; 100-2,15,30; 100-2,16,90; 100-4,11,40.1.3; 100-4,12,10; 100-4,12,30.6; 100-4,12,30.6.2

AMA: 2002,May,1; 1998,Nov,3-4; 1998,Jul,9; 1997,Aug,1; 1995,Spring,1; 1993,Spring,14, 34; 1992,Summer,1; 1992,Spring,24; 1991,Winter,11

26 Professional Component Only   80/80 Assist-at-Surgery Allowed/With Documentation   Unlisted   Not Covered

TC Technical Component Only   MED: Pub 100/NCD References   AMA: CPT Assistant References   1 - 9 ASC Group   ♂ Male Only   ♀ Female Only

22 — CPT Expert   CPT only © 2006 American Medical Association. All Rights Reserved. *(Black Ink)*   © 2006 Ingenix *(Blue Ink)*

ESTABLISHED PATIENT

99391 Periodic comprehensive preventive medicine reevaluation and management of an individual including an age and gender appropriate history, examination, counseling/anticipatory guidance/risk factor reduction interventions, and the ordering of appropriate immunization(s), laboratory/diagnostic procedures, established patient; infant (age younger than 1 year) Ⓐ Ⓔ

MED: 100-1,5,70; 100-2,15,30; 100-2,16,90; 100-4,11,40.1.3; 100-4,12,10; 100-4,12,30.6; 100-4,12,30.6.2

AMA: 2002,May,1; 1998,Nov,3-4; 1998,Jul,9; 1997,Aug,1; 1995,Spring,1; 1993,Spring,14, 34; 1992,Summer,1; 1992,Spring,24; 1991,Winter,11

99392 early childhood (age 1 through 4 years) Ⓐ Ⓔ

MED: 100-1,5,70; 100-2,15,30; 100-2,16,90; 100-4,11,40.1.3; 100-4,12,10; 100-4,12,30.6; 100-4,12,30.6.2

AMA: 2002,May,1; 1998,Nov,3-4; 1998,Jul,9; 1997,Aug,1; 1995,Spring,1; 1993,Spring,14, 34; 1992,Summer,1; 1992,Spring,24; 1991,Winter,11

99393 late childhood (age 5 through 11 years) Ⓐ Ⓔ

MED: 100-1,5,70; 100-2,15,30; 100-2,16,90; 100-4,11,40.1.3; 100-4,12,10; 100-4,12,30.6; 100-4,12,30.6.2

AMA: 2002,May,1; 1998,Nov,3-4; 1998,Jul,9; 1997,Aug,1; 1995,Spring,1; 1993,Spring,14, 34; 1992,Summer,1; 1992,Spring,24; 1991,Winter,11

99394 adolescent (age 12 through 17 years) Ⓐ Ⓔ

MED: 100-1,5,70; 100-2,15,30; 100-2,16,90; 100-4,11,40.1.3; 100-4,12,10; 100-4,12,30.6; 100-4,12,30.6.2

AMA: 2002,May,1; 1998,Nov,3-4; 1998,Jul,9; 1997,Aug,1; 1995,Spring,1; 1993,Spring,14, 34; 1992,Summer,1; 1992,Spring,24; 1991,Winter,11

99395 18-39 years Ⓐ Ⓔ

MED: 100-1,5,70; 100-2,15,30; 100-2,16,90; 100-4,11,40.1.3; 100-4,12,10; 100-4,12,30.6; 100-4,12,30.6.2

AMA: 2002,May,1; 1998,Nov,3-4; 1998,Jul,9; 1997,Aug,1; 1995,Spring,1; 1993,Spring,14, 34; 1992,Summer,1; 1992,Spring,24; 1991,Winter,11

99396 40-64 years Ⓐ Ⓔ

MED: 100-1,5,70; 100-2,15,30; 100-2,16,90; 100-4,11,40.1.3; 100-4,12,10; 100-4,12,30.6; 100-4,12,30.6.2

AMA: 2002,May,1; 1998,Nov,3-4; 1998,Jul,9; 1997,Aug,1; 1995,Spring,1; 1993,Spring,14, 34; 1992,Summer,1; 1992,Spring,24; 1991,Winter,11

99397 65 years and over Ⓐ Ⓔ

MED: 100-1,5,70; 100-2,15,30; 100-2,16,90; 100-4,11,40.1.3; 100-4,12,10; 100-4,12,30.6; 100-4,12,30.6.2

AMA: 2002,May,1; 1998,Nov,3-4; 1998,Jul,9; 1997,Aug,1; 1995,Spring,1; 1993,Spring,14, 34; 1992,Summer,1; 1992,Spring,24; 1991,Winter,11

COUNSELING AND/OR RISK FACTOR REDUCTION INTERVENTION

NEW OR ESTABLISHED PATIENT

Counseling and/or risk factor reduction intervention codes are used to report services provided at a separate encounter to promote health and prevent illness or injury. The services provided during the encounter will vary and should include issues such as family problems, diet and exercise, substance abuse, sexual practices, injury prevention, dental health, and diagnostic and laboratory tests that are available for review at the time of the visit. Report these codes for patients who do not have symptoms or a defined illness. Report the appropriate evaluation and management codes such as office, hospital, consultation for counseling patients with an illness or symptoms. For counseling of groups of patients with symptoms or defined illness, consult 99078.

PREVENTIVE MEDICINE, INDIVIDUAL COUNSELING

99401 Preventive medicine counseling and/or risk factor reduction intervention(s) provided to an individual (separate procedure); approximately 15 minutes Ⓔ

MED: 100-1,5,70; 100-2,15,30; 100-2,16,90; 100-4,11,40.1.3; 100-4,12,10; 100-4,12,30.6

AMA: 1998,Jan,12; 1997,Aug,1

99402 approximately 30 minutes Ⓔ

MED: 100-1,5,70; 100-2,15,30; 100-2,16,90; 100-4,11,40.1.3; 100-4,12,10; 100-4,12,30.6

AMA: 1997,Aug,1

99403 approximately 45 minutes Ⓔ

MED: 100-1,5,70; 100-2,15,30; 100-2,16,90; 100-4,11,40.1.3; 100-4,12,10; 100-4,12,30.6

AMA: 1997,Aug,1

99404 approximately 60 minutes Ⓔ

MED: 100-1,5,70; 100-2,15,30; 100-2,16,90; 100-4,11,40.1.3; 100-4,12,10; 100-4,12,30.6

AMA: 1997,Aug,1

PREVENTIVE MEDICINE, GROUP COUNSELING

99411 Preventive medicine counseling and/or risk factor reduction intervention(s) provided to individuals in a group setting (separate procedure); approximately 30 minutes Ⓔ

MED: 100-1,5,70; 100-2,15,30; 100-2,16,90; 100-4,11,40.1.3; 100-4,12,10; 100-4,12,30.6

AMA: 1997,Aug,1

99412 approximately 60 minutes Ⓔ

MED: 100-1,5,70; 100-2,15,30; 100-2,16,90; 100-4,11,40.1.3; 100-4,12,10; 100-4,12,30.6

AMA: 1998,Jan,12; 1997,Aug,1

OTHER PREVENTIVE MEDICINE SERVICES

99420 Administration and interpretation of health risk assessment instrument (eg, health hazard appraisal) Ⓔ

MED: 100-1,5,70; 100-2,15,30; 100-2,16,90; 100-4,11,40.1.3; 100-4,12,10; 100-4,12,30.6

99429 Unlisted preventive medicine service Ⓔ

MED: 100-1,5,70; 100-2,15,30; 100-2,16,90; 100-4,11,40.1.3; 100-4,12,10; 100-4,12,30.6

NEWBORN CARE

Codes 99431-99440 describe care provided to normal or high-risk newborns in several different settings. The codes identify specific locations, such as the hospital or birthing room, or other than hospital or birthing room.

Discharge services provided to newborns admitted and discharged on the same date should be reported with 99435. Discharge services to newborns discharged on a date subsequent to the admission date should be reported with 99238-99239.

99431 History and examination of the normal newborn infant, initiation of diagnostic and treatment programs and preparation of hospital records. (This code should also be used for birthing room deliveries.) Ⓐ Ⓥ 80 🄲

MED: 100-1,5,70; 100-2,15,30; 100-4,11,40.1.3; 100-4,12,10; 100-4,12,30.6

AMA: 1997,Apr,10

99432 Normal newborn care in other than hospital or birthing room setting, including physical examination of baby and conference(s) with parent(s) Ⓐ Ⓝ 80 🄲

MED: 100-1,5,70; 100-2,15,30; 100-4,11,40.1.3; 100-4,12,10; 100-4,12,30.6

AMA: 1999,May,11

99433 Subsequent hospital care, for the evaluation and management of a normal newborn, per day Ⓐ Ⓒ 80 🄲

Evaluation and Management

99435 — 99499

99435 History and examination of the normal newborn infant, including the preparation of medical records. (This code should only be used for newborns assessed and discharged from the hospital or birthing room on the same date.) [A][B][80][↩]

MED: 100-1,5,70; 100-2,15,30; 100-4,11,40.1.3; 100-4,12,10; 100-4,12,30.6

99436 Attendance at delivery (when requested by delivering physician) and initial stabilization of newborn [A][N][80][↩]

MED: 100-1,5,70; 100-2,15,30; 100-4,11,40.1.3; 100-4,12,10; 100-4,12,30.6
AMA: 1997,Nov,9-10
Note that this procedure may be reported in addition to 99431. However, this procedure cannot be reported in addition to 99440.

99440 Newborn resuscitation: provision of positive pressure ventilation and/or chest compressions in the presence of acute inadequate ventilation and/or cardiac output [A][S][80][↩]

MED: 100-1,5,70; 100-2,15,30; 100-4,4,20.5; 100-4,11,40.1.3; 100-4,12,10; 100-4,12,30.6
AMA: 1996,Mar,10; 1993,Summer,1

SPECIAL EVALUATION AND MANAGEMENT SERVICES

This group of codes (99450-99456) covers any purely evaluative services provided by a physician when no active management of the patient's problem is undertaken during the encounter.

Use these codes to report evaluations for life or disability insurance eligibility certificates and work-related medical disability. These services can be performed in the office or other setting, and no distinction is made between new or established patient.

These codes should not be used to indicate any active management of problems or conditions. If other E/M services and/or procedures are performed on the same date, report them with the appropriate E/M code in addition to the special evaluation code.

Code 99450 is a basic life or disability examination that includes a medical history; height, weight, and blood pressure measurement; collecting blood and urine specimens; and filling out the necessary forms and reports.

Codes 99455 and 99456 are used for work-related or medical disability. They include history, exam, formulation of a diagnosis, assessment of disability, impairment and capabilities, development of future medical treatment plans, and completion of necessary forms and reports. Use 99455 for the treating physician and 99456 for other than the treating physician.

BASIC LIFE AND/OR DISABILITY EVALUATION SERVICES

99450 Basic life and/or disability examination that includes: Measurement of height, weight and blood pressure; Completion of a medical history following a life insurance pro forma; Collection of blood sample and/or urinalysis complying with "chain of custody" protocols; and Completion of necessary documentation/certificates. [E]

MED: 100-1,5,70; 100-2,15,30; 100-4,11,40.1.3; 100-4,12,10; 100-4,12,30.6
AMA: 1995,Summer,14

WORK RELATED OR MEDICAL DISABILITY EVALUATION SERVICES

99455 Work related or medical disability examination by the treating physician that includes: Completion of a medical history commensurate with the patient's condition; Performance of an examination commensurate with the patient's condition; Formulation of a diagnosis, assessment of capabilities and stability, and calculation of impairment; Development of future medical treatment plan; and Completion of necessary documentation/certificates and report. [B][80][↩]

MED: 100-1,5,70; 100-2,15,30; 100-4,11,40.1.3; 100-4,12,10; 100-4,12,30.6
AMA: 1995,Summer,14
When completing workers' compensation forms, do not report CPT code 99080 with 99455.

99456 Work related or medical disability examination by other than the treating physician that includes: Completion of a medical history commensurate with the patient's condition; Performance of an examination commensurate with the patient's condition; Formulation of a diagnosis, assessment of capabilities and stability, and calculation of impairment; Development of future medical treatment plan; and Completion of necessary documentation/certificates and report. [B][80][↩]

MED: 100-1,5,70; 100-2,15,30; 100-4,11,40.1.3; 100-4,12,10; 100-4,12,30.6
AMA: 1995,Summer,14
When completing Workman's Compensation forms, do not report CPT code 99080 with 99456.

OTHER EVALUATION AND MANAGEMENT SERVICES

Code 99499 is an unlisted code to report other E/M services not specifically defined in the CPT manual.

99499 Unlisted evaluation and management service [B][80]

MED: 100-4,12,30.6
AMA: 1996,Apr,10

---

[26] Professional Component Only [80]/[80] Assist-at-Surgery Allowed/With Documentation Unlisted Not Covered

[TC] Technical Component Only **MED:** Pub 100/NCD References **AMA:** CPT Assistant References [1]-[9] ASC Group ♂ Male Only ♀ Female Only

24 — CPT Expert CPT only © 2006 American Medical Association. All Rights Reserved. *(Black Ink)* © 2006 Ingenix *(Blue Ink)*

Anesthesia

CODING INFORMATION

Two organizations are responsible for developing anesthesia codes and guidelines: the American Medical Association (AMA) and the American Society of Anesthesiologists (ASA). The AMA includes a section on anesthesia codes (00100–01999) in the CPT book immediately following the evaluation and management (E/M) section. In addition, the CPT book includes four codes (99100–99140) to report qualifying circumstances for anesthesia. Although categorized as medicine codes, the four codes can be found in the anesthesia section as part of the guidelines, as well as in the medicine section. The ASA publishes a Relative Value Guide (RVG) that contains codes from the anesthesia section of the CPT book but also includes 1) codes to supplement those in the CPT anesthesia section and 2) codes from other sections of the CPT book for services frequently provided by anesthesiologists.

The CPT book and ASA guidelines are similar. Guidelines are as follows:

1. Both specify that reporting of anesthesia services is appropriate when provided by or under the medical supervision of a physician. The ASA further specifies that a physician anesthesiologist should supervise anesthesia services.

2. According to both sets of guidelines, anesthesia services include but are not limited to general, regional, supplementation of local anesthesia, and other supportive services required to afford the patient optimal anesthesia care. The ASA includes monitored anesthesia care in the service and also states that you report any professional anesthesia services as if an anesthetic was administered.

3. The ASA publication is a relative value guide. A relative value is a numeric ranking assigned to a procedure in relation to other procedures in terms of work and cost. Therefore, in addition to codes and descriptions, the ASA relative value guide provides information on the value of each anesthesia service. The ASA relative value guide is not a fee schedule, but only a guide intended to assist physicians in developing consistent and equitable fees for their services.

ORGANIZATION OF ANESTHESIA CODES

THE CPT BOOK

The anesthesia section of the CPT book is organized into 15 anatomical sites followed by four additional categories for radiological and other procedures. Codes are organized by type of procedure (open, closed, endoscopic, etc.), and each code relates to specific surgical procedures, though there is no direct one-to-one correspondence. One anesthesia code may be used to report several surgical procedures that share similar anesthesia requirements.

Example

01202	**Anesthesia for arthroscopic procedures of hip joint**

This procedure code would be selected to report anesthesia services related to the following surgical procedures:

29860	**Arthroscopy, hip, diagnostic with or without synovial biopsy (separate procedure)**
29861	**Arthroscopy, hip, surgical; with removal of loose body or foreign body**
29862	**with debridement/shaving of articular cartilage (chondroplasty), abrasion arthroplasty, and/or resection of labrum**
29863	**with synovectomy**

ASA RELATIVE VALUE GUIDE

The codes in the main section of the ASA Relative Value Guide (RVG) are the same as those in the CPT book with two exceptions: The ASA includes a few codes not found in the CPT book and excludes a few codes found in the CPT book. In addition, some of the narrative descriptions used by the ASA differ slightly from those found in the CPT book.

The ASA RVG also lists codes for other services frequently provided by anesthesiologists. These codes are CPT codes found in the evaluation and management, medicine, and surgery sections of the CPT book. The services include: pulmonary function testing, evaluation and management services, pain management and nerve blocks, and placement of venous catheters and monitoring devices. In all cases, the ASA provides a relative value designation for each code.

REPORTING ANESTHESIA SERVICES

The anesthesia codes should be used only by physicians not performing the surgical procedures. Reporting anesthesia services differs from reporting other types of physician services. Reporting other physician services typically involves selecting the correct CPT code and submitting a specific fee for that CPT code. The fee is the same every time the service is provided. For example, a problem focused established patient exam and history is reported with code 99212 and the fee assigned to that procedure by a given physician is $30. The physician submits the fee of $30 every time he or she performs procedure 99212.

However, anesthesia billing is based on several variables specific to the particular anesthesia service. The fee submitted for a specific anesthesia code varies each time the code is reported.

The key terms described next are essential to the correct reporting of anesthesia services.

KEY TERMS

Basic value or base unit: the basic value, also referred to as the base unit or relative value, has two components. One component reflects all usual services included in the anesthesia service. Usual services include: pre-operative and postoperative visits, administration of fluids and/or blood products incident to the procedure, and interpretation of non-invasive monitoring (ECG, temperature, blood pressure, oximetry, capnography, and mass spectrometry). The second component reflects the relative work or cost of the specific anesthesia service. Cost in this context refers to the physician's cost of doing business. For anesthesiologists, the majority of the cost goes to malpractice insurance. For example, the basic value for the anesthesia service related to a closed reduction of a radius fracture might be three, as it has a relatively low level of work or cost. The basic value for an anesthesia service associated with an intrathoracic coronary artery bypass graft procedure might be 20, reflecting a high level of work or cost.

The ASA lists two exceptions to using the basic value listed in the RVG. A minimum basic value of five is allowed for all procedures of the head, neck or shoulder girdle, requiring field avoidance. In addition, any procedure performed in any position other than lithotomy or supine has a minimum basic value of five. If the anesthesia code associated with the surgical procedure carries a basic value greater than five the higher basic value is reported.

Base units for anesthesia listed in the RVG are widely accepted across the United States by both physicians and payers. However, some payers, especially government agency payers, may use different relative value scales developed exclusively for their use. Other payers may use national relative value guides based on the RVG, with some modification.

Time: Time is the actual time spent providing the anesthesia service. Time begins as the anesthesiologist prepares the patient for anesthesia care. Time ends when the personal attendance of the anesthesiologist is no longer required and the patient can be safely placed in post-anesthesia recovery under the supervision of nursing or other trained personnel.

Time is reported in units based on defined time increments. The most commonly used time increment is 15 minutes, with one unit being reported for each 15-minute increment. However, time units for anesthesia vary across the country. Both ASA and the CPT book suggest reporting time increments as customary in the geographic area.

The same holds for reporting fractions of time units. For example, a procedure requiring 65 minutes of anesthesia time, reported in 15-minute time increments, results in total time units of 4.33. In some areas, this is reported as the fractional amount 4.33; other areas might round to the nearest whole number four; or another geographical area might allow reporting of another full unit for any fractional amount to five.

For some anesthesia services, time is not reported additionally. The ASA RVG designates a +TM after the base unit for procedures requiring time reported separately. Do not list time separately for procedures without the designation.

Physical status modifiers: Physical status modifiers reflect the patient's state of health. Individuals undergoing surgery may be healthy or may have varying degrees of systemic disease. A patient's health status affects the work related to providing the anesthesia service. The CPT book states that physical status modifiers reflect the level of complexity associated with the anesthesia service.

Physical status modifiers in the CPT book and ASA RVG are represented with the letter P followed by a single digit (e.g., P1, P2). ASA RVG lists the number of additional anesthesia units allowed with each physical status modifier to the right in the column titled "units."

Anesthesia

Modifier	Description	Units
P1	Normal healthy patient	0
P2	Patient with mild systemic disease	0
P3	Patient with severe systemic disease	1
P4	Patient with severe systemic disease that is a constant threat to life	2
P5	Moribund patient who is not expected to survive without the operation	3
P6	A declared brain-dead patient whose organs are being removed for donor purposes	0

Qualifying circumstances: Many anesthesia services are provided under particularly difficult circumstances depending on factors such as extraordinary condition of patient, notable operative conditions, and unusual risk factors. The information provided by both the CPT book and the ASA RVG includes a list of important qualifying circumstances that significantly impact the character of the anesthesia service provided. These procedures are not be reported alone but as additional procedure numbers to qualify an anesthesia procedure or service. The ASA provides modifying units that may be added to the basic unit values, as follows:

Code	Description	ASA RVG Units
99100	Anesthesia for patient of extreme age, under one year and over seventy	1
99116	Anesthesia complicated by utilization of total body hypothermia	5
99135	Anesthesia complicated by utilization of controlled hypotension	5
99140	Anesthesia complicated by emergency conditions (specify)	2

An emergency exists when a delay in treatment poses a significant increase in the threat to the patient's life or to a body part, as defined in both the CPT book and ASA RVG.

Conversion factor: Anesthesia charges must be calculated by means of a conversion factor since the charges are not based on fixed amounts. A conversion factor is the dollar value associated with each unit of anesthesia. The dollar conversion factor is multiplied by the total number of anesthesia units for a given anesthesia service to arrive at the total charges for the anesthesia service.

The dollar conversion factor may vary significantly between geographical regions and to a lesser degree between physicians in a given geographic area. However, the standard formula to calculate total anesthesia units and anesthesia fees is basically the same both among regions and physicians as illustrated in the examples below.

Standard formula: Now that the basic elements of the anesthesia service have been defined, total anesthesia units for a given anesthesia service can be determined. Using the total units and the conversion factor, the fee for a specific anesthesia service can then be calculated.

The total charge for a specific anesthesia service is calculated by means of the following formula:

Basic Value + Time Units + Modifying Units = Total Units

Total Units X Conversion Factor = Total Fee

Example

A closed reduction of a distal radius fracture is accomplished under general anesthesia. The patient is a healthy 10-year-old. The procedure is not performed on an emergency basis. The anesthesiologist reports procedure 01820 that has a basic value of three. Total time for the procedure is 45 minutes. The anesthesiologist reports time units in 15-minute increments. The total units reported for the procedure are as follows:

Basic Value		3
Time Units (45 divided by 15)	+	3
Physical Status (P1)	+	0
Qualifying Circumstances (none)	+	0
Total Units	=	6

The anesthesiologist uses a conversion factor of $45 per unit of anesthesia.

Total Units		6
Conversion Factor	x	$45
Total Fee	=	$270

SPECIAL CODING SITUATIONS

Multiple Procedures

When multiple surgical procedures are performed during a single anesthetic administration, the ASA recommends reporting only the anesthesia procedure with the highest unit value. In other words, only one basic value is assigned per single surgical session. The time reported should be the combined total for all procedures performed.

Additional Procedures

Services not included in the usual anesthesia services may be reported separately. These services include unusual forms of monitoring, prolonged physician services, and provision of additional anesthesia services such as postoperative pain management. These additional services are reported in terms of units with the appropriate CPT or ASA codes under the designation "other procedures." They are calculated as an additional variable in the standard formula.

Unusual monitoring: Unusual forms of monitoring anesthesia are reported by most anesthesiologists and many payers allow benefits beyond the basic anesthesia service. For example, codes 36555–36558, 36568–36569 for insertion of a central venous catheter; 36620–36625 for insertion of an intra-arterial catheter, and 93503 Swan-Ganz insertion, represent unusual forms of monitoring that may be rendered by an anesthesiologist.

Prolonged physician services: Extended pre- or postoperative care provided to a patient whose condition requires services beyond the usual may be reported additionally. These services would be billed with prolonged service codes (99354–99359).

Moderate (conscious) sedation: To report moderate sedation provided by the same physician performing the procedure, consult codes 99143–99145.

When a physician other than a physician performing the procedure administers the moderate sedation in the facility setting, the second physician reports his/her services with codes 99148–99150. In the non-facility setting, codes 99148–99150 would not be used. Moderate sedation does not include minimal sedation (anxiolysis), deep sedation, or monitored anesthesia care (00100–01999).

Postoperative pain management: Normally postoperative pain management is provided or supervised by the surgeon by oral, intramuscular or intravenous medications. Postoperative pain management provided by the surgeon is included in the global fee for the surgical procedure. Some procedures and/or patients require more than the usual type of postoperative pain management, and this is frequently provided or supervised by an anesthesiologist. These services are additional procedures and are reported as follows:

- Epidural or subarachnoid pain management is reported with procedure codes 62310–62319 for placement of the epidural or subarachnoid catheter that includes the initial day of pain management. Subsequent management is reported with 01996 and is reported per day.

- Patient-controlled analgesia is reported with 01997 on a per day basis. Code 01997 is included only in the ASA Relative Value Guide not in the CPT book, but is recognized by most payers as a valid code for this anesthesia service.

- Postoperative pain management services are not calculated based on time. These services are reported as a single, daily charge.

Monitored (Stand-By) Anesthesia

Monitored anesthesia care is defined in the ASA RVG as those instances when an anesthesiologist has been requested to provide specific services to a patient undergoing a planned procedure. The patient receives either local anesthesia or no anesthesia. However, the anesthesiologist is required to provide pre-operative assessment, to remain in attendance during the procedure to monitor the patient and to administer additional anesthetics should they be required, and to provide postoperative services as required.

Monitored care, as described above, is reported as is customary for any other anesthesia procedure. The procedure should be assigned the applicable anesthesia code with time and modifying units being added as is customary in the local area.

Obstetrical Anesthesia

The formula for reporting of epidural analgesia for labor and delivery may differ from the standard formula in some geographical areas. When epidural analgesia is administered, an anesthesiologist may attend to more than one patient. The anesthesiologist may insert the epidural catheter, start the continuous anesthetic, and leave the patient's bedside. The anesthesiologist periodically returns to check on the patient or to increase the amount of anesthetic while attending to other patients who are also receiving epidurals for vaginal deliveries. For this reason epidural analgesia for labor and delivery may be reimbursed at a reduced rate.

The following are some variations in reporting anesthesia services when the anesthesiologist is not required to be in constant attendance:

1. Basic value and modifying units are reported as usual. The first hour of anesthesia is reported at the usual rate, but subsequent hours are reported at a reduced rate. For example, total units for the first hour would be reported in full, but units for the second hour would be reported at 50 percent and units for all subsequent hours at 25 percent. If 15-minute time increments were being used the first hour units would be reported as four units, the second hour as two, and third and subsequent hours as one unit each.

2. A flat rate may be established and reported regardless of the actual epidural time. Basic value units are included in the flat rate. For example, the anesthesiologist may bill $500 for anesthesia services provided at every vaginal delivery. Modifying units may or may not be reported separately.

3. Basic value and modifying units are reported as usual. Actual time spent in attendance of the patient may be used and reported at the usual rate. For example, a patient who received epidural analgesia for four hours might have required the anesthesiologist's presence for only two hours of the total time. If 15-minute time increments were used, the anesthesiologist would report eight units.

These are examples of possible variations and should not be adopted without evaluating current practices in the geographic area. Payers should be queried as to their rules for reporting anesthesia services related to obstetrical care.

Unusual Anesthesia

The CPT book defines unusual anesthesia as follows:

23 Unusual anesthesia: Occasionally, a procedure that usually requires either no anesthesia or local anesthesia must be done under general anesthesia due to unusual circumstances. This circumstance may be reported by adding modifier 23 to the procedure code of the basic service.

Although it is generally inappropriate to report anesthesia with some E/M, medicine, surgery, and radiology codes, there are situations where medical necessity requires anesthesia (e.g. a baby, small child, or hard-to-control patient needing dressings and/or debridement). Under these unusual circumstances, payers will usually allow the anesthesia charge. Submit an operative report and cover letter with the claim explaining the need for any unusual anesthesia.

Chronic Pain Management Services

Chronic pain management services are not anesthesia services. These are distinct services frequently performed by anesthesiologists who have additional training in pain management procedures. Pain management services are reported following the same rules as those for surgical procedures.

Pain management services include initial and subsequent evaluation and management (E/M) services, trigger point injections, spine and spinal cord injections, and nerve blocks.

E/M services may be reported with outpatient/office codes 99201–99215 or outpatient consultation codes 99241–99245 depending on the nature of the E/M service.

Tendon injections are reported with codes 20550 and 20551 Trigger point injections are reported with codes 20552 and 20553 for injections of single or multiple points in one or two, or three or more muscles, respectively. Codes 62280–62284 and 62290–62319 are used to report spine and spinal cord injections.

Nerve blocks are reported with codes 64400–64530. Nerve blocks are defined as the introduction or injection of an anesthetic agent into a nerve or nerve branch.

Home infusion procedures (99601–99602) report home infusion for pain therapy. Use 99601 for the first two hours and 99602 for each additional hour.

Each code for pain management services should have a specific fee and the fee should be the same each time that specific code is reported. In other words, no adjustments are made based on time, physical status, or qualifying circumstances.

SPECIAL REPORT

A service that is rarely provided, unusual, variable, or new may require a special report to help the payer determine the medical appropriateness of the service. Pertinent information should include an adequate definition or description of the nature, extent, and need for the procedure; and the time, effort, and equipment necessary to provide the service.

COMMON BILLING ERRORS

Incorrect ICD-9-CM or CPT coding is a frequent problem encountered in anesthesia reporting. The code may be incorrect because it does not match the diagnosis or procedure reported by the surgeon. Claims must reflect the same diagnosis and procedure by the anesthesiologist and surgeon, with the exception of listing a global surgery code when only part of the service is provided.

There are codes in the surgery section of the CPT book designated as "add on" codes. These add-on codes, however, are not used for coding anesthesia services.

For example, 11001 is an "add on" code. The primary procedure code is 11000 Debridement of extensive eczematous or infected skin; up to 10% of body surface. Always report 11001 with "in addition to" code 11000 because its description states each additional 10 percent of the body surface. In this case, the appropriate CPT code for determining anesthesia base units and guidelines is 11000.

HEAD

00100 Anesthesia for procedures on salivary glands, including biopsy N ◘

MED: 100-4,3,100.2; 100-4,4,10.4; 100-4,4,10.5; 100-4,4,10.10; 100-4,4,20.5; 100-4,4,20.6; 100-4,4,20.6.4; 100-4,4,61.2; 100-4,4,250.1.3; 100-4,4,250.3.1; 100-4,4,250.3.2; 100-4,4,250.3.3; 100-4,12,50; 100-4,12,140; 100-4,12,140.2; 100-4,12,140.3.2

AMA: 1999,Nov,6; 1997,Feb,4

00102 Anesthesia for procedures involving plastic repair of cleft lip N ◘

MED: 100-4,3,100.2; 100-4,4,10.4; 100-4,4,10.5; 100-4,4,10.10; 100-4,4,20.5; 100-4,4,20.6; 100-4,4,20.6.4; 100-4,4,61.2; 100-4,4,250.1.3; 100-4,4,250.3.1; 100-4,4,250.3.2; 100-4,4,250.3.3; 100-4,12,50; 100-4,12,140; 100-4,12,140.2; 100-4,12,140.3.2

AMA: 1999,Nov,6

00103 Anesthesia for reconstructive procedures of eyelid (eg, blepharoplasty, ptosis surgery) N ◘

MED: 100-4,3,100.2; 100-4,4,10.4; 100-4,4,10.5; 100-4,4,10.10; 100-4,4,20.5; 100-4,4,20.6; 100-4,4,20.6.4; 100-4,4,61.2; 100-4,4,250.1.3; 100-4,4,250.3.1; 100-4,4,250.3.2; 100-4,4,250.3.3; 100-4,12,50; 100-4,12,140; 100-4,12,140.2; 100-4,12,140.3.2

AMA: 1999,Nov,6

00104 Anesthesia for electroconvulsive therapy N ◘

MED: 100-4,3,100.2; 100-4,4,10.4; 100-4,4,10.5; 100-4,4,10.10; 100-4,4,20.5; 100-4,4,20.6; 100-4,4,20.6.4; 100-4,4,61.2; 100-4,4,250.1.3; 100-4,4,250.3.1; 100-4,4,250.3.2; 100-4,4,250.3.3; 100-4,12,50; 100-4,12,140; 100-4,12,140.2; 100-4,12,140.3.2

00120 Anesthesia for procedures on external, middle, and inner ear including biopsy; not otherwise specified N ◘

MED: 100-4,3,100.2; 100-4,4,10.4; 100-4,4,10.5; 100-4,4,10.10; 100-4,4,20.5; 100-4,4,20.6; 100-4,4,20.6.4; 100-4,4,61.2; 100-4,4,250.1.3; 100-4,4,250.3.1; 100-4,4,250.3.2; 100-4,4,250.3.3; 100-4,12,50; 100-4,12,140; 100-4,12,140.2; 100-4,12,140.3.2

00124 otoscopy N ◘

MED: 100-4,3,100.2; 100-4,4,10.4; 100-4,4,10.5; 100-4,4,10.10; 100-4,4,20.5; 100-4,4,20.6; 100-4,4,20.6.4; 100-4,4,61.2; 100-4,4,250.1.3; 100-4,4,250.3.1; 100-4,4,250.3.2; 100-4,4,250.3.3; 100-4,12,50; 100-4,12,140; 100-4,12,140.2; 100-4,12,140.3.2

AMA: 1999,Nov,7

00126 tympanotomy N ◘

MED: 100-4,3,100.2; 100-4,4,10.4; 100-4,4,10.5; 100-4,4,10.10; 100-4,4,20.5; 100-4,4,20.6; 100-4,4,20.6.4; 100-4,4,61.2; 100-4,4,250.1.3; 100-4,4,250.3.1; 100-4,4,250.3.2; 100-4,4,250.3.3; 100-4,12,50; 100-4,12,140; 100-4,12,140.2; 100-4,12,140.3.2

00140 Anesthesia for procedures on eye; not otherwise specified N ◘

MED: 100-4,3,100.2; 100-4,4,10.4; 100-4,4,10.5; 100-4,4,10.10; 100-4,4,20.5; 100-4,4,20.6; 100-4,4,20.6.4; 100-4,4,61.2; 100-4,4,250.1.3; 100-4,4,250.3.1; 100-4,4,250.3.2; 100-4,4,250.3.3; 100-4,12,50; 100-4,12,140; 100-4,12,140.2; 100-4,12,140.3.2

00142 lens surgery N ◘

MED: 100-3,10.1; 100-4,3,100.2; 100-4,4,10.4; 100-4,4,10.5; 100-4,4,10.10; 100-4,4,20.5; 100-4,4,20.6; 100-4,4,20.6.4; 100-4,4,61.2; 100-4,4,250.1.3; 100-4,4,250.3.1; 100-4,4,250.3.2; 100-4,4,250.3.3; 100-4,12,50; 100-4,12,140; 100-4,12,140.2; 100-4,12,140.3.2

00144 corneal transplant N ◘

MED: 100-4,3,100.2; 100-4,4,10.4; 100-4,4,10.5; 100-4,4,10.10; 100-4,4,20.5; 100-4,4,20.6; 100-4,4,20.6.4; 100-4,4,61.2; 100-4,4,250.1.3; 100-4,4,250.3.1; 100-4,4,250.3.2; 100-4,4,250.3.3; 100-4,12,50; 100-4,12,140; 100-4,12,140.2; 100-4,12,140.3.2

00145 vitreoretinal surgery N ◘

MED: 100-4,3,100.2; 100-4,4,10.4; 100-4,4,10.5; 100-4,4,10.10; 100-4,4,20.5; 100-4,4,20.6; 100-4,4,20.6.4; 100-4,4,61.2; 100-4,4,250.1.3; 100-4,4,250.3.1; 100-4,4,250.3.2; 100-4,4,250.3.3; 100-4,12,50; 100-4,12,140; 100-4,12,140.2; 100-4,12,140.3.2

00147 iridectomy N ◘

MED: 100-4,3,100.2; 100-4,4,10.4; 100-4,4,10.5; 100-4,4,10.10; 100-4,4,20.5; 100-4,4,20.6; 100-4,4,20.6.4; 100-4,4,61.2; 100-4,4,250.1.3; 100-4,4,250.3.1; 100-4,4,250.3.2; 100-4,4,250.3.3; 100-4,12,50; 100-4,12,140; 100-4,12,140.2; 100-4,12,140.3.2

00148 ophthalmoscopy N ◘

MED: 100-4,3,100.2; 100-4,4,10.4; 100-4,4,10.5; 100-4,4,10.10; 100-4,4,20.5; 100-4,4,20.6; 100-4,4,20.6.4; 100-4,4,61.2; 100-4,4,250.1.3; 100-4,4,250.3.1; 100-4,4,250.3.2; 100-4,4,250.3.3; 100-4,12,50; 100-4,12,140; 100-4,12,140.2; 100-4,12,140.3.2

00160 Anesthesia for procedures on nose and accessory sinuses; not otherwise specified N ◘

MED: 100-4,3,100.2; 100-4,4,10.4; 100-4,4,10.5; 100-4,4,10.10; 100-4,4,20.5; 100-4,4,20.6; 100-4,4,20.6.4; 100-4,4,61.2; 100-4,4,250.1.3; 100-4,4,250.3.1; 100-4,4,250.3.2; 100-4,4,250.3.3; 100-4,12,50; 100-4,12,140; 100-4,12,140.2; 100-4,12,140.3.2

00162 radical surgery N ◘

MED: 100-4,3,100.2; 100-4,4,10.4; 100-4,4,10.5; 100-4,4,10.10; 100-4,4,20.5; 100-4,4,20.6; 100-4,4,20.6.4; 100-4,4,61.2; 100-4,4,250.1.3; 100-4,4,250.3.1; 100-4,4,250.3.2; 100-4,4,250.3.3; 100-4,12,50; 100-4,12,140; 100-4,12,140.2; 100-4,12,140.3.2

00164 biopsy, soft tissue N ◘

MED: 100-4,3,100.2; 100-4,4,10.4; 100-4,4,10.5; 100-4,4,10.10; 100-4,4,20.5; 100-4,4,20.6; 100-4,4,20.6.4; 100-4,4,61.2; 100-4,4,250.1.3; 100-4,4,250.3.1; 100-4,4,250.3.2; 100-4,4,250.3.3; 100-4,12,50; 100-4,12,140; 100-4,12,140.2; 100-4,12,140.3.2

00170 Anesthesia for intraoral procedures, including biopsy; not otherwise specified N ◘

MED: 100-4,3,100.2; 100-4,4,10.4; 100-4,4,10.5; 100-4,4,10.10; 100-4,4,20.5; 100-4,4,20.6; 100-4,4,20.6.4; 100-4,4,61.2; 100-4,4,250.1.3; 100-4,4,250.3.1; 100-4,4,250.3.2; 100-4,4,250.3.3; 100-4,12,50; 100-4,12,140; 100-4,12,140.2; 100-4,12,140.3.2

00172 repair of cleft palate N ◘

MED: 100-4,3,100.2; 100-4,4,10.4; 100-4,4,10.5; 100-4,4,10.10; 100-4,4,20.5; 100-4,4,20.6; 100-4,4,20.6.4; 100-4,4,61.2; 100-4,4,250.1.3; 100-4,4,250.3.1; 100-4,4,250.3.2; 100-4,4,250.3.3; 100-4,12,50; 100-4,12,140; 100-4,12,140.2; 100-4,12,140.3.2

00174 excision of retropharyngeal tumor N ◘

MED: 100-4,3,100.2; 100-4,4,10.4; 100-4,4,10.5; 100-4,4,10.10; 100-4,4,20.5; 100-4,4,20.6; 100-4,4,20.6.4; 100-4,4,61.2; 100-4,4,250.1.3; 100-4,4,250.3.1; 100-4,4,250.3.2; 100-4,4,250.3.3; 100-4,12,50; 100-4,12,140; 100-4,12,140.2; 100-4,12,140.3.2

00176 radical surgery C ◘

MED: 100-4,3,100.2; 100-4,4,10.4; 100-4,4,10.5; 100-4,4,10.10; 100-4,4,20.5; 100-4,4,20.6; 100-4,4,20.6.4; 100-4,4,61.2; 100-4,4,250.1.3; 100-4,4,250.3.1; 100-4,4,250.3.2; 100-4,4,250.3.3; 100-4,12,50; 100-4,12,140; 100-4,12,140.2; 100-4,12,140.3.2

00190 Anesthesia for procedures on facial bones or skull; not otherwise specified N ◘

MED: 100-4,3,100.2; 100-4,4,10.4; 100-4,4,10.5; 100-4,4,10.10; 100-4,4,20.5; 100-4,4,20.6; 100-4,4,20.6.4; 100-4,4,61.2; 100-4,4,250.1.3; 100-4,4,250.3.1; 100-4,4,250.3.2; 100-4,4,250.3.3; 100-4,12,50; 100-4,12,140; 100-4,12,140.2; 100-4,12,140.3.2

00192 radical surgery (including prognathism) C ◘

MED: 100-4,3,100.2; 100-4,4,10.4; 100-4,4,10.5; 100-4,4,10.10; 100-4,4,20.5; 100-4,4,20.6; 100-4,4,20.6.4; 100-4,4,61.2; 100-4,4,250.1.3; 100-4,4,250.3.1; 100-4,4,250.3.2; 100-4,4,250.3.3; 100-4,12,50; 100-4,12,140; 100-4,12,140.2; 100-4,12,140.3.2

00210 Anesthesia for intracranial procedures; not otherwise specified N ◘

MED: 100-4,3,100.2; 100-4,4,10.4; 100-4,4,10.5; 100-4,4,10.10; 100-4,4,20.5; 100-4,4,20.6; 100-4,4,20.6.4; 100-4,4,61.2; 100-4,4,250.1.3; 100-4,4,250.3.1; 100-4,4,250.3.2; 100-4,4,250.3.3; 100-4,12,50; 100-4,12,140; 100-4,12,140.2; 100-4,12,140.3.2

00212 subdural taps N ◘

MED: 100-4,3,100.2; 100-4,4,10.4; 100-4,4,10.5; 100-4,4,10.10; 100-4,4,20.5; 100-4,4,20.6; 100-4,4,20.6.4; 100-4,4,61.2; 100-4,4,250.1.3; 100-4,4,250.3.1; 100-4,4,250.3.2; 100-4,4,250.3.3; 100-4,12,50; 100-4,12,140; 100-4,12,140.2; 100-4,12,140.3.2

⬢ Modifier 63 Exempt Code ⊙ Conscious Sedation + CPT Add-on Code ⊘ Modifier 51 Exempt Code ● New Code ▲ Revised Code

M Maternity Edit A Age Edit A-Y APC Status Indicators ◘ CCI Comprehensive Code 50 Bilateral Procedure

00214	burr holes, including ventriculography	C ◨

MED: 100-4,3,100.2; 100-4,4,10.4; 100-4,4,10.5; 100-4,4,10.10; 100-4,4,20.5; 100-4,4,20.6; 100-4,4,20.6.4; 100-4,4,61.2; 100-4,4,250.1.3; 100-4,4,250.3.1; 100-4,4,250.3.2; 100-4,4,250.3.3; 100-4,12,50; 100-4,12,140; 100-4,12,140.2; 100-4,12,140.3.2

AMA: 1999,Nov,7

00215	cranioplasty or elevation of depressed skull fracture, extradural (simple or compound)	C ◨

MED: 100-4,3,100.2; 100-4,4,10.4; 100-4,4,10.5; 100-4,4,10.10; 100-4,4,20.5; 100-4,4,20.6; 100-4,4,20.6.4; 100-4,4,61.2; 100-4,4,250.1.3; 100-4,4,250.3.1; 100-4,4,250.3.2; 100-4,4,250.3.3; 100-4,12,50; 100-4,12,140; 100-4,12,140.2; 100-4,12,140.3.2

00216	vascular procedures	N ◨

MED: 100-4,3,100.2; 100-4,4,10.4; 100-4,4,10.5; 100-4,4,10.10; 100-4,4,20.5; 100-4,4,20.6; 100-4,4,20.6.4; 100-4,4,61.2; 100-4,4,250.1.3; 100-4,4,250.3.1; 100-4,4,250.3.2; 100-4,4,250.3.3; 100-4,12,50; 100-4,12,140; 100-4,12,140.2; 100-4,12,140.3.2

00218	procedures in sitting position	N ◨

MED: 100-4,3,100.2; 100-4,4,10.4; 100-4,4,10.5; 100-4,4,10.10; 100-4,4,20.5; 100-4,4,20.6; 100-4,4,20.6.4; 100-4,4,61.2; 100-4,4,250.1.3; 100-4,4,250.3.1; 100-4,4,250.3.2; 100-4,4,250.3.3; 100-4,12,50; 100-4,12,140; 100-4,12,140.2; 100-4,12,140.3.2

00220	cerebrospinal fluid shunting procedures	N ◨

MED: 100-4,3,100.2; 100-4,4,10.4; 100-4,4,10.5; 100-4,4,10.10; 100-4,4,20.5; 100-4,4,20.6; 100-4,4,20.6.4; 100-4,4,61.2; 100-4,4,250.1.3; 100-4,4,250.3.1; 100-4,4,250.3.2; 100-4,4,250.3.3; 100-4,12,50; 100-4,12,140; 100-4,12,140.2; 100-4,12,140.3.2

00222	electrocoagulation of intracranial nerve	N ◨

MED: 100-4,3,100.2; 100-4,4,10.4; 100-4,4,10.5; 100-4,4,10.10; 100-4,4,20.5; 100-4,4,20.6; 100-4,4,20.6.4; 100-4,4,61.2; 100-4,4,250.1.3; 100-4,4,250.3.1; 100-4,4,250.3.2; 100-4,4,250.3.3; 100-4,12,50; 100-4,12,140; 100-4,12,140.2; 100-4,12,140.3.2

NECK

00300	Anesthesia for all procedures on the integumentary system, muscles and nerves of head, neck, and posterior trunk, not otherwise specified	N ◨

MED: 100-4,3,100.2; 100-4,4,10.4; 100-4,4,10.5; 100-4,4,10.10; 100-4,4,20.5; 100-4,4,20.6; 100-4,4,20.6.4; 100-4,4,61.2; 100-4,4,250.1.3; 100-4,4,250.3.1; 100-4,4,250.3.2; 100-4,4,250.3.3; 100-4,12,50; 100-4,12,140; 100-4,12,140.2; 100-4,12,140.3.2

AMA: 1999,Nov,7

00320	Anesthesia for all procedures on esophagus, thyroid, larynx, trachea and lymphatic system of neck; not otherwise specified, age 1 year or older	N ◨

MED: 100-4,3,100.2; 100-4,4,10.4; 100-4,4,10.5; 100-4,4,10.10; 100-4,4,20.5; 100-4,4,20.6; 100-4,4,20.6.4; 100-4,4,61.2; 100-4,4,250.1.3; 100-4,4,250.3.1; 100-4,4,250.3.2; 100-4,4,250.3.3; 100-4,12,50; 100-4,12,140; 100-4,12,140.2; 100-4,12,140.3.2

00322	needle biopsy of thyroid	N ◨

MED: 100-4,3,100.2; 100-4,4,10.4; 100-4,4,10.5; 100-4,4,10.10; 100-4,4,20.5; 100-4,4,20.6; 100-4,4,20.6.4; 100-4,4,61.2; 100-4,4,250.1.3; 100-4,4,250.3.1; 100-4,4,250.3.2; 100-4,4,250.3.3; 100-4,12,50; 100-4,12,140; 100-4,12,140.2; 100-4,12,140.3.2

To report anesthesia for procedures on the cervical spine and cord, consult CPT codes 00600, 00604, 00670.

▲ 00326	Anesthesia for all procedures on the larynx and trachea in children younger than 1 year of age	A N ◨

MED: 100-4,3,100.2

Note that code 00326 cannot be reported with CPT code 99100.

00350	Anesthesia for procedures on major vessels of neck; not otherwise specified	N ◨

MED: 100-4,3,100.2; 100-4,4,10.4; 100-4,4,10.5; 100-4,4,10.10; 100-4,4,20.5; 100-4,4,20.6; 100-4,4,20.6.4; 100-4,4,61.2; 100-4,4,250.1.3; 100-4,4,250.3.1; 100-4,4,250.3.2; 100-4,4,250.3.3; 100-4,12,50; 100-4,12,140; 100-4,12,140.2; 100-4,12,140.3.2

00352	simple ligation	N ◨

MED: 100-4,3,100.2; 100-4,4,10.4; 100-4,4,10.5; 100-4,4,10.10; 100-4,4,20.5; 100-4,4,20.6; 100-4,4,20.6.4; 100-4,4,61.2; 100-4,4,250.1.3; 100-4,4,250.3.1; 100-4,4,250.3.2; 100-4,4,250.3.3; 100-4,12,50; 100-4,12,140; 100-4,12,140.2; 100-4,12,140.3.2

To report anesthesia for arteriograms, consult CPT code 01916.

THORAX (CHEST WALL AND SHOULDER GIRDLE)

00400	Anesthesia for procedures on the integumentary system on the extremities, anterior trunk and perineum; not otherwise specified	N ◨

MED: 100-4,3,100.2; 100-4,4,10.4; 100-4,4,10.5; 100-4,4,10.10; 100-4,4,20.5; 100-4,4,20.6; 100-4,4,20.6.4; 100-4,4,61.2; 100-4,4,250.1.3; 100-4,4,250.3.1; 100-4,4,250.3.2; 100-4,4,250.3.3; 100-4,12,50; 100-4,12,140; 100-4,12,140.2; 100-4,12,140.3.2

00402	reconstructive procedures on breast (eg, reduction or augmentation mammoplasty, muscle flaps)	N ◨

MED: 100-4,3,100.2; 100-4,4,10.4; 100-4,4,10.5; 100-4,4,10.10; 100-4,4,20.5; 100-4,4,20.6; 100-4,4,20.6.4; 100-4,4,61.2; 100-4,4,250.1.3; 100-4,4,250.3.1; 100-4,4,250.3.2; 100-4,4,250.3.3; 100-4,12,50; 100-4,12,140; 100-4,12,140.2; 100-4,12,140.3.2

00404	radical or modified radical procedures on breast	N ◨

MED: 100-4,3,100.2; 100-4,4,10.4; 100-4,4,10.5; 100-4,4,10.10; 100-4,4,20.5; 100-4,4,20.6; 100-4,4,20.6.4; 100-4,4,61.2; 100-4,4,250.1.3; 100-4,4,250.3.1; 100-4,4,250.3.2; 100-4,4,250.3.3; 100-4,12,50; 100-4,12,140; 100-4,12,140.2; 100-4,12,140.3.2

00406	radical or modified radical procedures on breast with internal mammary node dissection	N ◨

MED: 100-4,3,100.2; 100-4,4,10.4; 100-4,4,10.5; 100-4,4,10.10; 100-4,4,20.5; 100-4,4,20.6; 100-4,4,20.6.4; 100-4,4,61.2; 100-4,4,250.1.3; 100-4,4,250.3.1; 100-4,4,250.3.2; 100-4,4,250.3.3; 100-4,12,50; 100-4,12,140; 100-4,12,140.2; 100-4,12,140.3.2

00410	electrical conversion of arrhythmias	N ◨

MED: 100-4,3,100.2; 100-4,4,10.4; 100-4,4,10.5; 100-4,4,10.10; 100-4,4,20.5; 100-4,4,20.6; 100-4,4,20.6.4; 100-4,4,61.2; 100-4,4,250.1.3; 100-4,4,250.3.1; 100-4,4,250.3.2; 100-4,4,250.3.3; 100-4,12,50; 100-4,12,140; 100-4,12,140.2; 100-4,12,140.3.2

00450	Anesthesia for procedures on clavicle and scapula; not otherwise specified	N ◨

MED: 100-4,3,100.2; 100-4,4,10.4; 100-4,4,10.5; 100-4,4,10.10; 100-4,4,20.5; 100-4,4,20.6; 100-4,4,20.6.4; 100-4,4,61.2; 100-4,4,250.1.3; 100-4,4,250.3.1; 100-4,4,250.3.2; 100-4,4,250.3.3; 100-4,12,50; 100-4,12,140; 100-4,12,140.2; 100-4,12,140.3.2

00452	radical surgery	C ◨

MED: 100-4,3,100.2; 100-4,4,10.4; 100-4,4,10.5; 100-4,4,10.10; 100-4,4,20.5; 100-4,4,20.6; 100-4,4,20.6.4; 100-4,4,61.2; 100-4,4,250.1.3; 100-4,4,250.3.1; 100-4,4,250.3.2; 100-4,4,250.3.3; 100-4,12,50; 100-4,12,140; 100-4,12,140.2; 100-4,12,140.3.2

00454	biopsy of clavicle	N ◨

MED: 100-4,3,100.2; 100-4,4,10.4; 100-4,4,10.5; 100-4,4,10.10; 100-4,4,20.5; 100-4,4,20.6; 100-4,4,20.6.4; 100-4,4,61.2; 100-4,4,250.1.3; 100-4,4,250.3.1; 100-4,4,250.3.2; 100-4,4,250.3.3; 100-4,12,50; 100-4,12,140; 100-4,12,140.2; 100-4,12,140.3.2

00470	Anesthesia for partial rib resection; not otherwise specified	N ◨

MED: 100-4,3,100.2; 100-4,4,10.4; 100-4,4,10.5; 100-4,4,10.10; 100-4,4,20.5; 100-4,4,20.6; 100-4,4,20.6.4; 100-4,4,61.2; 100-4,4,250.1.3; 100-4,4,250.3.1; 100-4,4,250.3.2; 100-4,4,250.3.3; 100-4,12,50; 100-4,12,140; 100-4,12,140.2; 100-4,12,140.3.2

00472	thoracoplasty (any type)	N ◨

MED: 100-4,3,100.2; 100-4,4,10.4; 100-4,4,10.5; 100-4,4,10.10; 100-4,4,20.5; 100-4,4,20.6; 100-4,4,20.6.4; 100-4,4,61.2; 100-4,4,250.1.3; 100-4,4,250.3.1; 100-4,4,250.3.2; 100-4,4,250.3.3; 100-4,12,50; 100-4,12,140; 100-4,12,140.2; 100-4,12,140.3.2

| 00474 | radical procedures (eg, pectus excavatum) ⒸⓄ |

MED: 100-4,3,100.2; 100-4,4,10.4; 100-4,4,10.5; 100-4,4,10.10; 100-4,4,20.5; 100-4,4,20.6; 100-4,4,20.6.4; 100-4,4,61.2; 100-4,4,250.1.3; 100-4,4,250.3.1; 100-4,4,250.3.2; 100-4,4,250.3.3; 100-4,12,50; 100-4,12,140; 100-4,12,140.2; 100-4,12,140.3.2

INTRATHORACIC

| 00500 | Anesthesia for all procedures on esophagus ⒶⓄ |

MED: 100-4,3,100.2; 100-4,4,10.4; 100-4,4,10.5; 100-4,4,10.10; 100-4,4,20.5; 100-4,4,20.6; 100-4,4,20.6.4; 100-4,4,61.2; 100-4,4,250.1.3; 100-4,4,250.3.1; 100-4,4,250.3.2; 100-4,4,250.3.3; 100-4,12,50; 100-4,12,140; 100-4,12,140.2; 100-4,12,140.3.2

| 00520 | Anesthesia for closed chest procedures; (including bronchoscopy) not otherwise specified ⒶⓄ |

MED: 100-4,3,100.2; 100-4,4,10.4; 100-4,4,10.5; 100-4,4,10.10; 100-4,4,20.5; 100-4,4,20.6; 100-4,4,20.6.4; 100-4,4,61.2; 100-4,4,250.1.3; 100-4,4,250.3.1; 100-4,4,250.3.2; 100-4,4,250.3.3; 100-4,12,50; 100-4,12,140; 100-4,12,140.2; 100-4,12,140.3.2

AMA: 1999,Nov,7

| 00522 | needle biopsy of pleura ⒶⓄ |

MED: 100-4,3,100.2; 100-4,4,10.4; 100-4,4,10.5; 100-4,4,10.10; 100-4,4,20.5; 100-4,4,20.6; 100-4,4,20.6.4; 100-4,4,61.2; 100-4,4,250.1.3; 100-4,4,250.3.1; 100-4,4,250.3.2; 100-4,4,250.3.3; 100-4,12,50; 100-4,12,140; 100-4,12,140.2; 100-4,12,140.3.2

| 00524 | pneumocentesis ⒸⓄ |

MED: 100-4,3,100.2; 100-4,4,10.4; 100-4,4,10.5; 100-4,4,10.10; 100-4,4,20.5; 100-4,4,20.6; 100-4,4,20.6.4; 100-4,4,61.2; 100-4,4,250.1.3; 100-4,4,250.3.1; 100-4,4,250.3.2; 100-4,4,250.3.3; 100-4,12,50; 100-4,12,140; 100-4,12,140.2; 100-4,12,140.3.2

| 00528 | mediastinoscopy and diagnostic thoracoscopy not utilizing one lung ventilation ⒶⓄ |

MED: 100-4,3,100.2; 100-4,4,10.4; 100-4,4,10.5; 100-4,4,10.10; 100-4,4,20.5; 100-4,4,20.6; 100-4,4,20.6.4; 100-4,4,61.2; 100-4,4,250.1.3; 100-4,4,250.3.1; 100-4,4,250.3.2; 100-4,4,250.3.3; 100-4,12,50; 100-4,12,140; 100-4,12,140.2; 100-4,12,140.3.2

AMA: 1999,Nov,7
To report anesthesia for tracheobronchial reconstruction, consult CPT code 00539.

| 00529 | mediastinoscopy and diagnostic thoracoscopy utilizing one lung ventilation ⒶⓄ |

MED: 100-4,3,100.2

| 00530 | Anesthesia for permanent transvenous pacemaker insertion ⒶⓄ |

MED: 100-3,20.8.3; 100-4,3,100.2; 100-4,4,10.4; 100-4,4,10.5; 100-4,4,10.10; 100-4,4,20.5; 100-4,4,20.6; 100-4,4,20.6.4; 100-4,4,61.2; 100-4,4,250.1.3; 100-4,4,250.3.1; 100-4,4,250.3.2; 100-4,4,250.3.3; 100-4,12,50; 100-4,12,140; 100-4,12,140.2; 100-4,12,140.3.2

| 00532 | Anesthesia for access to central venous circulation ⒶⓄ |

MED: 100-4,3,100.2; 100-4,4,10.4; 100-4,4,10.5; 100-4,4,10.10; 100-4,4,20.5; 100-4,4,20.6; 100-4,4,20.6.4; 100-4,4,61.2; 100-4,4,250.1.3; 100-4,4,250.3.1; 100-4,4,250.3.2; 100-4,4,250.3.3; 100-4,12,50; 100-4,12,140; 100-4,12,140.2; 100-4,12,140.3.2

| 00534 | Anesthesia for transvenous insertion or replacement of pacing cardioverter-defibrillator ⒶⓄ |

MED: 100-3,20.8.3; 100-4,3,100.2; 100-4,4,10.4; 100-4,4,10.5; 100-4,4,10.10; 100-4,4,20.5; 100-4,4,20.6; 100-4,4,20.6.4; 100-4,4,61.2; 100-4,4,250.1.3; 100-4,4,250.3.1; 100-4,4,250.3.2; 100-4,4,250.3.3; 100-4,12,50; 100-4,12,140; 100-4,12,140.2; 100-4,12,140.3.2
To report anesthesia in transthoracic approach, consult CPT code 00560.

| 00537 | Anesthesia for cardiac electrophysiologic procedures including radiofrequency ablation ⒶⓄ |

MED: 100-4,3,100.2

| 00539 | Anesthesia for tracheobronchial reconstruction ⒶⓄ |

MED: 100-4,3,100.2

| 00540 | Anesthesia for thoracotomy procedures involving lungs, pleura, diaphragm, and mediastinum (including surgical thoracoscopy); not otherwise specified ⒸⓄ |

MED: 100-4,3,100.2; 100-4,4,10.4; 100-4,4,10.5; 100-4,4,10.10; 100-4,4,20.5; 100-4,4,20.6; 100-4,4,20.6.4; 100-4,4,61.2; 100-4,4,250.1.3; 100-4,4,250.3.1; 100-4,4,250.3.2; 100-4,4,250.3.3; 100-4,12,50; 100-4,12,140; 100-4,12,140.2; 100-4,12,140.3.2

| 00541 | utilizing one lung ventilation ⒶⓄ |

MED: 100-4,3,100.2

| 00542 | decortication ⒸⓄ |

MED: 100-4,3,100.2; 100-4,4,10.4; 100-4,4,10.5; 100-4,4,10.10; 100-4,4,20.5; 100-4,4,20.6; 100-4,4,20.6.4; 100-4,4,61.2; 100-4,4,250.1.3; 100-4,4,250.3.1; 100-4,4,250.3.2; 100-4,4,250.3.3; 100-4,12,50; 100-4,12,140; 100-4,12,140.2; 100-4,12,140.3.2

| 00546 | pulmonary resection with thoracoplasty ⒸⓄ |

MED: 100-4,3,100.2; 100-4,4,10.4; 100-4,4,10.5; 100-4,4,10.10; 100-4,4,20.5; 100-4,4,20.6; 100-4,4,20.6.4; 100-4,4,61.2; 100-4,4,250.3.1; 100-4,4,250.3.2; 100-4,4,250.3.3; 100-4,12,50; 100-4,12,140; 100-4,12,140.2; 100-4,12,140.3.2

| 00548 | intrathoracic procedures on the trachea and bronchi ⒶⓄ |

MED: 100-4,3,100.2; 100-4,4,10.4; 100-4,4,10.5; 100-4,4,10.10; 100-4,4,20.5; 100-4,4,20.6; 100-4,4,20.6.4; 100-4,4,61.2; 100-4,4,250.1.3; 100-4,4,250.3.1; 100-4,4,250.3.2; 100-4,4,250.3.3; 100-4,12,50; 100-4,12,140; 100-4,12,140.2; 100-4,12,140.3.2

AMA: 1997,Nov,10

| 00550 | Anesthesia for sternal debridement ⒶⓄ |

MED: 100-4,3,100.2

| 00560 | Anesthesia for procedures on heart, pericardial sac, and great vessels of chest; without pump oxygenator ⒸⓄ |

MED: 100-3,160.8; 100-3,160.9; 100-4,3,100.2; 100-4,4,10.4; 100-4,4,10.5; 100-4,4,10.10; 100-4,4,20.5; 100-4,4,20.6; 100-4,4,20.6.4; 100-4,4,61.2; 100-4,4,250.1.3; 100-4,4,250.3.1; 100-4,4,250.3.2; 100-4,4,250.3.3; 100-4,12,50; 100-4,12,140; 100-4,12,140.2; 100-4,12,140.3.2

| ▲ 00561 | with pump oxygenator, under one year of age ⒶⒸⓄ |

MED: 100-4,3,100.2
Do not report 00561 with 99100, 99115, and 99135.

| 00562 | with pump oxygenator ⒸⓄ |

MED: 100-3,160.8; 100-3,160.9; 100-4,3,100.2; 100-4,4,10.4; 100-4,4,10.5; 100-4,4,10.10; 100-4,4,20.5; 100-4,4,20.6; 100-4,4,20.6.4; 100-4,4,61.2; 100-4,4,250.1.3; 100-4,4,250.3.1; 100-4,4,250.3.2; 100-4,4,250.3.3; 100-4,12,50; 100-4,12,140; 100-4,12,140.2; 100-4,12,140.3.2

| 00563 | with pump oxygenator with hypothermic circulatory arrest ⒶⓄ |

MED: 100-3,160.8; 100-3,160.9; 100-4,3,100.2

| 00566 | Anesthesia for direct coronary artery bypass grafting without pump oxygenator ⒶⓄ |

MED: 100-3,160.9; 100-4,3,100.2

| 00580 | Anesthesia for heart transplant or heart/lung transplant ⒸⓄ |

MED: 100-4,3,100.2; 100-4,4,10.4; 100-4,4,10.5; 100-4,4,10.10; 100-4,4,20.5; 100-4,4,20.6; 100-4,4,20.6.4; 100-4,4,61.2; 100-4,4,250.1.3; 100-4,4,250.3.1; 100-4,4,250.3.2; 100-4,4,250.3.3; 100-4,12,50; 100-4,12,140; 100-4,12,140.2; 100-4,12,140.3.2

---

⑬ Modifier 63 Exempt Code ⊙ Conscious Sedation ＋ CPT Add-on Code ⃠ Modifier 51 Exempt Code ● New Code ▲ Revised Code
Ⓜ Maternity Edit Ⓐ Age Edit Ⓐ-Ⓨ APC Status Indicators ⓄⓄ CCI Comprehensive Code ㊿ Bilateral Procedure

SPINE AND SPINAL CORD

00600 **Anesthesia for procedures on cervical spine and cord; not otherwise specified** N

MED: 100-4,3,100.2; 100-4,4,10.4; 100-4,4,10.5; 100-4,4,10.10; 100-4,4,20.5; 100-4,4,20.6; 100-4,4,20.6.4; 100-4,4,61.2; 100-4,4,250.1.3; 100-4,4,250.3.1; 100-4,4,250.3.2; 100-4,4,250.3.3; 100-4,12,50; 100-4,12,140; 100-4,12,140.2; 100-4,12,140.3.2

To report anesthesia for myelography, discography, or vertebroplasty, consult CPT code 01905.

00604 **procedures with patient in the sitting position** C

MED: 100-4,3,100.2; 100-4,4,10.4; 100-4,4,10.5; 100-4,4,10.10; 100-4,4,20.5; 100-4,4,20.6; 100-4,4,20.6.4; 100-4,4,61.2; 100-4,4,250.1.3; 100-4,4,250.3.1; 100-4,4,250.3.2; 100-4,4,250.3.3; 100-4,12,50; 100-4,12,140; 100-4,12,140.2; 100-4,12,140.3.2

00620 **Anesthesia for procedures on thoracic spine and cord; not otherwise specified** N

MED: 100-4,3,100.2

To report anesthesia for myelography, discography, or vertebroplasty, consult CPT code 01905.

00622 **thoracolumbar sympathectomy** C

MED: 100-4,3,100.2; 100-4,4,10.4; 100-4,4,10.5; 100-4,4,10.10; 100-4,4,20.5; 100-4,4,20.6; 100-4,4,20.6.4; 100-4,4,61.2; 100-4,4,250.1.3; 100-4,4,250.3.1; 100-4,4,250.3.2; 100-4,4,250.3.3; 100-4,12,50; 100-4,12,140; 100-4,12,140.2; 100-4,12,140.3.2

● **00625** **Anesthesia for procedures on the thoracic spine and cord, via an anterior transthoracic approach; not utilizing one lung ventilation** N

Use 00540-00541 for anesthesia for thoracotomy procedures other than spinal.

● **00626** **utilizing one lung ventilation** N

For anesthesia for thoracotomy procedures other than spinal, see 00540-00541.

00630 **Anesthesia for procedures in lumbar region; not otherwise specified** N

MED: 100-4,3,100.2; 100-4,4,10.4; 100-4,4,10.5; 100-4,4,10.10; 100-4,4,20.5; 100-4,4,20.6; 100-4,4,20.6.4; 100-4,4,61.2; 100-4,4,250.1.3; 100-4,4,250.3.1; 100-4,4,250.3.2; 100-4,4,250.3.3; 100-4,12,50; 100-4,12,140; 100-4,12,140.2; 100-4,12,140.3.2

To report anesthesia for myelography, discography, or vertebroplasty, consult CPT code 01905.

00632 **lumbar sympathectomy** C

MED: 100-4,3,100.2; 100-4,4,10.4; 100-4,4,10.5; 100-4,4,10.10; 100-4,4,20.5; 100-4,4,20.6; 100-4,4,20.6.4; 100-4,4,61.2; 100-4,4,250.1.3; 100-4,4,250.3.1; 100-4,4,250.3.2; 100-4,4,250.3.3; 100-4,12,50; 100-4,12,140; 100-4,12,140.2; 100-4,12,140.3.2

00634 **chemonucleolysis** N

MED: 100-4,3,100.2; 100-4,4,10.4; 100-4,4,10.5; 100-4,4,10.10; 100-4,4,20.5; 100-4,4,20.6; 100-4,4,20.6.4; 100-4,4,61.2; 100-4,4,250.1.3; 100-4,4,250.3.1; 100-4,4,250.3.2; 100-4,4,250.3.3; 100-4,12,50; 100-4,12,140; 100-4,12,140.2; 100-4,12,140.3.2

00635 **diagnostic or therapeutic lumbar puncture** N

MED: 100-4,3,100.2

00640 **Anesthesia for manipulation of the spine or for closed procedures on the cervical, thoracic or lumbar spine** N

MED: 100-4,3,100.2

00670 **Anesthesia for extensive spine and spinal cord procedures (eg, spinal instrumentation or vascular procedures)** C

MED: 100-4,3,100.2; 100-4,4,10.4; 100-4,4,10.5; 100-4,4,10.10; 100-4,4,20.5; 100-4,4,20.6; 100-4,4,20.6.4; 100-4,4,61.2; 100-4,4,250.1.3; 100-4,4,250.3.1; 100-4,4,250.3.2; 100-4,4,250.3.3; 100-4,12,50; 100-4,12,140; 100-4,12,140.2; 100-4,12,140.3.2

UPPER ABDOMEN

00700 **Anesthesia for procedures on upper anterior abdominal wall; not otherwise specified** N

MED: 100-4,3,100.2; 100-4,4,10.4; 100-4,4,10.5; 100-4,4,10.10; 100-4,4,20.5; 100-4,4,20.6; 100-4,4,20.6.4; 100-4,4,61.2; 100-4,4,250.1.3; 100-4,4,250.3.1; 100-4,4,250.3.2; 100-4,4,250.3.3; 100-4,12,50; 100-4,12,140; 100-4,12,140.2; 100-4,12,140.3.2

Note 0070T must be used with code 93010.

00702 **percutaneous liver biopsy** N

MED: 100-4,3,100.2; 100-4,4,10.4; 100-4,4,10.5; 100-4,4,10.10; 100-4,4,20.5; 100-4,4,20.6; 100-4,4,20.6.4; 100-4,4,61.2; 100-4,4,250.1.3; 100-4,4,250.3.1; 100-4,4,250.3.2; 100-4,4,250.3.3; 100-4,12,50; 100-4,12,140; 100-4,12,140.2; 100-4,12,140.3.2

00730 **Anesthesia for procedures on upper posterior abdominal wall** N

MED: 100-4,3,100.2; 100-4,4,10.4; 100-4,4,10.5; 100-4,4,10.10; 100-4,4,20.5; 100-4,4,20.6; 100-4,4,20.6.4; 100-4,4,61.2; 100-4,4,250.1.3; 100-4,4,250.3.1; 100-4,4,250.3.2; 100-4,4,250.3.3; 100-4,12,50; 100-4,12,140; 100-4,12,140.2; 100-4,12,140.3.2

00740 **Anesthesia for upper gastrointestinal endoscopic procedures, endoscope introduced proximal to duodenum** N

MED: 100-4,3,100.2; 100-4,4,10.4; 100-4,4,10.5; 100-4,4,10.10; 100-4,4,20.5; 100-4,4,20.6; 100-4,4,20.6.4; 100-4,4,61.2; 100-4,4,250.1.3; 100-4,4,250.3.1; 100-4,4,250.3.2; 100-4,4,250.3.3; 100-4,12,50; 100-4,12,140; 100-4,12,140.2; 100-4,12,140.3.2

AMA: 1999,Nov,7

00750 **Anesthesia for hernia repairs in upper abdomen; not otherwise specified** N

MED: 100-4,3,100.2; 100-4,4,10.4; 100-4,4,10.5; 100-4,4,10.10; 100-4,4,20.5; 100-4,4,20.6; 100-4,4,20.6.4; 100-4,4,61.2; 100-4,4,250.1.3; 100-4,4,250.3.1; 100-4,4,250.3.2; 100-4,4,250.3.3; 100-4,12,50; 100-4,12,140; 100-4,12,140.2; 100-4,12,140.3.2

00752 **lumbar and ventral (incisional) hernias and/or wound dehiscence** N

MED: 100-4,3,100.2; 100-4,4,10.4; 100-4,4,10.5; 100-4,4,10.10; 100-4,4,20.5; 100-4,4,20.6; 100-4,4,20.6.4; 100-4,4,61.2; 100-4,4,250.1.3; 100-4,4,250.3.1; 100-4,4,250.3.2; 100-4,4,250.3.3; 100-4,12,50; 100-4,12,140; 100-4,12,140.2; 100-4,12,140.3.2

00754 **omphalocele** N

MED: 100-4,3,100.2; 100-4,4,10.4; 100-4,4,10.5; 100-4,4,10.10; 100-4,4,20.5; 100-4,4,20.6; 100-4,4,20.6.4; 100-4,4,61.2; 100-4,4,250.1.3; 100-4,4,250.3.1; 100-4,4,250.3.2; 100-4,4,250.3.3; 100-4,12,50; 100-4,12,140; 100-4,12,140.2; 100-4,12,140.3.2

00756 **transabdominal repair of diaphragmatic hernia** N

MED: 100-4,3,100.2; 100-4,4,10.4; 100-4,4,10.5; 100-4,4,10.10; 100-4,4,20.5; 100-4,4,20.6; 100-4,4,20.6.4; 100-4,4,61.2; 100-4,4,250.1.3; 100-4,4,250.3.1; 100-4,4,250.3.2; 100-4,4,250.3.3; 100-4,12,50; 100-4,12,140; 100-4,12,140.2; 100-4,12,140.3.2

00770 **Anesthesia for all procedures on major abdominal blood vessels** N

MED: 100-4,3,100.2; 100-4,4,10.4; 100-4,4,10.5; 100-4,4,10.10; 100-4,4,20.5; 100-4,4,20.6; 100-4,4,20.6.4; 100-4,4,61.2; 100-4,4,250.1.3; 100-4,4,250.3.1; 100-4,4,250.3.2; 100-4,4,250.3.3; 100-4,12,50; 100-4,12,140; 100-4,12,140.2; 100-4,12,140.3.2

00790 Anesthesia for intraperitoneal procedures in upper abdomen including laparoscopy; not otherwise specified Ⓝ ⟷

MED: 100-4,3,100.2; 100-4,4,10.4; 100-4,4,10.5; 100-4,4,10.10; 100-4,4,20.5; 100-4,4,20.6; 100-4,4,20.6.4; 100-4,4,61.2; 100-4,4,250.1.3; 100-4,4,250.3.1; 100-4,4,250.3.2; 100-4,4,250.3.3; 100-4,12,50; 100-4,12,140; 100-4,12,140.2; 100-4,12,140.3.2

00792 partial hepatectomy or management of liver hemorrhage (excluding liver biopsy) Ⓒ ⟷

MED: 100-4,3,100.2; 100-4,4,10.4; 100-4,4,10.5; 100-4,4,10.10; 100-4,4,20.5; 100-4,4,20.6; 100-4,4,20.6.4; 100-4,4,61.2; 100-4,4,250.1.3; 100-4,4,250.3.1; 100-4,4,250.3.2; 100-4,4,250.3.3; 100-4,12,50; 100-4,12,140; 100-4,12,140.2; 100-4,12,140.3.2

00794 pancreatectomy, partial or total (eg, Whipple procedure) Ⓒ ⟷

MED: 100-4,3,100.2; 100-4,4,10.4; 100-4,4,10.5; 100-4,4,10.10; 100-4,4,20.5; 100-4,4,20.6; 100-4,4,20.6.4; 100-4,4,61.2; 100-4,4,250.1.3; 100-4,4,250.3.1; 100-4,4,250.3.2; 100-4,4,250.3.3; 100-4,12,50; 100-4,12,140; 100-4,12,140.2; 100-4,12,140.3.2

00796 liver transplant (recipient) Ⓒ ⟷

MED: 100-4,3,100.2; 100-4,4,10.4; 100-4,4,10.5; 100-4,4,10.10; 100-4,4,20.5; 100-4,4,20.6; 100-4,4,20.6.4; 100-4,4,61.2; 100-4,4,250.1.3; 100-4,4,250.3.2; 100-4,4,250.3.3; 100-4,12,50; 100-4,12,140; 100-4,12,140.2; 100-4,12,140.3.2

To report anesthesia for harvesting of the liver, consult CPT code 01990.

00797 gastric restrictive procedure for morbid obesity Ⓝ ⟷

MED: 100-4,3,100.2

LOWER ABDOMEN

00800 Anesthesia for procedures on lower anterior abdominal wall; not otherwise specified Ⓝ ⟷

MED: 100-4,3,100.2; 100-4,4,10.4; 100-4,4,10.5; 100-4,4,10.10; 100-4,4,20.5; 100-4,4,20.6; 100-4,4,20.6.4; 100-4,4,61.2; 100-4,4,250.1.3; 100-4,4,250.3.1; 100-4,4,250.3.2; 100-4,4,250.3.3; 100-4,12,50; 100-4,12,140; 100-4,12,140.2; 100-4,12,140.3.2

00802 panniculectomy Ⓒ ⟷

MED: 100-4,3,100.2; 100-4,4,10.4; 100-4,4,10.5; 100-4,4,10.10; 100-4,4,20.5; 100-4,4,20.6; 100-4,4,20.6.4; 100-4,4,61.2; 100-4,4,250.1.3; 100-4,4,250.3.1; 100-4,4,250.3.2; 100-4,4,250.3.3; 100-4,12,50; 100-4,12,140; 100-4,12,140.2; 100-4,12,140.3.2

00810 Anesthesia for lower intestinal endoscopic procedures, endoscope introduced distal to duodenum Ⓝ ⟷

MED: 100-4,3,100.2; 100-4,4,10.4; 100-4,4,10.5; 100-4,4,10.10; 100-4,4,20.5; 100-4,4,20.6; 100-4,4,20.6.4; 100-4,4,61.2; 100-4,4,250.1.3; 100-4,4,250.3.1; 100-4,4,250.3.2; 100-4,4,250.3.3; 100-4,12,50; 100-4,12,140; 100-4,12,140.2; 100-4,12,140.3.2

AMA: 1999,Nov,7

00820 Anesthesia for procedures on lower posterior abdominal wall Ⓝ ⟷

MED: 100-4,3,100.2; 100-4,4,10.4; 100-4,4,10.5; 100-4,4,10.10; 100-4,4,20.5; 100-4,4,20.6; 100-4,4,20.6.4; 100-4,4,61.2; 100-4,4,250.1.3; 100-4,4,250.3.1; 100-4,4,250.3.2; 100-4,4,250.3.3; 100-4,12,50; 100-4,12,140; 100-4,12,140.2; 100-4,12,140.3.2

00830 Anesthesia for hernia repairs in lower abdomen; not otherwise specified Ⓝ ⟷

MED: 100-4,3,100.2; 100-4,4,10.4; 100-4,4,10.5; 100-4,4,10.10; 100-4,4,20.5; 100-4,4,20.6; 100-4,4,20.6.4; 100-4,4,61.2; 100-4,4,250.1.3; 100-4,4,250.3.1; 100-4,4,250.3.2; 100-4,4,250.3.3; 100-4,12,50; 100-4,12,140; 100-4,12,140.2; 100-4,12,140.3.2

00832 ventral and incisional hernias Ⓝ ⟷

MED: 100-4,3,100.2; 100-4,4,10.4; 100-4,4,10.5; 100-4,4,10.10; 100-4,4,20.5; 100-4,4,20.6; 100-4,4,20.6.4; 100-4,4,61.2; 100-4,4,250.1.3; 100-4,4,250.3.1; 100-4,4,250.3.2; 100-4,4,250.3.3; 100-4,12,50; 100-4,12,140; 100-4,12,140.2; 100-4,12,140.3.2

To report anesthesia for hernia repairs, infant age 1 year or less, consult CPT codes 00834, 00836.

▲ **00834** Anesthesia for hernia repairs in the lower abdomen not otherwise specified, younger than 1 year of age Ⓐ Ⓝ ⟷

MED: 100-4,3,100.2

Note that code 00834 cannot be reported with CPT code 99100.

▲ **00836** Anesthesia for hernia repairs in the lower abdomen not otherwise specified, infants younger than 37 weeks gestational age at birth and younger than 50 weeks gestational age at time of surgery Ⓐ Ⓝ ⟷

MED: 100-4,3,100.2

Note that code 00836 cannot be reported with CPT code 99100.

00840 Anesthesia for intraperitoneal procedures in lower abdomen including laparoscopy; not otherwise specified Ⓝ ⟷

MED: 100-4,3,100.2; 100-4,4,10.4; 100-4,4,10.5; 100-4,4,10.10; 100-4,4,20.5; 100-4,4,20.6; 100-4,4,20.6.4; 100-4,4,61.2; 100-4,4,250.1.3; 100-4,4,250.3.1; 100-4,4,250.3.2; 100-4,4,250.3.3; 100-4,12,50; 100-4,12,140; 100-4,12,140.2; 100-4,12,140.3.2

00842 amniocentesis Ⓜ ♀ Ⓝ ⟷

MED: 100-4,3,100.2; 100-4,4,10.4; 100-4,4,10.5; 100-4,4,10.10; 100-4,4,20.5; 100-4,4,20.6; 100-4,4,20.6.4; 100-4,4,61.2; 100-4,4,250.1.3; 100-4,4,250.3.1; 100-4,4,250.3.2; 100-4,4,250.3.3; 100-4,12,50; 100-4,12,140; 100-4,12,140.2; 100-4,12,140.3.2

00844 abdominoperineal resection Ⓒ ⟷

MED: 100-4,3,100.2; 100-4,4,10.4; 100-4,4,10.5; 100-4,4,10.10; 100-4,4,20.5; 100-4,4,20.6; 100-4,4,20.6.4; 100-4,4,61.2; 100-4,4,250.1.3; 100-4,4,250.3.1; 100-4,4,250.3.2; 100-4,4,250.3.3; 100-4,12,50; 100-4,12,140; 100-4,12,140.2; 100-4,12,140.3.2

00846 radical hysterectomy ♀ Ⓒ ⟷

MED: 100-4,3,100.2; 100-4,4,10.4; 100-4,4,10.5; 100-4,4,10.10; 100-4,4,20.5; 100-4,4,20.6; 100-4,4,20.6.4; 100-4,4,61.2; 100-4,4,250.1.3; 100-4,4,250.3.1; 100-4,4,250.3.2; 100-4,4,250.3.3; 100-4,12,50; 100-4,12,140; 100-4,12,140.2; 100-4,12,140.3.2

00848 pelvic exenteration Ⓒ ⟷

MED: 100-4,3,100.2; 100-4,4,10.4; 100-4,4,10.5; 100-4,4,10.10; 100-4,4,20.5; 100-4,4,20.6; 100-4,4,20.6.4; 100-4,4,61.2; 100-4,4,250.1.3; 100-4,4,250.3.1; 100-4,4,250.3.2; 100-4,4,250.3.3; 100-4,12,50; 100-4,12,140; 100-4,12,140.2; 100-4,12,140.3.2

00851 tubal ligation/transection ♀ Ⓝ ⟷

MED: 100-4,3,100.2

00860 Anesthesia for extraperitoneal procedures in lower abdomen, including urinary tract; not otherwise specified Ⓝ ⟷

MED: 100-4,3,100.2; 100-4,4,10.4; 100-4,4,10.5; 100-4,4,10.10; 100-4,4,20.5; 100-4,4,20.6; 100-4,4,20.6.4; 100-4,4,61.2; 100-4,4,250.1.3; 100-4,4,250.3.1; 100-4,4,250.3.2; 100-4,4,250.3.3; 100-4,12,50; 100-4,12,140; 100-4,12,140.2; 100-4,12,140.3.2

▲ **00862** renal procedures, including upper one-third of ureter, or donor nephrectomy Ⓝ ⟷

MED: 100-4,3,100.2; 100-4,4,10.4; 100-4,4,10.5; 100-4,4,10.10; 100-4,4,20.5; 100-4,4,20.6; 100-4,4,20.6.4; 100-4,4,61.2; 100-4,4,250.1.3; 100-4,4,250.3.1; 100-4,4,250.3.2; 100-4,4,250.3.3; 100-4,12,50; 100-4,12,140; 100-4,12,140.2; 100-4,12,140.3.2

00864 total cystectomy Ⓒ ⟷

MED: 100-4,3,100.2; 100-4,4,10.4; 100-4,4,10.5; 100-4,4,10.10; 100-4,4,20.5; 100-4,4,20.6; 100-4,4,20.6.4; 100-4,4,61.2; 100-4,4,250.1.3; 100-4,4,250.3.1; 100-4,4,250.3.2; 100-4,4,250.3.3; 100-4,12,50; 100-4,12,140; 100-4,12,140.2; 100-4,12,140.3.2

00865 radical prostatectomy (suprapubic, retropubic) ♂ Ⓒ ⟷

00866 adrenalectomy Ⓒ ⟷

MED: 100-4,3,100.2; 100-4,4,10.4; 100-4,4,10.5; 100-4,4,10.10; 100-4,4,20.5; 100-4,4,20.6; 100-4,4,20.6.4; 100-4,4,61.2; 100-4,4,250.1.3; 100-4,4,250.3.1; 100-4,4,250.3.2; 100-4,4,250.3.3; 100-4,12,50; 100-4,12,140; 100-4,12,140.2; 100-4,12,140.3.2

00868	renal transplant (recipient)	C ⟷

MED: 100-4,3,100.2; 100-4,4,10.4; 100-4,4,10.5; 100-4,4,10.10; 100-4,4,20.5; 100-4,4,20.6; 100-4,4,20.6.4; 100-4,4,61.2; 100-4,4,250.1.3; 100-4,4,250.3.1; 100-4,4,250.3.2; 100-4,4,250.3.3; 100-4,12,50; 100-4,12,140; 100-4,12,140.2; 100-4,12,140.3.2

To report anesthesia for donor nephrectomy, consult CPT code 00862. To report anesthesia for harvesting a kidney from a brain-dead patient, consult CPT code 01990.

00870	cystolithotomy	N ⟷

MED: 100-4,3,100.2; 100-4,4,10.4; 100-4,4,10.5; 100-4,4,10.10; 100-4,4,20.5; 100-4,4,20.6; 100-4,4,20.6.4; 100-4,4,61.2; 100-4,4,250.1.3; 100-4,4,250.3.1; 100-4,4,250.3.2; 100-4,4,250.3.3; 100-4,12,50; 100-4,12,140; 100-4,12,140.2; 100-4,12,140.3.2

00872	Anesthesia for lithotripsy, extracorporeal shock wave; with water bath	N ⟷

MED: 100-4,3,100.2; 100-4,4,10.4; 100-4,4,10.5; 100-4,4,10.10; 100-4,4,20.5; 100-4,4,20.6; 100-4,4,20.6.4; 100-4,4,61.2; 100-4,4,250.1.3; 100-4,4,250.3.1; 100-4,4,250.3.2; 100-4,4,250.3.3; 100-4,12,50; 100-4,12,140; 100-4,12,140.2; 100-4,12,140.3.2

00873	without water bath	N ⟷

MED: 100-4,3,100.2; 100-4,4,10.4; 100-4,4,10.5; 100-4,4,10.10; 100-4,4,20.5; 100-4,4,20.6; 100-4,4,20.6.4; 100-4,4,61.2; 100-4,4,250.1.3; 100-4,4,250.3.1; 100-4,4,250.3.2; 100-4,4,250.3.3; 100-4,12,50; 100-4,12,140; 100-4,12,140.2; 100-4,12,140.3.2

00880	Anesthesia for procedures on major lower abdominal vessels; not otherwise specified	N ⟷

MED: 100-4,3,100.2; 100-4,4,10.4; 100-4,4,10.5; 100-4,4,10.10; 100-4,4,20.5; 100-4,4,20.6; 100-4,4,20.6.4; 100-4,4,61.2; 100-4,4,250.1.3; 100-4,4,250.3.1; 100-4,4,250.3.2; 100-4,4,250.3.3; 100-4,12,50; 100-4,12,140; 100-4,12,140.2; 100-4,12,140.3.2

00882	inferior vena cava ligation	C ⟷

MED: 100-4,3,100.2; 100-4,4,10.4; 100-4,4,10.5; 100-4,4,10.10; 100-4,4,20.5; 100-4,4,20.6; 100-4,4,20.6.4; 100-4,4,61.2; 100-4,4,250.1.3; 100-4,4,250.3.1; 100-4,4,250.3.2; 100-4,4,250.3.3; 100-4,12,50; 100-4,12,140; 100-4,12,140.2; 100-4,12,140.3.2

PERINEUM

00902	Anesthesia for; anorectal procedure	N ⟷

MED: 100-4,3,100.2; 100-4,4,10.4; 100-4,4,10.5; 100-4,4,10.10; 100-4,4,20.5; 100-4,4,20.6; 100-4,4,20.6.4; 100-4,4,61.2; 100-4,4,250.1.3; 100-4,4,250.3.1; 100-4,4,250.3.2; 100-4,4,250.3.3; 100-4,12,50; 100-4,12,140; 100-4,12,140.2; 100-4,12,140.3.2

00904	radical perineal procedure	C ⟷

MED: 100-4,3,100.2; 100-4,4,10.4; 100-4,4,10.5; 100-4,4,10.10; 100-4,4,20.5; 100-4,4,20.6; 100-4,4,20.6.4; 100-4,4,61.2; 100-4,4,250.1.3; 100-4,4,250.3.1; 100-4,4,250.3.2; 100-4,4,250.3.3; 100-4,12,50; 100-4,12,140; 100-4,12,140.2; 100-4,12,140.3.2

00906	vulvectomy	♀ N ⟷

MED: 100-4,3,100.2; 100-4,4,10.4; 100-4,4,10.5; 100-4,4,10.10; 100-4,4,20.5; 100-4,4,20.6; 100-4,4,20.6.4; 100-4,4,61.2; 100-4,4,250.1.3; 100-4,4,250.3.1; 100-4,4,250.3.2; 100-4,4,250.3.3; 100-4,12,50; 100-4,12,140; 100-4,12,140.2; 100-4,12,140.3.2

00908	perineal prostatectomy	♂ C ⟷

MED: 100-4,3,100.2; 100-4,4,10.4; 100-4,4,10.5; 100-4,4,10.10; 100-4,4,20.5; 100-4,4,20.6; 100-4,4,20.6.4; 100-4,4,61.2; 100-4,4,250.1.3; 100-4,4,250.3.1; 100-4,4,250.3.2; 100-4,4,250.3.3; 100-4,12,50; 100-4,12,140; 100-4,12,140.2; 100-4,12,140.3.2

00910	Anesthesia for transurethral procedures (including urethrocystoscopy); not otherwise specified	N ⟷

MED: 100-4,3,100.2; 100-4,4,10.4; 100-4,4,10.5; 100-4,4,10.10; 100-4,4,20.5; 100-4,4,20.6; 100-4,4,20.6.4; 100-4,4,61.2; 100-4,4,250.1.3; 100-4,4,250.3.1; 100-4,4,250.3.2; 100-4,4,250.3.3; 100-4,12,50; 100-4,12,140; 100-4,12,140.2; 100-4,12,140.3.2

00912	transurethral resection of bladder tumor(s)	N ⟷

MED: 100-4,3,100.2; 100-4,4,10.4; 100-4,4,10.5; 100-4,4,10.10; 100-4,4,20.5; 100-4,4,20.6; 100-4,4,20.6.4; 100-4,4,61.2; 100-4,4,250.1.3; 100-4,4,250.3.1; 100-4,4,250.3.2; 100-4,4,250.3.3; 100-4,12,50; 100-4,12,140; 100-4,12,140.2; 100-4,12,140.3.2

00914	transurethral resection of prostate	♂ N ⟷

MED: 100-4,3,100.2; 100-4,4,10.4; 100-4,4,10.5; 100-4,4,10.10; 100-4,4,20.5; 100-4,4,20.6; 100-4,4,20.6.4; 100-4,4,61.2; 100-4,4,250.1.3; 100-4,4,250.3.1; 100-4,4,250.3.2; 100-4,4,250.3.3; 100-4,12,50; 100-4,12,140; 100-4,12,140.2; 100-4,12,140.3.2

00916	post-transurethral resection bleeding	N ⟷

MED: 100-4,3,100.2; 100-4,4,10.4; 100-4,4,10.5; 100-4,4,10.10; 100-4,4,20.5; 100-4,4,20.6; 100-4,4,20.6.4; 100-4,4,61.2; 100-4,4,250.1.3; 100-4,4,250.3.1; 100-4,4,250.3.2; 100-4,4,250.3.3; 100-4,12,50; 100-4,12,140; 100-4,12,140.2; 100-4,12,140.3.2

00918	with fragmentation, manipulation and/or removal of ureteral calculus	N ⟷

MED: 100-4,3,100.2; 100-4,4,10.4; 100-4,4,10.5; 100-4,4,10.10; 100-4,4,20.5; 100-4,4,20.6; 100-4,4,20.6.4; 100-4,4,61.2; 100-4,4,250.1.3; 100-4,4,250.3.1; 100-4,4,250.3.2; 100-4,4,250.3.3; 100-4,12,50; 100-4,12,140; 100-4,12,140.2; 100-4,12,140.3.2

AMA: 1999,Nov,8

00920	Anesthesia for procedures on male genitalia (including open urethral procedures); not otherwise specified	♂ N ⟷

MED: 100-4,3,100.2; 100-4,4,10.4; 100-4,4,10.5; 100-4,4,10.10; 100-4,4,20.5; 100-4,4,20.6; 100-4,4,20.6.4; 100-4,4,61.2; 100-4,4,250.1.3; 100-4,4,250.3.1; 100-4,4,250.3.2; 100-4,4,250.3.3; 100-4,12,50; 100-4,12,140; 100-4,12,140.2; 100-4,12,140.3.2

00921	vasectomy, unilateral or bilateral	♂ N ⟷

MED: 100-4,3,100.2

00922	seminal vesicles	♂ N ⟷

MED: 100-4,3,100.2; 100-4,4,10.4; 100-4,4,10.5; 100-4,4,10.10; 100-4,4,20.5; 100-4,4,20.6; 100-4,4,20.6.4; 100-4,4,61.2; 100-4,4,250.1.3; 100-4,4,250.3.1; 100-4,4,250.3.2; 100-4,4,250.3.3; 100-4,12,50; 100-4,12,140; 100-4,12,140.2; 100-4,12,140.3.2

00924	undescended testis, unilateral or bilateral	♂ N ⟷

MED: 100-4,3,100.2; 100-4,4,10.4; 100-4,4,10.5; 100-4,4,10.10; 100-4,4,20.5; 100-4,4,20.6; 100-4,4,20.6.4; 100-4,4,61.2; 100-4,4,250.1.3; 100-4,4,250.3.1; 100-4,4,250.3.2; 100-4,4,250.3.3; 100-4,12,50; 100-4,12,140; 100-4,12,140.2; 100-4,12,140.3.2

00926	radical orchiectomy, inguinal	♂ N ⟷

MED: 100-4,3,100.2; 100-4,4,10.4; 100-4,4,10.5; 100-4,4,10.10; 100-4,4,20.5; 100-4,4,20.6; 100-4,4,20.6.4; 100-4,4,61.2; 100-4,4,250.1.3; 100-4,4,250.3.1; 100-4,4,250.3.2; 100-4,4,250.3.3; 100-4,12,50; 100-4,12,140; 100-4,12,140.2; 100-4,12,140.3.2

00928	radical orchiectomy, abdominal	♂ N ⟷

MED: 100-4,3,100.2; 100-4,4,10.4; 100-4,4,10.5; 100-4,4,10.10; 100-4,4,20.5; 100-4,4,20.6; 100-4,4,20.6.4; 100-4,4,61.2; 100-4,4,250.1.3; 100-4,4,250.3.1; 100-4,4,250.3.2; 100-4,4,250.3.3; 100-4,12,50; 100-4,12,140; 100-4,12,140.2; 100-4,12,140.3.2

00930	orchiopexy, unilateral or bilateral	♂ N ⟷

MED: 100-4,3,100.2; 100-4,4,10.4; 100-4,4,10.5; 100-4,4,10.10; 100-4,4,20.5; 100-4,4,20.6; 100-4,4,20.6.4; 100-4,4,61.2; 100-4,4,250.1.3; 100-4,4,250.3.1; 100-4,4,250.3.2; 100-4,4,250.3.3; 100-4,12,50; 100-4,12,140; 100-4,12,140.2; 100-4,12,140.3.2

00932	complete amputation of penis	♂ C ⟷

MED: 100-4,3,100.2; 100-4,4,10.4; 100-4,4,10.5; 100-4,4,10.10; 100-4,4,20.5; 100-4,4,20.6; 100-4,4,20.6.4; 100-4,4,61.2; 100-4,4,250.1.3; 100-4,4,250.3.1; 100-4,4,250.3.2; 100-4,4,250.3.3; 100-4,12,50; 100-4,12,140; 100-4,12,140.2; 100-4,12,140.3.2

00934	radical amputation of penis with bilateral inguinal lymphadenectomy	♂ C ⟷

MED: 100-4,3,100.2; 100-4,4,10.4; 100-4,4,10.5; 100-4,4,10.10; 100-4,4,20.5; 100-4,4,20.6; 100-4,4,20.6.4; 100-4,4,61.2; 100-4,4,250.1.3; 100-4,4,250.3.1; 100-4,4,250.3.2; 100-4,4,250.3.3; 100-4,12,50; 100-4,12,140; 100-4,12,140.2; 100-4,12,140.3.2

00936   radical amputation of penis with bilateral inguinal and iliac lymphadenectomy   ♂ Ⓒ 🔲

MED: 100-4,3,100.2; 100-4,4,10.4; 100-4,4,10.5; 100-4,4,10.10; 100-4,4,20.5; 100-4,4,20.6; 100-4,4,20.6.4; 100-4,4,61.2; 100-4,4,250.1.3; 100-4,4,250.3.1; 100-4,4,250.3.2; 100-4,4,250.3.3; 100-4,12,50; 100-4,12,140; 100-4,12,140.2; 100-4,12,140.3.2

00938   insertion of penile prosthesis (perineal approach)   ♂ Ⓝ 🔲

MED: 100-4,3,100.2; 100-4,4,10.4; 100-4,4,10.5; 100-4,4,10.10; 100-4,4,20.5; 100-4,4,20.6; 100-4,4,20.6.4; 100-4,4,61.2; 100-4,4,250.1.3; 100-4,4,250.3.1; 100-4,4,250.3.2; 100-4,4,250.3.3; 100-4,12,50; 100-4,12,140; 100-4,12,140.2; 100-4,12,140.3.2

00940   Anesthesia for vaginal procedures (including biopsy of labia, vagina, cervix or endometrium); **not otherwise specified**   ♀ Ⓝ 🔲

MED: 100-4,3,100.2; 100-4,4,10.4; 100-4,4,10.5; 100-4,4,10.10; 100-4,4,20.5; 100-4,4,20.6; 100-4,4,20.6.4; 100-4,4,61.2; 100-4,4,250.1.3; 100-4,4,250.3.1; 100-4,4,250.3.2; 100-4,4,250.3.3; 100-4,12,50; 100-4,12,140; 100-4,12,140.2; 100-4,12,140.3.2

00942   colpotomy, vaginectomy, colporrhaphy, and open urethral procedures   ♀ Ⓝ 🔲

MED: 100-4,3,100.2; 100-4,4,10.4; 100-4,4,10.5; 100-4,4,10.10; 100-4,4,20.5; 100-4,4,20.6; 100-4,4,20.6.4; 100-4,4,61.2; 100-4,4,250.1.3; 100-4,4,250.3.1; 100-4,4,250.3.2; 100-4,4,250.3.3; 100-4,12,50; 100-4,12,140; 100-4,12,140.2; 100-4,12,140.3.2

00944   vaginal hysterectomy   ♀ Ⓒ 🔲

MED: 100-4,3,100.2; 100-4,4,10.4; 100-4,4,10.5; 100-4,4,10.10; 100-4,4,20.5; 100-4,4,20.6; 100-4,4,20.6.4; 100-4,4,61.2; 100-4,4,250.1.3; 100-4,4,250.3.1; 100-4,4,250.3.2; 100-4,4,250.3.3; 100-4,12,50; 100-4,12,140; 100-4,12,140.2; 100-4,12,140.3.2

00948   cervical cerclage   ♀ Ⓝ 🔲

MED: 100-4,3,100.2; 100-4,4,10.4; 100-4,4,10.5; 100-4,4,10.10; 100-4,4,20.5; 100-4,4,20.6; 100-4,4,20.6.4; 100-4,4,61.2; 100-4,4,250.1.3; 100-4,4,250.3.1; 100-4,4,250.3.2; 100-4,4,250.3.3; 100-4,12,50; 100-4,12,140; 100-4,12,140.2; 100-4,12,140.3.2

00950   culdoscopy   ♀ Ⓝ 🔲

MED: 100-4,3,100.2; 100-4,4,10.4; 100-4,4,10.5; 100-4,4,10.10; 100-4,4,20.5; 100-4,4,20.6; 100-4,4,20.6.4; 100-4,4,61.2; 100-4,4,250.1.3; 100-4,4,250.3.1; 100-4,4,250.3.2; 100-4,4,250.3.3; 100-4,12,50; 100-4,12,140; 100-4,12,140.2; 100-4,12,140.3.2

00952   hysteroscopy and/or hysterosalpingography   ♀ Ⓝ 🔲

MED: 100-4,3,100.2; 100-4,4,10.4; 100-4,4,10.5; 100-4,4,10.10; 100-4,4,20.5; 100-4,4,20.6; 100-4,4,20.6.4; 100-4,4,61.2; 100-4,4,250.1.3; 100-4,4,250.3.2; 100-4,4,250.3.3; 100-4,12,50; 100-4,12,140; 100-4,12,140.2; 100-4,12,140.3.2

AMA: 1999,Nov,8

PELVIS (EXCEPT HIP)

01112   Anesthesia for bone marrow aspiration and/or biopsy, anterior or posterior iliac crest   Ⓝ ⊙

MED: 100-1,5,90.2; 100-2,15,80; 100-2,15,80.1; 100-4,3,100.2; 100-4,16,10; 100-4,16,10.1; 100-4,16,110.4

01120   Anesthesia for procedures on bony pelvis   Ⓝ 🔲

MED: 100-4,3,100.2; 100-4,12,50; 100-4,12,140; 100-4,12,140.2; 100-4,12,140.3.2

01130   Anesthesia for body cast application or revision   Ⓝ 🔲

MED: 100-4,3,100.2; 100-4,12,50; 100-4,12,140; 100-4,12,140.2; 100-4,12,140.3.2

01140   Anesthesia for interpelviabdominal (hindquarter) amputation   Ⓒ 🔲

MED: 100-4,3,100.2; 100-4,12,50; 100-4,12,140; 100-4,12,140.2; 100-4,12,140.3.2

01150   Anesthesia for radical procedures for tumor of pelvis, except hindquarter amputation   Ⓒ 🔲

MED: 100-4,3,100.2; 100-4,12,50; 100-4,12,140; 100-4,12,140.2; 100-4,12,140.3.2

01160   Anesthesia for closed procedures involving symphysis pubis or sacroiliac joint   Ⓝ 🔲

MED: 100-4,3,100.2; 100-4,12,50; 100-4,12,140; 100-4,12,140.2; 100-4,12,140.3.2

01170   Anesthesia for open procedures involving symphysis pubis or sacroiliac joint   Ⓝ 🔲

MED: 100-4,3,100.2; 100-4,12,50; 100-4,12,140; 100-4,12,140.2; 100-4,12,140.3.2

01173   Anesthesia for open repair of fracture disruption of pelvis or column fracture involving acetabulum   Ⓝ 🔲

MED: 100-4,3,100.2

01180   Anesthesia for obturator neurectomy; extrapelvic   Ⓝ 🔲

MED: 100-4,3,100.2; 100-4,12,50; 100-4,12,140; 100-4,12,140.2; 100-4,12,140.3.2

01190   intrapelvic   Ⓝ 🔲

MED: 100-4,3,100.2; 100-4,12,50; 100-4,12,140; 100-4,12,140.2; 100-4,12,140.3.2

UPPER LEG (EXCEPT KNEE)

01200   Anesthesia for all closed procedures involving hip joint   Ⓝ 🔲

MED: 100-4,3,100.2; 100-4,12,50; 100-4,12,140; 100-4,12,140.2; 100-4,12,140.3.2

01202   Anesthesia for arthroscopic procedures of hip joint   Ⓝ 🔲

MED: 100-4,3,100.2; 100-4,12,50; 100-4,12,140; 100-4,12,140.2; 100-4,12,140.3.2

01210   Anesthesia for open procedures involving hip joint; not otherwise specified   Ⓝ 🔲

MED: 100-4,3,100.2; 100-4,12,50; 100-4,12,140; 100-4,12,140.2; 100-4,12,140.3.2

01212   hip disarticulation   Ⓒ 🔲

MED: 100-4,3,100.2; 100-4,12,50; 100-4,12,140; 100-4,12,140.2; 100-4,12,140.3.2

01214   total hip arthroplasty   Ⓒ 🔲

MED: 100-4,3,100.2; 100-4,12,50; 100-4,12,140; 100-4,12,140.2; 100-4,12,140.3.2

01215   revision of total hip arthroplasty   Ⓝ 🔲

MED: 100-4,3,100.2

01220   Anesthesia for all closed procedures involving upper two-thirds of femur   Ⓝ 🔲

MED: 100-4,3,100.2; 100-4,12,50; 100-4,12,140; 100-4,12,140.2; 100-4,12,140.3.2

▲ **01230**   Anesthesia for open procedures involving upper two-thirds of femur; not otherwise specified   Ⓝ 🔲

MED: 100-4,3,100.2; 100-4,12,50; 100-4,12,140; 100-4,12,140.2; 100-4,12,140.3.2

▲ **01232**   amputation   Ⓒ 🔲

MED: 100-4,3,100.2; 100-4,12,50; 100-4,12,140; 100-4,12,140.2; 100-4,12,140.3.2

▲ **01234**   radical resection   Ⓒ 🔲

MED: 100-4,3,100.2

01250   Anesthesia for all procedures on nerves, muscles, tendons, fascia, and bursae of upper leg   Ⓝ 🔲

MED: 100-4,3,100.2; 100-4,12,50; 100-4,12,140; 100-4,12,140.2; 100-4,12,140.3.2

Anesthesia

01260 — 01490

01260	Anesthesia for all procedures involving veins of upper leg, including exploration N ⬚

MED: 100-4,3,100.2; 100-4,12,50; 100-4,12,140; 100-4,12,140.2; 100-4,12,140.3.2

01270	Anesthesia for procedures involving arteries of upper leg, including bypass graft; not otherwise specified N ⬚

MED: 100-4,3,100.2

01272	femoral artery ligation C ⬚

MED: 100-4,3,100.2

01274	femoral artery embolectomy C ⬚

MED: 100-4,3,100.2; 100-4,12,50; 100-4,12,140; 100-4,12,140.2; 100-4,12,140.3.2

KNEE AND POPLITEAL AREA

Diagnostic endoscopy/arthroscopy is always included in surgical endoscopy/arthroscopy, do not report separately.

01320	Anesthesia for all procedures on nerves, muscles, tendons, fascia, and bursae of knee and/or popliteal area N ⬚

MED: 100-4,3,100.2; 100-4,12,50; 100-4,12,140; 100-4,12,140.2; 100-4,12,140.3.2

▲ 01340	Anesthesia for all closed procedures on lower one-third of femur N ⬚

MED: 100-4,3,100.2; 100-4,12,50; 100-4,12,140; 100-4,12,140.2; 100-4,12,140.3.2

▲ 01360	Anesthesia for all open procedures on lower one-third of femur N ⬚

MED: 100-4,3,100.2; 100-4,12,50; 100-4,12,140; 100-4,12,140.2; 100-4,12,140.3.2

01380	Anesthesia for all closed procedures on knee joint N ⬚

MED: 100-4,3,100.2; 100-4,12,50; 100-4,12,140; 100-4,12,140.2; 100-4,12,140.3.2

01382	Anesthesia for diagnostic arthroscopic procedures of knee joint N ⬚

MED: 100-4,3,100.2; 100-4,12,50; 100-4,12,140; 100-4,12,140.2; 100-4,12,140.3.2

01390	Anesthesia for all closed procedures on upper ends of tibia, fibula, and/or patella N ⬚

MED: 100-4,3,100.2; 100-4,12,50; 100-4,12,140; 100-4,12,140.2; 100-4,12,140.3.2

01392	Anesthesia for all open procedures on upper ends of tibia, fibula, and/or patella N ⬚

MED: 100-4,3,100.2; 100-4,12,50; 100-4,12,140; 100-4,12,140.2; 100-4,12,140.3.2

01400	Anesthesia for open or surgical arthroscopic procedures on knee joint; not otherwise specified N ⬚

MED: 100-4,3,100.2; 100-4,12,50; 100-4,12,140; 100-4,12,140.2; 100-4,12,140.3.2

01402	total knee arthroplasty C ⬚

MED: 100-4,3,100.2; 100-4,12,50; 100-4,12,140; 100-4,12,140.2; 100-4,12,140.3.2

01404	disarticulation at knee C ⬚

MED: 100-4,3,100.2; 100-4,12,50; 100-4,12,140; 100-4,12,140.2; 100-4,12,140.3.2

01420	Anesthesia for all cast applications, removal, or repair involving knee joint N ⬚

MED: 100-4,3,100.2; 100-4,12,50; 100-4,12,140; 100-4,12,140.2; 100-4,12,140.3.2

01430	Anesthesia for procedures on veins of knee and popliteal area; not otherwise specified N ⬚

MED: 100-4,3,100.2

01432	arteriovenous fistula N ⬚

MED: 100-4,3,100.2

01440	Anesthesia for procedures on arteries of knee and popliteal area; not otherwise specified N ⬚

MED: 100-4,3,100.2; 100-4,12,50; 100-4,12,140; 100-4,12,140.2; 100-4,12,140.3.2

01442	popliteal thromboendarterectomy, with or without patch graft C ⬚

MED: 100-4,3,100.2; 100-4,12,50; 100-4,12,140; 100-4,12,140.2; 100-4,12,140.3.2

01444	popliteal excision and graft or repair for occlusion or aneurysm C ⬚

MED: 100-4,3,100.2

LOWER LEG (BELOW KNEE, INCLUDES ANKLE AND FOOT)

Diagnostic endoscopy/arthroscopy is always included in surgical endoscopy/arthroscopy; do not report separately.

01462	Anesthesia for all closed procedures on lower leg, ankle, and foot N ⬚

MED: 100-4,3,100.2

01464	Anesthesia for arthroscopic procedures of ankle and/or foot N ⬚

MED: 100-4,3,100.2; 100-4,12,50; 100-4,12,140; 100-4,12,140.2; 100-4,12,140.3.2

01470	Anesthesia for procedures on nerves, muscles, tendons, and fascia of lower leg, ankle, and foot; not otherwise specified N ⬚

MED: 100-4,3,100.2; 100-4,12,50; 100-4,12,140; 100-4,12,140.2; 100-4,12,140.3.2

01472	repair of ruptured Achilles tendon, with or without graft N ⬚

MED: 100-4,3,100.2; 100-4,12,50; 100-4,12,140; 100-4,12,140.2; 100-4,12,140.3.2

01474	gastrocnemius recession (eg, Strayer procedure) N ⬚

MED: 100-4,3,100.2; 100-4,12,50; 100-4,12,140; 100-4,12,140.2; 100-4,12,140.3.2

01480	Anesthesia for open procedures on bones of lower leg, ankle, and foot; not otherwise specified N ⬚

MED: 100-4,3,100.2; 100-4,12,50; 100-4,12,140; 100-4,12,140.2; 100-4,12,140.3.2

01482	radical resection (including below knee amputation) N ⬚

MED: 100-4,3,100.2; 100-4,12,50; 100-4,12,140; 100-4,12,140.2; 100-4,12,140.3.2

01484	osteotomy or osteoplasty of tibia and/or fibula N ⬚

MED: 100-4,3,100.2; 100-4,12,50; 100-4,12,140; 100-4,12,140.2; 100-4,12,140.3.2

01486	total ankle replacement C ⬚

MED: 100-4,3,100.2; 100-4,12,50; 100-4,12,140; 100-4,12,140.2; 100-4,12,140.3.2

01490	Anesthesia for lower leg cast application, removal, or repair N ⬚

MED: 100-4,3,100.2; 100-4,12,50; 100-4,12,140; 100-4,12,140.2; 100-4,12,140.3.2

26 Professional Component Only   80/80 Assist-at-Surgery Allowed/With Documentation   Unlisted   Not Covered

TC Technical Component Only   MED: Pub 100/NCD References   AMA: CPT Assistant References   1-9 ASC Group   ♂ Male Only   ♀ Female Only

36 — CPT Expert   CPT only © 2006 American Medical Association. All Rights Reserved. (Black Ink)   © 2006 Ingenix (Blue Ink)

01500 Anesthesia for procedures on arteries of lower leg, including bypass graft; not otherwise specified N ⚡

MED: 100-4,3,100.2; 100-4,12,50; 100-4,12,140; 100-4,12,140.2; 100-4,12,140.3.2

01502 embolectomy, direct or with catheter C ⚡

MED: 100-4,3,100.2; 100-4,12,50; 100-4,12,140; 100-4,12,140.2; 100-4,12,140.3.2

01520 Anesthesia for procedures on veins of lower leg; not otherwise specified N ⚡

MED: 100-4,3,100.2; 100-4,12,50; 100-4,12,140; 100-4,12,140.2; 100-4,12,140.3.2

01522 venous thrombectomy, direct or with catheter N ⚡

MED: 100-4,3,100.2; 100-4,12,50; 100-4,12,140; 100-4,12,140.2; 100-4,12,140.3.2

SHOULDER AND AXILLA

Diagnostic endoscopy/arthroscopy is always included in surgical endoscopy/arthroscopy; do not report separately.

These codes include procedures performed on the humeral head and neck, sternoclavicular, acromioclavicular, and shoulder joints.

01610 Anesthesia for all procedures on nerves, muscles, tendons, fascia, and bursae of shoulder and axilla N ⚡

MED: 100-4,3,100.2; 100-4,12,50; 100-4,12,140; 100-4,12,140.2; 100-4,12,140.3.2

01620 Anesthesia for all closed procedures on humeral head and neck, sternoclavicular joint, acromioclavicular joint, and shoulder joint N ⚡

MED: 100-4,3,100.2; 100-4,12,50; 100-4,12,140; 100-4,12,140.2; 100-4,12,140.3.2

01622 Anesthesia for diagnostic arthroscopic procedures of shoulder joint N ⚡

MED: 100-4,3,100.2; 100-4,12,50; 100-4,12,140; 100-4,12,140.2; 100-4,12,140.3.2

01630 Anesthesia for open or surgical arthroscopic procedures on humeral head and neck, sternoclavicular joint, acromioclavicular joint, and shoulder joint; not otherwise specified N ⚡

MED: 100-4,3,100.2; 100-4,12,50; 100-4,12,140; 100-4,12,140.2; 100-4,12,140.3.2

01632 radical resection C ⚡

MED: 100-4,3,100.2; 100-4,12,50; 100-4,12,140; 100-4,12,140.2; 100-4,12,140.3.2

01634 shoulder disarticulation C ⚡

MED: 100-4,3,100.2; 100-4,12,50; 100-4,12,140; 100-4,12,140.2; 100-4,12,140.3.2

01636 interthoracoscapular (forequarter) amputation C ⚡

MED: 100-4,3,100.2; 100-4,12,50; 100-4,12,140; 100-4,12,140.2; 100-4,12,140.3.2

01638 total shoulder replacement C ⚡

MED: 100-4,3,100.2; 100-4,12,50; 100-4,12,140; 100-4,12,140.2; 100-4,12,140.3.2

01650 Anesthesia for procedures on arteries of shoulder and axilla; not otherwise specified N ⚡

MED: 100-4,3,100.2; 100-4,12,50; 100-4,12,140; 100-4,12,140.2; 100-4,12,140.3.2

01652 axillary-brachial aneurysm C ⚡

MED: 100-4,3,100.2; 100-4,12,50; 100-4,12,140; 100-4,12,140.2; 100-4,12,140.3.2

01654 bypass graft C ⚡

MED: 100-4,3,100.2; 100-4,12,50; 100-4,12,140; 100-4,12,140.2; 100-4,12,140.3.2

01656 axillary-femoral bypass graft C ⚡

MED: 100-4,3,100.2; 100-4,12,50; 100-4,12,140; 100-4,12,140.2; 100-4,12,140.3.2

01670 Anesthesia for all procedures on veins of shoulder and axilla N ⚡

MED: 100-4,3,100.2; 100-4,12,50; 100-4,12,140; 100-4,12,140.2; 100-4,12,140.3.2

01680 Anesthesia for shoulder cast application, removal or repair; not otherwise specified N ⚡

MED: 100-4,3,100.2; 100-4,12,50; 100-4,12,140; 100-4,12,140.2; 100-4,12,140.3.2

01682 shoulder spica N ⚡

MED: 100-4,3,100.2; 100-4,12,50; 100-4,12,140; 100-4,12,140.2; 100-4,12,140.3.2

UPPER ARM AND ELBOW

Diagnostic endoscopy/arthroscopy is always included in surgical endoscopy/arthroscopy; do not report separately.

01710 Anesthesia for procedures on nerves, muscles, tendons, fascia, and bursae of upper arm and elbow; not otherwise specified N ⚡

MED: 100-4,3,100.2; 100-4,12,50; 100-4,12,140; 100-4,12,140.2; 100-4,12,140.3.2

01712 tenotomy, elbow to shoulder, open N ⚡

MED: 100-4,3,100.2; 100-4,12,50; 100-4,12,140; 100-4,12,140.2; 100-4,12,140.3.2

01714 tenoplasty, elbow to shoulder N ⚡

MED: 100-4,3,100.2; 100-4,12,50; 100-4,12,140; 100-4,12,140.2; 100-4,12,140.3.2

01716 tenodesis, rupture of long tendon of biceps N ⚡

MED: 100-4,3,100.2; 100-4,12,50; 100-4,12,140; 100-4,12,140.2; 100-4,12,140.3.2

01730 Anesthesia for all closed procedures on humerus and elbow N ⚡

MED: 100-4,3,100.2; 100-4,12,50; 100-4,12,140; 100-4,12,140.2; 100-4,12,140.3.2

01732 Anesthesia for diagnostic arthroscopic procedures of elbow joint N ⚡

MED: 100-4,3,100.2; 100-4,12,50; 100-4,12,140; 100-4,12,140.2; 100-4,12,140.3.2

01740 Anesthesia for open or surgical arthroscopic procedures of the elbow; not otherwise specified N ⚡

MED: 100-4,3,100.2; 100-4,12,50; 100-4,12,140; 100-4,12,140.2; 100-4,12,140.3.2

01742 osteotomy of humerus N ⚡

MED: 100-4,3,100.2; 100-4,12,50; 100-4,12,140; 100-4,12,140.2; 100-4,12,140.3.2

01744 repair of nonunion or malunion of humerus N ⚡

MED: 100-4,3,100.2; 100-4,12,50; 100-4,12,140; 100-4,12,140.2; 100-4,12,140.3.2

01756 radical procedures C ⚡

MED: 100-4,3,100.2; 100-4,12,50; 100-4,12,140; 100-4,12,140.2; 100-4,12,140.3.2

01758 excision of cyst or tumor of humerus N ⚡

MED: 100-4,3,100.2; 100-4,12,50; 100-4,12,140; 100-4,12,140.2; 100-4,12,140.3.2

01760 total elbow replacement N ⚡

MED: 100-4,3,100.2; 100-4,12,50; 100-4,12,140; 100-4,12,140.2; 100-4,12,140.3.2

01770 Anesthesia for procedures on arteries of upper arm and elbow; not otherwise specified Ⓝ ☐
MED: 100-4,3,100.2; 100-4,12,50; 100-4,12,140; 100-4,12,140.2; 100-4,12,140.3.2

01772 embolectomy Ⓝ ☐
MED: 100-4,3,100.2; 100-4,12,50; 100-4,12,140; 100-4,12,140.2; 100-4,12,140.3.2

01780 Anesthesia for procedures on veins of upper arm and elbow; not otherwise specified Ⓝ ☐
MED: 100-4,3,100.2; 100-4,12,50; 100-4,12,140; 100-4,12,140.2; 100-4,12,140.3.2

01782 phleborrhaphy Ⓝ ☐
MED: 100-4,3,100.2; 100-4,12,50; 100-4,12,140; 100-4,12,140.2; 100-4,12,140.3.2

FOREARM, WRIST, AND HAND

Diagnostic endoscopy/arthroscopy is always included in surgical endoscopy/arthroscopy; do not report separately.

01810 Anesthesia for all procedures on nerves, muscles, tendons, fascia, and bursae of forearm, wrist, and hand Ⓝ ☐
MED: 100-4,3,100.2; 100-4,12,50; 100-4,12,140; 100-4,12,140.2; 100-4,12,140.3.2

01820 Anesthesia for all closed procedures on radius, ulna, wrist, or hand bones Ⓝ ☐
MED: 100-4,3,100.2; 100-4,12,50; 100-4,12,140; 100-4,12,140.2; 100-4,12,140.3.2

01829 Anesthesia for diagnostic arthroscopic procedures on the wrist Ⓝ ☐
MED: 100-4,3,100.2

01830 Anesthesia for open or surgical arthroscopic/endoscopic procedures on distal radius, distal ulna, wrist, or hand joints; not otherwise specified Ⓝ ☐
MED: 100-4,3,100.2; 100-4,12,50; 100-4,12,140; 100-4,12,140.2; 100-4,12,140.3.2

01832 total wrist replacement Ⓝ ☐
MED: 100-4,3,100.2; 100-4,12,50; 100-4,12,140; 100-4,12,140.2; 100-4,12,140.3.2

01840 Anesthesia for procedures on arteries of forearm, wrist, and hand; not otherwise specified Ⓝ ☐
MED: 100-4,3,100.2; 100-4,12,50; 100-4,12,140; 100-4,12,140.2; 100-4,12,140.3.2

01842 embolectomy Ⓝ ☐
MED: 100-4,3,100.2; 100-4,12,50; 100-4,12,140; 100-4,12,140.2; 100-4,12,140.3.2

01844 Anesthesia for vascular shunt, or shunt revision, any type (eg, dialysis) Ⓝ ☐
MED: 100-4,3,100.2; 100-4,12,50; 100-4,12,140; 100-4,12,140.2; 100-4,12,140.3.2

01850 Anesthesia for procedures on veins of forearm, wrist, and hand; not otherwise specified Ⓝ ☐
MED: 100-4,3,100.2; 100-4,12,50; 100-4,12,140; 100-4,12,140.2; 100-4,12,140.3.2

01852 phleborrhaphy Ⓝ ☐
MED: 100-4,3,100.2; 100-4,12,50; 100-4,12,140; 100-4,12,140.2; 100-4,12,140.3.2

01860 Anesthesia for forearm, wrist, or hand cast application, removal, or repair Ⓝ ☐
MED: 100-4,3,100.2; 100-4,12,50; 100-4,12,140; 100-4,12,140.2; 100-4,12,140.3.2

RADIOLOGICAL PROCEDURES

▲ **01905** Anesthesia for myelography, discography, vertebroplasty Ⓝ ☐
MED: 100-4,3,100.2

01916 Anesthesia for diagnostic arteriography/venography Ⓝ ☐
MED: 100-3,20.17; 100-4,3,100.2; 100-4,12,50; 100-4,12,140; 100-4,12,140.2; 100-4,12,140.3.2

Note that code 01916 cannot be reported with therapeutic codes 01924-01926, 01930-01933.

01920 Anesthesia for cardiac catheterization including coronary angiography and ventriculography (not to include Swan-Ganz catheter) Ⓝ ☐
MED: 100-4,3,100.2; 100-4,12,50; 100-4,12,140; 100-4,12,140.2; 100-4,12,140.3.2

01922 Anesthesia for non-invasive imaging or radiation therapy Ⓝ ☐
MED: 100-4,3,100.2; 100-4,12,50; 100-4,12,140; 100-4,12,140.2; 100-4,12,140.3.2

01924 Anesthesia for therapeutic interventional radiologic procedures involving the arterial system; not otherwise specified Ⓝ ☐
MED: 100-4,3,100.2

01925 carotid or coronary Ⓝ ☐
MED: 100-4,3,100.2

01926 intracranial, intracardiac, or aortic Ⓝ ☐
MED: 100-4,3,100.2

01930 Anesthesia for therapeutic interventional radiologic procedures involving the venous/lymphatic system (not to include access to the central circulation); not otherwise specified Ⓝ ☐
MED: 100-4,3,100.2

01931 intrahepatic or portal circulation (eg, transcutaneous porto-caval shunt (TIPS)) Ⓝ ☐
MED: 100-4,3,100.2

01932 intrathoracic or jugular Ⓝ ☐
MED: 100-4,3,100.2

01933 intracranial Ⓝ ☐
MED: 100-4,3,100.2

BURN EXCISIONS OR DEBRIDEMENT

01951 Anesthesia for second and third degree burn excision or debridement with or without skin grafting, any site, for total body surface area (TBSA) treated during anesthesia and surgery; less than four percent total body surface area Ⓝ ☐
MED: 100-3,270.5; 100-4,3,20.1.2.8; 100-4,3,100.2

01952 between four and nine percent of total body surface area Ⓝ ☐
MED: 100-4,3,20.1.2.8; 100-4,3,100.2

+ **01953** each additional nine percent total body surface area or part thereof (List separately in addition to code for primary procedure) Ⓝ ☐
MED: 100-4,3,20.1.2.8; 100-4,3,100.2

Note that 01953 is an add-on code and must be used in conjunction with code 01952.

🄿🄲 Professional Component Only 🄃🄲 Technical Component Only MED: Pub 100/NCD References AMA: CPT Assistant References 🔟/🔟 Assist-at-Surgery Allowed/With Documentation ❶-❾ ASC Group Unlisted ♂ Male Only Not Covered ♀ Female Only

38 — CPT Expert CPT only © 2006 American Medical Association. All Rights Reserved. *(Black Ink)* © 2006 Ingenix *(Blue Ink)*

OBSTETRIC

01958 Anesthesia for external cephalic version procedure

MED: 100-4,3,100.2

01960 Anesthesia for vaginal delivery only

MED: 100-4,3,100.2

01961 Anesthesia for cesarean delivery only

MED: 100-4,3,100.2

01962 Anesthesia for urgent hysterectomy following delivery

MED: 100-4,3,100.2

01963 Anesthesia for cesarean hysterectomy without any labor analgesia/anesthesia care

MED: 100-4,3,100.2

01965 Anesthesia for incomplete or missed abortion procedures

MED: 100-4,3,100.2

01966 Anesthesia for induced abortion procedures

MED: 100-4,3,100.2

01967 Neuraxial labor analgesia/anesthesia for planned vaginal delivery (this includes any repeat subarachnoid needle placement and drug injection and/or any necessary replacement of an epidural catheter during labor)

MED: 100-4,3,100.2

+ 01968 Anesthesia for cesarean delivery following neuraxial labor analgesia/anesthesia (List separately in addition to code for primary procedure performed)

MED: 100-4,3,100.2

Note that 01968 is an add-on code and must be used in conjunction with code 01967.

+ 01969 Anesthesia for cesarean hysterectomy following neuraxial labor analgesia/anesthesia (List separately in addition to code for primary procedure performed)

MED: 100-4,3,100.2

Note that 01969 is an add-on code and must be used in conjunction with code 01967.

OTHER PROCEDURES

01990 Physiological support for harvesting of organ(s) from brain-dead patient

MED: 100-4,3,100.2; 100-4,12,50; 100-4,12,140; 100-4,12,140.2; 100-4,12,140.3.2

01991 Anesthesia for diagnostic or therapeutic nerve blocks and injections (when block or injection is performed by a different provider); other than the prone position

MED: 100-4,3,100.2

Note that code 01991 cannot be reported with CPT codes 99143-99150.

01992 prone position

MED: 100-4,3,100.2

Note that code 01992 cannot be reported with CPT code 99141.

01995 ~~Regional intravenous administration of local anesthetic agent or other medication (upper or lower extremity)~~

01996 Daily hospital management of epidural or subarachnoid continuous drug administration

MED: 100-4,3,100.2; 100-4,12,50; 100-4,12,140; 100-4,12,140.2; 100-4,12,140.3.2

AMA: 1997,Nov,10

Use code 01996 to report services performed after insertion of an epidural or subarachnoid catheter placed primarily for anesthesia administration during an operative session, but retained for post-operative pain management.

01999 Unlisted anesthesia procedure(s)

MED: 100-4,3,100.2; 100-4,12,50; 100-4,12,140; 100-4,12,140.2; 100-4,12,140.3.2

AMA: 1997,Feb,4

QUALIFYING CIRCUMSTANCES FOR ANESTHESIA

If an explanation is needed for these services, consult the Anesthesia guidelines.

+ 99100 Anesthesia for patient of extreme age, younger than 1 year and older than 70 (List separately in addition to code for primary anesthesia procedure)

MED: 100-4,12,50; 100-4,12,140; 100-4,12,140.2; 100-4,12,140.3.2

To procedure performed on infant one year of age or younger, consult CPT codes 00326, 00561, 00834, 00836.

+ 99116 Anesthesia complicated by utilization of total body hypothermia (List separately in addition to code for primary anesthesia procedure)

MED: 100-4,12,50; 100-4,12,140; 100-4,12,140.2; 100-4,12,140.3.2

+ 99135 Anesthesia complicated by utilization of controlled hypotension (List separately in addition to code for primary anesthesia procedure)

MED: 100-4,12,50; 100-4,12,140; 100-4,12,140.2; 100-4,12,140.3.2

+ 99140 Anesthesia complicated by emergency conditions (specify) (List separately in addition to code for primary anesthesia procedure)

MED: 100-4,12,50; 100-4,12,140; 100-4,12,140.2; 100-4,12,140.3.2

AMA: 2001,Mar,10; 2001,Mar,10

An emergency exists when a delay in treatment would lead to a significant increase in the threat to life or body part.

Surgery

CODING INFORMATION

ORGANIZATION

The surgery section (10021–69990) is the largest section of the CPT book. It is divided into 18 subsections by body system (e.g., integumentary, endocrine), procedure site (e.g., mediastinum and diaphragm), or type of service (e.g., maternity care and delivery). The subsections are as follows:

- General
- Integumentary System
- Musculoskeletal System
- Respiratory System
- Cardiovascular System
- Hemic and Lymphatic Systems
- Mediastinum and Diaphragm
- Digestive System
- Urinary System
- Male Genital System
- Intersex Surgery
- Female Genital System
- Maternity Care and Delivery
- Endocrine System
- Nervous System
- Eye and Ocular Adnexa
- Auditory System
- Operating Microscope

Instructions that apply to all surgical codes are found at the beginning of the surgery section. In addition, information or notes, specific to subsections, groups of codes and single codes are found throughout the surgery section. Guidelines, including terms and concepts, important to all surgical codes will be explained first. Then guidelines and notes specific to subsections or codes will be reviewed.

FORMAT OF THE TERMINOLOGY

CPT guidelines state that some of the procedures are not printed in their entirety but refer back to a common portion of the procedure listed in a preceding entry. This space-saving format means that many "indented" codes within a code range repeat some common portion of a procedure's description.

While some procedures presented in this indented form are mutually exclusive (i.e., cannot be billed together), others are not. For procedures that are not mutually exclusive, payers may make special allowances. Knowing which procedures are mutually exclusive, however, is the key to avoiding unbundling.

GENERAL INFORMATION

Surgical procedures can generally be divided into two categories: diagnostic and therapeutic.

SURGICAL PACKAGE

The majority of the CPT surgery codes are "package" services. According to the CPT book, they include the actual surgical procedure, local infiltration, metacarpal, or digital block or topical anesthesia, writing orders, postanesthesia recovery evaluation and typical follow-up care such as talking with the family and writing orders. Also included is the evaluation and management service on the day of or the day prior to surgery unless that is the visit that led to the decision for surgery. When a patient is seen for a routine follow-up postoperative visit within the normal follow-up period, code 99024 may be reported for normal uncomplicated postoperative care. However, additional payment will not be provided for this service since normal postoperative care is included in the surgical package.

Post-procedure care for diagnostic procedures includes only the care related to recover from the procedure itself. Care for the condition that required the procedure and any other conditions is not included and should be reported separately.

Many payers have strict guidelines related to reimbursement for preoperative services. Additional reimbursement for preoperative evaluation and management services is usually allowed prior to the decision for surgery or to establish the need for surgery. Reimbursement may be denied for any care provided after the decision for surgical intervention However, some payers may identify a specific preoperative period (24 hours to 30 days), during which no additional reimbursement will be made for evaluation and management services. Because of these differing payer policies, it is important for individual providers to establish a policy related to the reporting of preoperative services. Patients should be made aware of this policy. Review contractual arrangements with payers to verify that your policy is not in violation of those contracts.

Postoperative complications, exacerbations, and recurrences are not included in the surgical package and should be reported separately. Postoperative complications include conditions such as wound dehiscence, infection, and bleeding. A diagnosis code should be assigned to reflect the nature of the complication when billing for services rendered to treat the complication.

Unrelated care is always coded. Report services unrelated to the operative problem, such as care for other diseases or injuries, with an appropriate inpatient or outpatient level of service modifier and a corresponding diagnostic code that identifies a problem other than the surgical diagnosis.

Fragmentation and Unbundling

Understanding unbundling and fragmentation can be accomplished by first defining the term, "bundle." A bundle is a defined set of items or services wrapped together in a group, bunch, or package. The items in the bundle can be related or unrelated, but all defined elements must be present to make a specific bundle. Unbundling or fragmentation occurs primarily two ways.

First, unbundling occurs when minor integral services are reported separately or in addition to a major procedure. Unfortunately, since all minor components of a procedure may not be listed explicitly, it is sometimes difficult to determine which services are integral to a given procedure. One way to approach this is to ask what services are normally performed with a given procedure. A simple example is an excision of a skin lesion. To excise the skin lesion, an incision must be made. An incision is always integral to an excision of a lesion and should not be billed separately. However, an incision is not described in the excision of skin lesion codes. It is implicit because it must be performed with every excision.

Second, unbundling occurs when a single procedure with two or more explicitly described components is broken into its component parts and reported with several CPT codes instead of the single CPT code for the combined service. A simple example of this type of unbundle can be illustrated with the procedure for a combined abdominal hysterectomy with colpo-urethrocystopexy. Since the two components of this procedure are frequently performed together, a combined code 58152 has been assigned to describe this service. However, it is also possible to perform each of the components separately (abdominal hysterectomy 58150 and colpo-urethrocystopexy 51840 or 51845). When the combined procedure is performed during a single surgical session, it must be reported with the bundled CPT code 58152. If it is reported with code 58150 in conjunction with 51840 or 58145, it is considered unbundled or fragmented.

Unbundling, whether intentional or not, is considered by payers to be a form of fraudulent or reckless billing. The rationale is simple. Unbundled services will frequently net more reimbursement than reporting the single bundled CPT code.

The Centers for Medicare and Medicaid Services (CMS) has adopted the Correct Coding Initiative (CCI) unbundling guidelines, an evolving list of codes that cannot be reported in combination with other codes for Medicare claims. The CPT book does not have a specific guideline for unbundling. Instead, payers and other interested parties have developed guidelines for bundled procedures from information that is listed in the CPT book. The most common areas of the CPT book used for these interpretations are the format of the listed surgical procedures, separate procedures, and subsection information in the surgery guidelines.

Prevention Tips

Your office can take some easy steps to avoid problems with fragmentation or unbundling.

- Use a current CPT book as well as the current rules, regulations, and provider manuals for Medicare and for the private payers with whom you have a contractual arrangement.

- Educate everyone on CPT guidelines as well as the rules and regulations of your payers. Educational sessions should occur any time changes are made.

- When using a preprinted charge ticket or routing sheet, specify the exact CPT code and description. Always have an area on the charge ticket for the physician to indicate that a service should be coded by hand and code from the operative report or medical record. Many providers feel reimbursement is better by coding directly from the record or operative report.

- Date the charge ticket and update codes annually.

- Create your charge tickets or routing sheets to avoid fragmented billing. Adding the abbreviation "SP" to separate procedure codes alerts the coder that a separate procedure should not be reported when related to, or integral to, a major procedure.

- Make sure physicians provide coders with complete documentation and concise information. Query the physician if documentation is not adequate to support the codes selected.

- Use the correct modifiers as appropriate to clarify or append circumstances that can arise within global package time periods.

Separate Procedures

Separate procedures are services that are commonly carried out as an integral part of a larger service, and as such do not warrant separate identification. These services are noted in the CPT book with the parenthetical phrase "separate procedure." When this phrase appears before the semicolon, all indented descriptions that follow include it.

Separate procedures are often improperly reported as related procedures, which are performed for the same diagnosis and within the same operative area. Reporting a separate procedure in addition to the larger procedure to which it is related is incorrect. A separate procedure can be a component of, or incidental to, a larger, related procedure.

Diagnostic Procedures

Diagnostic procedures are performed to evaluate the patient's complaints or symptoms. These procedures help the physician establish the nature of the patient's disease or condition so that definitive care can be provided. Diagnostic procedures include endoscopy, arthroscopy, injection procedures, and biopsies. Follow-up care for diagnostic procedures includes only care directly related to recovery from the diagnostic procedure itself. Care of the condition identified by the diagnostic procedures or other concomitant conditions is not included and may be listed separately.

Therapeutic Services

Therapeutic services are performed for treatment of a specific diagnosis. These services include performance of the procedure, various incidental elements, and normal, related follow-up care.

Sequencing

The code with the highest dollar value is always sequenced first when reporting multiple procedures. The second and subsequent codes are ordered and listed in decreasing dollar values with the correct modifier appended. When reporting multiple procedures, do not reduce the amount of secondary codes. However, if overpaid, reimburse the payer for the overpayment. Set a ceiling on nonactionable overpayments in policy or contracts (e.g., up to $10 need not be refunded). Overpayments that are not returned to the payer may target an office for an audit.

Materials Supplied by a Physician

Many payers reimburse only for supplies that are excessive or extraordinarily expensive. Do not report supplies that are customarily included in surgical packages, such as gauze, sponges, applicators, or Steri-strips. Surgical services do not include the supply of medications, which may be coded and billed separately.

SURGICAL PROCEDURES

Several subsections of the CPT book contain guidelines, notes, definitions, and special instructions. Following is a list of some of the subsections:

- Biopsy
- Removal of Skin Tags
- Shaving of Epidermal/Dermal Lesions
- Excision of Benign and Malignant Lesions
- Repair of Wounds
- Adjacent Tissue Transfers
- Skin Replacement Surgery and Skin Substitutes
- Flaps (Skin and/or Deep Tissue)
- Burns, Local Treatment
- Destruction of Lesions
- Mohs Micrographic Surgery
- Breast- Excision
- Musculoskeletal
- Wound Exploration-Trauma
- Grafts (or Implants)
- Introduction or Removal
- Spine Surgeries
- Cast and Splint Application
- Musculoskeletal Endoscopy/Arthroscopy
- Respiratory Endoscopy
- Cardiovascular System
- Pacemaker/Defibrillator Care
- Electrophysiologic Procedures
- Coronary Artery Bypass Grafts (CABG)
- Endovascular Procedures
- Transluminal Angioplasty
- Transluminal Atherectomy
- Bypass Graft
- Composite Grafts
- Adjuvant Techniques
- Vascular Catheterization/Injection
- Transcatheter Procedures Intravenous
- Intravascular Ultrasound
- Bone Marrow or Stem Cell Services/Procedures
- Hemic and Lymphatic Systems
- Digestive
- Endoscopy/Laparoscopy
- Pancreas Transplantation
- Hernia Repair
- Renal Transplantation
- Urodynamics
- Urinary, Male Genital, Female Genital, Endocrine Endoscopy/ Laparoscopy
- Maternity Care and Delivery
- Surgery of Skull Base
- Neurostimulators
- Secondary Implant(s)
- Cataract Procedures
- Reconstruction
- Operating Microscope

RESULTS/TESTING/REPORTS

Results indicate the technical component of a procedure or service. Testing is the service that leads to the report and interpretation. Reports provide interpretation of the tests.

GENERAL

10021 **Fine needle aspiration; without imaging guidance**   [T] [80] [↔]

AMA: 2002,Aug,10

10022   **with imaging guidance**   [T] [80] [↔]

If radiological supervision and interpretation is performed, consult CPT codes 76942, 77002, 77012, 77021.

If percutaneous needle biopsy, other than fine needle aspiration, is performed, consult CPT code 20206 for muscle, 32400 for pleura, 32405 for lung or mediastinum, 42400 for salivary gland, 47000, 47001 for liver, 48102 for pancreas, 49180 for abdominal or retroperitoneal mass, 60100 for thyroid, 62269 for spinal cord.

If evaluation of fine needle aspirate is performed, consult CPT codes 88172, 88173.

INTEGUMENTARY SYSTEM

SKIN, SUBCUTANEOUS AND ACCESSORY STRUCTURES

INCISION AND DRAINAGE

To report excision procedures, consult CPT code 11400 and subsequent codes.

10040 **Acne surgery (eg, marsupialization, opening or removal of multiple milia, comedones, cysts, pustules)**   [T]

MED: 100-4,4,20.5

AMA: 1992,Fall,1

10060 **Incision and drainage of abscess (eg, carbuncle, suppurative hidradenitis, cutaneous or subcutaneous abscess, cyst, furuncle, or paronychia); simple or single**   [T] [↔]

MED: 100-4,4,20.5

10061   **complicated or multiple**   [T] [↔]

MED: 100-4,4,20.5

10080 **Incision and drainage of pilonidal cyst; simple**   [T] [↔]

MED: 100-4,4,20.5

10081   **complicated**   [T] [↔]

MED: 100-4,4,20.5

If an excision of a pilonidal cyst or sinus is performed, consult CPT codes 11770-11772.

10120 **Incision and removal of foreign body, subcutaneous tissues; simple**   [T] [↔]

MED: 100-4,4,20.5

10121   **complicated**   [2] [T] [↔]

MED: 100-2,15,260; 100-4,4,20.5; 100-4,12,90.3; 100-4,14,10

If exploration of a penetrating wound, not requiring thoracotomy or laparotomy, is performed, consult CPT codes 20100-20103. If debridement related to an open fracture(s) and/or dislocation(s) is performed, consult CPT codes 11010-11012.

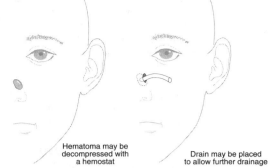

Hematoma may be decompressed with a hemostat

Drain may be placed to allow further drainage

10140 **Incision and drainage of hematoma, seroma or fluid collection**   [T] [↔]

To report imaging guidance, consult codes 76942, 77012, 77021.

10160 **Puncture aspiration of abscess, hematoma, bulla, or cyst**   [T] [↔]

To report imaging guidance, consult CPT codes 76942, 77012, 77021.

10180 **Incision and drainage, complex, postoperative wound infection**   [2] [T] [↔]

MED: 100-2,15,260; 100-4,4,20.5; 100-4,12,90.3; 100-4,14,10

If secondary closure of surgical wound is performed, consult CPT codes 12020, 12021, 13160.

EXCISION — DEBRIDEMENT

If dermabrasions are performed, consult CPT codes 15780-15811. If nail debridement is performed, consult CPT codes 11720-11721. If burns are being treated, consult CPT codes 16000-16035.

11000 **Debridement of extensive eczematous or infected skin; up to 10% of body surface**   [T] [↔]

+ 11001   **each additional 10% of the body surface (List separately in addition to code for primary procedure)**   [T]

Note that 11001 is an add-on code and must be used in conjunction with 11000.

11004 **Debridement of skin, subcutaneous tissue, muscle and fascia for necrotizing soft tissue infection; external genitalia and perineum**   [C] [↔]

11005   **abdominal wall, with or without fascial closure**   [C] [80]

11006   **external genitalia, perineum and abdominal wall, with or without fascial closure**   [C] [↔]

+ 11008 **Removal of prosthetic material or mesh, abdominal wall for necrotizing soft tissue infection (List separately in addition to code for primary procedure)**   [C] [80]

Note that 11008 must be used in conjunction with 11004-11006.

Do not report 11000-11001 and 11010-11044 together with 11008.

When skin grafts or flaps are performed separately for closure at the same session as 11004-11008, consult the relevant graft and flap codes.

For orchiectomy consult CPT code 54520.

For testicular transplantation consult CPT code 54680.

Integumentary System

11010 — 11313

11010 Debridement including removal of foreign material associated with open fracture(s) and/or dislocation(s); skin and subcutaneous tissues ☑ T ⬛

MED: 100-2,15,260; 100-4,4,20.5; 100-4,12,90.3; 100-4,14,10
AMA: 1997,Mar,1; 1997,Aug,6; 1997,Apr,10

11011 skin, subcutaneous tissue, muscle fascia, and muscle ☑ T ⬛

MED: 100-2,15,260; 100-4,4,20.5; 100-4,12,90.3; 100-4,14,10
AMA: 1997,Mar,1; 1997,Aug,6; 1997,Apr,10

11012 skin, subcutaneous tissue, muscle fascia, muscle, and bone ☑ T ⬛

MED: 100-2,15,260; 100-4,4,20.5; 100-4,12,90.3; 100-4,14,10
AMA: 1997,Mar,1; 1997,Aug,6; 1997,Apr,10

11040 Debridement; skin, partial thickness T ⬛

AMA: 1997,Feb,7; 1997,Aug,6; 1996,May,6; 1993,Fall,21

11041 skin, full thickness T ⬛

AMA: 1997,Feb,7; 1997,Aug,6; 1996,May,6; 1993,Fall,21

11042 skin, and subcutaneous tissue ☑ T ⬛

MED: 100-2,15,260; 100-4,4,20.5; 100-4,12,90.3; 100-4,14,10
AMA: 2000,Aug,5; 1997,Feb,7; 1997,Aug,6; 1996,May,6; 1992,Winter,10

11043 skin, subcutaneous tissue, and muscle ☑ T ⬛

MED: 100-2,15,260; 100-4,4,20.5; 100-4,12,90.3; 100-4,14,10
AMA: 1997,Feb,7; 1997,Aug,6; 1997,Apr,11; 1996,May,6

11044 skin, subcutaneous tissue, muscle, and bone ☑ T ⬛

MED: 100-2,15,260; 100-4,4,20.5; 100-4,12,90.3; 100-4,14,10
AMA: 1997,Feb,7; 1997,Aug,6; 1997,Apr,11; 1996,May,6; 1996,Mar,10; 1993,Fall,21
Do not report 11040-11044 with 97597-97602.

PARING OR CUTTING

To report lesion destruction, consult CPT codes 17000-17004.

11055 Paring or cutting of benign hyperkeratotic lesion (eg, corn or callus); single lesion T ⬛

AMA: 1999,Jan,11; 1997,Nov,11

11056 two to four lesions T ⬛

AMA: 1999,Jan,11; 1997,Nov,11

11057 more than four lesions T ⬛

AMA: 1999,Jan,11; 1997,Nov,11

BIOPSY

Often tissue obtained during certain skin procedures, such as excisions, destructions or removals is sent to pathology. This is considered a component of such procedures and should not be reported with codes 11100 or 11101.

Biopsies performed at different sites or on different lesions on the same date should be reported separately, append modifier 59.

11100 Biopsy of skin, subcutaneous tissue and/or mucous membrane (including simple closure), unless otherwise listed; single lesion T ⬛

AMA: 1997,Mar,4; 1997,Jun,5; 1994,Fall,18
If the conjunctiva is biopsied, consult CPT code 68100; if the eyelid is biopsied, consult CPT code 67810.

+ 11101 each separate/additional lesion (List separately in addition to code for primary procedure) T

AMA: 2000,Apr,6; 1994,Fall,18
Note that 11101 is an add-on code and must be used in conjunction with 11100.

REMOVAL OF SKIN TAGS

CPT codes 11200 and 11201 identify the use of scissors or any sharp methods, ligature strangulation, electrosurgical destruction or any combination of treatment methods including electrosurgical techniques or the use of chemicals. Local anesthesia is included in these services.

11200 Removal of skin tags, multiple fibrocutaneous tags, any area; up to and including 15 lesions T ⬛

AMA: 2002,Nov,11; 1997,Nov,11-12

+ 11201 each additional ten lesions (List separately in addition to code for primary procedure) T

AMA: 2002,Nov,11; 1997,Nov,11-12
Note that 11201 is an add-on code and must be used in conjunction with 11200.

SHAVING OF EPIDERMAL OR DERMAL LESIONS

Shaving is the removal of epidermal or dermal skin lesions without a full-thickness dermal excision by use of a transverse incision or horizontal slicing technique. Administration of local anesthesia and any chemical or electrocautery is included.

CPT codes 11300-11313, include local anesthesia, chemical or electrocauterization of the wound. These wounds do not require suture closure.

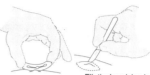

Shave excision of an elevated lesion; technique also used to biopsy

Eliptical excision is often used when tissue removal is larger than 4 mm or when deep pathology is suspected

A punch biopsy cuts a core of tissue as the tool is twisted downward

The skin is the largest organ of the human body and accounts for about 20 percent of total body weight. It serves mainly as a protective barrier, a temperature regulator, and as a sensory device. The epidermis is outermost and is the thinnest of the skin layers; the major part of the dermis is high in collagen and is notable for its great elasticity and strength; the major blood and nerve network is found in the middermis. Adnexal structures are the hair follicles, sebaceous glands, sweat glands, and the follicles that produce fingernails and toenails. Lesions are small areas of skin disease and may be solitary or multiple

11300 Shaving of epidermal or dermal lesion, single lesion, trunk, arms or legs; lesion diameter 0.5 cm or less T 80 ⬛

AMA: 2002,Nov,11; 2000,Feb,11

11301 lesion diameter 0.6 to 1.0 cm T 80 ⬛

AMA: 2000,Feb,11

11302 lesion diameter 1.1 to 2.0 cm T 80 ⬛

AMA: 2000,Feb,10

11303 lesion diameter over 2.0 cm T 80 ⬛

AMA: 2000,Feb,10

11305 Shaving of epidermal or dermal lesion, single lesion, scalp, neck, hands, feet, genitalia; lesion diameter 0.5 cm or less T 80 ⬛

AMA: 2000,Feb,10

11306 lesion diameter 0.6 to 1.0 cm T 80 ⬛

AMA: 2000,Feb,10

11307 lesion diameter 1.1 to 2.0 cm T 80 ⬛

AMA: 2000,Feb,10

11308 lesion diameter over 2.0 cm T 80 ⬛

AMA: 2000,Feb,10

11310 Shaving of epidermal or dermal lesion, single lesion, face, ears, eyelids, nose, lips, mucous membrane; lesion diameter 0.5 cm or less T 80 ⬛

AMA: 2000,Feb,10

11311 lesion diameter 0.6 to 1.0 cm T 80 ⬛

AMA: 2000,Feb,10

11312 lesion diameter 1.1 to 2.0 cm T 80 ⬛

AMA: 2000,Feb,10

11313 lesion diameter over 2.0 cm T 80 ⬛

AMA: 2000,Feb,10

EXCISION — BENIGN LESIONS

In the CPT book excision of benign lesions is defined as a full thickness removal of the lesion, including margins. Benign lesions may include neoplasms, cysts and growths caused by inflammation, fibrous tissue, and tissues present since

| 26 Professional Component Only | 80/80 Assist-at-Surgery Allowed/With Documentation | Unlisted | Not Covered |
| TC Technical Component Only | MED: Pub 100/NCD References AMA: CPT Assistant References | 1-9 ASC Group ♂ Male Only | ♀ Female Only |

44 — CPT Expert

CPT only © 2006 American Medical Association. All Rights Reserved. (Black Ink)

© 2006 Ingenix (Blue Ink)

birth. The lesions may occur in the skin or tissues below the skin. Non-layered closure and local anesthesia are included.

Layered, intermediate or complex closure of the defect created by the excision of the lesion is separately reported.

If an excision of a benign lesion(s) requiring more than simple closure (e.g., requiring intermediate, or complex closure) is performed, report the appropriate closure CPT codes (12031-12057 for intermediate, 13100-13153 for complex) in addition to appropriate lesion removal code (11400-11446). For reconstructive closure report CPT codes 14000-14300, 15002-15215776, and 15570-15770 in addition to appropriate lesion removal code. If electrosurgery, cryosurgery, laser, or chemical treatment is used, consult CPT codes 17000 and subsequent codes.

Each benign lesion excised should be reported separately. If the excision is unusual or complicated, append modifier 22 or 09922.

Code selection is based on excised diameter, which is defined as lesion diameter plus most narrow margins required to completely excise the lesion. Measurements should be taken prior to excision.

11400	**Excision, benign lesion including margins, except skin tag (unless listed elsewhere), trunk, arms or legs; excised diameter 0.5 cm or less**	T ◘
	AMA: 2002,Nov,5; 1996,May,11; 1995,Fall,3; 1993,Fall,7	
11401	**excised diameter 0.6 to 1.0 cm**	T ◘
	AMA: 2002,Nov,5; 1996,May,11; 1995,Fall,3; 1993,Fall,7	
11402	**excised diameter 1.1 to 2.0 cm**	T ◘
	AMA: 2002,Nov,5; 1996,May,11; 1995,Fall,3; 1993,Fall,7	
11403	**excised diameter 2.1 to 3.0 cm**	T ◘
	AMA: 2002,Nov,5; 1996,May,11; 1995,Fall,3; 1993,Fall,7	
11404	**excised diameter 3.1 to 4.0 cm**	1 T ◘
	MED: 100-2,15,260; 100-4,4,20.5; 100-4,12,90.3; 100-4,14,10	
	AMA: 2002,Nov,5; 1996,May,11; 1995,Fall,3; 1993,Fall,7	
11406	**excised diameter over 4.0 cm**	2 T ◘
	MED: 100-2,15,260; 100-4,4,20.5; 100-4,12,90.3; 100-4,14,10	
	AMA: 2002,Nov,5; 1996,May,11; 1995,Fall,3; 1993,Fall,7	
11420	**Excision, benign lesion including margins, except skin tag (unless listed elsewhere), scalp, neck, hands, feet, genitalia; excised diameter 0.5 cm or less**	T ◘
	AMA: 1995,Fall,3	
11421	**excised diameter 0.6 to 1.0 cm**	T ◘
	AMA: 1996,May,11; 1995,Fall,3	
11422	**excised diameter 1.1 to 2.0 cm**	T ◘
	AMA: 1996,May,11; 1995,Fall,3	
11423	**excised diameter 2.1 to 3.0 cm**	T ◘
	AMA: 1996,May,11; 1995,Fall,3	
11424	**excised diameter 3.1 to 4.0 cm**	2 T ◘
	MED: 100-2,15,260; 100-4,4,20.5; 100-4,12,90.3; 100-4,14,10	
	AMA: 1996,May,11; 1995,Fall,3	
11426	**excised diameter over 4.0 cm**	2 T ◘
	MED: 100-2,15,260; 100-4,4,20.5; 100-4,12,90.3; 100-4,14,10	
	AMA: 1996,May,11; 1995,Fall,3	

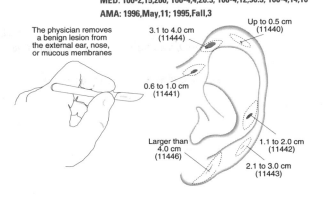

The physician removes a benign lesion from the external ear, nose, or mucous membranes

Up to 0.5 cm (11440)
3.1 to 4.0 cm (11444)
0.6 to 1.0 cm (11441)
Larger than 4.0 cm (11446)
1.1 to 2.0 cm (11442)
2.1 to 3.0 cm (11443)

11440	**Excision, other benign lesion including margins, except skin tag (unless listed elsewhere), face, ears, eyelids, nose, lips, mucous membrane; excised diameter 0.5 cm or less**	T ◘
	AMA: 1996,May,11; 1995,Fall,3	
11441	**excised diameter 0.6 to 1.0 cm**	T ◘
	AMA: 1996,May,11; 1995,Fall,3	
11442	**excised diameter 1.1 to 2.0 cm**	T ◘
	AMA: 2000,Aug,5; 1996,May,11; 1995,Fall,3	
11443	**excised diameter 2.1 to 3.0 cm**	T ◘
	AMA: 1996,May,11; 1995,Fall,3	
11444	**excised diameter 3.1 to 4.0 cm**	1 T ◘
	MED: 100-2,15,260; 100-4,4,20.5; 100-4,12,90.3; 100-4,14,10	
	AMA: 1996,May,11; 1995,Fall,3	
11446	**excised diameter over 4.0 cm**	2 T ◘
	MED: 100-2,15,260; 100-4,4,20.5; 100-4,12,90.3; 100-4,14,10	
	AMA: 1996,May,11; 1995,Fall,3	

If the excision on the eyelids involves more than skin, consult CPT code 67800 and subsequent codes.

11450	**Excision of skin and subcutaneous tissue for hidradenitis, axillary; with simple or intermediate repair**	2 T ◘
	MED: 100-2,15,260; 100-4,4,20.5; 100-4,12,90.3; 100-4,14,10	
11451	**with complex repair**	2 T 80 ◘
	MED: 100-2,15,260; 100-4,4,20.5; 100-4,12,90.3; 100-4,14,10	

If a skin graft or flap is used for closure, consult the appropriate CPT code and use in addition to 11451.

11462	**Excision of skin and subcutaneous tissue for hidradenitis, inguinal; with simple or intermediate repair**	2 T 80 ◘
	MED: 100-2,15,260; 100-4,4,20.5; 100-4,12,90.3; 100-4,14,10	
11463	**with complex repair**	2 T 80 ◘
	MED: 100-2,15,260; 100-4,4,20.5; 100-4,12,90.3; 100-4,14,10	

If a skin graft or flap is used for closure, consult the appropriate CPT code and use in addition to 11463.

11470	**Excision of skin and subcutaneous tissue for hidradenitis, perianal, perineal, or umbilical; with simple or intermediate repair**	2 T ◘
	MED: 100-2,15,260; 100-4,4,20.5; 100-4,12,90.3; 100-4,14,10	
11471	**with complex repair**	2 T 80 ◘
	MED: 100-2,15,260; 100-4,4,20.5; 100-4,12,90.3; 100-4,14,10	

If codes 11450-11471 are performed bilaterally, append modifier 50 or 09950.

If a skin graft or flap is used for closure, consult the appropriate CPT code and use in addition to 11471.

EXCISION — MALIGNANT LESIONS

Excision is defined as a full-thickness removal of lesion including simple closure of the wound. Excision codes are selected on the basis of the type of lesion (benign or malignant), anatomic site, and lesion diameter. Benign lesions include those described as cicatricial, fibrous, inflammatory, congenital and cystic as well as any other lesion that is noninvasive or nonmalignant. Malignant lesions are typically invasive or have the potential to metastasize. Examples of malignant lesions are basal cell carcinomas and melanomas of the skin.

Layered, intermediate or complex closure of the defect created by the excision of the lesion is separately reported.

If an excision of a malignant lesion(s) requiring more than simple closure (e.g., requiring intermediate, or complex closure) is performed, report the appropriate closure CPT codes (12031-12057 for intermediate, 13100-13153 for complex) in addition to appropriate lesion removal code (11600-11646). For reconstructive closure report CPT codes14000-14300, 15002-15776, and 15570-15770 in addition to appropriate lesion removal code.

Code selection is based on excised diameter, which is defined as lesion diameter plus most narrow margins required to completely excise the lesion. Measurements should be taken prior to excision.

If pathology shows margins were not large enough for complete lesion removal and an additional excision is performed at the same session, report only one code based on the greatest excised diameter. For re-excision at subsequent sessions, consult CPT codes 11600-11646, and append modifier 58 when appropriate.

11600　　**Excision, malignant lesion including margins, trunk, arms, or legs; excised diameter 0.5 cm or less**　T ◩

AMA: 2002,Nov,5; 1996,May,11; 1995,Fall,3

11601　　excised diameter 0.6 to 1.0 cm　T ◩

AMA: 1996,May,11; 1995,Fall,3

11602　　excised diameter 1.1 to 2.0 cm　T ◩

AMA: 1996,May,11; 1995,Fall,3

11603　　excised diameter 2.1 to 3.0 cm　T ◩

AMA: 1996,May,11; 1995,Fall,3

11604　　excised diameter 3.1 to 4.0 cm　2 T ◩

MED: 100-2,15,260; 100-4,4,20.5; 100-4,12,90.3; 100-4,14,10
AMA: 1996,May,11; 1995,Fall,3

11606　　excised diameter over 4.0 cm　2 T ◩

MED: 100-2,15,260; 100-4,4,20.5; 100-4,12,90.3; 100-4,14,10
AMA: 1996,May,11; 1995,Fall,3; 1991,Fall,6

11620　　**Excision, malignant lesion including margins, scalp, neck, hands, feet, genitalia; excised diameter 0.5 cm or less**　T ◩

AMA: 2002,Nov,5; 1995,Fall,3

11621　　excised diameter 0.6 to 1.0 cm　T ◩

AMA: 1996,May,11; 1995,Fall,3

11622　　excised diameter 1.1 to 2.0 cm　T ◩

AMA: 1996,May,11; 1995,Fall,3

11623　　excised diameter 2.1 to 3.0 cm　T ◩

AMA: 1996,May,11; 1995,Fall,3

11624　　excised diameter 3.1 to 4.0 cm　2 T ◩

MED: 100-2,15,260; 100-4,4,20.5; 100-4,12,90.3; 100-4,14,10
AMA: 1996,May,11; 1995,Fall,3

11626　　excised diameter over 4.0 cm　2 T ◩

MED: 100-2,15,260; 100-4,4,20.5; 100-4,12,90.3; 100-4,14,10
AMA: 1996,May,11; 1995,Fall,3

11640　　**Excision, malignant lesion including margins, face, ears, eyelids, nose, lips; excised diameter 0.5 cm or less**　T ◩

AMA: 2002,Nov,5; 1996,May,11; 1995,Fall,3

11641　　excised diameter 0.6 to 1.0 cm　T ◩

AMA: 1996,May,11; 1995,Fall,3

11642　　excised diameter 1.1 to 2.0 cm　T ◩

AMA: 1996,May,11; 1995,Fall,3

11643　　excised diameter 2.1 to 3.0 cm　T ◩

AMA: 1996,May,11; 1995,Fall,3

11644　　excised diameter 3.1 to 4.0 cm　2 T ◩

MED: 100-2,15,260; 100-4,4,20.5; 100-4,12,90.3; 100-4,14,10
AMA: 1996,May,11; 1995,Fall,3

11646　　excised diameter over 4.0 cm　2 T ◩

MED: 100-2,15,260; 100-4,4,20.5; 100-4,12,90.3; 100-4,14,10
AMA: 1996,May,11; 1995,Fall,3
If the excision on the eyelids involves more than skin, consult CPT code 67800 and subsequent codes.

NAILS

If drainage of a paronychia or onychia is performed, consult CPT codes 10060 and 10061.

11719　　**Trimming of nondystrophic nails, any number**　T ◩

MED: 100-2,16,100; 100-3,70.2.1; 100-4,4,20.5
AMA: 2002,Nov,5; 2002,Dec,4; 1997,Nov,12

11720　　**Debridement of nail(s) by any method(s); one to five**　T ◩

MED: 100-2,16,100; 100-3,70.2.1; 100-4,4,20.5
AMA: 2002,Nov,5; 2002,Dec,4

11721　　six or more　T ◩

MED: 100-2,16,100; 100-3,70.2.1; 100-4,4,20.5
AMA: 2002,Nov,5; 2002,Dec,4

11730　　**Avulsion of nail plate, partial or complete, simple; single**　T ◩

MED: 100-2,16,100; 100-3,70.2.1; 100-4,4,20.5
AMA: 2002,Nov,5; 2002,Dec,4; 1996,Mar,10

+ **11732**　　each additional nail plate (List separately in addition to code for primary procedure)　T ◩

MED: 100-2,16,100; 100-3,70.2.1; 100-4,4,20.5
AMA: 2002,Nov,5; 2002,Dec,4
Note that 11732 is an add-on code and must be used in conjunction with 11730.

11740　　**Evacuation of subungual hematoma**　T ◩

AMA: 2002,Nov,5; 2002,Dec,4

11750　　**Excision of nail and nail matrix, partial or complete, (eg, ingrown or deformed nail) for permanent removal;**　T ◩

MED: 100-2,16,100; 100-3,70.2.1; 100-4,4,20.5
AMA: 2002,Nov,5; 2002,Dec,4

11752　　with amputation of tuft of distal phalanx　T ◩

AMA: 2002,Nov,5
If a skin graft is performed, consult CPT code 15050.

11755　　**Biopsy of nail unit (eg, plate, bed, matrix, hyponychium, proximal and lateral nail folds) (separate procedure)**　T 80 ◩

AMA: 2002,Nov,5; 1996,Mar,11

11760　　**Repair of nail bed**　T ◩

AMA: 2002,Nov,5; 2002,Dec,4

11762　　**Reconstruction of nail bed with graft**　T ◩

AMA: 2002,Nov,5; 2002,Dec,4

11765　　**Wedge excision of skin of nail fold (eg, for ingrown toenail)**　T ◩

AMA: 2002,Nov,5; 2002,Dec,4
Cotting's operation

PILONIDAL CYST

11770　　**Excision of pilonidal cyst or sinus; simple**　3 T ◩

MED: 100-2,15,260; 100-4,4,20.5; 100-4,12,90.3; 100-4,14,10
If a pilonidal cyst is incised, consult CPT codes 10080 and 10081.

11771　　extensive　3 T ◩

MED: 100-2,15,260; 100-4,4,20.5; 100-4,12,90.3; 100-4,14,10

11772　　complicated　3 T ◩

MED: 100-2,15,260; 100-4,4,20.5; 100-4,12,90.3; 100-4,14,10

INTRODUCTION

11900　　**Injection, intralesional; up to and including seven lesions**　T ◩

AMA: 2000,Feb,11; 1998,May,10; 1996,Sep,5

26 Professional Component Only　　　　80/80 Assist-at-Surgery Allowed/With Documentation　　　Unlisted　　　Not Covered

TC Technical Component Only　　MED: Pub 100/NCD References　AMA: CPT Assistant References　1-9 ASC Group　♂ Male Only　♀ Female Only

46 — CPT Expert　　　　　CPT only © 2006 American Medical Association. All Rights Reserved. (Black Ink)　　　　© 2006 Ingenix (Blue Ink)

11901   more than seven lesions   T ⬚

AMA: 2000,Feb,11; 1998,May,10; 1996,Sep,5

If the injection of sclerosing solution is for a vein, consult CPT codes 36470-36471. If intralesional chemotherapy is administered, consult CPT codes 96405-96406.

Do not report 11900, 11901 for preoperative local anesthetic injections.

11920   Tattooing, intradermal introduction of insoluble opaque pigments to correct color defects of skin, including micropigmentation; 6.0 sq cm or less   T 80 ⬚

MED: 100-2,16,10; 100-2,16,120; 100-2,16,180; 100-4,4,20.5; 100-4,12,70; 100-4,13,20; 100-4,13,90

11921   6.1 to 20.0 sq cm   T 80 ⬚

MED: 100-2,16,10; 100-2,16,120; 100-2,16,180; 100-4,4,20.5; 100-4,12,70; 100-4,13,20; 100-4,13,90

+   **11922**   each additional 20.0 sq cm (List separately in addition to code for primary procedure)   T 80

MED: 100-2,16,10; 100-2,16,120; 100-2,16,180; 100-4,4,20.5

Note that 11922 is an add-on code and must be used in conjunction with 11921.

11950   Subcutaneous injection of filling material (eg, collagen); 1 cc or less   T 80 ⬚

MED: 100-2,16,10; 100-2,16,120; 100-2,16,180; 100-3,230.10; 100-4,4,20.5

11951   1.1 to 5.0 cc   T 80 ⬚

MED: 100-2,16,10; 100-2,16,120; 100-2,16,180; 100-3,230.10; 100-4,4,20.5

11952   5.1 to 10.0 cc   T 80 ⬚

MED: 100-2,16,10; 100-2,16,120; 100-2,16,180; 100-3,230.10; 100-4,4,20.5

11954   over 10.0 cc   T 80 ⬚

MED: 100-2,16,10; 100-2,16,120; 100-2,16,180; 100-3,230.10; 100-4,4,20.5

11960   Insertion of tissue expander(s) for other than breast, including subsequent expansion   2 T ⬚

MED: 100-2,15,260; 100-4,4,20.5; 100-4,12,90.3; 100-4,14,10

If the breast is reconstructed with a tissue expander(s), consult CPT code 19357.

11970   Replacement of tissue expander with permanent prosthesis   3 T ⬚

MED: 100-2,15,260; 100-4,4,20.5; 100-4,12,90.3; 100-4,14,10

11971   Removal of tissue expander(s) without insertion of prosthesis   1 T 80 ⬚

MED: 100-2,15,260; 100-4,4,20.5; 100-4,12,90.3; 100-4,14,10

11975   Insertion, implantable contraceptive capsules   ♀ E

11976   Removal, implantable contraceptive capsules   ♀ T 80 ⬚

11977   Removal with reinsertion, implantable contraceptive capsules   ♀ E

11980   Subcutaneous hormone pellet implantation (implantation of estradiol and/or testosterone pellets beneath the skin)   X ⬚

AMA: 1999,Nov,8

11981   Insertion, non-biodegradable drug delivery implant   X 80 ⬚

11982   Removal, non-biodegradable drug delivery implant   X 80 ⬚

11983   Removal with reinsertion, non-biodegradable drug delivery implant   X 80 ⬚

REPAIR (CLOSURE)

Repair is the surgical closure of a wound. The wound may be a result of injury/trauma or it may be a surgically created defect. Repairs can be any of the following:

- Stand alone procedures
- Separately reportable services when performed with certain other procedures as in the case of excisions requiring intermediate or complex repair
- An integral part of a more complex procedure and not separately reportable

Repairs are divided into three categories: simple, intermediate, and complex. They are further described by anatomic site and wound size.

Simple repair is performed when the wound is superficial, e.g., involving partial or full-thickness damage to the skin and/or subcutaneous tissues. There is no significant involvement of deeper structures and only simple, one layer, primary suturing is required. This procedure includes local anesthetic and chemical or electrocauterization of wounds not closed. Wounds closed with adhesive strips should be reported using the appropriate evaluation and management code.

Intermediate repair is performed for wounds and lacerations in which one or more of the deeper layers of subcutaneous tissue and non-muscle fascia are repaired in addition to the skin and subcutaneous tissue. Single-layer closure can also be coded as an intermediate repair if the wound is heavily contaminated and requires extensive cleaning or removal of particulate matter.

Complex repair includes repair of wounds requiring more than layered closure. Wounds coded from this category include those requiring revision, debridement, extensive undermining, and placement of stents or retention sutures. Complex repairs also include those requiring creation of a defect (e.g., extending excision) and special preparation of the site.

The following rules should be followed when reporting repairs:

- Measure the length of the repaired wound or wounds and report in centimeters. A centimeter is 0.39 inches.
- Add together the lengths of multiple wounds in the same classification and report as a single item. For example, a simple repair of a 2-centimeter scalp wound and a simple repair of a 1.5-centimeter wound of the forearm would be reported with a single code. 12002 Simple repair of superficial wounds of scalp, neck, axillae, external genitalia, trunk and/or extremities (including hands and feet); 2.6 cm to 7.5 cm This procedure is coded with a single procedure code because both wounds are classified as simple and both are in the same group of simple repairs (12001-12007). Total length of the two wounds is 3.5 centimeters so 12002 is reported.
- Wounds in more than one classification should be listed separately with the more complicated service listed as the primary procedure and the less complicated listed as the secondary procedure with modifier 51 Multiple procedures appended.
- Decontamination and debridement are considered integral to wound repair except when gross contamination requires prolonged cleansing or when appreciable amounts of devitalized contaminated tissue must be removed.
- Repair of nerves, blood vessels, and tendons should be reported under the appropriate system. Repair of associated skin wounds is considered integral to the repair of nerves, blood vessels, and tendons and is not reported separately unless the wound repair qualifies as complex. In these instances report the complex repair code.
- Simple exploration of nerves, blood vessels, and tendons exposed in an open wound is considered integral to the repair and should not be reported separately.
- Wounds resulting from penetrating trauma that require exploration, enlargement, extension, dissection, removal of foreign body, and/or ligation or coagulation of minor blood vessels of subcutaneous tissue, muscle fascia, or muscle should be reported with 20100-20103 as indicated.

REPAIR — SIMPLE

12001   Simple repair of superficial wounds of scalp, neck, axillae, external genitalia, trunk and/or extremities (including hands and feet); 2.5 cm or less   T ▢

AMA: 2002,Jan,10; 2000,Jul,10; 2000,Jan,11; 2000,Apr,8; 1998,Feb,11; 1996,Jun,7

12002   2.6 cm to 7.5 cm   T ▢

AMA: 2002,Jan,10

12004   7.6 cm to 12.5 cm   T ▢

AMA: 2002,Jan,10

12005   12.6 cm to 20.0 cm   2 T ▢

MED: 100-2,15,260; 100-4,4,20.5; 100-4,12,90.3; 100-4,14,10
AMA: 2002,Jan,10

12006   20.1 cm to 30.0 cm   2 T ▢

MED: 100-2,15,260; 100-4,4,20.5; 100-4,12,90.3; 100-4,14,10
AMA: 2002,Jan,10; 1998,Feb,11

12007   over 30.0 cm   2 T ▢

MED: 100-2,15,260; 100-4,4,20.5; 100-4,12,90.3; 100-4,14,10
AMA: 2002,Jan,10

12011   Simple repair of superficial wounds of face, ears, eyelids, nose, lips and/or mucous membranes; 2.5 cm or less   T ▢

AMA: 2002,Jan,10; 2000,May,8

12013   2.6 cm to 5.0 cm   T ▢

AMA: 2002,Jan,10

12014   5.1 cm to 7.5 cm   T ▢

AMA: 2002,Jan,10

12015   7.6 cm to 12.5 cm   T ▢

AMA: 2002,Jan,10

12016   12.6 cm to 20.0 cm   2 T ▢

MED: 100-2,15,260; 100-4,4,20.5; 100-4,12,90.3; 100-4,14,10
AMA: 2002,Jan,10

12017   20.1 cm to 30.0 cm   2 T 80 ▢

MED: 100-2,15,260; 100-4,4,20.5; 100-4,12,90.3; 100-4,14,10
AMA: 2002,Jan,10

12018   over 30.0 cm   2 T 80 ▢

MED: 100-2,15,260; 100-4,4,20.5; 100-4,12,90.3; 100-4,14,10
AMA: 2002,Jan,10

12020   Treatment of superficial wound dehiscence; simple closure   1 T ▢

MED: 100-2,15,260; 100-4,4,20.5; 100-4,12,90.3; 100-4,14,10
AMA: 2002,Jan,10

12021   with packing   1 T ▢

MED: 100-2,15,260; 100-4,4,20.5; 100-4,12,90.3; 100-4,14,10
AMA: 2002,Jan,10
If the secondary wound closure is extensive or complicated, consult CPT code 13160.

REPAIR — INTERMEDIATE

12031   Layer closure of wounds of scalp, axillae, trunk and/or extremities (excluding hands and feet); 2.5 cm or less   T ▢

AMA: 2002,Jan,10; 2000,Apr,8; 1997,Sep,11

12032   2.6 cm to 7.5 cm   T ▢

AMA: 2002,Jan,10; 1996,Jun,8

12034   7.6 cm to 12.5 cm   2 T ▢

MED: 100-2,15,260; 100-4,4,20.5; 100-4,12,90.3; 100-4,14,10
AMA: 2002,Jan,10; 1991,Fall,6

12035   12.6 cm to 20.0 cm   2 T ▢

MED: 100-2,15,260; 100-4,4,20.5; 100-4,12,90.3; 100-4,14,10
AMA: 2002,Jan,10

12036   20.1 cm to 30.0 cm   2 T ▢

MED: 100-2,15,260; 100-4,4,20.5; 100-4,12,90.3; 100-4,14,10
AMA: 2002,Jan,10

12037   over 30.0 cm   2 T 80 ▢

MED: 100-2,15,260; 100-4,4,20.5; 100-4,12,90.3; 100-4,14,10
AMA: 2002,Jan,10

12041   Layer closure of wounds of neck, hands, feet and/or external genitalia; 2.5 cm or less   T ▢

AMA: 2002,Jan,10; 2000,Apr,8; 1997,Sep,11

12042   2.6 cm to 7.5 cm   T ▢

AMA: 2002,Jan,10

12044   7.6 cm to 12.5 cm   2 T ▢

MED: 100-2,15,260; 100-4,4,20.5; 100-4,12,90.3; 100-4,14,10
AMA: 2002,Jan,10

12045   12.6 cm to 20.0 cm   2 T ▢

MED: 100-2,15,260; 100-4,4,20.5; 100-4,12,90.3; 100-4,14,10
AMA: 2002,Jan,10

12046   20.1 cm to 30.0 cm   2 T 80 ▢

MED: 100-2,15,260; 100-4,4,20.5; 100-4,12,90.3; 100-4,14,10
AMA: 2002,Jan,10

12047   over 30.0 cm   2 T 80 ▢

MED: 100-2,15,260; 100-4,4,20.5; 100-4,12,90.3; 100-4,14,10
AMA: 2002,Jan,10

12051   Layer closure of wounds of face, ears, eyelids, nose, lips and/or mucous membranes; 2.5 cm or less   T ▢

AMA: 2002,Jan,10; 2000,Apr,8; 1997,Sep,11

12052   2.6 cm to 5.0 cm   T ▢

AMA: 2002,Jan,10

12053   5.1 cm to 7.5 cm   T ▢

AMA: 2002,Jan,10

12054   7.6 cm to 12.5 cm   2 T ▢

MED: 100-2,15,260; 100-4,4,20.5; 100-4,12,90.3; 100-4,14,10
AMA: 2002,Jan,10

12055   12.6 cm to 20.0 cm   2 T ▢

MED: 100-2,15,260; 100-4,4,20.5; 100-4,12,90.3; 100-4,14,10
AMA: 2002,Jan,10

12056   20.1 cm to 30.0 cm   2 T 80 ▢

MED: 100-2,15,260; 100-4,4,20.5; 100-4,12,90.3; 100-4,14,10
AMA: 2002,Jan,10

12057   over 30.0 cm   2 T 80 ▢

MED: 100-2,15,260; 100-4,4,20.5; 100-4,12,90.3; 100-4,14,10
AMA: 2002,Jan,10

REPAIR — COMPLEX

13100   Repair, complex, trunk; 1.1 cm to 2.5 cm   2 T ▢

MED: 100-2,15,260; 100-4,4,20.5; 100-4,12,90.3; 100-4,14,10
AMA: 2000,Apr,8; 1999,Nov,9-10; 1998,Dec,5; 1997,Sep,11
If the repair is 1.0 cm or less, see simple or intermediate repairs.

13101   2.6 cm to 7.5 cm   3 T ▢

MED: 100-2,15,260; 100-4,4,20.5; 100-4,12,90.3; 100-4,14,10
AMA: 1999,Nov,9-10; 1998,Dec,5

+ 13102   each additional 5 cm or less (List separately in addition to code for primary procedure)   1 T ▢

AMA: 1999,Nov,9-10
Note that 13102 is an add-on code and must be used in conjunction with 13101.

26 Professional Component Only   80/80 Assist-at-Surgery Allowed/With Documentation   Unlisted   Not Covered

TC Technical Component Only   MED: Pub 100/NCD References   AMA: CPT Assistant References   1-9 ASC Group   ♂ Male Only   ♀ Female Only

48 — CPT Expert   CPT only © 2006 American Medical Association. All Rights Reserved. (Black Ink)   © 2006 Ingenix (Blue Ink)

13120   **Repair, complex, scalp, arms, and/or legs; 1.1 cm to 2.5 cm**   2 T ☐

MED: 100-2,15,260; 100-4,4,20.5; 100-4,12,90.3; 100-4,14,10
AMA: 2000,Apr,8; 1999,Nov,9-10; 1999,Apr,11; 1997,Sep,11
If the repair is 1.0 cm or less, see simple or intermediate repairs.

13121   **2.6 cm to 7.5 cm**   3 T ☐

MED: 100-2,15,260; 100-4,4,20.5; 100-4,12,90.3; 100-4,14,10
AMA: 2000,Feb,10; 1999,Nov,9-10; 1998,Dec,5

+ 13122   **each additional 5 cm or less (List separately in addition to code for primary procedure)**   1 T ☐

AMA: 1999,Nov,10
Note that 13122 is an add-on code and must be used in conjunction with 13121.

13131   **Repair, complex, forehead, cheeks, chin, mouth, neck, axillae, genitalia, hands and/or feet; 1.1 cm to 2.5 cm**   2 T ☐

MED: 100-2,15,260; 100-4,4,20.5; 100-4,12,90.3; 100-4,14,10
AMA: 2000,Apr,8; 1999,Nov,10; 1998,Dec,5; 1997,Sep,11; 1993,Fall,7
If the repair is 1.0 cm or less, see simple or intermediate repairs.

13132   **2.6 cm to 7.5 cm**   3 T ☐

MED: 100-2,15,260; 100-4,4,20.5; 100-4,12,90.3; 100-4,14,10
AMA: 1999,Nov,10; 1999,Dec,10; 1998,Dec,5; 1993,Fall,7

+ 13133   **each additional 5 cm or less (List separately in addition to code for primary procedure)**   1 T ☐

AMA: 1998,Nov,10
Note that 13133 is an add-on code and must be used in conjunction with 13132.

13150   **Repair, complex, eyelids, nose, ears and/or lips; 1.0 cm or less**   3 T ☐

MED: 100-2,15,260; 100-4,4,20.5; 100-4,12,90.3; 100-4,14,10
AMA: 2000,Apr,8; 1999,Nov,10; 1998,Dec,5; 1997,Sep,11
Consult also CPT codes 40650-40654, and 67961-67975.

13151   **1.1 cm to 2.5 cm**   3 T ☐

MED: 100-2,15,260; 100-4,4,20.5; 100-4,12,90.3; 100-4,14,10
AMA: 1999,Nov,10; 1998,Dec,5

13152   **2.6 cm to 7.5 cm**   3 T ☐

MED: 100-2,15,260; 100-4,4,20.5; 100-4,12,90.3; 100-4,14,10
AMA: 1999,Nov,10; 1998,Dec,5

+ 13153   **each additional 5 cm or less (List separately in addition to code for primary procedure)**   3 T ☐

AMA: 1999,Nov,10
If full thickness repair of the lip or the eyelid is required, consult relevant anatomical subsections.

Note that 13153 is an add-on code and must be used in conjunction with 13152.

13160   **Secondary closure of surgical wound or dehiscence, extensive or complicated**   2 T ☐

MED: 100-2,15,260; 100-4,4,20.5; 100-4,12,90.3; 100-4,14,10
AMA: 2000,Apr,8; 1998,Dec,5; 1997,Sep,11
To report packing or simple secondary wound closure, consult CPT codes 12020 and 12021.

ADJACENT TISSUE TRANSFER OR REARRANGEMENT

Anatomic site and size of the defect defines adjacent tissue transfer or rearrangement. Adjacent tissue transfers include excision of the defect or lesion so excision codes should not be reported additionally. For code selection, the term defect includes both primary and secondary defects. The primary defect results from the excision and the secondary defect results from the creation of the flap design. Measure both defects together to determine code selection.

Terms used to describe transfer or rearrangement procedures include: Z-plasty, W-plasty, V-Y-plasty, rotation flap, advancement flap, double pedicle flap. When applied to primary traumatic wound closure, the configuration listed must be developed by the surgeon to accomplish the repair. Transfer and rearrangement codes should not be applied when traumatic wounds incidentally result in these configurations.

Tissue transfer or rearrangement codes describe moving normal tissue from the donor site to the recipient site. The donor site is adjacent or next to the affected area, allowing the tissue to remain attached to its original location and blood supply, ensuring survival of the graft.

A skin graft that is needed to close a secondary defect is an additional procedure.

Refer to the specific anatomical subsections for CPT codes for full-thickness repairs of the lips and eyelids.

14000   **Adjacent tissue transfer or rearrangement, trunk; defect 10 sq cm or less**   2 T ☐

MED: 100-2,15,260; 100-4,4,20.5; 100-4,12,90.3; 100-4,14,10
AMA: 2000,Jul,10; 1999,Jul,3; 1996,Sep,11
Burrow's operation

14001   **defect 10.1 sq cm to 30.0 sq cm**   3 T ☐

MED: 100-2,15,260; 100-4,4,20.5; 100-4,12,90.3; 100-4,14,10
AMA: 1999,Jul,3

14020   **Adjacent tissue transfer or rearrangement, scalp, arms and/or legs; defect 10 sq cm or less**   3 T ☐

MED: 100-2,15,260; 100-4,4,20.5; 100-4,12,90.3; 100-4,14,10
AMA: 1999,Jul,3

14021   **defect 10.1 sq cm to 30.0 sq cm**   3 T ☐

MED: 100-2,15,260; 100-4,4,20.5; 100-4,12,90.3; 100-4,14,10
AMA: 1999,Jul,3

14040   **Adjacent tissue transfer or rearrangement, forehead, cheeks, chin, mouth, neck, axillae, genitalia, hands and/or feet; defect 10 sq cm or less**   2 T ☐

MED: 100-2,15,260; 100-4,4,20.5; 100-4,12,90.3; 100-4,14,10
AMA: 2000,Jul,10; 1999,Jul,3
Krimer's palatoplasty

14041   **defect 10.1 sq cm to 30.0 sq cm**   3 T ☐

MED: 100-2,15,260; 100-4,4,20.5; 100-4,12,90.3; 100-4,14,10
AMA: 1999,Jul,3

14060   **Adjacent tissue transfer or rearrangement, eyelids, nose, ears and/or lips; defect 10 sq cm or less**   3 T ☐

MED: 100-2,15,260; 100-4,4,20.5; 100-4,12,90.3; 100-4,14,10
AMA: 1999,Jul,3; 1999,Dec,10; 1993,Fall,7
Denonvillier's operation

14061   **defect 10.1 sq cm to 30.0 sq cm**   3 T ☐

MED: 100-2,15,260; 100-4,4,20.5; 100-4,12,90.3; 100-4,14,10
AMA: 1999,Jul,3

14300   **Adjacent tissue transfer or rearrangement, more than 30 sq cm, unusual or complicated, any area**   4 T ☐

MED: 100-2,15,260; 100-4,4,20.5; 100-4,12,90.3; 100-4,14,10
AMA: 1996,Sep,11

14350   **Filleted finger or toe flap, including preparation of recipient site**   3 T 86

MED: 100-2,15,260; 100-4,4,20.5; 100-4,12,90.3; 100-4,14,10

SKIN REPLACEMENT SURGERY AND SKIN SUBSTITUTES

The site where the tissue originates is referred to as the donor site, while the site where the tissue is being relocated is referred to as the recipient site.

Skin replacement surgery and skin substitute codes are chosen by the size and location of the defect (recipient site) and the type of graft or skin substitute. The codes include uncomplicated debridement of granulation tissue or recent avulsion.

Integumentary System

15000 — 15130

Surgical preparation of the recipient site should be reported separately with codes 15002-15005. These codes should also be used for burn and wound preparation or incisional or excisional scar contracture release that requires a skin graft.

Use 100 square cm for children age 10 and older and percentages of body surface area for infants and children younger than the age of 10.

Report codes 15100-15261 by recipient site for autologous skin grafts. For autologous tissue-cultured epidermal grafts, consult 15150-15157. Report 15040 for harvesting of autologous keratinocytes and dermal tissue for tissue-cultured skin grafts. Report 15170-15176 for acellular dermal replacement. Add modifier 58 for staged application procedures.

These codes require that the graft be anchored and not just stabilized with dressings.

SURGICAL PREPARATION

~~15000~~   ~~Surgical preparation or creation of recipient site by excision of open wounds, burn eschar, or scar (including subcutaneous tissues), or incisional release of scar contracture; first 100 sq cm or one percent of body area of infants and children~~

MED: 100-3,270.5
Use 15002-15005.

~~15001~~   ~~each additional 100 sq cm or each additional one percent of body area of infants and children (List separately in addition to code for primary procedure)~~
Use 15002-15005.

● 15002   Surgical preparation or creation of recipient site by excision of open wounds, burn eschar, or scar (including subcutaneous tissues), or incisional release of scar contracture, trunk, arms, legs; first 100 sq cm or 1% of body area of infants and children   2 T

+ ● 15003   each additional 100 sq cm or each additional 1% of body area of infants and children (List separately in addition to code for primary procedure)   1 T

Note that 15003 is an add-on code and must be with 15002.

● 15004   Surgical preparation or creation of recipient site by excision of open wounds, burn eschar, or scar (including subcutaneous tissues), or incisional release of scar contracture, face, scalp, eyelids, mouth, neck, ears, orbits, genitalia, hands, feet and/or multiple digits; first 100 sq cm or 1% of body area of infants and children   2 T

+ ● 15005   each additional 100 sq cm or each additional 1% of body area of infants and children (List separately in addition to code for primary procedure)   1 T

Note that 15005 is an add-on code and must be used in conjunction with 15004.

Use 15002-15005 in conjunction with the code for appropriate skin grafts or replacements, codes 15050-15261 or 15330-15336. List the graft or replacement separately by its procedure code when the graft, whether immediate or delayed, is applied.

GRAFTS

AUTOGRAFT/TISSUE CULTURED AUTOGRAFT

15040   Harvest of skin for tissue cultured skin autograft, 100 sq cm or less   2 T

MED: 100-4,3,20.1.2.8

15050   Pinch graft, single or multiple, to cover small ulcer, tip of digit, or other minimal open area (except on face), up to defect size 2 cm diameter   2 T ⬚

MED: 100-2,15,260; 100-4,3,20.1.2.8; 100-4,4,20.5; 100-4,12,90.3; 100-4,14,10
AMA: 1998,Nov,6; 1997,Sep,1; 1997,Apr,4

15100   Split-thickness autograft, trunk, arms, legs; first 100 sq cm or less, or 1% of body area of infants and children (except 15050)   2 T

MED: 100-2,15,260; 100-4,3,20.1.2.8; 100-4,4,20.5; 100-4,12,90.3; 100-4,14,10
AMA: 2002,Sep,3; 1998,Nov,6; 1997,Sep,1; 1997,Aug,6; 1997,Apr,4; 1993,Fall,7

+ 15101   each additional 100 sq cm, or each additional 1% of body area of infants and children, or part thereof (List separately in addition to code for primary procedure)   3 T

MED: 100-2,15,260; 100-4,3,20.1.2.8; 100-4,4,20.5; 100-4,12,90.3; 100-4,14,10
AMA: 2002,Sep,3; 1998,Nov,6; 1997,Apr,4
Note that 15101 is an add-on code and must be used in conjunction with 15100.

▲ 15110   Epidermal autograft, trunk, arms, legs; first 100 sq cm or less, or 1% of body area of infants and children   2 T

MED: 100-4,3,20.1.2.8

+ ▲ 15111   each additional 100 sq cm, or each additional 1% of body area of infants and children, or part thereof (List separately in addition to code for primary procedure)   1 T

MED: 100-4,3,20.1.2.8
Note that 15111 is an add-on code and must be used in conjunction with 15110.

▲ 15115   Epidermal autograft, face, scalp, eyelids, mouth, neck, ears, orbits, genitalia, hands, feet, and/or multiple digits; first 100 sq cm or less, or 1% of body area of infants and children   2 T

MED: 100-4,3,20.1.2.8

+ ▲ 15116   each additional 100 sq cm, or each additional 1% of body area of infants and children, or part thereof (List separately in addition to code for primary procedure)   1 T

MED: 100-4,3,20.1.2.8
Note that 15116 is an add-on code and must be used in conjunction with 15115.

▲ 15120   Split-thickness autograft, face, scalp, eyelids, mouth, neck, ears, orbits, genitalia, hands, feet, and/or multiple digits; first 100 sq cm or less, or 1% of body area of infants and children (except 15050)   2 T ⬚

MED: 100-2,15,260; 100-4,3,20.1.2.8; 100-4,4,20.5; 100-4,12,90.3; 100-4,14,10
AMA: 2002,Sep,3; 1999,Jan,4; 1998,Nov,6; 1997,Sep,1; 1997,Aug,6; 1997,Apr,4

+ ▲ 15121   each additional 100 sq cm, or each additional 1% of body area of infants and children, or part thereof (List separately in addition to code for primary procedure)   3 T

MED: 100-2,15,260; 100-4,3,20.1.2.8; 100-4,4,20.5; 100-4,12,90.3; 100-4,14,10
AMA: 2002,Sep,3; 1999,Jan,4; 1998,Nov,6; 1997,Sep,1; 1997,Aug,6; 1997,Apr,4
Note that 15121 is an add-on code and must be used in conjunction with 15120. If the split graft is performed on the eyelids, consult also CPT codes 67961 and subsequent codes.

▲ 15130   Dermal autograft, trunk, arms, legs; first 100 sq cm or less, or 1% of body area of infants and children   2 T

MED: 100-4,3,20.1.2.8; 100-4,4,20.5

26 Professional Component Only

80/80 Assist-at-Surgery Allowed/With Documentation   Unlisted   Not Covered

TC Technical Component Only   MED: Pub 100/NCD References   AMA: CPT Assistant References   1-9 ASC Group   ♂ Male Only   ♀ Female Only

50 — CPT Expert   CPT only © 2006 American Medical Association. All Rights Reserved. *(Black Ink)*   © 2006 Ingenix *(Blue Ink)*

+ ▲ **15131** each additional 100 sq cm, or each additional 1% of body area of infants and children, or part thereof (List separately in addition to code for primary procedure) 🔟 Ⓣ

MED: 100-4,3,20.1.2.8; 100-4,4,20.5
Note that 15131 is an add-on code and must be used in conjunction with 15130.

▲ **15135** Dermal autograft, face, scalp, eyelids, mouth, neck, ears, orbits, genitalia, hands, feet, and/or multiple digits; first 100 sq cm or less, or 1% of body area of infants and children 🔢 Ⓣ

MED: 100-4,3,20.1.2.8; 100-4,4,20.5

+ ▲ **15136** each additional 100 sq cm, or each additional 1% of body area of infants and children, or part thereof (List separately in addition to code for primary procedure) 🔟 Ⓣ

MED: 100-4,3,20.1.2.8; 100-4,4,20.5
Note that 15136 is an add-on code and must be used in conjunction with 15135.

15150 Tissue cultured epidermal autograft, trunk, arms, legs; first 25 sq cm or less 🔢 Ⓣ

MED: 100-4,3,20.1.2.8; 100-4,4,20.5

+ **15151** additional 1 sq cm to 75 sq cm (List separately in addition to code for primary procedure) 🔟 Ⓣ

MED: 100-4,3,20.1.2.8; 100-4,4,20.5
Code 15151 cannot be reported more than once per session.

Note that 15151 is an add-on code and must be used in conjunction with 15150.

+ ▲ **15152** each additional 100 sq cm, or each additional 1% of body area of infants and children, or part thereof (List separately in addition to code for primary procedure) 🔟 Ⓣ

MED: 100-4,3,20.1.2.8; 100-4,4,20.5
Note that 15152 is an add-on code and must be used in conjunction with 15151.

15155 Tissue cultured epidermal autograft, face, scalp, eyelids, mouth, neck, ears, orbits, genitalia, hands, feet, and/or multiple digits; first 25 sq cm or less 🔢 Ⓣ

MED: 100-4,3,20.1.2.8; 100-4,4,20.5

+ **15156** additional 1 sq cm to 75 sq cm (List separately in addition to code for primary procedure) 🔟 Ⓣ

MED: 100-4,3,20.1.2.8; 100-4,4,20.5
Code 15156 should not be reported more than once per session.

Note that 15156 is an add-on code and must be used in conjunction with 15155.

+ ▲ **15157** each additional 100 sq cm, or each additional 1% of body area of infants and children, or part thereof (List separately in addition to code for primary procedure) 🔟 Ⓣ

MED: 100-4,3,20.1.2.8; 100-4,4,20.5
Note that 15157 is an add-on code and must be used in conjunction with 15156.

ACELLULAR DERMAL REPLACEMENT

▲ **15170** Acellular dermal replacement, trunk, arms, legs; first 100 sq cm or less, or 1% of body area of infants and children Ⓣ

MED: 100-4,3,20.1.2.8; 100-4,4,20.5

+ ▲ **15171** each additional 100 sq cm, or each additional 1% of body area of infants and children, or part thereof (List separately in addition to code for primary procedure) Ⓣ

MED: 100-4,3,20.1.2.8; 100-4,4,20.5
Note that 15171 is an add-on code and must be used in conjunction with 15170.

▲ **15175** Acellular dermal replacement, face, scalp, eyelids, mouth, neck, ears, orbits, genitalia, hands, feet, and/or multiple digits; first 100 sq cm or less, or 1% of body area of infants and children Ⓣ

MED: 100-4,3,20.1.2.8; 100-4,4,20.5

+ ▲ **15176** each additional 100 sq cm, or each additional 1% of body area of infants and children, or part thereof (List separately in addition to code for primary procedure) Ⓣ

MED: 100-4,3,20.1.2.8; 100-4,4,20.5
Note that 15176 is an add-on code and must be used in conjunction with 15175.

15200 Full thickness graft, free, including direct closure of donor site, trunk; 20 sq cm or less 🔢 Ⓣ ◪

MED: 100-2,15,260; 100-4,3,20.1.2.8; 100-4,4,20.5; 100-4,12,90.3; 100-4,14,10
AMA: 1997,Sep,1; 1997,Aug,6; 1996,Aug,11

+ **15201** each additional 20 sq cm (List separately in addition to code for primary procedure) 🔢 Ⓣ 🔠

MED: 100-2,15,260; 100-4,3,20.1.2.8; 100-4,4,20.5; 100-4,12,90.3; 100-4,14,10
AMA: 1997,Sep,1; 1997,Aug,6; 1997,Apr,4
Note that 15201 is an add-on code and must be used in conjunction with 15200.

15220 Full thickness graft, free, including direct closure of donor site, scalp, arms, and/or legs; 20 sq cm or less 🔢 Ⓣ ◪

MED: 100-2,15,260; 100-4,3,20.1.2.8; 100-4,4,20.5; 100-4,12,90.3; 100-4,14,10
AMA: 1997,Sep,1; 1997,Aug,6; 1997,Apr,4

+ **15221** each additional 20 sq cm (List separately in addition to code for primary procedure) 🔢 Ⓣ

MED: 100-2,15,260; 100-4,3,20.1.2.8; 100-4,4,20.5; 100-4,12,90.3; 100-4,14,10
AMA: 1997,Sep,1; 1997,Aug,6; 1997,Apr,4
Note that 15221 is an add-on code and must be used in conjunction with 15220.

15240 Full thickness graft, free, including direct closure of donor site, forehead, cheeks, chin, mouth, neck, axillae, genitalia, hands, and/or feet; 20 sq cm or less 🔢 Ⓣ ◪

MED: 100-2,15,260; 100-4,3,20.1.2.8; 100-4,4,20.5; 100-4,12,90.3; 100-4,14,10
AMA: 2000,Nov,10; 1997,Sep,1; 1997,Aug,6; 1997,Apr,4
If the flap is microvascular, consult CPT codes 15756-15758.

If the graft is performed on the fingertip, consult CPT code 15050. If the repair is performed on a web finger (syndactyly), consult CPT codes 26560-26562.

+ **15241** each additional 20 sq cm (List separately in addition to code for primary procedure) 🔢 Ⓣ

MED: 100-2,15,260; 100-4,3,20.1.2.8; 100-4,4,20.5; 100-4,12,90.3; 100-4,14,10
AMA: 1997,Sep,1; 1997,Aug,6; 1997,Apr,4
Note that 15241 is an add-on code and must be used in conjunction with 15240.

15260   **Full thickness graft, free, including direct closure of donor site, nose, ears, eyelids, and/or lips; 20 sq cm or less** 🄬 Ⓣ ▣

> MED: 100-2,15,260; 100-4,3,20.1.2.8; 100-4,4,20.5; 100-4,12,90.3; 100-4,14,10
>
> AMA: 1999,Jul,3; 1997,Sep,1; 1997,Aug,6; 1997,Apr,4; 1993,Fall,7; 1991,Fall,7

+ **15261**   **each additional 20 sq cm (List separately in addition to code for primary procedure)** 🄬 Ⓣ

> MED: 100-2,15,260; 100-4,3,20.1.2.8; 100-4,4,20.5; 100-4,12,90.3; 100-4,14,10
>
> AMA: 1997,Sep,1; 1997,Aug,6; 1997,Apr,4; 1991,Fall,7
>
> Note that 15261 is an add-on code and must be used in conjunction with 15260. If a full-thickness graft is performed on the eyelids, consult also 67961 and subsequent codes. If the donor site repair requires a skin graft or local flaps, the procedure is to be added as an additional separate procedure.

ALLOGRAFT/TISSUE CULTURED ALLOGENIC SKIN SUBSTITUTE

These codes are used to report a non-autologous human skin graft from a donor to the recipient's body to resurface tissue damaged by burns, injury, infection, necrosis or surgery.

▲ **15300**   **Allograft skin for temporary wound closure, trunk, arms, legs; first 100 sq cm or less, or 1% of body area of infants and children** 🄬 Ⓣ

> MED: 100-4,3,20.1.2.8; 100-4,4,20.5

+ ▲ **15301**   **each additional 100 sq cm, or each additional 1% of body area of infants and children, or part thereof (List separately in addition to code for primary procedure)** 🄵 Ⓣ

> MED: 100-4,3,20.1.2.8; 100-4,4,20.5
>
> Note that 15301 is an add-on code and must be used in conjunction with 15300.

▲ **15320**   **Allograft skin for temporary wound closure, face, scalp, eyelids, mouth, neck, ears, orbits, genitalia, hands, feet, and/or multiple digits; first 100 sq cm or less, or 1% of body area of infants and children** 🄬 Ⓣ

> MED: 100-4,3,20.1.2.8; 100-4,4,20.5

+ ▲ **15321**   **each additional 100 sq cm, or each additional 1% of body area of infants and children, or part thereof (List separately in addition to code for primary procedure)** 🄵 Ⓣ

> MED: 100-4,3,20.1.2.8; 100-4,4,20.5
>
> Note that 15321 is an add-on code and must be used in conjunction with 15320.

▲ **15330**   **Acellular dermal allograft, trunk, arms, legs; first 100 sq cm or less, or 1% of body area of infants and children** 🄬 Ⓣ

> MED: 100-4,3,20.1.2.8; 100-4,4,20.5

+ ▲ **15331**   **each additional 100 sq cm, or each additional 1% of body area of infants and children, or part thereof (List separately in addition to code for primary procedure)** 🄵 Ⓣ

> MED: 100-4,3,20.1.2.8; 100-4,4,20.5
>
> Note that 15331 is an add-on code and must be used in conjunction with 15330.

▲ **15335**   **Acellular dermal allograft, face, scalp, eyelids, mouth, neck, ears, orbits, genitalia, hands, feet, and/or multiple digits; first 100 sq cm or less, or 1% of body area of infants and children** 🄬 Ⓣ

> MED: 100-4,3,20.1.2.8; 100-4,4,20.5

+ ▲ **15336**   **each additional 100 sq cm, or each additional 1% of body area of infants and children, or part thereof (List separately in addition to code for primary procedure)** 🄵 Ⓣ

> MED: 100-4,3,20.1.2.8; 100-4,4,20.5
>
> Note that 15336 is an add-on code and must be used in conjunction with 15335.

15340   **Tissue cultured allogeneic skin substitute; first 25 sq cm or less** Ⓣ

> MED: 100-4,3,20.1.2.8; 100-4,4,20.5

+ **15341**   **each additional 25 sq cm** Ⓣ

> MED: 100-4,3,20.1.2.8; 100-4,4,20.5
>
> Note that 15341 is an add-on code and must be used in conjunction with 15340. Codes 15340 and 15341 should not be reported with 11040-11042, 15002-15005.

▲ **15360**   **Tissue cultured allogeneic dermal substitute, trunk, arms, legs; first 100 sq cm or less, or 1% of body area of infants and children** Ⓣ

> MED: 100-4,3,20.1.2.8; 100-4,4,20.5

+ ▲ **15361**   **each additional 100 sq cm, or each additional 1% of body area of infants and children, or part thereof (List separately in addition to code for primary procedure)** Ⓣ

> MED: 100-4,3,20.1.2.8; 100-4,4,20.5
>
> Note that 15361 is an add-on code and must be used in conjunction with 15360.

▲ **15365**   **Tissue cultured allogeneic dermal substitute, face, scalp, eyelids, mouth, neck, ears, orbits, genitalia, hands, feet, and/or multiple digits; first 100 sq cm or less, or 1% of body area of infants and children** Ⓣ

> MED: 100-4,3,20.1.2.8; 100-4,4,20.5

+ ▲ **15366**   **each additional 100 sq cm, or each additional 1% of body area of infants and children, or part thereof (List separately in addition to code for primary procedure)** Ⓣ

> MED: 100-4,3,20.1.2.8; 100-4,4,20.5
>
> Note that 15366 is an add-on code and must be used in conjunction with 15365.

XENOGRAFT

▲ **15400**   **Xenograft, skin (dermal), for temporary wound closure, trunk, arms, legs; first 100 sq cm or less, or 1% of body area of infants and children** 🄬 Ⓣ ▣

> MED: 100-2,15,260; 100-4,3,20.1.2.8; 100-4,4,20.5; 100-4,12,90.3; 100-4,14,10
>
> AMA: 2001,Apr,10; 1999,Jan,4; 1998,Nov,6; 1997,Sep,1; 1997,Apr,4

+ ▲ **15401**   **each additional 100 sq cm, or each additional 1% of body area of infants and children, or part thereof (List separately in addition to code for primary procedure)** 🄬 Ⓣ

> MED: 100-2,15,260; 100-4,3,20.1.2.8; 100-4,4,20.5; 100-4,12,90.3; 100-4,14,10
>
> AMA: 1999,Jan,4; 1998,Nov,6
>
> Note that 15401 is an add-on code and must be used in conjunction with 15440.

▲ **15420**   **Xenograft skin (dermal), for temporary wound closure, face, scalp, eyelids, mouth, neck, ears, orbits, genitalia, hands, and/or multiple digits; first 100 sq cm or less, or 1% of body area of infants and children** 🄬 Ⓣ

> MED: 100-4,3,20.1.2.8; 100-4,4,20.5

🄬 Professional Component Only   🄼/🄼 Assist-at-Surgery Allowed/With Documentation   Unlisted   Not Covered

🄣 Technical Component Only   **MED:** Pub 100/NCD References   **AMA:** CPT Assistant References   🄵-🄹 ASC Group   ♂ Male Only   ♀ Female Only

52 — CPT Expert

+ ▲ 15421 each additional 100 sq cm, or each additional 1% of body area of infants and children, or part thereof (List separately in addition to code for primary procedure) **1 T**

MED: 100-4,3,20.1.2.8; 100-4,4,20.5;

Note that 15421 is an add-on code and must be used in conjunction with 15420.

▲ 15430 Acellular xenograft implant; first 100 sq cm or less, or 1% of body area of infants and children **2 T**

MED: 100-4,3,20.1.2.8; 100-4,4,20.5;

+ ▲ 15431 each additional 100 sq cm, or each additional 1% of body area of infants and children, or part thereof (List separately in addition to code for primary procedure) **1 T 80**

MED: 100-4,3,20.1.2.8; 100-4,4,20.5;

Note that 15431 is an add-on code and must be used in conjunction with 15430.

Codes 15430 and 15431 cannot be reported with 11040-11042, 15002-15005, or 0170T.

FLAPS (SKIN AND/OR DEEP TISSUES)

If the physician is attaching the flap in transfer or to a final site, select these codes by recipient site. If the physician is forming a tube for later or there will be a delay of the flap, report these codes by donor site.

If repair of the donor site requires skin grafts or local flaps, code as an additional procedure.

If the flap is microvascular, consult CPT codes 15756-15758.

Extensive immobilization (e.g., large casts and other devices) is not included in CPT codes 15570-15738 and should be reported separately.

Pedicle Flap

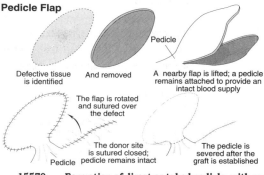

Defective tissue is identified

And removed

Pedicle

A nearby flap is lifted; a pedicle remains attached to provide an intact blood supply

The flap is rotated and sutured over the defect

The donor site is sutured closed; pedicle remains intact

Pedicle

The pedicle is severed after the graft is established

15570 Formation of direct or tubed pedicle, with or without transfer; trunk **3 T**

MED: 100-2,15,260; 100-4,3,20.1.2.8; 100-4,4,20.5; 100-4,12,90.3;
100-4,14,10
AMA: 2002,Nov,5

15572 scalp, arms, or legs **3 T**

MED: 100-2,15,260; 100-4,3,20.1.2.8; 100-4,4,20.5; 100-4,12,90.3;
100-4,14,10

15574 forehead, cheeks, chin, mouth, neck, axillae, genitalia, hands or feet **3 T**

MED: 100-2,15,260; 100-4,3,20.1.2.8; 100-4,4,20.5; 100-4,12,90.3;
100-4,14,10

15576 eyelids, nose, ears, lips, or intraoral **3 T**

MED: 100-2,15,260; 100-4,3,20.1.2.8; 100-4,4,20.5; 100-4,12,90.3;
100-4,14,10

15600 Delay of flap or sectioning of flap (division and inset); at trunk **3 T 80**

MED: 100-2,15,260; 100-4,3,20.1.2.8; 100-4,4,20.5; 100-4,12,90.3;
100-4,14,10
AMA: 1999,Nov,10

15610 at scalp, arms, or legs **3 T 80**

MED: 100-2,15,260; 100-4,3,20.1.2.8; 100-4,4,20.5; 100-4,12,90.3;
100-4,14,10

15620 at forehead, cheeks, chin, neck, axillae, genitalia, hands, or feet **4 T**

MED: 100-2,15,260; 100-4,3,20.1.2.8; 100-4,4,20.5; 100-4,12,90.3;
100-4,14,10

15630 at eyelids, nose, ears, or lips **3 T**

MED: 100-2,15,260; 100-4,3,20.1.2.8; 100-4,4,20.5; 100-4,12,90.3;
100-4,14,10

15650 Transfer, intermediate, of any pedicle flap (eg, abdomen to wrist, Walking tube), any location **5 T 80**

MED: 100-2,15,260; 100-4,3,20.1.2.8; 100-4,4,20.5; 100-4,12,90.3;
100-4,14,10

If the transfer is performed on the eyelids, nose, ears, or lips, consult also the anatomical area.

If a pedicle flap or skin graft is revised, defatted, or rearranged, consult CPT codes 13100-14300.

● 15731 Forehead flap with preservation of vascular pedicle (eg, axial pattern flap, paramedian forehead flap) **3 T**

Use 15732 for muscle, myocutaneous, or fasciocutaneous flap of the head or neck.

15732 Muscle, myocutaneous, or fasciocutaneous flap; head and neck (eg, temporalis, masseter muscle, sternocleidomastoid, levator scapulae) **3 T 80**

MED: 100-2,15,260; 100-4,3,20.1.2.8; 100-4,4,20.5; 100-4,12,90.3;
100-4,14,10

To report forehead flap with preservation of vascular pedicle, consult 15731.

15734 trunk **3 T 80**

MED: 100-2,15,260; 100-4,3,20.1.2.8; 100-4,4,20.5; 100-4,12,90.3;
100-4,14,10

15736 upper extremity **3 T**

MED: 100-2,15,260; 100-4,3,20.1.2.8; 100-4,4,20.5; 100-4,12,90.3;
100-4,14,10

15738 lower extremity **3 T 80**

MED: 100-2,15,260; 100-4,3,20.1.2.8; 100-4,4,20.5; 100-4,12,90.3;
100-4,14,10

OTHER FLAPS AND GRAFTS

If repair of the donor site requires skin grafts or local flaps, code as an additional procedure.

15740 Flap; island pedicle **2 T**

MED: 100-2,15,260; 100-4,3,20.1.2.8; 100-4,4,20.5; 100-4,12,90.3;
100-4,14,10

15750 neurovascular pedicle **2 T 80**

MED: 100-2,15,260; 100-4,3,20.1.2.8; 100-4,4,20.5; 100-4,12,90.3;
100-4,14,10

15756 Free muscle or myocutaneous flap with microvascular anastomosis **C 80**

AMA: 1998,Nov,6; 1997,Nov,12; 1997,Apr,5
Do not report 69990 in addition to code 15756 as the operating microscope is considered an inclusive component of the surgery.

15757 Free skin flap with microvascular anastomosis **C 80**

AMA: 1998,Nov,6; 1997,Apr,5
Do not report 69990 in addition to code 15757 as the operating microscope is considered an inclusive component of the surgery.

⊛ Modifier 63 Exempt Code   ⊙ Conscious Sedation   + CPT Add-on Code   ⊘ Modifier 51 Exempt Code   ● New Code   ▲ Revised Code

M Maternity Edit   **A** Age Edit   **A-Y** APC Status Indicators   **C** CCI Comprehensive Code   **50** Bilateral Procedure

Integumentary System

15758 — 15838

15758   **Free fascial flap with microvascular anastomosis**   C 80

AMA: 1998,Nov,6; 1997,Apr,5

Do not report 69990 in addition to code 15758 as the operating microscope is considered an inclusive component of the surgery.

15760   **Graft; composite (eg, full thickness of external ear or nasal ala), including primary closure, donor area**   2 T

MED: 100-2,15,260; 100-4,3,20.1.2.8; 100-4,4,20.5; 100-4,12,90.3; 100-4,14,10

AMA: 1997,Sep,1

15770   **derma-fat-fascia**   3 T 80

MED: 100-2,15,260; 100-4,3,20.1.2.8; 100-4,4,20.5; 100-4,12,90.3; 100-4,14,10

AMA: 1997,Sep,1

Hair shaft within follicle

Epidermis

Sebaceous gland attached to hair follicle

Ecrine sweat gland with duct open directly to surface

Apocrine sweat gland connected by duct to a hair follicle

Typical male pattern hair loss

Alopecia means hair loss and the condition is separated into two major categories: that which occurs with associated, visable scalp disease, and that which occurs in the absence of visible disease. Male and female pattern hair loss is of the latter category. Hirsutism is excess hair growth, particularly in women, and is often a sign of a systemic medical syndrome

15775   **Punch graft for hair transplant; 1 to 15 punch grafts**   3 T 80

MED: 100-2,15,260; 100-2,16,10; 100-2,16,120; 100-2,16,180; 100-4,4,20.5; 100-4,12,90.3; 100-4,14,10

AMA: 1997,Sep,1

15776   **more than 15 punch grafts**   3 T 80

MED: 100-2,15,260; 100-2,16,10; 100-2,16,120; 100-2,16,180; 100-4,4,20.5; 100-4,12,90.3; 100-4,14,10

AMA: 1997,Sep,1

If the procedure is a strip transplant, consult CPT code 15220.

OTHER PROCEDURES

15780   **Dermabrasion; total face (eg, for acne scarring, fine wrinkling, rhytids, general keratosis)**   T 80

15781   **segmental, face**   T

15782   **regional, other than face**   T 80

15783   **superficial, any site, (eg, tattoo removal)**   T 80

15786   **Abrasion; single lesion (eg, keratosis, scar)**   T

+ **15787**   **each additional four lesions or less (List separately in addition to code for primary procedure)**   T

Note that 15787 is an add-on code and must be used in conjunction with 15786.

15788   **Chemical peel, facial; epidermal**   T

15789   **dermal**   T

15792   **Chemical peel, nonfacial; epidermal**   T 80

15793   **dermal**   T 80

15819   **Cervicoplasty**   T 80

15820   **Blepharoplasty, lower eyelid;**   3 T 80 50

MED: 100-2,15,260; 100-4,4,20.5; 100-4,12,90.3; 100-4,14,10

15821   **with extensive herniated fat pad**   3 T 80 50

MED: 100-2,15,260; 100-4,4,20.5; 100-4,12,90.3; 100-4,14,10

15822   **Blepharoplasty, upper eyelid;**   3 T 80 50

MED: 100-2,15,260; 100-4,4,20.5; 100-4,12,90.3; 100-4,14,10

15823   **with excessive skin weighting down lid**   5 T 50

MED: 100-2,15,260; 100-4,4,20.5; 100-4,12,90.3; 100-4,14,10

AMA: 2000,Sep,7

If procedures 15820-15823 are performed bilaterally, append modifier 50 or 09950.

Frontalis (elevates brow)

Forehead rhytidectomy incision (15824)

A rhytidectomy is an excision to eliminate wrinkles. This procedure in the forehead region typically involves an incision just inside the scalp line. Skin and underlying tissues are then manipulated to eliminate wrinkles in the forehead

Procerus (wrinkles nose)

Corrugators (move brows medially)

15824   **Rhytidectomy; forehead**   3 T 80 50

MED: 100-2,15,260; 100-2,16,10; 100-2,16,120; 100-2,16,180; 100-4,4,20.5; 100-4,12,90.3; 100-4,14,10

If the brow ptosis is repaired, consult CPT code 67900.

15825   **neck with platysmal tightening (platysmal flap, P-flap)**   3 T 80 50

MED: 100-2,15,260; 100-2,16,10; 100-2,16,120; 100-2,16,180; 100-4,4,20.5; 100-4,12,90.3; 100-4,14,10

15826   **glabellar frown lines**   3 T 80 50

MED: 100-2,15,260; 100-4,4,20.5; 100-4,12,90.3; 100-4,14,10

15828   **cheek, chin, and neck**   3 T 80 50

MED: 100-2,15,260; 100-2,16,10; 100-2,16,120; 100-2,16,180; 100-4,4,20.5; 100-4,12,90.3; 100-4,14,10

15829   **superficial musculoaponeurotic system (SMAS) flap**   5 T 80 50

MED: 100-2,15,260; 100-2,16,10; 100-2,16,120; 100-2,16,180; 100-4,4,20.5; 100-4,12,90.3; 100-4,14,10

If rhytidectomy is performed bilaterally, append modifier 50.

● **15830**   **Excision, excessive skin and subcutaneous tissue (includes lipectomy); abdomen, infraumbilical panniculectomy**   3 T

Do not report 15830 in conjunction with 12031-12037, 13100-13102, 14000-14001 or 14300.

~~15831~~   ~~Excision, excessive skin and subcutaneous tissue (including lipectomy); abdomen (abdominoplasty)~~

▲ **15832**   **thigh**   3 T 80

MED: 100-2,15,260; 100-4,4,20.5; 100-4,12,90.3; 100-4,14,10

▲ **15833**   **leg**   3 T 80

MED: 100-2,15,260; 100-4,4,20.5; 100-4,12,90.3; 100-4,14,10

▲ **15834**   **hip**   3 T 80

MED: 100-2,15,260; 100-4,4,20.5; 100-4,12,90.3; 100-4,14,10

▲ **15835**   **buttock**   3 T 80

MED: 100-2,15,260; 100-4,4,20.5; 100-4,12,90.3; 100-4,14,10

▲ **15836**   **arm**   3 T 80

▲ **15837**   **forearm or hand**   T 80

▲ **15838**   **submental fat pad**   T 80

---

26 Professional Component Only   80/80 Assist-at-Surgery Allowed/With Documentation   Unlisted   Not Covered

TC Technical Component Only   MED: Pub 100/NCD References   AMA: CPT Assistant References   1-9 ASC Group   ♂ Male Only   ♀ Female Only

54 — CPT Expert   CPT only © 2006 American Medical Association. All Rights Reserved. (Black Ink)   © 2006 Ingenix (Blue Ink)

▲ 15839   **other area**   3 T 80 ▢

MED: 100-2,15,260; 100-4,4,20.5; 100-4,12,90.3; 100-4,14,10

If procedures 15832-15839 are performed bilaterally, append modifier 50.

15840   **Graft for facial nerve paralysis; free fascia graft (including obtaining fascia)**   4 T ▢

If the facial nerve graft is performed bilaterally, append modifier 50.

15841   **free muscle graft (including obtaining graft)**   4 T 80 ▢

MED: 100-2,15,260; 100-4,4,20.5; 100-4,12,90.3; 100-4,14,10

15842   **free muscle flap by microsurgical technique**   T 80 ▢

Do not report CPT code 69990 together with 15842.

15845   **regional muscle transfer**   4 T 80 ▢

MED: 100-2,15,260; 100-4,4,20.5; 100-4,12,90.3; 100-4,14,10

+ ● 15847   **Excision, excessive skin and subcutaneous tissue (includes lipectomy), abdomen (eg, abdominoplasty) (includes umbilical transposition and fascial plication) (List separately in addition to code for primary procedure)**   3 T

Note that 15847 is an add-on code and must be used in conjunction with 15830.

Use 49491-49587 for abdominal wall hernia repair.

Use 17999 for other abdominoplasty.

15850   **Removal of sutures under anesthesia (other than local), same surgeon**   T

AMA: 1993,Spring,34

15851   **Removal of sutures under anesthesia (other than local), other surgeon**   T ▢

AMA: 1993,Spring,34

15852   **Dressing change (for other than burns) under anesthesia (other than local)**   X ▢

15860   **Intravenous injection of agent (eg, fluorescein) to test vascular flow in flap or graft**   X 80 ▢

Cannula typically inserted through incision in front of ear

In 15876, a liposuction cannula is inserted through fat deposits creating tunnels and removing excess deposits

15876   **Suction assisted lipectomy; head and neck**   3 T 80 ▢

MED: 100-2,15,260; 100-2,16,10; 100-2,16,120; 100-2,16,180; 100-3,140.4; 100-4,4,20.5; 100-4,12,90.3; 100-4,14,10

15877   **trunk**   3 T 80 ▢

MED: 100-2,15,260; 100-2,16,10; 100-2,16,120; 100-2,16,180; 100-4,4,20.5; 100-4,12,90.3; 100-4,14,10

AMA: 1999,Oct,10

15878   **upper extremity**   3 T 80 ▢

MED: 100-2,15,260; 100-2,16,10; 100-2,16,120; 100-2,16,180; 100-4,4,20.5; 100-4,12,90.3; 100-4,14,10

15879   **lower extremity**   3 T 80 ▢

MED: 100-2,15,260; 100-2,16,10; 100-2,16,120; 100-2,16,180; 100-4,4,20.5; 100-4,12,90.3; 100-4,14,10

PRESSURE ULCERS (DECUBITUS ULCERS)

15920   **Excision, coccygeal pressure ulcer, with coccygectomy; with primary suture**   3 T 80 ▢

MED: 100-2,15,260; 100-3,270.5; 100-4,4,20.5; 100-4,12,90.3; 100-4,14,10

If a free skin graft is used to close an ulcer or the donor site, consult CPT codes 15002 and subsequent codes.

15922   **with flap closure**   4 T 80 ▢

MED: 100-2,15,260; 100-3,270.5; 100-4,4,20.5; 100-4,12,90.3; 100-4,14,10

15931   **Excision, sacral pressure ulcer, with primary suture;**   3 T ▢

MED: 100-2,15,260; 100-3,270.5; 100-4,4,20.5; 100-4,12,90.3; 100-4,14,10

15933   **with ostectomy**   3 T 80 ▢

MED: 100-2,15,260; 100-3,270.5; 100-4,4,20.5; 100-4,12,90.3; 100-4,14,10

15934   **Excision, sacral pressure ulcer, with skin flap closure;**   3 T ▢

MED: 100-2,15,260; 100-3,270.5; 100-4,4,20.5; 100-4,12,90.3; 100-4,14,10

15935   **with ostectomy**   4 T 80 ▢

MED: 100-2,15,260; 100-3,270.5; 100-4,4,20.5; 100-4,12,90.3; 100-4,14,10

15936   **Excision, sacral pressure ulcer, in preparation for muscle or myocutaneous flap or skin graft closure;**   4 T ▢

MED: 100-2,15,260; 100-3,270.5; 100-4,4,20.5; 100-4,12,90.3; 100-4,14,10

AMA: 1998,Nov,6-7

15937   **with ostectomy**   4 T 80 ▢

MED: 100-2,15,260; 100-3,270.5; 100-4,4,20.5; 100-4,12,90.3; 100-4,14,10

If a defect is repaired using a muscle or a myocutaneous flap, consult CPT code(s) 15734 and/or 15738 in addition to 15936 and 15937. If a defect is repaired using a split skin graft, consult CPT code(s) 15100 and/or 15101 in addition to 15936 and 15937.

15940   **Excision, ischial pressure ulcer, with primary suture;**   3 T ▢

MED: 100-2,15,260; 100-3,270.5; 100-4,4,20.5; 100-4,12,90.3; 100-4,14,10

15941   **with ostectomy (ischiectomy)**   3 T 80 ▢

MED: 100-2,15,260; 100-4,4,20.5; 100-4,12,90.3; 100-4,14,10

15944   **Excision, ischial pressure ulcer, with skin flap closure;**   3 T 80 ▢

MED: 100-2,15,260; 100-3,270.5; 100-4,4,20.5; 100-4,12,90.3; 100-4,14,10

15945   **with ostectomy**   4 T 80 ▢

MED: 100-2,15,260; 100-3,270.5; 100-4,4,20.5; 100-4,12,90.3; 100-4,14,10

15946   **Excision, ischial pressure ulcer, with ostectomy, in preparation for muscle or myocutaneous flap or skin graft closure**   4 T 80 ▢

MED: 100-2,15,260; 100-3,270.5; 100-4,4,20.5; 100-4,12,90.3; 100-4,14,10

AMA: 2003,Jan,23; 2002,Jun,10; 1998,Nov,6-7

If a defect is repaired using a muscle or a myocutaneous flap, consult CPT code(s) 15734 and/or 15738 in addition to 15946. If a defect is repaired using a split skin graft, consult CPT code(s) 15100 and/or 15101 in addition to 15946.

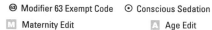

15950 Excision, trochanteric pressure ulcer, with primary suture; **3** T **↵**

MED: 100-2,15,260; 100-3,270.5; 100-4,4,20.5; 100-4,12,90.3; 100-4,14,10

15951 with ostectomy **4** T **80** **↵**

MED: 100-2,15,260; 100-3,270.5; 100-4,4,20.5; 100-4,12,90.3; 100-4,14,10

15952 Excision, trochanteric pressure ulcer, with skin flap closure; **3** T **80** **↵**

MED: 100-2,15,260; 100-3,270.5; 100-4,4,20.5; 100-4,12,90.3; 100-4,14,10

15953 with ostectomy **4** T **↵**

MED: 100-2,15,260; 100-3,270.5; 100-4,4,20.5; 100-4,12,90.3; 100-4,14,10

15956 Excision, trochanteric pressure ulcer, in preparation for muscle or myocutaneous flap or skin graft closure; **3** T **↵**

MED: 100-2,15,260; 100-3,270.5; 100-4,4,20.5; 100-4,12,90.3; 100-4,14,10

AMA: 1998,Nov,6-7

15958 with ostectomy **4** T **80** **↵**

MED: 100-2,15,260; 100-3,270.5; 100-4,4,20.5; 100-4,12,90.3; 100-4,14,10

AMA: 1998,Nov,6-7

If a defect is repaired using a muscle or a myocutaneous flap, consult CPT codes 15734 and/or 15738 in addition to 15956 and 15958. If a defect is repaired using a split skin graft, consult CPT codes 15100 and/or 15101 in addition to 15956 and 15958.

15999 Unlisted procedure, excision pressure ulcer **T** **80**

MED: 100-3,270.5; 100-4,4,20.5; 100-4,4,180.3

If a free skin graft is used to close an ulcer or the donor site, consult CPT codes 15002 and subsequent codes.

BURNS, LOCAL TREATMENT

CPT codes 16000-16036 identify local treatment of burned surface only. For management of burn patients (e.g., prolonged detention, hospital visits) and related medical services, consult appropriate services in the Medicine or Evaluation and Management chapters.

Codes 16020-16030 include the application of dressings that are not described in codes 15100-15431.

If the application of skin grafts or skin substitutes is performed, consult CPT codes 15100-15650.

The percentage of body surface and the depth of the burn should be listed.

Rule of Nines for Burns

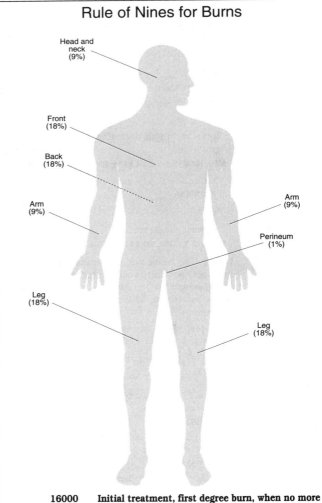

Head and neck (9%)

Front (18%)

Back (18%)

Arm (9%)

Arm (9%)

Perineum (1%)

Leg (18%)

Leg (18%)

16000 Initial treatment, first degree burn, when no more than local treatment is required **T** **↵**

MED: 100-4,3,20.1.2.8; 100-4,4,20.5; 100-4,12,70; 100-4,13,20; 100-4,13,90

AMA: 1997,Aug,6

16020 Dressings and/or debridement of partial-thickness burns, initial or subsequent; small (less than 5% total body surface area) **T** **↵**

MED: 100-3,270.5; 100-4,3,20.1.2.8; 100-4,4,20.5; 100-4,12,70; 100-4,13,20; 100-4,13,90

AMA: 1997,Aug,6

16025 medium (eg, whole face or whole extremity, or 5% to 10% total body surface area) **2** T **↵**

MED: 100-3,270.5; 100-4,3,20.1.2.8; 100-4,4,20.5; 100-4,12,70; 100-4,13,20; 100-4,13,90

AMA: 1997,Aug,6

16030 large (eg, more than one extremity, or greater than 10% total body surface area) **2** T **↵**

MED: 100-3,270.5; 100-4,3,20.1.2.8; 100-4,4,20.5; 100-4,12,70; 100-4,13,20; 100-4,13,90

AMA: 1997,Aug,6

16035 Escharotomy; initial incision **T** **↵**

MED: 100-4,3,20.1.2.8; 100-4,4,20.5

AMA: 1997,Aug,6

26 Professional Component Only   **80**/**80** Assist-at-Surgery Allowed/With Documentation   Unlisted   Not Covered

TC Technical Component Only   **MED:** Pub 100/NCD References   **AMA:** CPT Assistant References   **1**-**9** ASC Group   ♂ Male Only   ♀ Female Only

56 — CPT Expert

+ **16036** each additional incision (List separately in addition to code for primary procedure) [c]

MED: 100-4,3,20.1.2.8; 100-4,4,20.5

If a debridement, curettement of burn wound is performed, consult CPT codes 16020-16030.

Note that 16036 is an add-on code and must be used in conjunction with 16035.

DESTRUCTION

Destruction is defined as the ablation of benign, premalignant, or malignant tissue by any of the following methods used alone or in combination: electrosurgery, cryosurgery, laser, and chemical treatment. Lesions include condylomata, papillomata, molluscum contagiosum, herpetic lesions, warts, milia, actinic keratosis, or other benign, premalignant or malignant lesions. Destruction includes administration of local anesthesia. Codes from this section should not be used when a more specific destruction code is listed under the particular anatomical site. For example, code 40820 should be used for destruction of lesions of the vestibule of the mouth.

Consult CPT codes 40820, 46900-46917, 46924, 54050-54057, 54065, 56501, 56515, 57061, 57065, 67850, and 68135 for destruction of lesion(s) of specified anatomical sites.

To report the paring or cutting of benign hyperkeratotic lesions (e.g., corns or calluses), consult CPT codes 11055-11057. To report sharp removal or electrosurgical destruction of skin tags and fibrocutaneous tags, consult CPT codes 11200 and 11201. If cryotherapy is used for acne, consult CPT code 17340. If destruction is performed on malignant skin lesions, consult CPT codes 17260-17286. If epidermal or dermal lesions are shaved, consult CPT codes 11300-11313. To report the initiation or follow-up care of topical chemotherapy (e.g., 5-FU or comparable agents), consult the appropriate evaluation and management codes.

DESTRUCTION BENIGN OR PREMALIGNANT LESIONS

▲ **17000** Destruction (eg, laser surgery, electrosurgery, cryosurgery, chemosurgery, surgical curettement), premalignant lesions (eg, actinic keratoses); first lesion [T] [↺]

MED: 100-3,140.5; 100-4,4,20.5; 100-4,12,40.6
AMA: 1999,Jun,10; 1997,Nov,12

+ ▲ **17003** second through 14 lesions, each (List separately in addition to code for first lesion) [T]

MED: 100-3,140.5; 100-4,4,20.5; 100-4,12,40.6
AMA: 1999,Jun,10; 1997,Nov,12

Note that 17003 is an add-on code and must be used in conjunction with 17000.

See 17110, 17111 for destruction of common or plantar warts.

⊘ ▲ **17004** Destruction (eg, laser surgery, electrosurgery, cryosurgery, chemosurgery, surgical curettement), premalignant lesions (eg, actinic keratoses), 15 or more lesions [T] [↺]

MED: 100-3,140.5; 100-4,4,20.5; 100-4,12,40.6
AMA: 1999,Jun,10; 1998,Nov,7; 1997,Nov,12
Do not report 17004 with 17000-17003.

17106 Destruction of cutaneous vascular proliferative lesions (eg, laser technique); less than 10 sq cm [T] [↺]

MED: 100-3,140.5

17107 10.0 to 50.0 sq cm [T] [↺]

MED: 100-3,140.5

17108 over 50.0 sq cm [T] [80] [↺]

MED: 100-3,140.5

▲ **17110** Destruction (eg, laser surgery, electrosurgery, cryosurgery, chemosurgery, surgical curettement), of benign lesions other than skin tags or cutaneous vascular lesions; up to 14 lesions [T] [↺]

MED: 100-3,140.5
AMA: 1997,Nov,13

▲ **17111** 15 or more lesions [T] [↺]

MED: 100-3,140.5
AMA: 1997,Nov,13

To report the destruction of common or plantar warts, consult CPT codes 17000, 17003, and 17004.

17250 Chemical cauterization of granulation tissue (proud flesh, sinus or fistula) [T] [↺]

AMA: 1997,Nov,14

Do not report this service with removal/excision codes of the same lesion.

DESTRUCTION MALIGNANT LESIONS, ANY METHOD

17260 Destruction, malignant lesion (eg, laser surgery, electrosurgery, cryosurgery, chemosurgery, surgical curettement), trunk, arms or legs; lesion diameter 0.5 cm or less [T] [↺]

MED: 100-3,140.5

17261 lesion diameter 0.6 to 1.0 cm [T] [↺]

MED: 100-3,140.5

17262 lesion diameter 1.1 to 2.0 cm [T] [↺]

MED: 100-3,140.5

17263 lesion diameter 2.1 to 3.0 cm [T] [↺]

MED: 100-3,140.5

17264 lesion diameter 3.1 to 4.0 cm [T] [↺]

MED: 100-3,140.5

17266 lesion diameter over 4.0 cm [T] [↺]

MED: 100-3,140.5

17270 Destruction, malignant lesion (eg, laser surgery, electrosurgery, cryosurgery, chemosurgery, surgical curettement), scalp, neck, hands, feet, genitalia; lesion diameter 0.5 cm or less [T] [↺]

MED: 100-3,140.5

17271 lesion diameter 0.6 to 1.0 cm [T] [↺]

MED: 100-3,140.5

17272 lesion diameter 1.1 to 2.0 cm [T] [↺]

MED: 100-3,140.5

17273 lesion diameter 2.1 to 3.0 cm [T] [↺]

MED: 100-3,140.5

17274 lesion diameter 3.1 to 4.0 cm [T] [↺]

MED: 100-3,140.5

17276 lesion diameter over 4.0 cm [T] [↺]

MED: 100-3,140.5

17280 Destruction, malignant lesion (eg, laser surgery, electrosurgery, cryosurgery, chemosurgery, surgical curettement), face, ears, eyelids, nose, lips, mucous membrane; lesion diameter 0.5 cm or less [T] [↺]

MED: 100-3,140.5

17281 lesion diameter 0.6 to 1.0 cm [T] [↺]

MED: 100-3,140.5

17282 lesion diameter 1.1 to 2.0 cm [T] [↺]

MED: 100-3,140.5

17283 lesion diameter 2.1 to 3.0 cm [T] [↺]

MED: 100-3,140.5

---

⑥③ Modifier 63 Exempt Code ⊙ Conscious Sedation + CPT Add-on Code ⊘ Modifier 51 Exempt Code ● New Code ▲ Revised Code

[M] Maternity Edit [A] Age Edit [A]-[Y] APC Status Indicators [↺] CCI Comprehensive Code [50] Bilateral Procedure

17284	lesion diameter 3.1 to 4.0 cm	T ⬚

MED: 100-3,140.5

17286	lesion diameter over 4.0 cm	T ⬚

MED: 100-3,140.5

MOHS MICROGRAPHIC SURGERY

Mohs micrographic surgery is a special technique used to treat complex or ill-defined skin cancer and requires a single physician to provide two distinct services, surgery and pathology. The service is involves the removal of the lesion and an examination of 100% of the surgical margins. The surgeon also acts as the pathologist and performs mapping, color coding of specimens, microscopic examination of specimens, and complete histopathologic preparation. The physician separates the tumor specimen into pieces, and creates individual tissue blocks in a mounting medium for sectioning. Each individual embedded in a mounting medium is considered a block. Mohs microsurgery surgery codes should be used only when one physician is functioning as both the surgeon and the pathologist.

If a single physician is not acting as both the surgeon and the pathologist for these procedures, this group of CPT codes should not be used. When repair is performed, consult appropriate CPT codes for the type of repair (e.g., graft, wound repair).

If a skin biopsy is performed on the same day, and there was not prior pathology confirmation of a diagnosis, consult CPT codes 11100, 11101, and 88331 to report frozen section pathology performed on the same day with modifier 59.

~~17304~~	~~Chemosurgery (Mohs micrographic technique), including removal of all gross tumor, surgical excision of tissue specimens, mapping, color coding of specimens, microscopic examination of specimens by the surgeon, and complete histopathologic preparation including the first routine stain (eg, hematoxylin and eosin, toluidine blue); first stage, fresh tissue technique, up to 5 specimens~~

Use 17311-17313.

~~17305~~	~~second stage, fixed or fresh tissue, up to 5 specimens~~

Use 17311-17315.

~~17306~~	~~third stage, fixed or fresh tissue, up to 5 specimens~~

Use 17311-17315.

~~17307~~	~~additional stage(s), up to 5 specimens, each stage~~

Use 17311-17315.

~~17310~~	~~each additional specimen, after the first 5 specimens, fixed or fresh tissue, any stage (List separately in addition to code for primary procedure)~~

Use 17311-17315.

● 17311	Mohs micrographic technique, including removal of all gross tumor, surgical excision of tissue specimens, mapping, color coding of specimens, microscopic examination of specimens by the surgeon, and histopathologic preparation including routine stain(s) (eg, hematoxylin and eosin, toluidine blue), head, neck, hands, feet, genitalia, or any location with surgery directly involving muscle, cartilage, bone, tendon, major nerves, or vessels; first stage, up to 5 tissue blocks	T

+ ● 17312	each additional stage after the first stage, up to 5 tissue blocks (List separately in addition to code for primary procedure)	T

Note that 17312 is an add-on code and must be reported with 17311.

● 17313	Mohs micrographic technique, including removal of all gross tumor, surgical excision of tissue specimens, mapping, color coding of specimens, microscopic examination of specimens by the surgeon, and histopathologic preparation including routine stain(s) (eg, hematoxylin and eosin, toluidine blue), of the trunk, arms, or legs; first stage, up to 5 tissue blocks	T

+ ● 17314	each additional stage after the first stage, up to 5 tissue blocks (List separately in addition to code for primary procedure)	T

Note 17314 is an add-on code and must be reported with 17313.

+ ● 17315	Mohs micrographic technique, including removal of all gross tumor, surgical excision of tissue specimens, mapping, color coding of specimens, microscopic examination of specimens by the surgeon, and histopathologic preparation including routine stain(s) (eg, hematoxylin and eosin, toluidine blue), each additional block after the first 5 tissue blocks, any stage (List separately in addition to code for primary procedure)	T

Note that 17315 is an add-on code and must be reported with 17311-17314.

OTHER PROCEDURES

17340	Cryotherapy (CO2 slush, liquid N2) for acne	T ⬚

17360	Chemical exfoliation for acne (eg, acne paste, acid)	T ⬚

▲ 17380	Electrolysis epilation, each 30 minutes	T 80 ⬚

MED: 100-2,16,10; 100-2,16,120; 100-2,16,180; 100-4,4,20.5

To report actinotherapy, consult CPT code 96900.

17999	Unlisted procedure, skin, mucous membrane and subcutaneous tissue	T 80

MED: 100-4,4,180.3

AMA: 1998,Dec,9

BREAST

INCISION

19000	Puncture aspiration of cyst of breast;	T ⬚

AMA: 1994,Fall,18

+ 19001	each additional cyst (List separately in addition to code for primary procedure)	T ⬚

AMA: 1994,Fall,18

Note that 19001 is an add-on code and must be used in conjunction with 19000. To report imaging guidance, consult CPT codes 76942, 77021, 77031, 77032.

19020	Mastotomy with exploration or drainage of abscess, deep	2 T 50 ⬚

MED: 100-2,15,260; 100-4,4,20.5; 100-4,12,90.3; 100-4,14,10

19030	Injection procedure only for mammary ductogram or galactogram	N 50 ⬚

To report radiological supervision and interpretation, consult CPT codes 77053 and 77054. To report catheter lavage of mammary ducts for cytology specimen collection, consult CPT Category III codes 0046T and 0047T.

EXCISION

Breast biopsies include excision of cysts, tumors or lesions and may involve different amounts of tissue removed for evaluation or treatment.

Excisional breast procedures may include biopsy and may be open or percutaneous. This includes the excision of cysts, benign or malignant lesions of the breast and chest wall.

A biopsy is a procedure in which a lesion is removed without regard for surgical margins and is reported with codes 19100-19103.

Partial mastectomy procedures include lumpectomy, tylectomy, segmentectomy and quadrantectomy.

Partial mastectomy codes are reported with codes 19301 or 19302. A partial mastectomy should be reported when the surgeon pays particular attention to assuring adequate surgical margins surrounding the lesion are excised.

Total mastectomy procedures are reported with codes 19303-19307. These procedures include simple mastectomy, complete mastectomy, subcutaneous mastectomy, modified radical mastectomy, radical mastectomy, and more extensive procedures.

Codes 19260, 19271 or 19272 are used to report excision or resection of chest wall tumors. This includes ribs with or without reconstruction and with or without mediastinal lymphadenectomy. Codes 19260-19272 are not only to report breast tumors. Use these codes to report resection of chest wall tumors that originate from any chest wall component. (To report lung or pleural excisions , consult 32310 et seq.) To report bilateral procedures, append modifier 50.

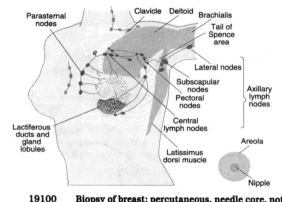

Labels: Parasternal nodes, Clavicle, Deltoid, Brachialis, Tail of Spence area, Lateral nodes, Subscapular nodes, Pectoral nodes, Axillary lymph nodes, Central lymph nodes, Lactiferous ducts and gland lobules, Latissimus dorsi muscle, Areola, Nipple

19100   **Biopsy of breast; percutaneous, needle core, not using imaging guidance**   1 T 50 ☐

MED: 100-2,15,260; 100-3,220.13; 100-4,4,20.5; 100-4,12,90.3; 100-4,14,10

AMA: 2002,May,18; 2001,Jan,8; 1998,Nov,7; 1997,Mar,4; 1996,Apr,8; 1994,Fall,18

To report fine needle aspiration, consult CPT code 10021.

To report image guided breast biopsy, consult CPT codes 10022, 19102, 19103.

19101   **open, incisional**   2 T 50 ☐

MED: 100-2,15,260; 100-3,220.13; 100-4,3,20.2.1; 100-4,4,20.5; 100-4,12,90.3; 100-4,14,10

AMA: 2002,May,18; 2001,Jan,8; 1994,Fall,19

19102   **percutaneous, needle core, using imaging guidance**   2 T 50 ☐

MED: 100-2,15,260; 100-3,220.13; 100-4,4,20.5; 100-4,12,90.3; 100-4,14,10

AMA: 2002,May,18; 2001,Jan,8

To report placement of percutaneous localization clip, report 19295 in conjunction with 19102.

To report the radiologic guidance in conjunction with a breast biopsy, consult CPT codes 76942, 77012, 77021, 77031, and 77032.

19103   **percutaneous, automated vacuum assisted or rotating biopsy device, using imaging guidance**   2 T 50 ☐

MED: 100-2,15,260; 100-3,220.13; 100-4,4,20.5; 100-4,12,90.3; 100-4,14,10

AMA: 2002,May,18; 2001,Jan,8

To report the radiologic guidance in conjunction with a breast biopsy, consult CPT codes 76942, 77012, 77021, 77031, and 77032. For placement of percutaneous localization clip, report 19295 in conjunction with 19103.

● **19105**   **Ablation, cryosurgical, of fibroadenoma, including ultrasound guidance, each fibroadenoma**   T

Do not report 19105 in conjunction with 76940, 76942.

Report only once when adjacent lesions are treated with one cryoprobe insertion.

19110   **Nipple exploration, with or without excision of a solitary lactiferous duct or a papilloma lactiferous duct**   2 T 50 ☐

MED: 100-2,15,260; 100-4,4,20.5; 100-4,12,90.3; 100-4,14,10

19112   **Excision of lactiferous duct fistula**   3 T 80 50 ☐

MED: 100-2,15,260; 100-4,4,20.5; 100-4,12,90.3; 100-4,14,10

▲ **19120**   **Excision of cyst, fibroadenoma, or other benign or malignant tumor, aberrant breast tissue, duct lesion, nipple or areolar lesion (except 19300), open, male or female, one or more lesions**   3 T 50 ☐

MED: 100-2,15,260; 100-4,4,20.5; 100-4,12,90.3; 100-4,14,10

AMA: 2001,May,10; 2001,Jan,8; 1997,Nov,14; 1996,Feb,9

19125   **Excision of breast lesion identified by preoperative placement of radiological marker, open; single lesion**   3 T 50 ☐

MED: 100-2,15,260; 100-4,4,20.5; 100-4,12,90.3; 100-4,14,10

AMA: 2001,Jan,8; 1998,Mar,10; 1994,Fall,18

19126   **each additional lesion separately identified by a preoperative radiological marker (List separately in addition to code for primary procedure)**   3 T ☐

MED: 100-2,15,260; 100-4,4,20.5; 100-4,12,90.3; 100-4,14,10

AMA: 2001,Jan,8; 1998,Mar,10; 1994,Fall,18

Note that 19126 is an add-on code and must be used in conjunction with 19125.

~~**19140**~~   ~~Mastectomy for gynecomastia~~

Use 19300-19307.

~~**19160**~~   ~~Mastectomy, partial (eg, lumpectomy, tylectomy, quadrantectomy, segmentectomy);~~

Use 19300-19307.

~~**19162**~~   ~~with axillary lymphadenectomy~~

Use 19300-19307.

~~**19180**~~   ~~Mastectomy, simple, complete~~

Use 19300-19307.

~~**19182**~~   ~~Mastectomy, subcutaneous~~

Use 19300-19307.

~~**19200**~~   ~~Mastectomy, radical, including pectoral muscles, axillary lymph nodes~~

Use 19300-19307.

~~**19220**~~   ~~Mastectomy, radical, including pectoral muscles, axillary and internal mammary lymph nodes (Urban type operation)~~

Use 19300-19307.

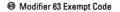

Integumentary System

19240 — 19340

Location and incidence of breast cancer

Upper inner 15 percent

Upper outer quadrant 50 percent

Each breast is divided into four quadrants: upper inner; upper outer; lower inner; and lower outer

Pectoralis muscle and axillary tail area

Inner lower 6 percent

Lower outer 11 percent

Fat

Nipple 18 percent

One of every 10 American women will develop breast cancer; about 150,000 cases are diagnosed annually; about 70 percent of invasive breast cancers are ductal carcinomas

Lactiferous ducts and gland lobules

Midline

~~19240~~   ~~Mastectomy, modified radical, including axillary lymph nodes, with or without pectoralis minor muscle, but excluding pectoralis major muscle~~

     Use 19300-19307.

19260   Excision of chest wall tumor including ribs   T 80 ◨

19271   Excision of chest wall tumor involving ribs, with plastic reconstruction; without mediastinal lymphadenectomy   C 80 ◨

19272   with mediastinal lymphadenectomy   C 80 ◨

     Codes 19260, 19271, and 19272 should not be reported in conjunction with code 32002, 32020, 32100, 32503, or 32504.

INTRODUCTION

19290   Preoperative placement of needle localization wire, breast;   1 N 50 ◨

     MED: 100-2,15,260; 100-4,4,20.5; 100-4,12,90.3; 100-4,14,10

     AMA: 1994,Fall,19

     To report radiological supervision and interpretation, consult CPT codes 76942, 77031, and 77032.

+   **19291**   each additional lesion (List separately in addition to code for primary procedure)   1 N 80

     MED: 100-2,15,260; 100-4,4,20.5; 100-4,12,90.3; 100-4,14,10

     AMA: 1994,Fall,19

     Note that 19291 is an add-on code and must be used in conjunction with 19290.

     For radiologic supervision and interpretation, use 76942, 77031, 77032.

+   **19295**   Image guided placement, metallic localization clip, percutaneous, during breast biopsy (List separately in addition to code for primary procedure)   1 S 80

     AMA: 2001,Jan,8

     Note that 19295 is an add-on code and must be used in conjunction with 19102, 19103.

19296   Placement of radiotherapy afterloading balloon catheter into the breast for interstitial radioelement application following partial mastectomy, includes imaging guidance; on date separate from partial mastectomy   9 T 80 50 ◨

+   **19297**   concurrent with partial mastectomy (List separately in addition to code for primary procedure)   9 T 80

     Note that 19297 must be used with 19301-19302.

⊙   **19298**   Placement of radiotherapy afterloading brachytherapy catheters (multiple tube and button type) into the breast for interstitial radioelement application following (at the time of or subsequent to) partial mastectomy, includes imaging guidance   9 S 80 50 ◨

MASTECTOMY PROCEDURES

●   **19300**   Mastectomy for gynecomastia   4 T

●   **19301**   Mastectomy, partial (eg, lumpectomy, tylectomy, quadrantectomy, segmentectomy);   3 T

●   **19302**   Mastectomy, partial (eg, lumpectomy, tylectomy, quadrantectomy, segmentectomy); with axillary lymphadenectomy   7 T

     See 19296-19298 for placement of radiotherapy afterloading balloon or brachytherapy catheters.

●   **19303**   Mastectomy, simple, complete   4 T

     Consult 19340, 19342 for immediate or delayed insertion of implant.

     Use 19300 for gynecomastia.

●   **19304**   Mastectomy, subcutaneous   4 T

     See 19340, 19342 for immediate or delayed insertion of implant.

●   **19305**   Mastectomy, radical, including pectoral muscles, axillary lymph nodes   C

     See 19340, 19342 for immediate or delayed insertion of implant.

●   **19306**   Mastectomy, radical, including pectoral muscles, axillary and internal mammary lymph nodes (Urban type operation)   C

     See 19340, 19342 for immediate or delayed insertion of implant.

●   **19307**   Mastectomy, modified radical, including axillary lymph nodes, with or without pectoralis minor muscle, but excluding pectoralis major muscle   T

     See 19340, 19342 for immediate or delayed insertion of implant.

REPAIR AND/OR RECONSTRUCTION

19316   Mastopexy   4 T 80 50 ◨

     MED: 100-2,15,260; 100-4,4,20.5; 100-4,12,90.3; 100-4,14,10

19318   Reduction mammaplasty   ♀ 4 T 80 50 ◨

     MED: 100-2,15,260; 100-4,4,20.5; 100-4,12,90.3; 100-4,14,10

     Aries-Pitanguy mammaplasty

19324   Mammaplasty, augmentation; without prosthetic implant   4 T 80 50 ◨

     MED: 100-2,15,260; 100-4,4,20.5; 100-4,12,90.3; 100-4,14,10

     If a flap or graft is needed, consult also appropriate number.

19325   with prosthetic implant   9 T 80 50 ◨

     MED: 100-2,15,260; 100-4,4,20.5; 100-4,12,90.3; 100-4,14,10

     Consult CPT code 99070 for supply of implant.

     If a flap or graft is needed, consult also appropriate number.

19328   Removal of intact mammary implant   1 T 50 ◨

     MED: 100-2,15,260; 100-4,4,20.5; 100-4,12,90.3; 100-4,14,10

19330   Removal of mammary implant material   1 T 50 ◨

     MED: 100-2,15,260; 100-4,4,20.5; 100-4,12,90.3; 100-4,14,10

     AMA: 2001,Nov,11

19340   Immediate insertion of breast prosthesis following mastopexy, mastectomy or in reconstruction   2 T 50 ◨

     MED: 100-2,15,260; 100-3,140.2; 100-4,4,20.5; 100-4,12,90.3; 100-4,14,10

     AMA: 1996,Aug,8

---

26 Professional Component Only   80/80 Assist-at-Surgery Allowed/With Documentation   Unlisted   Not Covered

TC Technical Component Only   **MED:** Pub 100/NCD References   **AMA:** CPT Assistant References   1-9 ASC Group   ♂ Male Only   ♀ Female Only

60 — CPT Expert   CPT only © 2006 American Medical Association. All Rights Reserved. (Black Ink)   © 2006 Ingenix (Blue Ink)

19342	Delayed insertion of breast prosthesis following mastopexy, mastectomy or in reconstruction ♀ **3** T 80 50 ◨	

MED: 100-2,15,260; 100-3,140.2; 100-4,4,20.5; 100-4,12,90.3; 100-4,14,10

AMA: 1996,Aug,8

Consult CPT code 99070 for supply of implant. If a custom breast implant is prepared, consult CPT code 19396.

19350	Nipple/areola reconstruction **4** T 50 ◨

MED: 100-2,15,260; 100-3,140.2; 100-4,4,20.5; 100-4,12,90.3; 100-4,14,10

AMA: 1996,Aug,11

19355	Correction of inverted nipples **4** T 80 50 ◨

MED: 100-2,15,260; 100-3,140.2; 100-4,4,20.5; 100-4,12,90.3; 100-4,14,10

19357	Breast reconstruction, immediate or delayed, with tissue expander, including subsequent expansion ♀ **5** T 80 50 ◨

MED: 100-2,15,260; 100-3,140.2; 100-4,4,20.5; 100-4,12,90.3; 100-4,14,10

▲ 19361	Breast reconstruction with latissimus dorsi flap, without prosthetic implant ♀ C 80 50 ◨

MED: 100-3,140.2

Also report 19340 for insertion of prosthesis.

19364	Breast reconstruction with free flap C 80 50 ◨

MED: 100-3,140.2

AMA: 1998,Nov,7; 1996,Aug,8

Do not report 69990 in addition to code 19364 as the operating microscope is considered an inclusive component of the surgery. Note that 19364 includes harvesting of the flap, microvascular transfer, closure of the donor site, and inset shaping the flap into a breast.

19366	Breast reconstruction with other technique **5** T 80 50 ◨

MED: 100-2,15,260; 100-3,140.2; 100-4,4,20.5; 100-4,12,90.3; 100-4,14,10

AMA: 1998,Nov,7; 1996,Aug,8

If an operating microscope is used, consult CPT code 69990. If a prosthesis is inserted, consult also CPT code 19340 or 19342.

19367	Breast reconstruction with transverse rectus abdominis myocutaneous flap (TRAM), single pedicle, including closure of donor site; ♀ C 80 50 ◨

MED: 100-3,140.2

AMA: 1998,Nov,7

19368	with microvascular anastomosis (supercharging) ♀ C 80 50 ◨

MED: 100-3,140.2

AMA: 1998,Nov,7

Do not report 69990 in addition to code 19368 as the operating microscope is considered an inclusive component of the surgery.

19369	Breast reconstruction with transverse rectus abdominis myocutaneous flap (TRAM), double pedicle, including closure of donor site ♀ C 80 50 ◨

MED: 100-3,140.2

AMA: 2000,Oct,1

19370	Open periprosthetic capsulotomy, breast **4** T 50 ◨

MED: 100-2,15,260; 100-3,140.2; 100-4,4,20.5; 100-4,12,90.3; 100-4,14,10

AMA: 1996,Aug,8

19371	Periprosthetic capsulectomy, breast **4** T 50 ◨

MED: 100-2,15,260; 100-3,140.2; 100-4,4,20.5; 100-4,12,90.3; 100-4,14,10

AMA: 2001,Nov,11; 1996,Aug,8

19380	Revision of reconstructed breast **5** T 50 ◨

MED: 100-2,15,260; 100-3,140.2; 100-4,4,20.5; 100-4,12,90.3; 100-4,14,10

19396	Preparation of moulage for custom breast implant T 80 50 ◨

MED: 100-3,140.2

AMA: 2003,Jan,1

OTHER PROCEDURES

To report microwave thermotherapy of breast, consult CPT Category III code 0061T.

19499	Unlisted procedure, breast T 80 50

MED: 100-4,4,20.5; 100-4,4,180.3

MUSCULOSKELETAL SYSTEM

Codes listed in the Musculoskeletal chapter include the application and removal of the first cast or traction device. Replacement of casts and/or traction devices subsequent to the first should be reported separately. CPT codes for other additional procedures, such as obtaining grafts and external fixation, should only be used if the procedure is not already listed as included as part of the basic procedure. Consult the glossary for terms and definitions and the front matter of this chapter for additional information.

To report computer assisted musculoskeletal surgical navigational orthopedic procedures, consult CPT Category III codes 0054T-0056T.

Fracture management codes are package services and include percutaneous pinning and open or closed treatment of the fracture, application and removal of the initial cast or splint, and normal, uncomplicated follow-up care.

Two types of fixation-internal and external-are described in the CPT book. Internal skeletal fixation involves wires, pins, screws, and/or plates placed through or within the fractured area to stabilize and immobilize the injury. This procedure is generally accomplished through an incision over the fracture site. It is commonly described as an open reduction with internal fixation (ORIF). Internal fixation may also be accomplished by percutaneous technique. In this case, a pin is inserted through the skin without an incision. Deep internal devices are usually left in place even after the fracture has healed. If the hardware is removed, report codes 20670 or 20680. Use modifier 78 Return to the operating room for a related procedure, or modifier 58 Staged or related procedure by the same physician during the postoperative period, if removal is performed during the initial hospital care or during the postoperative follow-up period. The ICD-9-CM code is assigned according to the reason for the removal (e.g., pain, infection). The codes describing internal fixation are placed throughout the fracture care codes according to anatomical site.

External fixation (20690-20694) is hardware passing through bone and skin and held rigid by cross-braces outside the body. External fixation is always removed after the fracture has healed and removal usually is considered part of the global service. However, if required to remain in place beyond the usual postoperative period, its removal should be reported (20694).

GENERAL

INCISION

| 20000 | Incision of soft tissue abscess (eg, secondary to osteomyelitis); superficial   T ◳ |
| 20005 | deep or complicated   2 T ◳ |

MED: 100-2,15,260; 100-4,4,20.5; 100-4,12,90.3; 100-4,14,10

WOUND EXPLORATION — TRAUMA (EG, PENETRATING GUNSHOT, STAB WOUND)

Use these codes to describe the physician's surgical treatment of a traumatic penetrating wound resulting from knives, guns, or other sources. The physician may explore or enlarge the wound, dissect the wound to determine penetration, remove foreign bodies, debridement, and repair minor blood vessels. When a thoracotomy or laparotomy is necessary to repair major structures or blood vessels, the code for that procedure is used instead of the 20100-20103 series.

20100	Exploration of penetrating wound (separate procedure); neck T 80 50 ◳
	AMA: 1996,Jun,7; 1996,Aug,10
20101	chest T ◳
	AMA: 1996,Jun,7
20102	abdomen/flank/back T 80 ◳
	AMA: 1996,Jun,7
20103	extremity T 80 ◳
	AMA: 1996,Jun,7; 1996,Aug,10

EXCISION

To report sequestrectomy, osteomyelitis, or drainage of bone abscess, consult CPT codes for appropriate anatomical area.

| 20150 | Excision of epiphyseal bar, with or without autogenous soft tissue graft obtained through same fascial incision   T 80 50 ◳ |

If bone marrow is aspirated, consult CPT code 38220.

| 20200 | Biopsy, muscle; superficial   2 T ◳ |

MED: 100-2,15,260; 100-4,4,20.5; 100-4,12,90.3; 100-4,14,10

If excision of a muscle tumor, deep, is included, consult specific anatomical section.

| 20205 | deep   3 T ◳ |

MED: 100-2,15,260; 100-4,4,20.5; 100-4,12,90.3; 100-4,14,10

| 20206 | Biopsy, muscle, percutaneous needle   1 T ◳ |

MED: 100-2,15,260; 100-4,4,20.5; 100-4,12,90.3; 100-4,14,10

To report imaging guidance, consult CPT codes 76942, 77012, 77021.

To report fine needle aspiration, consult CPT codes 10021 or 10022.

To report evaluation of fine needle aspirate, consult CPT codes 88172-88173.

| 20220 | Biopsy, bone, trocar, or needle; superficial (eg, ilium, sternum, spinous process, ribs)   1 T ◳ |

MED: 100-2,15,260; 100-3,150.3; 100-4,4,20.5; 100-4,12,90.3; 100-4,14,10
AMA: 1998,Jul,4; 1992,Winter,17

| 20225 | deep (eg, vertebral body, femur)   2 T ◳ |

MED: 100-2,15,260; 100-3,150.3; 100-4,4,20.5; 100-4,12,90.3; 100-4,14,10
AMA: 1998,Jul,4; 1992,Winter,17

If bone marrow is biopsied, consult CPT code 38221.

To report radiologic supervision and interpretation, see 77002, 77012, 77021.

| 20240 | Biopsy, bone, open; superficial (eg, ilium, sternum, spinous process, ribs, trochanter of femur)   2 T ◳ |

MED: 100-2,15,260; 100-3,150.3; 100-4,3,20.2.1; 100-4,4,20.5; 100-4,12,90.3; 100-4,14,10
AMA: 1998,Jul,4; 1992,Winter,17

| 20245 | deep (eg, humerus, ischium, femur)   3 T ◳ |

MED: 100-2,15,260; 100-3,150.3; 100-4,3,20.2.1; 100-4,4,20.5; 100-4,12,90.3; 100-4,14,10
AMA: 1998,Jul,4; 1992,Winter,17

| 20250 | Biopsy, vertebral body, open; thoracic   3 T ◳ |

MED: 100-2,15,260; 100-4,3,20.2.1; 100-4,4,20.5; 100-4,12,90.3; 100-4,14,10
AMA: 1998,Jul,4; 1992,Winter,17

| 20251 | lumbar or cervical   3 T 80 ◳ |

MED: 100-2,15,260; 100-4,3,20.2.1; 100-4,4,20.5; 100-4,12,90.3; 100-4,14,10
AMA: 1998,Jul,4; 1992,Winter,17

INTRODUCTION OR REMOVAL

If an injection procedure for arthrography is performed, consult appropriate anatomical area.

| 20500 | Injection of sinus tract; therapeutic (separate procedure)   T ◳ |
| 20501 | diagnostic (sinogram)   N ◳ |

To report radiologic supervision and interpretation, consult CPT code 76080.

| 20520 | Removal of foreign body in muscle or tendon sheath; simple   T ◳ |
| 20525 | deep or complicated   3 T ◳ |

MED: 100-2,15,260; 100-4,4,20.5; 100-4,12,90.3; 100-4,14,10

Musculoskeletal System

20526 — 20900

20526	Injection, therapeutic (eg, local anesthetic, corticosteroid), carpal tunnel [T] [50]	

AMA: 2002,Mar,7

20550 Injection(s); single tendon sheath, or ligament, aponeurosis (eg, plantar "fascia") [T]

MED: 100-3,150.7

AMA: 2002,Mar,7; 1998,Jun,10; 1996,Jan,7
To report imaging guidance, consult CPT codes 76003, 76393, 76942.

20551 single tendon origin/insertion [T]

MED: 100-3,150.7

AMA: 2002,Mar,7

20552 single or multiple trigger point(s), one or two muscle(s) [T]

MED: 100-3,150.7

AMA: 2002,Mar,7

20553 single or multiple trigger point(s), three or more muscle(s) [T]

MED: 100-3,150.7

AMA: 2002,Mar,7
To report imaging guidance, consult CPT codes 76942, 77002, 77021.

20600 Arthrocentesis, aspiration and/or injection; small joint or bursa (eg, fingers, toes) [T] [50]

MED: 100-3,150.6; 100-3,150.7

20605 intermediate joint or bursa (eg, temporomandibular, acromioclavicular, wrist, elbow or ankle, olecranon bursa) [T] [50]

MED: 100-3,150.6; 100-3,150.7

20610 major joint or bursa (eg, shoulder, hip, knee joint, subacromial bursa) [T] [50]

MED: 100-3,150.6; 100-3,150.7

AMA: 2001,Mar,10; 1992,Spring,8
To report imaging guidance, consult CPT codes 76942, 77002, 77012, 77021. To report procedure performed on ganglion cyst, consult CPT code 20612.

20612 Aspiration and/or injection of ganglion cyst(s) any location [T]

To report procedure performed on multiple cysts, append modifier 59.

20615 Aspiration and injection for treatment of bone cyst [T]

20650 Insertion of wire or pin with application of skeletal traction, including removal (separate procedure) [3] [T]

MED: 100-2,15,260; 100-4,4,20.5; 100-4,12,90.3; 100-4,14,10

⊘ **20660** Application of cranial tongs, caliper, or stereotactic frame, including removal (separate procedure) [C]

MED: 100-4,4,20.5; 100-4,4,220.4

AMA: 1997,Nov,14; 1996,Jun,10

20661 Application of halo, including removal; cranial [C]

20662 pelvic [T] [80]

20663 femoral [T] [80]

20664 Application of halo, including removal, cranial, 6 or more pins placed, for thin skull osteology (eg, pediatric patients, hydrocephalus, osteogenesis imperfecta), requiring general anesthesia [C]

20665 Removal of tongs or halo applied by another physician [X] [80]

20670 Removal of implant; superficial, (eg, buried wire, pin or rod) (separate procedure) [1] [T]

MED: 100-2,15,260; 100-4,4,20.5; 100-4,12,90.3; 100-4,14,10

20680 deep (eg, buried wire, pin, screw, metal band, nail, rod or plate) [3] [T] [80]

MED: 100-2,15,260; 100-4,4,20.5; 100-4,12,90.3; 100-4,14,10
AMA: 1992,Spring,11

⊘ **20690** Application of a uniplane (pins or wires in one plane), unilateral, external fixation system [2] [T] [50]

MED: 100-2,15,260; 100-4,4,20.5; 100-4,12,90.3; 100-4,14,10
AMA: 1999,Oct,4; 1993,Fall,21

⊘ **20692** Application of a multiplane (pins or wires in more than one plane), unilateral, external fixation system (eg, Ilizarov, Monticelli type) [3] [T] [80]

MED: 100-2,15,260; 100-4,4,20.5; 100-4,12,90.3; 100-4,14,10
AMA: 2000,Jul,11; 1999,Oct,4; 1993,Fall,21

20693 Adjustment or revision of external fixation system requiring anesthesia (eg, new pin(s) or wire(s) and/or new ring(s) or bar(s)) [3] [T]

MED: 100-2,15,260; 100-4,4,20.5; 100-4,12,90.3; 100-4,14,10
AMA: 2000,Jul,11; 1999,Oct,4; 1993,Fall,21

20694 Removal, under anesthesia, of external fixation system [1] [T]

MED: 100-2,15,260; 100-4,4,20.5; 100-4,12,90.3; 100-4,14,10
AMA: 2000,Jul,11; 1999,Oct,4; 1993,Fall,21; 1992,Winter,10

REPLANTATION

To report repair of bone(s), ligament(s), tendon(s), nerve(s), or blood vessel(s) with replantation, consult appropriate anatomic area, and append modifier 52.

20802 Replantation, arm (includes surgical neck of humerus through elbow joint), complete amputation [C] [80] [50]

20805 Replantation, forearm (includes radius and ulna to radial carpal joint), complete amputation [C] [80] [50]

20808 Replantation, hand (includes hand through metacarpophalangeal joints), complete amputation [C] [80] [50]

20816 Replantation, digit, excluding thumb (includes metacarpophalangeal joint to insertion of flexor sublimis tendon), complete amputation [C] [80]

AMA: 1996,Oct,11

20822 Replantation, digit, excluding thumb (includes distal tip to sublimis tendon insertion), complete amputation [T] [80]

20824 Replantation, thumb (includes carpometacarpal joint to MP joint), complete amputation [C] [80] [50]

20827 Replantation, thumb (includes distal tip to MP joint), complete amputation [C] [80] [50]

20838 Replantation, foot, complete amputation [C] [80] [50]

GRAFTS (OR IMPLANTS)

If spinal surgery bone graft(s) is needed, consult CPT codes 20930-20938. If needle aspiration of bone marrow for the purpose of bone grafting is needed, consult CPT code 38220. Do not report modifier 62 with any codes in range 20900-20938.

The harvesting of grafts through separate incisions should be reported separately unless the primary procedure code narrative states that it already includes obtaining grafts.

⊘ **20900** Bone graft, any donor area; minor or small (eg, dowel or button) [3] [T] [80]

MED: 100-2,15,260; 100-4,4,20.5; 100-4,12,90.3; 100-4,14,10
AMA: 2000,Dec,15

⊘ **20902**   major or large   4️⃣ T 80 ↻

MED: 100-2,15,260; 100-4,4,20.5; 100-4,12,90.3; 100-4,14,10

AMA: 2000,Dec,15

⊘ **20910**   Cartilage graft; costochondral   3️⃣ T 80 ↻

MED: 100-2,15,260; 100-4,4,20.5; 100-4,12,90.3; 100-4,14,10

⊘ **20912**   nasal septum   3️⃣ T 80 ↻

MED: 100-2,15,260; 100-4,4,20.5; 100-4,12,90.3; 100-4,14,10

To report ear cartilage, consult CPT code 21235.

⊘ **20920**   Fascia lata graft; by stripper   4️⃣ T ↻

MED: 100-2,15,260; 100-4,4,20.5; 100-4,12,90.3; 100-4,14,10

AMA: 1999,Aug,5

⊘ **20922**   by incision and area exposure, complex or sheet   3️⃣ T 80 ↻

MED: 100-2,15,260; 100-4,4,20.5; 100-4,12,90.3; 100-4,14,10

⊘ **20924**   Tendon graft, from a distance (eg, palmaris, toe extensor, plantaris)   4️⃣ T 80 ↻

MED: 100-2,15,260; 100-4,4,20.5; 100-4,12,90.3; 100-4,14,10

⊘ **20926**   Tissue grafts, other (eg, paratenon, fat, dermis)   4️⃣ T ↻

MED: 100-2,15,260; 100-4,4,20.5; 100-4,12,90.3; 100-4,14,10

AMA: 1999,Nov,10; 1999,Aug,5; 1991,Summer,12

CPT states that codes 20930-20938 should be reported, without modifier 51, in addition to the definitive procedure. Individual payer policies may differ, check with your specific payer.

⊘ **20930**   Allograft for spine surgery only; morselized   C

AMA: 1999,Nov,10; 1997,Sep,8; 1996,Mar,4; 1996,Feb,6

⊘ **20931**   structural   C ↻

AMA: 1996,Feb,6

⊘ **20936**   Autograft for spine surgery only (includes harvesting the graft); local (eg, ribs, spinous process, or laminar fragments) obtained from same incision   C

AMA: 1997,Sep,8; 1996,Feb,6

⊘ **20937**   morselized (through separate skin or fascial incision)   C 80 ↻

AMA: 1999,Dec,2; 1997,Sep,8; 1996,Feb,6

⊘ **20938**   structural, bicortical or tricortical (through separate skin or fascial incision)   C 80 ↻

AMA: 1997,Sep,8; 1996,Mar,5; 1996,Feb,6

OTHER PROCEDURES

20950   Monitoring of interstitial fluid pressure (includes insertion of device, eg, wick catheter technique, needle manometer technique) in detection of muscle compartment syndrome   T 80 ↻

Do not report 69990 in addition to codes 20955-20962 as the operating microscope is considered an inclusive component of these procedures.

20955   Bone graft with microvascular anastomosis; fibula   C 80 ↻

AMA: 1997,Apr,4

20956   iliac crest   C 80 ↻

AMA: 1997,Apr,4

20957   metatarsal   C 80 ↻

AMA: 1997,Apr,4

20962   other than fibula, iliac crest, or metatarsal   C 80 ↻

AMA: 1997,Apr,4

Do not report 69990 in addition to codes 20969-20973 as the operating microscope is considered an inclusive component of these procedures.

20969   Free osteocutaneous flap with microvascular anastomosis; other than iliac crest, metatarsal, or great toe   C 80 ↻

AMA: 1997,Apr,4

20970   iliac crest   C 80 ↻

AMA: 1997,Apr,4

20972   metatarsal   T 80 ↻

AMA: 1997,Apr,4

20973   great toe with web space   T 80 ↻

MED: 100-3,150.2

AMA: 1997,Apr,4

If a great toe wrap-around procedure is performed, consult CPT code 26551.

⊘ **20974**   Electrical stimulation to aid bone healing; noninvasive (nonoperative)   A ↻

MED: 100-3,150.2

AMA: 1996,Sep,11

⊘ **20975**   invasive (operative)   2️⃣ X 80 ↻

MED: 100-2,15,260; 100-3,150.2; 100-4,4,20.5; 100-4,12,90.3; 100-4,14,10

20979   Low intensity ultrasound stimulation to aid bone healing, noninvasive (nonoperative)   X ↻

MED: 100-3,220.5

AMA: 2000,Nov,8; 1999,Nov,10

⊙ **20982**   Ablation, bone tumor(s) (eg, osteoid osteoma, metastasis) radiofrequency, percutaneous, including computed tomographic guidance   T 80 50 ↻

Do not report 20982 with 77013.

20999   Unlisted procedure, musculoskeletal system, general   T 80

MED: 100-4,4,20.5; 100-4,4,180.3

HEAD

Codes listed in the Musculoskeletal chapter include the application and removal of the first cast or traction device. Replacement of casts and/or traction devices subsequent to the first should be reported separately. CPT codes for other additional procedures, such as obtaining grafts and external fixation, should only be used if the procedure is not already listed as included as part of the basic procedure. Consult the glossary for terms and definitions and the front matter of this chapter for additional information.

This section includes the skull, facial bones and the temporomandibular joint.

INCISION

21010   Arthrotomy, temporomandibular joint   2️⃣ T 80 50 ↻

MED: 100-2,15,260; 100-4,4,20.5; 100-4,12,90.3; 100-4,14,10

If a superficial abscess and hematoma is drained, consult CPT code 20000. If an embedded foreign body is removed from dentoalveolar structures, consult CPT codes 41805 and 41806.

If procedure 21010 is performed bilaterally, append modifier 50.

EXCISION

21015   Radical resection of tumor (eg, malignant neoplasm), soft tissue of face or scalp   3️⃣ T ↻

MED: 100-2,15,260; 100-4,4,20.5; 100-4,12,90.3; 100-4,14,10

If only a biopsy is done, consult CPT codes 20220 and 20240.

Consult CPT code 61501 for the excision of a skull tumor for osteomyelitis.

Musculoskeletal System

21025 — 21116

21025   Excision of bone (eg, for osteomyelitis or bone abscess); mandible   2 T ▣
MED: 100-2,15,260; 100-4,4,20.5; 100-4,12,90.3; 100-4,14,10

21026   facial bone(s)   2 T ▣
MED: 100-2,15,260; 100-4,4,20.5; 100-4,12,90.3; 100-4,14,10

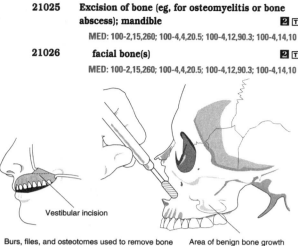

Vestibular incision

Burs, files, and osteotomes used to remove bone   Area of benign bone growth

21029   Removal by contouring of benign tumor of facial bone (eg, fibrous dysplasia)   2 T 80 ▣
MED: 100-2,15,260; 100-4,4,20.5; 100-4,12,90.3; 100-4,14,10

21030   Excision of benign tumor or cyst of maxilla or zygoma by enucleation and curettage   T ▣

21031   Excision of torus mandibularis   T ▣

21032   Excision of maxillary torus palatinus   T ▣

21034   Excision of malignant tumor of maxilla or zygoma   3 T 80 ▣
MED: 100-2,15,260; 100-4,4,20.5; 100-4,12,90.3; 100-4,14,10

21040   Excision of benign tumor or cyst of mandible, by enucleation and/or curettage   2 T ▣
MED: 100-2,15,260; 100-4,4,20.5; 100-4,12,90.3; 100-4,14,10
To report excision requiring osteotomy, consult CPT codes 21046, 21047.

21044   Excision of malignant tumor of mandible;   2 T 80 ▣
MED: 100-2,15,260; 100-4,4,20.5; 100-4,12,90.3; 100-4,14,10

21045   radical resection   C 80 ▣
If a bone graft is done, consult CPT code 21215.

21046   Excision of benign tumor or cyst of mandible; requiring intra-oral osteotomy (eg, locally aggressive or destructive lesion(s))   2 T 80 ▣
MED: 100-2,15,260; 100-4,4,20.5; 100-4,12,90.3; 100-4,14,10

21047   requiring extra-oral osteotomy and partial mandibulectomy (eg, locally aggressive or destructive lesion(s))   2 T 80 ▣
MED: 100-2,15,260; 100-4,4,20.5; 100-4,12,90.3; 100-4,14,10

21048   Excision of benign tumor or cyst of maxilla; requiring intra-oral osteotomy (eg, locally aggressive or destructive lesion(s))   T 80 ▣

21049   Excision of benign tumor or cyst of maxilla; requiring extra-oral osteotomy and partial maxillectomy (eg, locally aggressive or destructive lesion(s))   T 80 ▣

21050   Condylectomy, temporomandibular joint (separate procedure)   3 T 80 50 ▣
MED: 100-2,15,260; 100-4,4,20.5; 100-4,12,90.3; 100-4,14,10
If procedure 21050 is performed bilaterally, append modifier 50.

21060   Meniscectomy, partial or complete, temporomandibular joint (separate procedure)   2 T 80 50 ▣
MED: 100-2,15,260; 100-4,4,20.5; 100-4,12,90.3; 100-4,14,10
If procedure 21060 is performed bilaterally, append modifier 50.

21070   Coronoidectomy (separate procedure)   3 T 80 50 ▣
MED: 100-2,15,260; 100-4,4,20.5; 100-4,12,90.3; 100-4,14,10
If procedure 21070 is performed bilaterally, append modifier 50.

HEAD PROSTHESIS

Report codes 21076-21089 for professional services for the rehabilitation of patients with oral, facial, or other anatomical problems that require the use of a prosthesis such as an artificial eye, ear, or nose or intraoral obturator to close a cleft. Report these codes only when the physician designs, and constructs the graft and it is not built by an outside laboratory. For application or removal of calper or tons, consult 20660, 20665.

21076   Impression and custom preparation; surgical obturator prosthesis   T 80 ▣

21077   orbital prosthesis   T 80 50 ▣

21079   interim obturator prosthesis   T ▣

21080   definitive obturator prosthesis   T ▣

21081   mandibular resection prosthesis   T 80 ▣

21082   palatal augmentation prosthesis   T 80 ▣

21083   palatal lift prosthesis   T 80 ▣

21084   speech aid prosthesis   T 80 ▣

21085   oral surgical splint   T 80 ▣

21086   auricular prosthesis   T 80 50 ▣

21087   nasal prosthesis   T 80 ▣

21088   facial prosthesis   T 80 ▣

OTHER PROCEDURES

21089   Unlisted maxillofacial prosthetic procedure   T

INTRODUCTION OR REMOVAL

Codes listed in the Musculoskeletal chapter include the application and removal of the first cast or traction device. Replacement of casts and/or traction devices subsequent to the first should be reported separately. CPT codes for other additional procedures, such as obtaining grafts and external fixation, should only be used if the procedure is not already listed as included as part of the basic procedure. Consult the glossary for terms and definitions.

CPT codes 21076-21089 are reported only if the physician (not an outside lab) actually designs, prepares, and supplies the prosthesis.

21100   Application of halo type appliance for maxillofacial fixation, includes removal (separate procedure)   2 T 80 ▣
MED: 100-2,15,260; 100-4,4,20.5; 100-4,12,90.3; 100-4,14,10

21110   Application of interdental fixation device for conditions other than fracture or dislocation, includes removal   T ▣
AMA: 1997,Mar,10
If another physician removes an interdental fixation, consult CPT codes 20670-20680.

21116   Injection procedure for temporomandibular joint arthrography   N ▣
If radiological supervision and interpretation is performed, consult CPT code 70332. Code 77002 cannot be reported in addition to 70332.

26 Professional Component Only

80/80 Assist-at-Surgery Allowed/With Documentation

TC Technical Component Only   MED: Pub 100/NCD References   AMA: CPT Assistant References   1-9 ASC Group   Unlisted   Not Covered   ♂ Male Only   ♀ Female Only

66 — CPT Expert   CPT only © 2006 American Medical Association. All Rights Reserved. (Black Ink)   © 2006 Ingenix (Blue Ink)

Musculoskeletal System

21120 — 21188

REPAIR, REVISION, AND/OR RECONSTRUCTION

If cranioplasty is performed, consult CPT codes 21179, 21180, 62116, 62120, and 62140-62147.

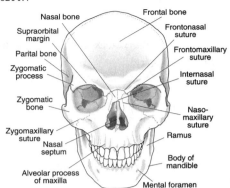

21120 Genioplasty; augmentation (autograft, allograft, prosthetic material) 🟦 T 🔲

21121 sliding osteotomy, single piece 🟦 T 80 🔲

MED: 100-2,15,260; 100-4,4,20.5; 100-4,12,90.3; 100-4,14,10

21122 sliding osteotomies, two or more osteotomies (eg, wedge excision or bone wedge reversal for asymmetrical chin) 🟦 T 80 🔲

MED: 100-2,15,260; 100-4,4,20.5; 100-4,12,90.3; 100-4,14,10

21123 sliding, augmentation with interpositional bone grafts (includes obtaining autografts) 🟦 T 80 🔲

MED: 100-2,15,260; 100-4,4,20.5; 100-4,12,90.3; 100-4,14,10

21125 Augmentation, mandibular body or angle; prosthetic material 🟦 T 80 🔲

21127 with bone graft, onlay or interpositional (includes obtaining autograft) 🟩 T 80 🔲

MED: 100-2,15,260; 100-4,4,20.5; 100-4,12,90.3; 100-4,14,10

21137 Reduction forehead; contouring only T 80 🔲

MED: 100-2,16,10; 100-2,16,120; 100-2,16,180; 100-4,4,20.5

21138 contouring and application of prosthetic material or bone graft (includes obtaining autograft) T 80 🔲

21139 contouring and setback of anterior frontal sinus wall T 80 🔲

21141 Reconstruction midface, LeFort I; single piece, segment movement in any direction (eg, for Long Face Syndrome), without bone graft C 80 🔲

21142 two pieces, segment movement in any direction, without bone graft C 80 🔲

21143 three or more pieces, segment movement in any direction, without bone graft C 80 🔲

21145 single piece, segment movement in any direction, requiring bone grafts (includes obtaining autografts) C 80 🔲

21146 two pieces, segment movement in any direction, requiring bone grafts (includes obtaining autografts) (eg, ungrafted unilateral alveolar cleft) C 80 🔲

21147 three or more pieces, segment movement in any direction, requiring bone grafts (includes obtaining autografts) (eg, ungrafted bilateral alveolar cleft or multiple osteotomies) C 80 🔲

21150 Reconstruction midface, LeFort II; anterior intrusion (eg, Treacher-Collins Syndrome) T 80 🔲

21151 any direction, requiring bone grafts (includes obtaining autografts) C 80 🔲

21154 Reconstruction midface, LeFort III (extracranial), any type, requiring bone grafts (includes obtaining autografts); without LeFort I C 80 🔲

21155 with LeFort I C 80 🔲

21159 Reconstruction midface, LeFort III (extra and intracranial) with forehead advancement (eg, mono bloc), requiring bone grafts (includes obtaining autografts); without LeFort I C 80 🔲

21160 with LeFort I C 80 🔲

21172 Reconstruction superior-lateral orbital rim and lower forehead, advancement or alteration, with or without grafts (includes obtaining autografts) C 80 🔲

If frontal or parietal craniotomy is performed for craniosynostosis, consult CPT code 61556.

21175 Reconstruction, bifrontal, superior-lateral orbital rims and lower forehead, advancement or alteration (eg, plagiocephaly, trigonocephaly, brachycephaly), with or without grafts (includes obtaining autografts) T 80 🔲

If bifrontal craniotomy is performed for craniosynostosis, consult CPT code 61557.

21179 Reconstruction, entire or majority of forehead and/or supraorbital rims; with grafts (allograft or prosthetic material) C 80 🔲

21180 with autograft (includes obtaining grafts) C 80 🔲

If an extensive craniectomy for multiple suture craniosynostosis is performed, consult CPT code 61558 or 61559.

21181 Reconstruction by contouring of benign tumor of cranial bones (eg, fibrous dysplasia), extracranial 🟦 T 80 🔲

MED: 100-2,15,260; 100-4,4,20.5; 100-4,12,90.3; 100-4,14,10

21182 Reconstruction of orbital walls, rims, forehead, nasoethmoid complex following intra- and extracranial excision of benign tumor of cranial bone (eg, fibrous dysplasia), with multiple autografts (includes obtaining grafts); total area of bone grafting less than 40 sq cm C 80 🔲

21183 total area of bone grafting greater than 40 sq cm but less than 80 sq cm C 80 🔲

21184 total area of bone grafting greater than 80 sq cm C 80 🔲

If a benign tumor of the cranial bones is excised, consult CPT codes 61563 and 61564.

21188 Reconstruction midface, osteotomies (other than LeFort type) and bone grafts (includes obtaining autografts) C 80 🔲

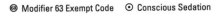

21193 Reconstruction of mandibular rami, horizontal, vertical, C, or L osteotomy; without bone graft `C` `80` `▢`

AMA: 1996,Apr,11
If cranioplasty is performed, consult CPT codes 21179, 21180, 62116, 62120, and 62140-62147.

21194 with bone graft (includes obtaining graft) `C` `80` `▢`

AMA: 1996,Apr,11

21195 Reconstruction of mandibular rami and/or body, sagittal split; without internal rigid fixation `T` `80` `▢`

AMA: 1996,Apr,11

21196 with internal rigid fixation `C` `80` `▢`

AMA: 1997,Mar,11; 1996,Apr,11

21198 Osteotomy, mandible, segmental; `T` `80` `▢`

21199 with genioglossus advancement `T` `80` `▢`

21206 Osteotomy, maxilla, segmental (eg, Wassmund or Schuchard) `5` `T` `80` `▢`

MED: 100-2,15,260; 100-4,4,20.5; 100-4,12,90.3; 100-4,14,10

21208 Osteoplasty, facial bones; augmentation (autograft, allograft, or prosthetic implant) `7` `T` `80` `▢`

MED: 100-2,15,260; 100-4,4,20.5; 100-4,12,90.3; 100-4,14,10

21209 reduction `5` `T` `80` `▢`

MED: 100-2,15,260; 100-4,4,20.5; 100-4,12,90.3; 100-4,14,10

21210 Graft, bone; nasal, maxillary or malar areas (includes obtaining graft) `7` `T` `▢`

MED: 100-2,15,260; 100-4,4,20.5; 100-4,12,90.3; 100-4,14,10
If cleft palate is repaired, consult CPT codes 42200-42225.

21215 mandible (includes obtaining graft) `7` `T` `▢`

MED: 100-2,15,260; 100-4,4,20.5; 100-4,12,90.3; 100-4,14,10

21230 Graft; rib cartilage, autogenous, to face, chin, nose or ear (includes obtaining graft) `7` `T` `80` `▢`

MED: 100-2,15,260; 100-4,4,20.5; 100-4,12,90.3; 100-4,14,10

21235 ear cartilage, autogenous, to nose or ear (includes obtaining graft) `7` `T` `▢`

MED: 100-2,15,260; 100-4,4,20.5; 100-4,12,90.3; 100-4,14,10

TMJ syndrome is often related to stress and tooth-grinding; in other cases, arthritis, injury, poorly aligned teeth, or ill-fitting dentures may be the cause

Upper joint space
Lower joint space
Articular disc (meniscus)
Cutaway detail
Condyle
Mandible
Cutaway view of temporomandibular joint (TMJ)
Symptoms include facial pain and chewing problems; TMJ syndrome occurs more frequently in women

21240 Arthroplasty, temporomandibular joint, with or without autograft (includes obtaining graft) `4` `T` `80` `50` `▢`

MED: 100-2,15,260; 100-4,4,20.5; 100-4,12,90.3; 100-4,14,10

21242 Arthroplasty, temporomandibular joint, with allograft `5` `T` `80` `50` `▢`

MED: 100-2,15,260; 100-4,4,20.5; 100-4,12,90.3; 100-4,14,10

21243 Arthroplasty, temporomandibular joint, with prosthetic joint replacement `5` `T` `80` `50` `▢`

MED: 100-2,15,260; 100-4,4,20.5; 100-4,12,90.3; 100-4,14,10

21244 Reconstruction of mandible, extraoral, with transosteal bone plate (eg, mandibular staple bone plate) `7` `T` `80` `▢`

MED: 100-2,15,260; 100-4,4,20.5; 100-4,12,90.3; 100-4,14,10

21245 Reconstruction of mandible or maxilla, subperiosteal implant; partial `7` `T` `80` `▢`

MED: 100-2,15,260; 100-4,4,20.5; 100-4,12,90.3; 100-4,14,10

21246 complete `7` `T` `80` `▢`

MED: 100-2,15,260; 100-4,4,20.5; 100-4,12,90.3; 100-4,14,10

21247 Reconstruction of mandibular condyle with bone and cartilage autografts (includes obtaining grafts) (eg, for hemifacial microsomia) `C` `80` `▢`

21248 Reconstruction of mandible or maxilla, endosteal implant (eg, blade, cylinder); partial `7` `T` `▢`

MED: 100-2,15,260; 100-4,4,20.5; 100-4,12,90.3; 100-4,14,10

21249 complete `7` `T` `80` `▢`

MED: 100-2,15,260; 100-4,4,20.5; 100-4,12,90.3; 100-4,14,10
If a reconstruction of the midface is performed, consult CPT codes 21141-21160.

21255 Reconstruction of zygomatic arch and glenoid fossa with bone and cartilage (includes obtaining autografts) `C` `80` `▢`

21256 Reconstruction of orbit with osteotomies (extracranial) and with bone grafts (includes obtaining autografts) (eg, micro-ophthalmia) `C` `80` `▢`

21260 Periorbital osteotomies for orbital hypertelorism, with bone grafts; extracranial approach `T` `80` `▢`

21261 combined intra- and extracranial approach `T` `80` `▢`

Grafts

In 21263, a frontal craniotomy is performed, the brain retracted, and the orbit approached from inside the skull; frontal bone is advanced and secured

Osteotomies are cut 360 degrees around the orbit; portions of nasal and ethmoid bones are removed

Grafts are placed and the bony orbits realigned

21263 with forehead advancement `T` `80` `▢`

21267 Orbital repositioning, periorbital osteotomies, unilateral, with bone grafts; extracranial approach `7` `T` `80` `▢`

MED: 100-2,15,260; 100-4,4,20.5; 100-4,12,90.3; 100-4,14,10

21268 combined intra- and extracranial approach `C` `80` `▢`

21270 Malar augmentation, prosthetic material `5` `T` `80` `▢`

MED: 100-2,15,260; 100-4,4,20.5; 100-4,12,90.3; 100-4,14,10
If malar augmentation with a bone graft is performed, consult CPT code 21210.

21275 Secondary revision of orbitocraniofacial reconstruction `7` `T` `80` `▢`

MED: 100-2,15,260; 100-4,4,20.5; 100-4,12,90.3; 100-4,14,10

21280 Medial canthopexy (separate procedure) `5` `T` `80` `50` `▢`

MED: 100-2,15,260; 100-4,4,20.5; 100-4,12,90.3; 100-4,14,10
If medial canthoplasty is performed, consult CPT code 67950.

21282	Lateral canthopexy 5 T 50 ⚏

MED: 100-2,15,260; 100-4,4,20.5; 100-4,12,90.3; 100-4,14,10

21295	Reduction of masseter muscle and bone (eg, for treatment of benign masseteric hypertrophy); extraoral approach 1 T 80 ⚏

MED: 100-2,15,260; 100-4,4,20.5; 100-4,12,90.3; 100-4,14,10

21296	intraoral approach 1 T 80 ⚏

MED: 100-2,15,260; 100-4,4,20.5; 100-4,12,90.3; 100-4,14,10

OTHER PROCEDURES

21299	Unlisted craniofacial and maxillofacial procedure T 80

MED: 100-4,4,20.5; 100-4,4,180.3

FRACTURE AND/OR DISLOCATION

To report operative repair of skull fracture, consult 62000-62010. To report closed treatment of skull fracture, consult the appropriate evaluation and management code.

~~21300~~	~~Closed treatment of skull fracture without operation~~

21310	Closed treatment of nasal bone fracture without manipulation 2 T ⚏

MED: 100-2,15,260; 100-4,4,20.5; 100-4,12,90.3; 100-4,14,10

21315	Closed treatment of nasal bone fracture; without stabilization 2 T ⚏

MED: 100-2,15,260; 100-4,4,20.5; 100-4,12,90.3; 100-4,14,10

21320	with stabilization 2 T ⚏

MED: 100-2,15,260; 100-4,4,20.5; 100-4,12,90.3; 100-4,14,10

21325	Open treatment of nasal fracture; uncomplicated 4 T 80 ⚏

MED: 100-2,15,260; 100-4,4,20.5; 100-4,12,90.3; 100-4,14,10

21330	complicated, with internal and/or external skeletal fixation 5 T 80 ⚏

MED: 100-2,15,260; 100-4,4,20.5; 100-4,12,90.3; 100-4,14,10

21335	with concomitant open treatment of fractured septum 7 T ⚏

MED: 100-2,15,260; 100-4,4,20.5; 100-4,12,90.3; 100-4,14,10

21336	Open treatment of nasal septal fracture, with or without stabilization 4 T 80 ⚏

MED: 100-2,15,260; 100-4,4,20.5; 100-4,12,90.3; 100-4,14,10

21337	Closed treatment of nasal septal fracture, with or without stabilization 2 T 80 ⚏

MED: 100-2,15,260; 100-4,4,20.5; 100-4,12,90.3; 100-4,14,10

21338	Open treatment of nasoethmoid fracture; without external fixation 4 T 80 ⚏

MED: 100-2,15,260; 100-4,4,20.5; 100-4,12,90.3; 100-4,14,10

21339	with external fixation 5 T 80 ⚏

MED: 100-2,15,260; 100-4,4,20.5; 100-4,12,90.3; 100-4,14,10

21340	Percutaneous treatment of nasoethmoid complex fracture, with splint, wire or headcap fixation, including repair of canthal ligaments and/or the nasolacrimal apparatus 4 T 80 ⚏

MED: 100-2,15,260; 100-4,4,20.5; 100-4,12,90.3; 100-4,14,10

21343	Open treatment of depressed frontal sinus fracture C 80 ⚏

21344	Open treatment of complicated (eg, comminuted or involving posterior wall) frontal sinus fracture, via coronal or multiple approaches C 80 ⚏

21345	Closed treatment of nasomaxillary complex fracture (LeFort II type), with interdental wire fixation or fixation of denture or splint 7 T 80 ⚏

MED: 100-2,15,260; 100-4,4,20.5; 100-4,12,90.3; 100-4,14,10

21346	Open treatment of nasomaxillary complex fracture (LeFort II type); with wiring and/or local fixation C ⚏

21347	requiring multiple open approaches C 80 ⚏

21348	with bone grafting (includes obtaining graft) C 80 ⚏

21355	Percutaneous treatment of fracture of malar area, including zygomatic arch and malar tripod, with manipulation 3 T 80 ⚏

MED: 100-2,15,260; 100-4,4,20.5; 100-4,12,90.3; 100-4,14,10

21356	Open treatment of depressed zygomatic arch fracture (eg, Gillies approach) 3 T 80 ⚏

21360	Open treatment of depressed malar fracture, including zygomatic arch and malar tripod C 80 ⚏

21365	Open treatment of complicated (eg, comminuted or involving cranial nerve foramina) fracture(s) of malar area, including zygomatic arch and malar tripod; with internal fixation and multiple surgical approaches C 80 ⚏

21366	with bone grafting (includes obtaining graft) C 80 ⚏

21385	Open treatment of orbital floor blowout fracture; transantral approach (Caldwell-Luc type operation) C 80 ⚏

21386	periorbital approach C 80 ⚏

21387	combined approach C 80 ⚏

21390	periorbital approach, with alloplastic or other implant T 80 ⚏

21395	periorbital approach with bone graft (includes obtaining graft) C 80 ⚏

21400	Closed treatment of fracture of orbit, except blowout; without manipulation 2 T 80 ⚏

MED: 100-2,15,260; 100-4,4,20.5; 100-4,12,90.3; 100-4,14,10

21401	with manipulation 3 T 80 ⚏

MED: 100-2,15,260; 100-4,4,20.5; 100-4,12,90.3; 100-4,14,10

21406	Open treatment of fracture of orbit, except blowout; without implant T 80 ⚏

21407	with implant T 80 ⚏

21408	with bone grafting (includes obtaining graft) T 80 ⚏

21421	Closed treatment of palatal or maxillary fracture (LeFort I type), with interdental wire fixation or fixation of denture or splint 4 T 80 ⚏

MED: 100-2,15,260; 100-4,4,20.5; 100-4,12,90.3; 100-4,14,10

21422	Open treatment of palatal or maxillary fracture (LeFort I type); C 80 ⚏

21423	complicated (comminuted or involving cranial nerve foramina), multiple approaches C 80 ⚏

21431	Closed treatment of craniofacial separation (LeFort III type) using interdental wire fixation of denture or splint C 80 ⚏

21432	Open treatment of craniofacial separation (LeFort III type); with wiring and/or internal fixation C 80 ⚏

Musculoskeletal System

21433 — 21557

21433	complicated (eg, comminuted or involving cranial nerve foramina), multiple surgical approaches	C 80 ◄

21435	complicated, utilizing internal and/or external fixation techniques (eg, head cap, halo device, and/or intermaxillary fixation)	C 80 ◄

If an internal or an external fixation device is removed, consult CPT code 20670.

21436	complicated, multiple surgical approaches, internal fixation, with bone grafting (includes obtaining graft)	C 80 ◄

21440	Closed treatment of mandibular or maxillary alveolar ridge fracture (separate procedure)	T 80 ◄

MED: 100-2,15,260; 100-4,4,20.5; 100-4,12,90.3; 100-4,14,10

21445	Open treatment of mandibular or maxillary alveolar ridge fracture (separate procedure)	4 T 80 ◄

MED: 100-2,15,260; 100-4,4,20.5; 100-4,12,90.3; 100-4,14,10

21450	Closed treatment of mandibular fracture; without manipulation	3 T 80 ◄

MED: 100-2,15,260; 100-4,4,20.5; 100-4,12,90.3; 100-4,14,10

21451	with manipulation	4 T 80 ◄

MED: 100-2,15,260; 100-4,4,20.5; 100-4,12,90.3; 100-4,14,10

In 21452, external fixation is necessary

Comminuted fractures

Metal or acrylic bar

Rods and pins placed in drilled holes

21452	Percutaneous treatment of mandibular fracture, with external fixation	2 T 80 ◄

MED: 100-2,15,260; 100-4,4,20.5; 100-4,12,90.3; 100-4,14,10

21453	Closed treatment of mandibular fracture with interdental fixation	3 T 80 ◄

MED: 100-2,15,260; 100-4,4,20.5; 100-4,12,90.3; 100-4,14,10

21454	Open treatment of mandibular fracture with external fixation	5 T 80 ◄

MED: 100-2,15,260; 100-4,4,20.5; 100-4,12,90.3; 100-4,14,10

21461	Open treatment of mandibular fracture; without interdental fixation	4 T 80 ◄

MED: 100-2,15,260; 100-4,4,20.5; 100-4,12,90.3; 100-4,14,10

21462	with interdental fixation	5 T 80 ◄

MED: 100-2,15,260; 100-4,4,20.5; 100-4,12,90.3; 100-4,14,10

21465	Open treatment of mandibular condylar fracture	4 T 80 ◄

MED: 100-2,15,260; 100-4,4,20.5; 100-4,12,90.3; 100-4,14,10

21470	Open treatment of complicated mandibular fracture by multiple surgical approaches including internal fixation, interdental fixation, and/or wiring of dentures or splints	T 80 ◄

AMA: 2002,Nov,10

21480	Closed treatment of temporomandibular dislocation; initial or subsequent	1 T 50 ◄

MED: 100-2,15,260; 100-4,4,20.5; 100-4,12,90.3; 100-4,14,10

21485	complicated (eg, recurrent requiring intermaxillary fixation or splinting), initial or subsequent	2 T 80 50 ◄

MED: 100-2,15,260; 100-4,4,20.5; 100-4,12,90.3; 100-4,14,10

21490	Open treatment of temporomandibular dislocation	3 T 80 50 ◄

MED: 100-2,15,260; 100-4,4,20.5; 100-4,12,90.3; 100-4,14,10

To report interdental wire fixation, consult CPT code 21497.

21495	Open treatment of hyoid fracture	T 80 ◄

If laryngoplasty with open reduction of a fracture is performed, consult CPT code 31584. For treatment of a closed fracture of the larynx, consult the appropriate evaluation and management codes.

21497	Interdental wiring, for condition other than fracture	2 T 80 ◄

MED: 100-2,15,260; 100-4,4,20.5; 100-4,12,90.3; 100-4,14,10

AMA: 1997,Mar,10

OTHER PROCEDURES

21499	Unlisted musculoskeletal procedure, head	T 80

MED: 100-4,4,20.5; 100-4,4,180.3

If a craniofacial or a maxillofacial procedure is unlisted, consult CPT code 21299.

NECK (SOFT TISSUES) AND THORAX

If these procedures are being performed on the cervical spine and back, consult CPT codes 21920 and others. If an injection is needed at the fracture site or trigger point, consult CPT code 20550.

INCISION

If a superficial abscess or hematoma is incised and drained, consult CPT codes 10060 and 10140.

21501	Incision and drainage, deep abscess or hematoma, soft tissues of neck or thorax;	2 T ◄

MED: 100-2,15,260; 100-4,4,20.5; 100-4,12,90.3; 100-4,14,10

If a subfascial incision and drainage is performed on the posterior spine, consult CPT codes 22010-22015.

21502	with partial rib ostectomy	2 T 80 ◄

MED: 100-2,15,260; 100-4,4,20.5; 100-4,12,90.3; 100-4,14,10

21510	Incision, deep, with opening of bone cortex (eg, for osteomyelitis or bone abscess), thorax	C 80 ◄

EXCISION

If bone biopsy is needed, consult CPT codes 20220-20251.

21550	Biopsy, soft tissue of neck or thorax	T ◄

If a needle biopsy of soft tissue is needed, consult CPT code 20206.

21555	Excision tumor, soft tissue of neck or thorax; subcutaneous	2 T ◄

MED: 100-2,15,260; 100-4,4,20.5; 100-4,12,90.3; 100-4,14,10

AMA: 2002,Oct,11

21556	deep, subfascial, intramuscular	2 T ◄

MED: 100-2,15,260; 100-4,4,20.5; 100-4,12,90.3; 100-4,14,10

21557	Radical resection of tumor (eg, malignant neoplasm), soft tissue of neck or thorax	T 80 ◄

PC Professional Component Only   **80/80** Assist-at-Surgery Allowed/With Documentation   Unlisted   Not Covered

TC Technical Component Only   **MED:** Pub 100/NCD References   **AMA:** CPT Assistant References   **1**-**9** ASC Group   ♂ Male Only   ♀ Female Only

70 — CPT Expert   CPT only © 2006 American Medical Association. All Rights Reserved. *(Black Ink)*   © *2006 Ingenix (Blue Ink)*

21600	**Excision of rib, partial**	② T 80

MED: 100-2,15,260; 100-4,4,20.5; 100-4,12,90.3; 100-4,14,10

If a radical resection for a tumor is performed, consult CPT code 19260.

If radical debridement due to injury is performed, consult CPT codes 11040-11044.

21610	**Costotransversectomy (separate procedure)**	② T 80 ☒

MED: 100-2,15,260; 100-4,4,20.5; 100-4,12,90.3; 100-4,14,10

21615	**Excision first and/or cervical rib;**	C 80 50 ☒
21616	**with sympathectomy**	C 80 50 ☒
21620	**Ostectomy of sternum, partial**	C 80 ☒
21627	**Sternal debridement**	C 80 ☒

If both debridement and closure are performed, consult CPT code 21750.

21630	**Radical resection of sternum;**	C 80 ☒
21632	**with mediastinal lymphadenectomy**	C 80 ☒

REPAIR, REVISION, AND/OR RECONSTRUCTION

If the wound is superficial, consult the Integumentary System section under Repair, Simple.

21685	**Hyoid myotomy and suspension**	T 80 ☒
21700	**Division of scalenus anticus; without resection of cervical rib**	② T 80 ☒

MED: 100-2,15,260; 100-4,4,20.5; 100-4,12,90.3; 100-4,14,10

21705	**with resection of cervical rib**	C 80 ☒
21720	**Division of sternocleidomastoid for torticollis, open operation; without cast application**	③ T 80 ☒

MED: 100-2,15,260; 100-4,4,20.5; 100-4,12,90.3; 100-4,14,10

If nerve transsection is performed, consult CPT codes 63191 and 64722.

21725	**with cast application**	③ T 80 ☒

MED: 100-2,15,260; 100-4,4,20.5; 100-4,12,90.3; 100-4,14,10

21740	**Reconstructive repair of pectus excavatum or carinatum; open**	C 80 ☒
21742	**minimally invasive approach (Nuss procedure), without thoracoscopy**	T 80 ☒
21743	**minimally invasive approach (Nuss procedure), with thoracoscopy**	T 80 ☒
21750	**Closure of median sternotomy separation with or without debridement (separate procedure)**	C 80 ☒

FRACTURE AND/OR DISLOCATION

21800	**Closed treatment of rib fracture, uncomplicated, each**	① T ☒

MED: 100-2,15,260; 100-4,4,20.5; 100-4,12,90.3; 100-4,14,10

21805	**Open treatment of rib fracture without fixation, each**	② T 80 ☒

MED: 100-2,15,260; 100-4,4,20.5; 100-4,12,90.3; 100-4,14,10

21810	**Treatment of rib fracture requiring external fixation (flail chest)**	C 80 ☒
21820	**Closed treatment of sternum fracture**	① T ☒

MED: 100-2,15,260; 100-4,4,20.5; 100-4,12,90.3; 100-4,14,10

21825	**Open treatment of sternum fracture with or without skeletal fixation**	C 80 ☒

If a sternoclavicular dislocation is treated, consult CPT codes 23520-23532.

OTHER PROCEDURES

21899	**Unlisted procedure, neck or thorax**	T 80

MED: 100-4,4,20.5; 100-4,4,180.3

BACK AND FLANK, EXCISION

21920	**Biopsy, soft tissue of back or flank; superficial**	T ☒
21925	**deep**	② T ☒

MED: 100-2,15,260; 100-4,4,20.5; 100-4,12,90.3; 100-4,14,10

If soft tissue needle biopsy is performed, consult CPT code 20206.

21930	**Excision, tumor, soft tissue of back or flank**	② T ☒

MED: 100-2,15,260; 100-4,4,20.5; 100-4,12,90.3; 100-4,14,10

21935	**Radical resection of tumor (eg, malignant neoplasm), soft tissue of back or flank**	③ T ☒

MED: 100-2,15,260; 100-4,4,20.5; 100-4,12,90.3; 100-4,14,10

SPINE (VERTEBRAL COLUMN)

Procedure codes for reporting spine surgeries are found in two sections of the CPT book. Fracture/dislocation, spinal fusion/instrumentation, and treatment of scoliosis/kyphosis are reported with codes from the musculoskeletal section. Procedures of the spine with spinal cord involvement are reported with codes from the nervous system section (62263-63746). It is not unusual for procedures to require a procedure from the musculoskeletal section (arthrodesis, instrumentation) with a procedure from the nervous system section (laminectomy, hemilaminectomy, diskectomy), and it is appropriate to report both procedures separately.

Arthrodesis is a joint fusion and spinal arthrodesis is reported with 22548-22632. These codes are assigned based on technique (anterior/anterolateral, posterior/posterolateral, or lateral). Codes 22548-22558, 22590-22612, and 22630 are for single interspace arthrodesis-two adjacent vertebral segments. When the surgery is performed on more than one interspace, each additional interspace is reported with 22585, 22614, or 22632. These procedures are considered "add on" services and are not reported with modifier 51.

Procedures for scoliosis and kyphosis (22800-22819) also include arthrodesis procedures. The arthrodesis procedures in this section differ since they involve multiple vertebral segments, and the code is assigned based on the number of segments treated.

Spinal instrumentation (22840-22855) involves placement of rods, hooks, and/or wires to stabilize the fusion or fracture. Instrumentation codes are assigned based on the type of instrumentation (segmental, non-segmental), the approach (anterior, posterior) and the number of vertebral segments involved. Instrumentation codes are exempt from modifier 51 and are reported in addition to the definitive procedure. However, if instrumentation reinsertion or removal or exploration of fusion is performed in conjunction with other definitive procedures including arthrodesis, modifier 51 should be appended.

Bone allografts and autografts should be reported separately with codes 20930-20938. These codes are exempt from modifier 51 and are reported in addition to the definitive procedure. Procedures of the spine with spinal cord are found in the nervous system section (62263-63746).

Diskectomy is the excision of intervertebral disk material. Codes 63075-63078 are specific to this surgery; however, many other codes from this section of the nervous system include diskectomies as a component of the procedure. Laminectomy is the removal of the entire lamina on both sides, inclusive of the spinous process. Hemilaminectomy is the excision of the right or left lamina, the posterior bony covering of the spinal cord. Laminotomy is the process of creating a hole in the lamina to achieve the required result, for example, excising a herniated intervertebral disk.

For the injection procedure of a myelography, consult CPT code 62284. For the injection procedure of a diskography, consult CPT codes 62290 and 62291. For the injection procedure for chemonucleolysis, single or multiple levels, consult CPT code 62292. For the injection procedure of facet joints, consult CPT codes 64470-64476 and 64622-64627.

For needle or trocar biopsy, consult CPT codes 20220-20225.

⊛ **Modifier 63 Exempt Code**   ⊙ **Conscious Sedation**   + **CPT Add-on Code**   ⊘ **Modifier 51 Exempt Code**   ● **New Code**   ▲ **Revised Code**

Ⓜ **Maternity Edit**   Ⓐ **Age Edit**   Ⓐ-Ⓨ **APC Status Indicators**   ☒ **CCI Comprehensive Code**   50 **Bilateral Procedure**

© *2006 Ingenix (Blue Ink)*   CPT only © 2006 American Medical Association. All Rights Reserved. *(Black Ink)*   **Musculoskeletal System — 71**

For bone biopsy, consult CPT code 20220-20251.

Report bone grafting procedure separately in addition to spinal arthrodesis. Consult codes 20930-20938. Do not use modifier 51 with these codes. Do not report modifier 62 with codes 20900-20938.

Spinal instrumentation codes are reported separately in addition to spinal arthrodesis. Consult codes 22840-22855 for spinal instrumentation codes performed with definitive vertebral procedures. Do not report modifier 51 with codes 22840-22848 and 22851. Do not report modifier 62 with instrumentation codes 22840-22848 and 22850-22852.

In some instances vertebral procedures are followed by arthrodesis and may also include bone grafts and instrumentation.

When arthrodesis is performed with another procedure, the arthrodesis should be reported in addition to the vertebral procedure with modifier 51. Because bone grafts and instrumentation are never performed without arthrodesis, modifier 51 is not used.

If arthrodesis is performed without other procedures and is combined with another definitive procedure, use modifier 51.

Surgeons that work together, each performing distinct parts of a single surgery, should report the procedure code and use modifier 62.

INCISION

	22010	**Incision and drainage, open, of deep abscess (subfascial), posterior spine; cervical, thoracic, or cervicothoracic**	C 80
	22015	**lumbar, sacral, or lumbosacral**	C

        Code 22015 cannot be reported with 22010.

        Code 22015 cannot be reported with instrumentation removal, codes 10180, 22850, and 22852.

        To report incision and drainage of a superficial abscess or hematoma, consult codes 10060 and 10140.

EXCISION

Surgeons, each performing distinct parts of a single surgery, should report the procedure code and use modifier 62. Modifier 62 may be used with code(s) 22100-22102, 22110-22114 and as appropriate to the related additional vertebral segment add-on code(s) 22103 and 22116 when both surgeons continue to perform distinct components of the surgery, working together as primary surgeons.

	22100	**Partial excision of posterior vertebral component (eg, spinous process, lamina or facet) for intrinsic bony lesion, single vertebral segment; cervical**	T 80
	22101	**thoracic**	T 80
	22102	**lumbar**	T 80
+	22103	**each additional segment (List separately in addition to code for primary procedure)**	T 80

        Note that 22103 is an add-on code and must be used in conjunction with 22100, 22101, and 22102.

	22110	**Partial excision of vertebral body, for intrinsic bony lesion, without decompression of spinal cord or nerve root(s), single vertebral segment; cervical**	C 80
	22112	**thoracic**	C 80
	22114	**lumbar**	C 80
+	22116	**each additional vertebral segment (List separately in addition to code for primary procedure)**	C 80

        Note that 22116 is in add-on code and must be used in conjunction with 22110, 22112 and 22114.

OSTEOTOMY

Surgeons each performing distinct parts of a single surgery when working together as primary surgeons should report the procedure code and use modifier 62. Modifier 62 may be used with code(s) 22210-22214, 22220-22224 and, as

appropriate to the related segment, add-on code(s) 22216 and 22226 if both surgeons continue to perform distinct components of the surgery. Modifier 62 should not be reported with codes 20900-20938.

Additional procedures, such as arthrodesis (CPT codes 22590-22632), bone grafting (CPT codes 20930-20938), and instrumentation (CPT codes 22840-22855), are reported in addition to the CPT codes for the definitive procedure. Do not report modifier 51 with instrumentation procedures, codes 22840-22855, or with bone graft procedures, codes 20930-20938.

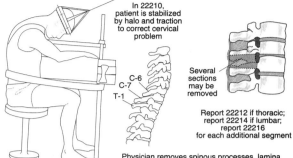

In 22210, patient is stabilized by halo and traction to correct cervical problem

C-6
C-7
T-1

Several sections may be removed

Report 22212 if thoracic; report 22214 if lumbar; report 22216 for each additional segment

Physician removes spinous processes, lamina

	22210	**Osteotomy of spine, posterior or posterolateral approach, one vertebral segment; cervical**	C 80 ▢
	22212	**thoracic**	C 80 ▢
	22214	**lumbar**	C 80 ▢
+	22216	**each additional vertebral segment (List separately in addition to primary procedure)**	C 80 ▢

        Note that 22216 is an add-on code and must be used in conjunction with 22210, 22212, and 22214.

▲	22220	**Osteotomy of spine, including discectomy, anterior approach, single vertebral segment; cervical**	C 80 ▢
▲	22222	**thoracic**	T 80 ▢
▲	22224	**lumbar**	C 80 ▢
+ ▲	22226	**each additional vertebral segment (List separately in addition to code for primary procedure)**	C 80 ▢

        Note that 22226 is an add-on code and must be used in conjunction with 22220, 22222, and 22224.

FRACTURE AND/OR DISLOCATION

Surgeons, each performing distinct parts of a single surgery, when working together as primary surgeons should report the procedure code and use modifier 62. Modifier 62 may be used with code(s) 22318-22327 and, as appropriate to the related additional fractured vertebra or dislocated segment, add-on code 22328 if both surgeons continue to perform distinct components of the surgery.

Additional procedures, such as arthrodesis (CPT codes 22590-22632), bone grafting (CPT codes 20930-20938), and instrumentation (CPT codes 22840-22855), are reported in addition to the CPT codes for the definitive procedure. Do not append modifier 51 with instrumentation procedures, codes 22840-22855, or with bone graft procedures, codes 20930-20938.

	22305	**Closed treatment of vertebral process fracture(s)**	1 T ▢

        MED: 100-2,15,260; 100-4,4,20.5; 100-4,12,90.3; 100-4,14,10

	22310	**Closed treatment of vertebral body fracture(s), without manipulation, requiring and including casting or bracing**	1 T ▢

        MED: 100-2,15,260; 100-4,4,20.5; 100-4,12,90.3; 100-4,14,10

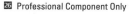

26 Professional Component Only   80/80 Assist-at-Surgery Allowed/With Documentation   **Unlisted**   **Not Covered**

TC Technical Component Only   **MED:** Pub 100/NCD References   **AMA:** CPT Assistant References   1-9 ASC Group   ♂ Male Only   ♀ Female Only

72 — CPT Expert   CPT only © 2006 American Medical Association. All Rights Reserved. *(Black Ink)*   © *2006* Ingenix *(Blue Ink)*

22315 Closed treatment of vertebral fracture(s) and/or dislocation(s) requiring casting or bracing, with and including casting and/or bracing, with or without anesthesia, by manipulation or traction [2] [T] [CCI]

> MED: 100-2,15,260; 100-4,4,20.5; 100-4,12,90.3; 100-4,14,10
> If spinal subluxation is performed, consult CPT code 97140.

22318 Open treatment and/or reduction of odontoid fracture(s) and or dislocation(s) (including os odontoideum), anterior approach, including placement of internal fixation; without grafting [C] [80] [CCI]

> AMA: 1999,Nov,11

22319 with grafting [C] [80] [CCI]

> AMA: 1999,Nov,11

22325 Open treatment and/or reduction of vertebral fracture(s) and/or dislocation(s), posterior approach, one fractured vertebrae or dislocated segment; lumbar [C] [80] [CCI]

> AMA: 1997,Sep,8

22326 cervical [C] [80] [CCI]

> AMA: 1997,Sep,8

22327 thoracic [C] [80] [CCI]

> AMA: 1997,Sep,8

+ 22328 each additional fractured vertebrae or dislocated segment (List separately in addition to code for primary procedure) [C] [80] [CCI]

> Note that 22328 is an add-on code and must be used in conjunction with 22325, 22326, and 22327.
>
> For anterior approach, consult CPT codes 63081-63091, and appropriate arthrodesis, bone graft and instrumentation codes.

MANIPULATION

22505 Manipulation of spine requiring anesthesia, any region [2] [T] [CCI]

> MED: 100-2,15,260; 100-4,4,20.5; 100-4,12,90.3; 100-4,14,10
> AMA: 1999,Jan,11; 1997,Mar,11
> For manipulation of the spine without anesthesia, consult CPT code 97140.

VERTEBRAL BODY, EMBOLIZATION OR INJECTION

These CPT codes describe the injection of a fixative into the vertebral body to bond bone fragments.

22520 Percutaneous vertebroplasty, one vertebral body, unilateral or bilateral injection; thoracic [9] [T] [CCI]

> AMA: 2001,Mar,1

22521 lumbar [9] [T] [CCI]

> AMA: 2001,Mar,1

+ 22522 each additional thoracic or lumbar vertebral body (List separately in addition to code for primary procedure) [9] [T] [CCI]

> AMA: 2001,Mar,1
> Note that 22522 is an add-on code and must be used in conjunction with 22520 and 22521.
>
> To report radiological supervision and interpretation, consult codes 72291 and 72292.

22523 Percutaneous vertebral augmentation, including cavity creation (fracture reduction and bone biopsy included when performed) using mechanical device, one vertebral body, unilateral or bilateral cannulation (eg, kyphoplasty); thoracic [T]

22524 lumbar [T]

+ 22525 each additional thoracic or lumbar vertebral body (List separately in addition to code for primary procedure) [T]

> Code 22525 cannot be reported with 20225 when performed at the same level as 22523-22525.
>
> Note that 22525 is an add-on code and must be used in conjunction with 22523 and 22524.
>
> To report radiological supervision and interpretation, consult CPT codes 72291 and 72292.

⊙ ● 22526 Percutaneous intradiscal electrothermal annuloplasty, unilateral or bilateral including fluoroscopic guidance; single level [T]

+ ⊙ ● 22527 one or more additional levels (List separately in addition to code for primary procedure) [T]

> Do not report 22526 or 22527 in conjunction with 77002 or 77003.
>
> See 0062T and 0063T when percutaneous intradiscal annuloplasty is performed using a method other than electrothemal.

ARTHRODESIS

Arthrodesis may be performed without other procedures so when it is performed in addition to other procedures such as osteotomy, fracture care, vertebral corpectomy or laminectomy, append modifier 51. Codes 22585, 22614 and 22632 are add-on procedures and should not be reported with the 51 modifier.

Instrumentation procedures should be reported with codes 22840-22855. Report codes 22840-22848 and 22851 with the code(s) for the definitive procedure(s) without appending modifier 51. Report modifier 51 with codes 22849, 22850, 22852 and 22855 when instrumentation reinsertion or removal codes are used with the other definitive procedures. This includes arthrodesis, decompression, and exploration of fusion. Do not report modifier 62, to spinal instrumentation codes 22840-22848 and 22850-22852.

Bone graft codes, 20930-20938, are reported in addition to the code for the definitive procedure without modifier 51. Modifier 62 should not be appended to codes 20900-20938.

LATERAL EXTRACAVITARY APPROACH TECHNIQUE

▲ 22532 Arthrodesis, lateral extracavitary technique, including minimal discectomy to prepare interspace (other than for decompression); thoracic [C] [80] [CCI]

▲ 22533 lumbar [C] [80] [CCI]

+ ▲ 22534 thoracic or lumbar, each additional vertebral segment (List separately in addition to code for primary procedure) [C] [80] [CCI]

> Note that 22534 is an add-on code and must be used in conjunction with 22532 and 22533.

ANTERIOR OR ANTEROLATERAL APPROACH TECHNIQUE

These codes address surgical approaches to the spine from the front or to the side of the front. CPT codes 22554-22558 are used to report arthrodesis of a single vertebral interspace. Consult CPT code 22585 for additional interspaces. The non-bony compartment between two adjacent vertebral bodies that contain the intervertebral disk, the nucleus pulposus, annulus fibrosus and two cartilagenous endplates is considered the vertebral interspace.

22548   **Arthrodesis, anterior transoral or extraoral technique, clivus-C1-C2 (atlas-axis), with or without excision of odontoid process** C 80

MED: 100-3,150.2

AMA: 2000,Sep,10; 1997,Sep,8; 1996,Feb,7; 1993,Spring,36

To report the injection procedure for myelography and/or computed tomography, consult CPT code 62284. To report the injection procedure of a diskography, consult CPT codes 62290 and 62291. To report the injection procedure To report chemonucleolysis, single or multiple levels, consult CPT code 62292. To report the injection procedure of facet joints, consult CPT codes 64470-64476 and 64622-64627.

22554   **Arthrodesis, anterior interbody technique, including minimal discectomy to prepare interspace (other than for decompression); cervical below C2** C 80

MED: 100-3,150.2

AMA: 2002,Feb,4; 2001,Jan,12; 2000,Sep,10; 1997,Sep,8; 1993,Spring,36

22556   **thoracic** C 80

MED: 100-3,150.2

AMA: 2002,Feb,4; 2000,Sep,10; 1997,Sep,8; 1996,Jul,7; 1993,Spring,36

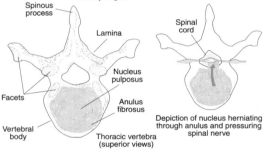

Intervertebral disc displacement and prolapse are major causes of disability among working people. When a disc prolapses, nuclear material bursts through the anulus fibrosus damaging ligaments, nerve roots, and other structures. The herniated matter usually fibroses and shrinks over time

22558   **lumbar** C 80

MED: 100-3,150.2

AMA: 2000,Sep,10; 1997,Sep,8; 1996,Mar,6; 1996,Jul,7; 1993,Spring,36

+   **22585**   **each additional interspace (List separately in addition to code for primary procedure)** C 80

MED: 100-3,150.2

AMA: 2000,Sep,10; 1997,Sep,8; 1996,Mar,6; 1993,Spring,36

Note that 22585 is an add-on code and must be used in conjunction with 22554, 22556, and 22558.

POSTERIOR, POSTEROLATERAL OR LATERAL TRANSVERSE PROCESS TECHNIQUE

These codes address surgical approaches to the spine from the back and side. The non-bony compartment between two adjacent vertebral bodies that contain the intervertebral disk, the nucleus pulposus, annulus fibrosus, and two cartilagenous endplates is considered the vertebral interspace.

Additional procedures, such as bone grafting (CPT codes 20930-20938) and instrumentation (CPT codes 22840-22855), are reported in addition to the CPT codes for the definitive procedure. Do not append modifier 51.

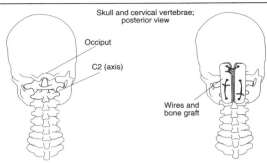

In 22590, the physician fuses skull to C2 (axis) to stabilize cervical vertebrae; anchor holes are drilled in the occiput of the skull

22590   **Arthrodesis, posterior technique, craniocervical (occiput-C2)** C 80

MED: 100-3,150.2

AMA: 1997,Sep,8; 1993,Spring,36

To report the injection procedure for myelography and/or computed tomography, consult CPT code 62284. To report the injection procedure of a diskography, consult CPT codes 62290 and 62291. To report the injection procedure To report chemonucleolysis, single or multiple levels, consult CPT code 62292. To report the injection procedure of facet joints, consult CPT codes 64470-64476 and 64622-64627.

22595   **Arthrodesis, posterior technique, atlas-axis (C1-C2)** C 80

MED: 100-3,150.2

AMA: 1997,Sep,8; 1993,Spring,36

To report the injection procedure for myelography and/or computed tomography, consult CPT code 62284. To report the injection procedure of a diskography, consult CPT codes 62290 and 62291. To report the injection procedure To report chemonucleolysis, single or multiple levels, consult CPT code 62292. To report the injection procedure of facet joints, consult CPT codes 64470-64476 and 64622-64627.

22600   **Arthrodesis, posterior or posterolateral technique, single level; cervical below C2 segment** C 80

MED: 100-3,150.2

AMA: 1997,Sep,8; 1993,Spring,36

22610   **thoracic (with or without lateral transverse technique)** C 80

MED: 100-3,150.2

AMA: 1997,Sep,8; 1993,Spring,36

22612   **lumbar (with or without lateral transverse technique)** T 80

MED: 100-3,150.2

AMA: 1997,Sep,8, 11; 1996,Mar,7; 1993,Spring,36

+   **22614**   **each additional vertebral segment (List separately in addition to code for primary procedure)** T 80

MED: 100-3,150.2

AMA: 1996,Mar,7

Note that 22614 is an add-on code and must be used in conjunction with 22600, 22610, and 22612.

22630   **Arthrodesis, posterior interbody technique, including laminectomy and/or discectomy to prepare interspace (other than for decompression), single interspace; lumbar** C 80

MED: 100-3,150.2

AMA: 2001,Jan,12; 1999,Nov,11; 1999,Dec,2; 1997,Sep,8; 1993,Spring,36

+ **22632** **each additional interspace (List separately in addition to code for primary procedure)** C 80

MED: 100-3,150.2

AMA: 1999,Dec,2; 1997,Sep,8

Note that 22632 is an add-on code and must be used in conjunction with 22630.

SPINE DEFORMITY (EG, SCOLIOSIS, KYPHOSIS)

To report bone graft procedures, consult CPT codes 20930-20938. Bone graft codes should be reported in addition to code(s) for the definitive procedure(s) without modifier 51. Modifier 62 should not be used with bone graft codes 20900-20938.

A vertebral segment describes the basic element into which the spine may be divided. It represents one complete vertebral bone and its associated articular processes and laminae.

Surgeons, each performing distinct parts of an arthrodesis for spinal deformity, when working together as primary surgeons, should report the procedure code and use modifier 62. Modifier 62 may be used with code(s) 22800-22819 if both surgeons continue to perform distinct components of the surgery.

Additional procedures, such as bone grafting (CPT codes 20930-20938) and instrumentation (CPT codes 22840-22855), are reported in addition to the CPT codes for the definitive procedure. Do not append modifier 51.

22800 **Arthrodesis, posterior, for spinal deformity, with or without cast; up to 6 vertebral segments** C 80

MED: 100-3,150.2

22802 **7 to 12 vertebral segments** C 80

MED: 100-3,150.2

AMA: 1996,Mar,10

22804 **13 or more vertebral segments** C 80

MED: 100-3,150.2

22808 **Arthrodesis, anterior, for spinal deformity, with or without cast; 2 to 3 vertebral segments** C 80

MED: 100-3,150.2

Smith-Robinson arthrodesis

22810 **4 to 7 vertebral segments** C 80

MED: 100-3,150.2

AMA: 1997,Sep,8; 1996,Mar,10

22812 **8 or more vertebral segments** C 80

MED: 100-3,150.2

22818 **Kyphectomy, circumferential exposure of spine and resection of vertebral segment(s) (including body and posterior elements); single or 2 segments** C 80

MED: 100-3,150.2

AMA: 1997,Nov,14

Excessively kyphotic thoracic spine may be caused by Scheuermann's disease or juvenile kyphosis

Excessive convexity in the thoracic region is known as kyphosis

Excessive concavity in the lumbar region is known as lordosis

Scoliosis is the lateral curvature of the spine; most commonly diagnosed during adolescence; occurrence is higher among females

22819 **3 or more segments** C 80

MED: 100-3,150.2

AMA: 1997,Nov,14

If arthrodesis is performed, consult CPT codes 22800-22804 and append modifier 51.

EXPLORATION

For instrumentation procedures, consult codes 22840-22855. Report 22840-22848 and 22851 with the codes(s) for the definitive procedure(s) without appending modifier 51. Report modifier 51 with 22849, 22850, 22852 and 22855 when instrumentation reinsertion or removal is reported with other definitive procedures such as arthrodesis, decompression, and exploration of fusion. For exploration of fusion, consult 22830. Report modifier 51 with code 22830 when exploration is reported with other definitive procedures such as arthrodesis and decompression.

22830 **Exploration of spinal fusion** C 80

MED: 100-3,150.2

AMA: 1997,Sep,11

SPINAL INSTRUMENTATION

This section describes the instruments affixed to the spine to correct defects resulting from injury or deformity. The instrumentation may correct the spine's anatomic position or help support injured vertebrae. Instrumentation is divided into segmental and non-segmental. Segmental instrumentation connects to each or most vertebra(e) it spans. Non-segmental instrumentation may span several vertebrae between fixation.

Spinal instrumentation and additional procedures, such as bone grafting (CPT codes 20930-20938) are reported in addition to the CPT code(s) for the primary procedure. Do not append modifier 51.

Report codes 22840-22855 when used with code(s) for fracture dislocation, arthrodesis, or exploration of fusion of the spine 22325-22328, 22532-22534, 22548-22812, and 22830. Do not append modifier 51 to codes 22840-22848, or 22851 when reported with code(s) for the definitive procedure(s). Append modifier 51 to codes 22849, 22850, 22852, and 22855 if they are used with other definitive procedure(s). This includes arthrodesis, decompression, and exploration of fusion. Do not report code 22849 with CPT codes 22850, 22852, and 22855 at the same spinal levels.

⊘ **22840** **Posterior non-segmental instrumentation (eg, Harrington rod technique, pedicle fixation across one interspace, atlantoaxial transarticular screw fixation, sublaminar wiring at C1, facet screw fixation)** C 80

AMA: 1999,Nov,12; 1997,Sep,8; 1996,Jul,10; 1996,Feb,6

⊘ **22841** **Internal spinal fixation by wiring of spinous processes** C

AMA: 1997,Sep,8; 1996,Feb,6

Hibb's fusion

⊘ **22842** **Posterior segmental instrumentation (eg, pedicle fixation, dual rods with multiple hooks and sublaminar wires); 3 to 6 vertebral segments** C 80

AMA: 1997,Sep,8; 1996,Mar,7; 1996,Feb,6

⊘ **22843** **7 to 12 vertebral segments** C 80

AMA: 1997,Sep,8; 1996,Feb,6

⊘ **22844** **13 or more vertebral segments** C 80

AMA: 1997,Sep,8; 1996,Feb,6

⊘ **22845** **Anterior instrumentation; 2 to 3 vertebral segments** C 80

AMA: 1997,Sep,8; 1996,Mar,10; 1996,Jul,7,10; 1996,Feb,6

Dwyer instrumentation technique

⊘ **22846** **4 to 7 vertebral segments** C 80

AMA: 1997,Sep,8; 1996,Feb,6

⊘ **22847** **8 or more vertebral segments** C 80

AMA: 1997,Sep,8; 1996,Feb,6

⊘ **22848** **Pelvic fixation (attachment of caudal end of instrumentation to pelvic bony structures) other than sacrum** C 80

AMA: 1997,Sep,8; 1996,Feb,6

22849 **Reinsertion of spinal fixation device** C 80

AMA: 2002,Nov,1; 1997,Sep,8; 1996,Feb,6

⊛ Modifier 63 Exempt Code ⊙ Conscious Sedation + CPT Add-on Code ⊘ Modifier 51 Exempt Code ● New Code ▲ Revised Code

M Maternity Edit A Age Edit A-Y APC Status Indicators CCI Comprehensive Code 50 Bilateral Procedure

22850 Removal of posterior nonsegmental instrumentation (eg, Harrington rod) C 80 🔄

AMA: 1997,Sep,8; 1996,Feb,6

⊘ **22851** Application of intervertebral biomechanical device(s) (eg, synthetic cage(s), threaded bone dowel(s), methylmethacrylate) to vertebral defect or interspace T 80 🔄

AMA: 2001,Mar,1; 1999,Nov,12; 1999,Dec,2; 1997,Sep,8; 1996,Feb,6

22852 Removal of posterior segmental instrumentation C 80 🔄

AMA: 1997,Sep,8; 1996,Feb,6

22855 Removal of anterior instrumentation C 80 🔄

AMA: 2002,Nov,1; 1997,Sep,8; 1996,Feb,6

● **22857** Total disc arthroplasty (artificial disc), anterior approach, including discectomy to prepare interspace (other than for decompression), lumbar, single interspace C

When performed at the same level, do not report 22857 with 22558, 22845, 22851, or 49010.

Use 0163T for additional interspace.

● **22862** Revision including replacement of total disc arthroplasty (artificial disc) anterior approach, lumbar, single interspace C

When performed at the same level, do not report 22862 with 22558, 22845, 22851, 22865, or 49010.

Use 0165T for additional interspace.

● **22865** Removal of total disc arthroplasty (artificial disc), anterior approach, lumbar, single interspace C

Do not report 22865 with 49010.

Use 0164T for additional interspace.

22857-22865 include fluoroscopy when used. To report decompression, consult 63001-63048.

OTHER PROCEDURES

22899 Unlisted procedure, spine T 80

MED: 100-4,4,20.5; 100-4,4,180.3
AMA: 2000,Sep,10; 2000,May,11

ABDOMEN

Replacement of casts and/or traction devices subsequent to the first should be reported separately. CPT codes for other additional procedures, such as obtaining grafts and external fixation, should only be used if the procedure is not already listed as included as part of the basic procedure. Consult the glossary for terms and definitions and the front matter of this chapter for additional information.

EXCISION

22900 Excision, abdominal wall tumor, subfascial (eg, desmoid) 4 T 80 🔄

MED: 100-2,15,260; 100-4,4,20.5; 100-4,12,90.3; 100-4,14,10

OTHER PROCEDURES

22999 Unlisted procedure, abdomen, musculoskeletal system T 80

MED: 100-4,4,20.5; 100-4,4,180.3

SHOULDER

Codes listed in the Musculoskeletal chapter include the application and removal of the first cast or traction device. Replacement of casts and/or traction devices subsequent to the first should be reported separately. CPT codes for other additional procedures, such as obtaining grafts and external fixation, should only be used if the procedure is not already listed as included as part of the basic procedure. Consult the glossary for terms and definitions.

This section includes the acromioclavicular joint, clavicle, head and neck of the humerus, shoulder joint, and sternoclavicular joint.

INCISION

23000 Removal of subdeltoid calcareous deposits, open 2 T 80 🔄

MED: 100-2,15,260; 100-4,4,20.5; 100-4,12,90.3; 100-4,14,10

To report arthroscopic removal of bursal deposits, consult CPT code 29999.

23020 Capsular contracture release (eg, Sever type procedure) 2 T 80 50 🔄

MED: 100-2,15,260; 100-4,4,20.5; 100-4,12,90.3; 100-4,14,10

If superficial incision and drainage is performed, consult CPT codes 10040-10160.

23030 Incision and drainage, shoulder area; deep abscess or hematoma 1 T 🔄

MED: 100-2,15,260; 100-4,4,20.5; 100-4,12,90.3; 100-4,14,10

Calcium deposits on the supraspinatus tendon are common and cause impingement of the bursa and pain upon raising the arm

Section of left shoulder

The fibrous capsule enclosing the shoulder is thin and loose to allow freedom of movement; four rotator cuff muscles (supraspinatous, infraspinatous, teres minor, and scapularis) work together to hold the head of the humerus in the glenoid cavity

23031 infected bursa 3 T 50 🔄

MED: 100-2,15,260; 100-4,4,20.5; 100-4,12,90.3; 100-4,14,10

23035 Incision, bone cortex (eg, osteomyelitis or bone abscess), shoulder area 3 T 80 50 🔄

MED: 100-2,15,260; 100-4,4,20.5; 100-4,12,90.3; 100-4,14,10

23040 Arthrotomy, glenohumeral joint, including exploration, drainage, or removal of foreign body 3 T 80 50 🔄

MED: 100-2,15,260; 100-4,4,20.5; 100-4,12,90.3; 100-4,14,10
AMA: 1998,Nov,8

23044 Arthrotomy, acromioclavicular, sternoclavicular joint, including exploration, drainage, or removal of foreign body 4 T 50 🔄

MED: 100-2,15,260; 100-4,4,20.5; 100-4,12,90.3; 100-4,14,10
AMA: 1998,Nov,8

EXCISION

23065 Biopsy, soft tissue of shoulder area; superficial T 50 🔄

23066 deep 2 T 50 🔄

MED: 100-2,15,260; 100-4,4,20.5; 100-4,12,90.3; 100-4,14,10

If a needle biopsy of soft tissue is performed, consult CPT code 20206.

23075 Excision, soft tissue tumor, shoulder area; subcutaneous 2 T 50 🔄

MED: 100-2,15,260; 100-4,4,20.5; 100-4,12,90.3; 100-4,14,10
AMA: 1998,Nov,8; 1992,Summer,22

23076 deep, subfascial, or intramuscular 2 T 50 🔄

MED: 100-2,15,260; 100-4,4,20.5; 100-4,12,90.3; 100-4,14,10
AMA: 1992,Summer,22

26 Professional Component Only 80/80 Assist-at-Surgery Allowed/With Documentation Unlisted Not Covered

TC Technical Component Only MED: Pub 100/NCD References AMA: CPT Assistant References 1-9 ASC Group ♂ Male Only ♀ Female Only

76 — CPT Expert CPT only © 2006 American Medical Association. All Rights Reserved. (Black Ink) © 2006 Ingenix (Blue Ink)

| 23077 | Radical resection of tumor (eg, malignant neoplasm), soft tissue of shoulder area | 3 T 80 50 ▣ |
| | MED: 100-2,15,260; 100-4,4,20.5; 100-4,12,90.3; 100-4,14,10 | |

23100	Arthrotomy, glenohumeral joint, including biopsy	2 T 80 50 ▣
	MED: 100-2,15,260; 100-4,4,20.5; 100-4,12,90.3; 100-4,14,10	
	AMA: 1998,Nov,8	

23101	Arthrotomy, acromioclavicular joint or sternoclavicular joint, including biopsy and/or excision of torn cartilage	7 T 50 ▣
	MED: 100-2,15,260; 100-4,4,20.5; 100-4,12,90.3; 100-4,14,10	
	AMA: 1998,Nov,8	

23105	Arthrotomy; glenohumeral joint, with synovectomy, with or without biopsy	4 T 80 50 ▣
	MED: 100-2,15,260; 100-4,4,20.5; 100-4,12,90.3; 100-4,14,10	
	AMA: 1998,Nov,8	

| 23106 | sternoclavicular joint, with synovectomy, with or without biopsy | 4 T 50 ▣ |
| | MED: 100-2,15,260; 100-4,4,20.5; 100-4,12,90.3; 100-4,14,10 | |

| 23107 | Arthrotomy, glenohumeral joint, with joint exploration, with or without removal of loose or foreign body | 4 T 80 50 ▣ |
| | MED: 100-2,15,260; 100-4,4,20.5; 100-4,12,90.3; 100-4,14,10 | |

23120	Claviculectomy; partial	5 T 80 ▣
	MED: 100-2,15,260; 100-4,4,20.5; 100-4,12,90.3; 100-4,14,10	
	If performed arthroscopically consult CPT code 29824.	
	Mumford claviculectomy	

| 23125 | total | 5 T 80 50 ▣ |
| | MED: 100-2,15,260; 100-4,4,20.5; 100-4,12,90.3; 100-4,14,10 | |

23130	Acromioplasty or acromionectomy, partial, with or without coracoacromial ligament release	5 T 50 ▣
	MED: 100-2,15,260; 100-4,4,20.5; 100-4,12,90.3; 100-4,14,10	
	AMA: 2001,Aug,11	

| 23140 | Excision or curettage of bone cyst or benign tumor of clavicle or scapula; | 4 T 50 ▣ |
| | MED: 100-2,15,260; 100-4,4,20.5; 100-4,12,90.3; 100-4,14,10 | |

| 23145 | with autograft (includes obtaining graft) | 5 T 80 50 ▣ |
| | MED: 100-2,15,260; 100-4,4,20.5; 100-4,12,90.3; 100-4,14,10 | |

| 23146 | with allograft | 5 T 80 50 ▣ |
| | MED: 100-2,15,260; 100-4,4,20.5; 100-4,12,90.3; 100-4,14,10 | |

| 23150 | Excision or curettage of bone cyst or benign tumor of proximal humerus; | 4 T 80 50 ▣ |
| | MED: 100-2,15,260; 100-4,4,20.5; 100-4,12,90.3; 100-4,14,10 | |

| 23155 | with autograft (includes obtaining graft) | 5 T 80 50 ▣ |
| | MED: 100-2,15,260; 100-4,4,20.5; 100-4,12,90.3; 100-4,14,10 | |

| 23156 | with allograft | 5 T 80 50 ▣ |
| | MED: 100-2,15,260; 100-4,4,20.5; 100-4,12,90.3; 100-4,14,10 | |

| 23170 | Sequestrectomy (eg, for osteomyelitis or bone abscess), clavicle | 2 T 50 ▣ |
| | MED: 100-2,15,260; 100-4,4,20.5; 100-4,12,90.3; 100-4,14,10 | |

| 23172 | Sequestrectomy (eg, for osteomyelitis or bone abscess), scapula | 2 T 80 50 ▣ |
| | MED: 100-2,15,260; 100-4,4,20.5; 100-4,12,90.3; 100-4,14,10 | |

| 23174 | Sequestrectomy (eg, for osteomyelitis or bone abscess), humeral head to surgical neck | 2 T 80 50 ▣ |
| | MED: 100-2,15,260; 100-4,4,20.5; 100-4,12,90.3; 100-4,14,10 | |

23180	Partial excision (craterization, saucerization, or diaphysectomy) bone (eg, osteomyelitis), clavicle	4 T 50 ▣
	MED: 100-2,15,260; 100-4,4,20.5; 100-4,12,90.3; 100-4,14,10	
	AMA: 1998,Nov,9	

23182	Partial excision (craterization, saucerization, or diaphysectomy) bone (eg, osteomyelitis), scapula	4 T 80 50 ▣
	MED: 100-2,15,260; 100-4,4,20.5; 100-4,12,90.3; 100-4,14,10	
	AMA: 1998,Nov,9	

23184	Partial excision (craterization, saucerization, or diaphysectomy) bone (eg, osteomyelitis), proximal humerus	4 T 80 50 ▣
	MED: 100-2,15,260; 100-4,4,20.5; 100-4,12,90.3; 100-4,14,10	
	AMA: 1998,Nov,9	

| 23190 | Ostectomy of scapula, partial (eg, superior medial angle) | 4 T 80 50 ▣ |
| | MED: 100-2,15,260; 100-4,4,20.5; 100-4,12,90.3; 100-4,14,10 | |

23195	Resection, humeral head	5 T 80 50 ▣
	MED: 100-2,15,260; 100-4,4,20.5; 100-4,12,90.3; 100-4,14,10	
	If replacement is needed with an implant, consult CPT code 23470.	

23200	Radical resection for tumor; clavicle	C 80 50 ▣
23210	scapula	C 80 50 ▣
23220	Radical resection of bone tumor, proximal humerus;	C 80 50 ▣
	AMA: 1998,Nov,8	
23221	with autograft (includes obtaining graft)	C 80 50 ▣
23222	with prosthetic replacement	C 80 50 ▣

INTRODUCTION OR REMOVAL

If arthrocentesis or needling of bursa is needed, consult CPT code 20610. If a K-wire or a pin is inserted or removed, consult CPT codes 20650, 20670, and 20680.

23330	Removal of foreign body, shoulder; subcutaneous	1 T 80 50 ▣
	MED: 100-2,15,260; 100-4,4,20.5; 100-4,12,90.3; 100-4,14,10	
	AMA: 1999,Aug,3	

23331	deep (eg, Neer hemiarthroplasty removal)	1 T 80 50 ▣
	MED: 100-2,15,260; 100-4,4,20.5; 100-4,12,90.3; 100-4,14,10	
	AMA: 1999,Aug,3	

| 23332 | complicated (eg, total shoulder) | C 80 50 ▣ |
| | AMA: 1999,Aug,3; 1998,Nov,8; 1996,Jun,10 | |

| 23350 | Injection procedure for shoulder arthrography or enhanced CT/MRI shoulder arthrography | N 50 ▣ |
| | AMA: 2001,Jul,3 | |

If radiological supervision and interpretation is performed, use code 73040. Fluoroscopy (77002) is inclusive of radiographic arthrography.

If fluoroscopic guided injection is performed for enhanced CT arthrography, use codes 23350, 77002, and 73201 or 73202. If fluoroscopic guided injection is performed for enhanced MR arthrography, use codes 23350, 77002, and 73222 or 73223.

For enhanced CT or enhanced MRI arthrography, use 77002 and either 73201, 73202, 73222, or 73223.

To report biopsy of the shoulder and joint, consult 29805-29826.

Musculoskeletal System

23395 — 23545

REPAIR, REVISION, AND/OR RECONSTRUCTION

23395 Muscle transfer, any type, shoulder or upper arm; single `5` `T` `80` `◨`
MED: 100-2,15,260; 100-4,4,20.5; 100-4,12,90.3; 100-4,14,10

23397 multiple `7` `T` `80` `◨`
MED: 100-2,15,260; 100-4,4,20.5; 100-4,12,90.3; 100-4,14,10

23400 Scapulopexy (eg, Sprengels deformity or for paralysis) `7` `T` `80` `50` `◨`
MED: 100-2,15,260; 100-4,4,20.5; 100-4,12,90.3; 100-4,14,10

23405 Tenotomy, shoulder area; single tendon `2` `T` `80` `◨`
MED: 100-2,15,260; 100-4,4,20.5; 100-4,12,90.3; 100-4,14,10
AMA: 1998,Nov,8

23406 multiple tendons through same incision `2` `T` `80` `◨`
MED: 100-2,15,260; 100-4,4,20.5; 100-4,12,90.3; 100-4,14,10
AMA: 1998,Nov,8

23410 Repair of ruptured musculotendinous cuff (eg, rotator cuff) open; acute `5` `T` `80` `50` `◨`
MED: 100-2,15,260; 100-4,4,20.5; 100-4,12,90.3; 100-4,14,10
AMA: 2002,Feb,11; 2001,Aug,11

23412 chronic `7` `T` `80` `50` `◨`
MED: 100-2,15,260; 100-4,4,20.5; 100-4,12,90.3; 100-4,14,10
AMA: 2002,Feb,11
To report arthroscopic procedure, consult CPT code 29827.

23415 Coracoacromial ligament release, with or without acromioplasty `5` `T` `50` `◨`
MED: 100-2,15,260; 100-4,4,20.5; 100-4,12,90.3; 100-4,14,10
If performed arthroscopically consult CPT code 29826.

23420 Reconstruction of complete shoulder (rotator) cuff avulsion, chronic (includes acromioplasty) `7` `T` `80` `50` `◨`
MED: 100-2,15,260; 100-4,4,20.5; 100-4,12,90.3; 100-4,14,10
AMA: 2002,Feb,11

23430 Tenodesis of long tendon of biceps `4` `T` `80` `50` `◨`
MED: 100-2,15,260; 100-4,4,20.5; 100-4,12,90.3; 100-4,14,10

23440 Resection or transplantation of long tendon of biceps `4` `T` `80` `50` `◨`
MED: 100-2,15,260; 100-4,4,20.5; 100-4,12,90.3; 100-4,14,10

23450 Capsulorrhaphy, anterior; Putti-Platt procedure or Magnuson type operation `5` `T` `80` `50` `◨`
MED: 100-2,15,260; 100-4,4,20.5; 100-4,12,90.3; 100-4,14,10
If arthroscopic thermal capsulorrhaphy is performed, consult CPT code 29999.

23455 with labral repair (eg, Bankart procedure) `7` `T` `80` `50` `◨`
MED: 100-2,15,260; 100-4,4,20.5; 100-4,12,90.3; 100-4,14,10
AMA: 1998,Nov,8
If performed arthroscopically, consult CPT code 29806.

23460 Capsulorrhaphy, anterior, any type; with bone block `5` `T` `80` `50` `◨`
MED: 100-2,15,260; 100-4,4,20.5; 100-4,12,90.3; 100-4,14,10
Bristow procedure

23462 with coracoid process transfer `7` `T` `80` `50` `◨`
MED: 100-2,15,260; 100-4,4,20.5; 100-4,12,90.3; 100-4,14,10
If open thermal capsulorrhaphy is performed, consult CPT code 23929.

23465 Capsulorrhaphy, glenohumeral joint, posterior, with or without bone block `5` `T` `80` `50` `◨`
MED: 100-2,15,260; 100-4,4,20.5; 100-4,12,90.3; 100-4,14,10
AMA: 1998,Nov,8
If sternoclavicular and acromioclavicular reconstruction is performed, consult CPT codes 23530 and 23550.

23466 Capsulorrhaphy, glenohumeral joint, any type multi-directional instability `7` `T` `80` `50` `◨`
MED: 100-2,15,260; 100-4,4,20.5; 100-4,12,90.3; 100-4,14,10
AMA: 1998,Nov,8

23470 Arthroplasty, glenohumeral joint; hemiarthroplasty `T` `80` `50` `◨`
AMA: 1998,Nov,8

23472 total shoulder (glenoid and proximal humeral replacement (eg, total shoulder)) `C` `80` `50` `◨`
AMA: 1998,Nov,8; 1996,Jun,10
If the total shoulder implant is removed, consult CPT codes 23331 and 23332. If an osteotomy of the proximal humerus is needed, consult CPT code 24400.

23480 Osteotomy, clavicle, with or without internal fixation; `4` `T` `50` `◨`
MED: 100-2,15,260; 100-4,4,20.5; 100-4,12,90.3; 100-4,14,10

23485 with bone graft for nonunion or malunion (includes obtaining graft and/or necessary fixation) `7` `T` `80` `50` `◨`
MED: 100-2,15,260; 100-4,4,20.5; 100-4,12,90.3; 100-4,14,10

23490 Prophylactic treatment (nailing, pinning, plating or wiring) with or without methylmethacrylate; clavicle `3` `T` `80` `50` `◨`
MED: 100-2,15,260; 100-4,4,20.5; 100-4,12,90.3; 100-4,14,10

23491 proximal humerus `3` `T` `80` `50` `◨`
MED: 100-2,15,260; 100-4,4,20.5; 100-4,12,90.3; 100-4,14,10
AMA: 1998,Nov,8

FRACTURE AND/OR DISLOCATION

23500 Closed treatment of clavicular fracture; without manipulation `1` `T` `50` `◨`
MED: 100-2,15,260; 100-4,4,20.5; 100-4,12,90.3; 100-4,14,10

23505 with manipulation `1` `T` `50` `◨`
MED: 100-2,15,260; 100-4,4,20.5; 100-4,12,90.3; 100-4,14,10

23515 Open treatment of clavicular fracture, with or without internal or external fixation `3` `T` `80` `50` `◨`
MED: 100-2,15,260; 100-4,4,20.5; 100-4,12,90.3; 100-4,14,10

23520 Closed treatment of sternoclavicular dislocation; without manipulation `1` `T` `80` `50` `◨`
MED: 100-2,15,260; 100-4,4,20.5; 100-4,12,90.3; 100-4,14,10

23525 with manipulation `1` `T` `80` `50` `◨`
MED: 100-2,15,260; 100-4,4,20.5; 100-4,12,90.3; 100-4,14,10

23530 Open treatment of sternoclavicular dislocation, acute or chronic; `3` `T` `80` `50` `◨`
MED: 100-2,15,260; 100-4,4,20.5; 100-4,12,90.3; 100-4,14,10

23532 with fascial graft (includes obtaining graft) `4` `T` `80` `50` `◨`
MED: 100-2,15,260; 100-4,4,20.5; 100-4,12,90.3; 100-4,14,10

23540 Closed treatment of acromioclavicular dislocation; without manipulation `1` `T` `50` `◨`
MED: 100-2,15,260; 100-4,4,20.5; 100-4,12,90.3; 100-4,14,10

23545 with manipulation `1` `T` `80` `50` `◨`
MED: 100-2,15,260; 100-4,4,20.5; 100-4,12,90.3; 100-4,14,10

23550 Open treatment of acromioclavicular dislocation, acute or chronic; ③ T 80 50 ⊡
MED: 100-2,15,260; 100-4,4,20.5; 100-4,12,90.3; 100-4,14,10

23552 with fascial graft (includes obtaining graft) ④ T 80 50 ⊡
MED: 100-2,15,260; 100-4,4,20.5; 100-4,12,90.3; 100-4,14,10

23570 Closed treatment of scapular fracture; without manipulation ① T 50 ⊡
MED: 100-2,15,260; 100-4,4,20.5; 100-4,12,90.3; 100-4,14,10

23575 with manipulation, with or without skeletal traction (with or without shoulder joint involvement) ① T 80 50 ⊡
MED: 100-2,15,260; 100-4,4,20.5; 100-4,12,90.3; 100-4,14,10

23585 Open treatment of scapular fracture (body, glenoid or acromion) with or without internal fixation ③ T 80 50 ⊡
MED: 100-2,15,260; 100-4,4,20.5; 100-4,12,90.3; 100-4,14,10

23600 Closed treatment of proximal humeral (surgical or anatomical neck) fracture; without manipulation T 50 ⊡
MED: 100-2,15,260; 100-4,4,20.5; 100-4,12,90.3; 100-4,14,10

23605 with manipulation, with or without skeletal traction ② T 50 ⊡
MED: 100-2,15,260; 100-4,4,20.5; 100-4,12,90.3; 100-4,14,10

23615 Open treatment of proximal humeral (surgical or anatomical neck) fracture, with or without internal or external fixation, with or without repair of tuberosity(s); ④ T 80 50 ⊡
MED: 100-2,15,260; 100-4,4,20.5; 100-4,12,90.3; 100-4,14,10

23616 with proximal humeral prosthetic replacement ④ T 80 50 ⊡
MED: 100-2,15,260; 100-4,4,20.5; 100-4,12,90.3; 100-4,14,10

23620 Closed treatment of greater humeral tuberosity fracture; without manipulation T 50 ⊡
MED: 100-2,15,260; 100-4,4,20.5; 100-4,12,90.3; 100-4,14,10
AMA: 1998,Nov,8

23625 with manipulation ② T 50 ⊡
MED: 100-2,15,260; 100-4,4,20.5; 100-4,12,90.3; 100-4,14,10

23630 Open treatment of greater humeral tuberosity fracture, with or without internal or external fixation ⑤ T 80 50 ⊡
MED: 100-2,15,260; 100-4,4,20.5; 100-4,12,90.3; 100-4,14,10
AMA: 1998,Nov,8

23650 Closed treatment of shoulder dislocation, with manipulation; without anesthesia ① T 50 ⊡
MED: 100-2,15,260; 100-4,4,20.5; 100-4,12,90.3; 100-4,14,10

23655 requiring anesthesia ① T 50 ⊡
MED: 100-2,15,260; 100-4,4,20.5; 100-4,12,90.3; 100-4,14,10

23660 Open treatment of acute shoulder dislocation ③ T 80 50 ⊡
MED: 100-2,15,260; 100-4,4,20.5; 100-4,12,90.3; 100-4,14,10
AMA: 1996,Feb,5
If recurrent dislocations are repaired, consult CPT codes 23450-23466.

23665 Closed treatment of shoulder dislocation, with fracture of greater humeral tuberosity, with manipulation ② T 50 ⊡
MED: 100-2,15,260; 100-4,4,20.5; 100-4,12,90.3; 100-4,14,10
AMA: 1998,Nov,8

23670 Open treatment of shoulder dislocation, with fracture of greater humeral tuberosity, with or without internal or external fixation ③ T 80 50 ⊡
MED: 100-2,15,260; 100-4,4,20.5; 100-4,12,90.3; 100-4,14,10
AMA: 1998,Nov,8

23675 Closed treatment of shoulder dislocation, with surgical or anatomical neck fracture, with manipulation ② T 50 ⊡
MED: 100-2,15,260; 100-4,4,20.5; 100-4,12,90.3; 100-4,14,10

23680 Open treatment of shoulder dislocation, with surgical or anatomical neck fracture, with or without internal or external fixation ③ T 80 50 ⊡
MED: 100-2,15,260; 100-4,4,20.5; 100-4,12,90.3; 100-4,14,10

MANIPULATION

23700 Manipulation under anesthesia, shoulder joint, including application of fixation apparatus (dislocation excluded) ① T ⊡
MED: 100-2,15,260; 100-4,4,20.5; 100-4,12,90.3; 100-4,14,10
AMA: 1999,Jan,1

ARTHRODESIS

23800 Arthrodesis, glenohumeral joint; ④ T 80 50 ⊡
MED: 100-2,15,260; 100-4,4,20.5; 100-4,12,90.3; 100-4,14,10
AMA: 1998,Nov,8

23802 with autogenous graft (includes obtaining graft) ⑦ T 80 ⊡
MED: 100-2,15,260; 100-4,4,20.5; 100-4,12,90.3; 100-4,14,10

AMPUTATION

23900 Interthoracoscapular amputation (forequarter) C 80 ⊡

23920 Disarticulation of shoulder; C 80 ⊡

23921 secondary closure or scar revision ③ T ⊡
MED: 100-2,15,260; 100-4,4,20.5; 100-4,12,90.3; 100-4,14,10

OTHER PROCEDURES

23929 Unlisted procedure, shoulder T 80
MED: 100-4,4,20.5; 100-4,4,180.3

HUMERUS (UPPER ARM) AND ELBOW

Codes listed in the Musculoskeletal chapter include the application and removal of the first cast or traction device. Replacement of casts and/or traction devices subsequent to the first should be reported separately. CPT codes for other additional procedures, such as obtaining grafts and external fixation, should only be used if the procedure is not already listed as included as part of the basic procedure. Consult the glossary for terms and definitions and the front matter of this chapter for additional information.

The elbow is considered to include the olecranon process and the radius head and neck.

INCISION

If superficial incision and drainage procedures are performed, consult CPT codes 10040-10160.

23930 Incision and drainage, upper arm or elbow area; deep abscess or hematoma ① T 50 ⊡
MED: 100-2,15,260; 100-4,4,20.5; 100-4,12,90.3; 100-4,14,10

23931 bursa ② T 50 ⊡
MED: 100-2,15,260; 100-4,4,20.5; 100-4,12,90.3; 100-4,14,10
AMA: 1998,Nov,8

23935 Incision, deep, with opening of bone cortex (eg, for osteomyelitis or bone abscess), humerus or elbow [2] [T] [80] [50] [⟷]
MED: 100-2,15,260; 100-4,4,20.5; 100-4,12,90.3; 100-4,14,10

24000 Arthrotomy, elbow, including exploration, drainage, or removal of foreign body [4] [T] [80] [50] [⟷]
MED: 100-2,15,260; 100-4,4,20.5; 100-4,12,90.3; 100-4,14,10
AMA: 1998,Nov,8-9

24006 Arthrotomy of the elbow, with capsular excision for capsular release (separate procedure) [4] [T] [80] [50] [⟷]
MED: 100-2,15,260; 100-4,4,20.5; 100-4,12,90.3; 100-4,14,10

EXCISION

24065 Biopsy, soft tissue of upper arm or elbow area; superficial [T] [50] [⟷]

24066 deep (subfascial or intramuscular) [2] [T] [50] [⟷]
MED: 100-2,15,260; 100-4,4,20.5; 100-4,12,90.3; 100-4,14,10
If needle biopsy of soft tissue is performed, consult CPT code 20206.

24075 Excision, tumor, soft tissue of upper arm or elbow area; subcutaneous [2] [T] [50] [⟷]
MED: 100-2,15,260; 100-4,4,20.5; 100-4,12,90.3; 100-4,14,10

24076 deep, subfascial or intramuscular [2] [T] [50] [⟷]
MED: 100-2,15,260; 100-4,4,20.5; 100-4,12,90.3; 100-4,14,10

24077 Radical resection of tumor (eg, malignant neoplasm), soft tissue of upper arm or elbow area [3] [T] [80] [50] [⟷]
MED: 100-2,15,260; 100-4,4,20.5; 100-4,12,90.3; 100-4,14,10

24100 Arthrotomy, elbow; with synovial biopsy only [1] [T] [80] [50] [⟷]
MED: 100-2,15,260; 100-4,4,20.5; 100-4,12,90.3; 100-4,14,10

24101 with joint exploration, with or without biopsy, with or without removal of loose or foreign body [4] [T] [80] [50] [⟷]
MED: 100-2,15,260; 100-4,4,20.5; 100-4,12,90.3; 100-4,14,10

24102 with synovectomy [4] [T] [80] [50] [⟷]
MED: 100-2,15,260; 100-4,4,20.5; 100-4,12,90.3; 100-4,14,10

24105 Excision, olecranon bursa [3] [T] [50] [⟷]
MED: 100-2,15,260; 100-4,4,20.5; 100-4,12,90.3; 100-4,14,10

24110 Excision or curettage of bone cyst or benign tumor, humerus; [2] [T] [50] [⟷]
MED: 100-2,15,260; 100-4,4,20.5; 100-4,12,90.3; 100-4,14,10

24115 with autograft (includes obtaining graft) [3] [T] [80] [50] [⟷]
MED: 100-2,15,260; 100-4,4,20.5; 100-4,12,90.3; 100-4,14,10

24116 with allograft [3] [T] [80] [50] [⟷]
MED: 100-2,15,260; 100-4,4,20.5; 100-4,12,90.3; 100-4,14,10

24120 Excision or curettage of bone cyst or benign tumor of head or neck of radius or olecranon process; [3] [T] [80] [50] [⟷]
MED: 100-2,15,260; 100-4,4,20.5; 100-4,12,90.3; 100-4,14,10

24125 with autograft (includes obtaining graft) [3] [T] [80] [50] [⟷]
MED: 100-2,15,260; 100-4,4,20.5; 100-4,12,90.3; 100-4,14,10

24126 with allograft [3] [T] [80] [50] [⟷]
MED: 100-2,15,260; 100-4,4,20.5; 100-4,12,90.3; 100-4,14,10

24130 Excision, radial head [3] [T] [50] [⟷]
MED: 100-2,15,260; 100-4,4,20.5; 100-4,12,90.3; 100-4,14,10
If replacement is performed with an implant, consult CPT code 24366.

24134 Sequestrectomy (eg, for osteomyelitis or bone abscess), shaft or distal humerus [2] [T] [80] [50] [⟷]
MED: 100-2,15,260; 100-4,4,20.5; 100-4,12,90.3; 100-4,14,10

24136 Sequestrectomy (eg, for osteomyelitis or bone abscess), radial head or neck [2] [T] [50] [⟷]
MED: 100-2,15,260; 100-4,4,20.5; 100-4,12,90.3; 100-4,14,10

24138 Sequestrectomy (eg, for osteomyelitis or bone abscess), olecranon process [2] [T] [80] [50] [⟷]
MED: 100-2,15,260; 100-4,4,20.5; 100-4,12,90.3; 100-4,14,10

24140 Partial excision (craterization, saucerization, or diaphysectomy) bone (eg, osteomyelitis), humerus [3] [T] [80] [50] [⟷]
MED: 100-2,15,260; 100-4,4,20.5; 100-4,12,90.3; 100-4,14,10
AMA: 1998,Nov,9

24145 Partial excision (craterization, saucerization, or diaphysectomy) bone (eg, osteomyelitis), radial head or neck [3] [T] [50] [⟷]
MED: 100-2,15,260; 100-4,4,20.5; 100-4,12,90.3; 100-4,14,10
AMA: 1998,Nov,9

24147 Partial excision (craterization, saucerization, or diaphysectomy) bone (eg, osteomyelitis), olecranon process [2] [T] [50] [⟷]
MED: 100-2,15,260; 100-4,4,20.5; 100-4,12,90.3; 100-4,14,10
AMA: 1998,Nov,9

24149 Radical resection of capsule, soft tissue, and heterotopic bone, elbow, with contracture release (separate procedure) [T] [80] [50] [⟷]
If only capsular and soft tissue is released, consult CPT code 24006.

24150 Radical resection for tumor, shaft or distal humerus; [T] [80] [50] [⟷]

24151 with autograft (includes obtaining graft) [T] [80] [50] [⟷]

24152 Radical resection for tumor, radial head or neck; [T] [80] [50] [⟷]

24153 with autograft (includes obtaining graft) [T] [80] [50] [⟷]

24155 Resection of elbow joint (arthrectomy) [3] [T] [80] [50] [⟷]
MED: 100-2,15,260; 100-4,4,20.5; 100-4,12,90.3; 100-4,14,10

INTRODUCTION OR REMOVAL

If a K-wire or a pin is inserted or removed, consult CPT codes 20650, 20670, and 20680. If arthrocentesis or needling of a bursa or a joint is performed, consult CPT code 20605.

24160 Implant removal; elbow joint [2] [T] [50] [⟷]
MED: 100-2,15,260; 100-4,4,20.5; 100-4,12,90.3; 100-4,14,10

24164 radial head [3] [T] [50] [⟷]
MED: 100-2,15,260; 100-4,4,20.5; 100-4,12,90.3; 100-4,14,10

24200 Removal of foreign body, upper arm or elbow area; subcutaneous [T] [80] [50] [⟷]

24201 deep (subfascial or intramuscular) [2] [T] [50] [⟷]
MED: 100-2,15,260; 100-4,4,20.5; 100-4,12,90.3; 100-4,14,10
AMA: 1998,Nov,8

24220 Injection procedure for elbow arthrography [N] [80] [50] [⟷]
If radiological supervision and interpretation is performed, use 73085. Do not report 77002 with 73085.
If an injection is performed for tennis elbow, consult CPT code 20550.

[26] Professional Component Only
[TC] Technical Component Only
[80]/[80] Assist-at-Surgery Allowed/With Documentation
MED: Pub 100/NCD References   AMA: CPT Assistant References
[1]-[9] ASC Group   ♂ Male Only   ♀ Female Only
Unlisted   Not Covered

80 — CPT Expert

REPAIR, REVISION, AND/OR RECONSTRUCTION

24300 Manipulation, elbow, under anesthesia [T] [50] [CCI]

If external fixation is applied, consult CPT codes 20690 or 20692.

24301 Muscle or tendon transfer, any type, upper arm or elbow, single (excluding 24320-24331) [4] [T] [80] [CCI]
MED: 100-2,15,260; 100-4,4,20.5; 100-4,12,90.3; 100-4,14,10

24305 Tendon lengthening, upper arm or elbow, each tendon [4] [T] [80] [CCI]
MED: 100-2,15,260; 100-4,4,20.5; 100-4,12,90.3; 100-4,14,10
AMA: 1998,Nov,8

24310 Tenotomy, open, elbow to shoulder, each tendon [3] [T] [80] [CCI]
MED: 100-2,15,260; 100-4,4,20.5; 100-4,12,90.3; 100-4,14,10
AMA: 1998,Nov,8

24320 Tenoplasty, with muscle transfer, with or without free graft, elbow to shoulder, single (Seddon-Brookes type procedure) [3] [T] [80] [CCI]
MED: 100-2,15,260; 100-4,4,20.5; 100-4,12,90.3; 100-4,14,10

24330 Flexor-plasty, elbow (eg, Steindler type advancement); [3] [T] [80] [50] [CCI]
MED: 100-2,15,260; 100-4,4,20.5; 100-4,12,90.3; 100-4,14,10

24331 with extensor advancement [3] [T] [80] [50] [CCI]
MED: 100-2,15,260; 100-4,4,20.5; 100-4,12,90.3; 100-4,14,10

24332 Tenolysis, triceps [T] [50] [CCI]

24340 Tenodesis of biceps tendon at elbow (separate procedure) [3] [T] [80] [50] [CCI]
MED: 100-2,15,260; 100-4,4,20.5; 100-4,12,90.3; 100-4,14,10

24341 Repair, tendon or muscle, upper arm or elbow, each tendon or muscle, primary or secondary (excludes rotator cuff) [3] [T] [80] [50] [CCI]
MED: 100-2,15,260; 100-4,4,20.5; 100-4,12,90.3; 100-4,14,10

24342 Reinsertion of ruptured biceps or triceps tendon, distal, with or without tendon graft [3] [T] [80] [50] [CCI]
MED: 100-2,15,260; 100-4,4,20.5; 100-4,12,90.3; 100-4,14,10

24343 Repair lateral collateral ligament, elbow, with local tissue [T] [80] [50] [CCI]

24344 Reconstruction lateral collateral ligament, elbow, with tendon graft (includes harvesting of graft) [T] [80] [50] [CCI]

24345 Repair medial collateral ligament, elbow, with local tissue [2] [T] [80] [50] [CCI]
MED: 100-2,15,260; 100-4,4,20.5; 100-4,12,90.3; 100-4,14,10

24346 Reconstruction medial collateral ligament, elbow, with tendon graft (includes harvesting of graft) [T] [80] [50] [CCI]

24350 Fasciotomy, lateral or medial (eg, tennis elbow or epicondylitis); [3] [T] [80] [50] [CCI]
MED: 100-2,15,260; 100-4,4,20.5; 100-4,12,90.3; 100-4,14,10

24351 with extensor origin detachment [3] [T] [80] [50] [CCI]
MED: 100-2,15,260; 100-4,4,20.5; 100-4,12,90.3; 100-4,14,10

24352 with annular ligament resection [3] [T] [80] [50] [CCI]
MED: 100-2,15,260; 100-4,4,20.5; 100-4,12,90.3; 100-4,14,10

24354 with stripping [3] [T] [50] [CCI]
MED: 100-2,15,260; 100-4,4,20.5; 100-4,12,90.3; 100-4,14,10

24356 with partial ostectomy [3] [T] [80] [50] [CCI]
MED: 100-2,15,260; 100-4,4,20.5; 100-4,12,90.3; 100-4,14,10

24360 Arthroplasty, elbow; with membrane (eg, fascial) [5] [T] [80] [50] [CCI]
MED: 100-2,15,260; 100-4,4,20.5; 100-4,12,90.3; 100-4,14,10
AMA: 1998,Nov,8

24361 with distal humeral prosthetic replacement [5] [T] [80] [50] [CCI]
MED: 100-2,15,260; 100-4,4,20.5; 100-4,4,61.2; 100-4,12,90.3; 100-4,14,10

24362 with implant and fascia lata ligament reconstruction [5] [T] [80] [50] [CCI]
MED: 100-2,15,260; 100-4,4,20.5; 100-4,12,90.3; 100-4,14,10

24363 with distal humerus and proximal ulnar prosthetic replacement (eg, total elbow) [7] [T] [80] [50] [CCI]
MED: 100-2,15,260; 100-4,4,20.5; 100-4,4,61.2; 100-4,12,90.3; 100-4,14,10

24365 Arthroplasty, radial head; [5] [T] [80] [50] [CCI]
MED: 100-2,15,260; 100-4,4,20.5; 100-4,12,90.3; 100-4,14,10

24366 with implant [5] [T] [80] [50] [CCI]
MED: 100-2,15,260; 100-4,4,20.5; 100-4,12,90.3; 100-4,14,10

24400 Osteotomy, humerus, with or without internal fixation [4] [T] [80] [50] [CCI]
MED: 100-2,15,260; 100-4,4,20.5; 100-4,12,90.3; 100-4,14,10

24410 Multiple osteotomies with realignment on intramedullary rod, humeral shaft (Sofield type procedure) [4] [T] [80] [50] [CCI]
MED: 100-2,15,260; 100-4,4,20.5; 100-4,12,90.3; 100-4,14,10

24420 Osteoplasty, humerus (eg, shortening or lengthening) (excluding 64876) [3] [T] [80] [50] [CCI]
MED: 100-2,15,260; 100-4,4,20.5; 100-4,12,90.3; 100-4,14,10

24430 Repair of nonunion or malunion, humerus; without graft (eg, compression technique) [3] [T] [80] [50] [CCI]
MED: 100-2,15,260; 100-4,4,20.5; 100-4,12,90.3; 100-4,14,10

24435 with iliac or other autograft (includes obtaining graft) [4] [T] [80] [50] [CCI]
MED: 100-2,15,260; 100-4,4,20.5; 100-4,12,90.3; 100-4,14,10

If a nonunion or malunion repair of the proximal radius and/or ulna is performed, consult CPT codes 25400-25420.

24470 Hemiepiphyseal arrest (eg, cubitus varus or valgus, distal humerus) [3] [T] [80] [50] [CCI]
MED: 100-2,15,260; 100-4,4,20.5; 100-4,12,90.3; 100-4,14,10

24495 Decompression fasciotomy, forearm, with brachial artery exploration [2] [T] [80] [50] [CCI]
MED: 100-2,15,260; 100-4,4,20.5; 100-4,12,90.3; 100-4,14,10

24498 Prophylactic treatment (nailing, pinning, plating or wiring), with or without methylmethacrylate, humeral shaft [3] [T] [80] [50] [CCI]
MED: 100-2,15,260; 100-4,4,20.5; 100-4,12,90.3; 100-4,14,10
AMA: 1998,Nov,8

FRACTURE AND/OR DISLOCATION

24500 Closed treatment of humeral shaft fracture; without manipulation [1] [T] [50] [CCI]
MED: 100-2,15,260; 100-4,4,20.5; 100-4,12,90.3; 100-4,14,10

24505 with manipulation, with or without skeletal traction [1] [T] [50] [CCI]
MED: 100-2,15,260; 100-4,4,20.5; 100-4,12,90.3; 100-4,14,10

24515 Open treatment of humeral shaft fracture with plate/screws, with or without cerclage [4] [T] [80] [50] [CCI]
MED: 100-2,15,260; 100-4,4,20.5; 100-4,12,90.3; 100-4,14,10

24516 Treatment of humeral shaft fracture, with insertion of intramedullary implant, with or without cerclage and/or locking screws 4 T 80 50
MED: 100-2,15,260; 100-4,4,20.5; 100-4,12,90.3; 100-4,14,10
AMA: 1996,Feb,4

24530 Closed treatment of supracondylar or transcondylar humeral fracture, with or without intercondylar extension; without manipulation 1 T 50
MED: 100-2,15,260; 100-4,4,20.5; 100-4,12,90.3; 100-4,14,10

24535 with manipulation, with or without skin or skeletal traction 1 T 50
MED: 100-2,15,260; 100-4,4,20.5; 100-4,12,90.3; 100-4,14,10

24538 Percutaneous skeletal fixation of supracondylar or transcondylar humeral fracture, with or without intercondylar extension 2 T 50
MED: 100-2,15,260; 100-4,4,20.5; 100-4,12,90.3; 100-4,14,10
AMA: 1992,Winter,10

24545 Open treatment of humeral supracondylar or transcondylar fracture, with or without internal or external fixation; without intercondylar extension 4 T 80 50
MED: 100-2,15,260; 100-4,4,20.5; 100-4,12,90.3; 100-4,14,10

24546 with intercondylar extension 5 T 80 50
MED: 100-2,15,260; 100-4,4,20.5; 100-4,12,90.3; 100-4,14,10

24560 Closed treatment of humeral epicondylar fracture, medial or lateral; without manipulation 1 T 50
MED: 100-2,15,260; 100-4,4,20.5; 100-4,12,90.3; 100-4,14,10

24565 with manipulation 2 T 50
MED: 100-2,15,260; 100-4,4,20.5; 100-4,12,90.3; 100-4,14,10

24566 Percutaneous skeletal fixation of humeral epicondylar fracture, medial or lateral, with manipulation 2 T 50
MED: 100-2,15,260; 100-4,4,20.5; 100-4,12,90.3; 100-4,14,10

24575 Open treatment of humeral epicondylar fracture, medial or lateral, with or without internal or external fixation 3 T 80 50
MED: 100-2,15,260; 100-4,4,20.5; 100-4,12,90.3; 100-4,14,10

24576 Closed treatment of humeral condylar fracture, medial or lateral; without manipulation 1 T 50
MED: 100-2,15,260; 100-4,4,20.5; 100-4,12,90.3; 100-4,14,10

24577 with manipulation 1 T 50
MED: 100-2,15,260; 100-4,4,20.5; 100-4,12,90.3; 100-4,14,10

24579 Open treatment of humeral condylar fracture, medial or lateral, with or without internal or external fixation 3 T 80 50
MED: 100-2,15,260; 100-4,4,20.5; 100-4,12,90.3; 100-4,14,10

24582 Percutaneous skeletal fixation of humeral condylar fracture, medial or lateral, with manipulation 2 T 50
MED: 100-2,15,260; 100-4,4,20.5; 100-4,12,90.3; 100-4,14,10

24586 Open treatment of periarticular fracture and/or dislocation of the elbow (fracture distal humerus and proximal ulna and/or proximal radius); 4 T 80 50
MED: 100-2,15,260; 100-4,4,20.5; 100-4,12,90.3; 100-4,14,10

24587 with implant arthroplasty 5 T 80 50
MED: 100-2,15,260; 100-4,4,20.5; 100-4,12,90.3; 100-4,14,10
Consult also CPT code 24361.

24600 Treatment of closed elbow dislocation; without anesthesia 1 T 50
MED: 100-2,15,260; 100-4,4,20.5; 100-4,12,90.3; 100-4,14,10

24605 requiring anesthesia 2 T 50
MED: 100-2,15,260; 100-4,4,20.5; 100-4,12,90.3; 100-4,14,10

24615 Open treatment of acute or chronic elbow dislocation 3 T 80 50
MED: 100-2,15,260; 100-4,4,20.5; 100-4,12,90.3; 100-4,14,10

24620 Closed treatment of Monteggia type of fracture dislocation at elbow (fracture proximal end of ulna with dislocation of radial head), with manipulation 2 T 80 50
MED: 100-2,15,260; 100-4,4,20.5; 100-4,12,90.3; 100-4,14,10

24635 Open treatment of Monteggia type of fracture dislocation at elbow (fracture proximal end of ulna with dislocation of radial head), with or without internal or external fixation 3 T 80 50
MED: 100-2,15,260; 100-4,4,20.5; 100-4,12,90.3; 100-4,14,10

24640 Closed treatment of radial head subluxation in child, nursemaid elbow, with manipulation A 80 50

24650 Closed treatment of radial head or neck fracture; without manipulation T 50

24655 with manipulation 1 T 50
MED: 100-2,15,260; 100-4,4,20.5; 100-4,12,90.3; 100-4,14,10

24665 Open treatment of radial head or neck fracture, with or without internal fixation or radial head excision; 4 T 80 50
MED: 100-2,15,260; 100-4,4,20.5; 100-4,12,90.3; 100-4,14,10

24666 with radial head prosthetic replacement 4 T 80 50
MED: 100-2,15,260; 100-4,4,20.5; 100-4,12,90.3; 100-4,14,10

24670 Closed treatment of ulnar fracture, proximal end (olecranon process); without manipulation 1 T 50
MED: 100-2,15,260; 100-4,4,20.5; 100-4,12,90.3; 100-4,14,10

24675 with manipulation 1 T 50
MED: 100-2,15,260; 100-4,4,20.5; 100-4,12,90.3; 100-4,14,10

24685 Open treatment of ulnar fracture proximal end (olecranon process), with or without internal or external fixation 3 T 80 50
MED: 100-2,15,260; 100-4,4,20.5; 100-4,12,90.3; 100-4,14,10

ARTHRODESIS

24800 Arthrodesis, elbow joint; local 4 T 80 50
MED: 100-2,15,260; 100-4,4,20.5; 100-4,12,90.3; 100-4,14,10

24802 with autogenous graft (includes obtaining graft) 5 T 80 50
MED: 100-2,15,260; 100-4,4,20.5; 100-4,12,90.3; 100-4,14,10

AMPUTATION

24900 Amputation, arm through humerus; with primary closure C 80 50

24920 open, circular (guillotine) C 80 50

24925 secondary closure or scar revision 3 T 80 50
MED: 100-2,15,260; 100-4,4,20.5; 100-4,12,90.3; 100-4,14,10

24930 re-amputation C 80 50

24931 with implant C 80 50

24935 Stump elongation, upper extremity T 80 50

---

26 Professional Component Only   80/80 Assist-at-Surgery Allowed/With Documentation   Unlisted   Not Covered

TC Technical Component Only   MED: Pub 100/NCD References   AMA: CPT Assistant References   1-9 ASC Group   ♂ Male Only   ♀ Female Only

24940   **Cineplasty, upper extremity, complete procedure**   ☒ 80 50 ↻

OTHER PROCEDURES

24999   **Unlisted procedure, humerus or elbow**   ☒ 80 50
MED: 100-4,4,20.5; 100-4,4,180.3

FOREARM AND WRIST

Codes listed in the Musculoskeletal chapter include the application and removal of the first cast or traction device. Replacement of casts and/or traction devices subsequent to the first should be reported separately. CPT codes for other additional procedures, such as obtaining grafts and external fixation, should only be used if the procedure is not already listed as included as part of the basic procedure. Consult the glossary for terms and definitions and the front matter of this chapter for additional information.

Forearm and wrist procedures include those performed on the radius, ulna, carpal bones, and joints.

To report application of external fixation in addition to internal fixation, consult 20690 and the appropriate internal fixation code.

INCISION

25000   **Incision, extensor tendon sheath, wrist (eg, deQuervains disease)**   ☒ ☒ 50 ↻
MED: 100-2,15,260; 100-4,4,20.5; 100-4,12,90.3; 100-4,14,10
AMA: 1998,Nov,8
If decompression of a median nerve is performed or for carpal tunnel syndrome, consult CPT code 64721.

25001   **Incision, flexor tendon sheath, wrist (eg, flexor carpi radialis)**   ☒ 50 ↻

25020   **Decompression fasciotomy, forearm and/or wrist, flexor OR extensor compartment; without debridement of nonviable muscle and/or nerve**   ☒ ☒ 50 ↻
MED: 100-2,15,260; 100-4,4,20.5; 100-4,12,90.3; 100-4,14,10

25023   **with debridement of nonviable muscle and/or nerve**   ☒ ☒ 80 50 ↻
MED: 100-2,15,260; 100-4,4,20.5; 100-4,12,90.3; 100-4,14,10
For superficial incision and drainage procedures, consult codes 10060-10160. If debridement is performed, consult also CPT codes 11000-11044.

If decompression fasciotomy with brachial artery exploration is performed, consult CPT code 24495.

25024   **Decompression fasciotomy, forearm and/or wrist, flexor AND extensor compartment; without debridement of nonviable muscle and/or nerve**   ☒ ☒ 50 ↻
MED: 100-2,15,260; 100-4,4,20.5; 100-4,12,90.3; 100-4,14,10

25025   **with debridement of nonviable muscle and/or nerve**   ☒ ☒ 80 50 ↻
MED: 100-2,15,260; 100-4,4,20.5; 100-4,12,90.3; 100-4,14,10

25028   **Incision and drainage, forearm and/or wrist; deep abscess or hematoma**   ☒ ☒ 50 ↻
MED: 100-2,15,260; 100-4,4,20.5; 100-4,12,90.3; 100-4,14,10

25031   **bursa**   ☒ ☒ 80 50 ↻
MED: 100-2,15,260; 100-4,4,20.5; 100-4,12,90.3; 100-4,14,10
AMA: 1998,Nov,9

25035   **Incision, deep, bone cortex, forearm and/or wrist (eg, osteomyelitis or bone abscess)**   ☒ ☒ 80 50 ↻
MED: 100-2,15,260; 100-4,4,20.5; 100-4,12,90.3; 100-4,14,10

25040   **Arthrotomy, radiocarpal or midcarpal joint, with exploration, drainage, or removal of foreign body**   ☒ ☒ 80 50 ↻
MED: 100-2,15,260; 100-4,4,20.5; 100-4,12,90.3; 100-4,14,10

EXCISION

25065   **Biopsy, soft tissue of forearm and/or wrist; superficial**   ☒ 50 ↻
If a needle biopsy of soft tissue is needed, consult CPT code 20206.

25066   **deep (subfascial or intramuscular)**   ☒ ☒ 50 ↻
MED: 100-2,15,260; 100-4,4,20.5; 100-4,12,90.3; 100-4,14,10
AMA: 1998,Nov,8
If a needle biopsy of soft tissue is needed, consult CPT code 20206.

25075   **Excision, tumor, soft tissue of forearm and/or wrist area; subcutaneous**   ☒ ☒ 50 ↻
MED: 100-2,15,260; 100-4,4,20.5; 100-4,12,90.3; 100-4,14,10

25076   **deep, (subfascial or intramuscular)**   ☒ ☒ 50 ↻
MED: 100-2,15,260; 100-4,4,20.5; 100-4,12,90.3; 100-4,14,10

25077   **Radical resection of tumor (eg, malignant neoplasm), soft tissue of forearm and/or wrist area**   ☒ ☒ 50 ↻
MED: 100-2,15,260; 100-4,4,20.5; 100-4,12,90.3; 100-4,14,10

25085   **Capsulotomy, wrist (eg, contracture)**   ☒ ☒ 80 50 ↻
MED: 100-2,15,260; 100-4,4,20.5; 100-4,12,90.3; 100-4,14,10

25100   **Arthrotomy, wrist joint; with biopsy**   ☒ ☒ 80 50 ↻
MED: 100-2,15,260; 100-4,4,20.5; 100-4,12,90.3; 100-4,14,10

25101   **with joint exploration, with or without biopsy, with or without removal of loose or foreign body**   ☒ ☒ 80 50 ↻
MED: 100-2,15,260; 100-4,4,20.5; 100-4,12,90.3; 100-4,14,10

25105   **with synovectomy**   ☒ ☒ 80 50 ↻
MED: 100-2,15,260; 100-4,4,20.5; 100-4,12,90.3; 100-4,14,10

25107   **Arthrotomy, distal radioulnar joint including repair of triangular cartilage, complex**   ☒ ☒ 80 50 ↻
MED: 100-2,15,260; 100-4,4,20.5; 100-4,12,90.3; 100-4,14,10

● 25109   **Excision of tendon, forearm and/or wrist, flexor or extensor, each**   ☒

25110   **Excision, lesion of tendon sheath, forearm and/or wrist**   ☒ ☒ 50 ↻
MED: 100-2,15,260; 100-4,4,20.5; 100-4,12,90.3; 100-4,14,10

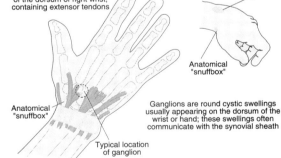

Synovial sheaths (blue) of the dorsum of right wrist, containing extensor tendons

Ganglion

Anatomical "snuffbox"

Anatomical "snuffbox"

Ganglions are round cystic swellings usually appearing on the dorsum of the wrist or hand; these swellings often communicate with the synovial sheath

Typical location of ganglion

25111   **Excision of ganglion, wrist (dorsal or volar); primary**   ☒ ☒ 50 ↻
MED: 100-2,15,260; 100-4,4,20.5; 100-4,12,90.3; 100-4,14,10
If this procedure involves the hand or finger, consult CPT code 26160.

25112   **recurrent**   ☒ ☒ 50 ↻
MED: 100-2,15,260; 100-4,4,20.5; 100-4,12,90.3; 100-4,14,10
If this procedure involves the hand or finger, consult CPT code 26160.

25115 Radical excision of bursa, synovia of wrist, or forearm tendon sheaths (eg, tenosynovitis, fungus, Tbc, or other granulomas, rheumatoid arthritis); flexors   4 T 50 ▣

MED: 100-2,15,260; 100-4,4,20.5; 100-4,12,90.3; 100-4,14,10

25116 extensors, with or without transposition of dorsal retinaculum   4 T 80 50 ▣

MED: 100-2,15,260; 100-4,4,20.5; 100-4,12,90.3; 100-4,14,10

If finger synovectomies are performed, consult CPT code 26145.

25118 Synovectomy, extensor tendon sheath, wrist, single compartment;   2 T 50 ▣

MED: 100-2,15,260; 100-4,4,20.5; 100-4,12,90.3; 100-4,14,10

25119 with resection of distal ulna   3 T 80 50 ▣

MED: 100-2,15,260; 100-4,4,20.5; 100-4,12,90.3; 100-4,14,10

25120 Excision or curettage of bone cyst or benign tumor of radius or ulna (excluding head or neck of radius and olecranon process);   3 T 80 50 ▣

MED: 100-2,15,260; 100-4,4,20.5; 100-4,12,90.3; 100-4,14,10

If this procedure involves the head or the neck of the radius or the olecranon process, consult CPT codes 24120-24126.

25125 with autograft (includes obtaining graft)   3 T 80 50 ▣

MED: 100-2,15,260; 100-4,4,20.5; 100-4,12,90.3; 100-4,14,10

25126 with allograft   3 T 80 50 ▣

MED: 100-2,15,260; 100-4,4,20.5; 100-4,12,90.3; 100-4,14,10

25130 Excision or curettage of bone cyst or benign tumor of carpal bones;   3 T 80 50 ▣

MED: 100-2,15,260; 100-4,4,20.5; 100-4,12,90.3; 100-4,14,10

25135 with autograft (includes obtaining graft)   3 T 80 50 ▣

MED: 100-2,15,260; 100-4,4,20.5; 100-4,12,90.3; 100-4,14,10

25136 with allograft   3 T 80 50 ▣

MED: 100-2,15,260; 100-4,4,20.5; 100-4,12,90.3; 100-4,14,10

25145 Sequestrectomy (eg, for osteomyelitis or bone abscess), forearm and/or wrist   2 T 80 50 ▣

MED: 100-2,15,260; 100-4,4,20.5; 100-4,12,90.3; 100-4,14,10

25150 Partial excision (craterization, saucerization, or diaphysectomy) of bone (eg, for osteomyelitis); ulna   2 T 50 ▣

MED: 100-2,15,260; 100-4,4,20.5; 100-4,12,90.3; 100-4,14,10

25151 radius   2 T 80 50 ▣

MED: 100-2,15,260; 100-4,4,20.5; 100-4,12,90.3; 100-4,14,10

If this procedure involves the head or the neck of the radius or the olecranon process, consult CPT codes 24145 and 24147.

25170 Radical resection for tumor, radius or ulna   T 80 50 ▣

25210 Carpectomy; one bone   3 T 80 ▣

MED: 100-2,15,260; 100-4,12,90.3; 100-4,14,10

If carpectomy is performed with an implant, consult CPT codes 25441-25445.

25215 all bones of proximal row   4 T 80 ▣

MED: 100-2,15,260; 100-4,4,20.5; 100-4,12,90.3; 100-4,14,10

25230 Radial styloidectomy (separate procedure)   4 T 50 ▣

MED: 100-2,15,260; 100-4,4,20.5; 100-4,12,90.3; 100-4,14,10

25240 Excision distal ulna partial or complete (eg, Darrach type or matched resection)   4 T 80 50 ▣

MED: 100-2,15,260; 100-4,4,20.5; 100-4,12,90.3; 100-4,14,10

If an implant replacement is performed for the distal ulna, consult CPT code 25442. If obtaining fascia for interposition, consult CPT codes 20920 and 20922.

INTRODUCTION OR REMOVAL

If a K-wire, a pin, or a rod is inserted or removed, consult CPT codes 20650, 20670, and 20680.

25246 Injection procedure for wrist arthrography   N 50 ▣

If radiological supervision and interpretation is needed, consult CPT code 73115. Code 77002 cannot be reported in addition to 73115.

If a superficial foreign body is removed, consult CPT code 20520.

25248 Exploration with removal of deep foreign body, forearm or wrist   2 T 50 ▣

MED: 100-2,15,260; 100-4,4,20.5; 100-4,12,90.3; 100-4,14,10

25250 Removal of wrist prosthesis; (separate procedure)   1 T 80 50 ▣

MED: 100-2,15,260; 100-4,4,20.5; 100-4,12,90.3; 100-4,14,10

25251 complicated, including total wrist   1 T 80 ▣

MED: 100-2,15,260; 100-4,4,20.5; 100-4,12,90.3; 100-4,14,10

25259 Manipulation, wrist, under anesthesia   T 50 ▣

If external fixation is applied, consult CPT code 20690 or 20692.

REPAIR, REVISION, AND/OR RECONSTRUCTION

25260 Repair, tendon or muscle, flexor, forearm and/or wrist; primary, single, each tendon or muscle   4 T ▣

MED: 100-2,15,260; 100-4,4,20.5; 100-4,12,90.3; 100-4,14,10

25263 secondary, single, each tendon or muscle   2 T 80 ▣

MED: 100-2,15,260; 100-4,4,20.5; 100-4,12,90.3; 100-4,14,10

25265 secondary, with free graft (includes obtaining graft), each tendon or muscle   3 T 80 ▣

MED: 100-2,15,260; 100-4,4,20.5; 100-4,12,90.3; 100-4,14,10

25270 Repair, tendon or muscle, extensor, forearm and/or wrist; primary, single, each tendon or muscle   4 T 80 ▣

MED: 100-2,15,260; 100-4,4,20.5; 100-4,12,90.3; 100-4,14,10

25272 secondary, single, each tendon or muscle   3 T 80 ▣

MED: 100-2,15,260; 100-4,4,20.5; 100-4,12,90.3; 100-4,14,10

25274 secondary, with free graft (includes obtaining graft), each tendon or muscle   4 T 80 ▣

MED: 100-2,15,260; 100-4,4,20.5; 100-4,12,90.3; 100-4,14,10

25275 Repair, tendon sheath, extensor, forearm and/or wrist, with free graft (includes obtaining graft) (eg, for extensor carpi ulnaris subluxation)   4 T 80 50 ▣

MED: 100-2,15,260; 100-4,4,20.5; 100-4,12,90.3; 100-4,14,10

25280 Lengthening or shortening of flexor or extensor tendon, forearm and/or wrist, single, each tendon   4 T 80 ▣

MED: 100-2,15,260; 100-4,4,20.5; 100-4,12,90.3; 100-4,14,10

25290 Tenotomy, open, flexor or extensor tendon, forearm and/or wrist, single, each tendon   3 T ▣

MED: 100-2,15,260; 100-4,4,20.5; 100-4,12,90.3; 100-4,14,10

25295 Tenolysis, flexor or extensor tendon, forearm and/or wrist, single, each tendon ③ T ▣
MED: 100-2,15,260; 100-4,4,20.5; 100-4,12,90.3; 100-4,14,10
AMA: 1998,Aug,10; 1997,Apr,11

25300 Tenodesis at wrist; flexors of fingers ③ T 80 50 ▣
MED: 100-2,15,260; 100-4,4,20.5; 100-4,12,90.3; 100-4,14,10

25301 extensors of fingers ③ T 80 50 ▣
MED: 100-2,15,260; 100-4,4,20.5; 100-4,12,90.3; 100-4,14,10

25310 Tendon transplantation or transfer, flexor or extensor, forearm and/or wrist, single; each tendon ③ T 80 ▣
MED: 100-2,15,260; 100-4,4,20.5; 100-4,12,90.3; 100-4,14,10
AMA: 2002,Jun,11

25312 with tendon graft(s) (includes obtaining graft), each tendon ④ T 80 ▣
MED: 100-2,15,260; 100-4,4,20.5; 100-4,12,90.3; 100-4,14,10

25315 Flexor origin slide (eg, for cerebral palsy, Volkmann contracture), forearm and/or wrist; ③ T 80 50 ▣
MED: 100-2,15,260; 100-4,4,20.5; 100-4,12,90.3; 100-4,14,10

25316 with tendon(s) transfer ③ T 80 50 ▣
MED: 100-2,15,260; 100-4,4,20.5; 100-4,12,90.3; 100-4,14,10

25320 Capsulorrhaphy or reconstruction, wrist, open (eg, capsulodesis, ligament repair, tendon transfer or graft) (includes synovectomy, capsulotomy and open reduction) for carpal instability ③ T 80 50 ▣
MED: 100-2,15,260; 100-4,4,20.5; 100-4,12,90.3; 100-4,14,10

25332 Arthroplasty, wrist, with or without interposition, with or without external or internal fixation ⑤ T 80 50 ▣
MED: 100-2,15,260; 100-4,4,20.5; 100-4,12,90.3; 100-4,14,10
If obtaining fascia for interposition, consult CPT codes 20920 and 20992. If arthroplasty with a prosthetic replacement is performed, consult CPT codes 25441-25446.

25335 Centralization of wrist on ulna (eg, radial club hand) ③ T 80 50 ▣
MED: 100-2,15,260; 100-4,4,20.5; 100-4,12,90.3; 100-4,14,10

25337 Reconstruction for stabilization of unstable distal ulna or distal radioulnar joint, secondary by soft tissue stabilization (eg, tendon transfer, tendon graft or weave, or tenodesis) with or without open reduction of distal radioulnar joint ⑤ T 50 ▣
MED: 100-2,15,260; 100-4,4,20.5; 100-4,12,90.3; 100-4,14,10
If a fascia lata graft is harvested, consult CPT codes 20920 and 20922.

25350 Osteotomy, radius; distal third ③ T 80 50 ▣
MED: 100-2,15,260; 100-4,4,20.5; 100-4,12,90.3; 100-4,14,10

25355 middle or proximal third ③ T 80 50 ▣
MED: 100-2,15,260; 100-4,4,20.5; 100-4,12,90.3; 100-4,14,10

25360 Osteotomy; ulna ③ T 80 50 ▣
MED: 100-2,15,260; 100-4,4,20.5; 100-4,12,90.3; 100-4,14,10

25365 radius AND ulna ③ T 80 50 ▣
MED: 100-2,15,260; 100-4,4,20.5; 100-4,12,90.3; 100-4,14,10

25370 Multiple osteotomies, with realignment on intramedullary rod (Sofield type procedure); radius OR ulna ③ T 80 50 ▣
MED: 100-2,15,260; 100-4,4,20.5; 100-4,12,90.3; 100-4,14,10

25375 radius AND ulna ④ T 80 50 ▣
MED: 100-2,15,260; 100-4,4,20.5; 100-4,12,90.3; 100-4,14,10

25390 Osteoplasty, radius OR ulna; shortening ③ T 80 50 ▣
MED: 100-2,15,260; 100-4,4,20.5; 100-4,12,90.3; 100-4,14,10

25391 lengthening with autograft ④ T 80 50 ▣
MED: 100-2,15,260; 100-4,4,20.5; 100-4,12,90.3; 100-4,14,10

25392 Osteoplasty, radius AND ulna; shortening (excluding 64876) ③ T 80 50 ▣
MED: 100-2,15,260; 100-4,4,20.5; 100-4,12,90.3; 100-4,14,10

25393 lengthening with autograft ④ T 80 50 ▣
MED: 100-2,15,260; 100-4,4,20.5; 100-4,12,90.3; 100-4,14,10

25394 Osteoplasty, carpal bone, shortening T 80 50 ▣

25400 Repair of nonunion or malunion, radius OR ulna; without graft (eg, compression technique) ③ T 80 50 ▣
MED: 100-2,15,260; 100-4,4,20.5; 100-4,12,90.3; 100-4,14,10

25405 with autograft (includes obtaining graft) ④ T 80 50 ▣
MED: 100-2,15,260; 100-4,4,20.5; 100-4,12,90.3; 100-4,14,10

25415 Repair of nonunion or malunion, radius AND ulna; without graft (eg, compression technique) ③ T 80 50 ▣
MED: 100-2,15,260; 100-4,12,90.3; 100-4,14,10

25420 with autograft (includes obtaining graft) ④ T 80 50 ▣
MED: 100-2,15,260; 100-4,4,20.5; 100-4,12,90.3; 100-4,14,10

25425 Repair of defect with autograft; radius OR ulna ③ T 80 50 ▣
MED: 100-2,15,260; 100-4,4,20.5; 100-4,12,90.3; 100-4,14,10

25426 radius AND ulna ④ T 80 50 ▣
MED: 100-2,15,260; 100-4,4,20.5; 100-4,12,90.3; 100-4,14,10

25430 Insertion of vascular pedicle into carpal bone (eg, Hori procedure) T 50

25431 Repair of nonunion of carpal bone (excluding carpal scaphoid (navicular)) (includes obtaining graft and necessary fixation), each bone T 80 50

25440 Repair of nonunion, scaphoid carpal (navicular) bone, with or without radial styloidectomy (includes obtaining graft and necessary fixation) ④ T 80 50
MED: 100-2,15,260; 100-4,4,20.5; 100-4,12,90.3; 100-4,14,10

25441 Arthroplasty with prosthetic replacement; distal radius ⑤ T 80 50 ▣
MED: 100-2,15,260; 100-4,4,20.5; 100-4,4,61.2; 100-4,12,90.3; 100-4,14,10

25442 distal ulna ⑤ T 80 50 ▣
MED: 100-2,15,260; 100-4,4,20.5; 100-4,4,61.2; 100-4,12,90.3; 100-4,14,10

25443 scaphoid carpal (navicular) ⑤ T 80 50 ▣
MED: 100-2,15,260; 100-4,4,20.5; 100-4,12,90.3; 100-4,14,10

25444 lunate ⑤ T 80 50 ▣
MED: 100-2,15,260; 100-4,4,20.5; 100-4,12,90.3; 100-4,14,10

25445 trapezium ⑤ T 50 ▣
MED: 100-2,15,260; 100-4,4,20.5; 100-4,12,90.3; 100-4,14,10

25446 distal radius and partial or entire carpus (total wrist) ⑦ T 80 50 ▣
MED: 100-2,15,260; 100-4,4,20.5; 100-4,4,61.2; 100-4,12,90.3; 100-4,14,10

Musculoskeletal System

25447 — 25635

25447 Arthroplasty, interposition, intercarpal or carpometacarpal joints [5][T][80][50][⬛]

MED: 100-2,15,260; 100-4,4,20.5; 100-4,12,90.3; 100-4,14,10
AMA: 1998,Nov,8
If wrist arthroplasty is performed, consult CPT code 25332.

25449 Revision of arthroplasty, including removal of implant, wrist joint [5][T][80][50][⬛]

MED: 100-2,15,260; 100-4,4,20.5; 100-4,12,90.3; 100-4,14,10

25450 Epiphyseal arrest by epiphysiodesis or stapling; distal radius OR ulna [3][T][50][⬛]

MED: 100-2,15,260; 100-4,4,20.5; 100-4,12,90.3; 100-4,14,10

25455 distal radius AND ulna [3][T][50][⬛]

MED: 100-2,15,260; 100-4,4,20.5; 100-4,12,90.3; 100-4,14,10

25490 Prophylactic treatment (nailing, pinning, plating or wiring) with or without methylmethacrylate; radius [3][T][80][50][⬛]

MED: 100-2,15,260; 100-4,4,20.5; 100-4,12,90.3; 100-4,14,10

25491 ulna [3][T][80][50][⬛]

MED: 100-2,15,260; 100-4,4,20.5; 100-4,12,90.3; 100-4,14,10

25492 radius AND ulna [3][T][80][50][⬛]

MED: 100-2,15,260; 100-4,4,20.5; 100-4,12,90.3; 100-4,14,10

FRACTURE AND/OR DISLOCATION

25500 Closed treatment of radial shaft fracture; without manipulation [T][50][⬛]

25505 with manipulation [1][T][50][⬛]

MED: 100-2,15,260; 100-4,4,20.5; 100-4,12,90.3; 100-4,14,10

25515 Open treatment of radial shaft fracture, with or without internal or external fixation [3][T][80][50][⬛]

MED: 100-2,15,260; 100-4,4,20.5; 100-4,12,90.3; 100-4,14,10

25520 Closed treatment of radial shaft fracture and closed treatment of dislocation of distal radioulnar joint (Galeazzi fracture/dislocation) [1][T][50][⬛]

MED: 100-2,15,260; 100-4,4,20.5; 100-4,12,90.3; 100-4,14,10

25525 Open treatment of radial shaft fracture, with internal and/or external fixation and closed treatment of dislocation of distal radioulnar joint (Galeazzi fracture/dislocation), with or without percutaneous skeletal fixation [4][T][80][50][⬛]

MED: 100-2,15,260; 100-4,4,20.5; 100-4,12,90.3; 100-4,14,10

25526 Open treatment of radial shaft fracture, with internal and/or external fixation and open treatment, with or without internal or external fixation of distal radioulnar joint (Galeazzi fracture/dislocation), includes repair of triangular fibrocartilage complex [5][T][80][50][⬛]

MED: 100-2,15,260; 100-4,4,20.5; 100-4,12,90.3; 100-4,14,10

25530 Closed treatment of ulnar shaft fracture; without manipulation [T][50][⬛]

25535 with manipulation [1][T][50][⬛]

MED: 100-2,15,260; 100-4,4,20.5; 100-4,12,90.3; 100-4,14,10

25545 Open treatment of ulnar shaft fracture, with or without internal or external fixation [3][T][80][50][⬛]

MED: 100-2,15,260; 100-4,4,20.5; 100-4,12,90.3; 100-4,14,10
AMA: 1999,Oct,4; 1993,Fall,23

25560 Closed treatment of radial and ulnar shaft fractures; without manipulation [T][50][⬛]

25565 with manipulation [2][T][50][⬛]

MED: 100-2,15,260; 100-4,4,20.5; 100-4,12,90.3; 100-4,14,10

25574 Open treatment of radial AND ulnar shaft fractures, with internal or external fixation; of radius OR ulna [3][T][80][50][⬛]

MED: 100-2,15,260; 100-4,4,20.5; 100-4,12,90.3; 100-4,14,10
AMA: 1999,Oct,4; 1993,Fall,23

25575 of radius AND ulna [3][T][80][50][⬛]

MED: 100-2,15,260; 100-4,4,20.5; 100-4,12,90.3; 100-4,14,10

▲ **25600** Closed treatment of distal radial fracture (eg, Colles or Smith type) or epiphyseal separation, includes closed treatment of fracture of ulnar styloid, when performed; without manipulation [T][50][⬛]

25605 with manipulation [3][T][50][⬛]

MED: 100-2,15,260; 100-4,4,20.5; 100-4,12,90.3; 100-4,14,10
Do not report 25600 or 26505 in conjunction with 25650.

● **25606** Percutaneous skeletal fixation of distal radial fracture or epiphyseal separation [3][T]

Do not report 25606 with 25650.

Use 25651 for percutaneous treatment and 25652 for open treatment of ulnar styloid fracture.

● **25607** Open treatment of distal radial extra-articular fracture or epiphyseal separation, with internal fixation [5][T]

Do not report 25607 with 25650.

Use 25651 for percutaneous treatment and 25652 for open treatment of ulnar styloid fracture.

● **25608** Open treatment of distal radial intra-articular fracture or epiphyseal separation; with internal fixation of 2 fragments [5][T]

Do not report 25608 with 25609.

● **25609** with internal fixation of 3 or more fragments [5][T]

Do not report 25608 or 25609 with 25650.

Use 25651 for percutaneous treatment and 25652 for open treatment of ulnar styloid fracture.

~~25611~~ ~~Percutaneous skeletal fixation of distal radial fracture (eg, Colles or Smith type) or epiphyseal separation, with or without fracture of ulnar styloid, requiring manipulation, with or without external fixation~~

Use 25606.

~~25620~~ ~~Open treatment of distal radial fracture (eg, Colles or Smith type) or epiphyseal separation, with or without fracture of ulnar styloid, with or without internal or external fixation~~

Use 25606-25609.

25622 Closed treatment of carpal scaphoid (navicular) fracture; without manipulation [T][50][⬛]

25624 with manipulation [2][T][80][50][⬛]

MED: 100-2,15,260; 100-4,4,20.5; 100-4,12,90.3; 100-4,14,10

25628 Open treatment of carpal scaphoid (navicular) fracture, with or without internal or external fixation [3][T][80][50][⬛]

MED: 100-2,15,260; 100-4,4,20.5; 100-4,12,90.3; 100-4,14,10

25630 Closed treatment of carpal bone fracture (excluding carpal scaphoid (navicular)); without manipulation, each bone [T][50][⬛]

25635 with manipulation, each bone [1][T][80][50][⬛]

MED: 100-2,15,260; 100-4,4,20.5; 100-4,12,90.3; 100-4,14,10

CPT only © 2006 American Medical Association. All Rights Reserved. (Black Ink)   © 2006 Ingenix (Blue Ink)

25645   Open treatment of carpal bone fracture (other than carpal scaphoid (navicular)), each bone **3** T 80 50 🗖

MED: 100-2,15,260; 100-4,4,20.5; 100-4,12,90.3; 100-4,14,10

25650   Closed treatment of ulnar styloid fracture   T 50 🗖

Do not report 25650 with 25600, 25605, or 25607-25609.

25651   Percutaneous skeletal fixation of ulnar styloid fracture   T 80 50 🗖

25652   Open treatment of ulnar styloid fracture   T 50 🗖

25660   Closed treatment of radiocarpal or intercarpal dislocation, one or more bones, with manipulation **1** T 80 50 🗖

MED: 100-2,15,260; 100-4,4,20.5; 100-4,12,90.3; 100-4,14,10

25670   Open treatment of radiocarpal or intercarpal dislocation, one or more bones **3** T 80 50 🗖

MED: 100-2,15,260; 100-4,4,20.5; 100-4,12,90.3; 100-4,14,10

25671   Percutaneous skeletal fixation of distal radioulnar dislocation **1** T 50 🗖

MED: 100-2,15,260; 100-4,4,20.5; 100-4,12,90.3; 100-4,14,10

25675   Closed treatment of distal radioulnar dislocation with manipulation **1** T 80 50 🗖

MED: 100-2,15,260; 100-4,4,20.5; 100-4,12,90.3; 100-4,14,10

25676   Open treatment of distal radioulnar dislocation, acute or chronic **2** T 80 50 🗖

MED: 100-2,15,260; 100-4,4,20.5; 100-4,12,90.3; 100-4,14,10

25680   Closed treatment of trans-scaphoperilunar type of fracture dislocation, with manipulation **2** T 80 50 🗖

MED: 100-2,15,260; 100-4,4,20.5; 100-4,12,90.3; 100-4,14,10

25685   Open treatment of trans-scaphoperilunar type of fracture dislocation **3** T 80 50 🗖

MED: 100-2,15,260; 100-4,4,20.5; 100-4,12,90.3; 100-4,14,10

25690   Closed treatment of lunate dislocation, with manipulation **1** T 80 50 🗖

MED: 100-2,15,260; 100-4,4,20.5; 100-4,12,90.3; 100-4,14,10

25695   Open treatment of lunate dislocation **2** T 80 50 🗖

MED: 100-2,15,260; 100-4,4,20.5; 100-4,12,90.3; 100-4,14,10

ARTHRODESIS

25800   Arthrodesis, wrist; complete, without bone graft (includes radiocarpal and/or intercarpal and/or carpometacarpal joints) **4** T 80 50 🗖

MED: 100-2,15,260; 100-4,4,20.5; 100-4,12,90.3; 100-4,14,10
AMA: 1998,Nov,8

25805   with sliding graft **5** T 80 50 🗖

MED: 100-2,15,260; 100-4,4,20.5; 100-4,12,90.3; 100-4,14,10

25810   with iliac or other autograft (includes obtaining graft) **5** T 80 50 🗖

MED: 100-2,15,260; 100-4,4,20.5; 100-4,12,90.3; 100-4,14,10

25820   Arthrodesis, wrist; limited, without bone graft (eg, intercarpal or radiocarpal) **4** T 80 50 🗖

MED: 100-2,15,260; 100-4,4,20.5; 100-4,12,90.3; 100-4,14,10
AMA: 1998,Nov,8

25825   with autograft (includes obtaining graft) **5** T 80 50 🗖

MED: 100-2,15,260; 100-4,4,20.5; 100-4,12,90.3; 100-4,14,10

25830   Arthrodesis, distal radioulnar joint with segmental resection of ulna, with or without bone graft (eg, Sauve-Kapandji procedure) **5** T 80 50 🗖

MED: 100-2,15,260; 100-4,4,20.5; 100-4,12,90.3; 100-4,14,10
AMA: 1998,Nov,8

AMPUTATION

25900   Amputation, forearm, through radius and ulna; C 80 50 🗖

25905   open, circular (guillotine) C 80 50 🗖

25907   secondary closure or scar revision **3** T 80 50 🗖

MED: 100-2,15,260; 100-4,4,20.5; 100-4,12,90.3; 100-4,14,10

25909   re-amputation C 80 50 🗖

25915   Krukenberg procedure C 80 50 🗖

25920   Disarticulation through wrist; C 80 50 🗖

25922   secondary closure or scar revision **3** T 80 50 🗖

MED: 100-2,15,260; 100-4,4,20.5; 100-4,12,90.3; 100-4,14,10

25924   re-amputation C 80 50 🗖

25927   Transmetacarpal amputation; C 80 50 🗖

25929   secondary closure or scar revision **3** T 80 50 🗖

MED: 100-2,15,260; 100-4,4,20.5; 100-4,12,90.3; 100-4,14,10

25931   re-amputation C 50 🗖

OTHER PROCEDURES

25999   Unlisted procedure, forearm or wrist   T 80 50

MED: 100-4,4,20.5; 100-4,4,180.3

HAND AND FINGERS

Codes listed in the Musculoskeletal chapter include the application and removal of the first cast or traction device. Replacement of casts and/or traction devices subsequent to the first should be reported separately. CPT codes for other additional procedures, such as obtaining grafts and external fixation, should only be used if the procedure is not already listed as included as part of the basic procedure. Consult the glossary for terms and definitions and the front matter of this chapter for additional information.

INCISION

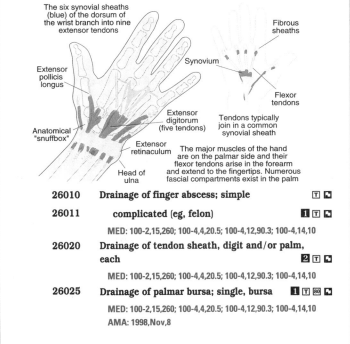

The six synovial sheaths (blue) of the dorsum of the wrist branch into nine extensor tendons

Fibrous sheaths

Synovium

Extensor pollicis longus

Flexor tendons

Anatomical "snuffbox"

Extensor digitorum (five tendons)

Tendons typically join in a common synovial sheath

Extensor retinaculum

Head of ulna

The major muscles of the hand are on the palmar side and their flexor tendons arise in the forearm and extend to the fingertips. Numerous fascial compartments exist in the palm

26010   Drainage of finger abscess; simple   T 🗖

26011   complicated (eg, felon) **1** T 🗖

MED: 100-2,15,260; 100-4,4,20.5; 100-4,12,90.3; 100-4,14,10

26020   Drainage of tendon sheath, digit and/or palm, each **2** T 🗖

MED: 100-2,15,260; 100-4,4,20.5; 100-4,12,90.3; 100-4,14,10

26025   Drainage of palmar bursa; single, bursa **1** T 80 🗖

MED: 100-2,15,260; 100-4,4,20.5; 100-4,12,90.3; 100-4,14,10
AMA: 1998,Nov,8

26030	multiple bursa	2 T 80
	MED: 100-2,15,260; 100-4,4,20.5; 100-4,12,90.3; 100-4,14,10	
	AMA: 1998,Nov,8	
26034	Incision, bone cortex, hand or finger (eg, osteomyelitis or bone abscess)	2 T
	MED: 100-2,15,260; 100-4,4,20.5; 100-4,12,90.3; 100-4,14,10	
	AMA: 1998,Nov,8	
26035	Decompression fingers and/or hand, injection injury (eg, grease gun)	T 80
26037	Decompressive fasciotomy, hand (excludes 26035)	T 80

If decompression of the fingers and/or hand for an injection injury is performed, consult CPT code 26035.

26040	Fasciotomy, palmar (eg, Dupuytren's contracture); percutaneous	4 T 50
	MED: 100-2,15,260; 100-4,4,20.5; 100-4,12,90.3; 100-4,14,10	
	AMA: 1998,Nov,8	
26045	open, partial	3 T 50
	MED: 100-2,15,260; 100-4,4,20.5; 100-4,12,90.3; 100-4,14,10	

If a fasciectomy is performed, consult CPT codes 26121-26125.

26055	Tendon sheath incision (eg, for trigger finger)	2 T
	MED: 100-2,15,260; 100-4,4,20.5; 100-4,12,90.3; 100-4,14,10	
26060	Tenotomy, percutaneous, single, each digit	2 T 80
	MED: 100-2,15,260; 100-4,4,20.5; 100-4,12,90.3; 100-4,14,10	
26070	Arthrotomy, with exploration, drainage, or removal of loose or foreign body; carpometacarpal joint	2 T 50
	MED: 100-2,15,260; 100-4,4,20.5; 100-4,12,90.3; 100-4,14,10	
	AMA: 1998,Nov,10	
26075	metacarpophalangeal joint, each	4 T 50
	MED: 100-2,15,260; 100-4,4,20.5; 100-4,12,90.3; 100-4,14,10	
26080	interphalangeal joint, each	4 T
	MED: 100-2,15,260; 100-4,4,20.5; 100-4,12,90.3; 100-4,14,10	

EXCISION

26100	Arthrotomy with biopsy; carpometacarpal joint, each	2 T 80 50
	MED: 100-2,15,260; 100-4,4,20.5; 100-4,12,90.3; 100-4,14,10	
26105	metacarpophalangeal joint, each	1 T 80 50
	MED: 100-2,15,260; 100-4,4,20.5; 100-4,12,90.3; 100-4,14,10	
26110	interphalangeal joint, each	1 T
	MED: 100-2,15,260; 100-4,4,20.5; 100-4,12,90.3; 100-4,14,10	
26115	Excision, tumor or vascular malformation, soft tissue of hand or finger; subcutaneous	2 T
	MED: 100-2,15,260; 100-4,4,20.5; 100-4,12,90.3; 100-4,14,10	
26116	deep (subfascial or intramuscular)	2 T
	MED: 100-2,15,260; 100-4,4,20.5; 100-4,12,90.3; 100-4,14,10	
26117	Radical resection of tumor (eg, malignant neoplasm), soft tissue of hand or finger	3 T
	MED: 100-2,15,260; 100-4,4,20.5; 100-4,12,90.3; 100-4,14,10	
26121	Fasciectomy, palm only, with or without Z-plasty, other local tissue rearrangement, or skin grafting (includes obtaining graft)	4 T 50
	MED: 100-2,15,260; 100-4,4,20.5; 100-4,12,90.3; 100-4,14,10	

If a fasciotomy is performed, consult CPT codes 26040 and 26045.

26123	Fasciectomy, partial palmar with release of single digit including proximal interphalangeal joint, with or without Z-plasty, other local tissue rearrangement, or skin grafting (includes obtaining graft);	4 T 50
	MED: 100-2,15,260; 100-4,4,20.5; 100-4,12,90.3; 100-4,14,10	

If a fasciotomy is performed, consult CPT codes 26040 and 26045.

+ 26125	each additional digit (List separately in addition to code for primary procedure)	4 T
	MED: 100-2,15,260; 100-4,4,20.5; 100-4,12,90.3; 100-4,14,10	

If a fasciotomy is performed, consult CPT codes 26040 and 26045.

Note that 26125 is an add-on code and must be used in conjunction with 26123.

26130	Synovectomy, carpometacarpal joint	3 T 50
	MED: 100-2,15,260; 100-4,4,20.5; 100-4,12,90.3; 100-4,14,10	
26135	Synovectomy, metacarpophalangeal joint including intrinsic release and extensor hood reconstruction, each digit	4 T 80
	MED: 100-2,15,260; 100-4,4,20.5; 100-4,12,90.3; 100-4,14,10	
26140	Synovectomy, proximal interphalangeal joint, including extensor reconstruction, each interphalangeal joint	2 T
	MED: 100-2,15,260; 100-4,4,20.5; 100-4,12,90.3; 100-4,14,10	
26145	Synovectomy, tendon sheath, radical (tenosynovectomy), flexor tendon, palm and/or finger, each tendon	3 T
	MED: 100-2,15,260; 100-4,4,20.5; 100-4,12,90.3; 100-4,14,10	
	AMA: 1998,Nov,8	

If a tendon sheath synovectomy is performed at the wrist, consult CPT codes 25115 and 25116.

26160	Excision of lesion of tendon sheath or joint capsule (eg, cyst, mucous cyst, or ganglion), hand or finger	3 T
	MED: 100-2,15,260; 100-4,4,20.5; 100-4,12,90.3; 100-4,14,10	

For a wrist ganglion, consult CPT codes 25111 and 25112. If this procedure is performed on a trigger digit, consult CPT code 26055.

▲ 26170	Excision of tendon, palm, flexor or extensor, single, each tendon	3 T 80
	MED: 100-2,15,260; 100-4,4,20.5; 100-4,12,90.3; 100-4,14,10	

Do not report 26170 with 26390, 26415.

▲ 26180	Excision of tendon, finger, flexor or extensor, each tendon	3 T 80
	MED: 100-2,15,260; 100-4,4,20.5; 100-4,12,90.3; 100-4,14,10	
	AMA: 1998,Nov,8	

Do not report 26180 with 26390, 26415.

26185	Sesamoidectomy, thumb or finger (separate procedure)	4 T 80 50
	MED: 100-2,15,260; 100-4,4,20.5; 100-4,12,90.3; 100-4,14,10	
26200	Excision or curettage of bone cyst or benign tumor of metacarpal;	2 T 80
	MED: 100-2,15,260; 100-4,4,20.5; 100-4,12,90.3; 100-4,14,10	
26205	with autograft (includes obtaining graft)	3 T
	MED: 100-2,15,260; 100-4,4,20.5; 100-4,12,90.3; 100-4,14,10	
26210	Excision or curettage of bone cyst or benign tumor of proximal, middle, or distal phalanx of finger;	2 T
	MED: 100-2,15,260; 100-4,4,20.5; 100-4,12,90.3; 100-4,14,10	

26215 with autograft (includes obtaining graft) ③ T ▯

MED: 100-2,15,260; 100-4,4,20.5; 100-4,12,90.3; 100-4,14,10

26230 Partial excision (craterization, saucerization, or diaphysectomy) bone (eg, osteomyelitis); metacarpal ⑦ T 80 ▯

MED: 100-2,15,260; 100-4,4,20.5; 100-4,12,90.3; 100-4,14,10

26235 proximal or middle phalanx of finger ③ T 80 ▯

MED: 100-2,15,260; 100-4,4,20.5; 100-4,12,90.3; 100-4,14,10

26236 distal phalanx of finger ③ T ▯

MED: 100-2,15,260; 100-4,12,90.3; 100-4,14,10

26250 Radical resection, metacarpal (eg, tumor); ③ T 80 ▯

MED: 100-2,15,260; 100-4,12,90.3; 100-4,14,10
AMA: 1998,Nov,8

26255 with autograft (includes obtaining graft) ③ T 80 ▯

MED: 100-2,15,260; 100-4,4,20.5; 100-4,12,90.3; 100-4,14,10

26260 Radical resection, proximal or middle phalanx of finger (eg, tumor); ③ T 80 ▯

MED: 100-2,15,260; 100-4,4,20.5; 100-4,12,90.3; 100-4,14,10
AMA: 1998,Nov,8

26261 with autograft (includes obtaining graft) ③ T 80 ▯

MED: 100-2,15,260; 100-4,4,20.5; 100-4,12,90.3; 100-4,14,10

26262 Radical resection, distal phalanx of finger (eg, tumor) ② T 80 ▯

MED: 100-2,15,260; 100-4,4,20.5; 100-4,12,90.3; 100-4,14,10
AMA: 1998,Nov,8

INTRODUCTION OR REMOVAL

26320 Removal of implant from finger or hand ② T ▯

MED: 100-2,15,260; 100-4,4,20.5; 100-4,12,90.3; 100-4,14,10

If a foreign body is removed from the hand or the finger, consult CPT codes 20520 and 20525.

REPAIR, REVISION, AND/OR RECONSTRUCTION

26340 Manipulation, finger joint, under anesthesia, each joint T 50 ▯

AMA: 2002,Nov,10

If external fixation is applied, consult CPT code 20690 or 20692.

26350 Repair or advancement, flexor tendon, not in zone 2 digital flexor tendon sheath (eg, no man's land); primary or secondary without free graft, each tendon ① T ▯

MED: 100-2,15,260; 100-4,4,20.5; 100-4,12,90.3; 100-4,14,10
AMA: 1998,Nov,8

26352 secondary with free graft (includes obtaining graft), each tendon ④ T 80 ▯

MED: 100-2,15,260; 100-4,4,20.5; 100-4,12,90.3; 100-4,14,10

26356 Repair or advancement, flexor tendon, in zone 2 digital flexor tendon sheath (eg, no man's land); primary, without free graft, each tendon ④ T ▯

MED: 100-2,15,260; 100-4,4,20.5; 100-4,12,90.3; 100-4,14,10
AMA: 1998,Nov,8; 1998,Dec,9

26357 secondary, without free graft, each tendon ④ T 80 ▯

MED: 100-2,15,260; 100-4,4,20.5; 100-4,12,90.3; 100-4,14,10

26358 secondary, with free graft (includes obtaining graft), each tendon ④ T 80 ▯

MED: 100-2,15,260; 100-4,4,20.5; 100-4,12,90.3; 100-4,14,10

26370 Repair or advancement of profundus tendon, with intact superficialis tendon; primary, each tendon ④ T 80 ▯

MED: 100-2,15,260; 100-4,4,20.5; 100-4,12,90.3; 100-4,14,10
AMA: 1998,Nov,8

26372 secondary with free graft (includes obtaining graft), each tendon ④ T 80 ▯

MED: 100-2,15,260; 100-4,4,20.5; 100-4,12,90.3; 100-4,14,10
AMA: 1998,Nov,8

26373 secondary without free graft, each tendon ③ T 80 ▯

MED: 100-2,15,260; 100-4,4,20.5; 100-4,12,90.3; 100-4,14,10

26390 Excision flexor tendon, with implantation of synthetic rod for delayed tendon graft, hand or finger, each rod ④ T 80 ▯

MED: 100-2,15,260; 100-4,4,20.5; 100-4,12,90.3; 100-4,14,10
AMA: 1998,Nov,8

26392 Removal of synthetic rod and insertion of flexor tendon graft, hand or finger (includes obtaining graft), each rod ③ T 80 ▯

MED: 100-2,15,260; 100-4,4,20.5; 100-4,12,90.3; 100-4,14,10
AMA: 1998,Nov,8

26410 Repair, extensor tendon, hand, primary or secondary; without free graft, each tendon ③ T ▯

MED: 100-2,15,260; 100-4,4,20.5; 100-4,12,90.3; 100-4,14,10
AMA: 1998,Nov,8

26412 with free graft (includes obtaining graft), each tendon ③ T 80 ▯

MED: 100-2,15,260; 100-4,4,20.5; 100-4,12,90.3; 100-4,14,10
AMA: 1998,Nov,8

26415 Excision of extensor tendon, with implantation of synthetic rod for delayed tendon graft, hand or finger, each rod ④ T 80 ▯

MED: 100-2,15,260; 100-4,4,20.5; 100-4,12,90.3; 100-4,14,10
AMA: 1998,Nov,8

26416 Removal of synthetic rod and insertion of extensor tendon graft (includes obtaining graft), hand or finger, each rod ③ T ▯

MED: 100-2,15,260; 100-4,4,20.5; 100-4,12,90.3; 100-4,14,10
AMA: 1999,Nov,12

26418 Repair, extensor tendon, finger, primary or secondary; without free graft, each tendon ④ T ▯

MED: 100-2,15,260; 100-4,4,20.5; 100-4,12,90.3; 100-4,14,10
AMA: 2000,Dec,14; 1999,Dec,10; 1998,Nov,8

26420 with free graft (includes obtaining graft) each tendon ④ T 80 ▯

MED: 100-2,15,260; 100-4,4,20.5; 100-4,12,90.3; 100-4,14,10

26426 Repair of extensor tendon, central slip, secondary (eg, boutonniere deformity); using local tissue(s), including lateral band(s), each finger ③ T ▯

MED: 100-2,15,260; 100-4,4,20.5; 100-4,12,90.3; 100-4,14,10
AMA: 1998,Nov,8

26428 with free graft (includes obtaining graft), each finger ③ T 80 ▯

MED: 100-2,15,260; 100-4,4,20.5; 100-4,12,90.3; 100-4,14,10

26432 Closed treatment of distal extensor tendon insertion, with or without percutaneous pinning (eg, mallet finger) ③ T ▯

MED: 100-2,15,260; 100-4,4,20.5; 100-4,12,90.3; 100-4,14,10
AMA: 1998,Nov,8

26433 Repair of extensor tendon, distal insertion, primary or secondary; without graft (eg, mallet finger) ③ Ⓣ ▣
MED: 100-2,15,260; 100-4,4,20.5; 100-4,12,90.3; 100-4,14,10
AMA: 1998,Nov,8

26434 with free graft (includes obtaining graft) ③ Ⓣ 80 ▣
MED: 100-2,15,260; 100-4,4,20.5; 100-4,12,90.3; 100-4,14,10
If a tenovaginotomy is performed on the trigger finger, consult CPT code 26055.

26437 Realignment of extensor tendon, hand, each tendon ③ Ⓣ ▣
MED: 100-2,15,260; 100-4,4,20.5; 100-4,12,90.3; 100-4,14,10
AMA: 1998,Nov,8

26440 Tenolysis, flexor tendon; palm OR finger, each tendon ③ Ⓣ ▣
MED: 100-2,15,260; 100-4,4,20.5; 100-4,12,90.3; 100-4,14,10
AMA: 2002,Apr,18

26442 palm AND finger, each tendon ③ Ⓣ ▣
MED: 100-2,15,260; 100-4,4,20.5; 100-4,12,90.3; 100-4,14,10

26445 Tenolysis, extensor tendon, hand OR finger, each tendon ③ Ⓣ ▣
MED: 100-2,15,260; 100-4,4,20.5; 100-4,12,90.3; 100-4,14,10
AMA: 2002,Dec,11; 1998,Nov,8

26449 Tenolysis, complex, extensor tendon, finger, including forearm, each tendon ③ Ⓣ 80 ▣
MED: 100-2,15,260; 100-4,4,20.5; 100-4,12,90.3; 100-4,14,10
AMA: 1998,Nov,8

26450 Tenotomy, flexor, palm, open, each tendon ③ Ⓣ 80 ▣
MED: 100-2,15,260; 100-4,4,20.5; 100-4,12,90.3; 100-4,14,10
AMA: 1998,Nov,8

26455 Tenotomy, flexor, finger, open, each tendon ③ Ⓣ 80 ▣
MED: 100-2,15,260; 100-4,4,20.5; 100-4,12,90.3; 100-4,14,10
AMA: 1998,Nov,8

26460 Tenotomy, extensor, hand or finger, open, each tendon ③ Ⓣ ▣
MED: 100-2,15,260; 100-4,4,20.5; 100-4,12,90.3; 100-4,14,10
AMA: 1998,Nov,8

26471 Tenodesis; of proximal interphalangeal joint, each joint ② Ⓣ 80 ▣
MED: 100-2,15,260; 100-4,4,20.5; 100-4,12,90.3; 100-4,14,10
AMA: 1998,Nov,8

26474 of distal joint, each joint ② Ⓣ 80 ▣
MED: 100-2,15,260; 100-4,4,20.5; 100-4,12,90.3; 100-4,14,10
AMA: 1998,Nov,8

26476 Lengthening of tendon, extensor, hand or finger, each tendon ① Ⓣ ▣
MED: 100-2,15,260; 100-4,4,20.5; 100-4,12,90.3; 100-4,14,10
AMA: 1998,Nov,8

26477 Shortening of tendon, extensor, hand or finger, each tendon ① Ⓣ ▣
MED: 100-2,15,260; 100-4,4,20.5; 100-4,12,90.3; 100-4,14,10
AMA: 1998,Nov,8

26478 Lengthening of tendon, flexor, hand or finger, each tendon ① Ⓣ 80 ▣
MED: 100-2,15,260; 100-4,4,20.5; 100-4,12,90.3; 100-4,14,10
AMA: 1998,Nov,8

26479 Shortening of tendon, flexor, hand or finger, each tendon ① Ⓣ 80 ▣
MED: 100-2,15,260; 100-4,4,20.5; 100-4,12,90.3; 100-4,14,10
AMA: 1998,Nov,8

26480 Transfer or transplant of tendon, carpometacarpal area or dorsum of hand; without free graft, each tendon ③ Ⓣ 80 ▣
MED: 100-2,15,260; 100-4,4,20.5; 100-4,12,90.3; 100-4,14,10
AMA: 1998,Nov,8

26483 with free tendon graft (includes obtaining graft), each tendon ③ Ⓣ 80 ▣
MED: 100-2,15,260; 100-4,4,20.5; 100-4,12,90.3; 100-4,14,10

26485 Transfer or transplant of tendon, palmar; without free tendon graft, each tendon ② Ⓣ 80 ▣
MED: 100-2,15,260; 100-4,4,20.5; 100-4,12,90.3; 100-4,14,10
AMA: 1998,Nov,8

26489 with free tendon graft (includes obtaining graft), each tendon ③ Ⓣ 80 ▣
MED: 100-2,15,260; 100-4,4,20.5; 100-4,12,90.3; 100-4,14,10

26490 Opponensplasty; superficialis tendon transfer type, each tendon ③ Ⓣ 80 ▣
MED: 100-2,15,260; 100-4,4,20.5; 100-4,12,90.3; 100-4,14,10

26492 tendon transfer with graft (includes obtaining graft), each tendon ③ Ⓣ 80 ▣
MED: 100-2,15,260; 100-4,4,20.5; 100-4,12,90.3; 100-4,14,10

26494 hypothenar muscle transfer ③ Ⓣ 80 ▣
MED: 100-2,15,260; 100-4,4,20.5; 100-4,12,90.3; 100-4,14,10

26496 other methods ③ Ⓣ 80 ▣
MED: 100-2,15,260; 100-4,4,20.5; 100-4,12,90.3; 100-4,14,10
If thumb fusion in opposition is performed, consult CPT code 26820.

26497 Transfer of tendon to restore intrinsic function; ring and small finger ③ Ⓣ 80 ▣
MED: 100-2,15,260; 100-4,4,20.5; 100-4,12,90.3; 100-4,14,10
AMA: 1998,Nov,8

26498 all four fingers ④ Ⓣ 80 ▣
MED: 100-2,15,260; 100-4,4,20.5; 100-4,12,90.3; 100-4,14,10

26499 Correction claw finger, other methods ③ Ⓣ 80 ▣
MED: 100-2,15,260; 100-4,4,20.5; 100-4,12,90.3; 100-4,14,10

26500 Reconstruction of tendon pulley, each tendon; with local tissues (separate procedure) ④ Ⓣ 80 ▣
MED: 100-2,15,260; 100-4,4,20.5; 100-4,12,90.3; 100-4,14,10
AMA: 1998,Nov,8

26502 with tendon or fascial graft (includes obtaining graft) (separate procedure) ④ Ⓣ 80 ▣
MED: 100-2,15,260; 100-4,4,20.5; 100-4,12,90.3; 100-4,14,10

~~**26504** with tendon prosthesis (separate procedure)~~
Use 26390.

26508 Release of thenar muscle(s) (eg, thumb contracture) ③ Ⓣ 80 ▣
MED: 100-2,15,260; 100-4,4,20.5; 100-4,12,90.3; 100-4,14,10
AMA: 1998,Nov,8

26510 Cross intrinsic transfer, each tendon ③ Ⓣ 80 ▣
MED: 100-2,15,260; 100-4,4,20.5; 100-4,12,90.3; 100-4,14,10

26516 Capsulodesis, metacarpophalangeal joint; single digit ① Ⓣ 80 ▣
MED: 100-2,15,260; 100-4,4,20.5; 100-4,12,90.3; 100-4,14,10
AMA: 1998,Nov,8

26517 two digits ③ Ⓣ 80 ▣
MED: 100-2,15,260; 100-4,4,20.5; 100-4,12,90.3; 100-4,14,10

26518 three or four digits 3 T 80 ▣

MED: 100-2,15,260; 100-4,4,20.5; 100-4,12,90.3; 100-4,14,10

26520 Capsulectomy or capsulotomy; metacarpophalangeal joint, each joint 3 T ▣

MED: 100-2,15,260; 100-4,4,20.5; 100-4,12,90.3; 100-4,14,10
AMA: 1998,Nov,8

26525 interphalangeal joint, each joint 3 T ▣

MED: 100-2,15,260; 100-4,4,20.5; 100-4,12,90.3; 100-4,14,10
AMA: 2002,Apr,18; 1998,Nov,8
To report a carpometacarpal joint arthroplasty, consult CPT code 25447.

26530 Arthroplasty, metacarpophalangeal joint; each joint 3 T 80 ▣

MED: 100-2,15,260; 100-4,4,20.5; 100-4,12,90.3; 100-4,14,10
AMA: 1998,Nov,8

26531 with prosthetic implant, each joint 7 T 80 ▣

MED: 100-2,15,260; 100-4,4,20.5; 100-4,12,90.3; 100-4,14,10
AMA: 1998,Nov,8

26535 Arthroplasty, interphalangeal joint; each joint 5 T ▣

MED: 100-2,15,260; 100-4,4,20.5; 100-4,12,90.3; 100-4,14,10
AMA: 1998,Nov,8

26536 with prosthetic implant, each joint 5 T 80 ▣

MED: 100-2,15,260; 100-4,4,20.5; 100-4,12,90.3; 100-4,14,10
AMA: 1998,Nov,8

26540 Repair of collateral ligament, metacarpophalangeal or interphalangeal joint 4 T 80 ▣

MED: 100-2,15,260; 100-4,4,20.5; 100-4,12,90.3; 100-4,14,10

26541 Reconstruction, collateral ligament, metacarpophalangeal joint, single; with tendon or fascial graft (includes obtaining graft) 7 T 80 ▣

MED: 100-2,15,260; 100-4,4,20.5; 100-4,12,90.3; 100-4,14,10
AMA: 1997,Jan,3

26542 with local tissue (eg, adductor advancement) 4 T 80 ▣

MED: 100-2,15,260; 100-4,4,20.5; 100-4,12,90.3; 100-4,14,10
AMA: 1997,Jan,3

26545 Reconstruction, collateral ligament, interphalangeal joint, single, including graft, each joint 4 T 80 ▣

MED: 100-2,15,260; 100-4,4,20.5; 100-4,12,90.3; 100-4,14,10

26546 Repair non-union, metacarpal or phalanx, (includes obtaining bone graft with or without external or internal fixation) 4 T 80 50 ▣

MED: 100-2,15,260; 100-4,4,20.5; 100-4,12,90.3; 100-4,14,10

26548 Repair and reconstruction, finger, volar plate, interphalangeal joint 4 T 80 ▣

MED: 100-2,15,260; 100-4,4,20.5; 100-4,12,90.3; 100-4,14,10

26550 Pollicization of a digit 2 T 80 ▣

MED: 100-2,15,260; 100-4,4,20.5; 100-4,12,90.3; 100-4,14,10

26551 Transfer, toe-to-hand with microvascular anastomosis; great toe wrap-around with bone graft C 80 ▣

AMA: 1998,Nov,8, 10-11; 1997,Jun,9; 1997,Apr,7
Do not report 69990 in addition to 26551-26554 as the operating microscope is considered an inclusive component of these procedures.

If a free osteocutaneous flap with microvascular anastomosis is performed on the great toe with web space, consult CPT code 20973.

26553 other than great toe, single C 80 ▣

AMA: 1998,Nov,8, 10-11; 1997,Jun,9; 1997,Apr,7

26554 other than great toe, double C 80 ▣

AMA: 1998,Nov,8, 10-11; 1997,Jun,9; 1997,Apr,7

26555 Transfer, finger to another position without microvascular anastomosis 3 T 80 ▣

MED: 100-2,15,260; 100-4,4,20.5; 100-4,12,90.3; 100-4,14,10
AMA: 1998,Nov,8, 10-11

26556 Transfer, free toe joint, with microvascular anastomosis C 80 ▣

AMA: 1998,Nov,8; 1997,Jun,9; 1997,Apr,7
Do not report 69990 in addition to 26556 as the operating microscope is considered an inclusive component of the surgery. If a great toe-to-hand transfer is performed, consult CPT code 20973.

26560 Repair of syndactyly (web finger) each web space; with skin flaps 2 T 80 ▣

MED: 100-2,15,260; 100-4,4,20.5; 100-4,12,90.3; 100-4,14,10

26561 with skin flaps and grafts 3 T 80 ▣

MED: 100-2,15,260; 100-4,4,20.5; 100-4,12,90.3; 100-4,14,10

26562 complex (eg, involving bone, nails) 4 T 80 ▣

MED: 100-2,15,260; 100-4,4,20.5; 100-4,12,90.3; 100-4,14,10

26565 Osteotomy; metacarpal, each 5 T 80 ▣

MED: 100-2,15,260; 100-4,4,20.5; 100-4,12,90.3; 100-4,14,10
AMA: 1998,Nov,9

26567 phalanx of finger, each 5 T 80 ▣

MED: 100-2,15,260; 100-4,4,20.5; 100-4,12,90.3; 100-4,14,10

26568 Osteoplasty, lengthening, metacarpal or phalanx 3 T 80 ▣

MED: 100-2,15,260; 100-4,4,20.5; 100-4,12,90.3; 100-4,14,10

26580 Repair cleft hand 5 T 80 ▣

MED: 100-2,15,260; 100-4,4,20.5; 100-4,12,90.3; 100-4,14,10
Barsky's procedure

26587 Reconstruction of polydactylous digit, soft tissue and bone 5 T 80 ▣

MED: 100-2,15,260; 100-4,4,20.5; 100-4,12,90.3; 100-4,14,10
AMA: 2001,Oct,10
If an excision is performed on the supernumerary digit, soft tissue only, consult CPT code 11200.

26590 Repair macrodactylia, each digit 5 T 80 ▣

MED: 100-2,15,260; 100-4,4,20.5; 100-4,12,90.3; 100-4,14,10
AMA: 2001,Oct,10

26591 Repair, intrinsic muscles of hand, each muscle 3 T 80 ▣

MED: 100-2,15,260; 100-4,4,20.5; 100-4,12,90.3; 100-4,14,10
AMA: 1998,Nov,8, 11; 1998,May,11; 1998,Jul,11

26593 Release, intrinsic muscles of hand, each muscle 3 T ▣

MED: 100-2,15,260; 100-4,4,20.5; 100-4,12,90.3; 100-4,14,10
AMA: 1998,Nov,8, 11

26596 Excision of constricting ring of finger, with multiple Z-plasties 2 T 80 ▣

MED: 100-2,15,260; 100-4,4,20.5; 100-4,12,90.3; 100-4,14,10
To report the release of scar contracture or graft repairs, consult CPT codes 11041-11042, 14040-14041, or 15120 and 15240.

FRACTURE AND/OR DISLOCATION

26600 Closed treatment of metacarpal fracture, single; without manipulation, each bone T ▣

26605 with manipulation, each bone 2 T ▣

MED: 100-2,15,260; 100-4,4,20.5; 100-4,12,90.3; 100-4,14,10

26607 Closed treatment of metacarpal fracture, with manipulation, with external fixation, each bone 2 T 80 ⬐

MED: 100-2,15,260; 100-4,4,20.5; 100-4,12,90.3; 100-4,14,10

26608 Percutaneous skeletal fixation of metacarpal fracture, each bone 4 T 80 ⬐

MED: 100-2,15,260; 100-4,4,20.5; 100-4,12,90.3; 100-4,14,10

26615 Open treatment of metacarpal fracture, single, with or without internal or external fixation, each bone 4 T ⬐

MED: 100-2,15,260; 100-4,4,20.5; 100-4,12,90.3; 100-4,14,10

26641 Closed treatment of carpometacarpal dislocation, thumb, with manipulation T 80 ⬐

26645 Closed treatment of carpometacarpal fracture dislocation, thumb (Bennett fracture), with manipulation 1 T 80 ⬐

MED: 100-2,15,260; 100-4,4,20.5; 100-4,12,90.3; 100-4,14,10

26650 Percutaneous skeletal fixation of carpometacarpal fracture dislocation, thumb (Bennett fracture), with manipulation, with or without external fixation 2 T ⬐

MED: 100-2,15,260; 100-4,4,20.5; 100-4,12,90.3; 100-4,14,10

26665 Open treatment of carpometacarpal fracture dislocation, thumb (Bennett fracture), with or without internal or external fixation 4 T ⬐

MED: 100-2,15,260; 100-4,4,20.5; 100-4,12,90.3; 100-4,14,10

26670 Closed treatment of carpometacarpal dislocation, other than thumb, with manipulation, each joint; without anesthesia T 80 ⬐

26675 requiring anesthesia 2 T 80 ⬐

MED: 100-2,15,260; 100-4,4,20.5; 100-4,12,90.3; 100-4,14,10

26676 Percutaneous skeletal fixation of carpometacarpal dislocation, other than thumb, with manipulation, each joint 2 T ⬐

MED: 100-2,15,260; 100-4,4,20.5; 100-4,12,90.3; 100-4,14,10

26685 Open treatment of carpometacarpal dislocation, other than thumb; with or without internal or external fixation, each joint 3 T ⬐

26686 complex, multiple or delayed reduction 3 T 80 ⬐

MED: 100-2,15,260; 100-4,4,20.5; 100-4,12,90.3; 100-4,14,10

26700 Closed treatment of metacarpophalangeal dislocation, single, with manipulation; without anesthesia T ⬐

26705 requiring anesthesia 2 T 80 ⬐

MED: 100-2,15,260; 100-4,4,20.5; 100-4,12,90.3; 100-4,14,10

26706 Percutaneous skeletal fixation of metacarpophalangeal dislocation, single, with manipulation 2 T ⬐

MED: 100-2,15,260; 100-4,4,20.5; 100-4,12,90.3; 100-4,14,10

26715 Open treatment of metacarpophalangeal dislocation, single, with or without internal or external fixation 4 T 80 ⬐

MED: 100-2,15,260; 100-4,4,20.5; 100-4,12,90.3; 100-4,14,10

26720 Closed treatment of phalangeal shaft fracture, proximal or middle phalanx, finger or thumb; without manipulation, each T ⬐

26725 with manipulation, with or without skin or skeletal traction, each T ⬐

26727 Percutaneous skeletal fixation of unstable phalangeal shaft fracture, proximal or middle phalanx, finger or thumb, with manipulation, each 7 T ⬐

MED: 100-2,15,260; 100-4,4,20.5; 100-4,12,90.3; 100-4,14,10

26735 Open treatment of phalangeal shaft fracture, proximal or middle phalanx, finger or thumb, with or without internal or external fixation, each 4 T ⬐

MED: 100-2,15,260; 100-4,4,20.5; 100-4,12,90.3; 100-4,14,10

26740 Closed treatment of articular fracture, involving metacarpophalangeal or interphalangeal joint; without manipulation, each T ⬐

26742 with manipulation, each 2 T ⬐

MED: 100-2,15,260; 100-4,4,20.5; 100-4,12,90.3; 100-4,14,10

26746 Open treatment of articular fracture, involving metacarpophalangeal or interphalangeal joint, with or without internal or external fixation, each 5 T ⬐

MED: 100-2,15,260; 100-4,4,20.5; 100-4,12,90.3; 100-4,14,10

26750 Closed treatment of distal phalangeal fracture, finger or thumb; without manipulation, each T ⬐

26755 with manipulation, each T ⬐

26756 Percutaneous skeletal fixation of distal phalangeal fracture, finger or thumb, each 2 T 80 ⬐

MED: 100-2,15,260; 100-4,4,20.5; 100-4,12,90.3; 100-4,14,10

26765 Open treatment of distal phalangeal fracture, finger or thumb, with or without internal or external fixation, each 4 T ⬐

MED: 100-2,15,260; 100-4,4,20.5; 100-4,12,90.3; 100-4,14,10

26770 Closed treatment of interphalangeal joint dislocation, single, with manipulation; without anesthesia T ⬐

26775 requiring anesthesia T ⬐

26776 Percutaneous skeletal fixation of interphalangeal joint dislocation, single, with manipulation 2 T ⬐

MED: 100-2,15,260; 100-4,4,20.5; 100-4,12,90.3; 100-4,14,10

26785 Open treatment of interphalangeal joint dislocation, with or without internal or external fixation, single 2 T ⬐

MED: 100-2,15,260; 100-4,4,20.5; 100-4,12,90.3; 100-4,14,10

ARTHRODESIS

26820 Fusion in opposition, thumb, with autogenous graft (includes obtaining graft) 5 T 80 ⬐

MED: 100-2,15,260; 100-4,4,20.5; 100-4,12,90.3; 100-4,14,10

26841 Arthrodesis, carpometacarpal joint, thumb, with or without internal fixation; 4 T 80 ⬐

MED: 100-2,15,260; 100-4,4,20.5; 100-4,12,90.3; 100-4,14,10

26842 with autograft (includes obtaining graft) 4 T 80 ⬐

MED: 100-2,15,260; 100-4,4,20.5; 100-4,12,90.3; 100-4,14,10

26843 Arthrodesis, carpometacarpal joint, digit, other than thumb, each; 3 T 80 ⬐

MED: 100-2,15,260; 100-4,4,20.5; 100-4,12,90.3; 100-4,14,10

26844 with autograft (includes obtaining graft) 3 T 80 ⬐

MED: 100-2,15,260; 100-4,4,20.5; 100-4,12,90.3; 100-4,14,10

26850 Arthrodesis, metacarpophalangeal joint, with or without internal fixation; 4 T 80 ⬐

MED: 100-2,15,260; 100-4,4,20.5; 100-4,12,90.3; 100-4,14,10

26852   with autograft (includes obtaining graft)   **4** T 80 ▣

MED: 100-2,15,260; 100-4,4,20.5; 100-4,12,90.3; 100-4,14,10

26860   **Arthrodesis, interphalangeal joint, with or without internal fixation;**   **3** T ▣

MED: 100-2,15,260; 100-4,4,20.5; 100-4,12,90.3; 100-4,14,10

+ 26861   each additional interphalangeal joint (List separately in addition to code for primary procedure)   **2** T ▣

MED: 100-2,15,260; 100-4,4,20.5; 100-4,12,90.3; 100-4,14,10

Note that 26861 is an add-on code and must be used in conjunction with 26860.

26862   with autograft (includes obtaining graft)   **4** T 80 ▣

MED: 100-2,15,260; 100-4,4,20.5; 100-4,12,90.3; 100-4,14,10

+ 26863   with autograft (includes obtaining graft), each additional joint (List separately in addition to code for primary procedure)   **3** T 80 ▣

MED: 100-2,15,260; 100-4,4,20.5; 100-4,12,90.3; 100-4,14,10

Note that 26863 is an add-on code and must be used in conjunction with 26862.

AMPUTATION

If the amputation is on the hand through metacarpal bones, consult CPT code 25927.

26910   **Amputation, metacarpal, with finger or thumb (ray amputation), single, with or without interosseous transfer**   **3** T ▣

MED: 100-2,15,260; 100-4,4,20.5; 100-4,12,90.3; 100-4,14,10

If repositioning is performed, consult CPT codes 26550 and 26555.

26951   **Amputation, finger or thumb, primary or secondary, any joint or phalanx, single, including neurectomies; with direct closure**   **2** T ▣

MED: 100-2,15,260; 100-4,4,20.5; 100-4,12,90.3; 100-4,14,10

26952   with local advancement flaps (V-Y, hood)   **4** T ▣

MED: 100-2,15,260; 100-4,4,20.5; 100-4,12,90.3; 100-4,14,10

If repair of a soft tissue defect requiring a split or a full thickness graft or other pedicle flaps is performed, consult CPT codes 15050-15758.

OTHER PROCEDURES

26989   Unlisted procedure, hands or fingers   T

MED: 100-4,4,20.5; 100-4,4,180.3

PELVIS AND HIP JOINT

Codes listed in the Musculoskeletal chapter include the application and removal of the first cast or traction device. Replacement of casts and/or traction devices subsequent to the first should be reported separately. CPT codes for other additional procedures, such as obtaining grafts and external fixation, should only be used if the procedure is not already listed as included as part of the basic procedure. Consult the glossary for terms and definitions and the front matter of this chapter for additional information.

This section includes procedures performed on the head and neck of the femur.

INCISION

If superficial incision and drainage procedures are performed, consult CPT codes 10040-10160.

26990   **Incision and drainage, pelvis or hip joint area; deep abscess or hematoma**   **1** T ▣

MED: 100-2,15,260; 100-4,4,20.5; 100-4,12,90.3; 100-4,14,10

26991   infected bursa   **1** T 80 ▣

MED: 100-2,15,260; 100-4,4,20.5; 100-4,12,90.3; 100-4,14,10

26992   **Incision, bone cortex, pelvis and/or hip joint (eg, osteomyelitis or bone abscess)**   C 80 ▣

AMA: 2002,Jan,10

27000   **Tenotomy, adductor of hip, percutaneous (separate procedure)**   **2** T 50 ▣

MED: 100-2,15,260; 100-4,4,20.5; 100-4,12,90.3; 100-4,14,10

27001   **Tenotomy, adductor of hip, open**   **3** T 80 50 ▣

MED: 100-2,15,260; 100-4,4,20.5; 100-4,12,90.3; 100-4,14,10

27003   **Tenotomy, adductor, subcutaneous, open, with obturator neurectomy**   **3** T 80 50 ▣

MED: 100-2,15,260; 100-4,4,20.5; 100-4,12,90.3; 100-4,14,10

27005   **Tenotomy, hip flexor(s), open (separate procedure)**   C 80 50 ▣

27006   **Tenotomy, abductors and/or extensor(s) of hip, open (separate procedure)**   C 80 50 ▣

27025   **Fasciotomy, hip or thigh, any type**   C 80 50 ▣

27030   **Arthrotomy, hip, with drainage (eg, infection)**   C 80 50 ▣

AMA: 1998,Nov,8

27033   **Arthrotomy, hip, including exploration or removal of loose or foreign body**   **3** T 80 50 ▣

MED: 100-2,15,260; 100-4,4,20.5; 100-4,12,90.3; 100-4,14,10

AMA: 1992,Spring,11

27035   **Denervation, hip joint, intrapelvic or extrapelvic intra-articular branches of sciatic, femoral, or obturator nerves**   **4** T 80 50 ▣

MED: 100-2,15,260; 100-3,160.1; 100-4,4,20.5; 100-4,12,90.3; 100-4,14,10

AMA: 1998,Nov,8

If an obturator neurectomy is performed, consult CPT codes 64763 and 64766.

27036   **Capsulectomy or capsulotomy, hip, with or without excision of heterotopic bone, with release of hip flexor muscles (ie, gluteus medius, gluteus minimus, tensor fascia latae, rectus femoris, sartorius, iliopsoas)**   C 80 50 ▣

EXCISION

27040   **Biopsy, soft tissue of pelvis and hip area; superficial**   **1** T 50 ▣

MED: 100-2,15,260; 100-4,4,20.5; 100-4,12,90.3; 100-4,14,10

27041   deep, subfascial or intramuscular   **2** T 50 ▣

MED: 100-2,15,260; 100-4,4,20.5; 100-4,12,90.3; 100-4,14,10

AMA: 1998,Nov,8

If a needle biopsy of the soft tissue is performed, consult CPT code 20206.

27047   **Excision, tumor, pelvis and hip area; subcutaneous tissue**   **2** T 50 ▣

MED: 100-2,15,260; 100-4,4,20.5; 100-4,12,90.3; 100-4,14,10

AMA: 1998,Nov,8

27048   deep, subfascial, intramuscular   **3** T 80 50 ▣

MED: 100-2,15,260; 100-4,4,20.5; 100-4,12,90.3; 100-4,14,10

27049   **Radical resection of tumor, soft tissue of pelvis and hip area (eg, malignant neoplasm)**   **3** T 80 50 ▣

MED: 100-2,15,260; 100-4,4,20.5; 100-4,12,90.3; 100-4,14,10

AMA: 1998,Nov,8

27050   **Arthrotomy, with biopsy; sacroiliac joint**   **3** T 80 50 ▣

MED: 100-2,15,260; 100-4,4,20.5; 100-4,12,90.3; 100-4,14,10

27052   hip joint   [3] [T] [80] [50]
MED: 100-2,15,260; 100-4,4,20.5; 100-4,12,90.3; 100-4,14,10

27054   Arthrotomy with synovectomy, hip joint   [C] [80] [50]

27060   Excision; ischial bursa   [5] [T] [50]
MED: 100-2,15,260; 100-4,4,20.5; 100-4,12,90.3; 100-4,14,10

27062   trochanteric bursa or calcification   [5] [T] [50]
MED: 100-2,15,260; 100-4,4,20.5; 100-4,12,90.3; 100-4,14,10

27065   Excision of bone cyst or benign tumor; superficial (wing of ilium, symphysis pubis, or greater trochanter of femur) with or without autograft   [5] [T] [80] [50]
MED: 100-2,15,260; 100-4,4,20.5; 100-4,12,90.3; 100-4,14,10

27066   deep, with or without autograft   [5] [T] [80] [50]
MED: 100-2,15,260; 100-4,4,20.5; 100-4,12,90.3; 100-4,14,10

27067   with autograft requiring separate incision   [5] [T] [80] [50]
MED: 100-2,15,260; 100-4,4,20.5; 100-4,12,90.3; 100-4,14,10

27070   Partial excision (craterization, saucerization) (eg, osteomyelitis or bone abscess); superficial (eg, wing of ilium, symphysis pubis, or greater trochanter of femur)   [C] [80] [50]

27071   deep (subfascial or intramuscular)   [C] [80] [50]

27075   Radical resection of tumor or infection; wing of ilium, one pubic or ischial ramus or symphysis pubis   [C] [80]

27076   ilium, including acetabulum, both pubic rami, or ischium and acetabulum   [C] [80]

27077   innominate bone, total   [C] [80]

27078   ischial tuberosity and greater trochanter of femur   [C] [80]

27079   ischial tuberosity and greater trochanter of femur, with skin flaps   [C] [80]

27080   Coccygectomy, primary   [2] [T] [80]
MED: 100-2,15,260; 100-4,4,20.5; 100-4,12,90.3; 100-4,14,10
If this procedure involves a pressure (decubitus) ulcer, consult CPT codes 15920, 15922, and 15931-15958.

INTRODUCTION OR REMOVAL

27086   Removal of foreign body, pelvis or hip; subcutaneous tissue   [1] [T] [80] [50]
MED: 100-2,15,260; 100-4,4,20.5; 100-4,12,90.3; 100-4,14,10
AMA: 1998,Jul,8

27087   deep (subfascial or intramuscular)   [3] [T] [80] [50]
MED: 100-2,15,260; 100-4,4,20.5; 100-4,12,90.3; 100-4,14,10
AMA: 1998,Nov,8

27090   Removal of hip prosthesis; (separate procedure)   [C] [80] [50]

27091   complicated, including total hip prosthesis, methylmethacrylate with or without insertion of spacer   [C] [80] [50]

27093   Injection procedure for hip arthrography; without anesthesia   [N] [50]
To report radiological supervision and interpretation of procedure, consult CPT code 73525. Do not report 77002 with 73525.

27095   with anesthesia   [N] [50]
To report radiological supervision and interpretation of procedure, consult CPT code 73525. Do not report 77002 in addition to 73525.

27096   Injection procedure for sacroiliac joint, arthrography and/or anesthetic/steroid   [B] [50]
AMA: 1999,Nov,12
Report 27096 only with imaging confirmation of intraarticular needle positioning.

To report radiological supervision and interpretation of sacroiliac joint arthrography, consult CPT code 73542.

To report fluoroscopic guidance without formal arthrography, use 77003.

Code 27096 is a unilateral procedure. For bilateral procedure, append modifier 50.

REPAIR, REVISION, AND/OR RECONSTRUCTION

27097   Release or recession, hamstring, proximal   [3] [T] [80] [50]
MED: 100-2,15,260; 100-4,4,20.5; 100-4,12,90.3; 100-4,14,10
AMA: 1998,Nov,8

27098   Transfer, adductor to ischium   [3] [T] [80] [50]
MED: 100-2,15,260; 100-4,4,20.5; 100-4,12,90.3; 100-4,14,10
AMA: 1998,Nov,8

27100   Transfer external oblique muscle to greater trochanter including fascial or tendon extension (graft)   [4] [T] [80] [50]
MED: 100-2,15,260; 100-4,4,20.5; 100-4,12,90.3; 100-4,14,10
Eggers procedure

27105   Transfer paraspinal muscle to hip (includes fascial or tendon extension graft)   [4] [T] [80]
MED: 100-2,15,260; 100-4,4,20.5; 100-4,12,90.3; 100-4,14,10

27110   Transfer iliopsoas; to greater trochanter of femur   [4] [T] [80] [50]
MED: 100-2,15,260; 100-4,4,20.5; 100-4,12,90.3; 100-4,14,10

27111   to femoral neck   [4] [T] [80] [50]
MED: 100-2,15,260; 100-4,4,20.5; 100-4,12,90.3; 100-4,14,10

27120   Acetabuloplasty; (eg, Whitman, Colonna, Haygroves, or cup type)   [C] [80] [50]

27122   resection, femoral head (eg, Girdlestone procedure)   [C] [80] [50]

27125   Hemiarthroplasty, hip, partial (eg, femoral stem prosthesis, bipolar arthroplasty)   [C] [80] [50]
AMA: 1998,Nov,8; 1998,Feb,11; 1992,Spring,8
If prosthetic replacement follows a fracture of the hip, consult CPT code 27236.

27130   Arthroplasty, acetabular and proximal femoral prosthetic replacement (total hip arthroplasty), with or without autograft or allograft   [C] [80] [50]
AMA: 1992,Spring,8

27132   Conversion of previous hip surgery to total hip arthroplasty, with or without autograft or allograft   [C] [80] [50]
AMA: 1992,Spring,11

27134   Revision of total hip arthroplasty; both components, with or without autograft or allograft   [C] [80] [50]

27137   acetabular component only, with or without autograft or allograft   [C] [80] [50]

27138   femoral component only, with or without allograft   [C] [80] [50]

27140   Osteotomy and transfer of greater trochanter of femur (separate procedure)   [C] [80] [50]

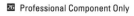 Professional Component Only
[TC] Technical Component Only
[80]/[80] Assist-at-Surgery Allowed/With Documentation
MED: Pub 100/NCD References   AMA: CPT Assistant References
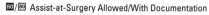 Unlisted   Not Covered
[1]-[9] ASC Group   ♂ Male Only   ♀ Female Only

94 — CPT Expert

27146 Osteotomy, iliac, acetabular or innominate bone; C 80 50 ☐

AMA: 1999,Feb,10
Salter osteotomy

27147 with open reduction of hip C 80 50 ☐

Pemberton osteotomy

27151 with femoral osteotomy C 80 50 ☐

27156 with femoral osteotomy and with open reduction of hip C 80 50 ☐

Chiari osteotomy

27158 Osteotomy, pelvis, bilateral (eg, congenital malformation) C 80 ☐

27161 Osteotomy, femoral neck (separate procedure) C 80 50 ☐

27165 Osteotomy, intertrochanteric or subtrochanteric including internal or external fixation and/or cast C 80 50 ☐

AMA: 1992,Spring,11

27170 Bone graft, femoral head, neck, intertrochanteric or subtrochanteric area (includes obtaining bone graft) C 80 50 ☐

AMA: 1992,Spring,11

27175 Treatment of slipped femoral epiphysis; by traction, without reduction C 80 50 ☐

27176 by single or multiple pinning, in situ C 80 50 ☐

27177 Open treatment of slipped femoral epiphysis; single or multiple pinning or bone graft (includes obtaining graft) C 80 50 ☐

27178 closed manipulation with single or multiple pinning C 80 50 ☐

27179 osteoplasty of femoral neck (Heyman type procedure) C 80 50 ☐

27181 osteotomy and internal fixation C 80 50 ☐

27185 Epiphyseal arrest by epiphysiodesis or stapling, greater trochanter of femur C 50 ☐

27187 Prophylactic treatment (nailing, pinning, plating or wiring) with or without methylmethacrylate, femoral neck and proximal femur C 80 50 ☐

FRACTURE AND/OR DISLOCATION

27193 Closed treatment of pelvic ring fracture, dislocation, diastasis or subluxation; without manipulation 1 T 50 ☐

MED: 100-2,15,260; 100-4,4,20.5; 100-4,12,90.3; 100-4,14,10

27194 with manipulation, requiring more than local anesthesia 2 T 80 ☐

MED: 100-2,15,260; 100-4,4,20.5; 100-4,12,90.3; 100-4,14,10

27200 Closed treatment of coccygeal fracture T ☐

27202 Open treatment of coccygeal fracture 2 T 80 ☐

MED: 100-2,15,260; 100-4,4,20.5; 100-4,12,90.3; 100-4,14,10

27215 Open treatment of iliac spine(s), tuberosity avulsion, or iliac wing fracture(s) (eg, pelvic fracture(s) which do not disrupt the pelvic ring), with internal fixation C 80 ☐

27216 Percutaneous skeletal fixation of posterior pelvic ring fracture and/or dislocation (includes ilium, sacroiliac joint and/or sacrum) T 80 ☐

27217 Open treatment of anterior ring fracture and/or dislocation with internal fixation (includes pubic symphysis and/or rami) C 80 ☐

27218 Open treatment of posterior ring fracture and/or dislocation with internal fixation (includes ilium, sacroiliac joint and/or sacrum) C 80 ☐

27220 Closed treatment of acetabulum (hip socket) fracture(s); without manipulation T 50 ☐

27222 with manipulation, with or without skeletal traction C 50 ☐

27226 Open treatment of posterior or anterior acetabular wall fracture, with internal fixation C 80 50 ☐

27227 Open treatment of acetabular fracture(s) involving anterior or posterior (one) column, or a fracture running transversely across the acetabulum, with internal fixation C 80 50 ☐

27228 Open treatment of acetabular fracture(s) involving anterior and posterior (two) columns, includes T-fracture and both column fracture with complete articular detachment, or single column or transverse fracture with associated acetabular wall fracture, with internal fixation C 80 50 ☐

27230 Closed treatment of femoral fracture, proximal end, neck; without manipulation 1 T 50 ☐

MED: 100-2,15,260; 100-4,4,20.5; 100-4,12,90.3; 100-4,14,10

27232 with manipulation, with or without skeletal traction C 50 ☐

27235 Percutaneous skeletal fixation of femoral fracture, proximal end, neck T 50 ☐

27236 Open treatment of femoral fracture, proximal end, neck, internal fixation or prosthetic replacement C 80 50 ☐

AMA: 1998,Feb,11; 1992,Spring,10

27238 Closed treatment of intertrochanteric, peritrochanteric, or subtrochanteric femoral fracture; without manipulation 1 T 50 ☐

MED: 100-2,15,260; 100-4,4,20.5; 100-4,12,90.3; 100-4,14,10

27240 with manipulation, with or without skin or skeletal traction C 50 ☐

27244 Treatment of intertrochanteric, peritrochanteric, or subtrochanteric femoral fracture; with plate/screw type implant, with or without cerclage C 80 50 ☐

27245 with intramedullary implant, with or without interlocking screws and/or cerclage C 80 50 ☐

27246 Closed treatment of greater trochanteric fracture, without manipulation 1 T 50 ☐

MED: 100-2,15,260; 100-4,4,20.5; 100-4,12,90.3; 100-4,14,10

27248 Open treatment of greater trochanteric fracture, with or without internal or external fixation C 80 50 ☐

27250 Closed treatment of hip dislocation, traumatic; without anesthesia 1 T 50 ☐

MED: 100-2,15,260; 100-4,4,20.5; 100-4,12,90.3; 100-4,14,10

27252 requiring anesthesia 2 T 50 ☐

MED: 100-2,15,260; 100-4,4,20.5; 100-4,12,90.3; 100-4,14,10

27253 Open treatment of hip dislocation, traumatic, without internal fixation C 80 50 ☐

27254 Open treatment of hip dislocation, traumatic, with acetabular wall and femoral head fracture, with or without internal or external fixation C 80 50 ☐

27256 Treatment of spontaneous hip dislocation (developmental, including congenital or pathological), by abduction, splint or traction; without anesthesia, without manipulation T 80 50 ☐

27257   with manipulation, requiring anesthesia   3 T 80 50

MED: 100-2,15,260; 100-4,4,20.5; 100-4,12,90.3; 100-4,14,10

27258   Open treatment of spontaneous hip dislocation (developmental, including congenital or pathological), replacement of femoral head in acetabulum (including tenotomy, etc);   C 80 50

Lorenz's operation

27259   with femoral shaft shortening   C 80 50

27265   Closed treatment of post hip arthroplasty dislocation; without anesthesia   1 T 50

MED: 100-2,15,260; 100-4,4,20.5; 100-4,12,90.3; 100-4,14,10

27266   requiring regional or general anesthesia   2 T 50

MED: 100-2,15,260; 100-4,4,20.5; 100-4,12,90.3; 100-4,14,10

MANIPULATION

27275   Manipulation, hip joint, requiring general anesthesia   2 T

MED: 100-2,15,260; 100-4,4,20.5; 100-4,12,90.3; 100-4,14,10

ARTHRODESIS

27280   Arthrodesis, sacroiliac joint (including obtaining graft)   C 80 50

27282   Arthrodesis, symphysis pubis (including obtaining graft)   C 80

27284   Arthrodesis, hip joint (including obtaining graft);   C 80 50

27286   with subtrochanteric osteotomy   C 80 50

AMPUTATION

27290   Interpelviabdominal amputation (hindquarter amputation)   C 80

Pean's amputation

27295   Disarticulation of hip   C 80

OTHER PROCEDURES

27299   Unlisted procedure, pelvis or hip joint   T 80 50

MED: 100-4,4,20.5; 100-4,4,180.3

FEMUR (THIGH REGION) AND KNEE JOINT

Codes listed in the Musculoskeletal chapter include the application and removal of the first cast or traction device. Replacement of casts and/or traction devices subsequent to the first should be reported separately. CPT codes for other additional procedures, such as obtaining grafts and external fixation, should only be used if the procedure is not already listed as included as part of the basic procedure. Consult the glossary for terms and definitions and the front matter of this chapter for additional information.

This section includes procedures performed on tibial plateaus.

INCISION

If a superficial abscess or hematoma is incised and drained, consult CPT codes 10040-10160.

27301   Incision and drainage, deep abscess, bursa, or hematoma, thigh or knee region   3 T 50

MED: 100-2,15,260; 100-4,4,20.5; 100-4,12,90.3; 100-4,14,10
AMA: 1998,Nov,9

27303   Incision, deep, with opening of bone cortex, femur or knee (eg, osteomyelitis or bone abscess)   C 80 50

AMA: 1998,Nov,8

27305   Fasciotomy, iliotibial (tenotomy), open   2 T 80 50

MED: 100-2,15,260; 100-4,4,20.5; 100-4,12,90.3; 100-4,14,10

If a combined Ober-Yount fasciotomy is performed, consult CPT code 27025.

27306   Tenotomy, percutaneous, adductor or hamstring; single tendon (separate procedure)   3 T 80 50

MED: 100-2,15,260; 100-4,4,20.5; 100-4,12,90.3; 100-4,14,10
AMA: 1998,Nov,8

27307   multiple tendons   3 T 80 50

MED: 100-2,15,260; 100-4,4,20.5; 100-4,12,90.3; 100-4,14,10
AMA: 1998,Nov,8

27310   Arthrotomy, knee, with exploration, drainage, or removal of foreign body (eg, infection)   4 T 80 50

MED: 100-2,15,260; 100-4,4,20.5; 100-4,12,90.3; 100-4,14,10
AMA: 1998,Nov,8

~~**27315**   Neurectomy, hamstring muscle~~

Use 27325.

~~**27320**   Neurectomy, popliteal (gastrocnemius)~~

Use 27326.

EXCISION

27323   Biopsy, soft tissue of thigh or knee area; superficial   1 T 50

MED: 100-2,15,260; 100-4,4,20.5; 100-4,12,90.3; 100-4,14,10
AMA: 1997,Jun,12

If a needle biopsy of soft tissue is performed, consult CPT code 20206.

27324   deep (subfascial or intramuscular)   1 T 50

MED: 100-2,15,260; 100-4,4,20.5; 100-4,12,90.3; 100-4,14,10
AMA: 1998,Nov,8; 1997,Mar,4

● **27325**   Neurectomy, hamstring muscle   2 T

● **27326**   Neurectomy, popliteal (gastrocnemius)   2 T

27327   Excision, tumor, thigh or knee area; subcutaneous   2 T 50

MED: 100-2,15,260; 100-4,4,20.5; 100-4,12,90.3; 100-4,14,10

27328   deep, subfascial, or intramuscular   3 T 50

MED: 100-2,15,260; 100-4,4,20.5; 100-4,12,90.3; 100-4,14,10

27329   Radical resection of tumor (eg, malignant neoplasm), soft tissue of thigh or knee area   4 T 80 50

MED: 100-2,15,260; 100-4,4,20.5; 100-4,12,90.3; 100-4,14,10

27330   Arthrotomy, knee; with synovial biopsy only   4 T 50

MED: 100-2,15,260; 100-4,4,20.5; 100-4,12,90.3; 100-4,14,10

27331   including joint exploration, biopsy, or removal of loose or foreign bodies   4 T 80 50

MED: 100-2,15,260; 100-4,4,20.5; 100-4,12,90.3; 100-4,14,10
AMA: 1998,Nov,8

---

26 Professional Component Only   80/80 Assist-at-Surgery Allowed/With Documentation   Unlisted   Not Covered

TC Technical Component Only   MED: Pub 100/NCD References   AMA: CPT Assistant References   1-9 ASC Group   ♂ Male Only   ♀ Female Only

96 — CPT Expert   CPT only © 2006 American Medical Association. All Rights Reserved. *(Black Ink)*   © *2006 Ingenix (Blue Ink)*

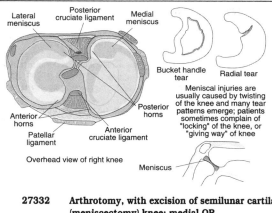

Lateral meniscus • Posterior cruciate ligament • Medial meniscus

Bucket handle tear — Radial tear

Meniscal injuries are usually caused by twisting of the knee and many tear patterns emerge; patients sometimes complain of "locking" of the knee, or "giving way" of knee

Anterior horns • Patellar ligament • Anterior cruciate ligament • Posterior horns

Overhead view of right knee

Meniscus

27332 Arthrotomy, with excision of semilunar cartilage (meniscectomy) knee; medial OR lateral ▪4▪ T 80 50 ▪
MED: 100-2,15,260; 100-4,4,20.5; 100-4,12,90.3; 100-4,14,10
AMA: 1998,Nov,8

27333 medial AND lateral ▪4▪ T 80 50 ▪
MED: 100-2,15,260; 100-4,4,20.5; 100-4,12,90.3; 100-4,14,10

27334 Arthrotomy, with synovectomy, knee; anterior OR posterior ▪4▪ T 80 50 ▪
MED: 100-2,15,260; 100-4,4,20.5; 100-4,12,90.3; 100-4,14,10
AMA: 1998,Nov,8

27335 anterior AND posterior including popliteal area ▪4▪ T 80 50 ▪
MED: 100-2,15,260; 100-4,4,20.5; 100-4,12,90.3; 100-4,14,10

27340 Excision, prepatellar bursa ▪3▪ T 50 ▪
MED: 100-2,15,260; 100-4,4,20.5; 100-4,12,90.3; 100-4,14,10

27345 Excision of synovial cyst of popliteal space (eg, Baker's cyst) ▪4▪ T 80 50 ▪
MED: 100-2,15,260; 100-4,4,20.5; 100-4,12,90.3; 100-4,14,10

27347 Excision of lesion of meniscus or capsule (eg, cyst, ganglion), knee ▪4▪ T 80 50 ▪
MED: 100-2,15,260; 100-4,4,20.5; 100-4,12,90.3; 100-4,14,10
AMA: 1998,Nov,11

27350 Patellectomy or hemipatellectomy ▪4▪ T 80 50 ▪
MED: 100-2,15,260; 100-4,4,20.5; 100-4,12,90.3; 100-4,14,10

27355 Excision or curettage of bone cyst or benign tumor of femur; ▪3▪ T 80 50 ▪
MED: 100-2,15,260; 100-4,4,20.5; 100-4,12,90.3; 100-4,14,10

27356 with allograft ▪4▪ T 80 50 ▪
MED: 100-2,15,260; 100-4,4,20.5; 100-4,12,90.3; 100-4,14,10

27357 with autograft (includes obtaining graft) ▪5▪ T 80 50 ▪
MED: 100-2,15,260; 100-4,4,20.5; 100-4,12,90.3; 100-4,14,10
AMA: 2002,Dec,11

+ **27358** with internal fixation (List in addition to code for primary procedure) ▪5▪ T 80 ▪
MED: 100-2,15,260; 100-4,4,20.5; 100-4,12,90.3; 100-4,14,10
Note that 27358 is an add-on code and must be used in conjunction with 27355, 27356, or 27357.

27360 Partial excision (craterization, saucerization, or diaphysectomy) bone, femur, proximal tibia and/or fibula (eg, osteomyelitis or bone abscess) ▪5▪ T 80 50 ▪
MED: 100-2,15,260; 100-4,4,20.5; 100-4,12,90.3; 100-4,14,10
AMA: 1998,Nov,8

27365 Radical resection of tumor, bone, femur or knee ▪C▪ 80 50 ▪
If a radical resection of a tumor, soft tissue, is performed, consult CPT code 27329.

INTRODUCTION OR REMOVAL

27370 Injection procedure for knee arthrography ▪N▪ 50 ▪
If radiological supervision and interpretation is performed, consult CPT code 73580. Code 77002 cannot be reported in addition to 73580.

27372 Removal of foreign body, deep, thigh region or knee area ▪7▪ T 80 50 ▪
MED: 100-2,15,260; 100-4,12,90.3; 100-4,14,10
If a knee prosthesis, including total knee, is removed, consult CPT code 27488. For arthroscopic knee procedures, consult CPT codes 29870-29887.

REPAIR, REVISION, AND/OR RECONSTRUCTION

27380 Suture of infrapatellar tendon; primary ▪1▪ T 80 50 ▪
MED: 100-2,15,260; 100-4,4,20.5; 100-4,12,90.3; 100-4,14,10

27381 secondary reconstruction, including fascial or tendon graft ▪3▪ T 80 50 ▪
MED: 100-2,15,260; 100-4,4,20.5; 100-4,12,90.3; 100-4,14,10

27385 Suture of quadriceps or hamstring muscle rupture; primary ▪3▪ T 80 50 ▪
MED: 100-2,15,260; 100-4,4,20.5; 100-4,12,90.3; 100-4,14,10

27386 secondary reconstruction, including fascial or tendon graft ▪3▪ T 80 50 ▪
MED: 100-2,15,260; 100-4,4,20.5; 100-4,12,90.3; 100-4,14,10

27390 Tenotomy, open, hamstring, knee to hip; single tendon ▪1▪ T 80 ▪
MED: 100-2,15,260; 100-4,4,20.5; 100-4,12,90.3; 100-4,14,10
AMA: 1998,Nov,8

27391 multiple tendons, one leg ▪2▪ T 80 ▪
MED: 100-2,15,260; 100-4,4,20.5; 100-4,12,90.3; 100-4,14,10
AMA: 1998,Nov,8

27392 multiple tendons, bilateral ▪3▪ T 80 ▪
MED: 100-2,15,260; 100-4,4,20.5; 100-4,12,40.7; 100-4,12,90.3; 100-4,14,10
AMA: 1998,Nov,8

27393 Lengthening of hamstring tendon; single tendon ▪2▪ T 80 ▪
MED: 100-2,15,260; 100-4,4,20.5; 100-4,12,90.3; 100-4,14,10
AMA: 1998,Nov,8

27394 multiple tendons, one leg ▪3▪ T 80 ▪
MED: 100-2,15,260; 100-4,4,20.5; 100-4,12,90.3; 100-4,14,10
AMA: 1998,Nov,8

27395 multiple tendons, bilateral ▪3▪ T 80 ▪
MED: 100-2,15,260; 100-4,4,20.5; 100-4,12,40.7; 100-4,12,90.3; 100-4,14,10
AMA: 1998,Nov,8

27396 Transplant, hamstring tendon to patella; single tendon ▪3▪ T 80 ▪
MED: 100-2,15,260; 100-4,4,20.5; 100-4,12,90.3; 100-4,14,10
AMA: 1998,Nov,8

27397 multiple tendons ▪3▪ T 80 ▪
MED: 100-2,15,260; 100-4,4,20.5; 100-4,12,90.3; 100-4,14,10
AMA: 1998,Nov,8

⊕ Modifier 63 Exempt Code   ⊙ Conscious Sedation   + CPT Add-on Code   ⊘ Modifier 51 Exempt Code   ● New Code   ▲ Revised Code

M Maternity Edit   A Age Edit   A-Y APC Status Indicators   ▪ CCI Comprehensive Code   50 Bilateral Procedure

   CPT only © 2006 American Medical Association. All Rights Reserved. (Black Ink)

27400 Transfer, tendon or muscle, hamstrings to femur (eg, Egger's type procedure) ▣ T 80 50 ▣

MED: 100-2,15,260; 100-4,4,20.5; 100-4,12,90.3; 100-4,14,10
AMA: 1998,Nov,8

27403 Arthrotomy with meniscus repair, knee ▣ T 80 50 ▣

MED: 100-2,15,260; 100-4,4,20.5; 100-4,12,90.3; 100-4,14,10
AMA: 1998,Nov,8

If arthroscopic repair is performed, consult CPT code 29882.

27405 Repair, primary, torn ligament and/or capsule, knee; collateral ▣ T 80 50 ▣

MED: 100-2,15,260; 100-4,4,20.5; 100-4,12,90.3; 100-4,14,10

27407 cruciate ▣ T 80 50 ▣

MED: 100-2,15,260; 100-4,4,20.5; 100-4,12,90.3; 100-4,14,10

27409 collateral and cruciate ligaments ▣ T 80 50 ▣

MED: 100-2,15,260; 100-4,4,20.5; 100-4,12,90.3; 100-4,14,10

To report ligament reconstruction, consult CPT codes 27427-27429

27412 Autologous chondrocyte implantation, knee T 80 50 ▣

Code 27412 cannot be reported with CPT codes 20926, 27331, or 27570.

For harvesting of chondrocytes, consult CPT code 29870.

27415 Osteochondral allograft, knee, open T 80 50 ▣

To report arthroscopic implant of osteochondral allograft, consult CPT code 29867.

27418 Anterior tibial tubercleplasty (eg, Maquet type procedure) ▣ T 80 50 ▣

MED: 100-2,15,260; 100-4,4,20.5; 100-4,12,90.3; 100-4,14,10

27420 Reconstruction of dislocating patella; (eg, Hauser type procedure) ▣ T 80 50 ▣

MED: 100-2,15,260; 100-4,4,20.5; 100-4,12,90.3; 100-4,14,10

27422 with extensor realignment and/or muscle advancement or release (eg, Campbell, Goldwaite type procedure) ▣ T 80 50 ▣

MED: 100-2,15,260; 100-4,4,20.5; 100-4,12,90.3; 100-4,14,10

27424 with patellectomy ▣ T 80 50 ▣

MED: 100-2,15,260; 100-4,4,20.5; 100-4,12,90.3; 100-4,14,10

27425 Lateral retinacular release, open ▣ T 50 ▣

MED: 100-2,15,260; 100-4,4,20.5; 100-4,12,90.3; 100-4,14,10
AMA: 2000,Nov,11

To report arthroscopic lateral release, consult CPT code 29873.

27427 Ligamentous reconstruction (augmentation), knee; extra-articular ▣ T 80 50 ▣

MED: 100-2,15,260; 100-4,4,20.5; 100-4,12,90.3; 100-4,14,10
AMA: 1999,Nov,13

If a primary repair of ligament(s) is performed in addition to reconstruction, report CPT code 27405, 27407, or 27409 in addition to 27427, 27428, or 27429.

27428 intra-articular (open) ▣ T 80 50 ▣

MED: 100-2,15,260; 100-4,4,20.5; 100-4,12,90.3; 100-4,14,10
AMA: 1999,Nov,13

If a primary repair of ligament(s) is performed in addition to reconstruction, report CPT code 27405, 27407, or 27409 in addition to 27427, 27428, or 27429.

27429 intra-articular (open) and extra-articular ▣ T 80 50 ▣

MED: 100-2,15,260; 100-4,4,20.5; 100-4,12,90.3; 100-4,14,10
AMA: 1999,Nov,13

If a primary repair of ligament(s) is performed in addition to reconstruction, report CPT code 27405, 27407, or 27409 in addition to 27427, 27428, or 27429.

27430 Quadricepsplasty (eg, Bennett or Thompson type) ▣ T 80 50 ▣

MED: 100-2,15,260; 100-4,4,20.5; 100-4,12,90.3; 100-4,14,10

27435 Capsulotomy, posterior capsular release, knee ▣ T 80 50 ▣

MED: 100-2,15,260; 100-4,4,20.5; 100-4,12,90.3; 100-4,14,10
AMA: 1998,Nov,8

27437 Arthroplasty, patella; without prosthesis ▣ T 50 ▣

MED: 100-2,15,260; 100-4,4,20.5; 100-4,12,90.3; 100-4,14,10

27438 with prosthesis ▣ T 80 50 ▣

MED: 100-2,15,260; 100-4,4,20.5; 100-4,12,90.3; 100-4,14,10

27440 Arthroplasty, knee, tibial plateau; T 80 50 ▣

27441 with debridement and partial synovectomy ▣ T 80 50 ▣

MED: 100-2,15,260; 100-4,4,20.5; 100-4,12,90.3; 100-4,14,10

27442 Arthroplasty, femoral condyles or tibial plateau(s), knee; ▣ T 80 50 ▣

MED: 100-2,15,260; 100-4,4,20.5; 100-4,12,90.3; 100-4,14,10
AMA: 1999,Nov,13

27443 with debridement and partial synovectomy ▣ T 80 50 ▣

MED: 100-2,15,260; 100-4,4,20.5; 100-4,12,90.3; 100-4,14,10

27445 Arthroplasty, knee, hinge prosthesis (eg, Walldius type) C 80 50 ▣

AMA: 1998,Nov,8

27446 Arthroplasty, knee, condyle and plateau; medial OR lateral compartment T 80 50 ▣

27447 medial AND lateral compartments with or without patella resurfacing (total knee arthroplasty) C 80 50 ▣

If a total knee arthroplasty is revised, consult CPT code 27487. If a total knee prosthesis is removed, consult CPT code 27488.

27448 Osteotomy, femur, shaft or supracondylar; without fixation C 80 50 ▣

27450 with fixation C 80 50 ▣

27454 Osteotomy, multiple, with realignment on intramedullary rod, femoral shaft (eg, Sofield type procedure) C 80 50 ▣

AMA: 1998,Nov,8

27455 Osteotomy, proximal tibia, including fibular excision or osteotomy (includes correction of genu varus (bowleg) or genu valgus (knock-knee)); before epiphyseal closure C 80 50 ▣

27457 after epiphyseal closure C 80 50 ▣

27465 Osteoplasty, femur; shortening (excluding 64876) C 80 50 ▣

27466 lengthening C 80 50 ▣

27468 combined, lengthening and shortening with femoral segment transfer C 80 50 ▣

27470 Repair, nonunion or malunion, femur, distal to head and neck; without graft (eg, compression technique) C 80 50 ▣

▣ Professional Component Only   80/80 Assist-at-Surgery Allowed/With Documentation   ▭ Unlisted ▭   ▭ Not Covered ▭

▣ Technical Component Only   MED: Pub 100/NCD References   AMA: CPT Assistant References   ▣-▣ ASC Group   ♂ Male Only   ♀ Female Only

98 — CPT Expert   CPT only © 2006 American Medical Association. All Rights Reserved. (Black Ink)   © 2006 Ingenix (Blue Ink)

27472   with iliac or other autogenous bone graft (includes obtaining graft)   C 80 50 ▣

27475   Arrest, epiphyseal, any method (eg, epiphysiodesis); distal femur   T 50 ▣

     AMA: 1998,Nov,8

27477   tibia and fibula, proximal   C 50 ▣

27479   combined distal femur, proximal tibia and fibula   C 80 50 ▣

27485   Arrest, hemiepiphyseal, distal femur or proximal tibia or fibula (eg, genu varus or valgus)   C 50 ▣

     AMA: 1998,Nov,8

27486   Revision of total knee arthroplasty, with or without allograft; one component   C 80 50 ▣

27487   femoral and entire tibial component   C 80 50 ▣

     AMA: 1998,Nov,8

27488   Removal of prosthesis, including total knee prosthesis, methylmethacrylate with or without insertion of spacer, knee   C 80 50 ▣

     AMA: 1998,Nov,8

27495   Prophylactic treatment (nailing, pinning, plating or wiring) with or without methylmethacrylate, femur   C 80 50 ▣

27496   Decompression fasciotomy, thigh and/or knee, one compartment (flexor or extensor or adductor);   5 T 50 ▣

     MED: 100-2,15,260; 100-4,4,20.5; 100-4,12,90.3; 100-4,14,10

27497   with debridement of nonviable muscle and/or nerve   3 T 80 50 ▣

     MED: 100-2,15,260; 100-4,4,20.5; 100-4,12,90.3; 100-4,14,10

27498   Decompression fasciotomy, thigh and/or knee, multiple compartments;   3 T 80 50 ▣

27499   with debridement of nonviable muscle and/or nerve   3 T 80 50 ▣

     MED: 100-2,15,260; 100-4,4,20.5; 100-4,12,90.3; 100-4,14,10

FRACTURE AND/OR DISLOCATION

If arthroscopic treatment of the intercondylar spine(s) and tuberosity fracture(s) of the knee is performed, consult CPT codes 29850 and 29851. If arthroscopic treatment of tibial fracture(s) is performed, consult CPT codes 29855 and 29856.

27500   Closed treatment of femoral shaft fracture, without manipulation   1 T 50 ▣

     MED: 100-2,15,260; 100-4,4,20.5; 100-4,12,90.3; 100-4,14,10

27501   Closed treatment of supracondylar or transcondylar femoral fracture with or without intercondylar extension, without manipulation   2 T 80 50 ▣

     MED: 100-2,15,260; 100-4,4,20.5; 100-4,12,90.3; 100-4,14,10

27502   Closed treatment of femoral shaft fracture, with manipulation, with or without skin or skeletal traction   2 T 50 ▣

     MED: 100-2,15,260; 100-4,4,20.5; 100-4,12,90.3; 100-4,14,10
     AMA: 1999,Oct,4; 1993,Fall,22

27503   Closed treatment of supracondylar or transcondylar femoral fracture with or without intercondylar extension, with manipulation, with or without skin or skeletal traction   3 T 80 50 ▣

     MED: 100-2,15,260; 100-4,4,20.5; 100-4,12,90.3; 100-4,14,10

27506   Open treatment of femoral shaft fracture, with or without external fixation, with insertion of intramedullary implant, with or without cerclage and/or locking screws   C 80 50 ▣

     AMA: 1992,Winter,10

27507   Open treatment of femoral shaft fracture with plate/screws, with or without cerclage   C 80 50 ▣

27508   Closed treatment of femoral fracture, distal end, medial or lateral condyle, without manipulation   1 T 50 ▣

     MED: 100-2,15,260; 100-4,4,20.5; 100-4,12,90.3; 100-4,14,10

27509   Percutaneous skeletal fixation of femoral fracture, distal end, medial or lateral condyle, or supracondylar or transcondylar, with or without intercondylar extension, or distal femoral epiphyseal separation   3 T 80 50 ▣

     MED: 100-2,15,260; 100-4,4,20.5; 100-4,12,90.3; 100-4,14,10

27510   Closed treatment of femoral fracture, distal end, medial or lateral condyle, with manipulation   1 T 50 ▣

     MED: 100-2,15,260; 100-4,4,20.5; 100-4,12,90.3; 100-4,14,10

27511   Open treatment of femoral supracondylar or transcondylar fracture without intercondylar extension, with or without internal or external fixation   C 80 50 ▣

27513   Open treatment of femoral supracondylar or transcondylar fracture with intercondylar extension, with or without internal or external fixation   C 80 50 ▣

27514   Open treatment of femoral fracture, distal end, medial or lateral condyle, with or without internal or external fixation   C 80 50 ▣

27516   Closed treatment of distal femoral epiphyseal separation; without manipulation   1 T 50 ▣

     MED: 100-2,15,260; 100-4,4,20.5; 100-4,12,90.3; 100-4,14,10

27517   with manipulation, with or without skin or skeletal traction   1 T 80 50 ▣

     MED: 100-2,15,260; 100-4,4,20.5; 100-4,12,90.3; 100-4,14,10

27519   Open treatment of distal femoral epiphyseal separation, with or without internal or external fixation   C 80 50 ▣

27520   Closed treatment of patellar fracture, without manipulation   1 T 50 ▣

     MED: 100-2,15,260; 100-4,4,20.5; 100-4,12,90.3; 100-4,14,10

27524   Open treatment of patellar fracture, with internal fixation and/or partial or complete patellectomy and soft tissue repair   T 80 50 ▣

27530   Closed treatment of tibial fracture, proximal (plateau); without manipulation   1 T 50 ▣

     MED: 100-2,15,260; 100-4,4,20.5; 100-4,12,90.3; 100-4,14,10

27532   with or without manipulation, with skeletal traction   1 T 50 ▣

     MED: 100-2,15,260; 100-4,4,20.5; 100-4,12,90.3; 100-4,14,10
     If arthroscopic treatment of a tibial fracture is performed, consult CPT codes 29855 and 29856.

27535   Open treatment of tibial fracture, proximal (plateau); unicondylar, with or without internal or external fixation   C 80 50 ▣

     If arthroscopic treatment of a tibial fracture is performed, consult CPT codes 29855 and 29856.

27536   bicondylar, with or without internal fixation   C 80 50 ▣

     If arthroscopic treatment of a tibial fracture is performed, consult CPT codes 29855 and 29856.

Musculoskeletal System

27538 — 27618

27538   Closed treatment of intercondylar spine(s) and/or tuberosity fracture(s) of knee, with or without manipulation   **1** T 80 50 ▣

MED: 100-2,15,260; 100-4,4,20.5; 100-4,12,90.3; 100-4,14,10

If treated arthroscopically, consult CPT codes 29850 and 29851.

27540   Open treatment of intercondylar spine(s) and/or tuberosity fracture(s) of the knee, with or without internal or external fixation   C 80 50 ▣

27550   Closed treatment of knee dislocation; without anesthesia   **1** T 80 50 ▣

MED: 100-2,15,260; 100-4,4,20.5; 100-4,12,90.3; 100-4,14,10

27552   requiring anesthesia   **1** T 80 50 ▣

MED: 100-2,15,260; 100-4,4,20.5; 100-4,12,90.3; 100-4,14,10

27556   Open treatment of knee dislocation, with or without internal or external fixation; without primary ligamentous repair or augmentation/reconstruction   C 80 50 ▣

27557   with primary ligamentous repair   C 80 50 ▣

27558   with primary ligamentous repair, with augmentation/reconstruction   C 80 50 ▣

27560   Closed treatment of patellar dislocation; without anesthesia   **1** T 50 ▣

MED: 100-2,15,260; 100-4,4,20.5; 100-4,12,90.3; 100-4,14,10

If this is a recurrent dislocation, consult CPT codes 27420-27424.

27562   requiring anesthesia   **1** T 80 50 ▣

MED: 100-2,15,260; 100-4,4,20.5; 100-4,12,90.3; 100-4,14,10

27566   Open treatment of patellar dislocation, with or without partial or total patellectomy   **2** T 80 50 ▣

MED: 100-2,15,260; 100-4,4,20.5; 100-4,12,90.3; 100-4,14,10

MANIPULATION

27570   Manipulation of knee joint under general anesthesia (includes application of traction or other fixation devices)   **1** T ▣

MED: 100-2,15,260; 100-4,4,20.5; 100-4,12,90.3; 100-4,14,10

ARTHRODESIS

27580   Arthrodesis, knee, any technique   C 80 50 ▣

Albert's operation

AMPUTATION

27590   Amputation, thigh, through femur, any level;   C 80 50 ▣

27591   immediate fitting technique including first cast   C 80 50 ▣

27592   open, circular (guillotine)   C 80 50 ▣

27594   secondary closure or scar revision   **3** T 50 ▣

MED: 100-2,15,260; 100-4,4,20.5; 100-4,12,90.3; 100-4,14,10

27596   re-amputation   C 50 ▣

27598   Disarticulation at knee   C 80 50 ▣

MED: 100-4,4,20.5; 100-4,4,180.3

Batch-Spittler-McFaddin operation

OTHER PROCEDURES

27599   Unlisted procedure, femur or knee   T 80 50

LEG (TIBIA AND FIBULA) AND ANKLE JOINT

Codes listed in the Musculoskeletal chapter include the application and removal of the first cast or traction device. Replacement of casts and/or traction devices subsequent to the first should be reported separately. CPT codes for other additional procedures, such as obtaining grafts and external fixation, should only be used if the procedure is not already listed as included as part of the basic procedure. Consult the glossary for terms and definitions and the front matter of this chapter for additional information.

INCISION

27600   Decompression fasciotomy, leg; anterior and/or lateral compartments only   **3** T 50 ▣

MED: 100-2,15,260; 100-4,4,20.5; 100-4,12,90.3; 100-4,14,10

If a decompression fasciotomy is performed with debridement, consult CPT codes 27892-27894. If superficial incision and drainage procedures are performed, consult CPT codes 10040-10160.

27601   posterior compartment(s) only   **3** T 50 ▣

MED: 100-2,15,260; 100-4,4,20.5; 100-4,12,90.3; 100-4,14,10

27602   anterior and/or lateral, and posterior compartment(s)   **3** T 80 50 ▣

MED: 100-2,15,260; 100-4,4,20.5; 100-4,12,90.3; 100-4,14,10

27603   Incision and drainage, leg or ankle; deep abscess or hematoma   **2** T 50 ▣

MED: 100-2,15,260; 100-4,4,20.5; 100-4,12,90.3; 100-4,14,10

27604   infected bursa   **2** T 80 50 ▣

MED: 100-2,15,260; 100-4,4,20.5; 100-4,12,90.3; 100-4,14,10

27605   Tenotomy, percutaneous, Achilles tendon (separate procedure); local anesthesia   **1** T 80 50 ▣

MED: 100-2,15,260; 100-4,4,20.5; 100-4,12,90.3; 100-4,14,10

27606   general anesthesia   **1** T 50 ▣

MED: 100-2,15,260; 100-4,4,20.5; 100-4,12,90.3; 100-4,14,10

27607   Incision (eg, osteomyelitis or bone abscess), leg or ankle   **2** T 50 ▣

MED: 100-2,15,260; 100-4,4,20.5; 100-4,12,90.3; 100-4,14,10

27610   Arthrotomy, ankle, including exploration, drainage, or removal of foreign body   **2** T 50 ▣

MED: 100-2,15,260; 100-4,4,20.5; 100-4,12,90.3; 100-4,14,10
AMA: 1998,Nov,9

27612   Arthrotomy, posterior capsular release, ankle, with or without Achilles tendon lengthening   **3** T 80 50 ▣

MED: 100-2,15,260; 100-4,4,20.5; 100-4,12,90.3; 100-4,14,10
AMA: 1998,Nov,8
Consult also CPT code 27685.

EXCISION

27613   Biopsy, soft tissue of leg or ankle area; superficial   T 50 ▣

If a needle biopsy is performed on soft tissue, consult CPT code 20206.

27614   deep (subfascial or intramuscular)   **2** T 50 ▣

MED: 100-2,15,260; 100-4,4,20.5; 100-4,12,90.3; 100-4,14,10
AMA: 1998,Nov,8

27615   Radical resection of tumor (eg, malignant neoplasm), soft tissue of leg or ankle area   **3** T 80 50 ▣

MED: 100-2,15,260; 100-4,4,20.5; 100-4,12,90.3; 100-4,14,10

27618   Excision, tumor, leg or ankle area; subcutaneous tissue   **2** T 50 ▣

MED: 100-2,15,260; 100-4,4,20.5; 100-4,12,90.3; 100-4,14,10

26 Professional Component Only   **80/80** Assist-at-Surgery Allowed/With Documentation   Unlisted   Not Covered

TC Technical Component Only   MED: Pub 100/NCD References   AMA: CPT Assistant References   **1**-**9** ASC Group   ♂ Male Only   ♀ Female Only

100 — CPT Expert   CPT only © 2006 American Medical Association. All Rights Reserved. (Black Ink)   © 2006 Ingenix (Blue Ink)

27619   deep (subfascial or intramuscular) ③ T 50 ▣
MED: 100-2,15,260; 100-4,4,20.5; 100-4,12,90.3; 100-4,14,10

27620   Arthrotomy, ankle, with joint exploration, with or without biopsy, with or without removal of loose or foreign body ④ T 80 50 ▣
MED: 100-2,15,260; 100-4,4,20.5; 100-4,12,90.3; 100-4,14,10

27625   Arthrotomy, with synovectomy, ankle; ④ 80 50 ▣
MED: 100-2,15,260; 100-4,4,20.5; 100-4,12,90.3; 100-4,14,10
AMA: 1998,Nov,8

27626   including tenosynovectomy ④ T 80 50 ▣
MED: 100-2,15,260; 100-4,4,20.5; 100-4,12,90.3; 100-4,14,10

27630   Excision of lesion of tendon sheath or capsule (eg, cyst or ganglion), leg and/or ankle ③ T 50 ▣
MED: 100-2,15,260; 100-4,4,20.5; 100-4,12,90.3; 100-4,14,10

27635   Excision or curettage of bone cyst or benign tumor, tibia or fibula; ③ T 50 ▣
MED: 100-2,15,260; 100-4,4,20.5; 100-4,12,90.3; 100-4,14,10

27637   with autograft (includes obtaining graft) ③ T 80 50 ▣
MED: 100-2,15,260; 100-4,4,20.5; 100-4,12,90.3; 100-4,14,10

27638   with allograft ③ T 80 50 ▣
MED: 100-2,15,260; 100-4,4,20.5; 100-4,12,90.3; 100-4,14,10

27640   Partial excision (craterization, saucerization, or diaphysectomy) bone (eg, osteomyelitis or exostosis); tibia ② T 50 ▣
MED: 100-2,15,260; 100-4,4,20.5; 100-4,12,90.3; 100-4,14,10

27641   fibula ② T 50 ▣
MED: 100-2,15,260; 100-4,4,20.5; 100-4,12,90.3; 100-4,14,10

27645   Radical resection of tumor, bone; tibia C 80 50 ▣

27646   fibula C 80 50 ▣

27647   talus or calcaneus ③ T 80 50 ▣
MED: 100-2,15,260; 100-4,4,20.5; 100-4,12,90.3; 100-4,14,10

INTRODUCTION OR REMOVAL

27648   Injection procedure for ankle arthrography N 80 50 ▣

If radiological supervision and interpretation is performed, consult CPT code 73615. Do not report 77002 with 73615.

If ankle arthroscopy is performed, consult CPT codes 29894-29898.

REPAIR, REVISION, AND/OR RECONSTRUCTION

27650   Repair, primary, open or percutaneous, ruptured Achilles tendon; ③ T 80 50 ▣
MED: 100-2,15,260; 100-4,4,20.5; 100-4,12,90.3; 100-4,14,10

27652   with graft (includes obtaining graft) ③ T 50 ▣
MED: 100-2,15,260; 100-4,4,20.5; 100-4,12,90.3; 100-4,14,10

27654   Repair, secondary, Achilles tendon, with or without graft ③ T 80 50 ▣
MED: 100-2,15,260; 100-4,4,20.5; 100-4,12,90.3; 100-4,14,10

27656   Repair, fascial defect of leg ② T 80 50 ▣
MED: 100-2,15,260; 100-4,4,20.5; 100-4,12,90.3; 100-4,14,10

27658   Repair, flexor tendon, leg; primary, without graft, each tendon ① T 80 ▣
MED: 100-2,15,260; 100-4,4,20.5; 100-4,12,90.3; 100-4,14,10
AMA: 1998,Nov,8

27659   secondary, with or without graft, each tendon ② T 80 ▣
MED: 100-2,15,260; 100-4,4,20.5; 100-4,12,90.3; 100-4,14,10

27664   Repair, extensor tendon, leg; primary, without graft, each tendon ② T 80 ▣
MED: 100-2,15,260; 100-4,4,20.5; 100-4,12,90.3; 100-4,14,10
AMA: 1998,Nov,8

27665   secondary, with or without graft, each tendon ② T 80 ▣
MED: 100-2,15,260; 100-4,4,20.5; 100-4,12,90.3; 100-4,14,10
AMA: 1998,Nov,8

27675   Repair, dislocating peroneal tendons; without fibular osteotomy ② T 80 50 ▣
MED: 100-2,15,260; 100-4,4,20.5; 100-4,12,90.3; 100-4,14,10

27676   with fibular osteotomy ③ T 80 50 ▣
MED: 100-2,15,260; 100-4,4,20.5; 100-4,12,90.3; 100-4,14,10

27680   Tenolysis, flexor or extensor tendon, leg and/or ankle; single, each tendon ③ T ▣
MED: 100-2,15,260; 100-4,4,20.5; 100-4,12,90.3; 100-4,14,10
AMA: 1998,Nov,8

27681   multiple tendons (through separate incision(s)) ② T ▣
MED: 100-2,15,260; 100-4,4,20.5; 100-4,12,90.3; 100-4,14,10
AMA: 1998,Nov,8

27685   Lengthening or shortening of tendon, leg or ankle; single tendon (separate procedure) ③ T 80 ▣
MED: 100-2,15,260; 100-4,4,20.5; 100-4,12,90.3; 100-4,14,10
AMA: 1998,Nov,8

27686   multiple tendons (through same incision), each ③ T ▣
MED: 100-2,15,260; 100-4,4,20.5; 100-4,12,90.3; 100-4,14,10
AMA: 1998,Nov,8

27687   Gastrocnemius recession (eg, Strayer procedure) ③ T 80 50 ▣
MED: 100-2,15,260; 100-4,4,20.5; 100-4,12,90.3; 100-4,14,10
Toe extensors as a group are considered a single tendon when transplanted into midfoot.

27690   Transfer or transplant of single tendon (with muscle redirection or rerouting); superficial (eg, anterior tibial extensors into midfoot) ④ T 80 50 ▣
MED: 100-2,15,260; 100-4,4,20.5; 100-4,12,90.3; 100-4,14,10

27691   deep (eg, anterior tibial or posterior tibial through interosseous space, flexor digitorum longus, flexor hallucis longus, or peroneal tendon to midfoot or hindfoot) ④ T 80 50 ▣
MED: 100-2,15,260; 100-4,4,20.5; 100-4,12,90.3; 100-4,14,10
Barr procedure

+ **27692**   each additional tendon (List separately in addition to code for primary procedure) ③ T 80
MED: 100-2,15,260; 100-4,4,20.5; 100-4,12,90.3; 100-4,14,10
Note that 27692 is an add-on code and must be used in conjunction with 27690 and 27691.

27695   Repair, primary, disrupted ligament, ankle; collateral ② T 50 ▣
MED: 100-2,15,260; 100-4,4,20.5; 100-4,12,90.3; 100-4,14,10

27696   both collateral ligaments ② T 50 ▣
MED: 100-2,15,260; 100-4,4,20.5; 100-4,12,90.3; 100-4,14,10

27698   Repair, secondary, disrupted ligament, ankle, collateral (eg, Watson-Jones procedure) ② T 80 50 ▣
MED: 100-2,15,260; 100-4,4,20.5; 100-4,12,90.3; 100-4,14,10

Musculoskeletal System

27700 — 27816

27700 Arthroplasty, ankle; 5 T 80 50
MED: 100-2,15,260; 100-4,4,20.5; 100-4,12,90.3; 100-4,14,10

27702 with implant (total ankle) C 80 50
27703 revision, total ankle C 80 50

27704 Removal of ankle implant 2 T 50
MED: 100-2,15,260; 100-4,4,20.5; 100-4,12,90.3; 100-4,14,10

27705 Osteotomy; tibia 2 T 80 50
MED: 100-2,15,260; 100-4,4,20.5; 100-4,12,90.3; 100-4,14,10

27707 fibula 2 T 50
MED: 100-2,15,260; 100-4,4,20.5; 100-4,12,90.3; 100-4,14,10

27709 tibia and fibula 2 T 80 50
MED: 100-2,15,260; 100-4,4,20.5; 100-4,12,90.3; 100-4,14,10

27712 multiple, with realignment on intramedullary rod (eg, Sofield type procedure) C 80 50

If an osteotomy is performed to correct genu varus (bowleg) or genu valgus (knock-knee), consult CPT codes 27455-27457.

27715 Osteoplasty, tibia and fibula, lengthening or shortening C 80 50
Anderson tibial lengthening

27720 Repair of nonunion or malunion, tibia; without graft, (eg, compression technique) C 80 50

27722 with sliding graft C 80 50

27724 with iliac or other autograft (includes obtaining graft) C 80 50

27725 by synostosis, with fibula, any method C 80 50

27727 Repair of congenital pseudarthrosis, tibia C 80 50

27730 Arrest, epiphyseal (epiphysiodesis), open; distal tibia 2 T 50
MED: 100-2,15,260; 100-4,4,20.5; 100-4,12,90.3; 100-4,14,10
AMA: 1998,Nov,8

27732 distal fibula 2 T 50
MED: 100-2,15,260; 100-4,4,20.5; 100-4,12,90.3; 100-4,14,10

27734 distal tibia and fibula 2 T 50
MED: 100-2,15,260; 100-4,4,20.5; 100-4,12,90.3; 100-4,14,10

27740 Arrest, epiphyseal (epiphysiodesis), any method, combined, proximal and distal tibia and fibula; 2 T 80 50
MED: 100-2,15,260; 100-4,4,20.5; 100-4,12,90.3; 100-4,14,10
AMA: 1998,Nov,8

27742 and distal femur 2 T 80 50
MED: 100-2,15,260; 100-4,4,20.5; 100-4,12,90.3; 100-4,14,10
If epiphyseal arrest of proximal tibia and fibula is performed, consult CPT code 27477.

27745 Prophylactic treatment (nailing, pinning, plating or wiring) with or without methylmethacrylate, tibia 3 T 80 50
MED: 100-2,15,260; 100-4,4,20.5; 100-4,12,90.3; 100-4,14,10

FRACTURE AND/OR DISLOCATION

27750 Closed treatment of tibial shaft fracture (with or without fibular fracture); without manipulation 1 T 50
MED: 100-2,15,260; 100-4,4,20.5; 100-4,12,90.3; 100-4,14,10
AMA: 1996,Mar,10; 1993,Fall,21; 1992,Winter,10

27752 with manipulation, with or without skeletal traction 1 T 50
MED: 100-2,15,260; 100-4,4,20.5; 100-4,12,90.3; 100-4,14,10
AMA: 1996,Mar,10; 1996,Feb,3; 1993,Fall,21; 1992,Winter,10

27756 Percutaneous skeletal fixation of tibial shaft fracture (with or without fibular fracture) (eg, pins or screws) 3 T 80 50
MED: 100-2,15,260; 100-4,4,20.5; 100-4,12,90.3; 100-4,14,10
AMA: 1992,Winter,10

27758 Open treatment of tibial shaft fracture, (with or without fibular fracture) with plate/screws, with or without cerclage 4 T 80 50
MED: 100-2,15,260; 100-4,4,20.5; 100-4,12,90.3; 100-4,14,10
AMA: 2000,Mar,11; 1992,Winter,10

27759 Treatment of tibial shaft fracture (with or without fibular fracture) by intramedullary implant, with or without interlocking screws and/or cerclage 4 T 80 50
MED: 100-2,15,260; 100-4,4,20.5; 100-4,12,90.3; 100-4,14,10
AMA: 1992,Winter,10

27760 Closed treatment of medial malleolus fracture; without manipulation 1 T 50
MED: 100-2,15,260; 100-4,4,20.5; 100-4,12,90.3; 100-4,14,10

27762 with manipulation, with or without skin or skeletal traction 1 T 50
MED: 100-2,15,260; 100-4,4,20.5; 100-4,12,90.3; 100-4,14,10

27766 Open treatment of medial malleolus fracture, with or without internal or external fixation 3 T 50
MED: 100-2,15,260; 100-4,4,20.5; 100-4,12,90.3; 100-4,14,10

27780 Closed treatment of proximal fibula or shaft fracture; without manipulation 1 T 50
MED: 100-2,15,260; 100-4,4,20.5; 100-4,12,90.3; 100-4,14,10
AMA: 1992,Winter,11

27781 with manipulation 1 T 50
MED: 100-2,15,260; 100-4,4,20.5; 100-4,12,90.3; 100-4,14,10

27784 Open treatment of proximal fibula or shaft fracture, with or without internal or external fixation 3 T 50
MED: 100-2,15,260; 100-4,4,20.5; 100-4,12,90.3; 100-4,14,10
AMA: 2000,Mar,11

27786 Closed treatment of distal fibular fracture (lateral malleolus); without manipulation 1 T 50
MED: 100-2,15,260; 100-4,4,20.5; 100-4,12,90.3; 100-4,14,10

27788 with manipulation 1 T 50
MED: 100-2,15,260; 100-4,4,20.5; 100-4,12,90.3; 100-4,14,10

27792 Open treatment of distal fibular fracture (lateral malleolus), with or without internal or external fixation 3 T 50
MED: 100-2,15,260; 100-4,4,20.5; 100-4,12,90.3; 100-4,14,10

27808 Closed treatment of bimalleolar ankle fracture, (including Potts); without manipulation 1 T 50
MED: 100-2,15,260; 100-4,4,20.5; 100-4,12,90.3; 100-4,14,10

27810 with manipulation 1 T 50
MED: 100-2,15,260; 100-4,4,20.5; 100-4,12,90.3; 100-4,14,10

27814 Open treatment of bimalleolar ankle fracture, with or without internal or external fixation 3 T 80 50
MED: 100-2,15,260; 100-4,4,20.5; 100-4,12,90.3; 100-4,14,10

27816 Closed treatment of trimalleolar ankle fracture; without manipulation 1 T 50
MED: 100-2,15,260; 100-4,4,20.5; 100-4,12,90.3; 100-4,14,10

26 Professional Component Only
TC Technical Component Only

80/80 Assist-at-Surgery Allowed/With Documentation
MED: Pub 100/NCD References **AMA:** CPT Assistant References

Unlisted
Not Covered

1-9 ASC Group ♂ Male Only ♀ Female Only

102 — CPT Expert
CPT only © 2006 American Medical Association. All Rights Reserved. *(Black Ink)*
© 2006 Ingenix *(Blue Ink)*

27818   with manipulation   **1** T 50 ☒
MED: 100-2,15,260; 100-4,4,20.5; 100-4,12,90.3; 100-4,14,10

27822   Open treatment of trimalleolar ankle fracture, with or without internal or external fixation, medial and/or lateral malleolus; without fixation of posterior lip   **3** T 80 50 ☒
MED: 100-2,15,260; 100-4,4,20.5; 100-4,12,90.3; 100-4,14,10

27823   with fixation of posterior lip   **3** T 80 50 ☒
MED: 100-2,15,260; 100-4,4,20.5; 100-4,12,90.3; 100-4,14,10

27824   Closed treatment of fracture of weight bearing articular portion of distal tibia (eg, pilon or tibial plafond), with or without anesthesia; without manipulation   **1** T 50 ☒
MED: 100-2,15,260; 100-4,4,20.5; 100-4,12,90.3; 100-4,14,10

27825   with skeletal traction and/or requiring manipulation   **2** T 80 50 ☒
MED: 100-2,15,260; 100-4,4,20.5; 100-4,12,90.3; 100-4,14,10

27826   Open treatment of fracture of weight bearing articular surface/portion of distal tibia (eg, pilon or tibial plafond), with internal or external fixation; of fibula only   **3** T 80 50 ☒
MED: 100-2,15,260; 100-4,4,20.5; 100-4,12,90.3; 100-4,14,10

27827   of tibia only   **3** T 80 50 ☒
MED: 100-2,15,260; 100-4,4,20.5; 100-4,12,90.3; 100-4,14,10

27828   of both tibia and fibula   **4** T 80 50 ☒
MED: 100-2,15,260; 100-4,4,20.5; 100-4,12,90.3; 100-4,14,10

27829   Open treatment of distal tibiofibular joint (syndesmosis) disruption, with or without internal or external fixation   **2** T 80 50 ☒
MED: 100-2,15,260; 100-4,4,20.5; 100-4,12,90.3; 100-4,14,10
AMA: 1992,Winter,11

27830   Closed treatment of proximal tibiofibular joint dislocation; without anesthesia   **1** T 80 50 ☒
MED: 100-2,15,260; 100-4,4,20.5; 100-4,12,90.3; 100-4,14,10

27831   requiring anesthesia   **1** T 80 50 ☒
MED: 100-2,15,260; 100-4,4,20.5; 100-4,12,90.3; 100-4,14,10

27832   Open treatment of proximal tibiofibular joint dislocation, with or without internal or external fixation, or with excision of proximal fibula   **2** T 80 50 ☒
MED: 100-2,15,260; 100-4,4,20.5; 100-4,12,90.3; 100-4,14,10

27840   Closed treatment of ankle dislocation; without anesthesia   **1** T 50 ☒
MED: 100-2,15,260; 100-4,4,20.5; 100-4,12,90.3; 100-4,14,10

27842   requiring anesthesia, with or without percutaneous skeletal fixation   **1** T 50 ☒
MED: 100-2,15,260; 100-4,4,20.5; 100-4,12,90.3; 100-4,14,10

27846   Open treatment of ankle dislocation, with or without percutaneous skeletal fixation; without repair or internal fixation   **3** T 80 50 ☒
MED: 100-2,15,260; 100-4,4,20.5; 100-4,12,90.3; 100-4,14,10

27848   with repair or internal or external fixation   **3** T 80 50 ☒
MED: 100-2,15,260; 100-4,4,20.5; 100-4,12,90.3; 100-4,14,10

MANIPULATION

27860   Manipulation of ankle under general anesthesia (includes application of traction or other fixation apparatus)   **1** T 80 ☒
MED: 100-2,15,260; 100-4,4,20.5; 100-4,12,90.3; 100-4,14,10

ARTHRODESIS

27870   Arthrodesis, ankle, open   **4** T 80 50 ☒
MED: 100-2,15,260; 100-4,4,20.5; 100-4,12,90.3; 100-4,14,10
To report arthroscopic ankle arthrodesis, consult CPT code 29899.

27871   Arthrodesis, tibiofibular joint, proximal or distal   **4** T 80 50 ☒
MED: 100-2,15,260; 100-4,4,20.5; 100-4,12,90.3; 100-4,14,10

AMPUTATION

27880   Amputation, leg, through tibia and fibula;   C 80 70 ☒
Burgess amputation

27881   with immediate fitting technique including application of first cast   C 80 70 ☒

27882   open, circular (guillotine)   C 80 70 ☒

27884   secondary closure or scar revision   **3** T 70 ☒
MED: 100-2,15,260; 100-4,4,20.5; 100-4,12,90.3; 100-4,14,10

27886   re-amputation   C 50 ☒

27888   Amputation, ankle, through malleoli of tibia and fibula (eg, Syme, Pirogoff type procedures), with plastic closure and resection of nerves   C 80 70 ☒

27889   Ankle disarticulation   **3** T 70 ☒
MED: 100-2,15,260; 100-4,4,20.5; 100-4,12,90.3; 100-4,14,10

OTHER PROCEDURES

27892   Decompression fasciotomy, leg; anterior and/or lateral compartments only, with debridement of nonviable muscle and/or nerve   **3** T 80 50 ☒
MED: 100-2,15,260; 100-4,4,20.5; 100-4,12,90.3; 100-4,14,10
If decompression fasciotomy without debridement, is performed on the leg, consult CPT code 27600.

27893   posterior compartment(s) only, with debridement of nonviable muscle and/or nerve   **3** T 80 50 ☒
MED: 100-2,15,260; 100-4,4,20.5; 100-4,12,90.3; 100-4,14,10
If decompression fasciotomy without debridement, is performed on the leg, consult CPT code 27601.

27894   anterior and/or lateral, and posterior compartment(s), with debridement of nonviable muscle and/or nerve   **3** T 80 50 ☒
MED: 100-2,15,260; 100-4,4,20.5; 100-4,12,90.3; 100-4,14,10
If decompression fasciotomy without debridement, is performed on the leg, consult CPT code 27602.

27899   Unlisted procedure, leg or ankle   T 80 50
AMA: 2000,Aug,11

FOOT AND TOES

Codes listed in the Musculoskeletal chapter include the application and removal of the first cast or traction device. Replacement of casts and/or traction devices subsequent to the first should be reported separately. CPT codes for other additional procedures, such as obtaining grafts and external fixation, should only be used if the procedure is not already listed as included as part of the basic procedure. Consult the glossary for terms and definitions and the front matter of this chapter for additional information.

INCISION

If superficial incision and drainage procedures are performed, consult CPT codes 10040-10160

28001   Incision and drainage, bursa, foot   T ☒
AMA: 1998,Nov,9

28002 Incision and drainage below fascia, with or without tendon sheath involvement, foot; single bursal space ▨ T ▨
MED: 100-2,15,260; 100-4,4,20.5; 100-4,12,90.3; 100-4,14,10
AMA: 1998,Nov,8

28003 multiple areas ▨ T ▨
MED: 100-2,15,260; 100-4,4,20.5; 100-4,12,90.3; 100-4,14,10
AMA: 1998,Nov,9

28005 Incision, bone cortex (eg, osteomyelitis or bone abscess), foot ▨ T ▨
MED: 100-2,15,260; 100-4,4,20.5; 100-4,12,90.3; 100-4,14,10
AMA: 1998,Nov,9

28008 Fasciotomy, foot and/or toe ▨ T ▨ ▨
MED: 100-2,15,260; 100-4,4,20.5; 100-4,12,90.3; 100-4,14,10
Consult also CPT codes 28060, 28062, and 28250.

28010 Tenotomy, percutaneous, toe; single tendon T ▨
AMA: 1998,Nov,8

28011 multiple tendons ▨ T ▨
MED: 100-2,15,260; 100-4,4,20.5; 100-4,12,90.3; 100-4,14,10
AMA: 1998,Nov,8
If an open tenotomy is performed, consult CPT codes 28230-28234.

28020 Arthrotomy, including exploration, drainage, or removal of loose or foreign body; intertarsal or tarsometatarsal joint ▨ T ▨
MED: 100-2,15,260; 100-4,4,20.5; 100-4,12,90.3; 100-4,14,10

28022 metatarsophalangeal joint ▨ T ▨
MED: 100-2,15,260; 100-4,4,20.5; 100-4,12,90.3; 100-4,14,10

28024 interphalangeal joint ▨ T ▨
MED: 100-2,15,260; 100-4,4,20.5; 100-4,12,90.3; 100-4,14,10

~~**28030** Neurectomy, intrinsic musculature of foot~~
Use 28055.

28035 Release, tarsal tunnel (posterior tibial nerve decompression) ▨ T ▨
MED: 100-2,15,260; 100-4,4,20.5; 100-4,12,90.3; 100-4,14,10
AMA: 1998,Nov,8
If other nerves are entrapped, consult CPT codes 64704 and 64722.

EXCISION

28043 Excision, tumor, foot; subcutaneous tissue ▨ T ▨
MED: 100-2,15,260; 100-4,4,20.5; 100-4,12,90.3; 100-4,14,10

28045 deep, subfascial, intramuscular ▨ T ▨ ▨ ▨
MED: 100-2,15,260; 100-4,4,20.5; 100-4,12,90.3; 100-4,14,10

28046 Radical resection of tumor (eg, malignant neoplasm), soft tissue of foot ▨ T ▨ ▨
MED: 100-2,15,260; 100-4,4,20.5; 100-4,12,90.3; 100-4,14,10

28050 Arthrotomy with biopsy; intertarsal or tarsometatarsal joint ▨ T ▨ ▨
MED: 100-2,15,260; 100-4,4,20.5; 100-4,12,90.3; 100-4,14,10

28052 metatarsophalangeal joint ▨ T ▨ ▨
MED: 100-2,15,260; 100-4,4,20.5; 100-4,12,90.3; 100-4,14,10

28054 interphalangeal joint ▨ T ▨ ▨ ▨
MED: 100-2,15,260; 100-4,4,20.5; 100-4,12,90.3; 100-4,14,10

● **28055** Neurectomy, intrinsic musculature of foot ▨ T

28060 Fasciectomy, plantar fascia; partial (separate procedure) ▨ T ▨ ▨
MED: 100-2,15,260; 100-4,4,20.5; 100-4,12,90.3; 100-4,14,10

28062 radical (separate procedure) ▨ T ▨
MED: 100-2,15,260; 100-4,4,20.5; 100-4,12,90.3; 100-4,14,10
If a plantar fasciotomy is performed, consult CPT codes 28008 and 28250.

28070 Synovectomy; intertarsal or tarsometatarsal joint, each ▨ T ▨
MED: 100-2,15,260; 100-4,4,20.5; 100-4,12,90.3; 100-4,14,10

28072 metatarsophalangeal joint, each ▨ T ▨
MED: 100-2,15,260; 100-4,4,20.5; 100-4,12,90.3; 100-4,14,10

Plantar view of right foot showing common location of Morton neuroma

Morton neuroma is a chronic inflammation or irritation of the nerves in the web space between the heads of the metatarsals and phalanges

28080 Excision, interdigital (Morton) neuroma, single, each ▨ T ▨ ▨
MED: 100-2,15,260; 100-4,4,20.5; 100-4,12,90.3; 100-4,14,10

28086 Synovectomy, tendon sheath, foot; flexor ▨ T ▨ ▨ ▨
MED: 100-2,15,260; 100-4,4,20.5; 100-4,12,90.3; 100-4,14,10

28088 extensor ▨ T ▨ ▨ ▨
MED: 100-2,15,260; 100-4,4,20.5; 100-4,12,90.3; 100-4,14,10

28090 Excision of lesion, tendon, tendon sheath, or capsule (including synovectomy) (eg, cyst or ganglion); foot ▨ T ▨ ▨
MED: 100-2,15,260; 100-4,4,20.5; 100-4,12,90.3; 100-4,14,10
AMA: 1998,Nov,8

28092 toe(s), each ▨ T ▨
MED: 100-2,15,260; 100-4,4,20.5; 100-4,12,90.3; 100-4,14,10

28100 Excision or curettage of bone cyst or benign tumor, talus or calcaneus; ▨ T ▨ ▨ ▨
MED: 100-2,15,260; 100-4,4,20.5; 100-4,12,90.3; 100-4,14,10

28102 with iliac or other autograft (includes obtaining graft) ▨ T ▨ ▨ ▨
MED: 100-2,15,260; 100-4,4,20.5; 100-4,12,90.3; 100-4,14,10

28103 with allograft ▨ T ▨ ▨ ▨
MED: 100-2,15,260; 100-4,4,20.5; 100-4,12,90.3; 100-4,14,10

28104 Excision or curettage of bone cyst or benign tumor, tarsal or metatarsal, except talus or calcaneus; ▨ T ▨ ▨
MED: 100-2,15,260; 100-4,4,20.5; 100-4,12,90.3; 100-4,14,10

28106 with iliac or other autograft (includes obtaining graft) ▨ T ▨ ▨
MED: 100-2,15,260; 100-4,4,20.5; 100-4,12,90.3; 100-4,14,10

28107 with allograft ▨ T ▨ ▨
MED: 100-2,15,260; 100-4,4,20.5; 100-4,12,90.3; 100-4,14,10

28108 Excision or curettage of bone cyst or benign tumor, phalanges of foot ▨ T ▨
If a partial ostectomy (e.g., hallux valgus, Silver type procedure) is performed, consult CPT code 28290.

28110 Ostectomy, partial excision, fifth metatarsal head (bunionette) (separate procedure) 3 T 50

MED: 100-2,15,260; 100-4,4,20.5; 100-4,12,90.3; 100-4,14,10
AMA: 2000,Sep,9; 1998,Oct,10

28111 Ostectomy, complete excision; first metatarsal head 3 T 50

MED: 100-2,15,260; 100-4,4,20.5; 100-4,12,90.3; 100-4,14,10

28112 other metatarsal head (second, third or fourth) 3 T 50

MED: 100-2,15,260; 100-4,4,20.5; 100-4,12,90.3; 100-4,14,10

28113 fifth metatarsal head 3 T 80 50

MED: 100-2,15,260; 100-4,4,20.5; 100-4,12,90.3; 100-4,14,10

28114 all metatarsal heads, with partial proximal phalangectomy, excluding first metatarsal (eg, Clayton type procedure) 3 T 80 50

MED: 100-2,15,260; 100-4,4,20.5; 100-4,12,90.3; 100-4,14,10

28116 Ostectomy, excision of tarsal coalition 3 T 50

MED: 100-2,15,260; 100-4,4,20.5; 100-4,12,90.3; 100-4,14,10

28118 Ostectomy, calcaneus; 4 T 80 50

MED: 100-2,15,260; 100-4,4,20.5; 100-4,12,90.3; 100-4,14,10

28119 for spur, with or without plantar fascial release 4 T 50

MED: 100-2,15,260; 100-4,4,20.5; 100-4,12,90.3; 100-4,14,10

28120 Partial excision (craterization, saucerization, sequestrectomy, or diaphysectomy) bone (eg, osteomyelitis or bossing); talus or calcaneus 7 T 50

MED: 100-2,15,260; 100-4,4,20.5; 100-4,12,90.3; 100-4,14,10
Barker operation

28122 tarsal or metatarsal bone, except talus or calcaneus 3 T 80 50

MED: 100-2,15,260; 100-4,4,20.5; 100-4,12,90.3; 100-4,14,10
AMA: 1998,Nov,11
If a partial excision of talus or calcaneus is performed, consult CPT code 28120. If a cheilectomy is performed for hallux rigidus, consult CPT code 28289.

28124 phalanx of toe T 50

28126 Resection, partial or complete, phalangeal base, each toe 3 T

MED: 100-2,15,260; 100-4,4,20.5; 100-4,12,90.3; 100-4,14,10
AMA: 1998,Nov,8

28130 Talectomy (astragalectomy) 3 T 80 50

MED: 100-2,15,260; 100-4,4,20.5; 100-4,12,90.3; 100-4,14,10
Whitman astragalectomy

28140 Metatarsectomy 3 T

MED: 100-2,15,260; 100-4,4,20.5; 100-4,12,90.3; 100-4,14,10

28150 Phalangectomy, toe, each toe 3 T

MED: 100-2,15,260; 100-4,4,20.5; 100-4,12,90.3; 100-4,14,10
AMA: 1998,Nov,8

28153 Resection, condyle(s), distal end of phalanx, each toe 3 T

MED: 100-2,15,260; 100-4,4,20.5; 100-4,12,90.3; 100-4,14,10
AMA: 1998,Nov,8

28160 Hemiphalangectomy or interphalangeal joint excision, toe, proximal end of phalanx, each 3 T

MED: 100-2,15,260; 100-4,4,20.5; 100-4,12,90.3; 100-4,14,10
AMA: 1998,Nov,8

28171 Radical resection of tumor, bone; tarsal (except talus or calcaneus) 3 T 80

MED: 100-2,15,260; 100-4,4,20.5; 100-4,12,90.3; 100-4,14,10

28173 metatarsal 3 T

MED: 100-2,15,260; 100-4,4,20.5; 100-4,12,90.3; 100-4,14,10

28175 phalanx of toe 3 T

MED: 100-2,15,260; 100-4,4,20.5; 100-4,12,90.3; 100-4,14,10
If a radical resection of a talus or a calcaneus tumor is performed, consult CPT code 27647.

INTRODUCTION OR REMOVAL

28190 Removal of foreign body, foot; subcutaneous T 50

28192 deep 2 T 50

MED: 100-2,15,260; 100-4,4,20.5; 100-4,12,90.3; 100-4,14,10

28193 complicated 4 T 50

MED: 100-2,15,260; 100-4,4,20.5; 100-4,12,90.3; 100-4,14,10

REPAIR, REVISION, AND/OR RECONSTRUCTION

28200 Repair, tendon, flexor, foot; primary or secondary, without free graft, each tendon 3 T

MED: 100-2,15,260; 100-4,4,20.5; 100-4,12,90.3; 100-4,14,10
AMA: 1998,Nov,8

28202 secondary with free graft, each tendon (includes obtaining graft) 3 T 80

MED: 100-2,15,260; 100-4,4,20.5; 100-4,12,90.3; 100-4,14,10

28208 Repair, tendon, extensor, foot; primary or secondary, each tendon 3 T

MED: 100-2,15,260; 100-4,4,20.5; 100-4,12,90.3; 100-4,14,10
AMA: 1998,Nov,8

28210 secondary with free graft, each tendon (includes obtaining graft) 3 T 80

MED: 100-2,15,260; 100-4,4,20.5; 100-4,12,90.3; 100-4,14,10

28220 Tenolysis, flexor, foot; single tendon T

AMA: 1998,Nov,8

28222 multiple tendons 1 T

MED: 100-2,15,260; 100-4,4,20.5; 100-4,12,90.3; 100-4,14,10
AMA: 1998,Nov,8

28225 Tenolysis, extensor, foot; single tendon 1 T

MED: 100-2,15,260; 100-4,4,20.5; 100-4,12,90.3; 100-4,14,10
AMA: 1998,Nov,8

28226 multiple tendons 1 T

MED: 100-2,15,260; 100-4,4,20.5; 100-4,12,90.3; 100-4,14,10
AMA: 1998,Nov,8

28230 Tenotomy, open, tendon flexor; foot, single or multiple tendon(s) (separate procedure) T

AMA: 1998,Nov,8

28232 toe, single tendon (separate procedure) T

AMA: 1998,Nov,8

28234 Tenotomy, open, extensor, foot or toe, each tendon 2 T

MED: 100-2,15,260; 100-4,4,20.5; 100-4,12,90.3; 100-4,14,10
AMA: 1998,Nov,8

28238 Reconstruction (advancement), posterior tibial tendon with excision of accessory tarsal navicular bone (eg, Kidner type procedure) 3 T 80 50

MED: 100-2,15,260; 100-4,4,20.5; 100-4,12,90.3; 100-4,14,10
If a subcutaneous tenotomy is performed, consult CPT codes 28010 and 28011. If a transfer or transplant of a tendon with muscle redirection or rerouting is performed, consult CPT codes 27690-27692. If an extensor hallucis longus transfer with a great toe IP fusion (Jones procedure) is performed, consult CPT code 28760.

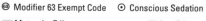

28240 Tenotomy, lengthening, or release, abductor hallucis muscle   2 T 50

MED: 100-2,15,260; 100-4,4,20.5; 100-4,12,90.3; 100-4,14,10

28250 Division of plantar fascia and muscle (eg, Steindler stripping) (separate procedure)   3 T 80 50

MED: 100-2,15,260; 100-4,4,20.5; 100-4,12,90.3; 100-4,14,10

28260 Capsulotomy, midfoot; medial release only (separate procedure)   3 T 80 50

MED: 100-2,15,260; 100-4,4,20.5; 100-4,12,90.3; 100-4,14,10

28261 with tendon lengthening   3 T 80 50

MED: 100-2,15,260; 100-4,4,20.5; 100-4,12,90.3; 100-4,14,10

28262 extensive, including posterior talotibial capsulotomy and tendon(s) lengthening (eg, resistant clubfoot deformity)   4 T 80 50

MED: 100-2,15,260; 100-4,4,20.5; 100-4,12,90.3; 100-4,14,10

28264 Capsulotomy, midtarsal (eg, Heyman type procedure)   1 T 80 50

MED: 100-2,15,260; 100-4,4,20.5; 100-4,12,90.3; 100-4,14,10

Cuneiform bones; Metatarsals; Phalanges; Cuboid; Metatarso-phalangeal joint; Metatarso-phalangeal joint; Interphalangeal joints; Tenorrhaphy

Tarsals, metatarsals, and phalanges

The metatarsophalangeal joint capsule is incised (capsulotomy)

28270 Capsulotomy; metatarsophalangeal joint, with or without tenorrhaphy, each joint (separate procedure)   3 T 50

MED: 100-2,15,260; 100-4,4,20.5; 100-4,12,90.3; 100-4,14,10

28272 interphalangeal joint, each joint (separate procedure)   T 50

AMA: 2002,Dec,11

28280 Syndactylization, toes (eg, webbing or Kelikian type procedure)   2 T 80 50

MED: 100-2,15,260; 100-4,4,20.5; 100-4,12,90.3; 100-4,14,10
AMA: 1998,Nov,8

28285 Correction, hammertoe (eg, interphalangeal fusion, partial or total phalangectomy)   3 T 50

MED: 100-2,15,260; 100-4,4,20.5; 100-4,12,90.3; 100-4,14,10
AMA: 1998,Nov,8

28286 Correction, cock-up fifth toe, with plastic skin closure (eg, Ruiz-Mora type procedure)   4 T

MED: 100-2,15,260; 100-4,4,20.5; 100-4,12,90.3; 100-4,14,10
AMA: 1998,Nov,8

28288 Ostectomy, partial, exostectomy or condylectomy, metatarsal head, each metatarsal head   3 T

MED: 100-2,15,260; 100-4,4,20.5; 100-4,12,90.3; 100-4,14,10

28289 Hallux rigidus correction with cheilectomy, debridement and capsular release of the first metatarsophalangeal joint   3 T 80 50

MED: 100-2,15,260; 100-4,4,20.5; 100-4,12,90.3; 100-4,14,10
AMA: 1998,Nov,11

Hallux valgus bunion; Medial emminence of metatarsal bone; Right foot; Base of proximal phalanx is resected; A portion of the metatarsal head is resected; Correction of hallux valgus bunion by resection of joint; Kirshner wires stabilize the osteotomy; Keller type approach; Prosthetic implant placed in the joint

28290 Correction, hallux valgus (bunion), with or without sesamoidectomy; simple exostectomy (eg, Silver type procedure)   2 T 50

MED: 100-2,15,260; 100-4,4,20.5; 100-4,12,90.3; 100-4,14,10
AMA: 1996,Dec,5

Hallux valgus bunion; Medial emminence of metatarsal bone; Right foot; Base of proximal phalanx is resected; A portion of the metatarsal head is resected; Correction of hallux valgus bunion by resection of joint; Kirshner wires stabilize the osteotomy; Keller type approach; Prosthetic implant placed in the joint

28292 Keller, McBride, or Mayo type procedure   2 T 80 50

MED: 100-2,15,260; 100-4,4,20.5; 100-4,12,90.3; 100-4,14,10
AMA: 2000,Sep,9; 1996,Dec,5

28293 resection of joint with implant   3 T 80 50

MED: 100-2,15,260; 100-4,4,20.5; 100-4,12,90.3; 100-4,14,10
AMA: 1996,Dec,6

28294 with tendon transplants (eg, Joplin type procedure)   3 T 80 50

MED: 100-2,15,260; 100-4,4,20.5; 100-4,12,90.3; 100-4,14,10
AMA: 1996,Dec,6

28296 with metatarsal osteotomy (eg, Mitchell, Chevron, or concentric type procedures)   3 T 80 50

MED: 100-2,15,260; 100-4,4,20.5; 100-4,12,90.3; 100-4,14,10
AMA: 1997,Jan,10; 1996,Dec,6

28297 Lapidus-type procedure   3 T 80 50

MED: 100-2,15,260; 100-4,4,20.5; 100-4,12,90.3; 100-4,14,10
AMA: 1996,Dec,6

28298 by phalanx osteotomy   3 T 80 50

MED: 100-2,15,260; 100-4,4,20.5; 100-4,12,90.3; 100-4,14,10
AMA: 1996,Dec,7

28299 by double osteotomy   5 T 80 50

MED: 100-2,15,260; 100-4,4,20.5; 100-4,12,90.3; 100-4,14,10
AMA: 1996,Dec,7

28300 Osteotomy; calcaneus (eg, Dwyer or Chambers type procedure), with or without internal fixation   2 T 80 50

MED: 100-2,15,260; 100-4,4,20.5; 100-4,12,90.3; 100-4,14,10

28302 talus   2 T 80 50

MED: 100-2,15,260; 100-4,4,20.5; 100-4,12,90.3; 100-4,14,10

28304 Osteotomy, tarsal bones, other than calcaneus or talus; ☑2 T 80 50 ▱

MED: 100-2,15,260; 100-4,4,20.5; 100-4,12,90.3; 100-4,14,10
AMA: 1998,Nov,8

28305 with autograft (includes obtaining graft) (eg, Fowler type) ☑3 T 80 50 ▱

MED: 100-2,15,260; 100-4,4,20.5; 100-4,12,90.3; 100-4,14,10

28306 Osteotomy, with or without lengthening, shortening or angular correction, metatarsal; first metatarsal ☑4 T 80 50 ▱

MED: 100-2,15,260; 100-4,4,20.5; 100-4,12,90.3; 100-4,14,10
AMA: 1999,Dec,7; 1998,Nov,8

28307 first metatarsal with autograft (other than first toe) ☑4 T 80 50 ▱

MED: 100-2,15,260; 100-4,4,20.5; 100-4,12,90.3; 100-4,14,10
AMA: 1998,Nov,9

28308 other than first metatarsal, each ☑2 T 80 50 ▱

MED: 100-2,15,260; 100-4,4,20.5; 100-4,12,90.3; 100-4,14,10

28309 multiple (eg, Swanson type cavus foot procedure) ☑4 T 80 50 ▱

MED: 100-2,15,260; 100-4,4,20.5; 100-4,12,90.3; 100-4,14,10
AMA: 1999,Dec,7; 1998,Nov,8

28310 Osteotomy, shortening, angular or rotational correction; proximal phalanx, first toe (separate procedure) ☑3 T ▱

MED: 100-2,15,260; 100-4,4,20.5; 100-4,12,90.3; 100-4,14,10

28312 other phalanges, any toe ☑3 T ▱

MED: 100-2,15,260; 100-4,4,20.5; 100-4,12,90.3; 100-4,14,10

28313 Reconstruction, angular deformity of toe, soft tissue procedures only (eg, overlapping second toe, fifth toe, curly toes) ☑2 T ▱

MED: 100-2,15,260; 100-4,4,20.5; 100-4,12,90.3; 100-4,14,10
AMA: 1998,Nov,8

28315 Sesamoidectomy, first toe (separate procedure) ☑4 T 50 ▱

MED: 100-2,15,260; 100-4,4,20.5; 100-4,12,90.3; 100-4,14,10

28320 Repair, nonunion or malunion; tarsal bones ☑4 T 80 ▱

MED: 100-2,15,260; 100-4,4,20.5; 100-4,12,90.3; 100-4,14,10
AMA: 1998,Nov,9

28322 metatarsal, with or without bone graft (includes obtaining graft) ☑4 T 80 ▱

MED: 100-2,15,260; 100-4,12,90.3; 100-4,14,10

28340 Reconstruction, toe, macrodactyly; soft tissue resection ☑4 T ▱

MED: 100-2,15,260; 100-4,12,90.3; 100-4,14,10

28341 requiring bone resection ☑4 T ▱

MED: 100-2,15,260; 100-4,12,90.3; 100-4,14,10

28344 Reconstruction, toe(s); polydactyly ☑4 T ▱

MED: 100-2,15,260; 100-4,12,90.3; 100-4,14,10

28345 syndactyly, with or without skin graft(s), each web ☑4 T 80 ▱

MED: 100-2,15,260; 100-4,12,90.3; 100-4,14,10

28360 Reconstruction, cleft foot T 80 ▱

FRACTURE AND/OR DISLOCATION

28400 Closed treatment of calcaneal fracture; without manipulation ☑1 T 50 ▱

MED: 100-2,15,260; 100-4,12,90.3; 100-4,14,10

28405 with manipulation ☑2 T 80 50 ▱

MED: 100-2,15,260; 100-4,12,90.3; 100-4,14,10
Bohler reduction

28406 Percutaneous skeletal fixation of calcaneal fracture, with manipulation ☑2 T 80 50 ▱

MED: 100-2,15,260; 100-4,12,90.3; 100-4,14,10

28415 Open treatment of calcaneal fracture, with or without internal or external fixation; ☑3 T 80 50 ▱

MED: 100-2,15,260; 100-4,12,90.3; 100-4,14,10

28420 with primary iliac or other autogenous bone graft (includes obtaining graft) ☑4 T 80 50 ▱

MED: 100-2,15,260; 100-4,12,90.3; 100-4,14,10

28430 Closed treatment of talus fracture; without manipulation T 50 ▱

28435 with manipulation ☑2 T 80 50 ▱

MED: 100-2,15,260; 100-4,12,90.3; 100-4,14,10

28436 Percutaneous skeletal fixation of talus fracture, with manipulation ☑2 T 50 ▱

MED: 100-2,15,260; 100-4,12,90.3; 100-4,14,10

28445 Open treatment of talus fracture, with or without internal or external fixation ☑3 T 80 50 ▱

MED: 100-2,15,260; 100-4,12,90.3; 100-4,14,10

28450 Treatment of tarsal bone fracture (except talus and calcaneus); without manipulation, each T ▱

AMA: 2001,Dec,7

28455 with manipulation, each T 80 ▱

28456 Percutaneous skeletal fixation of tarsal bone fracture (except talus and calcaneus), with manipulation, each ☑2 T ▱

MED: 100-2,15,260; 100-4,12,90.3; 100-4,14,10

28465 Open treatment of tarsal bone fracture (except talus and calcaneus), with or without internal or external fixation, each ☑3 T ▱

MED: 100-2,15,260; 100-4,12,90.3; 100-4,14,10

28470 Closed treatment of metatarsal fracture; without manipulation, each T ▱

28475 with manipulation, each T ▱

28476 Percutaneous skeletal fixation of metatarsal fracture, with manipulation, each ☑2 T 80 ▱

MED: 100-2,15,260; 100-4,12,90.3; 100-4,14,10

28485 Open treatment of metatarsal fracture, with or without internal or external fixation, each ☑4 T ▱

MED: 100-2,15,260; 100-4,12,90.3; 100-4,14,10

28490 Closed treatment of fracture great toe, phalanx or phalanges; without manipulation T ▱

28495 with manipulation T ▱

28496 Percutaneous skeletal fixation of fracture great toe, phalanx or phalanges, with manipulation ☑2 T ▱

MED: 100-2,15,260; 100-4,12,90.3; 100-4,14,10

28505 Open treatment of fracture great toe, phalanx or phalanges, with or without internal or external fixation ☑3 T ▱

MED: 100-2,15,260; 100-4,12,90.3; 100-4,14,10

28510 Closed treatment of fracture, phalanx or phalanges, other than great toe; without manipulation, each T ▱

28515 with manipulation, each T ▱

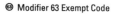

28525   Open treatment of fracture, phalanx or phalanges, other than great toe, with or without internal or external fixation, each   3 T 80 ▢

MED: 100-2,15,260; 100-4,12,90.3; 100-4,14,10

28530   Closed treatment of sesamoid fracture   T 80 ▢

28531   Open treatment of sesamoid fracture, with or without internal fixation   3 T ▢

MED: 100-2,15,260; 100-4,12,90.3; 100-4,14,10

28540   Closed treatment of tarsal bone dislocation, other than talotarsal; without anesthesia   T 80 ▢

28545   requiring anesthesia   1 T 80 ▢

MED: 100-2,15,260; 100-4,12,90.3; 100-4,14,10

28546   Percutaneous skeletal fixation of tarsal bone dislocation, other than talotarsal, with manipulation   2 T 80 ▢

MED: 100-2,15,260; 100-4,12,90.3; 100-4,14,10

28555   Open treatment of tarsal bone dislocation, with or without internal or external fixation   2 T 80 ▢

MED: 100-2,15,260; 100-4,12,90.3; 100-4,14,10

28570   Closed treatment of talotarsal joint dislocation; without anesthesia   T 80 ▢

28575   requiring anesthesia   1 T 80 ▢

MED: 100-2,15,260; 100-4,12,90.3; 100-4,14,10

28576   Percutaneous skeletal fixation of talotarsal joint dislocation, with manipulation   3 T 80 ▢

28585   Open treatment of talotarsal joint dislocation, with or without internal or external fixation   3 T 80 ▢

MED: 100-2,15,260; 100-4,12,90.3; 100-4,14,10

28600   Closed treatment of tarsometatarsal joint dislocation; without anesthesia   T 80 ▢

28605   requiring anesthesia   1 T 80 ▢

MED: 100-2,15,260; 100-4,12,90.3; 100-4,14,10

28606   Percutaneous skeletal fixation of tarsometatarsal joint dislocation, with manipulation   2 T ▢

MED: 100-2,15,260; 100-4,12,90.3; 100-4,14,10

28615   Open treatment of tarsometatarsal joint dislocation, with or without internal or external fixation   3 T 80 ▢

MED: 100-2,15,260; 100-4,12,90.3; 100-4,14,10

28630   Closed treatment of metatarsophalangeal joint dislocation; without anesthesia   T 80 ▢

28635   requiring anesthesia   1 T 80 ▢

MED: 100-2,15,260; 100-4,12,90.3; 100-4,14,10

28636   Percutaneous skeletal fixation of metatarsophalangeal joint dislocation, with manipulation   3 T ▢

MED: 100-2,15,260; 100-4,12,90.3; 100-4,14,10

28645   Open treatment of metatarsophalangeal joint dislocation, with or without internal or external fixation   3 T ▢

MED: 100-2,15,260; 100-4,12,90.3; 100-4,14,10

28660   Closed treatment of interphalangeal joint dislocation; without anesthesia   T ▢

28665   requiring anesthesia   1 T 80 ▢

MED: 100-2,15,260; 100-4,12,90.3; 100-4,14,10

28666   Percutaneous skeletal fixation of interphalangeal joint dislocation, with manipulation   3 T ▢

MED: 100-2,15,260; 100-4,12,90.3; 100-4,14,10

28675   Open treatment of interphalangeal joint dislocation, with or without internal or external fixation   3 T ▢

MED: 100-2,15,260; 100-4,12,90.3; 100-4,14,10

ARTHRODESIS

28705   Arthrodesis; pantalar   4 T 80 ▢

MED: 100-2,15,260; 100-4,12,90.3; 100-4,14,10

28715   triple   4 T 80 ▢

MED: 100-2,15,260; 100-4,12,90.3; 100-4,14,10

28725   subtalar   4 T 80 ▢

MED: 100-2,15,260; 100-4,12,90.3; 100-4,14,10
Dunn arthrodesis

28730   Arthrodesis, midtarsal or tarsometatarsal, multiple or transverse;   4 T 80 ▢

MED: 100-2,15,260; 100-4,12,90.3; 100-4,14,10
Lambrinudi arthrodesis

28735   with osteotomy (eg, flatfoot correction)   4 T 80 ▢

MED: 100-2,15,260; 100-4,12,90.3; 100-4,14,10

28737   Arthrodesis, with tendon lengthening and advancement, midtarsal, tarsal navicular-cuneiform (eg, Miller type procedure)   5 T 80 ▢

MED: 100-2,15,260; 100-4,12,90.3; 100-4,14,10

28740   Arthrodesis, midtarsal or tarsometatarsal, single joint   4 T 80 ▢

MED: 100-2,15,260; 100-4,12,90.3; 100-4,14,10

28750   Arthrodesis, great toe; metatarsophalangeal joint   4 T 80 50 ▢

MED: 100-2,15,260; 100-4,12,90.3; 100-4,14,10
AMA: 1996,Dec,7

28755   interphalangeal joint   4 T 50 ▢

MED: 100-2,15,260; 100-4,12,90.3; 100-4,14,10

28760   Arthrodesis, with extensor hallucis longus transfer to first metatarsal neck, great toe, interphalangeal joint (eg, Jones type procedure)   4 T 80 50 ▢

MED: 100-2,15,260; 100-4,12,90.3; 100-4,14,10
AMA: 1998,Nov,8
If a hammertoe operation or interphalangeal joint fusion is performed, consult CPT code 28285.

AMPUTATION

28800   Amputation, foot; midtarsal (eg, Chopart type procedure)   C 80 50 ▢

28805   transmetatarsal   C 80 50 ▢

28810   Amputation, metatarsal, with toe, single   2 T 80 ▢

MED: 100-2,15,260; 100-4,12,90.3; 100-4,14,10

28820   Amputation, toe; metatarsophalangeal joint   2 T ▢

MED: 100-2,15,260; 100-4,12,90.3; 100-4,14,10

28825   interphalangeal joint   2 T ▢

MED: 100-2,15,260; 100-4,12,90.3; 100-4,14,10
If the tuft of the distal phalanx is amputated, consult CPT code 11752.

OTHER PROCEDURES

To report extracorporeal shock wave therapy involving musculoskeletal system not otherwise specified, consult Category III codes 0019T, 0101T, 0102T.

---

26 Professional Component Only   80/80 Assist-at-Surgery Allowed/With Documentation   Unlisted   Not Covered

TC Technical Component Only   MED: Pub 100/NCD References   AMA: CPT Assistant References   1-9 ASC Group   ♂ Male Only   ♀ Female Only

108 — CPT Expert   CPT only © 2006 American Medical Association. All Rights Reserved. *(Black Ink)*   © 2006 Ingenix *(Blue Ink)*

28890 | Extracorporeal shock wave, high energy, performed by a physician, requiring anesthesia other than local, including ultrasound guidance, involving the plantar fascia T 80 50

> To report extracorporeal shock wave therapy involving musculoskeletal system not otherwise specified, consult Category III codes 0019T, 0101T, 0102T.

28899 | Unlisted procedure, foot or toes T 80
MED: 100-4,4,180.3

APPLICATION OF CASTS AND STRAPPING

Codes listed in the Musculoskeletal chapter include the application and removal of the first cast or traction device. Replacement of casts and/or traction devices subsequent to the first should be reported separately. CPT codes for other additional procedures, such as obtaining grafts and external fixation, should only be used if the procedure is not already listed as included as part of the basic procedure.

Codes found in the application of casts and strapping section (29000-29799) should be reported separately when:

- The cast application or strapping is a replacement procedure used during or after the period of follow-up care.
- The cast application or strapping is an initial service performed without restorative treatment or procedures to stabilize or protect a fracture, injury, or dislocation and/or to afford comfort to a patient.
- An initial casting or strapping when no other treatment or procedure is performed or will be performed by the same physician.
- A physician performs the initial application of a cast or strapping subsequent to another physician having performed a restorative treatment or procedure.
- A physician who applies the initial cast, strap, or splint and also assumes all of the subsequent fracture, dislocation, or injury care cannot use the application of casts and strapping codes as an initial service. The first cast, splint, or strap application is included in the treatment of the fracture and/or dislocation codes.
- A temporary cast, splint, or strap is not considered to be a part of the preoperative care. It is not necessary to use modifier 56.
- Report evaluation and management services only if they are separately identifiable from the application of the cast, splint, or strap.
- Do not report removal of the cast or strap separately.

Use these codes when replacing a cast or strap during or after follow-up care. They also apply when the application is an initial service without treatment or procedure to protect an injury.

Casts are rigid dressings, often made of fiberglass or plaster. Strapping is the application of tape to bind, correct, or protect an anatomical part.

If orthotics management and training are necessary, consult CPT code 97760-97762.

BODY AND UPPER EXTREMITY

CASTS

29000 | Application of halo type body cast (see 20661-20663 for insertion) S 80 CCI
MED: 100-4,4,240
AMA: 2002,Apr,13; 1996,Feb,3, 5

29010 | Application of Risser jacket, localizer, body; only S 80 CCI
MED: 100-4,4,240
AMA: 2002,Apr,13; 1996,Feb,3

29015 | including head S 80 CCI
MED: 100-4,4,240
AMA: 2002,Apr,13; 1996,Feb,3

29020 | Application of turnbuckle jacket, body; only S 80 CCI
MED: 100-4,4,240
AMA: 2002,Apr,13; 1996,Feb,3

29025 | including head S 80 CCI
MED: 100-4,4,240
AMA: 2002,Apr,13; 1996,Feb,3

29035 | Application of body cast, shoulder to hips; S 80 CCI
MED: 100-4,4,240
AMA: 2002,Apr,13; 1996,Feb,3

29040 | including head, Minerva type S 80 CCI
MED: 100-4,4,240
AMA: 2002,Apr,13; 1996,Feb,3

29044 | including one thigh S 80 CCI
MED: 100-4,4,240
AMA: 2002,Apr,13; 1996,Feb,3

29046 | including both thighs S 80 CCI
MED: 100-4,4,240
AMA: 2002,Apr,13; 1996,Feb,3

29049 | Application, cast; figure-of-eight S 80 CCI
MED: 100-2,15,100; 100-4,4,240
AMA: 2002,Apr,13; 1996,Feb,3

29055 | shoulder spica S 80 CCI
MED: 100-2,15,100; 100-4,4,240
AMA: 2002,Apr,13; 1996,Feb,3

29058 | plaster Velpeau S 80 CCI
MED: 100-2,15,100; 100-4,4,240
AMA: 2002,Apr,13; 1996,Feb,3

29065 | shoulder to hand (long arm) S 50 CCI
MED: 100-2,15,100; 100-4,4,240
AMA: 2002,Apr,13; 1996,Feb,3

29075 | elbow to finger (short arm) S 50 CCI
MED: 100-2,15,100; 100-4,4,240
AMA: 2002,Apr,13; 1996,Feb,3, 4

29085 | hand and lower forearm (gauntlet) S 50 CCI
MED: 100-2,15,100; 100-4,4,240
AMA: 2002,Dec,11; 2002,Apr,13; 1996,Feb,3

29086 | finger (eg, contracture) S 50 CCI
MED: 100-2,15,100; 100-4,4,240
AMA: 2002,Apr,13

SPLINTS

29105 | Application of long arm splint (shoulder to hand) S 50 CCI
MED: 100-2,15,100; 100-4,4,240
AMA: 2002,Apr,13; 1996,Feb,3

29125 | Application of short arm splint (forearm to hand); static S 50 CCI
MED: 100-2,15,100; 100-4,4,240
AMA: 2002,Apr,13; 1996,Feb,3, 4

29126 | dynamic S 50 CCI
MED: 100-2,15,100; 100-4,4,240
AMA: 2002,Apr,13; 1996,Feb,3

29130 | Application of finger splint; static S 50 CCI
MED: 100-2,15,100; 100-4,4,240
AMA: 2002,Apr,13; 1996,Feb,3

29131 | dynamic S 50 CCI
MED: 100-2,15,100; 100-4,4,240
AMA: 2002,Apr,13; 1996,Feb,3

STRAPPING — ANY AGE

29200 | Strapping; thorax S CCI
MED: 100-2,15,100
AMA: 2002,Apr,13; 1996,Feb,3

29220 | low back S CCI
MED: 100-2,15,100
AMA: 2002,Apr,13; 1996,Feb,3

Musculoskeletal System

29240 — 29805

29240	shoulder (eg, Velpeau)	S
	MED: 100-2,15,100	
	AMA: 2002,Apr,13; 1996,Feb,3	
29260	elbow or wrist	S 50
	MED: 100-2,15,100	
	AMA: 2002,Apr,13; 1996,Feb,3	
29280	hand or finger	S 50
	MED: 100-2,15,100	
	AMA: 2002,Apr,13; 1996,Feb,3	

LOWER EXTREMITY

CASTS

29305	Application of hip spica cast; one leg	S 80
	MED: 100-4,4,240	
	AMA: 2002,Apr,13; 1996,Feb,3	
29325	one and one-half spica or both legs	S 80
	MED: 100-4,4,240	
	AMA: 2002,Apr,13; 1996,Feb,3	

To report the application of a hip spica (body) cast, including thighs only, consult CPT code 29046.

29345	Application of long leg cast (thigh to toes);	S 50
	MED: 100-4,4,240	
	AMA: 2002,Apr,13; 1996,Feb,3	
29355	walker or ambulatory type	S 50
	MED: 100-4,4,240	
	AMA: 2002,Apr,13; 1996,Feb,3	
29358	Application of long leg cast brace	S 50
	MED: 100-4,4,240	
	AMA: 2002,Apr,13; 1996,Feb,3	
29365	Application of cylinder cast (thigh to ankle)	S 50
	MED: 100-4,4,240	
	AMA: 2002,Apr,13; 1996,Feb,3	
29405	Application of short leg cast (below knee to toes);	S 50
	MED: 100-2,15,100; 100-4,4,240	
	AMA: 2002,Apr,13; 1996,Feb,3	
29425	walking or ambulatory type	S 50
	MED: 100-2,15,100; 100-4,4,240	
	AMA: 2002,Apr,13; 1996,Feb,3	
29435	Application of patellar tendon bearing (PTB) cast	S 50
	MED: 100-4,4,240	
	AMA: 2002,Apr,13; 1996,Feb,3	
29440	Adding walker to previously applied cast	S 50
	MED: 100-2,15,100; 100-4,4,240	
	AMA: 2002,Apr,13; 1996,Feb,3	
29445	Application of rigid total contact leg cast	S 50
	MED: 100-4,4,240	
	AMA: 2002,Apr,13; 1996,Feb,3	
29450	Application of clubfoot cast with molding or manipulation, long or short leg	S 50
	MED: 100-4,4,240	
	AMA: 2002,Apr,13; 1996,Feb,3	

SPLINTS

29505	Application of long leg splint (thigh to ankle or toes)	S 50
	MED: 100-2,15,100; 100-4,4,240	
	AMA: 2002,Apr,13; 1996,Feb,3	
29515	Application of short leg splint (calf to foot)	S 50
	MED: 100-2,15,100; 100-4,4,240	
	AMA: 2002,Apr,13; 1996,Feb,3	

STRAPPING — ANY AGE

29520	Strapping; hip	S 80
	MED: 100-2,15,100	
	AMA: 2002,Apr,13; 1996,Feb,3	
29530	knee	S
	MED: 100-2,15,100	
	AMA: 2002,Apr,13; 1996,Feb,3	
29540	ankle and/or foot	S
	MED: 100-2,15,100	
	AMA: 2002,Apr,13; 1996,Feb,3	
29550	toes	S
	MED: 100-2,15,100	
	AMA: 2002,Apr,13; 1996,Feb,3	
29580	Unna boot	S 50
	MED: 100-2,15,100	
	AMA: 2002,Apr,13; 1999,Jul,10; 1996,Feb,3	
29590	Denis-Browne splint strapping	S
	AMA: 2002,Apr,13; 1996,Feb,3	

REMOVAL OR REPAIR

These codes are only used for casts applied by another physician.

29700	Removal or bivalving; gauntlet, boot or body cast	S
	AMA: 2002,Apr,13	
29705	full arm or full leg cast	S 50
	AMA: 2002,Apr,13	
29710	shoulder or hip spica, Minerva, or Risser jacket, etc.	S 80 50
	AMA: 2002,Apr,13	
29715	turnbuckle jacket	S 80
	AMA: 2002,Apr,13	
29720	Repair of spica, body cast or jacket	S
	AMA: 2002,Apr,13	
29730	Windowing of cast	S
	AMA: 2002,Apr,13	
29740	Wedging of cast (except clubfoot casts)	S
	AMA: 2002,Apr,13	
29750	Wedging of clubfoot cast	S 80 50
	AMA: 2002,Apr,13	

OTHER PROCEDURES

29799	Unlisted procedure, casting or strapping	S 80
	MED: 100-4,4,180.3	

ENDOSCOPY/ARTHROSCOPY

When arthrotomy is performed in addition to the arthroscopy, append with modifier 51.

Diagnostic endoscopy/arthroscopy is always included in surgical endoscopy/arthroscopy; do not report separately.

29800	Arthroscopy, temporomandibular joint, diagnostic, with or without synovial biopsy (separate procedure)	3 T 80 50
	MED: 100-2,15,260; 100-3,100.2; 100-4,12,90.3; 100-4,14,10	
29804	Arthroscopy, temporomandibular joint, surgical	3 T 80 50
	MED: 100-2,15,260; 100-3,100.2; 100-4,12,90.3; 100-4,14,10	

To report open procedure, consult CPT code 21010.

29805	Arthroscopy, shoulder, diagnostic, with or without synovial biopsy (separate procedure)	3 T 50
	MED: 100-2,15,260; 100-3,100.2; 100-4,12,90.3; 100-4,14,10	

To report open procedure, consult CPT codes 23065-23066, 23100-23101.

---

26 Professional Component Only   80/80 Assist-at-Surgery Allowed/With Documentation   Unlisted   Not Covered

TC Technical Component Only   MED: Pub 100/NCD References   AMA: CPT Assistant References   1-9 ASC Group   ♂ Male Only   ♀ Female Only

110 — CPT Expert   CPT only © 2006 American Medical Association. All Rights Reserved. (Black Ink)   © 2006 Ingenix (Blue Ink)

Musculoskeletal System

29806 — 29860

29806 Arthroscopy, shoulder, surgical; capsulorrhaphy   3 T 50 ⊠
MED: 100-2,15,260; 100-3,100.2; 100-4,12,90.3; 100-4,14,10

If an open procedure is performed, consult CPT codes 23450-23466.

If thermal capsulorrhaphy is performed, consult CPT code 29999.

29807 repair of SLAP lesion   3 T 50 ⊠
MED: 100-2,15,260; 100-3,100.2; 100-4,12,90.3; 100-4,14,10

29819 Arthroscopy, shoulder, surgical; with removal of loose body or foreign body   3 T 50 ⊠
MED: 100-2,15,260; 100-3,100.2; 100-4,12,90.3; 100-4,14,10

To report open procedure, consult CPT codes 23040-23044, 23107.

29820 synovectomy, partial   3 T 80 50 ⊠
MED: 100-2,15,260; 100-3,100.2; 100-4,12,90.3; 100-4,14,10
To report open procedure, consult CPT code 23105.

29821 synovectomy, complete   3 T 80 50 ⊠
MED: 100-2,15,260; 100-3,100.2; 100-4,12,90.3; 100-4,14,10
To report open procedure, consult CPT code 23105.

29822 debridement, limited   3 T 80 50 ⊠
MED: 100-2,15,260; 100-3,100.2; 100-4,12,90.3; 100-4,14,10
AMA: 2001,May,8
To report open procedure, consult the specific open shoulder procedure performed.

29823 debridement, extensive   3 T 80 50 ⊠
MED: 100-2,15,260; 100-3,100.2; 100-4,12,90.3; 100-4,14,10
To report open procedure, consult the specific open shoulder procedure performed.

29824 distal claviculectomy including distal articular surface (Mumford procedure)   5 T 80 50 ⊠
MED: 100-2,15,260; 100-3,100.2; 100-4,12,90.3; 100-4,14,10
To report open procedure, consult CPT code 23120.

29825 with lysis and resection of adhesions, with or without manipulation   3 T 80 50 ⊠
MED: 100-2,15,260; 100-3,100.2; 100-4,12,90.3; 100-4,14,10
To report open procedure, consult the specific open shoulder procedure performed.

29826 decompression of subacromial space with partial acromioplasty, with or without coracoacromial release   3 T 80 50 ⊠
MED: 100-2,15,260; 100-3,100.2; 100-4,12,90.3; 100-4,14,10
AMA: 2001,May,8
To report open procedure, consult CPT code 23130 or 23415.

29827 with rotator cuff repair   5 T 80 50 ⊠
MED: 100-2,15,260; 100-3,100.2; 100-4,12,90.3; 100-4,14,10
To report open or mini-open repair, consult CPT code 23412.

If arthroscopic subacromial decompression is performed at the same time, consult CPT code 29826, and append modifier 51.

If arthroscopic distal clavicle resection is performed at the same time, consult CPT code 29824, and append modifier 51.

29830 Arthroscopy, elbow, diagnostic, with or without synovial biopsy (separate procedure)   3 T 50 ⊠
MED: 100-2,15,260; 100-3,100.2; 100-4,12,90.3; 100-4,14,10

29834 Arthroscopy, elbow, surgical; with removal of loose body or foreign body   3 T 80 50 ⊠
MED: 100-2,15,260; 100-3,100.2; 100-4,12,90.3; 100-4,14,10

29835 synovectomy, partial   3 T 80 50 ⊠
MED: 100-2,15,260; 100-3,100.2; 100-4,12,90.3; 100-4,14,10

29836 synovectomy, complete   3 T 80 50 ⊠
MED: 100-2,15,260; 100-3,100.2; 100-4,12,90.3; 100-4,14,10

29837 debridement, limited   3 T 80 50 ⊠
MED: 100-2,15,260; 100-3,100.2; 100-4,12,90.3; 100-4,14,10

29838 debridement, extensive   3 T 80 50 ⊠
MED: 100-2,15,260; 100-3,100.2; 100-4,12,90.3; 100-4,14,10

29840 Arthroscopy, wrist, diagnostic, with or without synovial biopsy (separate procedure)   3 T 80 50 ⊠
MED: 100-2,15,260; 100-3,100.2; 100-4,12,90.3; 100-4,14,10

29843 Arthroscopy, wrist, surgical; for infection, lavage and drainage   3 T 80 50 ⊠
MED: 100-2,15,260; 100-3,100.2; 100-4,12,90.3; 100-4,14,10

29844 synovectomy, partial   3 T 80 50 ⊠
MED: 100-2,15,260; 100-3,100.2; 100-4,12,90.3; 100-4,14,10

29845 synovectomy, complete   3 T 80 50 ⊠
MED: 100-2,15,260; 100-3,100.2; 100-4,12,90.3; 100-4,14,10

29846 excision and/or repair of triangular fibrocartilage and/or joint debridement   3 T 80 50 ⊠
MED: 100-2,15,260; 100-3,100.2; 100-4,12,90.3; 100-4,14,10

29847 internal fixation for fracture or instability   3 T 80 50 ⊠
MED: 100-2,15,260; 100-3,100.2; 100-4,12,90.3; 100-4,14,10

29848 Endoscopy, wrist, surgical, with release of transverse carpal ligament   9 T 50 ⊠
MED: 100-2,15,260; 100-3,100.2; 100-4,12,90.3; 100-4,14,10
AMA: 1999,Dec,7
If this is an open procedure, consult CPT code 64721.

29850 Arthroscopically aided treatment of intercondylar spine(s) and/or tuberosity fracture(s) of the knee, with or without manipulation; without internal or external fixation (includes arthroscopy)   4 T 80 50 ⊠
MED: 100-2,15,260; 100-3,100.2; 100-4,12,90.3; 100-4,14,10

29851 with internal or external fixation (includes arthroscopy)   4 T 80 50 ⊠
MED: 100-2,15,260; 100-3,100.2; 100-4,12,90.3; 100-4,14,10
If a bone graft is performed, consult CPT codes 20900 and 20902.

29855 Arthroscopically aided treatment of tibial fracture, proximal (plateau); unicondylar, with or without internal or external fixation (includes arthroscopy)   4 T 80 50 ⊠
MED: 100-2,15,260; 100-3,100.2; 100-4,12,90.3; 100-4,14,10
If a bone graft is performed, consult CPT codes 20900 and 20902.

29856 bicondylar, with or without internal or external fixation (includes arthroscopy)   4 T 80 50 ⊠
MED: 100-2,15,260; 100-3,100.2; 100-4,12,90.3; 100-4,14,10

29860 Arthroscopy, hip, diagnostic with or without synovial biopsy (separate procedure)   4 T 80 50 ⊠
MED: 100-2,15,260; 100-3,100.2; 100-4,12,90.3; 100-4,14,10
AMA: 1998,Jul,8; 1997,Nov,15

Musculoskeletal System

29861 — 29887

29861 Arthroscopy, hip, surgical; with removal of loose body or foreign body 4 T 80 50 ▢

MED: 100-2,15,260; 100-3,100.2; 100-4,12,90.3; 100-4,14,10
AMA: 1998,Jul,8; 1997,Nov,15

29862 Arthroscopy, hip, surgical; with debridement/shaving of articular cartilage (chondroplasty), abrasion arthroplasty, and/or resection of labrum 9 T 80 50 ▢

MED: 100-2,15,260; 100-3,100.2; 100-4,12,90.3; 100-4,14,10
AMA: 1998,Jul,8; 1997,Nov,15

29863 with synovectomy 4 T 80 50 ▢

MED: 100-2,15,260; 100-3,100.2; 100-4,12,90.3; 100-4,14,10
AMA: 1998,Jul,8; 1997,Nov,15

Cylindrical plugs of healthy bone are harvested, usually from a non-weight bearing area of the femur

The technique employs arthroscopy

Recipient holes are drilled and the grafts tamped into position. Report 29867 when the donor bone comes from a tissue bank, rather than harvested from the patient

29866 Arthroscopy, knee, surgical; osteochondral autograft(s) (eg, mosaicplasty) (includes harvesting of the autograft) T 80 50 ▢

Code 29866 cannot be reported with CPT codes 29870, 29871, 29875, 29884 when performed at the same session and/or CPT codes 29874, 29877, 29879, 29885-29887 when performed in the same compartment.

29867 osteochondral allograft (eg, mosaicplasty) T 80 50 ▢

Code 29867 cannot be reported with CPT codes 27570, 29870, 29871, 29875, and 29884 when performed at the same session and/or CPT codes 29874, 29877, 29879, 29885-29887 when performed in the same compartment.

Code 29867 cannot be reported with CPT code 27415.

29868 meniscal transplantation (includes arthrotomy for meniscal insertion), medial or lateral T 80 50 ▢

Code 29868 cannot be reported with CPT codes 29870, 29871, 29875, 29880, 29883, 29884 when performed at the same session or CPT code 29874, 29877, 29881, or 29882 when performed in the same compartment.

29870 Arthroscopy, knee, diagnostic, with or without synovial biopsy (separate procedure) 3 T 50 ▢

MED: 100-2,15,260; 100-3,100.2; 100-4,12,90.3; 100-4,14,10
To report open autologous chondrocyte implantation of the knee, consult CPT code 27412.

29871 Arthroscopy, knee, surgical; for infection, lavage and drainage 3 T 50 ▢

MED: 100-2,15,260; 100-3,100.2; 100-4,12,90.3; 100-4,14,10
AMA: 2001,Aug,5
To report implantation of osteochondral graft to treat an articular surface defect, consult CPT codes 27412, 27415, 29866, and 29867.

29873 Arthroscopy, knee, surgical; with lateral release 3 T 50 ▢

MED: 100-3,100.2
To report open lateral release, consult CPT code 27425.

29874 for removal of loose body or foreign body (eg, osteochondritis dissecans fragmentation, chondral fragmentation) 3 T 80 50 ▢

MED: 100-2,15,260; 100-3,100.2; 100-4,12,90.3; 100-4,14,10
AMA: 2001,Aug,5

29875 synovectomy, limited (eg, plica or shelf resection) (separate procedure) 4 T 80 50 ▢

MED: 100-2,15,260; 100-3,100.2; 100-4,12,90.3; 100-4,14,10
AMA: 2001,Aug,5

29876 synovectomy, major, two or more compartments (eg, medial or lateral) 4 T 50 ▢

MED: 100-2,15,260; 100-3,100.2; 100-4,12,90.3; 100-4,14,10
AMA: 2001,Aug,5

29877 debridement/shaving of articular cartilage (chondroplasty) 4 T 80 50 ▢

MED: 100-2,15,260; 100-3,100.2; 100-4,12,90.3; 100-4,14,10
AMA: 2001,Aug,5; 1999,Jun,11; 1996,Feb,9

29879 abrasion arthroplasty (includes chondroplasty where necessary) or multiple drilling or microfracture 3 T 80 50 ▢

MED: 100-2,15,260; 100-3,100.2; 100-4,12,90.3; 100-4,14,10
AMA: 2001,Aug,5; 1999,Nov,13

29880 with meniscectomy (medial AND lateral, including any meniscal shaving) 4 T 80 50 ▢

MED: 100-2,15,260; 100-3,100.2; 100-4,12,90.3; 100-4,14,10
AMA: 2001,Aug,5; 1999,Jun,11

29881 with meniscectomy (medial OR lateral, including any meniscal shaving) 4 T 80 50 ▢

MED: 100-2,15,260; 100-3,100.2; 100-4,12,90.3; 100-4,14,10
AMA: 2001,Aug,5; 1999,Jun,11; 1996,Feb,9

29882 with meniscus repair (medial OR lateral) 3 T 50 ▢

MED: 100-2,15,260; 100-3,100.2; 100-4,12,90.3; 100-4,14,10
AMA: 2001,Aug,5

29883 with meniscus repair (medial AND lateral) 3 T 80 50 ▢

MED: 100-2,15,260; 100-3,100.2; 100-4,12,90.3; 100-4,14,10
AMA: 2001,Aug,5
To report meniscal transplantation, medial or lateral, knee, consult CPT code 29868.

29884 with lysis of adhesions, with or without manipulation (separate procedure) 3 T 80 50 ▢

MED: 100-2,15,260; 100-3,100.2; 100-4,12,90.3; 100-4,14,10
AMA: 2001,Aug,5

29885 drilling for osteochondritis dissecans with bone grafting, with or without internal fixation (including debridement of base of lesion) 3 T 80 50 ▢

MED: 100-2,15,260; 100-3,100.2; 100-4,12,90.3; 100-4,14,10
AMA: 2001,Aug,5

29886 drilling for intact osteochondritis dissecans lesion 3 T 50 ▢

MED: 100-2,15,260; 100-3,100.2; 100-4,12,90.3; 100-4,14,10
AMA: 2001,Aug,5

29887 drilling for intact osteochondritis dissecans lesion with internal fixation 3 T 80 50 ▢

MED: 100-2,15,260; 100-3,100.2; 100-4,12,90.3; 100-4,14,10
AMA: 2001,Aug,5

26 Professional Component Only
TC Technical Component Only
80/80 Assist-at-Surgery Allowed/With Documentation
MED: Pub 100/NCD References   AMA: CPT Assistant References
1-**9** ASC Group
Unlisted
♂ Male Only
Not Covered
♀ Female Only

112 — CPT Expert   CPT only © 2006 American Medical Association. All Rights Reserved. (Black Ink)   © 2006 Ingenix (Blue Ink)

29888   **Arthroscopically aided anterior cruciate ligament
repair/augmentation or
reconstruction**   3 T 80 50 ◨

MED: 100-2,15,260; 100-3,100.2; 100-4,12,90.3; 100-4,14,10

Note that 29888 and 29889 should not be reported in
conjunction with reconstructive procedures
27427-27429.

29889   **Arthroscopically aided posterior cruciate ligament
repair/augmentation or
reconstruction**   3 T 80 50 ◨

MED: 100-2,15,260; 100-3,100.2; 100-4,12,90.3; 100-4,14,10

AMA: 2001,Aug,8; 1998,Oct,11; 1996,Sep,9

29891   **Arthroscopy, ankle, surgical, excision of osteochondral
defect of talus and/or tibia, including drilling of the
defect**   3 T 80 50 ◨

MED: 100-2,15,260; 100-3,100.2; 100-4,12,90.3; 100-4,14,10

29892   **Arthroscopically aided repair of large osteochondritis
dissecans lesion, talar dome fracture, or tibial plafond
fracture, with or without internal fixation (includes
arthroscopy)**   3 T 80 50 ◨

MED: 100-2,15,260; 100-3,100.2; 100-4,12,90.3; 100-4,14,10

AMA: 1997,Nov,15

29893   **Endoscopic plantar fasciotomy**   9 T 80 50 ◨

MED: 100-2,15,260; 100-3,100.2; 100-4,12,90.3; 100-4,14,10

AMA: 1997,Nov,15

29894   **Arthroscopy, ankle (tibiotalar and fibulotalar joints),
surgical; with removal of loose body or foreign
body**   3 T 80 50 ◨

MED: 100-2,15,260; 100-3,100.2; 100-4,12,90.3; 100-4,14,10

29895   **synovectomy, partial**   3 T 80 50 ◨

MED: 100-2,15,260; 100-3,100.2; 100-4,12,90.3; 100-4,14,10

29897   **debridement, limited**   3 T 80 50 ◨

MED: 100-2,15,260; 100-3,100.2; 100-4,12,90.3; 100-4,14,10

29898   **debridement, extensive**   3 T 80 50 ◨

MED: 100-2,15,260; 100-3,100.2; 100-4,12,90.3; 100-4,14,10

29899   **with ankle arthrodesis**   3 T 80 50 ◨

MED: 100-2,15,260; 100-3,100.2; 100-4,12,90.3; 100-4,14,10

To report open ankle arthrodesis, consult CPT code
27870.

29900   **Arthroscopy, metacarpophalangeal joint, diagnostic,
includes synovial biopsy**   3 T 80 50 ◨

MED: 100-2,15,260; 100-3,100.2; 100-4,12,90.3; 100-4,14,10

Code 29900 should not be reported with CPT codes
29901, 29902.

29901   **Arthroscopy, metacarpophalangeal joint, surgical; with
debridement**   3 T 80 50 ◨

MED: 100-2,15,260; 100-3,100.2; 100-4,12,90.3; 100-4,14,10

29902   **with reduction of displaced ulnar collateral
ligament (eg, Stenar lesion)**   3 T 80 50 ◨

MED: 100-2,15,260; 100-3,100.2; 100-4,12,90.3; 100-4,14,10

29999   **Unlisted procedure, arthroscopy**   T 80 50 ◨

MED: 100-3,100.2; 100-4,4,180.3

RESPIRATORY SYSTEM

NOSE

INCISION

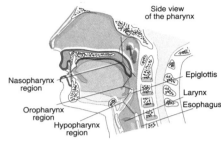

Side view of the pharynx

Nasopharynx region
Oropharynx region
Hypopharynx region
Epiglottis
Larynx
Esophagus

The nasopharynx is the membranous passage above the level of the soft palate; the oropharynx is the region between the soft palate and the upper edge of the epiglottis; the hypopharynx is the region of the epiglottis to the juncture of the larynx and esophagus; the three regions are collectively known as the pharynx

30000   **Drainage abscess or hematoma, nasal, internal approach**   T 80

If this procedure requires an external approach, consult CPT codes 10060 and 10140.

30020   **Drainage abscess or hematoma, nasal septum**   T

If a lateral rhinotomy is performed, consult specific application (eg, 30118, 30320).

EXCISION

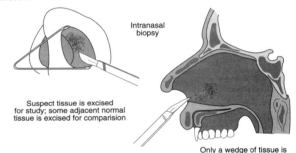

Intranasal biopsy

Suspect tissue is excised for study; some adjacent normal tissue is excised for comparision

Only a wedge of tissue is removed for larger lesions

30100   **Biopsy, intranasal**   T

If the skin of the nose is biopsied, consult CPT codes 11100 and 11101.

30110   **Excision, nasal polyp(s), simple**   T 50

Note that 30110 is generally performed in an office setting. If a bilateral procedure is performed, append modifier 50.

30115   **Excision, nasal polyp(s), extensive**   2 T 50

MED: 100-2,15,260; 100-4,12,90.3; 100-4,14,10

Note that 30115 generally requires the facilities available in a hospital setting. If a bilateral procedure is performed, append modifier 50.

30117   **Excision or destruction (eg, laser), intranasal lesion; internal approach**   3 T

MED: 100-2,15,260; 100-3,140.5; 100-4,12,90.3; 100-4,14,10

30118   **external approach (lateral rhinotomy)**   3 T 80

MED: 100-2,15,260; 100-3,140.5; 100-4,12,90.3; 100-4,14,10

30120   **Excision or surgical planing of skin of nose for rhinophyma**   1 T

MED: 100-2,15,260; 100-4,12,90.3; 100-4,14,10

30124   **Excision dermoid cyst, nose; simple, skin, subcutaneous**   T

30125   **complex, under bone or cartilage**   2 T 80

MED: 100-2,15,260; 100-4,12,90.3; 100-4,14,10

30130   **Excision inferior turbinate, partial or complete, any method**   3 T 50

MED: 100-2,15,260; 100-4,12,90.3; 100-4,14,10
AMA: 2001,Sep,10; 1998,Nov,11; 1998,Feb,11

To report excision of superior or middle turbinate, consult 30999.

30140   **Submucous resection inferior turbinate, partial or complete, any method**   2 T 50

MED: 100-2,15,260; 100-4,12,90.3; 100-4,14,10
AMA: 2002,Dec,10; 1998,Nov,11

30150   **Rhinectomy; partial**   3 T

MED: 100-2,15,260; 100-4,12,90.3; 100-4,14,10

If primary or delayed closure and/or reconstruction is performed, consult the Integumentary System (13150-13152, 14060-14300, 15120, 15121, 15260, 15261, 15760, and 20900-20912).

30160   **total**   4 T 80

MED: 100-2,15,260; 100-4,12,90.3; 100-4,14,10

If primary or delayed closure and/or reconstruction is needed, consult the Integumentary System codes (13150-13160, 14060-14300, 15120, 15121, 15260, 15261, 15760, and 20900-20912).

INTRODUCTION

30200   **Injection into turbinate(s), therapeutic**   T

30210   **Displacement therapy (Proetz type)**   T

30220   **Insertion, nasal septal prosthesis (button)**   3 T

REMOVAL OF FOREIGN BODY

30300   **Removal foreign body, intranasal; office type procedure**   X

30310   **requiring general anesthesia**   1 T 80

MED: 100-2,15,260; 100-4,12,90.3; 100-4,14,10

30320   **by lateral rhinotomy**   2 T 80

MED: 100-2,15,260; 100-4,12,90.3; 100-4,14,10

REPAIR

If obtaining tissues for a graft, consult CPT codes 20900-20926 and 21210.

30400   **Rhinoplasty, primary; lateral and alar cartilages and/or elevation of nasal tip**   4 T 80

MED: 100-2,15,260; 100-4,12,90.3; 100-4,14,10

If columellar reconstruction is performed, consult CPT codes 13150-13153.

     Carpue's operation

30410   **complete, external parts including bony pyramid, lateral and alar cartilages, and/or elevation of nasal tip**   5 T 80

MED: 100-2,15,260; 100-4,12,90.3; 100-4,14,10

30420   **including major septal repair**   5 T

MED: 100-2,15,260; 100-4,12,90.3; 100-4,14,10

30430   **Rhinoplasty, secondary; minor revision (small amount of nasal tip work)**   3 T 80

MED: 100-2,15,260; 100-4,12,90.3; 100-4,14,10

30435   **intermediate revision (bony work with osteotomies)**   5 T 80

MED: 100-2,15,260; 100-4,12,90.3; 100-4,14,10

30450	**major revision (nasal tip work and osteotomies)** 🅷 Ⓣ 🆂
	MED: 100-2,15,260; 100-4,12,90.3; 100-4,14,10

Cleft lip and cleft palate are described according to length of cleft and whether bilateral or unilateral

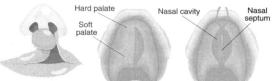

Complete unilateral cleft lip

Isolated unilateral complete cleft of palate

Bilateral complete cleft of lip and palate

Cleft lip with or without cleft palate is a common birth defect and is seen once or twice per 1000 live births; the condition is twice as common among boys than girls; isolated cleft palate is distinct from cleft lip with or without cleft palate and occurs about once in 2000 births; the condition is more common among girls than boys

30460	**Rhinoplasty for nasal deformity secondary to congenital cleft lip and/or palate, including columellar lengthening; tip only** 🅷 Ⓣ 🆂
	MED: 100-2,15,260; 100-4,12,90.3; 100-4,14,10
30462	**tip, septum, osteotomies** 🅹 Ⓣ 🆂
	MED: 100-2,15,260; 100-4,12,90.3; 100-4,14,10
30465	**Repair of nasal vestibular stenosis (eg, spreader grafting, lateral nasal wall reconstruction)** 🅹 Ⓣ 🆂
	MED: 100-2,15,260; 100-4,12,90.3; 100-4,14,10

Code 30465 is used to report a bilateral procedure. if the procedure is done as a unilateral procedure, append with modifier 52. If a graft procedure is performed, consult CPT codes 20900-20926 and 21210.

30520	**Septoplasty or submucous resection, with or without cartilage scoring, contouring or replacement with graft** 🄳 Ⓣ
	MED: 100-2,15,260; 100-4,12,90.3; 100-4,14,10
	AMA: 2002,Dec,10; 1997,Oct,11

If submucous resection of the turbinates is performed, consult CPT code 30140.

30540	**Repair choanal atresia; intranasal** 🄵 Ⓣ 🆂 ⊙
	MED: 100-2,15,260; 100-4,12,90.3; 100-4,14,10
30545	**transpalatine** 🄵 Ⓣ 🆂 ⊙
	MED: 100-2,15,260; 100-4,12,90.3; 100-4,14,10
30560	**Lysis intranasal synechia** 🄲 Ⓣ
	MED: 100-2,15,260; 100-4,12,90.3; 100-4,14,10
30580	**Repair fistula; oromaxillary (combine with 31030 if antrotomy is included)** 🄳 Ⓣ
	MED: 100-2,15,260; 100-4,12,90.3; 100-4,14,10
30600	**oronasal** 🄳 Ⓣ 🆂
	MED: 100-2,15,260; 100-4,12,90.3; 100-4,14,10

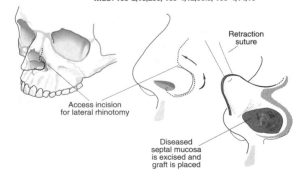

Retraction suture

Access incision for lateral rhinotomy

Diseased septal mucosa is excised and graft is placed

30620	**Septal or other intranasal dermatoplasty (does not include obtaining graft)** 🄷 Ⓣ
	MED: 100-2,15,260; 100-4,12,90.3; 100-4,14,10
30630	**Repair nasal septal perforations** 🄷 Ⓣ 🆂
	MED: 100-2,15,260; 100-4,12,90.3; 100-4,14,10

DESTRUCTION

30801	**Cautery and/or ablation, mucosa of inferior turbinates, unilateral or bilateral, any method; superficial** 🄸 Ⓣ
	MED: 100-2,15,260; 100-4,12,90.3; 100-4,14,10

To report cautery and ablation of the superior or middle turbinates, consult 30999.

30802	**intramural** 🄸 Ⓣ
	MED: 100-2,15,260; 100-4,12,90.3; 100-4,14,10

Codes 30801 and 30802, and 30930 cannot be reported with 30130 or 30140. Consult CPT codes 30901-30906 for cautery to control nasal hemorrhage.

OTHER PROCEDURES

30901	**Control nasal hemorrhage, anterior, simple (limited cautery and/or packing) any method** Ⓣ 🅅
30903	**Control nasal hemorrhage, anterior, complex (extensive cautery and/or packing) any method** 🄸 Ⓣ 🅅
	MED: 100-2,15,260; 100-4,12,90.3; 100-4,14,10
30905	**Control nasal hemorrhage, posterior, with posterior nasal packs and/or cautery, any method; initial** 🄸 Ⓣ
	MED: 100-2,15,260; 100-4,12,90.3; 100-4,14,10
30906	**subsequent** 🄸 Ⓣ
	MED: 100-2,15,260; 100-4,12,90.3; 100-4,14,10
30915	**Ligation arteries; ethmoidal** 🄲 Ⓣ
	MED: 100-2,15,260; 100-4,12,90.3; 100-4,14,10

If the external carotid artery is ligated, consult CPT code 37600.

30920	**internal maxillary artery, transantral** 🄳 Ⓣ
	MED: 100-2,15,260; 100-4,12,90.3; 100-4,14,10

If the external carotid artery is ligated, consult CPT code 37600.

30930	**Fracture nasal inferior turbinate(s), therapeutic** 🄳 Ⓣ 🅅
	MED: 100-2,15,260; 100-4,12,90.3; 100-4,14,10
	AMA: 2002,Dec,10; 2001,Jul,11

Codes 30801, 30802, 30930 cannot be reported with 30130 or 30140.

To report fracture of superior or middle turbinate(s), consult 30999.

30999	**Unlisted procedure, nose** Ⓣ 🆂
	MED: 100-4,4,180.3

Respiratory System

31000 — 31235

ACCESSORY SINUSES

INCISION

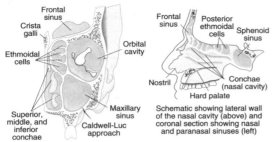

Frontal sinus · Crista galli · Ethmoidal cells · Orbital cavity · Superior, middle, and inferior conchae · Maxillary sinus · Caldwell-Luc approach

Frontal sinus · Posterior ethmoidal cells · Sphenoid sinus · Nostril · Conchae (nasal cavity) · Hard palate

Schematic showing lateral wall of the nasal cavity (above) and coronal section showing nasal and paranasal sinuses (left)

The nasal sinuses are air filled cavities in the cranial bones that bear their names; all are lined with mucous membrane continuous with the nasal cavity and all drain fluids into the nasal cavity. The ethmoid cells vary in size and number and feature very thin septa, or walls. The maxillary sinuses are the largest and are the most frequently infected.

31000 Lavage by cannulation; maxillary sinus (antrum puncture or natural ostium) T 50

> If a bilateral procedure is performed, append modifier 50.

31002 sphenoid sinus T 80 50

31020 Sinusotomy, maxillary (antrotomy); intranasal 2 T 50
MED: 100-2,15,260; 100-4,12,90.3; 100-4,14,10

> If a bilateral procedure is performed, append modifier 50.

31030 radical (Caldwell-Luc) without removal of antrochoanal polyps 3 T 50
MED: 100-2,15,260; 100-4,12,90.3; 100-4,14,10

> If a bilateral procedure is performed, append modifier 50.

31032 radical (Caldwell-Luc) with removal of antrochoanal polyps 4 T 50
MED: 100-2,15,260; 100-4,12,90.3; 100-4,14,10

> If a bilateral procedure is performed, append modifier 50.

31040 Pterygomaxillary fossa surgery, any approach T

> If a transantral ligation of the internal maxillary artery is performed, consult CPT code 30920.

31050 Sinusotomy, sphenoid, with or without biopsy; 2 T 50
MED: 100-2,15,260; 100-4,12,90.3; 100-4,14,10

31051 with mucosal stripping or removal of polyp(s) 4 T 50
MED: 100-2,15,260; 100-4,12,90.3; 100-4,14,10

31070 Sinusotomy frontal; external, simple (trephine operation) 2 T 50
MED: 100-2,15,260; 100-4,12,90.3; 100-4,14,10

> If a frontal intranasal sinusotomy is performed, consult CPT code 31726.

> **Killian operation**

31075 transorbital, unilateral (for mucocele or osteoma, Lynch type) 4 T 80 50
MED: 100-2,15,260; 100-4,12,90.3; 100-4,14,10

31080 obliterative without osteoplastic flap, brow incision (includes ablation) 4 T 80 50
MED: 100-2,15,260; 100-4,12,90.3; 100-4,14,10

> **Ridell sinusotomy**

31081 obliterative, without osteoplastic flap, coronal incision (includes ablation) 4 T 80 50
MED: 100-2,15,260; 100-4,12,90.3; 100-4,14,10

31084 obliterative, with osteoplastic flap, brow incision 4 T 80 50
MED: 100-2,15,260; 100-4,12,90.3; 100-4,14,10

31085 obliterative, with osteoplastic flap, coronal incision 4 T 80 50
MED: 100-2,15,260; 100-4,12,90.3; 100-4,14,10

31086 nonobliterative, with osteoplastic flap, brow incision 4 T 80 50
MED: 100-2,15,260; 100-4,12,90.3; 100-4,14,10

31087 nonobliterative, with osteoplastic flap, coronal incision 4 T 80 50
MED: 100-2,15,260; 100-4,12,90.3; 100-4,14,10

31090 Sinusotomy, unilateral, three or more paranasal sinuses (frontal, maxillary, ethmoid, sphenoid) 5 T 50
MED: 100-2,15,260; 100-4,12,90.3; 100-4,14,10
AMA: 1998,Nov,11; 1997,Nov,15

EXCISION

31200 Ethmoidectomy; intranasal, anterior 2 T 50
MED: 100-2,15,260; 100-4,12,90.3; 100-4,14,10

31201 intranasal, total 5 T 50
MED: 100-2,15,260; 100-4,12,90.3; 100-4,14,10

31205 extranasal, total 3 T 80 50
MED: 100-2,15,260; 100-4,12,90.3; 100-4,14,10

31225 Maxillectomy; without orbital exenteration C 80 50

31230 with orbital exenteration (en bloc) C 80 50

> If only orbital exenteration is performed, consult CPT codes 65110 and subsequent codes. If skin grafts are necessary, consult CPT codes 15120 and subsequent codes.

ENDOSCOPY

Sinus endoscopies include the examination of all parts of the sinuses, including the nasal cavity to the turbinates, and the spheno-ethmoid recess. Any sinusotomy performed during the examination is included in these codes.

Unless otherwise stated, CPT codes 31231-31294 report unilateral procedures. If these procedures are performed bilaterally, append modifier 50.

31231 Nasal endoscopy, diagnostic, unilateral or bilateral (separate procedure) T
MED: 100-3,100.2; 100-4,12,40.6
AMA: 1997,Jan,4

31233 Nasal/sinus endoscopy, diagnostic with maxillary sinusoscopy (via inferior meatus or canine fossa puncture) 2 T 50
MED: 100-2,15,260; 100-3,100.2; 100-4,12,40.6; 100-4,12,90.3; 100-4,14,10
AMA: 1997,Jan,4

31235 Nasal/sinus endoscopy, diagnostic with sphenoid sinusoscopy (via puncture of sphenoidal face or cannulation of ostium) 1 T 50
MED: 100-2,15,260; 100-3,100.2; 100-4,12,40.6; 100-4,12,90.3; 100-4,14,10
AMA: 1997,Jan,4

31237 Nasal/sinus endoscopy, surgical; with biopsy, polypectomy or debridement (separate procedure) 🄾 Ⓣ 🄼 🄲

MED: 100-2,15,260; 100-3,100.2; 100-4,12,40.6; 100-4,12,90.3; 100-4,14,10

AMA: 2001,Dec,6; 1997,Jan,4

31238 with control of nasal hemorrhage 🄸 Ⓣ 🄼 🄼 🄲

MED: 100-2,15,260; 100-4,12,40.6; 100-4,12,90.3; 100-4,14,10

AMA: 1997,Jan,4

31239 with dacryocystorhinostomy 🄴 Ⓣ 🄼 🄼 🄲

MED: 100-2,15,260; 100-4,12,40.6; 100-4,12,90.3; 100-4,14,10

AMA: 1997,Jan,4

31240 with concha bullosa resection 🄾 Ⓣ 🄼 🄼 🄲

MED: 100-2,15,260; 100-4,12,40.6; 100-4,12,90.3; 100-4,14,10

AMA: 1997,Jan,4

If an endoscopic osteomeatal complex (OMC) resection with antrostomy and/or anterior ethnoidectomy, with or without polyp removal is performed, consult CPT codes 31254 and 31256. For OMC resection with antrostomy, removal of antral mucosal disease, and/or anterior ethmoidectomy, with or without polyp removal, consult codes 31254 and 31267, For endoscopic frontal sinus exploration, OMC resection and/or anterior ethmoidectomy, with or without polyp removal, consult codes 31254 and 31276; and when antrostomy is also performed, consult codes 31254, 31256, and 31276. Consult codes 31231-31235 for an endoscopic nasal diagnostic endoscopy. For OMC resection, frontal sinus exploration, antrostomy, removal of antral mucosal disease, and/or anterior ethmoidectomy, with or without the removal of polyps, consult CPT codes 31254, 31267, and 31276.

31254 Nasal/sinus endoscopy, surgical; with ethmoidectomy, partial (anterior) 🄾 Ⓣ 🄼 🄲

MED: 100-2,15,260; 100-3,100.2; 100-4,12,40.6; 100-4,12,90.3; 100-4,14,10

AMA: 2001,Dec,6; 1997,Sep,10; 1997,Oct,5; 1997,Jan,4

31255 with ethmoidectomy, total (anterior and posterior) 🄵 Ⓣ 🄼 🄲

MED: 100-2,15,260; 100-4,12,40.6; 100-4,12,90.3; 100-4,14,10

AMA: 2002,Dec,10; 1997,Jan,4

Acute sinusitis refers to a single, short course of infection; chronic sinusitis refers to a continuing condition

Ethmoid air cells (sinus)
Orbit
Frontal sinus
Nasal cavity and middle turbinate
Middle turbinate
Inferior turbinate
Hard palate
Sphenoid sinus
Maxillary sinus
Soft palate

31256 Nasal/sinus endoscopy, surgical, with maxillary antrostomy; 🄾 Ⓣ 🄼 🄲

MED: 100-2,15,260; 100-3,100.2; 100-4,12,40.6; 100-4,12,90.3; 100-4,14,10

AMA: 1997,Jan,4

If an endoscopic anterior and posterior ethmoidectomy (APE), and antrostomy with or without polyp(s) removal is performed, consult CPT codes 31255 and 31256. When APE, antrostomy and removal of antral mucosal disease, with or without polyp(s) removal is performed, consult CPT codes 31255 and 31267. When APE, frontal sinus exploration, with or without polyp(s) removal is performed, consult CPT codes 31255 and 31276.

31267 with removal of tissue from maxillary sinus 🄾 Ⓣ 🄼 🄲

MED: 100-2,15,260; 100-4,12,40.6; 100-4,12,90.3; 100-4,14,10

AMA: 2001,Dec,6; 1997,Jan,4

If an endoscopic anterior and posterior ethmoidectomy (APE), frontal sinus exploration, and antrostomy, with or without polyp(s) removal is performed, consult CPT codes 31255, 31256,and 31276. When APE, frontal sinus exploration, antrostomy and removal of antral mucosal disease, with or without polyp(s) removal is performed, consult CPT codes 31255, 31267, and 31276.

31276 Nasal/sinus endoscopy, surgical with frontal sinus exploration, with or without removal of tissue from frontal sinus 🄾 Ⓣ 🄼 🄲

MED: 100-2,15,260; 100-3,100.2; 100-4,12,40.6; 100-4,12,90.3; 100-4,14,10

AMA: 1997,Jan,4

Consult CPT codes 31231-31235 for unilateral endoscopy of two or more sinuses. If an endoscopic anterior and posterior ethmoidectomy and spenoidotomy (APS), with or without polyp(s) removal is performed, consult CPT codes 31255, 31287, or 31288. For APS and antrostomy, with or without polyp(s) removal, consult codes 31255, 31256, and 31287 or 31288. For APS, antrostomy and removal of antral mucosal disease, without without polyp(s) removal, consult codes 31255, 31267 and 31287 or 31288. For APS and frontal sinus exploration with or without polyp(s) removal, consult codes 31255, 31287, or 31288, and 31276. For APS with or without polyp(s) removal, with frontal sinus exploration and antrostomy, consult codes 31255, 31256, 31287 or 31288, and 31276. For APS with frontal sinus exploration, antrostomy and removal of antral mucosal disease, with or without polyp(s) removal, consult codes 31255, 31267, 31287 or 31288, and 31276.

31287 Nasal/sinus endoscopy, surgical, with sphenoidotomy; 🄾 Ⓣ 🄼 🄼 🄲

MED: 100-2,15,260; 100-3,100.2; 100-4,12,40.6; 100-4,12,90.3; 100-4,14,10

AMA: 1997,Jan,4

31288 with removal of tissue from the sphenoid sinus 🄾 Ⓣ 🄼 🄼 🄲

MED: 100-2,15,260; 100-4,12,40.6; 100-4,12,90.3; 100-4,14,10

AMA: 1997,Jan,4

31290 Nasal/sinus endoscopy, surgical, with repair of cerebrospinal fluid leak; ethmoid region 🄲 🄼 🄼 🄲

MED: 100-3,100.2; 100-4,12,40.6

AMA: 1997,Jan,4

31291 sphenoid region 🄲 🄼 🄼 🄲

MED: 100-4,12,40.6

AMA: 1997,Jan,4

31292 Nasal/sinus endoscopy, surgical; with medial or inferior orbital wall decompression Ⓣ 🄼 🄼 🄲

MED: 100-3,100.2; 100-4,12,40.6

AMA: 1997,Jan,4

31293 with medial orbital wall and inferior orbital wall decompression Ⓣ 🄼 🄼 🄲

MED: 100-4,12,40.6

AMA: 1997,Jan,4

31294 with optic nerve decompression Ⓣ 🄼 🄼 🄲

MED: 100-4,12,40.6

AMA: 1997,Jan,4

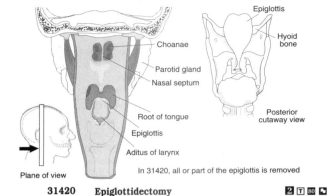

In 31420, all or part of the epiglottis is removed

OTHER PROCEDURES

31299 Unlisted procedure, accessory sinuses   T 80

MED: 100-4,4,180.3; 100-4,12,40.6

If a hypophysectomy is performed using a transantral or a transeptal approach, consult CPT code 61548. If a transcranial hypophysectomy is performed, consult CPT code 61546.

LARYNX

EXCISION

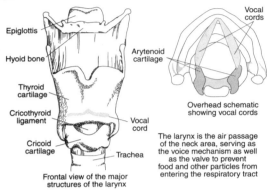

The larynx is the air passage of the neck area, serving as the voice mechanism as well as the valve to prevent food and other particles from entering the respiratory tract

Frontal view of the major structures of the larynx

31300 Laryngotomy (thyrotomy, laryngofissure); with removal of tumor or laryngocele, cordectomy   5 T 80

MED: 100-2,15,260; 100-4,12,90.3; 100-4,14,10

31320 diagnostic   2 T 80

MED: 100-2,15,260; 100-4,12,90.3; 100-4,14,10

31360 Laryngectomy; total, without radical neck dissection   C 80

31365 total, with radical neck dissection   C 80

AMA: 2001,Oct,10

31367 subtotal supraglottic, without radical neck dissection   C 80

31368 subtotal supraglottic, with radical neck dissection   C 80

31370 Partial laryngectomy (hemilaryngectomy); horizontal   C 80

31375 laterovertical   C 80

31380 anterovertical   C 80

31382 antero-latero-vertical   C 80

31390 Pharyngolaryngectomy, with radical neck dissection; without reconstruction   C 80

31395 with reconstruction   C 80

31400 Arytenoidectomy or arytenoidopexy, external approach   2 T 80

MED: 100-2,15,260; 100-4,12,90.3; 100-4,14,10

If performed endoscopically, consult CPT code 31560.

31420 Epiglottidectomy   2 T 80

MED: 100-2,15,260; 100-4,12,90.3; 100-4,14,10

INTRODUCTION

⊘ **31500** Intubation, endotracheal, emergency procedure   S

If an injection procedure is used for segmental bronchography, use 31656.

31502 Tracheotomy tube change prior to establishment of fistula tract   T

ENDOSCOPY

Code each anatomic site examined via endoscope.

31505 Laryngoscopy, indirect; diagnostic (separate procedure)   T

MED: 100-3,100.2; 100-4,12,40.6
AMA: 1999,Nov,13

31510 with biopsy   2 T 80

MED: 100-2,15,260; 100-3,100.2; 100-4,12,40.6; 100-4,12,90.3; 100-4,14,10
AMA: 1999,Nov,13

31511 with removal of foreign body   2 T

MED: 100-2,15,260; 100-3,100.2; 100-4,12,40.6; 100-4,12,90.3; 100-4,14,10
AMA: 1999,Nov,13

31512 with removal of lesion   2 T 80

MED: 100-2,15,260; 100-3,100.2; 100-4,12,40.6; 100-4,12,90.3; 100-4,14,10
AMA: 1999,Nov,13

31513 with vocal cord injection   2 T 80

MED: 100-2,15,260; 100-3,100.2; 100-4,12,40.6; 100-4,12,90.3; 100-4,14,10
AMA: 1999,Nov,13

31515 Laryngoscopy direct, with or without tracheoscopy; for aspiration   1 T

MED: 100-2,15,260; 100-3,100.2; 100-4,12,40.6; 100-4,12,90.3; 100-4,14,10

31520 diagnostic, newborn   A T 80 ⊛

MED: 100-3,100.2; 100-4,12,40.6

31525 diagnostic, except newborn   1 T

MED: 100-2,15,260; 100-3,100.2; 100-4,12,40.6; 100-4,12,90.3; 100-4,14,10

31526 diagnostic, with operating microscope or telescope   2 T

MED: 100-2,15,260; 100-3,100.2; 100-4,12,40.6; 100-4,12,90.3; 100-4,14,10
AMA: 1998,Nov,11-12
Do not report 69990 in addition to 31526 as the operating microscope is considered an inclusive component of the surgery.

31527   **with insertion of obturator**   🔟 Ⓣ 80 ⚡

MED: 100-2,15,260; 100-3,100.2; 100-4,12,40.6; 100-4,12,90.3;
100-4,14,10

31528   **with dilation, initial**   ➋ Ⓣ 80 ⚡

MED: 100-2,15,260; 100-3,100.2; 100-4,12,40.6; 100-4,12,90.3;
100-4,14,10

31529   **with dilation, subsequent**   ➋ Ⓣ 80 ⚡

MED: 100-2,15,260; 100-3,100.2; 100-4,12,40.6; 100-4,12,90.3;
100-4,14,10

31530   **Laryngoscopy, direct, operative, with foreign body removal;**   ➋ Ⓣ ⚡

MED: 100-2,15,260; 100-3,100.2; 100-4,12,40.6; 100-4,12,90.3;
100-4,14,10

31531   **with operating microscope or telescope**   ➌ Ⓣ 80 ⚡

MED: 100-2,15,260; 100-3,100.2; 100-4,12,40.6; 100-4,12,90.3;
100-4,14,10

AMA: 1998,Nov,11-12
Do not report 69990 in addition to 31531 as the operating microscope or telescope is considered an inclusive component of the surgery.

31535   **Laryngoscopy, direct, operative, with biopsy;**   ➋ Ⓣ ⚡

MED: 100-2,15,260; 100-3,100.2; 100-4,12,40.6; 100-4,12,90.3;
100-4,14,10

31536   **with operating microscope or telescope**   ➌ Ⓣ ⚡

MED: 100-2,15,260; 100-3,100.2; 100-4,12,40.6; 100-4,12,90.3;
100-4,14,10

AMA: 1998,Nov,11-12
Do not report 69990 in addition to 31536 as the operating microscope or telescope is considered an inclusive component of the surgery.

31540   **Laryngoscopy, direct, operative, with excision of tumor and/or stripping of vocal cords or epiglottis;**   ➌ Ⓣ ⚡

MED: 100-2,15,260; 100-3,100.2; 100-4,12,40.6; 100-4,12,90.3;
100-4,14,10

31541   **with operating microscope or telescope**   ➍ Ⓣ ⚡

MED: 100-2,15,260; 100-3,100.2; 100-4,12,40.6; 100-4,12,90.3;
100-4,14,10

AMA: 1998,Nov,11-12
Do not report 69990 in addition to 31541 as the operating microscope or telescope is considered an inclusive component of the surgery.

31545   **Laryngoscopy, direct, operative, with operating microscope or telescope, with submucosal removal of non-neoplastic lesion(s) of vocal cord; reconstruction with local tissue flap(s)**   ➍ Ⓣ ⚡

31546   **reconstruction with graft(s) (includes obtaining autograft)**   ➍ Ⓣ ⚡

Code 31546 cannot be reported with CPT code 20926 for graft harvest.

For reconstruction of vocal cord with allograft consult CPT code 31599.

Code 31545 or 31546 cannot be reported with CPT codes 31540, 31541, and 69990.

31560   **Laryngoscopy, direct, operative, with arytenoidectomy;**   ➎ Ⓣ 80 ⚡

MED: 100-2,15,260; 100-3,100.2; 100-4,12,40.6; 100-4,12,90.3;
100-4,14,10

31561   **with operating microscope or telescope**   ➎ Ⓣ 80 ⚡

MED: 100-2,15,260; 100-3,100.2; 100-4,12,40.6; 100-4,12,90.3;
100-4,14,10

AMA: 1998,Nov,11-12
Do not report 69990 in addition to 31561 as the operating microscope or telescope is considered an inclusive component of the surgery.

31570   **Laryngoscopy, direct, with injection into vocal cord(s), therapeutic;**   ➋ Ⓣ ⚡

MED: 100-2,15,260; 100-3,100.2; 100-4,12,40.6; 100-4,12,90.3;
100-4,14,10

31571   **with operating microscope or telescope**   ➋ Ⓣ ⚡

MED: 100-2,15,260; 100-3,100.2; 100-4,12,40.6; 100-4,12,90.3;
100-4,14,10

AMA: 1998,Nov,11-12
Do not report 69990 in addition to 31571 as the operating microscope or telescope is considered an inclusive component of the surgery.

31575   **Laryngoscopy, flexible fiberoptic; diagnostic**   Ⓣ ⚡

31576   **with biopsy**   ➋ Ⓣ ⚡

MED: 100-2,15,260; 100-4,12,90.3; 100-4,14,10

31577   **with removal of foreign body**   ➋ Ⓣ 80 ⚡

MED: 100-2,15,260; 100-4,12,90.3; 100-4,14,10

31578   **with removal of lesion**   ➋ Ⓣ 80 ⚡

MED: 100-2,15,260; 100-4,12,90.3; 100-4,14,10

If flexible fiberoptic endoscopic evaluation of swallowing is performed, consult CPT codes 92612-92613; for sensory testing, consult CPT code 92614-92615; for swallowing with sensory testing, consult CPT codes 92616-92617.

To report flexible fiberoptic laryngoscopy performed as part of a flexible fiberoptic endoscopic evaluation of swallowing and/or laryngeal sensory testing by cine or video recording, consult CPT codes 92612-92617.

31579   **Laryngoscopy, flexible or rigid fiberoptic, with stroboscopy**   Ⓣ ⚡

REPAIR

31580   **Laryngoplasty; for laryngeal web, two stage, with keel insertion and removal**   ➎ Ⓣ 80 ⚡

MED: 100-2,15,260; 100-4,12,90.3; 100-4,14,10

31582   **for laryngeal stenosis, with graft or core mold, including tracheotomy**   ➎ Ⓣ ⚡

MED: 100-2,15,260; 100-4,12,90.3; 100-4,14,10

31584   **with open reduction of fracture**   Ⓒ 80 ⚡

31587   **Laryngoplasty, cricoid split**   Ⓒ 80 ⚡

31588   **Laryngoplasty, not otherwise specified (eg, for burns, reconstruction after partial laryngectomy)**   ➎ Ⓣ 80 ⚡

MED: 100-2,15,260; 100-4,12,90.3; 100-4,14,10

31590   **Laryngeal reinnervation by neuromuscular pedicle**   ➎ Ⓣ 80 ⚡

MED: 100-2,15,260; 100-4,12,90.3; 100-4,14,10

Respiratory System

31527 — 31590

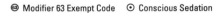

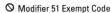
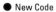
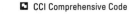

DESTRUCTION

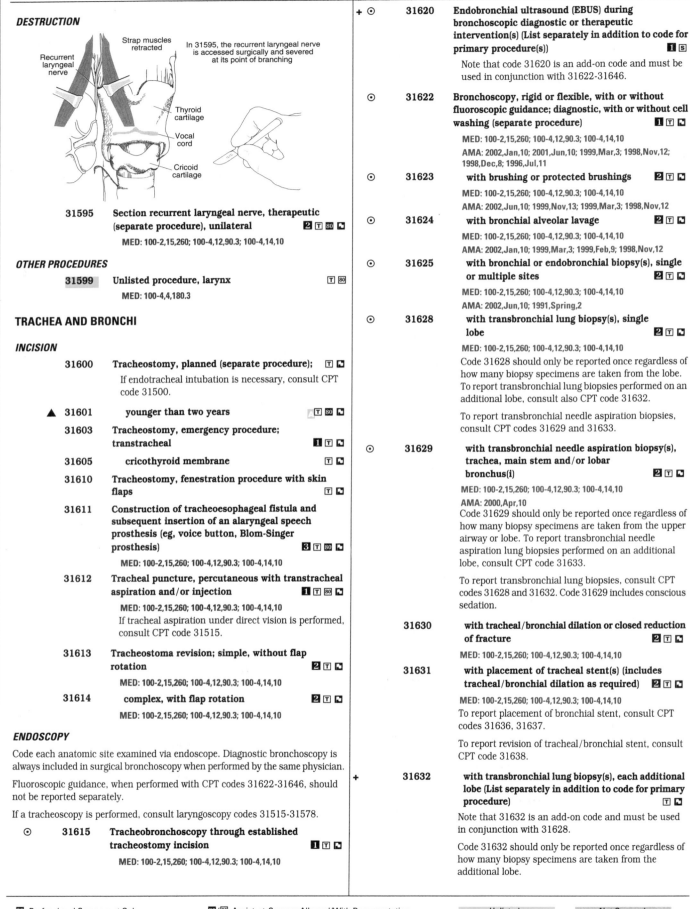

Strap muscles retracted

Recurrent laryngeal nerve

In 31595, the recurrent laryngeal nerve is accessed surgically and severed at its point of branching

Thyroid cartilage

Vocal cord

Cricoid cartilage

31595 Section recurrent laryngeal nerve, therapeutic (separate procedure), unilateral ☐2 ☐T ☐80 ☐

MED: 100-2,15,260; 100-4,12,90.3; 100-4,14,10

OTHER PROCEDURES

31599 Unlisted procedure, larynx ☐T ☐80

MED: 100-4,4,180.3

TRACHEA AND BRONCHI

INCISION

31600 Tracheostomy, planned (separate procedure); ☐T ☐

If endotracheal intubation is necessary, consult CPT code 31500.

▲ **31601** younger than two years ☐ ☐T ☐80 ☐

31603 Tracheostomy, emergency procedure; transtracheal ☐1 ☐T ☐

31605 cricothyroid membrane ☐T ☐

31610 Tracheostomy, fenestration procedure with skin flaps ☐T ☐

31611 Construction of tracheoesophageal fistula and subsequent insertion of an alaryngeal speech prosthesis (eg, voice button, Blom-Singer prosthesis) ☐3 ☐T ☐80 ☐

MED: 100-2,15,260; 100-4,12,90.3; 100-4,14,10

31612 Tracheal puncture, percutaneous with transtracheal aspiration and/or injection ☐1 ☐T ☐80 ☐

MED: 100-2,15,260; 100-4,12,90.3; 100-4,14,10

If tracheal aspiration under direct vision is performed, consult CPT code 31515.

31613 Tracheostoma revision; simple, without flap rotation ☐2 ☐T ☐

MED: 100-2,15,260; 100-4,12,90.3; 100-4,14,10

31614 complex, with flap rotation ☐2 ☐T ☐

MED: 100-2,15,260; 100-4,12,90.3; 100-4,14,10

ENDOSCOPY

Code each anatomic site examined via endoscope. Diagnostic bronchoscopy is always included in surgical bronchoscopy when performed by the same physician.

Fluoroscopic guidance, when performed with CPT codes 31622-31646, should not be reported separately.

If a tracheoscopy is performed, consult laryngoscopy codes 31515-31578.

⊙ **31615** Tracheobronchoscopy through established tracheostomy incision ☐1 ☐T ☐

MED: 100-2,15,260; 100-4,12,90.3; 100-4,14,10

+ ⊙ **31620** Endobronchial ultrasound (EBUS) during bronchoscopic diagnostic or therapeutic intervention(s) (List separately in addition to code for primary procedure(s)) ☐1 ☐S

Note that code 31620 is an add-on code and must be used in conjunction with 31622-31646.

⊙ **31622** Bronchoscopy, rigid or flexible, with or without fluoroscopic guidance; diagnostic, with or without cell washing (separate procedure) ☐1 ☐T ☐

MED: 100-2,15,260; 100-4,12,90.3; 100-4,14,10

AMA: 2002,Jan,10; 2001,Jun,10; 1999,Mar,3; 1998,Nov,12; 1998,Dec,8; 1996,Jul,11

⊙ **31623** with brushing or protected brushings ☐2 ☐T ☐

MED: 100-2,15,260; 100-4,12,90.3; 100-4,14,10

AMA: 2002,Jun,10; 1999,Nov,13; 1999,Mar,3; 1998,Nov,12

⊙ **31624** with bronchial alveolar lavage ☐2 ☐T ☐

MED: 100-2,15,260; 100-4,12,90.3; 100-4,14,10

AMA: 2002,Jan,10; 1999,Mar,3; 1999,Feb,9; 1998,Nov,12

⊙ **31625** with bronchial or endobronchial biopsy(s), single or multiple sites ☐2 ☐T ☐

MED: 100-2,15,260; 100-4,12,90.3; 100-4,14,10

AMA: 2002,Jun,10; 1991,Spring,2

⊙ **31628** with transbronchial lung biopsy(s), single lobe ☐2 ☐T ☐

MED: 100-2,15,260; 100-4,12,90.3; 100-4,14,10

Code 31628 should only be reported once regardless of how many biopsy specimens are taken from the lobe. To report transbronchial lung biopsies performed on an additional lobe, consult also CPT code 31632.

To report transbronchial needle aspiration biopsies, consult CPT codes 31629 and 31633.

⊙ **31629** with transbronchial needle aspiration biopsy(s), trachea, main stem and/or lobar bronchus(i) ☐2 ☐T ☐

MED: 100-2,15,260; 100-4,12,90.3; 100-4,14,10

AMA: 2000,Apr,10

Code 31629 should only be reported once regardless of how many biopsy specimens are taken from the upper airway or lobe. To report transbronchial needle aspiration lung biopsies performed on an additional lobe, consult CPT code 31633.

To report transbronchial lung biopsies, consult CPT codes 31628 and 31632. Code 31629 includes conscious sedation.

31630 with tracheal/bronchial dilation or closed reduction of fracture ☐2 ☐T ☐

MED: 100-2,15,260; 100-4,12,90.3; 100-4,14,10

31631 with placement of tracheal stent(s) (includes tracheal/bronchial dilation as required) ☐2 ☐T ☐

MED: 100-2,15,260; 100-4,12,90.3; 100-4,14,10

To report placement of bronchial stent, consult CPT codes 31636, 31637.

To report revision of tracheal/bronchial stent, consult CPT code 31638.

+ **31632** with transbronchial lung biopsy(s), each additional lobe (List separately in addition to code for primary procedure) ☐T ☐

Note that 31632 is an add-on code and must be used in conjunction with 31628.

Code 31632 should only be reported once regardless of how many biopsy specimens are taken from the additional lobe.

+   **31633**   **with transbronchial needle aspiration biopsy(s), each additional lobe (List separately in addition to code for primary procedure)**   T 🔲

Note that 31633 is an add-on code and must be used in conjunction with 31629.

Code 31633 should only be reported once regardless of how many needle aspiration biopsy specimens are taken from the additional lobe or trachea.

⊙   **31635**   **with removal of foreign body**   2 T 🔲

MED: 100-2,15,260; 100-4,12,90.3; 100-4,14,10
AMA: 2002,Jun,10

31636   **with placement of bronchial stent(s) (includes tracheal/bronchial dilation as required), initial bronchus**   2 T 🔲

+   **31637**   **each additional major bronchus stented (List separately in addition to code for primary procedure)**   1 T

Note that 31637 must be used with 31636.

31638   **with revision of tracheal or bronchial stent inserted at previous session (includes tracheal/bronchial dilation as required)**   2 T 🔲

31640   **with excision of tumor**   2 T 🔲

MED: 100-2,15,260; 100-4,12,90.3; 100-4,14,10

31641   **Bronchoscopy, (rigid or flexible); with destruction of tumor or relief of stenosis by any method other than excision (eg, laser therapy, cryotherapy)**   2 T 🔲

MED: 100-2,15,260; 100-4,12,90.3; 100-4,14,10
AMA: 2000,Sep,5; 1999,Nov,13

If bronchoscopic photodynamic therapy is performed, report CPT code 31641 in addition to 96570 and 96571 as appropriate.

31643   **with placement of catheter(s) for intracavitary radioelement application**   2 T 🔲

MED: 100-2,15,260; 100-4,12,90.3; 100-4,14,10
AMA: 1999,Mar,3; 1998,Nov,12

If intracavitary radioelement application is performed, consult CPT codes 77761-77763 and 77781-77784.

⊙   **31645**   **with therapeutic aspiration of tracheobronchial tree, initial (eg, drainage of lung abscess)**   1 T 🔲

MED: 100-2,15,260; 100-4,12,90.3; 100-4,14,10

If catheter aspiration of the tracheobronchial tree at bedside is performed, consult CPT code 31725. Code 31645 includes conscious sedation.

⊙   **31646**   **with therapeutic aspiration of tracheobronchial tree, subsequent**   1 T 🔲

MED: 100-2,15,260; 100-4,12,90.3; 100-4,14,10

If catheter aspiration of the tracheobronchial tree at bedside is performed, consult CPT code 31725. Code 31646 includes conscious sedation.

⊙   **31656**   **with injection of contrast material for segmental bronchography (fiberscope only)**   1 T 80 🔲

MED: 100-2,15,260; 100-4,12,90.3; 100-4,14,10

To report radiological supervision and interpretation, consult CPT codes 71040 and 71060.

INTRODUCTION

If endotracheal intubation is performed, consult CPT code 31500. If tracheal aspiration under direct vision is performed, consult CPT code 31515.

~~**31700**~~   ~~**Catheterization, transglottic (separate procedure)**~~

MED: 100-2,15,260; 100-4,12,90.3; 100-4,14,10

~~**31708**~~   ~~**Instillation of contrast material for laryngography or bronchography, without catheterization**~~

~~**31710**~~   ~~**Catheterization for bronchography, with or without instillation of contrast material**~~

31715   **Transtracheal injection for bronchography**   N 80 50 🔲

To report radiological supervision and interpretation, consult CPT codes 71040 and 71060. If prolonged services are necessary, consult CPT codes 99354-99360.

31717   **Catheterization with bronchial brush biopsy**   1 T 🔲

MED: 100-2,15,260; 100-4,12,90.3; 100-4,14,10
AMA: 2001,Feb,11

31720   **Catheter aspiration (separate procedure); nasotracheal**   1 T 🔲

MED: 100-2,15,260; 100-4,12,90.3; 100-4,14,10

⊙   **31725**   **tracheobronchial with fiberscope, bedside**   C 🔲

31730   **Transtracheal (percutaneous) introduction of needle wire dilator/stent or indwelling tube for oxygen therapy**   1 T 🔲

MED: 100-2,15,260; 100-4,12,90.3; 100-4,14,10

EXCISION, REPAIR

31750   **Tracheoplasty; cervical**   5 T 80 🔲

MED: 100-2,15,260; 100-4,12,90.3; 100-4,14,10

31755   **tracheopharyngeal fistulization, each stage**   2 T 80 🔲

MED: 100-2,15,260; 100-4,12,90.3; 100-4,14,10

31760   **intrathoracic**   C 80 🔲

31766   **Carinal reconstruction**   C 80 🔲

31770   **Bronchoplasty; graft repair**   C 80 🔲

If a lobectomy and bronchoplasty are performed, consult CPT code 32501.

31775   **excision stenosis and anastomosis**   C 80 🔲

31780   **Excision tracheal stenosis and anastomosis; cervical**   C 80 🔲

31781   **cervicothoracic**   C 80 🔲

31785   **Excision of tracheal tumor or carcinoma; cervical**   T 80 🔲

31786   **thoracic**   C 80 🔲

31800   **Suture of tracheal wound or injury; cervical**   C 80 🔲

31805   **intrathoracic**   C 80 🔲

31820   **Surgical closure tracheostomy or fistula; without plastic repair**   1 T 80 🔲

MED: 100-2,15,260; 100-4,12,90.3; 100-4,14,10

If a tracheoesophageal fistula is repaired, consult CPT codes 43305 and 43312.

31825   **with plastic repair**   2 T 80 🔲

MED: 100-2,15,260; 100-4,12,90.3; 100-4,14,10

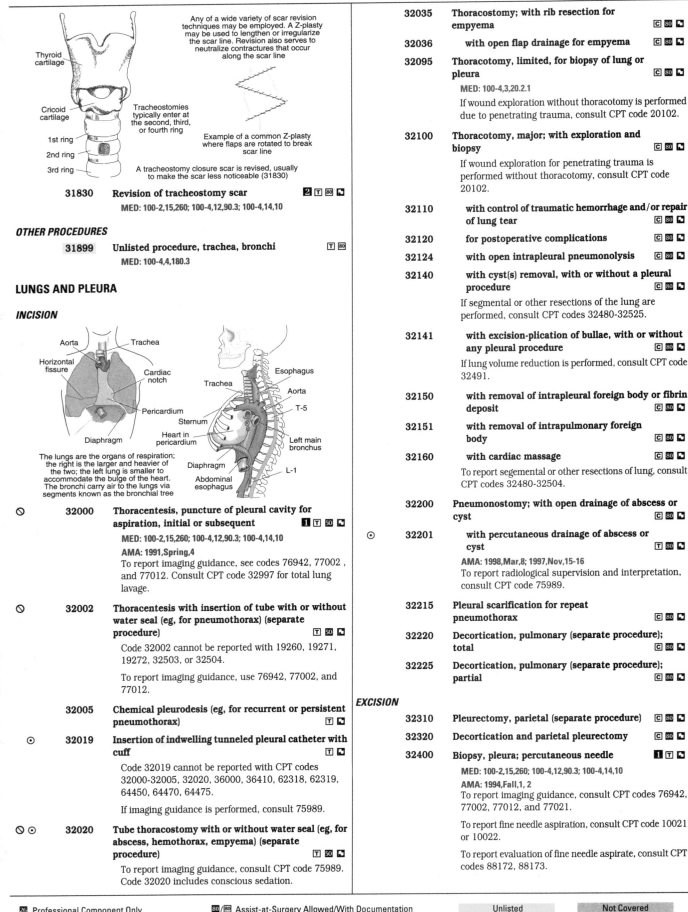

Any of a wide variety of scar revision techniques may be employed. A Z-plasty may be used to lengthen or irregularize the scar line. Revision also serves to neutralize contractures that occur along the scar line

Thyroid cartilage

Cricoid cartilage

1st ring

2nd ring

3rd ring

Tracheostomies typically enter at the second, third, or fourth ring

Example of a common Z-plasty where flaps are rotated to break scar line

A tracheostomy closure scar is revised, usually to make the scar less noticeable (31830)

31830　　**Revision of tracheostomy scar**　　🔲 Ⓣ 80 🔲
MED: 100-2,15,260; 100-4,12,90.3; 100-4,14,10

OTHER PROCEDURES

31899　　Unlisted procedure, trachea, bronchi　　Ⓣ 80
MED: 100-4,4,180.3

LUNGS AND PLEURA

INCISION

Aorta　Trachea

Horizontal fissure

Cardiac notch

Pericardium

Diaphragm

Trachea

Esophagus

Aorta

T-5

Sternum

Heart in pericardium

Diaphragm

Abdominal esophagus

Left main bronchus

L-1

The lungs are the organs of respiration; the right is the larger and heavier of the two; the left lung is smaller to accommodate the bulge of the heart. The bronchi carry air to the lungs via segments known as the bronchial tree

⊘　**32000**　　**Thoracentesis, puncture of pleural cavity for aspiration, initial or subsequent**　🔲 Ⓣ 50 🔲
MED: 100-2,15,260; 100-4,12,90.3; 100-4,14,10
AMA: 1991,Spring,4
To report imaging guidance, see codes 76942, 77002, and 77012. Consult CPT code 32997 for total lung lavage.

⊘　**32002**　　**Thoracentesis with insertion of tube with or without water seal (eg, for pneumothorax) (separate procedure)**　Ⓣ 50 🔲
Code 32002 cannot be reported with 19260, 19271, 19272, 32503, or 32504.

To report imaging guidance, use 76942, 77002, and 77012.

32005　　**Chemical pleurodesis (eg, for recurrent or persistent pneumothorax)**　Ⓣ 🔲

⊙　**32019**　　**Insertion of indwelling tunneled pleural catheter with cuff**　Ⓣ 🔲
Code 32019 cannot be reported with CPT codes 32000-32005, 32020, 36000, 36410, 62318, 62319, 64450, 64470, 64475.

If imaging guidance is performed, consult 75989.

⊘ ⊙　**32020**　　**Tube thoracostomy with or without water seal (eg, for abscess, hemothorax, empyema) (separate procedure)**　Ⓣ 50 🔲
To report imaging guidance, consult CPT code 75989. Code 32020 includes conscious sedation.

32035　　**Thoracostomy; with rib resection for empyema**　🅒 80 🔲

32036　　　　with open flap drainage for empyema　🅒 80 🔲

32095　　**Thoracotomy, limited, for biopsy of lung or pleura**　🅒 80 🔲
MED: 100-4,3,20.2.1
If wound exploration without thoracotomy is performed due to penetrating trauma, consult CPT code 20102.

32100　　**Thoracotomy, major; with exploration and biopsy**　🅒 80 🔲
If wound exploration for penetrating trauma is performed without thoracotomy, consult CPT code 20102.

32110　　　　with control of traumatic hemorrhage and/or repair of lung tear　🅒 80 🔲

32120　　　　for postoperative complications　🅒 80 🔲

32124　　　　with open intrapleural pneumonolysis　🅒 80 🔲

32140　　　　with cyst(s) removal, with or without a pleural procedure　🅒 80 🔲
If segmental or other resections of the lung are performed, consult CPT codes 32480-32525.

32141　　　　with excision-plication of bullae, with or without any pleural procedure　🅒 80 🔲
If lung volume reduction is performed, consult CPT code 32491.

32150　　　　with removal of intrapleural foreign body or fibrin deposit　🅒 80 🔲

32151　　　　with removal of intrapulmonary foreign body　🅒 80 🔲

32160　　　　with cardiac massage　🅒 80 🔲
To report segemental or other resections of lung, consult CPT codes 32480-32504.

32200　　**Pneumonostomy; with open drainage of abscess or cyst**　🅒 80 🔲

⊙　**32201**　　　　with percutaneous drainage of abscess or cyst　Ⓣ 80 🔲
AMA: 1998,Mar,8; 1997,Nov,15-16
To report radiological supervision and interpretation, consult CPT code 75989.

32215　　**Pleural scarification for repeat pneumothorax**　🅒 80 🔲

32220　　**Decortication, pulmonary (separate procedure); total**　🅒 80 🔲

32225　　**Decortication, pulmonary (separate procedure); partial**　🅒 80 🔲

EXCISION

32310　　**Pleurectomy, parietal (separate procedure)**　🅒 80 🔲

32320　　**Decortication and parietal pleurectomy**　🅒 80 🔲

32400　　**Biopsy, pleura; percutaneous needle**　🔲 Ⓣ 🔲
MED: 100-2,15,260; 100-4,12,90.3; 100-4,14,10
AMA: 1994,Fall,1, 2
To report imaging guidance, consult CPT codes 76942, 77002, 77012, and 77021.

To report fine needle aspiration, consult CPT code 10021 or 10022.

To report evaluation of fine needle aspirate, consult CPT codes 88172, 88173.

26 Professional Component Only　　　　**80/80** Assist-at-Surgery Allowed/With Documentation　　　Unlisted　　　　Not Covered

TC Technical Component Only　　**MED:** Pub 100/NCD References　**AMA:** CPT Assistant References　**1**-**9** ASC Group　♂ Male Only　♀ Female Only

122 — CPT Expert　　　　**CPT only © 2006 American Medical Association. All Rights Reserved.** *(Black Ink)*　　　**© 2006 Ingenix** *(Blue Ink)*

Respiratory System

31830 — 32400

32402	open	C 80
	MED: 100-4,3,20.2.1	
	AMA: 1994,Fall,1, 2	
32405	**Biopsy, lung or mediastinum, percutaneous needle**	1 T
	MED: 100-2,15,260; 100-4,12,90.3; 100-4,14,10	
	AMA: 2002,Aug,10; 1997,Mar,4; 1994,Fall,1, 2	

To report radiological supervision and interpretation, consult CPT codes 76942, 77002, 77012, and 77021.

To report fine needle aspiration, consult CPT code 10022.

To report evaluation of fine needle aspirate, consult CPT codes 88172, 88173.

REMOVAL

32420	**Pneumocentesis, puncture of lung for aspiration**	1 T
	MED: 100-2,15,260; 100-4,12,90.3; 100-4,14,10	
	AMA: 1994,Fall,1, 2	

Trachea
Aortic arch
Superior lobe bronchi
Lungs
Pericardium
Middle lobe bronchi
Pulmonary arterial trunk
Cardiac notch
Abdominal esophagus
Diaphragm
Inferior lobe bronchi

The right lung is larger and heavier than the left due to space lost to the bulge of the heart at the cardiac notch. The pulmonary arteries (blue at left) deliver venous blood to the lungs where it is oxygenated and converted into arterial blood

32440	**Removal of lung, total pneumonectomy;**	C 80
	AMA: 1994,Fall,1	
32442	**with resection of segment of trachea followed by broncho-tracheal anastomosis (sleeve pneumonectomy)**	C 80
	AMA: 1994,Fall,1, 3	
32445	**extrapleural**	C 80
	AMA: 1994,Fall,1, 3	

For extrapleural pneumonectomy with empyemectomy consult CPT codes 32445 and 32540.

To report lung resection performed with a chest wall tumor resection, report the code for the chest wall tumor resection, 19260-19272, as appropriate, in addition to the code for the lung resection, 32480-32500.

32480	**Removal of lung, other than total pneumonectomy; single lobe (lobectomy)**	C 80
	AMA: 1994,Fall,1, 4; 1991,Spring,5	
32482	**two lobes (bilobectomy)**	C 80
	AMA: 1994,Fall,1, 4	
32484	**single segment (segmentectomy)**	C 80
	AMA: 1994,Fall,1, 4	
32486	**with circumferential resection of segment of bronchus followed by broncho-bronchial anastomosis (sleeve lobectomy)**	C 80
	AMA: 1994,Fall,1, 4	
32488	**all remaining lung following previous removal of a portion of lung (completion pneumonectomy)**	C 80
	AMA: 1994,Fall,1, 4	

32491	**excision-plication of emphysematous lung(s) (bullous or non-bullous) for lung volume reduction, sternal split or transthoracic approach, with or without any pleural procedure**	C 80 50
	MED: 100-4,3,100.7	
32500	**wedge resection, single or multiple**	C 80
	AMA: 1997,Mar,4; 1994,Fall,1, 5	

To report lung resection performed with a chest wall tumor resection, report the code for the chest wall tumor resection, 19260-19272, as appropriate, in addition to the code for the lung resection, 32440-32445.

+ 32501	**Resection and repair of portion of bronchus (bronchoplasty) when performed at time of lobectomy or segmentectomy (List separately in addition to code for primary procedure)**	C 80

Note that 32501 is an add-on code and must be used in conjunction with 32480, 32482, and 32484. Note also that 32501 is to be used when a portion of the bronchus is removed in order to preserve the lung and consequently requires plastic closure to maintain function of that preserved lung. This code is not to be used when the proximal end of a resected bronchus is closed.

32503	**Resection of apical lung tumor (eg, Pancoast tumor), including chest wall resection, rib(s) resection(s), neurovascular dissection, when performed; without chest wall reconstruction(s)**	C 80
32504	**with chest wall reconstruction**	C 80

Codes 32503, 32504 cannot be reported with 19260, 19271, 19272, 32002, 32020, 32100.

To report performance of lung resection in conjunction with chest wall resection, consult 19260, 19271, 19272 and 32480-32500, 32503, 32504.

32540	**Extrapleural enucleation of empyema (empyemectomy)**	C 80

ENDOSCOPY

Surgical thoracoscopy always includes diagnostic thoracoscopy.

Code each anatomic site examined via endoscope.

32601	**Thoracoscopy, diagnostic (separate procedure); lungs and pleural space, without biopsy**	T 80
	MED: 100-3,100.2; 100-4,12,40.6	
	AMA: 1994,Fall,1, 4	
32602	**lungs and pleural space, with biopsy**	T 80
	MED: 100-3,100.2; 100-4,12,40.6	
	AMA: 1997,Jun,5; 1994,Fall,1, 4	
32603	**pericardial sac, without biopsy**	T 80
	MED: 100-3,100.2; 100-4,12,40.6	
	AMA: 1994,Fall,1, 4	
32604	**pericardial sac, with biopsy**	T 80
	MED: 100-3,100.2; 100-4,12,40.6	
	AMA: 1994,Fall,1, 4	
32605	**mediastinal space, without biopsy**	T 80
	MED: 100-3,100.2; 100-4,12,40.6	
	AMA: 1994,Fall,1, 4	
32606	**mediastinal space, with biopsy**	T 80
	MED: 100-3,100.2; 100-4,12,40.6	
	AMA: 1994,Fall,1, 5	
32650	**Thoracoscopy, surgical; with pleurodesis (eg, mechanical or chemical)**	C 80
	MED: 100-3,100.2; 100-4,12,40.6	
	AMA: 1994,Fall,1, 6	

32402 — 32650

Respiratory System

32651 — 32960

32651 with partial pulmonary decortication © 80 ↻

MED: 100-3,100.2; 100-4,12,40.6

AMA: 1994,Fall,1, 6

32652 with total pulmonary decortication, including intrapleural pneumonolysis © 80 ↻

MED: 100-3,100.2; 100-4,12,40.6

AMA: 1994,Fall,1, 6

32653 with removal of intrapleural foreign body or fibrin deposit © 80 ↻

MED: 100-3,100.2; 100-4,12,40.6

AMA: 1994,Fall,1, 6

32654 with control of traumatic hemorrhage © 80 ↻

MED: 100-3,100.2; 100-4,12,40.6

AMA: 1994,Fall,1, 6

32655 with excision-plication of bullae, including any pleural procedure © 80 ↻

MED: 100-3,100.2; 100-4,12,40.6

AMA: 1994,Fall,1, 6

32656 with parietal pleurectomy © 80 ↻

MED: 100-3,100.2; 100-4,12,40.6

AMA: 1994,Fall,1, 6

32657 with wedge resection of lung, single or multiple © 80 ↻

MED: 100-3,100.2; 100-4,12,40.6

AMA: 1994,Fall,1, 6

32658 with removal of clot or foreign body from pericardial sac © 80 ↻

MED: 100-3,100.2; 100-4,12,40.6

AMA: 1994,Fall,1, 6

32659 with creation of pericardial window or partial resection of pericardial sac for drainage © 80 ↻

MED: 100-3,100.2; 100-4,12,40.6

AMA: 1994,Fall,1, 6

32660 with total pericardiectomy © 80 ↻

MED: 100-3,100.2; 100-4,12,40.6

AMA: 1994,Fall,1, 6

32661 with excision of pericardial cyst, tumor, or mass © 80 ↻

MED: 100-3,100.2; 100-4,12,40.6

AMA: 1994,Fall,1, 6

32662 with excision of mediastinal cyst, tumor, or mass © 80 ↻

MED: 100-3,100.2; 100-4,12,40.6

AMA: 1994,Fall,1, 6

32663 with lobectomy, total or segmental © 80 ↻

MED: 100-3,100.2; 100-4,12,40.6

AMA: 1994,Fall,1, 6

32664 with thoracic sympathectomy © 80 50 ↻

MED: 100-3,100.2; 100-4,12,40.6

AMA: 1994,Fall,1, 6

32665 with esophagomyotomy (Heller type) © 80 ↻

MED: 100-3,100.2; 100-4,12,40.6

AMA: 1994,Fall,1, 6

REPAIR

32800 Repair lung hernia through chest wall © 80 ↻

MED: 100-3,100.2; 100-4,12,40.6

32810 Closure of chest wall following open flap drainage for empyema (Clagett type procedure) © 80 ↻

MED: 100-3,100.2; 100-4,12,40.6

32815 Open closure of major bronchial fistula © 80 ↻

MED: 100-3,100.2; 100-4,12,40.6

32820 Major reconstruction, chest wall (posttraumatic) © 80 ↻

MED: 100-3,100.2; 100-4,12,40.6

LUNG TRANSPLANTATION

Lung transplantation involves three different components:

- Harvesting of the lung and cold preservation (See 32850).
- Backbench work consists of preparation of cadaver donor single lung or both lungs prior to transplantation. This includes dissection of the lung from tissue around it and preparation of the pulmonary venous/atrial cuff, pulmonary artery and bronchus bilaterally (see codes 32855, 32856).
- Recipient transplantation which includes transplanting a single lung or both lungs into the patient (See 32851-32854).

32850 Donor pneumonectomy(s) (including cold preservation), from cadaver donor © ↻

MED: 100-3,100.2; 100-4,12,40.6

32851 Lung transplant, single; without cardiopulmonary bypass © 80 ↻

MED: 100-3,100.2; 100-4,12,40.6

32852 with cardiopulmonary bypass © 80 ↻

MED: 100-3,100.2; 100-4,12,40.6

32853 Lung transplant, double (bilateral sequential or en bloc); without cardiopulmonary bypass © 80 ↻

MED: 100-3,100.2; 100-4,12,40.6

32854 with cardiopulmonary bypass © 80 ↻

MED: 100-3,100.2; 100-4,12,40.6

32855 Backbench standard preparation of cadaver donor lung allograft prior to transplantation, including dissection of allograft from surrounding soft tissues to prepare pulmonary venous/atrial cuff, pulmonary artery, and bronchus; unilateral © 80 ↻

32856 bilateral © 80 ↻

To report resection or repair procedures on the donor lung, consult CPT codes 32491, 32500, 35216, or 35278.

SURGICAL COLLAPSE THERAPY; THORACOPLASTY

Consult also CPT codes 32503 and 32504

32900 Resection of ribs, extrapleural, all stages © 80 ↻

MED: 100-3,100.2; 100-4,12,40.6

32905 Thoracoplasty, Schede type or extrapleural (all stages); © 80 ↻

MED: 100-3,100.2; 100-4,12,40.6

32906 with closure of bronchopleural fistula © 80 ↻

MED: 100-3,100.2; 100-4,12,40.6

If the first rib for thoracic outer compression is resected, consult CPT codes 21615 and 21616.

If the major bronchial fistula required open closure, consult CPT code 32815.

32940 Pneumonolysis, extraperiosteal, including filling or packing procedures © 80 ↻

MED: 100-3,100.2; 100-4,12,40.6

32960 Pneumothorax, therapeutic, intrapleural injection of air Ⓣ ↻

MED: 100-3,100.2; 100-4,12,40.6

---

26 Professional Component Only   80/80 Assist-at-Surgery Allowed/With Documentation   Unlisted   Not Covered

TC Technical Component Only   **MED:** Pub 100/NCD References   **AMA:** CPT Assistant References   1-9 ASC Group   ♂ Male Only   ♀ Female Only

124 — CPT Expert   CPT only © 2006 American Medical Association. All Rights Reserved. *(Black Ink)*   © *2006 Ingenix (Blue Ink)*

OTHER PROCEDURES

32997   **Total lung lavage (unilateral)**   ⓒ 🔄
  MED: 100-3,100.2; 100-4,12,40.6
  AMA: 1999,Nov,14; 1998,Nov,13
  If a bronchoscopic bronchial alveolar lavage is
  performed, consult CPT code 31624.

● **32998**   **Ablation therapy for reduction or eradication of one
  or more pulmonary tumor(s) including pleura or chest
  wall when involved by tumor extension, percutaneous,
  radiofrequency, unilateral**   Ⓣ
  For imaging guidance and monitoring, consult codes
  76940, 77013, and 77022.

32999   **Unlisted procedure, lungs and pleura**   Ⓣ 80
  MED: 100-3,100.2; 100-4,4,180.3; 100-4,12,40.6
  AMA: 2002,Jan,11

CARDIOVASCULAR SYSTEM

HEART AND PERICARDIUM

Code vascular catheterization to include introduction and all lesser order catheterization used in the approach. Consult 36218 and 36248 to report additional second and third order arterial catheterization within the same family of arteries. Code separately catheterization in first order vessels different from the family originally coded.

If monitoring and the operation of pump and other nonsurgical services are performed, consult CPT codes 99190-99192, 99291, 99292, and 99354-99360. If other medical or laboratory related services are performed, consult the appropriate section of CPT. If radiological supervision and interpretation are performed, consult CPT codes 75600-75978.

PERICARDIUM

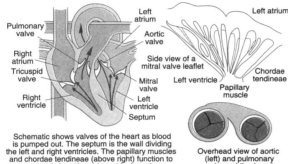

Pulmonary valve · Right atrium · Tricuspid valve · Right ventricle · Left atrium · Aortic valve · Side view of a mitral valve leaflet · Mitral valve · Left ventricle · Left ventricle · Septum · Papillary muscle · Chordae tendineae · Left atrium

Schematic shows valves of the heart as blood is pumped out. The septum is the wall dividing the left and right ventricles. The papillary muscles and chordae tendineae (above right) function to open and close the atrioventricular valves

Overhead view of aortic (left) and pulmonary valves while closed

⊙ **33010**   **Pericardiocentesis; initial**   2 T ▫

MED: 100-2,15,260; 100-4,12,90.3; 100-4,14,10
If radiological supervision and interpretation is performed, consult CPT code 76930.

⊙ **33011**   **subsequent**   2 T 80 ▫

MED: 100-2,15,260; 100-4,12,90.3; 100-4,14,10
If radiological supervision and interpretation is performed, consult CPT code 76930.

33015   **Tube pericardiostomy**   C ▫

33020   **Pericardiotomy for removal of clot or foreign body (primary procedure)**   C 80 ▫

33025   **Creation of pericardial window or partial resection for drainage**   C 80 ▫

33030   **Pericardiectomy, subtotal or complete; without cardiopulmonary bypass**   C 80 ▫

     Delorme pericardiectomy

33031   **with cardiopulmonary bypass**   C 80 ▫

33050   **Excision of pericardial cyst or tumor**   C 80 ▫

CARDIAC TUMOR

33120   **Excision of intracardiac tumor, resection with cardiopulmonary bypass**   C 80 ▫

33130   **Resection of external cardiac tumor**   C 80 ▫

TRANSMYOCARDIAL REVASCULARIZATION

33140   **Transmyocardial laser revascularization, by thoracotomy; (separate procedure)**   C 80 ▫

MED: 100-3,20.6
AMA: 2001,Apr,7; 2000,Nov,5; 1999,Nov,14

\+   **33141**   **performed at the time of other open cardiac procedure(s) (List separately in addition to code for primary procedure)**   C 80

MED: 100-3,20.6
AMA: 2001,Apr,7
Note that 33141 is an add-on code and must be used in conjunction with 33400-33496, 33510-33536, and 33542.

PACEMAKER OR PACING CARDIOVERTER-DEFIBRILLATOR

Pacemakers differ from pacing cardioverter-defibrillator pulse generators. In their simplicity, pacemakers maintain the rhythm of the heart through electrodes placed on the heart or in an artery. The electronics within stimulate one or more chambers in the heart. Pacing cardioverter-defibrillators also include a generator that stimulates the heart but also applies defibrillating shocks to treat ventricular tachycardia or ventricular fibrillation. Most are placed in a subcutaneous "pocket" below the clavicle or below the ribcage.

A single chamber pacemaker includes a pulse generator and one electrode. A dual chamber includes a pulse generator and two electrodes. If an additional electrode is inserted in the left ventricle (biventricular pacing), report separately with code 33224 or 33225. For epicardial placement of the electrode, consult 33202-33203. Electrodes are inserted through a vein (transvenous) or on the surface of the heart (epicardial). Pacemaker systems are either single or dual chamber systems. In a single chamber system a single electrode is placed in either the atrium or ventricle. In a dual chamber system two electrodes are placed, one into the atrium and one into the ventricle.

Electrode positioning on the the epicardial surface of the heart requires thoracotomy, or thorascopic placement of the leads. The physician may first try by transvenous extraction. If this is unsuccessful a thoracotomy may be necessary. In this event consult codes 33212, 33213, 33240 in addition to the thoracotomy or endoscopic placement of the epicardial lead to report the insertion of the generator if it is performed by the same physician at the same operative session.

Replacement of a pulse generator requires assignment of two codes, one for the removal and another for the insertion. This may also be referred to as a pacemaker battery change.

When an additional electrode is required to achieve left ventricular pacing, report CPT code 33224 or 33225.

Repositioning of a previously implanted electrode should be reported with CPT code 33215 or 33226. Consult 33206-33208, 33210-33213, or 33224 for replacement of an electrode.

If an electronic, telephonic analysis of the internal pacemaker system is performed, consult CPT codes 93731-93736.

If radiological supervision and interpretation with insertion of pacemaker is performed, consult CPT code 71090.

~~**33200**~~   ~~**Insertion of permanent pacemaker with epicardial electrode(s); by thoracotomy**~~

MED: 100-3,20.8; 100-3,20.8.1

~~**33201**~~   ~~**by xiphoid approach**~~

MED: 100-3,20.8; 100-3,20.8.1; 100-3,20.8.3

● **33202**   **Insertion of epicardial electrode(s); open incision (eg, thoracotomy, median sternotomy, subxiphoid approach)**   C

● **33203**   **endoscopic approach (eg, thoracoscopy, pericardioscopy)**   C

When epicardial lead placement is performemd by the same physician at the same session as the insertion of the generator, report 33202, 33203 in conjunction with 33212, 33213, as appropriate.

⊙ **33206**   **Insertion or replacement of permanent pacemaker with transvenous electrode(s); atrial**   T ▫

MED: 100-3,20.8; 100-3,20.8.1; 100-3,20.8.3
AMA: 1999,Nov,15; 1996,Oct,9; 1994,Summer,10, 17

⊙ **33207** ventricular ⊤ ☐

MED: 100-3,20.8; 100-3,20.8.1; 100-3,20.8.3

AMA: 1999,Nov,15; 1996,Oct,9; 1994,Summer,10, 17

⊙ **33208** **atrial and ventricular** ⊤ ☐

MED: 100-3,20.8; 100-3,20.8.1; 100-3,20.8.3

AMA: 1999,Nov,15; 1996,Jul,10; 1994,Summer,10, 17
Subcutaneous insertion of pulse generator and transvenous placement of electrode(s) are included in codes 33206-33208, do not report separately.

⊙ **33210** **Insertion or replacement of temporary transvenous single chamber cardiac electrode or pacemaker catheter (separate procedure)** ⊤ ☐

MED: 100-3,20.8; 100-3,20.8.1; 100-3,20.8.3

AMA: 1994,Summer,10, 17

⊙ **33211** **Insertion or replacement of temporary transvenous dual chamber pacing electrodes (separate procedure)** ⊤ ☐

MED: 100-3,20.8; 100-3,20.8.1; 100-3,20.8.3; 100-4,4,61.2

AMA: 1994,Summer,10, 17

⊙ **33212** **Insertion or replacement of pacemaker pulse generator only; single chamber, atrial or ventricular** ③ ⊤ ☐

MED: 100-3,20.8; 100-3,20.8.1; 100-4,4,61.2

AMA: 1994,Summer,10, 18; 1994,Fall,24

⊙ **33213** dual chamber ③ ⊤ ☐

MED: 100-3,20.8; 100-3,20.8.1

AMA: 1998,Feb,11; 1996,Oct,10; 1994,Summer,10, 18
Use 33212, 33213, as appropriate, in conjunction with the epicardial lead placement codes 33202, 33203 to report the insertion of the generator when done by the same physician during the same session.

⊙ **33214** **Upgrade of implanted pacemaker system, conversion of single chamber system to dual chamber system (includes removal of previously placed pulse generator, testing of existing lead, insertion of new lead, insertion of new pulse generator)** ⊤ 80 ☐

MED: 100-3,20.8; 100-3,20.8.1

AMA: 1994,Summer,10, 18; 1994,Fall,24
Report 33214 with 33202, 33203 when epicardial electrode placement is performed.

33215 **Repositioning of previously implanted transvenous pacemaker or pacing cardioverter-defibrillator (right atrial or right ventricular) electrode** ⊤ ☐

MED: 100-3,20.4; 100-3,20.8; 100-3,20.8.1

⊙ **33216** **Insertion of a transvenous electrode; single chamber (one electrode) permanent pacemaker or single chamber pacing cardioverter-defibrillator** ⊤ ☐

MED: 100-3,20.4; 100-3,20.8; 100-3,20.8.1; 100-3,20.8.3; 100-4,4,61.2

AMA: 1999,Nov,15-16; 1996,Jul,10; 1994,Summer,10, 18

⊙ **33217** dual chamber (two electrodes) permanent pacemaker or dual chamber pacing cardioverter-defibrillator ⊤ ☐

MED: 100-3,20.4; 100-3,20.8; 100-3,20.8.1; 100-3,20.8.3; 100-4,4,61.2

AMA: 1999,Nov,15-16; 1996,Jul,10; 1994,Summer,10, 18
Codes 33216-33217 should not be reported with 33214.

⊙ **33218** **Repair of single transvenous electrode for a single chamber, permanent pacemaker or single chamber pacing cardioverter-defibrillator** ⊤ ☐

MED: 100-3,20.4; 100-3,20.8; 100-3,20.8.1; 100-3,20.8.3

AMA: 1999,Nov,15-16; 1996,Oct,1, 9; 1994,Summer,10, 19
If atrial or ventricular single chamber single transvenous electrode is repaired with the replacement of a pulse generator, consult CPT codes 33212 or 33213 and 33218 or 33220.

⊙ **33220** **Repair of two transvenous electrodes for a dual chamber permanent pacemaker or dual chamber pacing cardioverter-defibrillator** ⊤ ☐

MED: 100-3,20.4; 100-3,20.8; 100-3,20.8.1; 100-3,20.8.3

AMA: 1999,Nov,15-16; 1996,Oct,9; 1994,Summer,10, 19

⊙ **33222** **Revision or relocation of skin pocket for pacemaker** ② ⊤ ☐

MED: 100-2,15,260; 100-3,20.8; 100-3,20.8.1; 100-3,20.8.3; 100-4,12,90.3; 100-4,14,10

AMA: 1999,Nov,15-16; 1994,Summer,10; 1994,Spring,30

⊙ **33223** **Revision of skin pocket for single or dual chamber pacing cardioverter-defibrillator** ② ⊤ 80 ☐

MED: 100-2,15,260; 100-3,20.4; 100-3,20.8; 100-3,20.8.1; 100-4,12,90.3; 100-4,14,10

AMA: 1999,Nov,15-16; 1994,Summer,10, 19

33224 **Insertion of pacing electrode, cardiac venous system, for left ventricular pacing, with attachment to previously placed pacemaker or pacing cardioverter-defibrillator pulse generator (including revision of pocket, removal, insertion, and/or replacement of generator)** ⊤ ☐

MED: 100-3,20.4; 100-3,20.8; 100-3,20.8.1; 100-4,4,61.2
Report 33224 with 33202, 33203 when epicardial electrode placement is performed.

+ **33225** **Insertion of pacing electrode, cardiac venous system, for left ventricular pacing, at time of insertion of pacing cardioverter-defibrillator or pacemaker pulse generator (including upgrade to dual chamber system) (List separately in addition to code for primary procedure)** ⊤ ☐

MED: 100-3,20.4; 100-3,20.8; 100-3,20.8.1; 100-4,4,61.2
Note that 33225 is an add-on code and must be used in conjunction with 33206-33208, 33212-33214, 33216-33217, 33222, 33233-33235, 33240, and 33249.

33226 **Repositioning of previously implanted cardiac venous system (left ventricular) electrode (including removal, insertion and/or replacement of generator)** ⊤ ☐

MED: 100-3,20.8; 100-3,20.8.1

⊙ **33233** **Removal of permanent pacemaker pulse generator** ② ⊤ ☐

MED: 100-3,20.8; 100-3,20.8.1

AMA: 1996,Oct,10; 1994,Summer,10, 19; 1994,Fall,24

⊙ **33234** **Removal of transvenous pacemaker electrode(s); single lead system, atrial or ventricular** ⊤ ☐

MED: 100-3,20.8; 100-3,20.8.1; 100-3,20.8.3

AMA: 1999,Nov,16; 1994,Summer,10, 19

⊙ **33235** dual lead system ⊤ ☐

MED: 100-3,20.8; 100-3,20.8.1; 100-3,20.8.3

AMA: 1999,Nov,16; 1994,Summer,10, 19

33236 **Removal of permanent epicardial pacemaker and electrodes by thoracotomy; single lead system, atrial or ventricular** ⓒ 80 ☐

MED: 100-3,20.8; 100-3,20.8.1; 100-3,20.8.3

AMA: 1999,Nov,16; 1994,Summer,10, 19

33237 dual lead system ⓒ 80 ☐

MED: 100-3,20.8; 100-3,20.8.1; 100-3,20.8.3

AMA: 1999,Nov,16; 1994,Summer,10, 19

33238 **Removal of permanent transvenous electrode(s) by thoracotomy** ⓒ 80 ☐

MED: 100-3,20.4; 100-3,20.8; 100-3,20.8.1; 100-3,20.8.3

AMA: 1999,Nov,16; 1994,Summer,10, 19

⊕ Modifier 63 Exempt Code ⊙ Conscious Sedation + CPT Add-on Code ⊘ Modifier 51 Exempt Code ● New Code ▲ Revised Code

Ⓜ Maternity Edit Ⓐ Age Edit Ⓐ-Ⓥ APC Status Indicators ☐ CCI Comprehensive Code 50 Bilateral Procedure

⊙ **33240** **Insertion of single or dual chamber pacing cardioverter-defibrillator pulse generator** B

MED: 100-3,20.4; 100-3,20.8; 100-3,20.8.1; 100-3,20.8.3

AMA: 2000,Jul,5; 1999,Nov,16-17; 1996,Jun,10; 1994,Summer,40
Use 33240, as appropriate, in addition to the epicardial lead placement codes to report the insertion of the generator when done by the same physician during the same session.

⊙ **33241** **Subcutaneous removal of single or dual chamber pacing cardioverter-defibrillator pulse generator** T 80

MED: 100-3,20.4; 100-3,20.8; 100-3,20.8.1; 100-3,20.8.3

AMA: 1999,Nov,16-17; 1994,Summer,40
If an electrode(s) is removed by thoracotomy, consult CPT code 33243 in conjunction with 33241.

If an electrode(s) is removed transvenously, report 33244 in conjunction with 33241.

If the complete pacing defibrillator system is removed and replaced, report 33241 and 33243 or 33244 and 33249. If the implantable cardioverter-defibrillator pulse gnerator and/or leads are repaired, consult CPT codes 33218 and 33220.

33243 **Removal of single or dual chamber pacing cardioverter-defibrillator electrode(s); by thoracotomy** C 80

MED: 100-3,20.4; 100-3,20.8; 100-3,20.8.1; 100-3,20.8.3

AMA: 1999,Nov,16-17; 1994,Summer,40

⊙ **33244** **by transvenous extraction** T

MED: 100-3,20.4; 100-3,20.8; 100-3,20.8.1

AMA: 2000,Jul,5; 1999,Nov,16-17; 1994,Summer,40
To report subcutaneous removal of pulse generator, consult CPT code 33241, report in conjunction with 33243 or 33244.

~~33245~~ ~~Insertion of epicardial single or dual chamber pacing cardioverter-defibrillator electrodes by thoracotomy;~~

MED: 100-3,20.4; 100-3,20.8; 100-3,20.8.1; 100-3,20.8.3

~~33246~~ ~~with insertion of pulse generator~~

MED: 100-3,20.4; 100-3,20.8; 100-3,20.8.1; 100-3,20.8.3

⊙ **33249** **Insertion or repositioning of electrode lead(s) for single or dual chamber pacing cardioverter-defibrillator and insertion of pulse generator** B

MED: 100-3,20.4; 100-3,20.8; 100-3,20.8.1

AMA: 1999,Nov,16-17; 1994,Summer,21
To report removal and reinsertion of a complete pacing cardioverter-defibrillator system, consult CPT codes 33241 and 33243 or 33244 and 33249.

ELECTROPHYSIOLOGIC OPERATIVE PROCEDURES

The following code range are used to report the surgical treatment of supraventricular dysrhythmias. The procedure can be performed by a variety of methods including radiofrequency, cryotherapy, microwave, ultrasound, or laser. Codes 33254-33256, 33265-33266 is included in excision or isolation of the left arterial appendage. Codes 33254-33256 must only be reported when there is no concurrently performed procedure that requires a median sternotomy or cardiopulmonary bypass. If 33254-33256 are formed with a concurrent procedure that requires median sternotomy or cardiopulmonary bypass, report nonthoracoscopic electrophysiologic procedure code 33999.

Limited operative ablation and reconstruction includes the surgical isolation of triggers of the supraventricular dysrhythmias by operative ablation that isolates the pulmonary veins or other anatomically defined triggers in the left or right atrium.

Extensive operative ablation and reconstruction includes all the services included in the limited procedure plus additional ablation of atrial tissue to eliminate sustained supraventricular dysrhythmias. Operative ablation that involves either the right atrium, the atrial septum, or the left atrium in continuity with the arterioventricular annulus is required.

INCISION

33250 **Operative ablation of supraventricular arrhythmogenic focus or pathway (eg, Wolff-Parkinson-White, atrioventricular node re-entry), tract(s) and/or focus (foci); without cardiopulmonary bypass** C 80

AMA: 1999,Nov,17-18; 1994,Summer,16

33251 **with cardiopulmonary bypass** C 80

AMA: 1999,Nov,17-18; 1994,Summer,16

~~33253~~ ~~Operative incisions and reconstruction of atria for treatment of atrial fibrillation or atrial flutter (eg, maze procedure)~~

Use 33254-33256.

● **33254** **Operative tissue ablation and reconstruction of atria, limited (eg, modified maze procedure)** C

● **33255** **Operative tissue ablation and reconstruction of atria, extensive (eg, maze procedure); without cardiopulmonary bypass** C

● **33256** **with cardiopulmonary bypass** C

Do not report 33254-33258 with 32020, 32100, 33120, 33130, 33210, 33211, 33400-33507, 33510-33523, 33533-33548, 33600-33853, 33860-33863, 33910-33920.

33261 **Operative ablation of ventricular arrhythmogenic focus with cardiopulmonary bypass** C 80

AMA: 1994,Summer,16

ENDOSCOPY

● **33265** **Endoscopy, surgical; operative tissue ablation and reconstruction of atria, limited (eg, modified maze procedure), without cardiopulmonary bypass** C

● **33266** **operative tissue ablation and reconstruction of atria, extensive (eg, maze procedure), without cardiopulmonary bypass** C

Do not report 33265-33266 with 32020, 33210, or 33211.

PATIENT-ACTIVATED EVENT RECORDER

Note that initial implantation includes programming. If subsequent electronic analysis and/or reprogramming are performed, consult CPT code 93727.

33282 **Implantation of patient-activated cardiac event recorder** S

AMA: 2000,Jul,5; 1999,Nov,17-18

33284 **Removal of an implantable, patient-activated cardiac event recorder** T

AMA: 2000,Jul,5; 1999,Nov,17-18

WOUNDS OF THE HEART AND GREAT VESSELS

33300 **Repair of cardiac wound; without bypass** C 80

33305 **with cardiopulmonary bypass** C 80

33310 **Cardiotomy, exploratory (includes removal of foreign body, atrial or ventricular thrombus); without bypass** C 80

26 Professional Component Only

80/80 Assist-at-Surgery Allowed/With Documentation

Unlisted

Not Covered

TC Technical Component Only

MED: Pub 100/NCD References AMA: CPT Assistant References

1-9 ASC Group ♂ Male Only ♀ Female Only

128 — CPT Expert

CPT only © 2006 American Medical Association. All Rights Reserved. *(Black Ink)*

© 2006 Ingenix *(Blue Ink)*

33315   with cardiopulmonary bypass   C 80 ⊡

Unless a separate incision in the heart is made to remove the atrial or ventricular thrombus do not report CPT codes 33310 or 33315 in conjunction with other cardiac procedures.

If a separate heart incision is made to remove the thrombus append modifier 59 to code 33315 when reported with 33120, 33130, 33420-33468, 33496, 33542, 33545, 33641-33647, 33670, 33681, or 33975-33980.

33320   Suture repair of aorta or great vessels; without shunt or cardiopulmonary bypass   C 80 ⊡

33321   with shunt bypass   C 80 ⊡

33322   with cardiopulmonary bypass   C 80 ⊡

33330   Insertion of graft, aorta or great vessels; without shunt, or cardiopulmonary bypass   C 80 ⊡

33332   with shunt bypass   C 80 ⊡

33335   with cardiopulmonary bypass   C 80 ⊡

CARDIAC VALVES

AORTIC VALVE

Overhead detail of closed aortic valve showing three cusps

Aortic valve (closed)

The mitral valve gates the left atrium from the left ventricle. It has two leaflets operated by chordae tendineae attached to papillary muscle

Right ventricle

The aortic and pulmonary valves have three cusps and are open only when the ventricles are contracting

Septum between ventricles

Left atrium

Cutaway view of heart showing left-side valves

Mitral valve (opened)

Papillary muscle

Left ventricle

Stenosis means the cusps are fused, usually leaving a small central opening. When cusps become thick and inflexible, closure is incomplete (incompetent) and a back-rush or regurgitation results

Detail showing closed valve leaflet and chordae tendineae

33400   Valvuloplasty, aortic valve; open, with cardiopulmonary bypass   C 80 ⊡

33401   open, with inflow occlusion   C 80 ⊛ ⊡

33403   using transventricular dilation, with cardiopulmonary bypass   C 80 ⊛ ⊡

33404   Construction of apical-aortic conduit   C 80 ⊡

33405   Replacement, aortic valve, with cardiopulmonary bypass; with prosthetic valve other than homograft or stentless valve   C 80 ⊡

     AMA: 1999,Nov,18

33406   with allograft valve (freehand)   C 80 ⊡

     AMA: 1999,Nov,18

33410   with stentless tissue valve   C 80 ⊡

     AMA: 1999,Nov,18

33411   Replacement, aortic valve; with aortic annulus enlargement, noncoronary cusp   C 80 ⊡

33412   with transventricular aortic annulus enlargement (Konno procedure)   C 80 ⊡

33413   by translocation of autologous pulmonary valve with allograft replacement of pulmonary valve (Ross procedure)   C 80 ⊡

33414   Repair of left ventricular outflow tract obstruction by patch enlargement of the outflow tract   C 80 ⊡

33415   Resection or incision of subvalvular tissue for discrete subvalvular aortic stenosis   C 80 ⊡

33416   Ventriculomyotomy (-myectomy) for idiopathic hypertrophic subaortic stenosis (eg, asymmetric septal hypertrophy)   C 80 ⊡

33417   Aortoplasty (gusset) for supravalvular stenosis   C 80 ⊡

MITRAL VALVE

33420   Valvotomy, mitral valve; closed heart   C ⊡

33422   open heart, with cardiopulmonary bypass   C 80 ⊡

33425   Valvuloplasty, mitral valve, with cardiopulmonary bypass;   C 80 ⊡

33426   with prosthetic ring   C 80 ⊡

33427   radical reconstruction, with or without ring   C 80 ⊡

33430   Replacement, mitral valve, with cardiopulmonary bypass   C 80 ⊡

TRICUSPID VALVE

33460   Valvectomy, tricuspid valve, with cardiopulmonary bypass   C 80 ⊡

33463   Valvuloplasty, tricuspid valve; without ring insertion   C 80 ⊡

33464   with ring insertion   C 80 ⊡

33465   Replacement, tricuspid valve, with cardiopulmonary bypass   C 80 ⊡

33468   Tricuspid valve repositioning and plication for Ebstein anomaly   C 80 ⊡

PULMONARY VALVE

33470   Valvotomy, pulmonary valve, closed heart; transventricular   C 80 ⊛ ⊡

Note that modifier 63 cannot be reported with CPT code 33470.

     Brock's operation

33471   via pulmonary artery   C 80 ⊡

If percutaneous valvuloplasty of the pulmonary valve is performed, consult CPT code 92990.

     Brock's operation

33472   Valvotomy, pulmonary valve, open heart; with inflow occlusion   C 80 ⊛ ⊡

     Brock's operation

33474   with cardiopulmonary bypass   C 80 ⊡

     Brock's operation

33475   Replacement, pulmonary valve   C 80 ⊡

33476   Right ventricular resection for infundibular stenosis, with or without commissurotomy   C 80 ⊡

     Brock's operation

33478   Outflow tract augmentation (gusset), with or without commissurotomy or infundibular resection   C 80 ⊡

If a cavopulmonary anastomosis to a second superior vena cava is performed, report code 33478 in conjunction with 33768.

OTHER VALVULAR PROCEDURES

33496   Repair of non-structural prosthetic valve dysfunction with cardiopulmonary bypass (separate procedure)   C 80 ⊡

     AMA: 1997,Nov,16

If this procedure is a reoperation, use CPT code 33530 in addition to 33496.

CORONARY ARTERY ANOMALIES

Codes in this section include endarterectomy or angioplasty.

33500   Repair of coronary arteriovenous or arteriocardiac chamber fistula; with cardiopulmonary bypass   C 80 ▯

33501   without cardiopulmonary bypass   C 80 ▯

33502   Repair of anomalous coronary artery from pulmonary artery origin; by ligation   C 80 ⊚ ▯

33503   by graft, without cardiopulmonary bypass   C 80 ⊚ ▯

Modifier 63 should not be reported with codes 33502 and 33503.

33504   by graft, with cardiopulmonary bypass   C 80 ▯

33505   with construction of intrapulmonary artery tunnel (Takeuchi procedure)   C 80 ⊚ ▯

33506   by translocation from pulmonary artery to aorta   C 80 ⊚ ▯

33507   Repair of anomalous (eg, intramural) aortic origin of coronary artery by unroofing or translocation   C 80

ENDOSCOPY

Diagnostic endoscopy is always included in surgical endoscopy, do not report separately.

+   33508   Endoscopy, surgical, including video-assisted harvest of vein(s) for coronary artery bypass procedure (List separately in addition to code for primary procedure)   N 80 ▯

Note that 33508 is an add-on code and must be used in conjunction with 33510-33523.

To report harvest of upper extremity vein, open procedure, consult CPT code 35500.

CORONARY ARTERY BYPASS GRAFTS

Coronary artery bypass grafts (CABG) are coded by type of graft. Venous grafting alone is reported with 33510-33516. Arterial grafting alone is reported with 33533-33545. Combined arterial-venous grafting is reported with 33517-33523 in combination with 33533-33535. Codes 33517-33523 cannot be reported alone.

Procurement of saphenous vein grafts is included in CABG procedures and should not be reported separately. If a second surgeon procures the graft, report the services as assistant surgeon services with modifier 80 Assistant surgeon appended to the applicable CABG code.

To report harvesting of an upper extremity vein, consult CPT code 35500. To report harvesting of a femoropopliteal vein segment, consult CPT code 35572. These services should be reported in addition to the appropriate CABG procedure code.

VENOUS GRAFTING ONLY FOR CORONARY ARTERY BYPASS

Use the following codes to report coronary artery bypass procedures using venous grafts only. Do not use these codes to report coronary artery bypass procedures using arterial grafts and venous grafts during the same surgery. For combined arterial-venous graft surgery, consult CPT codes 33517-33523 and 33533-33536.

CPT codes 33510-33516 include the harvesting of the saphenous vein graft and it should not be reported separately. Harvesting of an upper extremity vein may be reported separately, consult CPT code 35500. Harvesting of a femoropopliteal vein segment may be reported separately, consult CPT code 35572. These codes report bypass procedures using venous grafts only.

33510   Coronary artery bypass, vein only; single coronary venous graft   C 80 ▯

AMA: 2001,Apr,7; 1999,Jul,11; 1992,Winter,12; 1991,Fall,5

33511   two coronary venous grafts   C 80 ▯

AMA: 2001,Apr,7; 1999,Jul,11; 1992,Winter,12; 1991,Fall,5

33512   three coronary venous grafts   C 80 ▯

AMA: 2001,Apr,7; 1992,Winter,12; 1991,Fall,5

33513   four coronary venous grafts   C 80 ▯

AMA: 2001,Apr,7; 1992,Winter,12; 1991,Fall,5

33514   five coronary venous grafts   C 80 ▯

AMA: 2001,Apr,7; 1992,Winter,12; 1991,Fall,5

33516   six or more coronary venous grafts   C 80 ▯

AMA: 2001,Apr,7; 1999,Jul,11; 1992,Winter,12; 1991,Fall,5

COMBINED ARTERIAL-VENOUS GRAFTING FOR CORONARY BYPASS

Use these codes to report coronary artery bypass procedures using both venous and arterial grafts during the same procedure, but do not use them alone. They must be reported with a code from range 33533-33536. Harvesting of an upper extremity vein may be reported separately, consult CPT code 35500. Harvesting of a femoropopliteal vein segment may be reported separately, consult CPT code 35572.

Two codes must be used to report arterial-venous grafts:

1. 33517-33523 for the combined arterial-venous graft code
2. 33533-33536 for the appropriate arterial graft code

Harvesting the artery for grafting is included in 33533-33536 and should not be reported separately except when an upper extremity artery is used. To report harvesting of an upper extremity artery, consult 35600. When a surgical assistant harvests the venous or arterial graft, add modifier 80 to codes 33517-33523, 33533-33536, as appropriate.

CPT codes 33517-33523 include the harvesting of the saphenous vein graft and it should not be reported separately.

⊘   **33517**   Coronary artery bypass, using venous graft(s) and arterial graft(s); single vein graft (List separately in addition to code for arterial graft)   C 80 ▯

AMA: 2001,Apr,7; 1999,Nov,18; 1992,Winter,13; 1991,Fall,5

⊘   **33518**   two venous grafts (List separately in addition to code for arterial graft)   C 80 ▯

AMA: 2001,Apr,7; 1992,Winter,13; 1991,Fall,5

⊘   **33519**   three venous grafts (List separately in addition to code for arterial graft)   C 80 ▯

AMA: 2001,Apr,7; 1992,Winter,13; 1991,Fall,5

⊘   **33521**   four venous grafts (List separately in addition to code for arterial graft)   C 80 ▯

AMA: 2001,Apr,7; 1992,Winter,13; 1991,Fall,5

⊘   **33522**   five venous grafts (List separately in addition to code for arterial graft)   C 80 ▯

AMA: 2001,Apr,7; 1992,Winter,13; 1991,Fall,5

⊘   **33523**   six or more venous grafts (List separately in addition to code for arterial graft)   C 80 ▯

AMA: 2001,Apr,7; 1992,Winter,13; 1991,Fall,5

+   33530   Reoperation, coronary artery bypass procedure or valve procedure, more than one month after original operation (List separately in addition to code for primary procedure)   C 80 ▯

AMA: 2001,Jul,11; 2001,Apr,7; 1992,Winter,13; 1991,Fall,5
Note that 33530 is an add-on code and must be used in conjunction with 33400-33496, 33510-33536, and 33863.

ARTERIAL GRAFTING FOR CORONARY ARTERY BYPASS

Use the following codes to report coronary artery bypass surgeries using either arterial grafts only or a combination of arterial-venous grafts. The codes include using the internal mammary artery, gastroepiploic artery, epigastric artery, radial artery, and arterial conduits procured from other sites.

Two codes must be used to report arterial-venous grafts:

1. 33533-33536 for the arterial graft code
2. 33517-33523 for the appropriate arterial-venous graft code

26 Professional Component Only   **80/80** Assist-at-Surgery Allowed/With Documentation   Unlisted   Not Covered

TC Technical Component Only   **MED:** Pub 100/NCD References   **AMA:** CPT Assistant References   **1-9** ASC Group   ♂ Male Only   ♀ Female Only

130 — CPT Expert   CPT only © 2006 American Medical Association. All Rights Reserved. *(Black Ink)*   © 2006 Ingenix *(Blue Ink)*

Harvesting the artery for grafting is included in the description for 33533-33536 and should not be reported separately except when an upper extremity artery is harvested. Harvesting of an upper extremity artery may be reported using code 35600. Report the harvesting of an upper extremity vein with code 35500. When a surgical assistant harvests the venous or arterial graft, add modifier 80 to codes 33517-33523, 33533-33536, as appropriate.

Harvesting of a femoropopliteal vein segment may be reported separately, consult CPT code 35572.

33533 Coronary artery bypass, using arterial graft(s); single arterial graft ⓒ 80 🔲

AMA: 2001,Apr,7; 1999,Nov,18; 1992,Winter,12

33534 two coronary arterial grafts ⓒ 80 🔲

AMA: 2001,Apr,7; 1992,Winter,12

33535 three coronary arterial grafts ⓒ 80 🔲

AMA: 2001,Apr,7; 1992,Winter,12

33536 four or more coronary arterial grafts ⓒ 80 🔲

AMA: 2001,Apr,7; 1992,Winter,12

33542 Myocardial resection (eg, ventricular aneurysmectomy) ⓒ 80 🔲

33545 Repair of postinfarction ventricular septal defect, with or without myocardial resection ⓒ 80 🔲

33548 Surgical ventricular restoration procedure, includes prosthetic patch, when performed (eg, ventricular remodeling, SVR, SAVER, Dor procedures) ⓒ 80

Code 33548 cannot be reported with 32020, 33210, 33211, 33310, 33315.

To report Batista procedure or pachopexy, consult 33999.

CORONARY ENDARTERECTOMY

+ **33572** Coronary endarterectomy, open, any method, of left anterior descending, circumflex, or right coronary artery performed in conjunction with coronary artery bypass graft procedure, each vessel (List separately in addition to primary procedure) ⓒ 80 🔲

Note that 33572 is an add-on code and must be used in conjunction with 33510-33516 and 33533-33536.

SINGLE VENTRICLE AND OTHER COMPLEX CARDIAC ANOMALIES

33600 Closure of atrioventricular valve (mitral or tricuspid) by suture or patch ⓒ 80 🔲

33602 Closure of semilunar valve (aortic or pulmonary) by suture or patch ⓒ 80 🔲

33606 Anastomosis of pulmonary artery to aorta (Damus-Kaye-Stansel procedure) ⓒ 80 🔲

33608 Repair of complex cardiac anomaly other than pulmonary atresia with ventricular septal defect by construction or replacement of conduit from right or left ventricle to pulmonary artery ⓒ 80 🔲

If pulmonary artery arborization anomalies are repaired by unifocalization, consult CPT codes 33925-33926.

33610 Repair of complex cardiac anomalies (eg, single ventricle with subaortic obstruction) by surgical enlargement of ventricular septal defect ⓒ 80 ㊦ 🔲

33611 Repair of double outlet right ventricle with intraventricular tunnel repair; ⓒ 80 ㊦ 🔲

33612 with repair of right ventricular outflow tract obstruction ⓒ 80 🔲

33615 Repair of complex cardiac anomalies (eg, tricuspid atresia) by closure of atrial septal defect and anastomosis of atria or vena cava to pulmonary artery (simple Fontan procedure) ⓒ 80 🔲

33617 Repair of complex cardiac anomalies (eg, single ventricle) by modified Fontan procedure ⓒ 80 🔲

If a cavopulmonary anastomosis to a second superior vena cava is performed, report code 33617 in conjunction with 33768.

33619 Repair of single ventricle with aortic outflow obstruction and aortic arch hypoplasia (hypoplastic left heart syndrome) (eg, Norwood procedure) ⓒ 80 ㊦ 🔲

SEPTAL DEFECT

33641 Repair atrial septal defect, secundum, with cardiopulmonary bypass, with or without patch ⓒ 80 🔲

33645 Direct or patch closure, sinus venosus, with or without anomalous pulmonary venous drainage ⓒ 80 🔲

33647 Repair of atrial septal defect and ventricular septal defect, with direct or patch closure ⓒ 80 ㊦ 🔲

Consult CPT code 33615 for the repair of tricuspid atresia.

33660 Repair of incomplete or partial atrioventricular canal (ostium primum atrial septal defect), with or without atrioventricular valve repair ⓒ 80 🔲

33665 Repair of intermediate or transitional atrioventricular canal, with or without atrioventricular valve repair ⓒ 80 🔲

33670 Repair of complete atrioventricular canal, with or without prosthetic valve ⓒ 80 ㊦ 🔲

● **33675** Closure of multiple ventricular septal defects; ⓒ

● **33676** with pulmonary valvotomy or infundibular resection (acyanotic) ⓒ

● **33677** with removal of pulmonary artery band, with or without gusset ⓒ

Do not report 33675-33677 with 32002, 32020, 32100, 33210, 33881, 33684, or 33688.

See 0166T and 0167T for transmyocardial closure.

Use 93581 for percutaneous closure.

▲ **33681** Closure of single ventricular septal defect, with or without patch; ⓒ 80 🔲

33684 with pulmonary valvotomy or infundibular resection (acyanotic) ⓒ 80 🔲

33688 with removal of pulmonary artery band, with or without gusset ⓒ 80 🔲

Use 33724 for pulomnary vein repair requiring creation of atrial septal defect.

33690 Banding of pulmonary artery ⓒ 80 ㊦ 🔲

33692 Complete repair tetralogy of Fallot without pulmonary atresia; ⓒ 80 🔲

33694 with transannular patch ⓒ 80 ㊦ 🔲

33697 Complete repair tetralogy of Fallot with pulmonary atresia including construction of conduit from right ventricle to pulmonary artery and closure of ventricular septal defect ⓒ 80 🔲

SINUS OF VALSALVA

33702 Repair sinus of Valsalva fistula, with cardiopulmonary bypass; ⓒ 80 🔲

33710 with repair of ventricular septal defect ⓒ 80 🔲

㊦ Modifier 63 Exempt Code · ⊙ Conscious Sedation · + CPT Add-on Code · ⊘ Modifier 51 Exempt Code · ● New Code · ▲ Revised Code

Ⓜ Maternity Edit · Age Edit · Ⓐ-Ⓨ APC Status Indicators · 🔲 CCI Comprehensive Code · 80 Bilateral Procedure

© 2006 Ingenix *(Blue Ink)* · CPT only © 2006 American Medical Association. All Rights Reserved. *(Black Ink)* · Cardiovascular System — 131

Cardiovascular System

33533 — 33710

Cardiovascular System

33720 — 33853

33720	Repair sinus of Valsalva aneurysm, with cardiopulmonary bypass	ⒸⒷⓄ
33722	Closure of aortico-left ventricular tunnel	ⒸⒷⓄ

VENOUS ANOMALIES

● 33724   Repair of isolated partial anomalous pulmonary venous return (eg, Scimitar Syndrome)   Ⓒ

Do not report 33724 with 32020, 33210, or 33211.

● 33726   Repair of pulmonary venous stenosis   Ⓒ

Do not report 33726 with 32020, 33210, or 33211.

33730   Complete repair of anomalous pulmonary venous return (supracardiac, intracardiac, or infracardiac types)   ⒸⒷⓈⓄ

To code a partial anomalous return, consult atrial septal defect.

See 33724 for partial anomalous pulmonary venous return. See 33726 for repair of pulmonary venous stenosis.

33732   Repair of cor triatriatum or supravalvular mitral ring by resection of left atrial membrane   ⒸⒷⓈⓄ

SHUNTING PROCEDURES

33735	Atrial septectomy or septostomy; closed heart (Blalock-Hanlon type operation)	ⒸⒷⓈⓄ
33736	open heart with cardiopulmonary bypass	ⒸⒷⓈⓄ
33737	open heart, with inflow occlusion	ⒸⒷⓄ
33750	Shunt; subclavian to pulmonary artery (Blalock-Taussig type operation)	ⒸⒷⓈⓄ
33755	ascending aorta to pulmonary artery (Waterston type operation)	ⒸⒷⓈⓄ
33762	descending aorta to pulmonary artery (Potts-Smith type operation)	ⒸⒷⓈⓄ
33764	central, with prosthetic graft	ⒸⒷⓄ
33766	superior vena cava to pulmonary artery for flow to one lung (classical Glenn procedure)	ⒸⒷⓄ
33767	superior vena cava to pulmonary artery for flow to both lungs (bidirectional Glenn procedure)	ⒸⒷⓄ
+ 33768	Anastomosis, cavopulmonary, second superior vena cava (List separately in addition to primary procedure)	ⒸⒷ

Report code 33768 with 33478, 33617, 33767.

Code 33768 cannot be reported with 32020, 33210, 33211.

TRANSPOSITION OF THE GREAT VESSELS

33770   Repair of transposition of the great arteries with ventricular septal defect and subpulmonary stenosis; without surgical enlargement of ventricular septal defect   ⒸⒷⓄ

33771   with surgical enlargement of ventricular septal defect   ⒸⒷⓄ

33774   Repair of transposition of the great arteries, atrial baffle procedure (eg, Mustard or Senning type) with cardiopulmonary bypass;   ⒸⒷⓄ

33775	with removal of pulmonary band	ⒸⒷⓄ
33776	with closure of ventricular septal defect	ⒸⒷⓄ
33777	with repair of subpulmonic obstruction	ⒸⒷⓄ

33778   Repair of transposition of the great arteries, aortic pulmonary artery reconstruction (eg, Jatene type);   ⒸⒷⓈⓄ

33779	with removal of pulmonary band	ⒸⒷⓄ
33780	with closure of ventricular septal defect	ⒸⒷⓄ
33781	with repair of subpulmonic obstruction	ⒸⒷⓄ

TRUNCUS ARTERIOSUS

33786   Total repair, truncus arteriosus (Rastelli type operation)   ⒸⒷⓈⓄ

33788   Reimplantation of an anomalous pulmonary artery   ⒸⒷⓄ

If banding of the pulmonary artery is performed, consult CPT code 33690.

AORTIC ANOMALIES

33800   Aortic suspension (aortopexy) for tracheal decompression (eg, for tracheomalacia) (separate procedure)   ⒸⒷⓄ

33802	Division of aberrant vessel (vascular ring);	ⒸⒷⓄ
33803	with reanastomosis	ⒸⒷⓄ

33813   Obliteration of aortopulmonary septal defect; without cardiopulmonary bypass   ⒸⒷⓄ

33814   with cardiopulmonary bypass   ⒸⒷⓄ

33820   Repair of patent ductus arteriosus; by ligation   ⒸⒷⓄ

33822	by division, younger than 18 years	ⒶⒸⒷⓄ
33824	by division, 18 years and older	ⒸⒷⓄ

33840   Excision of coarctation of aorta, with or without associated patent ductus arteriosus; with direct anastomosis   ⒸⒷⓄ

33845   with graft   ⒸⒷⓄ

33851   repair using either left subclavian artery or prosthetic material as gusset for enlargement   ⒸⒷⓄ

33852   Repair of hypoplastic or interrupted aortic arch using autogenous or prosthetic material; without cardiopulmonary bypass   ⒸⒷⓄ

Aortic valve   Left coronary artery   Left, right atria   Basal

Descending branch (anterior ventricular)

Apical

Right coronary artery   Descending branch (posterior interventricular)

Posterior wall

Intraventricular septum divides left and right ventricles

Coronary arterial branching patterns may vary widely; dead heart tissue, usually caused by arterial occlusion, is called a myocardial infarct and about 1.5 million cases are reported annually. Inadequate blood supply can lead to "angina pectoris," or chest pain

Interior heart schematic to locate a myocardial infarction; walls of the left ventrical are much thicker and more than half of MI occurrences will see some degree of transient impairment to the left ventricle

33853   with cardiopulmonary bypass   ⒸⒷⓄ

THORACIC AORTIC ANEURYSM

Codes 33880-33891 are used to report placement of an endovascular graft for repair of the descending thoracic aorta. These codes include all the device introduction, manipulation, positioning, and deployment. Do not report balloon angioplasty and/or stent deployment separately. Report open arterial exposure and associated closure of the arteriotomy sites (34812, 34820, 34833, 34834), introduction of guidewires and catheters (36140, 36200-36218), and extensive

㉖ Professional Component Only   ⑧⓪/⑧⓪ Assist-at-Surgery Allowed/With Documentation | Unlisted | | Not Covered |

ⓉⒸ Technical Component Only   **MED:** Pub 100/NCD References   **AMA:** CPT Assistant References   ❶-❾ ASC Group   ♂ Male Only   ♀ Female Only

132 — CPT Expert   CPT only © 2006 American Medical Association. All Rights Reserved. (*Black Ink*)   © 2006 Ingenix (*Blue Ink*)

repair or replacement of an artery (35226, 35286), and transposition of subclavian artery to carotid, and carotid-carotid bypass performed in conjunction with endovascular repair of the descending thoracic aorta (33889, 33891) separately. Codes 33880 and 33881 include placement of all distal extensions. However, if proximal extensions are needed, they should be reported separately.

Consult 75956-75959 for fluoroscopic guidance.

Report other interventional procedures performed at the time of the endovascular repair separately.

33860 **Ascending aorta graft, with cardiopulmonary bypass, with or without valve suspension;** Ⓒ 80 ▨

33861 **with coronary reconstruction** Ⓒ 80 ▨

33863 **with aortic root replacement using composite prosthesis and coronary reconstruction** Ⓒ 80 ▨

33870 **Transverse arch graft, with cardiopulmonary bypass** Ⓒ 80 ▨

33875 **Descending thoracic aorta graft, with or without bypass** Ⓒ 80 ▨

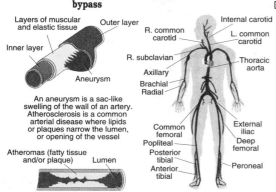

Layers of muscular and elastic tissue — Outer layer
Inner layer
Aneurysm

An aneurysm is a sac-like swelling of the wall of an artery. Atherosclerosis is a common arterial disease where lipids or plaques narrow the lumen, or opening of the vessel.

Atheromas (fatty tissue and/or plaque) — Lumen

Internal carotid
R. common carotid
L. common carotid
R. subclavian
Thoracic aorta
Axillary
Brachial
Radial
Common femoral
External iliac
Popliteal
Deep femoral
Posterior tibial
Peroneal
Anterior tibial

33877 **Repair of thoracoabdominal aortic aneurysm with graft, with or without cardiopulmonary bypass** Ⓒ 80 ▨

ENDOVASCULAR REPAIR OF DESCENDING THORACIC AORTA

33880 **Endovascular repair of descending thoracic aorta (eg, aneurysm, pseudoaneurysm, dissection, penetrating ulcer, intramural hematoma, or traumatic disruption); involving coverage of left subclavian artery origin, initial endoprosthesis plus descending thoracic aortic extension(s), if required, to level of celiac artery origin** Ⓒ 80

To report radiological supervision and interpretation, use 75956 with 33880.

33881 **not involving coverage of left subclavian artery origin, initial endoprosthesis plus descending thoracic aortic extension(s), if required, to level of celiac artery origin** Ⓒ 80

To report radiological supervision and interpretation, use 75957 with 33881.

33883 **Placement of proximal extension prosthesis for endovascular repair of descending thoracic aorta (eg, aneurysm, pseudoaneurysm, dissection, penetrating ulcer, intramural hematoma, or traumatic disruption); initial extension** Ⓒ 80

To report radiological supervision and interpretation, use 75958 with 33883.

Codes 33881, 33883 cannot be reported when extension placement converts repair to cover left subclavian origin. Use only 33880.

\+ **33884** **each additional proximal extension (List separately in addition to code for primary procedure)** Ⓒ 80

Note that 33884 is an add-on code and must be used in conjunction with 33883.

To report radiological supervision and interpretation, report 75958 with 33884.

33886 **Placement of distal extension prosthesis(s) delayed after endovascular repair of descending thoracic aorta** Ⓒ 80

Code 33886 cannot be reported with 33880, 33881.

Code 33886 can be reported only once, regardless of the number of modules deployed.

To report radiological supervision and interpretation, report 75959 with 33886.

33889 **Open subclavian to carotid artery transposition performed in conjunction with endovascular repair of descending thoracic aorta, by neck incision, unilateral** Ⓒ 80 50

Code 33889 cannot be reported with 35694.

33891 **Bypass graft, with other than vein, transcervical retropharyngeal carotid-carotid, performed in conjunction with endovascular repair of descending thoracic aorta, by neck incision** Ⓒ 80 50

Code 33891 cannot be reported with 35509, 35601.

PULMONARY ARTERY

33910 **Pulmonary artery embolectomy; with cardiopulmonary bypass** Ⓒ 80 ▨

MED: 100-3,240.6

33915 **without cardiopulmonary bypass** Ⓒ 80 ▨

MED: 100-3,240.6

33916 **Pulmonary endarterectomy, with or without embolectomy, with cardiopulmonary bypass** Ⓒ 80 ▨

MED: 100-3,240.6

33917 **Repair of pulmonary artery stenosis by reconstruction with patch or graft** Ⓒ 80 ▨

MED: 100-3,240.6

33920 **Repair of pulmonary atresia with ventricular septal defect, by construction or replacement of conduit from right or left ventricle to pulmonary artery** Ⓒ 80 ▨

MED: 100-3,240.6

If other complex cardiac anomalies by construction of right or left ventricle to pulmonary artery conduit are repaired, consult CPT code 33608.

33922 **Transection of pulmonary artery with cardiopulmonary bypass** Ⓒ 80 ⓺ ▨

MED: 100-3,240.6

\+ **33924** **Ligation and takedown of a systemic-to-pulmonary artery shunt, performed in conjunction with a congenital heart procedure (List separately in addition to code for primary procedure)** Ⓒ 80 ▨

MED: 100-3,240.6

Note that 33924 is an add-on code and must be used in conjunction with 33470-33475, 33600-33619, 33684-33688, 33692-33697, 33735-33767, 33770-33781, 33786, and 33920-33922.

33925 **Repair of pulmonary artery arborization anomalies by unifocalization; without cardiopulmonary bypass** Ⓒ 80

Cardiovascular System

33926 — 33999

33926   with cardiopulmonary bypass   © 80

Codes 33925, 33926 cannot be reported with 33697.

HEART/LUNG TRANSPLANTATION

Heart with or without lung transplantation involves three different components:

- Cadaver donor cardiectomy with or without pneumonectomy consists of harvesting and cold preservation of the graft prior to transport (see 33930, 33940).
- Backbench work includes dissection of the tissue around the heart and lungs and preparation of aorta, superior vena cava, inferior vena cava, and trachea for transplantation (see 33933, 33944). Repair or resection procedures of the donor heart should be reported using codes 33300, 33310, 33320, 33400, 33463, 33464, 33510, 33641, 35216, 35276, and 35685, as appropriate.
- Recipient transplantation which includes transplanting the heart/lungs into the patient (see 33935, 33945). To report implantation of an artificial heart system with recipient cardiectomy or heart replacement system components, consult CPT Category III codes 0051T-0053T.

33930   Donor cardiectomy-pneumonectomy (including cold preservation)   © ◘

33933   Backbench standard preparation of cadaver donor heart/lung allograft prior to transplantation, including dissection of allograft from surrounding soft tissues to prepare aorta, superior vena cava, inferior vena cava, and trachea for implantation   © 80 ◘

MED: 100-4,3,90.2; 100-4,3,90.2.1

33935   Heart-lung transplant with recipient cardiectomy-pneumonectomy   © 80 ◘

33940   Donor cardiectomy (including cold preservation)   © ◘

33944   Backbench standard preparation of cadaver donor heart allograft prior to transplantation, including dissection of allograft from surrounding soft tissues to prepare aorta, superior vena cava, inferior vena cava, pulmonary artery, and left atrium for implantation   © 80 ◘

MED: 100-4,3,90.2; 100-4,3,90.2.1

To report resection or repair of the donor heart, consult CPT codes 33300, 33310, 33320, 33400, 33463, 33464, 33510, 33641, 35216, 35276, 35685.

33945   Heart transplant, with or without recipient cardiectomy   © 80 ◘

CARDIAC ASSIST

To report percutaneous implantation of extracorporeal ventricular assist device or for removal of percutaneously implanted extracorporeal ventricular assist device, consult CPT Category III codes 0048T-0050T.

33960   Prolonged extracorporeal circulation for cardiopulmonary insufficiency; initial 24 hours   © 80 ❽ ◘

If an insertion of a cannula is performed for prolonged extracorporeal circulation, consult CPT code 36822.

+   **33961**   each additional 24 hours (List separately in addition to code for primar procedure)   © 80 ❽ ◘

If an insertion of a cannula is performed for prolonged extracorporeal circulation, consult CPT code 36822.

Note that 33961 is an add-on code and must be used in conjunction with 33960.

33967   Insertion of intra-aortic balloon assist device, percutaneous   © 80 ◘

AMA: 2002,Feb,1

33968   Removal of intra-aortic balloon assist device, percutaneous   © ◘

AMA: 2000,Jan,10; 1999,Nov,19

33970   Insertion of intra-aortic balloon assist device through the femoral artery, open approach   © 80 ◘

AMA: 1999,Nov,19

If the insertion is performed percutaneously, consult CPT code 33967.

33971   Removal of intra-aortic balloon assist device including repair of femoral artery, with or without graft   © ◘

33973   Insertion of intra-aortic balloon assist device through the ascending aorta   © 80 ◘

33974   Removal of intra-aortic balloon assist device from the ascending aorta, including repair of the ascending aorta, with or without graft   © ◘

33975   Insertion of ventricular assist device; extracorporeal, single ventricle   © 80 ◘

MED: 100-4,3,90.2.1

AMA: 2002,Feb,1

33976   extracorporeal, biventricular   © 80 ◘

MED: 100-4,3,90.2.1

AMA: 2002,Feb,1

33977   Removal of ventricular assist device; extracorporeal, single ventricle   © 80 ◘

MED: 100-4,3,90.2.1

AMA: 2002,Feb,1

33978   extracorporeal, biventricular   © 80 ◘

MED: 100-4,3,90.2.1

AMA: 2002,Feb,1

33979   Insertion of ventricular assist device, implantable intracorporeal, single ventricle   © 80 ◘

MED: 100-4,3,90.2.1

AMA: 2002,Feb,1

33980   Removal of ventricular assist device, implantable intracorporeal, single ventricle   © 80 ◘

MED: 100-4,3,90.2.1

AMA: 2002,Feb,1

OTHER PROCEDURES

33999   Unlisted procedure, cardiac surgery   Ⓣ 80

MED: 100-3,20.6; 100-4,4,180.3

AMA: 1999,Oct,11

ARTERIES AND VEINS

Primary vascular procedures include the establishment of both inflow and outflow. Also included is the portion of the operative arteriogram performed by the surgeon. When performed, sympathectomy is included in the listed aortic procedures. Report 37799 for unlisted vascular procedures.

26 Professional Component Only   80/80 Assist-at-Surgery Allowed/With Documentation   Unlisted   Not Covered

TC Technical Component Only   MED: Pub 100/NCD References   AMA: CPT Assistant References   1-9 ASC Group   ♂ Male Only   ♀ Female Only

134 — CPT Expert   CPT only © 2006 American Medical Association. All Rights Reserved. (Black Ink)   © 2006 Ingenix (Blue Ink)

EMBOLECTOMY/THROMBECTOMY

ARTERIAL, WITH OR WITHOUT CATHETER

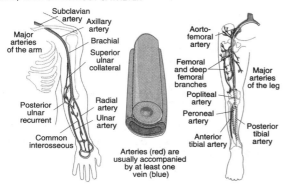

Arteries (red) are usually accompanied by at least one vein (blue)

34001 **Embolectomy or thrombectomy, with or without catheter; carotid, subclavian or innominate artery, by neck incision** 🄲 80 50 🄲
   MED: 100-3,160.8

34051 **innominate, subclavian artery, by thoracic incision** 🄲 80 50 🄲

34101 **axillary, brachial, innominate, subclavian artery, by arm incision** 🅃 80 50 🄲

34111 **radial or ulnar artery, by arm incision** 🅃 80 50 🄲

34151 **renal, celiac, mesentery, aortoiliac artery, by abdominal incision** 🄲 80 50 🄲

34201 **femoropopliteal, aortoiliac artery, by leg incision** 🅃 80 50 🄲

34203 **popliteal-tibio-peroneal artery, by leg incision** 🅃 80 50 🄲

VENOUS, DIRECT OR WITH CATHETER

34401 **Thrombectomy, direct or with catheter; vena cava, iliac vein, by abdominal incision** 🄲 80 50 🄲

34421 **vena cava, iliac, femoropopliteal vein, by leg incision** 🅃 80 50 🄲
   AMA: 1994,Spring,30

34451 **vena cava, iliac, femoropopliteal vein, by abdominal and leg incision** 🄲 80 50 🄲

34471 **subclavian vein, by neck incision** 🅃 50 🄲

34490 **axillary and subclavian vein, by arm incision** 🅃 50 🄲

VENOUS RECONSTRUCTION

34501 **Valvuloplasty, femoral vein** 🅃 80 50 🄲

34502 **Reconstruction of vena cava, any method** 🄲 80 🄲

34510 **Venous valve transposition, any vein donor** 🅃 80 50 🄲

34520 **Cross-over vein graft to venous system** 🅃 80 50 🄲

34530 **Saphenopopliteal vein anastomosis** 🅃 80 50 🄲

ENDOVASCULAR REPAIR OF ABDOMINAL AORTIC ANEURYSM

CPT codes 38000-34834 address the repair of a weakness of the aorta with an endovascular graft under fluoroscopic guidance. These codes include open femoral or iliac artery exposure, device manipulation and deployment, balloon angioplasty, stent deployment, and closure. Report introduction of guidewires and catheters separately.

If extensive repair or replacement of an artery is required, report as an additional procedure.

If fluoroscopic guidance is performed with endovascular aneurysm repair, consult 75952 or 75953. Angiography of the aorta and its branches for diagnostic imaging before deployment of the endovascular device, fluoroscopic guidance in the delivery of the endovascular components, and arterial angiography during the procedure are included in code 75952.

Report other interventional procedures such as renal transluminal angioplasty, arterial embolization, or intravascular ultrasound separately.

34800 **Endovascular repair of infrarenal abdominal aortic aneurysm or dissection; using aorto-aortic tube prosthesis** 🄲 80 🄲
   AMA: 2002,Sep,3; 2000,Dec,1

34802 **using modular bifurcated prosthesis (one docking limb)** 🄲 80 🄲
   AMA: 2002,Sep,3; 2000,Dec,1

34803 **using modular bifurcated prosthesis (two docking limbs)** 🄲 80 🄲

   To report endovascular repair of abdominal aortic aneurysm or dissection involving visceral vessels using a fenestrated modular bifurcated prosthesis with two docking limbs, consult Category III codes 0078T, 0079T.

34804 **using unibody bifurcated prosthesis** 🄲 80 🄲
   AMA: 2002,Sep,3; 2000,Dec,1

34805 **using aorto-uniiliac or aorto-unifemoral prosthesis** 🄲 80 🄲

+ **34808** **Endovascular placement of iliac artery occlusion device (List separately in addition to code for primary procedure)** 🄲 80 🄲
   AMA: 2002,Sep,3; 2000,Dec,1
   Note that 34808 is an add-on code and must be used in conjunction with codes 34800, 34805, 34813, 34825 and 34826.

   To report radiological supervision and interpretation, consult CPT code 75952, report with codes 34800-34808.

   To report open arterial exposure, consult CPT codes 34812, 34820, 34833, or 34834, in addition to codes 34800-34808.

34812 **Open femoral artery exposure for delivery of endovascular prosthesis, by groin incision, unilateral** 🄲 80 50 🄲
   AMA: 2003,Feb,1; 2002,Sep,3; 2000,Dec,1
   To report a procedure performed bilaterally, append modifier 50.

+ **34813** **Placement of femoral-femoral prosthetic graft during endovascular aortic aneurysm repair (List separately in addition to code for primary procedure)** 🄲 80 🄲
   AMA: 2002,Sep,3; 2000,Dec,1
   Note that 34813 is an add-on code and must be used in conjunction with 34812.

   If femoral artery grafting is performed, consult CPT codes 35521, 35533, 35539, 35540, 35551-35558, 35566, 35621, 35646, 35651-35661, 35666 and 35700.

34820 **Open iliac artery exposure for delivery of endovascular prosthesis or iliac occlusion during endovascular therapy, by abdominal or retroperitoneal incision, unilateral** 🄲 80 50 🄲
   AMA: 2003,Feb,1; 2002,Sep,3; 2000,Dec,1

⊗ Modifier 63 Exempt Code ⊙ Conscious Sedation ✛ CPT Add-on Code ⊘ Modifier 51 Exempt Code ● New Code ▲ Revised Code
Ⓜ Maternity Edit Ⓐ Age Edit Ⓐ-Ⓨ APC Status Indicators 🄲 CCI Comprehensive Code 50 Bilateral Procedure

© 2006 Ingenix *(Blue Ink)* CPT only © 2006 American Medical Association. All Rights Reserved. *(Black Ink)* Cardiovascular System — 135

Cardiovascular System

34825 — 35045

34825 Placement of proximal or distal extension prosthesis for endovascular repair of infrarenal abdominal aortic or iliac aneurysm, false aneurysm, or dissection; initial vessel ☐ ☐ ☐

AMA: 2003,Feb,1; 2002,Sep,3; 2000,Dec,1
Report codes 34825 and 34826 with codes 34800-34808 and 34900, when appropriate.

To report a staged procedure, append modifier 58.

To report radiological supervision and interpretation, consult CPT code 75953.

+ **34826** each additional vessel (List separately in addition to code for primary procedure) ☐ ☐ ☐

AMA: 2003,Feb,1; 2002,Sep,3; 2000,Dec,1
Note that 34826 is an add-on code and must be reported in conjunction with 34825.

34830 Open repair of infrarenal aortic aneurysm or dissection, plus repair of associated arterial trauma, following unsuccessful endovascular repair; tube prosthesis ☐ ☐ ☐

AMA: 2002,Sep,3; 2000,Dec,1

34831 aorto-bi-iliac prosthesis ☐ ☐ ☐

AMA: 2002,Sep,3; 2000,Dec,1

34832 aorto-bifemoral prosthesis ☐ ☐ ☐

AMA: 2002,Sep,3; 2000,Dec,1

34833 Open iliac artery exposure with creation of conduit for delivery of aortic or iliac endovascular prosthesis, by abdominal or retroperitoneal incision, unilateral ☐ ☐ ☐ ☐

AMA: 2003,Feb,1
Do not report 34833 in conjunction with CPT code 34820.

To report procedure performed bilaterally, append modifier 50.

34834 Open brachial artery exposure to assist in the deployment of aortic or iliac endovascular prosthesis by arm incision, unilateral ☐ ☐ ☐ ☐

AMA: 2003,Feb,1
To report procedure performed bilaterally, append modifier 50.

ENDOVASCULAR REPAIR OF ILIAC ANEURYSM

Code 34900 includes angioplasty and/or stent placements within the target treatment zone either before or after endograft vascular graft replacement, do not report separately. The following services should be reported in addition to 34900 when appropriate; open femoral or iliac artery exposure (34812, 34820), introduction of guidewires or catheters (36200, 36215-36218), extensive repair or artery replacement (35206-35286).

If fluoroscopic guidance is performed with endovascular iliac aneurysm repair, consult 75954. Angiography of the aorta and iliac arteries for diagnostic imaging before deployment of the endovascular device, fluoroscopic guidance in the delivery of the endovascular components, and angiography to verify for correct placement of the graft, check for endoleaks, and assess the status of the runoff vessels is included in 75954.

Report other interventional procedures performed at the time of the endovascular aortic aneurysm repair separately when appropriate.

34900 Endovascular graft placement for repair of iliac artery (eg, aneurysm, pseudoaneurysm, arteriovenous malformation, trauma) ☐ ☐ ☐

AMA: 2003,Feb,1
To report radiological supervision and interpretation, consult CPT code 75954.

To report placement of extension prosthesis during endovascular iliac artery repair, consult CPT code 34825.

To report procedure performed bilaterally, append modifier 50.

DIRECT REPAIR OF ANEURYSM OR EXCISION (PARTIAL OR TOTAL) AND GRAFT INSERTION FOR ANEURYSM, FALSE ANEURYSM, RUPTURED ANEURYSM, AND ASSOCIATED OCCLUSIVE DISEASE

Preparation of the artery for anastomosis, including endarterectomy is included in CPT codes 35001-35152.

If direct repairs associated with occlusive disease only are performed, consult CPT codes 35201-35286.

If a thoracic aortic aneurysm is repaired, consult CPT codes 33860-33875.

If an intracranial aneurysm is repaired, consult CPT code 61700 and subsequent codes.

To report endovascular repair of abdominal aortic aneurysm, consult CPT codes 34800-34826; of iliac artery aneurysm, consult CPT code 34900; thoracic aortic aneurysm, consult code 33880.

35001 Direct repair of aneurysm, pseudoaneurysm, or excision (partial or total) and graft insertion, with or without patch graft; for aneurysm and associated occlusive disease, carotid, subclavian artery, by neck incision ☐ ☐ ☐

35002 for ruptured aneurysm, carotid, subclavian artery, by neck incision ☐ ☐ ☐

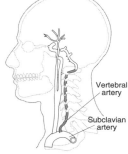
An incision is made in the back of the neck to directly approach an aneurysm or false aneurysm of the vertebral artery. The artery is either repaired directly or excised with a graft

Graft repair

Vertebral artery

Subclavian artery

35005 for aneurysm, pseudoaneurysm, and associated occlusive disease, vertebral artery ☐ ☐ ☐

35011 for aneurysm and associated occlusive disease, axillary-brachial artery, by arm incision ☐ ☐ ☐

35013 for ruptured aneurysm, axillary-brachial artery, by arm incision ☐ ☐ ☐

35021 for aneurysm, pseudoaneurysm, and associated occlusive disease, innominate, subclavian artery, by thoracic incision ☐ ☐ ☐

35022 for ruptured aneurysm, innominate, subclavian artery, by thoracic incision ☐ ☐ ☐

35045 for aneurysm, pseudoaneurysm, and associated occlusive disease, radial or ulnar artery ☐ ☐ ☐

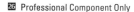

35081	for aneurysm, pseudoaneurysm, and associated occlusive disease, abdominal aorta	C 80 ⟷

MED: 100-3,20.23

AMA: 2001,Dec,7; 2000,Dec,1

35082	for ruptured aneurysm, abdominal aorta	C 80 ⟷

MED: 100-3,20.23

35091	for aneurysm, pseudoaneurysm, and associated occlusive disease, abdominal aorta involving visceral vessels (mesenteric, celiac, renal)	C 80 50 ⟷

MED: 100-3,20.23

AMA: 2000,Dec,1

35092	for ruptured aneurysm, abdominal aorta involving visceral vessels (mesenteric, celiac, renal)	C 80 50 ⟷
35102	for aneurysm, pseudoaneurysm, and associated occlusive disease, abdominal aorta involving iliac vessels (common, hypogastric, external)	C 80 50 ⟷
35103	for ruptured aneurysm, abdominal aorta involving iliac vessels (common, hypogastric, external)	C 80 50 ⟷
35111	for aneurysm, pseudoaneurysm, and associated occlusive disease, splenic artery	C 80 50 ⟷
35112	for ruptured aneurysm, splenic artery	C 80 50 ⟷
35121	for aneurysm, pseudoaneurysm, and associated occlusive disease, hepatic, celiac, renal, or mesenteric artery	C 80 50 ⟷
35122	for ruptured aneurysm, hepatic, celiac, renal, or mesenteric artery	C 80 50 ⟷
35131	for aneurysm, pseudoaneurysm, and associated occlusive disease, iliac artery (common, hypogastric, external)	C 80 50 ⟷

AMA: 2003,Feb,1

35132	for ruptured aneurysm, iliac artery (common, hypogastric, external)	C 80 50 ⟷
35141	for aneurysm, pseudoaneurysm, and associated occlusive disease, common femoral artery (profunda femoris, superficial femoral)	C 80 50 ⟷
35142	for ruptured aneurysm, common femoral artery (profunda femoris, superficial femoral)	C 80 50 ⟷
35151	for aneurysm, pseudoaneurysm, and associated occlusive disease, popliteal artery	C 80 50 ⟷
35152	for ruptured aneurysm, popliteal artery	C 80 50 ⟷

REPAIR ARTERIOVENOUS FISTULA

35180	Repair, congenital arteriovenous fistula; head and neck	T 80 ⟷
35182	thorax and abdomen	C 80 ⟷
35184	extremities	T 80 ⟷
35188	Repair, acquired or traumatic arteriovenous fistula; head and neck	4 T 80 ⟷

MED: 100-2,15,260; 100-4,12,90.3; 100-4,14,10

35189	thorax and abdomen	C 80 ⟷
35190	extremities	T 80 ⟷

REPAIR BLOOD VESSEL OTHER THAN FOR FISTULA, WITH OR WITHOUT PATCH ANGIOPLASTY

If an AV fistula is repaired, consult CPT codes 35180-35190.

35201	Repair blood vessel, direct; neck	T 80 50 ⟷
35206	upper extremity	T 80 50 ⟷

AMA: 2000,Oct,1

35207	hand, finger	4 T 50 ⟷

MED: 100-2,15,260; 100-4,12,90.3; 100-4,14,10

35211	intrathoracic, with bypass	C 80 50 ⟷
35216	intrathoracic, without bypass	C 80 50 ⟷
35221	intra-abdominal	C 80 50 ⟷
35226	lower extremity	T 80 50 ⟷
35231	Repair blood vessel with vein graft; neck	T 80 50 ⟷
35236	upper extremity	T 80 50 ⟷
35241	intrathoracic, with bypass	C 80 50 ⟷
35246	intrathoracic, without bypass	C 80 50 ⟷
35251	intra-abdominal	C 80 50 ⟷
35256	lower extremity	T 80 50 ⟷
35261	Repair blood vessel with graft other than vein; neck	T 80 50 ⟷
35266	upper extremity	T 80 50 ⟷
35271	intrathoracic, with bypass	C 80 50 ⟷
35276	intrathoracic, without bypass	C 80 50 ⟷
35281	intra-abdominal	C 80 50 ⟷
35286	lower extremity	T 80 50 ⟷

THROMBOENDARTERECTOMY

If a coronary artery bypass is performed, consult CPT codes 33510-33536 and 33572.

▲	35301	Thromboendarterectomy, including patch graft, if performed; carotid, vertebral, subclavian, by neck incision	C 80 50 ⟷

MED: 100-3,20.1; 100-3,160.8

●	35302	superficial femoral artery	C
●	35303	popliteal artery	C

Do not report 35302 or 35303 with 35483 or 35500.

●	35304	tibioperoneal trunk artery	C
●	35305	tibial or peroneal artery, initial vessel	C
+ ●	35306	each additional tibial or peroneal artery (List separately in addition to code for primary procedure)	C

Note that 35306 is an add-on code and must be reported with 35305.

Do not report 35304, 35305, or 35306 with 35485 or 35500.

35311	subclavian, innominate, by thoracic incision	C 80 50 ⟷

MED: 100-3,20.1

35321	axillary-brachial	T 80 50 ⟷
35331	abdominal aorta	C 80 50 ⟷
35341	mesenteric, celiac, or renal	C 80 50 ⟷
35351	iliac	C 80 50 ⟷
35355	iliofemoral	C 80 50 ⟷
35361	combined aortoiliac	C 80 50 ⟷
35363	combined aortoiliofemoral	C 80 50 ⟷
35371	common femoral	C 80 50 ⟷
35372	deep (profunda) femoral	C 80 50 ⟷

⊛ Modifier 63 Exempt Code	⊙ Conscious Sedation	+ CPT Add-on Code	⊘ Modifier 51 Exempt Code	● New Code	▲ Revised Code
M Maternity Edit	A Age Edit	A-Y APC Status Indicators	C CCI Comprehensive Code	50 Bilateral Procedure	

Cardiovascular System

~~35381~~   ~~femoral and/or popliteal, and/or tibioperoneal~~
Use 35302-35306.

+   **35390**   **Reoperation, carotid, thromboendarterectomy, more than one month after original operation (List separately in addition to code for primary procedure)** [C] [80] [↻]

AMA: 1997,Nov,16
Note that 35390 is an add-on code and must be used in conjunction with 35301.

ANGIOSCOPY

+   **35400**   **Angioscopy (non-coronary vessels or grafts) during therapeutic intervention (List separately in addition to code for primary procedure)** [C] [80] [↻]

Note that 35400 is an add-on code and must be used in conjunction with a code for the therapeutic intervention.

TRANSLUMINAL ANGIOPLASTY

OPEN

For radiological supervision and interpretation, consult CPT codes 75962-75968 and 75978.

When performed as part of another procedure, append modifier 51 or 52 as appropriate.

35450   **Transluminal balloon angioplasty, open; renal or other visceral artery** [C] [80] [50] [↻]

MED: 100-3,20.7
AMA: 2000,Dec,1; 1997,Feb,2, 3

35452   **aortic** [C] [80] [50] [↻]

AMA: 1997,Feb,2, 3

35454   **iliac** [C] [80] [50] [↻]

AMA: 2003,Feb,1; 2000,Dec,1; 1997,Feb,2, 3

35456   **femoral-popliteal** [C] [80] [50] [↻]

AMA: 1997,Feb,2, 3

35458   **brachiocephalic trunk or branches, each vessel** [T] [80] [50] [↻]

MED: 100-4,4,61.2
AMA: 2001,May,11; 1997,Feb,2, 3

35459   **tibioperoneal trunk and branches** [T] [80] [50] [↻]

MED: 100-4,4,61.2
AMA: 1997,Feb,2, 3

35460   **venous** [T] [50] [↻]

MED: 100-4,4,61.2
AMA: 1997,Feb,2, 3

PERCUTANEOUS

For radiological supervision and interpretation, consult CPT codes 75962-75968 and 75978.

Codes for catheter placement should also be reported.

⊙   **35470**   **Transluminal balloon angioplasty, percutaneous; tibioperoneal trunk or branches, each vessel** [T] [50] [↻]

MED: 100-3,20.7; 100-4,4,61.2
AMA: 1997,Feb,2, 3; 1996,Aug,3

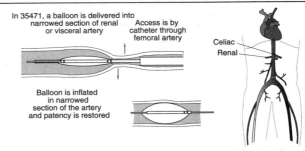

In 35471, a balloon is delivered into narrowed section of renal or visceral artery

Access is by catheter through femoral artery

Balloon is inflated in narrowed section of the artery and patency is restored

Celiac
Renal

A balloon angioplasty is performed on the renal or visceral artery in a percutaneous procedure

⊙   **35471**   **renal or visceral artery** [T] [50] [↻]

MED: 100-3,20.7; 100-4,4,61.2
AMA: 1997,Feb,2, 3; 1996,Aug,3

⊙   **35472**   **aortic** [T] [80] [50] [↻]

MED: 100-3,20.7; 100-4,4,61.2
AMA: 1997,Feb,2, 3; 1996,Aug,3

⊙   **35473**   **iliac** [T] [50] [↻]

MED: 100-3,20.7; 100-4,4,61.2
AMA: 2003,Feb,1; 2001,May,1; 1997,Feb,2, 3; 1996,Aug,3; 1993,Fall,11

⊙   **35474**   **femoral-popliteal** [T] [50] [↻]

MED: 100-3,20.7; 100-4,4,61.2
AMA: 2001,May,1; 1997,Feb,2, 3; 1996,Aug,3

⊙   **35475**   **brachiocephalic trunk or branches, each vessel** [T] [50] [↻]

MED: 100-3,20.7; 100-4,4,61.2
AMA: 2001,May,1; 1997,Feb,2, 3; 1996,Aug,3

⊙   **35476**   **venous** [T] [50] [↻]

MED: 100-3,20.7; 100-4,4,61.2
AMA: 2001,May,1; 1997,Feb,2, 3; 1996,Aug,3

TRANSLUMINAL ATHERECTOMY

OPEN

If radiological supervision and interpretation is needed, consult CPT codes 75992-75996.

When performed as part of another procedure, append modifier 51 or 52 as appropriate.

35480   **Transluminal peripheral atherectomy, open; renal or other visceral artery** [C] [80] [↻]

AMA: 1997,Feb,2, 3

35481   **aortic** [C] [80] [↻]

AMA: 1997,Feb,2

35482   **iliac** [C] [80] [↻]

AMA: 1997,Feb,2

35483   **femoral-popliteal** [C] [80] [↻]

AMA: 1997,Feb,2

35484   **brachiocephalic trunk or branches, each vessel** [T] [80] [↻]

MED: 100-4,4,61.2
AMA: 1997,Feb,2

35485   **tibioperoneal trunk and branches** [T] [80] [↻]

MED: 100-4,4,61.2
AMA: 1997,Feb,2

PERCUTANEOUS

For radiological supervision and interpretation, consult CPT codes 75992-75996.

Codes for catheter placement should also be reported.

35490   **Transluminal peripheral atherectomy, percutaneous; renal or other visceral artery** [T] [80] [↻]

MED: 100-4,4,61.2
AMA: 1997,Feb,2

35491	**aortic**	T 80 ↻

MED: 100-4,4,61.2
AMA: 1997,Feb,2

35492	**iliac**	T 80 ↻

MED: 100-4,4,61.2
AMA: 1997,Feb,2

35493	**femoral-popliteal**	T ↻

MED: 100-4,4,61.2
AMA: 1997,Feb,2

35494	**brachiocephalic trunk or branches, each vessel**	T ↻

MED: 100-4,4,61.2
AMA: 1997,Feb,2

35495	**tibioperoneal trunk and branches**	T 80 ↻

MED: 100-4,4,61.2
AMA: 1997,Feb,2

BYPASS GRAFT

VEIN

Harvesting of the saphenous vein graft is included in codes 35501-35587 and not reported separately or as co-surgery. To report vein harvesting; upper extremity, consult CPT code 35500; femoropopliteal vein segment, consult CPT code 35572; two segments from two distant sites, consult CPT code 35682; three or more segments from distant sites, consult CPT code 35683. These should be reported in addition to the bypass graft procedure.

+ 35500 Harvest of upper extremity vein, one segment, for lower extremity or coronary artery bypass procedure (List separately in addition to code for primary procedure) T 80 ↻

AMA: 1999,Nov,19; 1999,Mar,6; 1998,Nov,13
Note that 35500 is an add-on code and must be used in conjunction with CPT codes 33510-33536, 35556, 35566, 35571, 35583-35587.

If more than one vein segment is harvested, consult CPT codes 35682 and 35683.

To report endoscopic procedure, consult CPT code 35508.

▲ 35501 Bypass graft, with vein; common carotid-ipsilateral internal carotid C 80 50 ↻

AMA: 1999,Apr,11

▲ 35506	**carotid-subclavian or subclavian-carotid**	C 80 50 ↻

35507	~~subclavian-carotid~~	

Use 35506.

35508	**carotid-vertebral**	C 80 50 ↻

MED: 100-3,20.1

▲ 35509	**carotid-contralateral carotid**	C 80 50 ↻
35510	**carotid-brachial**	C 80 50 ↻
35511	**subclavian-subclavian**	C 80 50 ↻
35512	**subclavian-brachial**	C 80 50 ↻
35515	**subclavian-vertebral**	C 80 50 ↻

MED: 100-3,20.1

35516	**subclavian-axillary**	C 80 50 ↻
35518	**axillary-axillary**	C 80 50 ↻
35521	**axillary-femoral**	C 80 50 ↻

If a bypass graft is performed with a synthetic graft, consult CPT code 35621.

35522	**axillary-brachial**	C 80 50 ↻
35525	**brachial-brachial**	C 80 50 ↻

35526	**aortosubclavian or carotid**	C 80 50 ↻

If a bypass graft is performed with a synthetic graft, consult CPT code 35626.

35531	**aortoceliac or aortomesenteric**	C 80 50 ↻
35533	**axillary-femoral-femoral**	C 80 50 ↻

If a bypass graft is performed with a synthetic graft, consult CPT code 35654.

35536	**splenorenal**	C 80 50 ↻

AMA: 1999,Jun,10

● 35537	**aortoiliac**	C

Use 35637 for bypass graft performed with synthetic graft.

Do not report 35537 with 35538.

● 35538	**aortobi-iliac**	C

Use 35638 for bypass graft performed with synthetic graft.

Do not report 35538 with 35537.

● 35539	**aortofemoral**	C

Use 35647 for bypass graft performed with synthetic graft.

Do not report 35539 with 35540.

● 35540	**aortobifemoral**	C

Use 35646 for bypass graft performed with synthetic graft.

Do not report 35540 with 35539.

~~35541~~	~~aortoiliac or bi-iliac~~	

Use 35537 or 35538.

~~35546~~	~~aortofemoral or bifemoral~~	

Use 35539 or 35540.

35548	**aortoiliofemoral, unilateral**	C 80 ↻

If a bypass graft is performed with a synthetic graft, consult CPT code 37799.

35549	**aortoiliofemoral, bilateral**	C 80 ↻

If a bypass graft is performed with a synthetic graft, consult CPT code 37799.

35551	**aortofemoral-popliteal**	C 80 50 ↻
35556	**femoral-popliteal**	C 80 50 ↻
35558	**femoral-femoral**	C 80 50 ↻
35560	**aortorenal**	C 80 50 ↻

AMA: 1999,Jun,10

35563	**ilioiliac**	C 80 50 ↻
35565	**iliofemoral**	C 80 50 ↻
35566	**femoral-anterior tibial, posterior tibial, peroneal artery or other distal vessels**	C 80 50 ↻
35571	**popliteal-tibial, -peroneal artery or other distal vessels**	C 80 50 ↻

Cardiovascular System

35572 — 35691

+ 35572 **Harvest of femoropopliteal vein, one segment, for vascular reconstruction procedure (eg, aortic, vena caval, coronary, peripheral artery) (List separately in addition to code for primary procedure)** N 80 ⬚

Note that 35572 is an add-on code and must be used in conjunction with 33510-33516, 33517-33523, 33533-33536, 34502, 34520, 35001-35002, 35011-35022, 35102-35103, 35121-35152, 35231-35256, 35501-35587, 35879-35907.

To report procedure performed bilaterally, append modifier 50.

IN-SITU VEIN

35583 **In-situ vein bypass; femoral-popliteal** C 80 50 ⬚

To report aortobifemoral bypass using synthetic conduit, and femoral-popliteal bypass with vein conduit in-situ, consult CPT codes 35646 and 35583. To report aorto(uni)femoral bypass with synthetic conduit, and femoral-popliteal bypass with vein conduit in-situe, consult CPT codes 35647 and 35583. To report aortofemoral bypass using vein conduit, and femoral-popliteal bypass with vein conduit in-situ, consult CPT codes 35539 and 35583.

35585 **femoral-anterior tibial, posterior tibial, or peroneal artery** C 80 50 ⬚

35587 **popliteal-tibial, peroneal** C 80 50 ⬚
AMA: 1999,Apr,11

OTHER THAN VEIN

⊘ 35600 **Harvest of upper extremity artery, one segment, for coronary artery bypass procedure** C 80 ⬚

▲ 35601 **Bypass graft, with other than vein; common carotid-ipsilateral internal carotid** C 80 50 ⬚
MED: 100-3,20.1

35606 **carotid-subclavian** C 80 50 ⬚
MED: 100-3,20.1

35612 **subclavian-subclavian** C 80 50 ⬚

35616 **subclavian-axillary** C 80 50 ⬚

35621 **axillary-femoral** C 80 50 ⬚

35623 **axillary-popliteal or -tibial** C 80 50 ⬚

35626 **aortosubclavian or carotid** C 80 50 ⬚

Vena cava and renal veins — Celiac trunk — Superior mesenteric — Renal — Abdominal aorta — Synthetic graft — Abdominal aorta as it exits diaphragm — Blockage

In 35631, a bypass graft of material other than vein is surgically installed from the aorta to the celiac, mesenteric, or renal arteries. The graft is typically placed in an end-to-side fashion on both the aorta and the recipient vessel downstream from the blockage

35631 **aortoceliac, aortomesenteric, aortorenal** C 80 50 ⬚

35636 **splenorenal (splenic to renal arterial anastomosis)** C 80 50 ⬚

● 35637 **aortoiliac** C

● 35638 **aortobi-iliac** C

~~35641~~ ~~aortoiliac or bi-iliac~~
Use 35637 or 35638.

35642 **carotid-vertebral** C 80 50 ⬚
MED: 100-3,20.1

35645 **subclavian-vertebral** C 80 50 ⬚
MED: 100-3,20.1

35646 **aortobifemoral** C 80 ⬚

To report open placment of aortobifemoral prosthesis post unsuccessful endovascular repair, consult CPT code 34832.

35647 **aortofemoral** C 80 50 ⬚

35650 **axillary-axillary** C 80 50 ⬚

35651 **aortofemoral-popliteal** C 80 50 ⬚

35654 **axillary-femoral-femoral** C 80 ⬚

35656 **femoral-popliteal** C 80 50 ⬚

35661 **femoral-femoral** C 80 50 ⬚

35663 **ilioiliac** C 80 50 ⬚

35665 **iliofemoral** C 80 50 ⬚

35666 **femoral-anterior tibial, posterior tibial, or peroneal artery** C 80 50 ⬚

35671 **popliteal-tibial or -peroneal artery** C 80 50 ⬚

COMPOSITE GRAFTS

Use the following codes to report harvest and anastomosis of two or more vein segments from sites distant to that where the bypass is being performed.

+ 35681 **Bypass graft; composite, prosthetic and vein (List separately in addition to code for primary procedure)** C 80 ⬚
AMA: 1999,Mar,6; 1999,Apr,11; 1998,Nov,13-14
Note that 35681 is not to be reported in addition to 35682 and 35683.

+ 35682 **autogenous composite, two segments of veins from two locations (List separately in addition to code for primary procedure)** C 80 ⬚
AMA: 2002,Sep,3; 1999,Mar,6; 1999,Apr,11; 1998,Nov,13-14
Note that 35682 is not to be reported in addition to 35681 and 35683.

+ 35683 **autogenous composite, three or more segments of vein from two or more locations (List separately in addition to code for primary procedure)** C 80 ⬚
AMA: 2002,Sep,3; 1999,Mar,6; 1999,Apr,11; 1998,Nov,13-14
Note that 35683 is not to be reported in addition to 35681 and 35682.

ADJUVANT TECHNIQUES

To report composite graft(s), consult CPT codes 35681-35683.

+ 35685 **Placement of vein patch or cuff at distal anastomosis of bypass graft, synthetic conduit (List separately in addition to code for primary procedure)** T 80 ⬚
AMA: 2002,Sep,3
Note that 35685 is an add-on code and must be used in conjunction with CPT codes 35656, 35666, or 35671.

+ 35686 **Creation of distal arteriovenous fistula during lower extremity bypass surgery (non-hemodialysis) (List separately in addition to code for primary procedure)** T 80 ⬚
AMA: 2002,Sep,3
Note that 35686 is an add-on code and must be used in conjunction with CPT codes 35556, 35566, 35571, 35583-35587, 35656, 35666, or 35671.

ARTERIAL TRANSPOSITION

35691 **Transposition and/or reimplantation; vertebral to carotid artery** C 80 50 ⬚

---

26 Professional Component Only   80/80 Assist-at-Surgery Allowed/With Documentation   Unlisted   Not Covered
TC Technical Component Only   MED: Pub 100/NCD References   AMA: CPT Assistant References   1-9 ASC Group   ♂ Male Only   ♀ Female Only

| 35693 | vertebral to subclavian artery | C 80 50 ↔ |
| 35694 | subclavian to carotid artery | C 80 50 ↔ |

Report code 33889 for an open subclavian to carotid artery transposition performed with an endovascular repair of the descending thoracic aorta.

| 35695 | carotid to subclavian artery | C 80 50 ↔ |
| + 35697 | Reimplantation, visceral artery to infrarenal aortic prosthesis, each artery (List separately in addition to code for primary procedure) | C 80 ↔ |

Code 35697 should not be reported with CPT code 33877

EXCISION, EXPLORATION, REPAIR, REVISION

| + 35700 | Reoperation, femoral-popliteal or femoral (popliteal)-anterior tibial, posterior tibial, peroneal artery, or other distal vessels, more than one month after original operation (List separately in addition to code for primary procedure) | C 80 ↔ |

Note that 35700 is an add-on code and must be used in conjunction with 35556, 35566, 35571, 35583, 35585, 35587, 35656, 35666, and 35671.

| 35701 | Exploration (not followed by surgical repair), with or without lysis of artery; carotid artery | C 80 50 ↔ |
| 35721 | femoral artery | C 80 50 ↔ |

AMA: 1996,Jun,8

35741	popliteal artery	C 80 50 ↔
35761	other vessels	T 80 50 ↔
35800	Exploration for postoperative hemorrhage, thrombosis or infection; neck	C 80 ↔
35820	chest	C 80 ↔
35840	abdomen	C 80 ↔
35860	extremity	T 80 ↔
35870	Repair of graft-enteric fistula	C 80 ↔
35875	Thrombectomy of arterial or venous graft (other than hemodialysis graft or fistula);	9 T ↔

MED: 100-2,15,260; 100-4,12,90.3; 100-4,14,10
AMA: 2000,Apr,10; 1999,Mar,6; 1999,Feb,6; 1998,Nov,14

| 35876 | with revision of arterial or venous graft | 9 T 80 ↔ |

MED: 100-2,15,260; 100-4,12,90.3; 100-4,14,10
AMA: 1998,Nov,14

If thrombectomy of hemodialysis graft of fistula is performed, consult CPT codes 36831 and 36833.

If thrombectomy with revision of any non-coronary arterial or venous graft, including those of the lower extremity (other than hemodialysis graft of fistula) of a lower extremity blood vessel (with or without patch angioplasty), consult CPT code 35226. For repair (other than for a fistula) for a lower extremity blood vessel using a vein graft, consult CPT code 35256.

| 35879 | Revision, lower extremity arterial bypass, without thrombectomy, open; with vein patch angioplasty | T 80 50 ↔ |

AMA: 1999,Nov,19

| 35881 | with segmental vein interposition | T 80 50 ↔ |

AMA: 1999,Nov,19
To report open revision of previous autogenous vein bypass graft of lower extremity, use CPT code 35879 or 35881. Consult CPT codes 35901-35907 and the appropriate revascularization code for the excision of infected grafts.

| ● 35883 | Revision, femoral anastomosis of synthetic arterial bypass graft in groin, open; with nonautogenous patch graft (eg, Dacron, ePTFE, bovine pericardium) | T |
| ● 35884 | with autogenous vein patch graft | T |

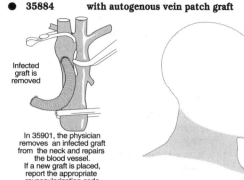

Infected graft is removed

In 35901, the physician removes an infected graft from the neck and repairs the blood vessel. If a new graft is placed, report the appropriate revascularization code

35901	Excision of infected graft; neck	C 80 ↔
35903	extremity	T 80 ↔
35905	thorax	C 80 ↔
35907	abdomen	C 80 ↔

VASCULAR INJECTION PROCEDURES

Vascular catheterization/injection services include local anesthesia, introduction of needle or catheter, injection of contrast media, and use of power injections. Since these are diagnostic procedures, only the pre-injection and post-injection care directly related to the procedure is included. Catheters, drugs, and contrast media should be reported separately.

Selective vascular catheterization codes include introduction and all lesser order vessels catheterized used in the approach. Selective catheterization of the right middle cerebral artery includes the introduction and placement catheterization of the right common and internal carotid arteries. Only code 36217 for the third order branch would be reported. Additional second or third order vessels supplied by the same first order branch are reported with "add on" procedure codes 36012, 36218, and 36248.

These procedures are reported by vascular family and, as such, any procedure performed on more than one vascular family is reported separately using the conventions described above. Bilateral procedures are reported as separate vascular families.

To report injection procedures with cardiac catheterizations, consult CPT codes 93541-93545.

To report chemotherapy administration for malignant disease, consult CPT codes 96401-96549.

INTRAVENOUS

| 36000 | Introduction of needle or intracatheter, vein | N 50 ↔ |

MED: 100-4,12,30.6.12
AMA: 1998,Jul,1; 1998,Apr,1, 3, 7

| 36002 | Injection procedures (eg, thrombin) for percutaneous treatment of extremity pseudoaneurysm | S 50 ↔ |

To report imaging guidance, consult CPT codes 76942, 77002, 77012, or 77021.

To report ultrasound guided compression repair of pseudoaneurysms, consult CPT code 76936.

Code 36002 should not be used to report vascular sealant of an arteriotomy site.

| 36005 | Injection procedure for extremity venography (including introduction of needle or intracatheter) | N 80 50 ↔ |

To report radiological supervision and interpretation, consult CPT codes 75820 and 75822.

36010   Introduction of catheter, superior or inferior vena cava   N 50 ⟷

AMA: 2001,May,10; 2000,Sep,11; 1998,Apr,1; 1996,Aug,2

36011   Selective catheter placement, venous system; first order branch (eg, renal vein, jugular vein)   N 50 ⟷

AMA: 1998,Apr,1; 1996,Aug,11

36012   second order, or more selective, branch (eg, left adrenal vein, petrosal sinus)   N 50 ⟷

AMA: 1996,Aug,11

36013   Introduction of catheter, right heart or main pulmonary artery   N ⟷

AMA: 1996,Aug,11

36014   Selective catheter placement, left or right pulmonary artery   N 50 ⟷

AMA: 1998,Apr,1; 1996,Aug,11

36015   Selective catheter placement, segmental or subsegmental pulmonary artery   N 50 ⟷

AMA: 2000,Sep,11; 1996,Aug,11
If a flow directed catheter is inserted (eg. Swan-Ganz), consult CPT code 93503. If venous catheterization is performed for selective organ blood sampling, consult CPT code 36500.

INTRA-ARTERIAL — INTRA-AORTIC

If angioplasty is performed, consult CPT codes 35470-35475. If transcatheter therapies are performed, consult CPT codes 37200-37208, 61624, and 61626.

If radiological supervision and interpretation is needed, see the Radiology section of CPT. If angiography is performed, consult CPT codes 75600-75790.

36100   Introduction of needle or intracatheter, carotid or vertebral artery   N 50 ⟷

AMA: 1996,Aug,11

36120   Introduction of needle or intracatheter; retrograde brachial artery   N ⟷

AMA: 1996,Aug,3; 1993,Fall,16

36140   extremity artery   N ⟷

AMA: 1996,Aug,3; 1993,Fall,16

36145   arteriovenous shunt created for dialysis (cannula, fistula, or graft)   N ⟷

AMA: 2001,May,1; 1997,Feb,2; 1996,Aug,3
To report insertion of arteriovenous cannula, consult CPT codes 36810-36821.

36160   Introduction of needle or intracatheter, aortic, translumbar   N ⟷

AMA: 1996,Aug,3

36200   Introduction of catheter, aorta   N 50 ⟷

AMA: 2003,Feb,1; 1996,Aug,3; 1993,Fall,16

36215   Selective catheter placement, arterial system; each first order thoracic or brachiocephalic branch, within a vascular family   N ⟷

AMA: 2003,Feb,1; 2000,Sep,11; 1998,Apr,1; 1997,Nov,16; 1996,Aug,3; 1993,Fall,15
To report catheter placement for coronary angiography, consult CPT code 93508.

36216   initial second order thoracic or brachiocephalic branch, within a vascular family   N ⟷

AMA: 2000,Oct,4; 1996,Aug,3; 1993,Fall,15

36217   initial third order or more selective thoracic or brachiocephalic branch, within a vascular family   N ⟷

AMA: 2000,Oct,4; 1996,Aug,3; 1993,Fall,15

+ 36218   additional second order, third order, and beyond, thoracic or brachiocephalic branch, within a vascular family (List in addition to code for initial second or third order vessel as appropriate)   N ⟷

AMA: 2000,Oct,4; 1996,Aug,3; 1993,Fall,15
Note that 36218 is an add-on code and must be used in conjunction with 36216 and 36217.

36245   Selective catheter placement, arterial system; each first order abdominal, pelvic, or lower extremity artery branch, within a vascular family   N 50 ⟷

AMA: 2001,Jan,14; 1996,Aug,3; 1993,Fall,15

36246   initial second order abdominal, pelvic, or lower extremity artery branch, within a vascular family   N 50 ⟷

AMA: 2001,Jan,14; 1996,Aug,3; 1993,Fall,15

36247   initial third order or more selective abdominal, pelvic, or lower extremity artery branch, within a vascular family   N 50 ⟷

AMA: 2001,Jan,14; 1996,Aug,3; 1993,Fall,15

+ 36248   additional second order, third order, and beyond, abdominal, pelvic, or lower extremity artery branch, within a vascular family (List in addition to code for initial second or third order vessel as appropriate)   N ⟷

AMA: 2001,Jan,14; 1998,Apr,1, 7; 1996,Aug,3; 1993,Fall,15
Note that 36248 is an add-on code and must be used in conjunction with 36246 and 36247.

36260   Insertion of implantable intra-arterial infusion pump (eg, for chemotherapy of liver)   3 T ⟷

MED: 100-2,15,260; 100-3,110.6; 100-3,280.14; 100-4,4,61.2; 100-4,12,90.3; 100-4,14,10
AMA: 1995,Fall,5

36261   Revision of implanted intra-arterial infusion pump   2 T 80 ⟷

MED: 100-2,15,260; 100-3,280.14; 100-4,12,90.3; 100-4,14,10

36262   Removal of implanted intra-arterial infusion pump   1 T ⟷

MED: 100-2,15,260; 100-3,280.14; 100-4,12,90.3; 100-4,14,10

36299   Unlisted procedure, vascular injection   N 80

MED: 100-4,4,180.3

VENOUS

▲ 36400   Venipuncture, younger than age 3 years, necessitating physician's skill, not to be used for routine venipuncture; femoral or jugular vein   A N ⟷

▲ 36405   scalp vein   A N ⟷

▲ 36406   other vein   A N ⟷

36410   Venipuncture, age 3 years or older, necessitating physician's skill (separate procedure), for diagnostic or therapeutic purposes (not to be used for routine venipuncture)   N ⟷

MED: 100-4,12,30.6.12
AMA: 2001,May,11
If venipuncture is performed as part of critical care services (99291-99292) do not report separately.

36415   Collection of venous blood by venipuncture   A ⊛

MED: 100-4,12,30.6.12
AMA: 1999,Oct,11; 1998,Mar,10; 1997,Feb,9; 1996,Jun,10

36416   Collection of capillary blood specimen (eg, finger, heel, ear stick)   N

▲ 36420   Venipuncture, cutdown; younger than age 1 year   A T 80 ⊛ ⟷

2G Professional Component Only   80/80 Assist-at-Surgery Allowed/With Documentation   Unlisted   Not Covered

TC Technical Component Only   MED: Pub 100/NCD References   AMA: CPT Assistant References   1-9 ASC Group   ♂ Male Only   ♀ Female Only

142 — CPT Expert   CPT only © 2006 American Medical Association. All Rights Reserved. (Black Ink)   © 2006 Ingenix (Blue Ink)

36425   age 1 or over   T ◪

MED: 100-3,20.18; 100-3,110.5; 100-3,110.7; 100-3,110.16; 100-4,12,70; 100-4,13,20; 100-4,13,90

36430   **Transfusion, blood or blood components**   S ◪

MED: 100-1,3,20.5; 100-1,3,20.5.2; 100-2,1,10; 100-3,110.5; 100-3,110.7; 100-3,110.8; 100-3,110.16; 100-4,3,40.2.2

AMA: 2001,Mar,10; 1997,Aug,18

▲ **36440**   **Push transfusion, blood, 2 years or younger**   A S 80 ◪

MED: 100-1,3,20.5; 100-1,3,20.5.2; 100-3,110.5; 100-3,110.7; 100-3,110.8; 100-3,110.16; 100-4,3,40.2.2

36450   **Exchange transfusion, blood; newborn**   A S 80 63 ◪

MED: 100-1,3,20.5; 100-1,3,20.5.2; 100-3,110.5; 100-3,110.7; 100-3,110.8; 100-3,110.16; 100-4,3,40.2.2

36455   other than newborn   S ◪

MED: 100-1,3,20.5.2; 100-3,110.5; 100-3,110.7; 100-3,110.16; 100-4,3,40.2.2

36460   **Transfusion, intrauterine, fetal**   ♀ S 80 63 ◪

MED: 100-1,3,20.5.2; 100-3,110.5; 100-3,110.7; 100-3,110.8; 100-4,3,40.2.2

If radiological supervision and interpretation is performed, consult CPT code 76941.

36468   **Single or multiple injections of sclerosing solutions, spider veins (telangiectasia); limb or trunk**   T 80 ◪

MED: 100-2,16,10; 100-2,16,120; 100-2,16,180

36469   face   T 80 ◪

MED: 100-2,16,10; 100-2,16,120; 100-2,16,180

36470   **Injection of sclerosing solution; single vein**   T 50 ◪

MED: 100-2,16,10; 100-2,16,120; 100-2,16,180; 100-3,150.7

36471   multiple veins, same leg   T 50 ◪

MED: 100-2,16,10; 100-2,16,120; 100-2,16,180; 100-3,150.7

36475   **Endovenous ablation therapy of incompetent vein, extremity, inclusive of all imaging guidance and monitoring, percutaneous, radiofrequency; first vein treated**   9 T 50 ◪

+ **36476**   second and subsequent veins treated in a single extremity, each through separate access sites (List separately in addition to code for primary procedure)   9 T 50

Note that 36476 must be used with 36475.

Codes 36475, 36476 cannot be reported with CPT codes 36000-36005, 36410, 36425, 36478, 36479, 37204, 75894, 76000-76001, 76937, 76942, 77002, 93970, and 93971.

36478   **Endovenous ablation therapy of incompetent vein, extremity, inclusive of all imaging guidance and monitoring, percutaneous, laser; first vein treated**   9 T 50 ◪

+ **36479**   second and subsequent veins treated in a single extremity, each through separate access sites (List separately in addition to code for primary procedure)   9 T 50

Note that 36479 must be used with 36478.

Codes 36478, 36479 cannot be reported with CPT codes 36000-36005, 36410, 36425, 36475, 36476, 37204, 75894, 76000-76001, 76937, 76942, 77002, 93970, 93971.

36481   **Percutaneous portal vein catheterization by any method**   N ◪

AMA: 2002,Mar,10; 1996,Oct,1

To report radiological supervision and interpretation, consult CPT codes 75885 and 75887.

36500   **Venous catheterization for selective organ blood sampling**   N ◪

If the superior or inferior vena cava is catheterized, consult CPT code 36010. If radiological supervision and interpretation is performed, consult CPT code 75893.

36510   **Catheterization of umbilical vein for diagnosis or therapy, newborn**   N 80 63 ◪

MED: 100-3,110.14

Modifier 63 should not be reported with code 36510.

36511   **Therapeutic apheresis; for white blood cells**   S ◪

MED: 100-1,3,20.5.2; 100-3,110.14; 100-4,4,231.9

36512   for red blood cells   S ◪

MED: 100-1,3,20.5.2; 100-3,110.14; 100-4,4,231.9

36513   for platelets   S ◪

MED: 100-1,3,20.5.2; 100-3,110.14; 100-4,4,231.9

36514   for plasma pheresis   S ◪

MED: 100-1,3,20.5.2; 100-3,110.14; 100-4,4,231.9

36515   with extracorporeal immunoadsorption and plasma reinfusion   S ◪

MED: 100-1,3,20.5.2; 100-3,110.14; 100-4,4,231.9

36516   with extracorporeal selective adsorption or selective filtration and plasma reinfusion   S ◪

MED: 100-1,3,20.5.2; 100-3,110.14; 100-4,4,231.9

To report physician evaluation, append modifier 26.

36522   **Photopheresis, extracorporeal**   S ◪

MED: 100-3,20.5; 100-3,110.4; 100-4,4,231.9

AMA: 1993,Fall,25

36540   **Collection of blood specimen from a completely implantable venous access device**   Q

AMA: 2002,Nov,1; 2002,Jan,11

Note that 36540 cannot be used in conjunction with CPT codes 36415, 36416.

To report venous blood specimen collection by venipuncture, consult CPT code 36415.

To report capillary blood specimen collection, consult CPT code 36416.

36550   **Declotting by thrombolytic agent of implanted vascular access device or catheter**   T 80 ◪

AMA: 1999,Nov,20

CENTRAL VENOUS ACCESS PROCEDURES

For coding purposes to qualify as a central venous access catheter or device, the tip must end in the subclavian, brachiocephalic (innominate) or iliac veins, the superior or inferior vena cava, or right atrium. The venous access device may be inserted centrally (jugular, subclavian, femoral vein or inferior vena cava) or peripherally (e.g., basilic or cephalic). There is no longer a coding distinction made between percutaneous venous access and that achieved via cutdown.

Procedures for the insertion of central venous access fall into the following categories:

- **Insertion:** Placement through a newly established venous access.
- **Repair:** Fixing of device without replacement of any components.
- **Partial replacement:** Replacement of only the catheter component, not the entire device.
- **Complete replacement:** Replacement of entire (all components) device via same access site.
- **Removal:** Removal of entire (all components) device.
- **Removal of obstruction:** Mechanical removal of obstructive material from device.

For the above categories of service rendered on a dual catheter system placed from separate venous access sites, report the appropriate procedure code with a frequency of two. If an existing device is entirely removed and a new device placed via a separate venous access site, then report both the removal and insertion.

Cardiovascular System

36555 — 36590

To report refilling and maintenance of an implantable pump or reservoir for intravenous or intra-arterial drug delivery, consult CPT code 96530.

To report radiological imaging used during these procedures, consult CPT codes 76937, 77001.

INSERTION OF CENTRAL VENOUS ACCESS DEVICE

(handwritten: DRU uses this most of time)

⊙ ▲ **36555** **Insertion of non-tunneled centrally inserted central venous catheter; younger than 5 years of age** Ⓐ 🔳 Ⓣ 🔳

To report peripherally inserted non-tunneled central venous catheter, under 5 years of age, consult CPT code 36568.

~ **36556** **age 5 years or older** 🔳 Ⓣ 🔳

To report peripherally inserted non-tunneled central venous catheter, age 5 years or older, consult CPT code 36569.

⊙ ▲ **36557** **Insertion of tunneled centrally inserted central venous catheter, without subcutaneous port or pump; younger than 5 years of age** Ⓐ 🔳 Ⓣ 🔳 🔳 🔳

MED: 100-4,4,61.2

⊙ **36558** **age 5 years or older** 🔳 Ⓣ 🔳 🔳 🔳

MED: 100-4,4,61.2

To report peripherally inserted central venous catheter with port, 5 years or older, consult CPT code 36571.

⊙ ▲ **36560** **Insertion of tunneled centrally inserted central venous access device, with subcutaneous port; younger than 5 years of age** Ⓐ 🔳 Ⓣ 🔳 🔳 🔳

To report peripherally inserted central venous access device with subcutaneous port, under 5 years of age, consult CPT code 36570.

⊙ **36561** **age 5 years or older** 🔳 Ⓣ 🔳 🔳 🔳

To report peripherally inserted central venous catheter with subcutaneous port, 5 years or older, consult CPT code 36571.

⊙ **36563** **Insertion of tunneled centrally inserted central venous access device with subcutaneous pump** 🔳 Ⓣ 🔳 🔳

MED: 100-4,4,61.2

⊙ **36565** **Insertion of tunneled centrally inserted central venous access device, requiring two catheters via two separate venous access sites; without subcutaneous port or pump (eg, Tesio type catheter)** 🔳 Ⓣ 🔳 🔳 🔳

⊙ **36566** **with subcutaneous port(s)** 🔳 Ⓣ 🔳 🔳 🔳

⊙ ▲ **36568** **Insertion of peripherally inserted central venous catheter (PICC), without subcutaneous port or pump; younger than 5 years of age** Ⓐ 🔳 Ⓣ 🔳

To report placement of centrally inserted non-tunneled central venous catheter, without subcutaneous port or pump, under 5 years of age, consult CPT code 36555.

36569 **age 5 years or older** 🔳 Ⓣ 🔳

To report placement of centrally inserted non-tunneled central venous catheter, without subcutaneous port or pump, age 5 years or older, consult CPT code 36556.

⊙ ▲ **36570** **Insertion of peripherally inserted central venous access device, with subcutaneous port; younger than 5 years of age** Ⓐ 🔳 Ⓣ 🔳 🔳 🔳

MED: 100-4,4,61.2

To report insertion of tunneled centrally inserted central venous access device with subcutaneous port, under 5 years of age, consult CPT code 36560.

⊙ **36571** **age 5 years or older** 🔳 Ⓣ 🔳 🔳 🔳

MED: 100-4,4,61.2

To report insertion of tunneled centrally inserted central venous access device with subcutaneous port, age 5 years or older, consult CPT code 36561.

REPAIR OF CENTRAL VENOUS ACCESS DEVICE

To report mechanical removal of pericatheter obstructive material, consult CPT code 36595.

To report mechanical removal of intracatheter obstructive material, consult CPT code 36596.

36575 **Repair of tunneled or non-tunneled central venous access catheter, without subcutaneous port or pump, central or peripheral insertion site** 🔳 Ⓣ 🔳 🔳

⊙ **36576** **Repair of central venous access device, with subcutaneous port or pump, central or peripheral insertion site** 🔳 Ⓣ 🔳 🔳

PARTIAL REPLACEMENT OF CENTRAL VENOUS ACCESS DEVICE (CATHETER ONLY)

⊙ **36578** **Replacement, catheter only, of central venous access device, with subcutaneous port or pump, central or peripheral insertion site** 🔳 Ⓣ 🔳 🔳

To report replacement of entire device through same venous access site, consult CPT codes 36582 or 36583.

COMPLETE REPLACEMENT OF CENTRAL VENOUS ACCESS DEVICE THROUGH SAME VENOUS ACCESS SITE

36580 **Replacement, complete, of a non-tunneled centrally inserted central venous catheter, without subcutaneous port or pump, through same venous access** 🔳 Ⓣ 🔳

⊙ **36581** **Replacement, complete, of a tunneled centrally inserted central venous catheter, without subcutaneous port or pump, through same venous access** 🔳 Ⓣ 🔳 🔳

MED: 100-4,4,61.2

⊙ **36582** **Replacement, complete, of a tunneled centrally inserted central venous access device, with subcutaneous port, through same venous access** 🔳 Ⓣ 🔳 🔳

⊙ **36583** **Replacement, complete, of a tunneled centrally inserted central venous access device, with subcutaneous pump, through same venous access** 🔳 Ⓣ 🔳 🔳

MED: 100-4,4,61.2

36584 **Replacement, complete, of a peripherally inserted central venous catheter (PICC), without subcutaneous port or pump, through same venous access** 🔳 Ⓣ 🔳

⊙ **36585** **Replacement, complete, of a peripherally inserted central venous access device, with subcutaneous port, through same venous access** 🔳 Ⓣ 🔳 🔳

MED: 100-4,4,61.2

REMOVAL OF CENTRAL VENOUS ACCESS DEVICE

36589 **Removal of tunneled central venous catheter, without subcutaneous port or pump** 🔳 Ⓣ 🔳 🔳 🔳

⊙ **36590** **Removal of tunneled central venous access device, with subcutaneous port or pump, central or peripheral insertion** 🔳 Ⓣ 🔳 🔳

Codes 36589 and 36590 cannot be reported for removal of non-tunneled central venous catheters.

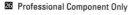 Professional Component Only
Ⓣ Technical Component Only

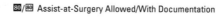 Assist-at-Surgery Allowed/With Documentation
MED: Pub 100/NCD References   **AMA:** CPT Assistant References
🔳-🔳 ASC Group   ♂ Male Only

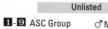 Unlisted   Not Covered
♀ Female Only

144 — CPT Expert   CPT only © 2006 American Medical Association. All Rights Reserved. *(Black Ink)*   © 2006 Ingenix *(Blue Ink)*

MECHANICAL REMOVAL OF OBSTRUCTIVE MATERIAL

36595 **Mechanical removal of pericatheter obstructive material (eg, fibrin sheath) from central venous device via separate venous access** ⓣ ▣

Code 36550 cannot be reported in addition to 36595.

To report venous catheterization, consult CPT codes 36010-36012.

To report radiological supervision and interpretation, consult CPT code 75901.

36596 **Mechanical removal of intraluminal (intracatheter) obstructive material from central venous device through device lumen** ⓣ ▣

Code 36550 cannot be reported in addition to 36596.

To report venous catheterization, consult CPT codes 36010-36012.

To report radiological supervision and interpretation, consult CPT code 75902.

OTHER CENTRAL VENOUS ACCESS PROCEDURES

36597 **Repositioning of previously placed central venous catheter under fluoroscopic guidance** ⓣ ▣

To report fluoroscopic guidance, consult CPT code 76000.

36598 **Contrast injection(s) for radiologic evaluation of existing central venous access device, including fluoroscopy, image documentation and report** ⓧ 80 50

Code 36598 cannot be reported with 36595, 36596, or 76000.

To report complete diagnostic studies, consult 75820, 75825, 75827.

ARTERIAL

36600 **Arterial puncture, withdrawal of blood for diagnosis** ⓠ ▣

MED: 100-4,12,30.6.12
AMA: 1995,Fall,7
If arterial puncture is performed as part of critical care services (99291-99292) do not report separately.

⊘ **36620** **Arterial catheterization or cannulation for sampling, monitoring or transfusion (separate procedure); percutaneous** ⓝ ▣

MED: 100-3,110.5; 100-3,110.7; 100-3,110.8
AMA: 1998,Apr,3; 1995,Fall,7

36625 **cutdown** ⓝ ▣

MED: 100-3,110.5; 100-3,110.8
AMA: 1995,Fall,7

36640 **Arterial catheterization for prolonged infusion therapy (chemotherapy), cutdown** ❶ ⓣ ▣

MED: 100-2,15,260; 100-3,110.6; 100-4,4,61.2; 100-4,12,90.3; 100-4,14,10
AMA: 1995,Fall,7
Consult also 96420-96425. If arterial catheterization is performed for occlusion therapy, consult CPT code 75894.

⊘ **36660** **Catheterization, umbilical artery, newborn, for diagnosis or therapy** Ⓐ ⓒ 80 63 ▣

AMA: 1995,Fall,8

INTRAOSSEOUS

36680 **Placement of needle for intraosseous infusion** ⓣ 80 ▣

HEMODIALYSIS ACCESS, INTERVASCULAR CANNULATION FOR EXTRACORPOREAL CIRCULATION, OR SHUNT INSERTION

36800 **Insertion of cannula for hemodialysis, other purpose (separate procedure); vein to vein** ❸ ⓣ ▣

MED: 100-2,15,260; 100-4,12,90.3; 100-4,14,10
AMA: 1993,Fall,3

36810 **arteriovenous, external (Scribner type)** ❸ ⓣ ▣

MED: 100-2,15,260; 100-4,12,90.3; 100-4,14,10
AMA: 1993,Fall,3

36815 **arteriovenous, external revision, or closure** ❸ ⓣ ▣

MED: 100-2,15,260; 100-4,12,90.3; 100-4,14,10
AMA: 1993,Fall,3

36818 **Arteriovenous anastomosis, open; by upper arm cephalic vein transposition** ❸ ⓣ 80 ▣

Code 36818 cannot be reported with CPT codes 36819, 36820, 36821, and 36830 during a unilateral upper extremity procedure. For an open arteriovenous anastomoses performed at the same operative session on both extremities, report modifier 50 or 59 as required.

36819 **by upper arm basilic vein transposition** ❸ ⓣ 80 ▣

MED: 100-2,15,260; 100-4,12,90.3; 100-4,14,10
AMA: 1999,Nov,20
Code 36819 cannot be reported with CPT codes 36818, 36820, 36821, and 36830 during a unilateral upper extremity procedure. For an open arteriovenous anastomoses performed at the same operative session on both extremities, report modifier 50 or 59 as required.

36820 **by forearm vein transposition** ❸ ⓣ 80 50 ▣

MED: 100-2,15,260; 100-4,12,90.3; 100-4,14,10

36821 **direct, any site (eg, Cimino type) (separate procedure)** ❸ ⓣ 80 ▣

MED: 100-2,15,260; 100-4,12,90.3; 100-4,14,10
AMA: 1999,Nov,20; 1997,Feb,2; 1993,Fall,3

36822 **Insertion of cannula(s) for prolonged extracorporeal circulation for cardiopulmonary insufficiency (ECMO) (separate procedure)** ⓒ ▣

AMA: 1997,Feb,11; 1993,Fall,3
If maintenance is performed for prolonged extracorporal circulation, consult CPT codes 33960 and 33961.

36823 **Insertion of arterial and venous cannula(s) for isolated extracorporeal circulation including regional chemotherapy perfusion to an extremity, with or without hyperthermia, with removal of cannula(s) and repair of arteriotomy and venotomy sites** ⓒ ▣

MED: 100-3,110.6
AMA: 1998,Nov,14-15
Code 36823 includes chemotherapy perfusion supported by a membrane oxygenator/perfusion pump. Do not report 96408-96425 with 36823.

36825 **Creation of arteriovenous fistula by other than direct arteriovenous anastomosis (separate procedure); autogenous graft** ❹ ⓣ 80 ▣

MED: 100-2,15,260; 100-4,12,90.3; 100-4,14,10
AMA: 1997,Feb,1; 1993,Fall,3
If direct arteriovenous anastomosis is performed, consult CPT code 36821.

---

⑬ Modifier 63 Exempt Code   ⊙ Conscious Sedation   ✛ CPT Add-on Code   ⊘ Modifier 51 Exempt Code   ● New Code   ▲ Revised Code

Ⓜ Maternity Edit   Ⓐ Age Edit   Ⓐ-Ⓨ APC Status Indicators   Ⓒ CCI Comprehensive Code   50 Bilateral Procedure

36830 nonautogenous graft (eg, biological collagen, thermoplastic graft) 🔳 Ⓣ 80 🔲

MED: 100-2,15,260; 100-4,12,90.3; 100-4,14,10

AMA: 1997,Feb,1; 1993,Fall,3

If direct arteriovenous anastomosis is performed, consult CPT code 36821.

36831 Thrombectomy, open, arteriovenous fistula without revision, autogenous or nonautogenous dialysis graft (separate procedure) 🔳 Ⓣ 80 🔲

MED: 100-2,15,260; 100-4,12,90.3; 100-4,14,10

AMA: 1999,Mar,6; 1999,Feb,6; 1999,Apr,11; 1998,Nov,14-15

36832 Revision, open, arteriovenous fistula; without thrombectomy, autogenous or nonautogenous dialysis graft (separate procedure) 🔳 Ⓣ 80 🔲

MED: 100-2,15,260; 100-4,12,90.3; 100-4,14,10

AMA: 1999,Nov,20; 1999,Mar,6; 1999,Feb,6; 1999,Apr,11; 1998,Nov,15; 1997,Feb,2; 1993,Fall,3

36833 with thrombectomy, autogenous or nonautogenous dialysis graft (separate procedure) 🔳 Ⓣ 80 🔲

MED: 100-2,15,260; 100-4,12,90.3; 100-4,14,10

AMA: 1999,Feb,6; 1999,Apr,11; 1998,Nov,15

36834 Plastic repair of arteriovenous aneurysm (separate procedure) 🔳 Ⓣ 80 🔲

AMA: 1993,Fall,3

36835 Insertion of Thomas shunt (separate procedure) 🔳 Ⓣ

MED: 100-2,15,260; 100-4,12,90.3; 100-4,14,10

36838 Distal revascularization and interval ligation (DRIL), upper extremity hemodialysis access (steal syndrome) Ⓣ 80 50 🔲

Code 36838 cannot be reported with CPT codes 35512, 35522, 36832, 37607, 37618.

36860 External cannula declotting (separate procedure); without balloon catheter 🔳 Ⓣ 🔲

MED: 100-2,15,260; 100-4,12,90.3; 100-4,14,10

AMA: 2001,May,1; 1999,Feb,6; 1998,Nov,15; 1997,Feb,2; 1993,Fall,3

36861 with balloon catheter 🔳 Ⓣ 🔲

MED: 100-2,15,260; 100-4,12,90.3; 100-4,14,10

AMA: 2001,May,1; 1997,Feb,2; 1993,Fall,3

To report imaging guidance is performed, consult CPT code 76000.

⊙ **36870** Thrombectomy, percutaneous, arteriovenous fistula, autogenous or nonautogenous graft (includes mechanical thrombus extraction and intra-graft thrombolysis) 🔳 Ⓣ 50 🔲

MED: 100-2,15,260; 100-4,12,90.3; 100-4,14,10

AMA: 2001,May,1

Do not report code 36550 with 36870. For catheterization, report code 36145.

To report radiological supervision and interpretation, consult CPT code 75790.

PORTAL DECOMPRESSION PROCEDURES

37140 Venous anastomosis, open; portocaval 🄲 🔲

If peritoneal-venous shunt is inserted, consult CPT code 49425.

37145 renoportal 🄲 80 🔲

37160 caval-mesenteric 🄲 80 🔲

37180 splenorenal, proximal 🄲 80 🔲

37181 splenorenal, distal (selective decompression of esophagogastric varices, any technique) 🄲 80 🔲

To report percutaneous procedure, consult CPT code 37182.

37182 Insertion of transvenous intrahepatic portosystemic shunt(s) (TIPS) (includes venous access, hepatic and portal vein catheterization, portography with hemodynamic evaluation, intrahepatic tract formation/dilatation, stent placement and all associated imaging guidance and documentation) 🄲 80 🔲

To report open procedure, consult CPT code 37140.

Note that 75885 and 75887 cannot be reported with CPT code 37182.

37183 Revision of transvenous intrahepatic portosystemic shunt(s) (TIPS) (includes venous access, hepatic and portal vein catheterization, portography with hemodynamic evaluation, intrahepatic tract recanulization/dilatation, stent placement and all associated imaging guidance and documentation) Ⓣ 80 🔲

Note that 75885 and 75887 cannot be reported with CPT code 37183.

TRANSCATHETER PROCEDURES

The appropriate CPT codes for placement of catheters and radiological supervision and interpretation should be reported in addition to the following therapeutic procedures.

Mechanical Thrombectomy

Report separately code(s) for catheter placement(s), diagnostic studies, and other percutaneous interventions.

Codes 37184-37188 include radiological supervision and interpretation during the procedure.

Injection(s) of a thrombolytic substance during the procedure is included and not separately reportable with a mechanical thrombectomy. However, continuous infusion before and after the procedure is not included and may be reported with codes 37201, 75896, 75989.

For coronary mechanical thrombectomy, consult 92973.

For mechanical thrombectomy for dialysis fistula, consult 36870.

Arterial Mechanical Thrombectomy

Arterial mechanical thrombectomy may be performed as a "primary" transcatheter procedure with planning before the procedure, the procedure itself, and evaluation after the procedure. Primary mechanical thrombectomy is reported per vascular family. Report 37184 for the initial vessel treated and 37185 for the second and all succeeding vessel(s) in the same vascular family. Report mechanical thrombectomy of an additional vascular family treated through a separate access site, by appending modifier 51 to 37184-37185, as appropriate.

Do not report 37184-37185 for mechanical thrombectomy performed for the treatment of a thrombus or embolus that complicates other percutaneous interventional procedures. Consult CPT code 37186 for these procedures. Arterial mechanical thrombectomy is considered a "secondary" transcatheter procedure for taking out short segments of thrombus or embolus when performed either before or after another percutaneous procedure. Report secondary mechanical thrombectomy with 37186. Do not report 37186 with 37184-37185.

Venous Mechanical Thrombectomy

Report the initial application of venous mechanical thrombectomy with code 37188. Use modifier 50 to report a bilateral procedure.

26 Professional Component Only — 80/80 Assist-at-Surgery Allowed/With Documentation — Unlisted — Not Covered

TC Technical Component Only — MED: Pub 100/NCD References — AMA: CPT Assistant References — 1-9 ASC Group — ♂ Male Only — ♀ Female Only

146 — CPT Expert — CPT only © 2006 American Medical Association. All Rights Reserved. (Black Ink) — © 2006 Ingenix (Blue Ink)

ARTERIAL MECHANICAL THROMBECTOMY

⊙ 37184 **Primary percutaneous transluminal mechanical thrombectomy, noncoronary, arterial or arterial bypass graft, including fluoroscopic guidance and intraprocedural pharmacological thrombolytic injection(s); initial vessel** T 50

MED: 100-4,4,61.2

Code 37184 cannot be reported with 76000, 76001, 90774, 99143-99150.

+ ⊙ 37185 **second and all subsequent vessel(s) within the same vascular family (List separately in addition to code for primary mechanical thrombectomy procedure)** T

Code 37185 cannot be reported with 76000, 76001, 90775.

+ ⊙ 37186 **Secondary percutaneous transluminal thrombectomy (eg, nonprimary mechanical, snare basket, suction technique), noncoronary, arterial or arterial bypass graft, including fluoroscopic guidance and intraprocedural pharmacological thrombolytic injections, provided in conjunction with another percutaneous intervention other than primary mechanical thrombectomy (List separately in addition to code for primary procedure)** T

Code 37186 cannot be reported with 76000, 76001, 90775.

VENOUS MECHANICAL THROMBECTOMY

⊙ 37187 **Percutaneous transluminal mechanical thrombectomy, vein(s), including intraprocedural pharmacological thrombolytic injections and fluoroscopic guidance** T 50

MED: 100-4,4,61.2

Code 37187 cannot be reported with 76000, 76001, 90775.

⊙ 37188 **Percutaneous transluminal mechanical thrombectomy, vein(s), including intraprocedural pharmacological thrombolytic injections and fluoroscopic guidance, repeat treatment on subsequent day during course of thrombolytic therapy** T 50

MED: 100-4,4,61.2

Code 37188 cannot be reported with 76000, 76001, 90775.

OTHER PROCEDURES

37195 **Thrombolysis, cerebral, by intravenous infusion** T 80

AMA: 1997,Nov,16

37200 **Transcatheter biopsy** T

To report radiological supervision and interpretation, consult CPT code 75970.

37201 **Transcatheter therapy, infusion for thrombolysis other than coronary** T

AMA: 2001,May,1; 2001,Feb,10; 1997,Feb,2
To report radiological supervision and interpretation, consult CPT code 75896.

If thrombolysis of the coronary vessels is performed, consult CPT codes 92975 and 92977.

37202 **Transcatheter therapy, infusion other than for thrombolysis, any type (eg, spasmolytic, vasoconstrictive)** T

AMA: 1998,Jan,11; 1998,Apr,3, 9; 1996,Oct,11
To report radiological supervision and interpretation, consult CPT code 75896.

⊙ 37203 **Transcatheter retrieval, percutaneous, of intravascular foreign body (eg, fractured venous or arterial catheter)** T

MED: 100-3,20.28

To report radiological supervision and interpretation, consult CPT code 75961.

37204 **Transcatheter occlusion or embolization (eg, for tumor destruction, to achieve hemostasis, to occlude a vascular malformation), percutaneous, any method, non-central nervous system, non-head or neck** T

MED: 100-3,20.28
AMA: 1998,Sep,7; 1998,Oct,10
To report radiological supervision and interpretation, consult CPT code 75894.

Consult also CPT codes 61624 and 61626.

37205 **Transcatheter placement of an intravascular stent(s), (except coronary, carotid, and vertebral vessel), percutaneous; initial vessel** T 80

AMA: 2003,Feb,1; 2001,May,1; 1993,Fall,18
To report radiological supervision and interpretation, consult CPT code 75960.

+ 37206 **each additional vessel (List separately in addition to code for primary procedure)** T 80

AMA: 2003,Feb,1; 1993,Fall,18
Note that 37206 is an add-on code and must be used in conjunction with 37205.

To report transcatheter placement of intravascular cervical carotid artery stent(s), consult CPT codes 37215, 37216.

To report transcatheter placement of extracranial vertebral or intrathoracic carotid artery stent(s), consult Category III codes 0075T, 0076T.

For radiological supervision and interpretation, consult CPT code 75960.

37207 **Transcatheter placement of an intravascular stent(s), (non-coronary vessel), open; initial vessel** T 80 50

AMA: 2003,Feb,1
To report radiological supervision and interpretation, consult CPT code 75960.

To report catheterizations, consult CPT codes 36215-36248.

To report transcatheter placement of intracoronary stent(s), consult CPT codes 92980, 92981.

+ 37208 **each additional vessel (List separately in addition to code for primary procedure)** T 80

AMA: 2003,Feb,1
To report radiological supervision and interpretation, consult CPT code 75960.

To report catheterizations, consult CPT codes 36215-36248.

To report transcatheter placement of intracoronary stent(s), consult CPT codes 92980, 92981.

Note that 37208 is an add-on code and must be used in conjunction with 37207.

37209 **Exchange of a previously placed intravascular catheter during thrombolytic therapy** T

To report radiological supervision and interpretation consult CPT code 75900.

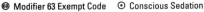 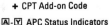 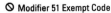

Cardiovascular System

⊙ ● **37210** **Uterine fibroid embolization (UFE, embolization of the uterine arteries to treat uterine fibroids, leiomyomata), percutaneous approach inclusive of vascular access, vessel selection, embolization, and all radiological supervision and interpretation, intraprocedural roadmapping, and imaging guidance necessary to complete the procedure** ⊤

⊙ **37215** **Transcatheter placement of intravascular stent(s), cervical carotid artery, percutaneous; with distal embolic protection** C 80 ⤴

⊙ **37216** **without distal embolic protection** E 80 ⤴

All diagnostic imaging for ipsilateral, cervical and cerebral carotid arteriography, all related radiological supervision and interpretation, and all ipsilateral selective carotid catheterization are included in 37215 and 37216. Codes 37215 and 37216 include stenting when ipsilateral carotid arteriogram verifies the need for the procedure. Report the appropriate code for catheterization and imaging if stenting is not required rather than 37215 and 37216.

Codes 37215 and 37216 cannot be reported with CPT codes 75671 and 75680.

For transcatheter placement of extracranial vertebral or intrathoracic carotid artery stent(s), consult Category III codes 0075T and 0076T.

For percutaneous transcatheter placement of intravascular stents other than coronary, carotid or vertebral, consult CPT codes 37205 and 37206.

INTRAVASCULAR ULTRASOUND SERVICES

Includes all manipulations and repositioning of the transducer with the specific vessel being examined, before and after treatment.

+ **37250** **Intravascular ultrasound (non-coronary vessel) during diagnostic evaluation and/or therapeutic intervention; initial vessel (List separately in addition to code for primary procedure)** S 80 ⤴

MED: 100-3,220.5
AMA: 1999,Nov,20; 1997,Nov,17
If catheterization is performed, consult CPT codes 36215-36248. If transcatheter therapies are performed, consult CPT codes 37200-37208, 61624, and 61626. For radiological supervision and interpretation, consult CPT codes 75945 and 75946.

Note that 37250 is an add-on code and must be used in conjunction with the appropriate CPT code for the diagnostic or therapeutic procedure performed.

+ **37251** **each additional vessel (List separately in addition to code for primary procedure)** S 80

MED: 100-3,220.5
AMA: 1999,Nov,20; 1997,Nov,17
Note that 37251 is an add-on code and must be used in conjunction with 37250.

ENDOSCOPY

Diagnostic endoscopy is always included in surgical endoscopy.

37500 **Vascular endoscopy, surgical, with ligation of perforator veins, subfascial (SEPS)** 3 ⊤ 50 ⤴

To report open procedure, consult CPT code 37760.

37501 **Unlisted vascular endoscopy procedure** ⊤ 50

LIGATION AND OTHER PROCEDURES

37565 **Ligation, internal jugular vein** ⊤ 80 ⤴
MED: 100-3,160.8

External carotid artery is ligated

External carotid artery
Internal carotid artery
Carotid artery
Sternocleidomastoid muscle

37600 **Ligation; external carotid artery** ⊤ 80 ⤴
MED: 100-3,160.8
If ligation is used to treat an intracranial aneurysm, consult CPT code 61703.

37605 **internal or common carotid artery** ⊤ 80 ⤴
MED: 100-3,160.8

37606 **internal or common carotid artery, with gradual occlusion, as with Selverstone or Crutchfield clamp** ⊤ 80 ⤴
MED: 100-3,160.8
To report permanent transcatheter arterial occlusion or embolization, consult CPT codes 31624-31626.

To report temporary endovascular arterial balloon occlusion, consult CPT code 61623.

37607 **Ligation or banding of angioaccess arteriovenous fistula** 3 ⊤ ⤴
MED: 100-2,15,260; 100-4,12,90.3; 100-4,14,10

37609 **Ligation or biopsy, temporal artery** 2 ⊤ 50 ⤴
MED: 100-2,15,260; 100-4,12,90.3; 100-4,14,10

37615 **Ligation, major artery (eg, post-traumatic, rupture); neck** ⊤ 80 ⤴
Touroff ligation

37616 **chest** C 80 ⤴
Bardenheurer operation

37617 **abdomen** C 80 ⤴

37618 **extremity** C 80 ⤴

37620 **Interruption, partial or complete, of inferior vena cava by suture, ligation, plication, clip, extravascular, intravascular (umbrella device)** ⊤ ⤴
AMA: 2001,May,10; 2000,Nov,10
To report radiological supervision and interpretation, consult CPT code 75940.

37650 **Ligation of femoral vein** 2 ⊤ 50 ⤴
MED: 100-2,15,260; 100-4,12,90.3; 100-4,14,10

37660 **Ligation of common iliac vein** C 80 ⤴

37700 **Ligation and division of long saphenous vein at saphenofemoral junction, or distal interruptions** 2 ⊤ 50 ⤴
MED: 100-2,15,260; 100-4,12,90.3; 100-4,14,10
AMA: 1996,Aug,10
Code 37700 should not be reported with 37718, 37722.

37718 **Ligation, division, and stripping, short saphenous vein** 3 ⊤ 50
To report bilateral procedure, use modifier 50.

Code 37718 cannot be reported with 37735, 37780.

37210 — 37718

37722 Ligation, division, and stripping, long (greater) saphenous veins from saphenofemoral junction to knee or below ⑤ T 50

> To report ligation and stripping of the short saphenous vein, consult CPT code 37718.
>
> To report bilateral procedure, use modifier 50.
>
> Code 37722 cannot be reported with 37700, 37735.

37735 Ligation and division and complete stripping of long or short saphenous veins with radical excision of ulcer and skin graft and/or interruption of communicating veins of lower leg, with excision of deep fascia ⑤ T 80 50

> MED: 100-2,15,260; 100-4,12,90.3; 100-4,14,10
>
> Code 37735 cannot be reported with 37700, 37718, 37722, 37780.

37760 Ligation of perforator veins, subfascial, radical (Linton type), with or without skin graft, open ⑤ T 80 🔲

> MED: 100-2,15,260; 100-4,12,90.3; 100-4,14,10
>
> To report endoscopic procedure, consult CPT code 37500.

37765 Stab phlebectomy of varicose veins, one extremity; 10-20 stab incisions T 50 🔲

> To report less than 10 incisions, use CPT code 37799. To report more than 20 incisions, use CPT code 37766.

37766 more than 20 incisions T 50 🔲

37780 Ligation and division of short saphenous vein at saphenopopliteal junction (separate procedure) ⑤ T 50 🔲

> MED: 100-2,15,260; 100-4,12,90.3; 100-4,14,10
>
> AMA: 1996,Aug,10

37785 Ligation, division, and/or excision of varicose vein cluster(s), one leg ⑤ T 50 🔲

> MED: 100-2,15,260; 100-4,12,90.3; 100-4,14,10

37788 Penile revascularization, artery, with or without vein graft ♂ C 80 🔲

37790 Penile venous occlusive procedure ♂ ⑤ T 80 🔲

> MED: 100-2,15,260; 100-4,12,90.3; 100-4,14,10

37799 Unlisted procedure, vascular surgery T 80

> MED: 100-4,4,180.3
>
> AMA: 2001,May,11; 1997,Sep,10; 1997,Feb,10; 1993,Spring,12; 1993,Fall,3

HEMIC AND LYMPHATIC SYSTEMS

SPLEEN

EXCISION

38100 Splenectomy; total (separate procedure) C 80 🔲

38101 partial (separate procedure) C 80 🔲

+ 38102 total, en bloc for extensive disease, in conjunction with other procedure (List in addition to code for primary procedure) C 80 🔲

REPAIR

38115 Repair of ruptured spleen (splenorrhaphy) with or without partial splenectomy C 80 🔲

LAPAROSCOPY

Surgical laparoscopy always includes diagnostic laparoscopy.

To report diagnostic laparoscopy, consult CPT code 49320.

38120 Laparoscopy, surgical, splenectomy T 80 🔲

> AMA: 2000,Mar,5; 1999,Nov,20-21

38129 Unlisted laparoscopy procedure, spleen T 80

> AMA: 2000,Mar,5; 1999,Nov,20-21

INTRODUCTION

38200 Injection procedure for splenoportography N 80 🔲

> To report radiological supervision and interpretation, consult CPT code 75810.

GENERAL

BONE MARROW OR STEM CELL SERVICES/PROCEDURES

CPT codes 38207-38215 should be reported only once per day.

38204 Management of recipient hematopoietic progenitor cell donor search and cell acquisition N

38205 Blood-derived hematopoietic progenitor cell harvesting for transplantation, per collection; allogenic S 80 🔲

38206 autologous S 80 🔲

> MED: 100-3,110.8.1

38207 Transplant preparation of hematopoietic progenitor cells; cryopreservation and storage E

> To report diagnostic cryopreservation and storage, consult CPT code 88240.

38208 thawing of previously frozen harvest, without washing E

> To report diagnostic thawing and expansion of frozen cells, consult CPT code 88241.

38209 thawing of previously frozen harvest, with washing E

38210 specific cell depletion within harvest, T-cell depletion E

38211 tumor cell depletion E

38212 red blood cell removal E

38213 platelet depletion E

38214 plasma (volume) depletion E

38215 cell concentration in plasma, mononuclear, or buffy coat layer E

> Codes 38207-38215 cannot be reported with CPT codes 88182, 88184-88189.

38220 Bone marrow; aspiration only T 80 50 🔲

> MED: 100-1,5,90.2; 100-2,15,80; 100-2,15,80.1; 100-4,16,10; 100-4,16,10.1; 100-4,16,110.4

38221 biopsy, needle or trocar T 80 50 🔲

> MED: 100-1,5,90.2; 100-2,15,80; 100-2,15,80.1; 100-4,16,10; 100-4,16,10.1; 100-4,16,110.4
>
> To report bone marrow biopsy interpretation, consult CPT code 88305.

38230 Bone marrow harvesting for transplantation S 80 🔲

> MED: 100-1,5,90.2; 100-2,15,80; 100-2,15,80.1; 100-3,190.1; 100-4,16,10; 100-4,16,10.1; 100-4,16,110.4

38240 Bone marrow or blood-derived peripheral stem cell transplantation; allogenic S 80 🔲

> MED: 100-2,15,80; 100-2,15,80.1; 100-3,110.8.1; 100-3,190.1; 100-4,3,90.3; 100-4,3,90.3.1; 100-4,3,90.3.3; 100-4,32,90
>
> AMA: 1999,Nov,21; 1998,Nov,15; 1996,Apr,1

Hemic And Lymphatic Systems

38241 — 38570

38241   **autologous**   9 80 ◨

MED: 100-2,15,80; 100-2,15,80.1; 100-3,110.8.1; 100-4,3,90.3; 100-4,3,90.3.2; 100-4,3,90.3.3; 100-4,32,90

AMA: 1999,Nov,21; 1998,Nov,15; 1996,Apr,1

38242   **allogeneic donor lymphocyte infusions**   9 80 ◨

MED: 100-3,190.1

If bone marrow aspiration is performed, consult CPT code 38220.

If modification, treatment, and processing of bone marrow or blood-derived stem cell specimens is performed for transplantation, consult CPT code 38210-38213.

If compatibility studies are performed, consult CPT codes 86812-86822.

If cryopreservation, freezing, and storage of blood-derived stem cells is performed for transplantation, consult CPT code 88240. If thawing and expansion of blood-derived stem cells is performed for transplantation, consult CPT code 88241.

LYMPH NODES AND LYMPHATIC CHANNELS

INCISION

38300   **Drainage of lymph node abscess or lymphadenitis; simple**   1 T ◨

MED: 100-2,15,260; 100-4,12,90.3; 100-4,14,10

38305   **extensive**   2 T ◨

MED: 100-2,15,260; 100-4,12,90.3; 100-4,14,10

Cancers of the lymphatic system are called lymphomas; they are more common after age 50 and occur most frequently in the groin (inguinal), neck (cervical), and armpit (axillary) nodes

About 14 percent of malignant lymphomas are Hodgkin's disease, a form of cancer distinguished by the presence of unique, large, R-S cells; incidence peaks in the late 20s. Because the malignant lymphomas occur early in life, they account for more years of potential life lost than many of the more common cancers

Cervical lymph nodes
Entrance of thoracic duct into subclavian vein
Intercostal lymph nodes
Cisterna chyli
Axillary nodes
Thymus
Spleen
Lumbar nodes
Thoracic duct
Mesenteric nodes
Retosacral nodes
Intestinal nodes
Iliac nodes
Mesocolic nodes
Inguinal nodes

38308   **Lymphangiotomy or other operations on lymphatic channels**   2 T 80 ◨

MED: 100-2,15,260; 100-4,12,90.3; 100-4,14,10

38380   **Suture and/or ligation of thoracic duct; cervical approach**   C 80 ◨

38381   **thoracic approach**   C 80 ◨

38382   **abdominal approach**   C 80 ◨

EXCISION

If injection is performed for sentinel node identification, consult CPT code 38792.

38500   **Biopsy or excision of lymph node(s); open, superficial**   2 T 50 ◨

MED: 100-2,15,260; 100-4,3,20.2.1; 100-4,12,90.3; 100-4,14,10

AMA: 1999,Jul,6; 1997,Jun,5

Do not report code 38500 in conjunction with 38700-38780.

38505   **by needle, superficial (eg, cervical, inguinal, axillary)**   1 T 50 ◨

MED: 100-2,15,260; 100-4,12,90.3; 100-4,14,10

To report imaging guidance, consult CPT codes 76942, 77012, or 77021.

If fine needle aspiration is performed, consult CPT code 10021 or 10022.

To report evaluation of fine needle aspirate, consult CPT codes 88172, 88173.

38510   **open, deep cervical node(s)**   2 T 50 ◨

MED: 100-2,15,260; 100-4,3,20.2.1; 100-4,12,90.3; 100-4,14,10

AMA: 1998,May,10

38520   **open, deep cervical node(s) with excision scalene fat pad**   2 T 50 ◨

MED: 100-2,15,260; 100-4,3,20.2.1; 100-4,12,90.3; 100-4,14,10

AMA: 1998,May,10

38525   **open, deep axillary node(s)**   2 T 50 ◨

MED: 100-2,15,260; 100-4,3,20.2.1; 100-4,12,90.3; 100-4,14,10

AMA: 1999,Jul,6; 1998,May,10

38530   **open, internal mammary node(s)**   2 T 80 50 ◨

MED: 100-2,15,260; 100-4,3,20.2.1; 100-4,12,90.3; 100-4,14,10

AMA: 1998,May,10

If percutaneous needle biopsy is performed on a retroperitoneal lymph node or mass, consult CPT code 49180; if fine needle aspiration is performed, consult CPT code 10022.

Do not report CPT code 38530 in conjuction with 38720-38746.

38542   **Dissection, deep jugular node(s)**   2 T 80 50 ◨

MED: 100-2,15,260; 100-4,12,90.3; 100-4,14,10

AMA: 1999,Jul,6

If radical cervical neck dissection is performed, consult CPT code 38720.

38550   **Excision of cystic hygroma, axillary or cervical; without deep neurovascular dissection**   3 T 80 ◨

MED: 100-2,15,260; 100-4,12,90.3; 100-4,14,10

38555   **with deep neurovascular dissection**   4 T 80 ◨

MED: 100-2,15,260; 100-4,12,90.3; 100-4,14,10

LIMITED LYMPHADENECTOMY FOR STAGING

38562   **Limited lymphadenectomy for staging (separate procedure); pelvic and para-aortic**   C 80 ◨

AMA: 2001,Mar,10

If this procedure is combined with prostatectomy, consult CPT code 55812 or 55842. If this procedure is combined with the insertion of a radioactive substance into the prostate, consult CPT code 55862.

38564   **retroperitoneal (aortic and/or splenic)**   C 80 ◨

LAPAROSCOPY

Diagnostic laparoscopy is always included in surgical laparoscopy. To report diagnostic laparoscopy, consult CPT code 49320.

38570   **Laparoscopy, surgical; with retroperitoneal lymph node sampling (biopsy), single or multiple**   9 T 80 ◨

MED: 100-2,15,260; 100-4,12,90.3; 100-4,14,10

AMA: 2000,Mar,5; 1999,Nov,21

If drainage of a lymphocele to the peritoneal cavity is performed, consult CPT code 49323.

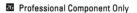

26 Professional Component Only   80/80 Assist-at-Surgery Allowed/With Documentation   Unlisted   Not Covered

TC Technical Component Only   MED: Pub 100/NCD References   AMA: CPT Assistant References   1-9 ASC Group   ♂ Male Only   ♀ Female Only

150 — CPT Expert   CPT only © 2006 American Medical Association. All Rights Reserved. *(Black Ink)*   © 2006 Ingenix *(Blue Ink)*

38571	with bilateral total pelvic lymphadenectomy	9 T 80 🔲

MED: 100-2,15,260; 100-4,12,90.3; 100-4,14,10
AMA: 2000,Mar,5; 1999,Nov,21

38572	with bilateral total pelvic lymphadenectomy and peri-aortic lymph node sampling (biopsy), single or multiple	9 T 80 🔲

MED: 100-2,15,260; 100-4,12,90.3; 100-4,14,10
AMA: 1999,Nov,21

38589	Unlisted laparoscopy procedure, lymphatic system	T 80 50

MED: 100-4,4,180.3
AMA: 2000,Mar,5; 1999,Nov,21

RADICAL LYMPHADENECTOMY (RADICAL RESECTION OF LYMPH NODES)

If limited pelvic and retroperitoneal lymphadenectomies are performed, consult CPT codes 38562 and 38564.

38700	Suprahyoid lymphadenectomy	T 80 50 🔲

AMA: 2002,Aug,8
To report a bilateral procedure, append modifier 50 to code 38700.

38720	Cervical lymphadenectomy (complete)	T 80 50 🔲

AMA: 2002,Aug,8; 2001,Oct,10
To report a bilateral procedure, append modifier 50 to code 38720.

38724	Cervical lymphadenectomy (modified radical neck dissection)	C 80 50 🔲

AMA: 2002,Aug,8; 2001,Jan,13

38740	Axillary lymphadenectomy; superficial	2 T 80 🔲

MED: 100-2,15,260; 100-4,12,90.3; 100-4,14,10

38745	complete	4 T 80 🔲

MED: 100-2,15,260; 100-4,12,90.3; 100-4,14,10

+ **38746**	Thoracic lymphadenectomy, regional, including mediastinal and peritracheal nodes (List separately in addition to code for primary procedure)	C 80 🔲

Note that 38746 is an add-on code that must be used in conjunction with the appropriate code for the primary procedure. This code cannot be reported alone.

+ **38747**	Abdominal lymphadenectomy, regional, including celiac, gastric, portal, peripancreatic, with or without para-aortic and vena caval nodes (List separately in addition to code for primary procedure)	C 80 🔲

AMA: 1998,Nov,15
Note that 38747 is an add-on code that must be used in conjunction with the appropriate code for the primary procedure. This code cannot be reported alone.

38760	Inguinofemoral lymphadenectomy, superficial, including Cloquets node (separate procedure)	2 T 80 50 🔲

MED: 100-2,15,260; 100-4,12,90.3; 100-4,14,10
To report a bilateral procedure, append modifier 50 to code 38760.

38765	Inguinofemoral lymphadenectomy, superficial, in continuity with pelvic lymphadenectomy, including external iliac, hypogastric, and obturator nodes (separate procedure)	C 80 50 🔲

To report a bilateral procedure, append modifier 50 to code 38765.

38770	Pelvic lymphadenectomy, including external iliac, hypogastric, and obturator nodes (separate procedure)	C 80 50 🔲

To report a bilateral procedure, append modifier 50 to code 38770.

38780	Retroperitoneal transabdominal lymphadenectomy, extensive, including pelvic, aortic, and renal nodes (separate procedure)	C 80 🔲

If lymphedematous skin and subcutaneous tissue are excised and repaired, consult CPT codes 15004, 15005, and 15570-15650.

INTRODUCTION

38790	Injection procedure; lymphangiography	N 50 🔲

If radiological supervision and interpretation is performed, consult CPT codes 75801-75807.

⊘	**38792**	for identification of sentinel node	Q 50 🔲

AMA: 1999,Jul,6; 1998,Nov,15
If the sentinel node is excised, consult CPT codes 38500-38542. If nuclear medicine lymphatics and lymph gland imaging is performed, consult CPT code 78195.

38794	Cannulation, thoracic duct	N 80 🔲

OTHER PROCEDURES

38999	Unlisted procedure, hemic or lymphatic system	S 80

AMA: 1998,May,10

MEDIASTINUM AND DIAPHRAGM

MEDIASTINUM

INCISION

39000	Mediastinotomy with exploration, drainage, removal of foreign body, or biopsy; cervical approach	C 80 🔲
39010	transthoracic approach, including either transthoracic or median sternotomy	C 80 🔲

EXCISION

39200	Excision of mediastinal cyst	C 80 🔲
39220	Excision of mediastinal tumor	C 80 🔲

If a substernal thyroidectomy is performed, consult CPT code 60270. If a thymectomy is performed, consult CPT code 60520.

ENDOSCOPY

39400	Mediastinoscopy, with or without biopsy	T 🔲

OTHER PROCEDURES

39499	Unlisted procedure, mediastinum	C 80

MED: 100-4,4,180.3

DIAPHRAGM

REPAIR

To report a transabdominal repair of diaphragmatic (esophageal hiatal) hernia, consult 43324, 43325.

39501	Repair, laceration of diaphragm, any approach	C 80 🔲

AMA: 2000,Nov,3

---

63 Modifier 63 Exempt Code	⊙ Conscious Sedation	+ CPT Add-on Code
M Maternity Edit	A Age Edit	A-Y APC Status Indicators

⊘ Modifier 51 Exempt Code	● New Code
🔲 CCI Comprehensive Code	▲ Revised Code
	50 Bilateral Procedure

39502   Repair, paraesophageal hiatus hernia, transabdominal, with or without fundoplasty, vagotomy, and/or pyloroplasty, except neonatal   C 80 ▣

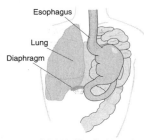

Esophagus

Lung

Diaphragm

A defect of the diaphragm
can allow abdominal contents
to herniate into the thoracic cavity

Code 39503 reports the repair of a diaphragmatic hernia in a neonate. The nature of the repair may necessitate the creation of a ventral hernia (an opening in the anterior abdomen to accommodate the viscera). A chest tube may or may not be required

The code is reserved for procedures on neonates

39503   Repair, neonatal diaphragmatic hernia, with or without chest tube insertion and with or without creation of ventral hernia   C 80 ⊗ ▣

39520   Repair, diaphragmatic hernia (esophageal hiatal); transthoracic   C 80 ▣

39530   combined, thoracoabdominal   C 80 ▣

39531   combined, thoracoabdominal, with dilation of stricture (with or without gastroplasty)   C 80 ▣

39540   Repair, diaphragmatic hernia (other than neonatal), traumatic; acute   C 80 ▣
      AMA: 2000,Nov,3

39541   chronic   C 80 ▣

39545   Imbrication of diaphragm for eventration, transthoracic or transabdominal, paralytic or nonparalytic·   C 80 ▣
      AMA: 2000,Nov,3

39560   Resection, diaphragm; with simple repair (eg, primary suture)   C 80 ▣
      AMA: 2000,Nov,3; 1999,Nov,21

39561   with complex repair (eg, prosthetic material, local muscle flap)   C 80 ▣
      AMA: 2000,Nov,3; 1999,Nov,21

OTHER PROCEDURES

39599   Unlisted procedure, diaphragm   C 80
      MED: 100-4,4,180.3

(side tab) Mediastinum and Diaphragm

(side tab) 39502 — 39599

---

26 Professional Component Only   80/80 Assist-at-Surgery Allowed/With Documentation   Unlisted   Not Covered

TC Technical Component Only   MED: Pub 100/NCD References   AMA: CPT Assistant References   1-9 ASC Group   ♂ Male Only   ♀ Female Only

DIGESTIVE SYSTEM

LIPS

To report procedures performed on the skin of the lips, consult CPT code 10040 and subsequent codes.

EXCISION

40490   **Biopsy of lip**   T ◨

40500   **Vermilionectomy (lip shave), with mucosal advancement**   2 T ◨

     MED: 100-2,15,260; 100-4,12,90.3; 100-4,14,10

40510   **Excision of lip; transverse wedge excision with primary closure**   2 T ◨

     MED: 100-2,15,260; 100-4,12,90.3; 100-4,14,10

     If mucous lesions are excised, consult CPT codes 40810-40816.

40520   **V-excision with primary direct linear closure**   2 T ◨

     MED: 100-2,15,260; 100-4,12,90.3; 100-4,14,10

     If mucous lesions are excised, consult CPT codes 40810-40816.

40525   **full thickness, reconstruction with local flap (eg, Estlander or fan)**   2 T ◨

     MED: 100-2,15,260; 100-4,12,90.3; 100-4,14,10

40527   **full thickness, reconstruction with cross lip flap (Abbe-Estlander)**   2 T 80 ◨

     MED: 100-2,15,260; 100-4,12,90.3; 100-4,14,10

40530   **Resection of lip, more than one-fourth, without reconstruction**   2 T ◨

     MED: 100-2,15,260; 100-4,12,90.3; 100-4,14,10

     If reconstruction is performed, consult CPT codes 13131 and subsequent codes.

REPAIR (CHEILOPLASTY)

If the cleft palate is repaired, consult CPT codes 42200 and subsequent codes. If other reconstructive procedures are performed, consult CPT codes 14060, 14061, 15120-15261, 15574, 15576, and 15630.

40650   **Repair lip, full thickness; vermilion only**   3 T 80 ◨

     MED: 100-2,15,260; 100-4,12,90.3; 100-4,14,10

     AMA: 2000,Jul,10

40652   **up to half vertical height**   3 T 80 ◨

     MED: 100-2,15,260; 100-4,12,90.3; 100-4,14,10

     AMA: 2000,Jul,10

40654   **over one-half vertical height, or complex**   3 T ◨

     MED: 100-2,15,260; 100-4,12,90.3; 100-4,14,10

40700   **Plastic repair of cleft lip/nasal deformity; primary, partial or complete, unilateral**   7 T 80 ◨

     MED: 100-2,15,260; 100-4,12,90.3; 100-4,14,10

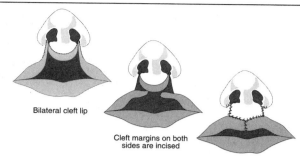

Bilateral cleft lip

Cleft margins on both sides are incised

Margins are closed, correcting cleft

40701   **primary bilateral, one stage procedure**   7 T 80 ◨

     MED: 100-2,15,260; 100-4,12,90.3; 100-4,14,10

40702   **primary bilateral, one of two stages**   T 80 ◨

40720   **secondary, by recreation of defect and reclosure**   7 T 80 50 ◨

     MED: 100-2,15,260; 100-4,12,90.3; 100-4,14,10

     If rhinoplasty only is performed for nasal deformity secondary to a congenital cleft lip, consult CPT codes 30460 and 30462.

     To report a bilateral procedure, append modifier 50 to code 40720. To report repair of a cleft lip, with cross pedicle flap (Abbe-Estlander types), consult 40527.

40761   **with cross lip pedicle flap (Abbe-Estlander type), including sectioning and inserting of pedicle**   3 T ◨

     MED: 100-2,15,260; 100-4,12,90.3; 100-4,14,10

OTHER PROCEDURES

40799   **Unlisted procedure, lips**   T 80

     MED: 100-4,4,180.3

VESTIBULE OF MOUTH

INCISION

Part of the oral cavity outside the dentoalveolar structures includes the mucosal and submucosal tissue of lips and cheeks.

40800   **Drainage of abscess, cyst, hematoma, vestibule of mouth; simple**   T ◨

40801   **complicated**   2 T ◨

     MED: 100-2,15,260; 100-4,12,90.3; 100-4,14,10

40804   **Removal of embedded foreign body, vestibule of mouth; simple**   X 80 ◨

40805   **complicated**   T 80 ◨

40806   **Incision of labial frenum (frenotomy)**   T 80 ◨

EXCISION, DESTRUCTION

40808   **Biopsy, vestibule of mouth**   T ◨

40810   **Excision of lesion of mucosa and submucosa, vestibule of mouth; without repair**   T ◨

40812   **with simple repair**   T ◨

40814   **with complex repair**   2 T ◨

     MED: 100-2,15,260; 100-4,12,90.3; 100-4,14,10

40816   **complex, with excision of underlying muscle**   2 T ◨

     MED: 100-2,15,260; 100-4,12,90.3; 100-4,14,10

40818   **Excision of mucosa of vestibule of mouth as donor graft**   1 T 80 ◨

     MED: 100-2,15,260; 100-4,12,90.3; 100-4,14,10

   CPT only © 2006 American Medical Association. All Rights Reserved. (Black Ink)

40819	Excision of frenum, labial or buccal (frenumectomy, frenulectomy, frenectomy)	**1** T 80 ◨
	MED: 100-2,15,150; 100-2,15,260; 100-4,12,90.3; 100-4,14,10	
40820	Destruction of lesion or scar of vestibule of mouth by physical methods (eg, laser, thermal, cryo, chemical)	T ◨
	MED: 100-3,140.5	

REPAIR

40830	Closure of laceration, vestibule of mouth; 2.5 cm or less	T 80 ◨
40831	over 2.5 cm or complex	**1** T 80 ◨
	MED: 100-2,15,260; 100-4,12,90.3; 100-4,14,10	
40840	Vestibuloplasty; anterior	**2** T 80 ◨
	MED: 100-2,15,260; 100-4,12,90.3; 100-4,14,10	
40842	posterior, unilateral	**3** T 80 ◨
	MED: 100-2,15,260; 100-4,12,90.3; 100-4,14,10	
40843	posterior, bilateral	**3** T 80 ◨
	MED: 100-2,15,260; 100-4,12,90.3; 100-4,14,10	
40844	entire arch	**5** T 80 ◨
	MED: 100-2,15,260; 100-4,12,90.3; 100-4,14,10	
40845	complex (including ridge extension, muscle repositioning)	**5** T 80 ◨
	MED: 100-2,15,260; 100-4,12,90.3; 100-4,14,10	

If skin grafts are performed, consult CPT codes 15002 and subsequent codes.

OTHER PROCEDURES

40899	Unlisted procedure, vestibule of mouth	T 80
	MED: 100-4,4,180.3	

TONGUE AND FLOOR OF MOUTH

INCISION

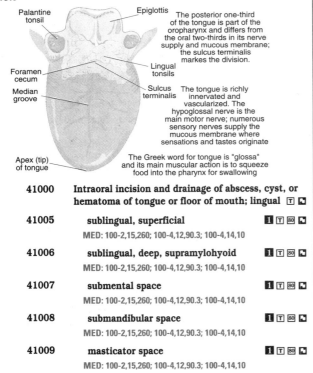

Palatine tonsil
Epiglottis
The posterior one-third of the tongue is part of the oropharynx and differs from the oral two-thirds in its nerve supply and mucous membrane; the sulcus terminalis markes the division.
Foramen cecum
Lingual tonsils
Median groove
Sulcus terminalis
The tongue is richly innervated and vascularized. The hypoglossal nerve is the main motor nerve; numerous sensory nerves supply the mucous membrane where sensations and tastes originate
Apex (tip) of tongue
The Greek word for tongue is "glossa" and its main muscular action is to squeeze food into the pharynx for swallowing

41000	Intraoral incision and drainage of abscess, cyst, or hematoma of tongue or floor of mouth; lingual	T ◨
41005	sublingual, superficial	**1** T 80 ◨
	MED: 100-2,15,260; 100-4,12,90.3; 100-4,14,10	
41006	sublingual, deep, supramylohyoid	**1** T 80 ◨
	MED: 100-2,15,260; 100-4,12,90.3; 100-4,14,10	
41007	submental space	**1** T 80 ◨
	MED: 100-2,15,260; 100-4,12,90.3; 100-4,14,10	
41008	submandibular space	**1** T 80 ◨
	MED: 100-2,15,260; 100-4,12,90.3; 100-4,14,10	
41009	masticator space	**1** T 80 ◨
	MED: 100-2,15,260; 100-4,12,90.3; 100-4,14,10	

41010	Incision of lingual frenum (frenotomy)	**1** T 80 ◨
	MED: 100-2,15,260; 100-4,12,90.3; 100-4,14,10	
41015	Extraoral incision and drainage of abscess, cyst, or hematoma of floor of mouth; sublingual	**1** T 80 ◨
	MED: 100-2,15,260; 100-4,12,90.3; 100-4,14,10	
41016	submental	**1** T 80 ◨
	MED: 100-2,15,260; 100-4,12,90.3; 100-4,14,10	
41017	submandibular	**1** T 80 ◨
	MED: 100-2,15,260; 100-4,12,90.3; 100-4,14,10	
41018	masticator space	**1** T 80 ◨
	MED: 100-2,15,260; 100-4,12,90.3; 100-4,14,10	

If a frenoplasty is performed, consult CPT code 41520.

EXCISION

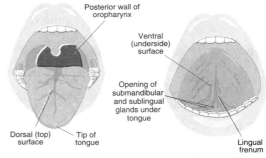

Posterior wall of oropharynx
Ventral (underside) surface
Opening of submandibular and sublingual glands under tongue
Dorsal (top) surface
Tip of tongue
Lingual frenum

Anterior (front) two-thirds of tongue comprises most of easily visible portions; the base, or root, comprises the remainder of tongue

41100	Biopsy of tongue; anterior two-thirds	T ◨
41105	posterior one-third	T ◨
41108	Biopsy of floor of mouth	T ◨
41110	Excision of lesion of tongue without closure	T ◨
41112	Excision of lesion of tongue with closure; anterior two-thirds	**2** T ◨
	MED: 100-2,15,260; 100-4,12,90.3; 100-4,14,10	
41113	posterior one-third	**2** T ◨
	MED: 100-2,15,260; 100-4,12,90.3; 100-4,14,10	
41114	with local tongue flap	**2** T 80 ◨
	MED: 100-2,15,260; 100-4,12,90.3; 100-4,14,10	

Note that 41114 must be listed in addition to 41112 or 41113.

41115	Excision of lingual frenum (frenectomy)	T 80 ◨
	MED: 100-2,15,150	
41116	Excision, lesion of floor of mouth	**1** T ◨
	MED: 100-2,15,260; 100-4,12,90.3; 100-4,14,10	
41120	Glossectomy; less than one-half tongue	**5** T 80 ◨
	MED: 100-2,15,260; 100-4,12,90.3; 100-4,14,10	
41130	hemiglossectomy	C 80 ◨
41135	partial, with unilateral radical neck dissection	C 80 ◨
41140	complete or total, with or without tracheostomy, without radical neck dissection	C 80 ◨

Regnolli's excision

41145	complete or total, with or without tracheostomy, with unilateral radical neck dissection	C 80 ◨
41150	composite procedure with resection floor of mouth and mandibular resection, without radical neck dissection	C 80 ◨

26 Professional Component Only   **80/80** Assist-at-Surgery Allowed/With Documentation   Unlisted   Not Covered

TC Technical Component Only   **MED:** Pub 100/NCD References   **AMA:** CPT Assistant References   **1-9** ASC Group   ♂ Male Only   ♀ Female Only

154 — CPT Expert   CPT only © 2006 American Medical Association. All Rights Reserved. (Black Ink)   © 2006 Ingenix (Blue Ink)

41153	composite procedure with resection floor of mouth, with suprahyoid neck dissection	C 80 ☑
41155	composite procedure with resection floor of mouth, mandibular resection, and radical neck dissection (Commando type)	C 80 ☑
	AMA: 2001,Jan,13	

REPAIR

41250	Repair of laceration 2.5 cm or less; floor of mouth and/or anterior two-thirds of tongue	2 T 80 ☑
	MED: 100-2,15,260; 100-4,12,90.3; 100-4,14,10	
41251	posterior one-third of tongue	2 T 80 ☑
	MED: 100-2,15,260; 100-4,12,90.3; 100-4,14,10	
41252	Repair of laceration of tongue, floor of mouth, over 2.6 cm or complex	2 T 80 ☑
	MED: 100-2,15,260; 100-4,12,90.3; 100-4,14,10	

OTHER PROCEDURES

41500	Fixation of tongue, mechanical, other than suture (eg, K-wire)	1 T 80 ☑
	MED: 100-2,15,260; 100-4,12,90.3; 100-4,14,10	
41510	Suture of tongue to lip for micrognathia (Douglas type procedure)	1 T 80 ☑
	MED: 100-2,15,260; 100-4,12,90.3; 100-4,14,10	
41520	Frenoplasty (surgical revision of frenum, eg, with Z-plasty)	2 T 80 ☑
	MED: 100-2,15,260; 100-4,12,90.3; 100-4,14,10	
	If a frenotomy is performed, consult CPT codes 40806 and 41010.	
41599	Unlisted procedure, tongue, floor of mouth	T 80
	MED: 100-4,4,180.3	
	AMA: 2000,Dec,14	

DENTOALVEOLAR STRUCTURES

INCISION

41800	Drainage of abscess, cyst, hematoma from dentoalveolar structures	1 T ☑
	MED: 100-2,15,260; 100-4,12,90.3; 100-4,14,10	
41805	Removal of embedded foreign body from dentoalveolar structures; soft tissues	T 80 ☑
41806	bone	T 80 ☑

EXCISION, DESTRUCTION

Gingival recession

Excessive mucosal growth

Gingivitis is an inflammatory response to bacteria on the teeth; it is characterized by tender, red, swollen gums and can lead to gingival recession

41820	Gingivectomy, excision gingiva, each quadrant	T 80 ☑
41821	Operculectomy, excision pericoronal tissues	T 80 ☑

41822	Excision of fibrous tuberosities, dentoalveolar structures	T 80 ☑
41823	Excision of osseous tuberosities, dentoalveolar structures	T 80 ☑
41825	Excision of lesion or tumor (except listed above), dentoalveolar structures; without repair	T ☑
41826	with simple repair	T ☑
41827	with complex repair	2 T ☑
	MED: 100-2,15,260; 100-4,12,90.3; 100-4,14,10	
	If the destruction of lesion is nonexcisional, consult CPT code 41850.	
41828	Excision of hyperplastic alveolar mucosa, each quadrant (specify)	T 80 ☑
41830	Alveolectomy, including curettage of osteitis or sequestrectomy	T 80 ☑
41850	Destruction of lesion (except excision), dentoalveolar structures	T 80 ☑

OTHER PROCEDURES

41870	Periodontal mucosal grafting	T 80 ☑
41872	Gingivoplasty, each quadrant (specify)	T 80 ☑
41874	Alveoloplasty, each quadrant (specify)	T 80 ☑
	MED: 100-2,15,150	
	If laceration closure is performed, consult CPT codes 40830 and 40831. If a segmental osteotomy is performed, consult CPT code 21206. If fractures are reduced, consult CPT codes 21421-21490.	
41899	Unlisted procedure, dentoalveolar structures	T 80
	MED: 100-4,4,180.3	

PALATE AND UVULA

INCISION

42000	Drainage of abscess of palate, uvula	2 T 80 ☑
	MED: 100-2,15,260; 100-4,12,90.3; 100-4,14,10	

EXCISION, DESTRUCTION

42100	Biopsy of palate, uvula	T ☑
42104	Excision, lesion of palate, uvula; without closure	T ☑
42106	with simple primary closure	T ☑
42107	with local flap closure	2 T ☑
	MED: 100-2,15,260; 100-4,12,90.3; 100-4,14,10	
	If a skin graft is performed, consult CPT codes 14040-14300. If a mucosal graft is performed, consult CPT code 40818.	
42120	Resection of palate or extensive resection of lesion	4 T 80 ☑
	MED: 100-2,15,260; 100-4,12,90.3; 100-4,14,10	
	If reconstruction of palate with extraoral tissue is performed, consult CPT codes 14040-14300, 15050, 15120, 15240, and 15576.	
42140	Uvulectomy, excision of uvula	2 T ☑
	MED: 100-2,15,260; 100-4,12,90.3; 100-4,14,10	
42145	Palatopharyngoplasty (eg, uvulopalatopharyngoplasty, uvulopharyngoplasty)	5 T ☑
	MED: 100-2,15,260; 100-4,12,90.3; 100-4,14,10	
42160	Destruction of lesion, palate or uvula (thermal, cryo or chemical)	T 80 ☑

---

⑥³ Modifier 63 Exempt Code   ⊙ Conscious Sedation   + CPT Add-on Code   ⊘ Modifier 51 Exempt Code   ● New Code   ▲ Revised Code

M Maternity Edit   A Age Edit   A-Y APC Status Indicators   ☑ CCI Comprehensive Code   50 Bilateral Procedure

REPAIR

42180	Repair, laceration of palate; up to 2 cm	**1** T 80 ◩
	MED: 100-2,15,260; 100-4,12,90.3; 100-4,14,10	
42182	over 2 cm or complex	**2** T 80 ◩
	MED: 100-2,15,260; 100-4,12,90.3; 100-4,14,10	
42200	Palatoplasty for cleft palate, soft and/or hard palate only	**5** T 80 ◩
	MED: 100-2,15,260; 100-4,12,90.3; 100-4,14,10	
42205	Palatoplasty for cleft palate, with closure of alveolar ridge; soft tissue only	**5** T 80 ◩
	MED: 100-2,15,260; 100-4,12,90.3; 100-4,14,10	
42210	with bone graft to alveolar ridge (includes obtaining graft)	**5** T 80 ◩
	MED: 100-2,15,260; 100-4,12,90.3; 100-4,14,10	
42215	Palatoplasty for cleft palate; major revision	**7** T 80 ◩
	MED: 100-2,15,260; 100-4,12,90.3; 100-4,14,10	
42220	secondary lengthening procedure	**5** T 80 ◩
	MED: 100-2,15,260; 100-4,12,90.3; 100-4,14,10	
42225	attachment pharyngeal flap	T 80 ◩
	AMA: 1997,Aug,18	
42226	Lengthening of palate, and pharyngeal flap	**5** T 80 ◩
	MED: 100-2,15,260; 100-4,12,90.3; 100-4,14,10	
42227	Lengthening of palate, with island flap	T 80 ◩
42235	Repair of anterior palate, including vomer flap	**5** T 80 ◩
	MED: 100-2,15,260; 100-4,12,90.3; 100-4,14,10	
42260	Repair of nasolabial fistula	**4** T 80 ◩
	MED: 100-2,15,260; 100-4,12,90.3; 100-4,14,10	

If a cleft lip is repaired, consult CPT codes 40700 and subsequent codes.

42280	Maxillary impression for palatal prosthesis	T 80 ◩
42281	Insertion of pin-retained palatal prosthesis	T 80 ◩

OTHER PROCEDURES

42299	Unlisted procedure, palate, uvula	T 80
	MED: 100-4,4,180.3	

SALIVARY GLAND AND DUCTS

INCISION

42300	Drainage of abscess; parotid, simple	**1** T ◩
	MED: 100-2,15,260; 100-4,12,90.3; 100-4,14,10	
42305	parotid, complicated	**2** T 80 ◩
	MED: 100-2,15,260; 100-4,12,90.3; 100-4,14,10	
42310	Drainage of abscess; submaxillary or sublingual, intraoral	**1** T 80 ◩
	MED: 100-2,15,260; 100-4,12,90.3; 100-4,14,10	
42320	submaxillary, external	**1** T 80 ◩
	MED: 100-2,15,260; 100-4,12,90.3; 100-4,14,10	
42330	Sialolithotomy; submandibular (submaxillary), sublingual or parotid, uncomplicated, intraoral	T ◩
42335	submandibular (submaxillary), complicated, intraoral	T ◩

42340	parotid, extraoral or complicated intraoral	**2** T 80 ◩
	MED: 100-2,15,260; 100-4,12,90.3; 100-4,14,10	

EXCISION

42400	Biopsy of salivary gland; needle	T ◩

To report fine needle aspiration, consult CPT codes 10021, 10022.

To report evaluation of fine needle aspirate, consult CPT codes 88172, 88173.

If imaging guidance is performed, see 76942, 77002, 77012, or 77021.

42405	incisional	**2** T ◩
	MED: 100-2,15,260; 100-4,12,90.3; 100-4,14,10	

If imaging guidance is performed, see 76942, 77002, 77012, or 77021.

42408	Excision of sublingual salivary cyst (ranula)	**3** T 80 ◩
	MED: 100-2,15,260; 100-4,12,90.3; 100-4,14,10	
42409	Marsupialization of sublingual salivary cyst (ranula)	**3** T 80 ◩
	MED: 100-2,15,260; 100-4,12,90.3; 100-4,14,10	

If fistulization of a sublingual salivary cyst is performed, consult CPT code 42325.

After the larynx, the oral cavity and oropharynx are the most common sites for squamous cell carcinoma of the head and neck

Hard palate
Soft palate
Sublingual gland and ducts
Wharton duct
Vestibule
Parotid gland and duct
Submandibular gland
Tonsils

The parotid gland is a common site for malignant lesions, occurring there several times more frequently than cancers of the other major salivary glands

42410	Excision of parotid tumor or parotid gland; lateral lobe, without nerve dissection	**3** T 80 ◩
	MED: 100-2,15,260; 100-4,12,90.3; 100-4,14,10	
42415	lateral lobe, with dissection and preservation of facial nerve	**7** T 80 ◩
	MED: 100-2,15,260; 100-4,12,90.3; 100-4,14,10	
42420	total, with dissection and preservation of facial nerve	**7** T 80 ◩
	MED: 100-2,15,260; 100-4,12,90.3; 100-4,14,10	
42425	total, en bloc removal with sacrifice of facial nerve	**7** T 80 ◩
	MED: 100-2,15,260; 100-4,12,90.3; 100-4,14,10	
42426	total, with unilateral radical neck dissection	C 80 ◩

If suture or grafting of a facial nerve is performed, consult CPT codes 64864, 64865, 69740, and 69745.

42440	Excision of submandibular (submaxillary) gland	**3** T 80 ◩
	MED: 100-2,15,260; 100-4,12,90.3; 100-4,14,10	
42450	Excision of sublingual gland	**2** T 80 ◩
	MED: 100-2,15,260; 100-4,12,90.3; 100-4,14,10	

26 Professional Component Only   **80**/**80** Assist-at-Surgery Allowed/With Documentation   Unlisted   Not Covered

TC Technical Component Only   **MED:** Pub 100/NCD References   **AMA:** CPT Assistant References   **1**-**9** ASC Group   ♂ Male Only   ♀ Female Only

156 — CPT Expert

REPAIR

42500	Plastic repair of salivary duct, sialodochoplasty; primary or simple	3 T 80 ⬙
	MED: 100-2,15,260; 100-4,12,90.3; 100-4,14,10	
42505	secondary or complicated	4 T ⬙
	MED: 100-2,15,260; 100-4,12,90.3; 100-4,14,10	
42507	Parotid duct diversion, bilateral (Wilke type procedure);	3 T 80 ⬙
	MED: 100-2,15,260; 100-4,12,90.3; 100-4,14,10	
42508	with excision of one submandibular gland	4 T 80 ⬙
	MED: 100-2,15,260; 100-4,12,90.3; 100-4,14,10	
42509	with excision of both submandibular glands	4 T 80 ⬙
	MED: 100-2,15,260; 100-4,12,90.3; 100-4,14,10	
42510	with ligation of both submandibular (Wharton's) ducts	4 T 80 ⬙
	MED: 100-2,15,260; 100-4,12,90.3; 100-4,14,10	

OTHER PROCEDURES

42550	Injection procedure for sialography	N ⬙
	If radiological supervision and interpretation is performed, consult CPT code 70390.	
42600	Closure salivary fistula	1 T 80 ⬙
	MED: 100-2,15,260; 100-4,12,90.3; 100-4,14,10	
42650	Dilation salivary duct	T ⬙
42660	Dilation and catheterization of salivary duct, with or without injection	T 80 ⬙
42665	Ligation salivary duct, intraoral	7 T 80 ⬙
42699	Unlisted procedure, salivary glands or ducts	T 80
	MED: 100-4,4,180.3	

PHARYNX, ADENOIDS, AND TONSILS

INCISION

42700	Incision and drainage abscess; peritonsillar	1 T ⬙
	MED: 100-2,15,260; 100-4,12,90.3; 100-4,14,10	
42720	retropharyngeal or parapharyngeal, intraoral approach	1 T 80 ⬙
	MED: 100-2,15,260; 100-4,12,90.3; 100-4,14,10	
42725	retropharyngeal or parapharyngeal, external approach	2 T 80 ⬙
	MED: 100-2,15,260; 100-4,12,90.3; 100-4,14,10	

EXCISION, DESTRUCTION

The nasal cavities and paranasal sinuses are lined with a continuous mucous membrane

Frontal coronal section of left side of skull showing sinuses

Orbit, Ethmoidal cells, Maxillary sinus, Middle and inferior meatus, Nasal cavity, Nasopharynx region, Oropharynx region, Hypopharynx region, Vocal cord and larynx, Auditory tube, Epiglottis, Trachea

The pharynx is a transitional zone between the oral cavity and the rest of the digestive canal. It is the common route for both air and food.

42800	Biopsy; oropharynx	T ⬙

42802	hypopharynx	1 T ⬙
	MED: 100-2,15,260; 100-4,12,90.3; 100-4,14,10	
42804	nasopharynx, visible lesion, simple	1 T ⬙
	MED: 100-2,15,260; 100-4,12,90.3; 100-4,14,10	
42806	nasopharynx, survey for unknown primary lesion	2 T ⬙
	MED: 100-2,15,260; 100-4,12,90.3; 100-4,14,10	
	If a laryngoscopic biopsy is performed, consult CPT codes 31510, 31535, and 31536.	
42808	Excision or destruction of lesion of pharynx, any method	2 T ⬙
	MED: 100-2,15,260; 100-4,12,90.3; 100-4,14,10	
42809	Removal of foreign body from pharynx	X ⬙
42810	Excision branchial cleft cyst or vestige, confined to skin and subcutaneous tissues	3 T 80 ⬙
	MED: 100-2,15,260; 100-4,12,90.3; 100-4,14,10	
42815	Excision branchial cleft cyst, vestige, or fistula, extending beneath subcutaneous tissues and/or into pharynx	5 T 80 ⬙
	MED: 100-2,15,260; 100-4,12,90.3; 100-4,14,10	
▲ 42820	Tonsillectomy and adenoidectomy; younger than age 12	A 3 T 80 ⬙
	MED: 100-2,15,260; 100-4,12,90.3; 100-4,14,10	
	AMA: 1998,Feb,11; 1997,Aug,18	
42821	age 12 or over	5 T 80 ⬙
	MED: 100-2,15,260; 100-4,12,90.3; 100-4,14,10	
	AMA: 1997,Aug,18	
▲ 42825	Tonsillectomy, primary or secondary; younger than age 12	A 4 T 80 ⬙
	MED: 100-2,15,260; 100-4,12,90.3; 100-4,14,10	
	AMA: 1997,Aug,18	
42826	age 12 or over	4 T ⬙
	MED: 100-2,15,260; 100-4,12,90.3; 100-4,14,10	
	AMA: 1997,Aug,18	
▲ 42830	Adenoidectomy, primary; younger than age 12	A 4 T 80 ⬙
	MED: 100-2,15,260; 100-4,12,90.3; 100-4,14,10	
42831	age 12 or over	4 T 80 ⬙
	MED: 100-2,15,260; 100-4,12,90.3; 100-4,14,10	
▲ 42835	Adenoidectomy, secondary; younger than age 12	A 4 T 80 ⬙
	MED: 100-2,15,260; 100-4,12,90.3; 100-4,14,10	
42836	age 12 or over	4 T 80 ⬙
	MED: 100-2,15,260; 100-4,12,90.3; 100-4,14,10	
	AMA: 1998,Feb,11	
42842	Radical resection of tonsil, tonsillar pillars, and/or retromolar trigone; without closure	T 80 ⬙
42844	closure with local flap (eg, tongue, buccal)	T 80 ⬙
42845	closure with other flap	C 80 ⬙
	If closure is performed with another flap(s), consult the appropriate CPT code for the flap(s). If this procedure is combined with a radical neck dissection, consult also CPT code 38720.	

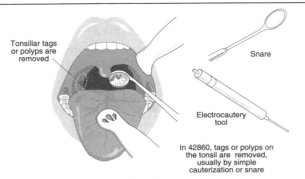

Tonsillar tags or polyps are removed

Snare

Electrocautery tool

In 42860, tags or polyps on the tonsil are removed, usually by simple cauterization or snare

42860	Excision of tonsil tags	3 T 80 ⬚

MED: 100-2,15,260; 100-4,12,90.3; 100-4,14,10

42870	Excision or destruction lingual tonsil, any method (separate procedure)	3 T 80 ⬚

MED: 100-2,15,260; 100-4,12,90.3; 100-4,14,10

If the nasopharynx is resected by bicoronal and/or transzygomatic approach, consult CPT codes 61586 and 61600.

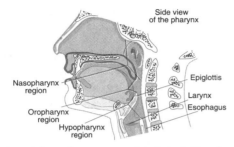

Side view of the pharynx

Nasopharynx region

Oropharynx region

Hypopharynx region

Epiglottis

Larynx

Esophagus

The nasopharynx is the membranous passage above the level of the soft palate; the oropharynx is the region between the soft palate and the upper edge of the epiglottis; the hypopharynx is the region of the epiglottis to the juncture of the larynx and esophagus; the three regions are collectively known as the pharynx

42890	Limited pharyngectomy	7 T 80 ⬚

MED: 100-2,15,260; 100-4,12,90.3; 100-4,14,10

42892	Resection of lateral pharyngeal wall or pyriform sinus, direct closure by advancement of lateral and posterior pharyngeal walls	7 T 80 ⬚

MED: 100-2,15,260; 100-4,12,90.3; 100-4,14,10

If this procedure is combined with a radical neck dissection, consult CPT code 38720.

42894	Resection of pharyngeal wall requiring closure with myocutaneous flap	C 80 ⬚

If this procedure is combined with a radical neck dissection, consult CPT code 38720.

REPAIR

42900	Suture pharynx for wound or injury	1 T 80 ⬚

MED: 100-2,15,260; 100-4,12,90.3; 100-4,14,10

42950	Pharyngoplasty (plastic or reconstructive operation on pharynx)	2 T 80 ⬚

MED: 100-2,15,260; 100-4,12,90.3; 100-4,14,10
If this procedure involves the pharyngeal flap, consult CPT code 42225.

42953	Pharyngoesophageal repair	C 80 ⬚

If closure with myocutaneous or other flap is performed, use the appropriate CPT code in addition to 42953.

OTHER PROCEDURES

42955	Pharyngostomy (fistulization of pharynx, external for feeding)	2 T 80 ⬚

MED: 100-2,15,260; 100-4,12,90.3; 100-4,14,10

42960	Control oropharyngeal hemorrhage, primary or secondary (eg, post-tonsillectomy); simple	1 T 80 ⬚

MED: 100-2,15,260; 100-4,12,90.3; 100-4,14,10

42961	complicated, requiring hospitalization	C 80 ⬚
42962	with secondary surgical intervention	2 T 80 ⬚

MED: 100-2,15,260; 100-4,12,90.3; 100-4,14,10

42970	Control of nasopharyngeal hemorrhage, primary or secondary (eg, postadenoidectomy); simple, with posterior nasal packs, with or without anterior packs and/or cautery	T ⬚
42971	complicated, requiring hospitalization	C 80 ⬚
42972	with secondary surgical intervention	3 T 80 ⬚

MED: 100-2,15,260; 100-4,12,90.3; 100-4,14,10

42999	Unlisted procedure, pharynx, adenoids, or tonsils	T 80

MED: 100-4,4,180.3

ESOPHAGUS

INCISION

If esophageal intubation is performed with a laparotomy, consult CPT code 43510.

43020	Esophagotomy, cervical approach, with removal of foreign body	T 80 ⬚
43030	Cricopharyngeal myotomy	T 80 ⬚
43045	Esophagotomy, thoracic approach, with removal of foreign body	C 80 ⬚

EXCISION

To report gastrointestinal reconstruction for previous esophagectomy, consult CPT codes 43360, 43361.

43100	Excision of lesion, esophagus, with primary repair; cervical approach	C 80 ⬚
43101	thoracic or abdominal approach	C 80 ⬚
43107	Total or near total esophagectomy, without thoracotomy; with pharyngogastrostomy or cervical esophagogastrostomy, with or without pyloroplasty (transhiatal)	C 80 ⬚
43108	with colon interposition or small intestine reconstruction, including intestine mobilization, preparation and anastomosis(es)	C 80 ⬚
43112	Total or near total esophagectomy, with thoracotomy; with pharyngogastrostomy or cervical esophagogastrostomy, with or without pyloroplasty	C 80 ⬚
43113	with colon interposition or small intestine reconstruction, including intestine mobilization, preparation, and anastomosis(es)	C 80 ⬚

26 Professional Component Only

TC Technical Component Only

80/**80** Assist-at-Surgery Allowed/With Documentation

MED: Pub 100/NCD References   **AMA:** CPT Assistant References

Unlisted   Not Covered

1-**9** ASC Group   ♂ Male Only   ♀ Female Only

158 — CPT Expert

43116 Partial esophagectomy, cervical, with free intestinal graft, including microvascular anastomosis, obtaining the graft and intestinal reconstruction ⓒ 80 ⌧

AMA: 1998,Nov,16; 1997,Nov,17
Do not report 69990 in addition to 43116 as the operating microscope is considered an inclusive component of the surgery. If another physician performs an intestinal or a free jejunal graft with microvascular anastomosis, append modifier 52 to this code. If a free jejunal graft with microvascular anastomosis is performed alone, consult CPT code 43496.

43117 Partial esophagectomy, distal two-thirds, with thoracotomy and separate abdominal incision, with or without proximal gastrectomy; with thoracic esophagogastrostomy, with or without pyloroplasty (Ivor Lewis) ⓒ 80 ⌧

43118 with colon interposition or small intestine reconstruction, including intestine mobilization, preparation, and anastomosis(es) ⓒ 80 ⌧

43121 Partial esophagectomy, distal two-thirds, with thoracotomy only, with or without proximal gastrectomy, with thoracic esophagogastrostomy, with or without pyloroplasty ⓒ 80 ⌧

43122 Partial esophagectomy, thoracoabdominal or abdominal approach, with or without proximal gastrectomy; with esophagogastrostomy, with or without pyloroplasty ⓒ 80 ⌧

43123 with colon interposition or small intestine reconstruction, including intestine mobilization, preparation, and anastomosis(es) ⓒ 80 ⌧

43124 Total or partial esophagectomy, without reconstruction (any approach), with cervical esophagostomy ⓒ 80 ⌧

43130 Diverticulectomy of hypopharynx or esophagus, with or without myotomy; cervical approach ⊤ 80 ⌧

43135 thoracic approach ⓒ 80 ⌧

ENDOSCOPY

Gastrointestinal endoscopy codes are reported by site and are listed as follows: esophagus (43200-43232), upper gastrointestinal (43234-43259), endoscopic retrograde cholangiopancreatography (ERCP) (43260-43272), other small intestine or stomal (44360-44397), and large intestine (45300-45392).

Endoscopic procedures may be diagnostic or surgical. The procedure is considered diagnostic when performed to visualize an abnormality or determine the extent of disease. When anything more than visualization is performed, the procedure is considered to be a surgical procedure. A surgical endoscopy always includes a diagnostic endoscopy.

For example, if the patient is to have a diagnostic flexible sigmoidoscopy with biopsy of a lesion during the same surgical session, the diagnostic portion of the procedure (45330) would not be reported separately. Only the surgical portion of the procedure (45331) would be reported.

Diagnostic endoscopic procedures can be reported with open or incisional procedures.

Diagnostic endoscopy is always included in surgical endoscopy.

⊙ **43200** Esophagoscopy, rigid or flexible; diagnostic, with or without collection of specimen(s) by brushing or washing (separate procedure) ❶ ⊤ ⌧

MED: 100-2,15,260; 100-3,100.2; 100-4,12,90.3; 100-4,14,10
AMA: 1999,Nov,21; 1998,Jun,10; 1994,Spring,1

⊙ **43201** with directed submucosal injection(s), any substance ❶ ⊤ ⌧

MED: 100-2,15,260; 100-4,12,90.3; 100-4,14,10
To report injection sclerosis of esophageal varices, consult CPT code 43204.

⊙ **43202** with biopsy, single or multiple ❶ ⊤ ⌧

MED: 100-2,15,260; 100-3,100.2; 100-4,12,40.6; 100-4,12,90.3; 100-4,14,10
AMA: 1994,Spring,1

⊙ **43204** with injection sclerosis of esophageal varices ❶ ⊤ ⌧

MED: 100-2,15,260; 100-3,100.2; 100-3,100.10; 100-4,12,90.3; 100-4,14,10
AMA: 1994,Spring,1

⊙ **43205** with band ligation of esophageal varices ❶ ⊤ 80 ⌧

MED: 100-2,15,260; 100-3,100.2; 100-4,12,90.3; 100-4,14,10
AMA: 1994,Spring,1

⊙ **43215** with removal of foreign body ❶ ⊤ ⌧

MED: 100-2,15,260; 100-3,100.2; 100-4,12,90.3; 100-4,14,10
AMA: 1994,Spring,1
To report radiological supervision and interpretation, consult CPT code 74235.

⊙ **43216** with removal of tumor(s), polyp(s), or other lesion(s) by hot biopsy forceps or bipolar cautery ❶ ⊤ 80 ⌧

MED: 100-2,15,260; 100-3,100.2; 100-4,12,90.3; 100-4,14,10
AMA: 1994,Spring,1

⊙ **43217** with removal of tumor(s), polyp(s), or other lesion(s) by snare technique ❶ ⊤ ⌧

MED: 100-2,15,260; 100-3,100.2; 100-4,12,40.6; 100-4,12,90.3; 100-4,14,10
AMA: 1994,Spring,1

⊙ **43219** with insertion of plastic tube or stent ❶ ⊤ ⌧

MED: 100-2,15,260; 100-3,100.2; 100-4,12,90.3; 100-4,14,10
AMA: 1994,Spring,2

⊙ **43220** with balloon dilation (less than 30 mm diameter) ❶ ⊤ ⌧

MED: 100-2,15,260; 100-3,100.2; 100-4,12,90.3; 100-4,14,10
AMA: 1997,Jan,10; 1994,Spring,2
If an endoscopic dilation is performed with a balloon 30 mm in diameter or larger, consult CPT code 43458. If dilation is performed without visualization, consult CPT codes 43450-43453.

If the procedure is performed with imaging guidance consult CPT code 74360.

⊙ **43226** with insertion of guide wire followed by dilation over guide wire ❶ ⊤ ⌧

MED: 100-2,15,260; 100-3,100.2; 100-4,12,90.3; 100-4,14,10
AMA: 1994,Spring,2
To report radiological supervision and interpretation, consult CPT code 74360.

⊙ **43227** with control of bleeding (eg, injection, bipolar cautery, unipolar cautery, laser, heater probe, stapler, plasma coagulator) ❷ ⊤ ⌧

MED: 100-2,15,260; 100-3,100.2; 100-4,12,90.3; 100-4,14,10
AMA: 1994,Spring,2

⊙ **43228** with ablation of tumor(s), polyp(s), or other lesion(s), not amenable to removal by hot biopsy forceps, bipolar cautery or snare technique ❷ ⊤ ⌧

MED: 100-2,15,260; 100-3,100.2; 100-4,12,90.3; 100-4,14,10
AMA: 1998,Nov,21; 1994,Spring,2
If esophagoscopic photodynamic therapy is performed, report 43228 in addition to CPT codes 96570 and 96571 as appropriate.

⊙ **43231** **with endoscopic ultrasound examination** 2 T 80 ↔

MED: 100-2,15,260; 100-3,220.5; 100-4,12,90.3; 100-4,14,10
AMA: 2001,Oct,4
Do not report CPT code 76975 when reporting 43231.

⊙ **43232** **with transendoscopic ultrasound-guided intramural or transmural fine needle aspiration/biopsy(s)** 2 T 80 ↔

MED: 100-2,15,260; 100-3,220.5; 100-4,12,90.3; 100-4,14,10
AMA: 2001,Oct,4
To report interpretation of specimen, consult CPT codes 88172 and 88173.

Code 76975 cannot be reported with CPT code 43232.

Code 43232 cannot be reported with CPT code 76942.

⊙ **43234** **Upper gastrointestinal endoscopy, simple primary examination (eg, with small diameter flexible endoscope) (separate procedure)** 1 T ↔

MED: 100-2,15,260; 100-3,100.2; 100-4,12,90.3; 100-4,14,10

⊙ **43235** **Upper gastrointestinal endoscopy including esophagus, stomach, and either the duodenum and/or jejunum as appropriate; diagnostic, with or without collection of specimen(s) by brushing or washing (separate procedure)** 1 T ↔

MED: 100-2,15,260; 100-3,100.2; 100-4,12,90.3; 100-4,14,10
AMA: 1997,Dec,11; 1994,Spring,4

⊙ **43236** **with directed submucosal injection(s), any substance** 2 T ↔

MED: 100-2,15,260; 100-4,12,90.3; 100-4,14,10
To report injection sclerosis of esophageal an/or gastric varices, consult CPT code 43243.

⊙ **43237** **with endoscopic ultrasound examination limited to the esophagus** 2 T 80 ↔

Code 43237 cannot be reported with CPT code 76975.

⊙ **43238** **with transendoscopic ultrasound-guided intramural or transmural fine needle aspiration/biopsy(s), esophagus (includes endoscopic ultrasound examination limited to the esophagus)** 2 T 80 ↔

Code 43238 cannot be reported with CPT codes 76942 or 76975.

⊙ **43239** **with biopsy, single or multiple** 2 T ↔

MED: 100-2,15,260; 100-3,100.2; 100-4,12,90.3; 100-4,14,10
AMA: 2001,Oct,4; 1999,Feb,11; 1998,Apr,14; 1994,Spring,4
To report upper gastrointestinal endoscopy with injection of implant material into and along the muscle of the lower esophageal sphincter, Category III code 0133T should be reported.

⊙ **43240** **with transmural drainage of pseudocyst** 2 T ↔

MED: 100-2,15,260; 100-4,12,90.3; 100-4,14,10
AMA: 2001,Oct,4

⊙ **43241** **with transendoscopic intraluminal tube or catheter placement** 2 T ↔

MED: 100-2,15,260; 100-3,100.2; 100-4,12,90.3; 100-4,14,10
AMA: 2001,Nov,7; 1994,Spring,4

⊙ **43242** **with transendoscopic ultrasound-guided intramural or transmural fine needle aspiration/biopsy(s) (includes endoscopic ultrasound examination of the esophagus, stomach, and either the duodenum and/or jejunum as appropriate)** 2 T 80 ↔

MED: 100-2,15,260; 100-3,220.5; 100-4,12,90.3; 100-4,14,10
AMA: 2001,Oct,4
To report interpretation of specimen, consult CPT codes 88172, 88173.

Code 43242 cannot be reported with CPT codes 76942 or 76975.

To report this procedure limited to the esophagus, consult CPT code 43238.

⊙ **43243** **with injection sclerosis of esophageal and/or gastric varices** 2 T ↔

MED: 100-2,15,260; 100-3,100.2; 100-3,100.10; 100-4,12,90.3; 100-4,14,10
AMA: 1994,Spring,4

⊙ **43244** **with band ligation of esophageal and/or gastric varices** 2 T 80 ↔

MED: 100-2,15,260; 100-3,100.2; 100-4,12,90.3; 100-4,14,10
AMA: 1994,Spring,4

⊙ **43245** **with dilation of gastric outlet for obstruction (eg, balloon, guide wire, bougie)** 2 T ↔

MED: 100-2,15,260; 100-3,100.2; 100-4,12,90.3; 100-4,14,10
AMA: 2001,Oct,4; 1994,Spring,4
Code 43245 cannot be reported with CPT code 43256.

⊙ **43246** **with directed placement of percutaneous gastrostomy tube** 2 T 80 ↔

MED: 100-2,15,260; 100-3,100.2; 100-4,12,90.3; 100-4,14,10; 100-4,20,50.3; 100-4,20,100.2.2
AMA: 1997,Feb,10; 1994,Spring,4
To report radiological supervision and interpretation, consult CPT code 74350.

⊙ **43247** **with removal of foreign body** 2 T ↔

MED: 100-2,15,260; 100-3,100.2; 100-4,12,90.3; 100-4,14,10
AMA: 1994,Spring,4
To report radiological supervision and interpretation, consult CPT code 74235.

⊙ **43248** **with insertion of guide wire followed by dilation of esophagus over guide wire** 2 T ↔

MED: 100-2,15,260; 100-3,100.2; 100-4,12,90.3; 100-4,14,10
AMA: 1997,Dec,11; 1994,Spring,4

⊙ **43249** **with balloon dilation of esophagus (less than 30 mm diameter)** 2 T ↔

MED: 100-2,15,260; 100-3,100.2; 100-4,12,90.3; 100-4,14,10

⊙ **43250** **with removal of tumor(s), polyp(s), or other lesion(s) by hot biopsy forceps or bipolar cautery** 2 T ↔

MED: 100-2,15,260; 100-3,100.2; 100-4,12,90.3; 100-4,14,10
AMA: 1999,Feb,11; 1994,Spring,4

⊙ **43251** **with removal of tumor(s), polyp(s), or other lesion(s) by snare technique** 2 T ↔

MED: 100-2,15,260; 100-3,100.2; 100-4,12,90.3; 100-4,14,10
AMA: 1994,Spring,4

⊙ **43255** **with control of bleeding, any method** 2 T ↔

MED: 100-2,15,260; 100-3,100.2; 100-4,12,90.3; 100-4,14,10
AMA: 1994,Spring,4

⊙ **43256** **with transendoscopic stent placement (includes predilation)** 3 T ↔

MED: 100-2,15,260; 100-3,100.2; 100-4,4,61.2; 100-4,12,90.3; 100-4,14,10

⊙ 43257   **with delivery of thermal energy to the muscle of lower esophageal sphincter and/or gastric cardia, for treatment of gastroesophageal reflux disease** 〔3〕〔T〕〔⊡〕

⊙ 43258   **with ablation of tumor(s), polyp(s), or other lesion(s) not amenable to removal by hot biopsy forceps, bipolar cautery or snare technique** 〔3〕〔T〕〔⊡〕

MED: 100-2,15,260; 100-3,100.2; 100-4,12,90.3; 100-4,14,10

AMA: 1994,Spring,4

If injection sclerosis of esophageal varices is performed, consult CPT code 43204 or 43243.

⊙ 43259   **with endoscopic ultrasound examination, including the esophagus, stomach, and either the duodenum and/or jejunum as appropriate** 〔3〕〔T〕〔80〕〔⊡〕

MED: 100-2,15,260; 100-3,100.2; 100-3,220.5; 100-4,12,30.1; 100-4,12,90.3; 100-4,14,10

AMA: 1994,Spring,4

Code 43259 cannot be reported with CPT code 76975.

⊙ 43260   **Endoscopic retrograde cholangiopancreatography (ERCP); diagnostic, with or without collection of specimen(s) by brushing or washing (separate procedure)** 〔2〕〔T〕〔⊡〕

MED: 100-2,15,260; 100-3,100.2; 100-4,12,90.3; 100-4,14,10

AMA: 1994,Spring,5

To report radiological supervision and interpretation performed with codes 46260-43272, consult CPT codes 74328, 74329 and 74330.

⊙ 43261   **with biopsy, single or multiple** 〔2〕〔T〕〔⊡〕

MED: 100-2,15,260; 100-3,100.2; 100-4,12,90.3; 100-4,14,10

AMA: 1994,Spring,5

⊙ 43262   **with sphincterotomy/papillotomy** 〔2〕〔T〕〔⊡〕

MED: 100-2,15,260; 100-3,100.2; 100-4,12,90.3; 100-4,14,10

AMA: 1994,Spring,5

⊙ 43263   **with pressure measurement of sphincter of Oddi (pancreatic duct or common bile duct)** 〔2〕〔T〕〔⊡〕

MED: 100-2,15,260; 100-3,100.2; 100-4,12,90.3; 100-4,14,10

AMA: 1994,Spring,5

To report radiological supervision and interpretation, consult CPT codes 74328, 74329, and 74330.

⊙ 43264   **with endoscopic retrograde removal of calculus/calculi from biliary and/or pancreatic ducts** 〔2〕〔T〕〔⊡〕

MED: 100-2,15,260; 100-3,100.2; 100-4,12,90.3; 100-4,14,10

AMA: 1994,Spring,5

If these procedures (43264-43271) are performed with a sphincterotomy, consult also CPT code 43262.

⊙ 43265   **with endoscopic retrograde destruction, lithotripsy of calculus/calculi, any method** 〔2〕〔T〕〔⊡〕

MED: 100-2,15,260; 100-3,100.2; 100-4,12,90.3; 100-4,14,10

AMA: 1994,Spring,5

⊙ 43267   **with endoscopic retrograde insertion of nasobiliary or nasopancreatic drainage tube** 〔2〕〔T〕〔⊡〕

MED: 100-2,15,260; 100-3,100.2; 100-4,12,90.3; 100-4,14,10

AMA: 1994,Spring,6

⊙ 43268   **with endoscopic retrograde insertion of tube or stent into bile or pancreatic duct** 〔2〕〔T〕〔⊡〕

MED: 100-2,15,260; 100-3,100.2; 100-4,12,90.3; 100-4,14,10

AMA: 1994,Spring,6

⊙ 43269   **with endoscopic retrograde removal of foreign body and/or change of tube or stent** 〔2〕〔T〕〔⊡〕

MED: 100-2,15,260; 100-3,100.2; 100-4,12,90.3; 100-4,14,10

AMA: 1994,Spring,6

⊙ 43271   **with endoscopic retrograde balloon dilation of ampulla, biliary and/or pancreatic duct(s)** 〔2〕〔T〕〔⊡〕

MED: 100-2,15,260; 100-3,100.2; 100-4,12,90.3; 100-4,14,10

AMA: 1994,Spring,6

⊙ 43272   **with ablation of tumor(s), polyp(s), or other lesion(s) not amenable to removal by hot biopsy forceps, bipolar cautery or snare technique** 〔2〕〔T〕〔80〕〔⊡〕

MED: 100-2,15,260; 100-3,100.2; 100-4,12,90.3; 100-4,14,10

LAPAROSCOPY

Diagnostic laparoscopy is always included in surgical laparoscopy.

To report only a diagnostic laparoscopy (peritoneoscopy), consult CPT code 49320.

43280   **Laparoscopy, surgical, esophagogastric fundoplasty (eg, Nissen, Toupet procedures)** 〔T〕〔80〕〔⊡〕

AMA: 2002,Dec,1; 2000,Mar,5; 1999,Nov,22

If an open approach is used, consult CPT code 43324.

43289   **Unlisted laparoscopy procedure, esophagus** 〔T〕〔80〕〔50〕

AMA: 2000,Mar,5; 1999,Nov,22

REPAIR

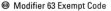

Proximal esophagus

Intestinal esophagus

Thyroid cartilage
Cricoid cartilage
Trachea
Esophagus

Diaphragm

Stomach

Sections of stomach or bowel are commonly used to repair a resected portion of the esophagus

The esophagus is a muscular tube that delivers food from the oral cavity to the stomach. It spans the cervical, thoracic, and abdominal regions and numerous surgical approaches may be used

43300   **Esophagoplasty (plastic repair or reconstruction), cervical approach; without repair of tracheoesophageal fistula** 〔C〕〔80〕〔⊡〕

43305   **with repair of tracheoesophageal fistula** 〔C〕〔80〕〔⊡〕

43310   **Esophagoplasty (plastic repair or reconstruction), thoracic approach; without repair of tracheoesophageal fistula** 〔C〕〔80〕〔⊡〕

43312   **with repair of tracheoesophageal fistula** 〔C〕〔80〕〔⊡〕

43313   **Esophagoplasty for congenital defect (plastic repair or reconstruction), thoracic approach; without repair of congenital tracheoesophageal fistula** 〔C〕〔80〕〔63〕〔⊡〕

43314   **with repair of congenital tracheoesophageal fistula** 〔C〕〔80〕〔63〕〔⊡〕

43320   **Esophagogastrostomy (cardioplasty), with or without vagotomy and pyloroplasty, transabdominal or transthoracic approach** 〔C〕〔80〕〔⊡〕

43324   **Esophagogastric fundoplasty (eg, Nissen, Belsey IV, Hill procedures)** 〔C〕〔80〕

AMA: 1999,Nov,22; 1996,Sep,10

If a laparoscopic approach is used, consult CPT code 43280.

43325   **Esophagogastric fundoplasty; with fundic patch (Thal-Nissen procedure)** 〔C〕〔80〕〔⊡〕

If a cricopharyngeal myotomy is performed, consult CPT code 43030.

43326   **with gastroplasty (eg, Collis)** 〔C〕〔80〕〔⊡〕

Digestive

43330 — 43610

43330 **Esophagomyotomy (Heller type); abdominal approach** ⓒ 80 ▣

AMA: 1999,Nov,22

43331 thoracic approach ⓒ 80 ▣

AMA: 1999,Nov,22
If a thoracoscopic esophagomyotomy is performed, consult CPT code 32665.

43340 **Esophagojejunostomy (without total gastrectomy); abdominal approach** ⓒ 80 ▣

43341 thoracic approach ⓒ 80 ▣

43350 **Esophagostomy, fistulization of esophagus, external; abdominal approach** ⓒ 80 ▣

43351 thoracic approach ⓒ 80 ▣

43352 cervical approach ⓒ 80 ▣

43360 **Gastrointestinal reconstruction for previous esophagectomy, for obstructing esophageal lesion or fistula, or for previous esophageal exclusion; with stomach, with or without pyloroplasty** ⓒ 80 ▣

43361 with colon interposition or small intestine reconstruction, including intestine mobilization, preparation, and anastomosis(es) ⓒ 80 ▣

43400 **Ligation, direct, esophageal varices** ⓒ 80 ▣

43401 **Transection of esophagus with repair, for esophageal varices** ⓒ 80 ▣

43405 **Ligation or stapling at gastroesophageal junction for pre-existing esophageal perforation** ⓒ 80 ▣

43410 **Suture of esophageal wound or injury; cervical approach** ⓒ 80 ▣

AMA: 1996,Jun,7

43415 transthoracic or transabdominal approach ⓒ 80 ▣

43420 **Closure of esophagostomy or fistula; cervical approach** ⓒ 80 ▣

43425 transthoracic or transabdominal approach ⓒ 80 ▣

If an esophageal hiatal hernia is repaired, consult CPT codes 39520 and subsequent codes.

MANIPULATION

If an associated esophagogram is performed, consult CPT code 74220.

43450 **Dilation of esophagus, by unguided sound or bougie, single or multiple passes** ❶ ⓣ ▣

MED: 100-2,15,260; 100-4,12,90.3; 100-4,14,10
AMA: 1998,Jun,10; 1998,Apr,14; 1997,Jan,10; 1994,Spring,1

⊙ **43453** **Dilation of esophagus, over guide wire** ❶ ⓣ ▣

MED: 100-2,15,260; 100-4,12,90.3; 100-4,14,10
AMA: 1997,Jan,10; 1997,Dec,11; 1994,Spring,1
If dilation is performed with direct visualization, consult CPT code 43220.

⊙ **43456** **Dilation of esophagus, by balloon or dilator, retrograde** ❷ ⓣ ▣

MED: 100-2,15,260; 100-4,12,90.3; 100-4,14,10
AMA: 1997,Jan,10; 1994,Spring,3

⊙ **43458** **Dilation of esophagus with balloon (30 mm diameter or larger) for achalasia** ❷ ⓣ ▣

MED: 100-2,15,260; 100-4,12,90.3; 100-4,14,10
AMA: 1997,Jan,10; 1994,Spring,3
If dilation is performed with a balloon less than 30 mm in diameter, consult CPT code 43220. If radiological supervision and interpretation is performed, consult CPT code 74360.

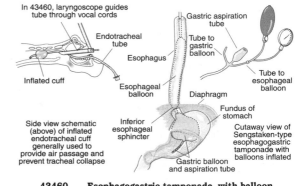

In 43460, laryngoscope guides tube through vocal cords
Endotracheal tube
Inflated cuff
Esophagus
Esophageal balloon
Side view schematic (above) of inflated endotracheal cuff generally used to provide air passage and prevent tracheal collapse
Gastric aspiration tube
Tube to gastric balloon
Tube to esophageal balloon
Diaphragm
Fundus of stomach
Inferior esophageal sphincter
Cutaway view of Sengstaken-type esophagogastric tamponade with balloons inflated
Gastric balloon and aspiration tube

43460 **Esophagogastric tamponade, with balloon (Sengstaaken type)** ⓒ ▣

If an esophageal foreign body is removed by balloon catheter, consult CPT codes 43215, 43247, and 74235.

OTHER PROCEDURES

43496 **Free jejunum transfer with microvascular anastomosis** ⓒ 80 ▣

AMA: 1998,Nov,16; 1997,Nov,17; 1997,Jun,10; 1997,Apr,4
Do not report 69990 in addition to 43496 as the operating microscope is considered an inclusive component of the surgery.

43499 **Unlisted procedure, esophagus** ⓣ 80

MED: 100-4,4,180.3

STOMACH

INCISION

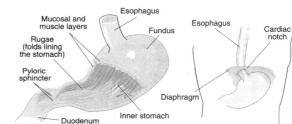

Mucosal and muscle layers
Esophagus
Fundus
Rugae (folds lining the stomach)
Pyloric sphincter
Duodenum
Inner stomach
Diaphragm
Esophagus
Cardiac notch

The stomach is a highly distensible organ that serves as a reservoir to mix food and break it down with digestive juices. The esophagus pierces the diaphragm at the cardiac notch, where the stomach begins. The pyloric sphincter marks the inferior border of the stomach. The vagal nerve trunks run down the front and back of the esophagus and serve the stomach by controlling secretion of digestive acids

43500 **Gastrotomy; with exploration or foreign body removal** ⓒ 80 ▣

43501 with suture repair of bleeding ulcer ⓒ 80 ▣

43502 with suture repair of pre-existing esophagogastric laceration (eg, Mallory-Weiss) ⓒ 80 ▣

43510 with esophageal dilation and insertion of permanent intraluminal tube (eg, Celestin or Mousseaux-Barbin) ⓣ 80 ▣

43520 **Pyloromyotomy, cutting of pyloric muscle (Fredet-Ramstedt type operation)** ⓒ 80 ⑨ ▣

EXCISION

43600 **Biopsy of stomach; by capsule, tube, peroral (one or more specimens)** ❶ ⓣ ▣

MED: 100-2,15,260; 100-4,12,90.3; 100-4,14,10

43605 by laparotomy ⓒ 80 ▣

43610 **Excision, local; ulcer or benign tumor of stomach** ⓒ 80 ▣

43611	malignant tumor of stomach	C 80 ↕
43620	Gastrectomy, total; with esophagoenterostomy	C 80 ↕
43621	with Roux-en-Y reconstruction	C 80 ↕
43622	with formation of intestinal pouch, any type	C 80 ↕
43631	Gastrectomy, partial, distal; with gastroduodenostomy	C 80 ↕

Billroth operation

| 43632 | with gastrojejunostomy | C 80 ↕ |

Polya anastomosis

| 43633 | with Roux-en-Y reconstruction | C 80 ↕ |
| 43634 | with formation of intestinal pouch | C 80 ↕ |

+ 43635 Vagotomy when performed with partial distal gastrectomy (List separately in addition to code(s) for primary procedure) C 80 ↕

AMA: 1997,Nov,17

Note that 43635 is an add-on code and must be used in conjunction with 43631, 43632, 43633, and 43634.

43640 Vagotomy including pyloroplasty, with or without gastrostomy; truncal or selective C 80 ↕

If pyloroplasty is performed, consult CPT code 43800. If a vagotomy is performed, consult CPT codes 64752-64760.

43641 parietal cell (highly selective) C 80 ↕

If an upper gastrointestinal endoscopy is performed, consult CPT codes 43234-43259.

LAPAROSCOPY

Diagnostic laparoscopy is always included in surgical endoscopy.

To report only a diagnostic laparoscopy (peritoneoscopy), consult CPT code 49320.

43644 Laparoscopy, surgical, gastric restrictive procedure; with gastric bypass and Roux-en-Y gastroenterostomy (roux limb 150 cm or less) C 80 ↕

Code 43644 cannot be reported with CPT codes 43846, 49320.

Report Esophagogastroduodenoscopy (EGD) performed for a different condition with modifier 59.

43645 with gastric bypass and small intestine reconstruction to limit absorption C 80 ↕

Code 43645 cannot be reported with CPT codes 49320, 43847.

● 43647 Laparoscopy, surgical; implantation or replacement of gastric neurostimulator electrodes, antrum T

● 43648 revision or removal of gastric neurostimulator electrodes, antrum T

Use 43881 or 43882 for open approach.

Use 64590 for insertion of gastric neurostimulator pulse generator. Use 64595 for revision or removal of the gastric neurostimulator pulse generator.

Use 95999 for electronic analysis and programming of gastric neurostimulator pulse generator.

Use codes 0155T or 0156T for laparoscopic implantation, revision or removal of gastric neurostimulator electrodes, lesser curvature (morbid obesity).

Use 0162T for electronic analysis and programming of gastric pulse generator, lesser curvature (morbid obesity).

43651	transection of vagus nerves, truncal	T 80 ↕

AMA: 2000,Mar,5; 1999,Nov,22

| 43652 | transection of vagus nerves, selective or highly selective | T 80 ↕ |

AMA: 2000,Mar,5; 1999,Nov,22

| 43653 | gastrostomy, without construction of gastric tube (eg, Stamm procedure) (separate procedure) | 9 T 80 ↕ |

MED: 100-2,15,260; 100-4,12,90.3; 100-4,14,10

AMA: 2000,Mar,5; 1999,Nov,22

43659 Unlisted laparoscopy procedure, stomach T 80 50

AMA: 2000,Mar,5; 1999,Nov,22

INTRODUCTION

⊙ **43750** Percutaneous placement of gastrostomy tube 2 T ↕

MED: 100-2,15,260; 100-3,30.7; 100-3,100.2; 100-4,12,90.3; 100-4,14,10; 100-4,20,50.3; 100-4,20,100.2.2

AMA: 1994,Spring,1

To report radiological supervision and interpretation, consult CPT code 74350.

43752 Naso- or oro-gastric tube placement, requiring physician's skill and fluoroscopic guidance (includes fluoroscopy, image documentation and report) ⊠ ↕

MED: 100-3,30.7; 100-3,100.2; 100-4,20,50.3; 100-4,20,100.2.2

AMA: 2002,Jan,11

To report enteric tube placement, consult CPT codes 44500, 74340.

Code 43752 cannot be reported with CPT codes 99291-99292, 99293-99294, 99295-99296 or 99298-99299.

43760 Change of gastrostomy tube 1 T ↕

MED: 100-2,15,260; 100-3,30.7; 100-3,100.2; 100-4,12,90.3; 100-4,14,10; 100-4,20,50.3; 100-4,20,100.2.2

If an endoscopic placement of a gastrostomy tube is performed, consult CPT code 43246. For radiological supervision and interpretation, consult CPT code 75984.

43761 Repositioning of the gastric feeding tube, any method, through the duodenum for enteric nutrition 1 T ↕

MED: 100-3,30.7; 100-3,100.2; 100-4,20,50.3; 100-4,20,100.2.2

AMA: 1999,Nov,22; 1996,Oct,9

If imaging guidance is performed, consult CPT code 75984.

BARIATRIC SURGERY

Bariatric surgery may include the stomach, duodenum, jejunum, and/or the ileum.

Band adjustments are included during the postoperative period after gastric restriction that utilizes the adjustable gastric band technique. Band adjustment refers to changing the gastric band diameter by injection or aspiration of fluid through the subcutaneous port component.

43770 Laparoscopy, surgical, gastric restrictive procedure; placement of adjustable gastric band (gastric band and subcutaneous port components) C 80

To report replacement of an individual component, use 43770 with modifier 52.

43771 revision of adjustable gastric band component only C 80

43772 removal of adjustable gastric band component only C 80

43773 removal and replacement of adjustable gastric band component only C 80

Code 43773 cannot be reported with 43772.

Digestive

43774 — 44010

43774   removal of adjustable gastric band and subcutaneous port components   Ⓒ 80

To report removal and replacement of both gastric band and subcutaneous port components, consult CPT code 43659.

OTHER PROCEDURES

43800   Pyloroplasty   Ⓒ 80 ◪

If pyloroplasty and vagotomy are performed, consult CPT code 43640.

43810   Gastroduodenostomy   Ⓒ 80 ◪

43820   Gastrojejunostomy; without vagotomy   Ⓒ 80 ◪

43825   with vagotomy, any type   Ⓒ 80 ◪

43830   Gastrostomy, open; without construction of gastric tube (eg, Stamm procedure) (separate procedure)   Ⓣ 80 ◪

AMA: 1999,Nov,22

43831   neonatal, for feeding   Ⓐ Ⓣ 80 ㊿ ◪

AMA: 1999,Nov,22

If a gastrostomy tube is changed, consult CPT code 43760.

43832   with construction of gastric tube (eg, Janeway procedure)   Ⓒ 80 ◪

AMA: 1999,Nov,22

43840   Gastrorrhaphy, suture of perforated duodenal or gastric ulcer, wound, or injury   Ⓒ 80 ◪

MED: 100-3,100.12

43842   Gastric restrictive procedure, without gastric bypass, for morbid obesity; vertical-banded gastroplasty   Ⓔ 80 ◪

MED: 100-3,40.5; 100-3,100.1; 100-3,100.8

AMA: 1998,May,5

43843   other than vertical-banded gastroplasty   Ⓒ 80 ◪

MED: 100-3,40.5; 100-3,100.1; 100-3,100.8

AMA: 1998,May,5

43845   Gastric restrictive procedure with partial gastrectomy, pylorus-preserving duodenoileostomy and ileoileostomy (50 to 100 cm common channel) to limit absorption (biliopancreatic diversion with duodenal switch)   Ⓒ 80 ◪

Code 43845 cannot be reported with CPT codes 43633, 43847, 44130, and 49000.

43846   Gastric restrictive procedure, with gastric bypass for morbid obesity; with short limb (150 cm or less) Roux-en-Y gastroenterostomy   Ⓒ 80 ◪

MED: 100-3,40.5; 100-3,100.1; 100-3,100.8

AMA: 1998,May,5

To report greater than 150 cm, consult CPT code 43847.

To report laparoscopic procedure, consult CPT code 43644.

43847   with small intestine reconstruction to limit absorption   Ⓒ 80 ◪

MED: 100-3,40.5; 100-3,100.1; 100-3,100.8

AMA: 1998,May,5

43848   Revision, open, of gastric restrictive procedure for morbid obesity, other than adjustable gastric band (separate procedure)   Ⓒ 80 ◪

MED: 100-3,40.5; 100-3,100.1; 100-3,100.8

AMA: 1998,May,5

For adjustable gastric band procedures, consult CPT codes 43770-43774, 43886-43888.

43850   Revision of gastroduodenal anastomosis (gastroduodenostomy) with reconstruction; without vagotomy   Ⓒ 80 ◪

43855   with vagotomy   Ⓒ 80 ◪

43860   Revision of gastrojejunal anastomosis (gastrojejunostomy) with reconstruction, with or without partial gastrectomy or intestine resection; without vagotomy   Ⓒ 80 ◪

MED: 100-3,100.1

43865   with vagotomy   Ⓒ 80 ◪

MED: 100-3,100.1

43870   Closure of gastrostomy, surgical   ❶ Ⓣ 80 ◪

MED: 100-2,15,260; 100-4,12,90.3; 100-4,14,10

43880   Closure of gastrocolic fistula   Ⓒ 80 ◪

● **43881**   Implantation or replacement of gastric neurostimulator electrodes, antrum, open   Ⓒ

● **43882**   Revision or removal of gastric neurostimulator electrodes, antrum, open   Ⓒ

Use 43647 or 43648 for laparoscopic approach.

Use 64590 for insertion of gastric neurostimulator pulse generator. Use 64595 for revision or removal of the gastric neurostimulator pulse generator.

Use 95999 for electronic analysis and programming of gastric neurostimulator pulse generator.

Use codes 0157T or 0158T for revision or removal of gastric neurostimulator electrodes, lesser curvature (morbid obesity).

Use 0162T for electronic analysis and programming of gastric neurostimulator pulse generator, lesser curvature (morbid obesity).

43886   Gastric restrictive procedure, open; revision of subcutaneous port component only   Ⓣ 80

43887   removal of subcutaneous port component only   Ⓣ 80

43888   removal and replacement of subcutaneous port component only   Ⓣ 80

Code 43888 cannot be reported with 43774, 43887.

To report the laparoscopic removal of both gastric band and subcutaneous port components, consult CPT code 43774.

To report removal and replacement of both gastric band and subcutaneous port components, consult code 43659.

43999   Unlisted procedure, stomach   Ⓣ 80

MED: 100-4,4,180.3

INTESTINES (EXCEPT RECTUM)

INCISION

44005   Enterolysis (freeing of intestinal adhesion) (separate procedure)   Ⓒ 80 ◪

AMA: 2000,Jan,11; 2000,Apr,10; 1999,Nov,23; 1997,Nov,17

Code 44005 is not to be used with CPT code 45136.

If a laparoscopic approach is used, consult CPT code 44180.

44010   Duodenotomy, for exploration, biopsy(s), or foreign body removal   Ⓒ 80 ◪

MED: 100-4,3,20.2.1

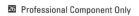

㉖ Professional Component Only   80/80 Assist-at-Surgery Allowed/With Documentation   Unlisted   Not Covered

Ⓣ Technical Component Only   **MED:** Pub 100/NCD References   **AMA:** CPT Assistant References   ❶-❾ ASC Group   ♂ Male Only   ♀ Female Only

164 — CPT Expert   CPT only © 2006 American Medical Association. All Rights Reserved. *(Black Ink)*   © *2006 Ingenix (Blue Ink)*

+ 44015 **Tube or needle catheter jejunostomy for enteral alimentation, intraoperative, any method (List separately in addition to primary procedure)** C 80 ⬚

AMA: 2002,Mar,10
Note that 44015 is an add-on code that must be used in conjunction with the appropriate code for the primary procedure. This code cannot be reported alone.

44020 **Enterotomy, small intestine, other than duodenum; for exploration, biopsy(s), or foreign body removal** C 80 ⬚

MED: 100-4,3,20.2.1

Anterior abdominal skin   Baker-type tube

Depicted at left is a tube threaded through intestine for decompression

Peritoneum

Bowel lumen

Note that the bowel is sutured to the abdominal wall

In 44021, a select portion of intestine is surgically approached and incised. A tube is inserted into the bowel lumen and threaded distally, often to a point of obstruction. The tube is used to decompress the bowel segment it passes through, often during or immediately following surgery for bowel obstruction.

44021 **for decompression (eg, Baker tube)** C 80 ⬚

44025 **Colotomy, for exploration, biopsy(s), or foreign body removal** C 80 ⬚

MED: 100-4,3,20.2.1

Amussat's operation

44050 **Reduction of volvulus, intussusception, internal hernia, by laparotomy** C 80 ⬚

44055 **Correction of malrotation by lysis of duodenal bands and/or reduction of midgut volvulus (eg, Ladd procedure)** C 80 ⊛ ⬚

EXCISION

Intestinal transplantation involves three different components:

- Cadaver or living donor enterectomy which consists of harvesting and cold preparation of the graft prior to transplantation and care of the donor (44132, 44133).
- Backbench work consists of preparation of donor intestine prior to transplantation. This includes mobilizing and developing the superior mesenteric artery and vein (44715). Also included is any additional reconstruction of graft including venous and arterial anastomosis(es) (44720-44721) prior to transplantation.
- Recipient transplantation which includes transplanting the intestine into the patient (codes 44135 and 44136).

44100 **Biopsy of intestine by capsule, tube, peroral (one or more specimens)** 1 T ⬚

MED: 100-2,15,260; 100-4,12,90.3; 100-4,14,10

44110 **Excision of one or more lesions of small or large intestine not requiring anastomosis, exteriorization, or fistulization; single enterotomy** C 80 ⬚

44111 **multiple enterotomies** C 80 ⬚

44120 **Enterectomy, resection of small intestine; single resection and anastomosis** C 80 ⬚

Code 44120 is not to be used with code 45136.

+ 44121 **each additional resection and anastomosis (List separately in addition to code for primary procedure)** C 80 ⬚

Note that 44121 is an add-on code and must be used in conjunction with 44120.

44125 **with enterostomy** C 80 ⬚

44126 **Enterectomy, resection of small intestine for congenital atresia, single resection and anastomosis of proximal segment of intestine; without tapering** C 80 ⊛ ⬚

44127 **with tapering** C 80 ⊛ ⬚

+ 44128 **each additional resection and anastomosis (List separately in addition to code for primary procedure)** C 80 ⊛ ⬚

Note that 44128 is an add-on code and must be used in conjunction with codes 44126 and 44127.

44130 **Enteroenterostomy, anastomosis of intestine, with or without cutaneous enterostomy (separate procedure)** C 80 ⬚

44132 **Donor enterectomy (including cold preservation), open; from cadaver donor** C 80 ⬚

MED: 100-4,3,90.6

To report backbench intestinal graft preparation or reconstruction, consult CPT codes 44715, 44720, 44721.

44133 **partial, from living donor** C 80 ⬚

MED: 100-4,3,90.6

44135 **Intestinal allotransplantation; from cadaver donor** C 80 ⬚

MED: 100-4,3,90.6

44136 **from living donor** C 80 ⬚

MED: 100-4,3,90.6

44137 **Removal of transplanted intestinal allograft, complete** C 80 ⬚

To report partial removal of transplant allograft, consult CPT codes 44120, 44121, and 44140.

+ 44139 **Mobilization (take-down) of splenic flexure performed in conjunction with partial colectomy (List separately in addition to primary procedure)** C 80 ⬚

Note that 44139 is an add-on code and must be used in conjunction with 44140-44147.

44140 **Colectomy, partial; with anastomosis** C 80 ⬚

If procedure is performed laparoscopically, consult CPT code 44204.

44141 **with skin level cecostomy or colostomy** C 80 ⬚

44143 **with end colostomy and closure of distal segment (Hartmann type procedure)** C 80 ⬚

To report laparoscopic procedure, consult CPT code 44206.

44144 **with resection, with colostomy or ileostomy and creation of mucofistula** C 80 ⬚

44145 **with coloproctostomy (low pelvic anastomosis)** C 80 ⬚

To report laparoscopic procedure, consult CPT code 44207.

44146 **with coloproctostomy (low pelvic anastomosis), with colostomy** C 80 ⬚

To report laparoscopic procedure, consult CPT code 44208.

⊛ Modifier 63 Exempt Code   ⊙ Conscious Sedation   + CPT Add-on Code   ⊘ Modifier 51 Exempt Code   ● New Code   ▲ Revised Code

M Maternity Edit   A Age Edit   A-Y APC Status Indicators   ⬚ CCI Comprehensive Code   50 Bilateral Procedure

Digestive

44147 — 44314

44147	abdominal and transanal approach	C 80 ◨

44150	Colectomy, total, abdominal, without proctectomy; with ileostomy or ileoproctostomy	C 80 ◨

To report laparoscopic procedure, consult CPT code 44210.

Lane's operation

44151	with continent ileostomy	C 80 ◨

~~44152~~	~~with rectal mucosectomy, ileoanal anastomosis, with or without loop ileostomy~~	

~~44153~~	~~with rectal mucosectomy, ileoanal anastomosis, creation of ileal reservoir (S or J), with or without loop ileostomy~~	

Use 44799.

44155	Colectomy, total, abdominal, with proctectomy; with ileostomy	C 80 ◨

To report laparoscopic procedure, consult CPT code 44212.

Miles' colectomy

44156	with continent ileostomy	C 80 ◨

● 44157	with ileoanal anastomosis, includes loop ileostomy, and rectal mucosectomy, when performed	C

● 44158	with ileoanal anastomosis, creation of ileal reservoir (S or J), includes loop ileostomy, and rectal mucosectomy, when performed	C

Use 44211 for laparoscopic procedure.

44160	Colectomy, partial, with removal of terminal ileum with ileocolostomy	C 80 ◨

To report laparoscopic procedure (peritoneoscopy), consult CPT code 44205.

LAPAROSCOPY

Diagnostic laparoscopy is always included in a surgical laparoscopy. To report only diagnostic laparoscopy, consult CPT code 49320.

INCISION

44180	Laparoscopy, surgical, enterolysis (freeing of intestinal adhesion) (separate procedure)	T 80

ENTEROSTOMY-EXTERNAL FISTULIZATION OF INTESTINES

44186	Laparoscopy, surgical; jejunostomy (eg, for decompression or feeding)	T 80

44187	ileostomy or jejunostomy, non-tube	C 80

To report open procedure, consult CPT code 44310.

44188	Laparoscopy, surgical, colostomy or skin level cecostomy	C 80

To report open procedure, consult CPT code 44320.

Do not report 44188 in conjunction with 44970.

EXCISION

44202	Laparoscopy, surgical; enterectomy, resection of small intestine, single resection and anastomosis	C 80 ◨

AMA: 2000,Mar,5; 1999,Nov,23

+ 44203	each additional small intestine resection and anastomosis (List separately in addition to code for primary procedure)	C 80 ◨

Note that 44203 is an add-on code and must be used in conjunction with CPT code 44202.

To report open procedure, consult CPT codes 44120, 44121.

44204	colectomy, partial, with anastomosis	C 80 ◨

To report open procedure, consult CPT code 44140.

44205	colectomy, partial, with removal of terminal ileum with ileocolostomy	C 80 ◨

To report open procedure, consult CPT code 44160.

44206	colectomy, partial, with end colostomy and closure of distal segment (Hartmann type procedure)	T 80 ◨

To report open procedure, consult CPT code 44143.

44207	colectomy, partial, with anastomosis, with coloproctostomy (low pelvic anastomosis)	T 80 ◨

To report open procedure, consult CPT code 44145.

44208	colectomy, partial, with anastomosis, with coloproctostomy (low pelvic anastomosis) with colostomy	T 80 ◨

To report open procedure, consult CPT code 44146.

44210	colectomy, total, abdominal, without proctectomy, with ileostomy or ileoproctostomy	C 80 ◨

To report open procedure, consult CPT code 44150.

▲ 44211	colectomy, total, abdominal, with proctectomy, with ileoanal anastomosis, creation of ileal reservoir (S or J), with loop ileostomy, includes rectal mucosectomy, when performed	C 80 ◨

To report open procedure, consult CPT codes 44157, 44158.

44212	colectomy, total, abdominal, with proctectomy, with ileostomy	C 80 ◨

To report open procedure, consult CPT code 44155.

+ 44213	Laparoscopy, surgical, mobilization (take-down) of splenic flexure performed in conjunction with partial colectomy (List separately in addition to primary procedure)	T 80

Note that 44213 is an add-on code and must be reported in conjunction with 44204-44208.

To report open procedure, consult CPT code 44139.

REPAIR

44227	Laparoscopy, surgical, closure of enterostomy, large or small intestine, with resection and anastomosis	C 80

To report open procedure, consult CPT codes 44625, 44626.

OTHER PROCEDURES

44238	Unlisted laparoscopy procedure, intestine (except rectum)	T 80 50 ◨

ENTEROSTOMY — EXTERNAL FISTULIZATION OF INTESTINES

44300	Enterostomy or cecostomy, tube (eg, for decompression or feeding) (separate procedure)	C 80 ◨

AMA: 2002,Mar,10

44310	Ileostomy or jejunostomy, non-tube	C 80 ◨

AMA: 2002,Mar,10

To report laparoscopic procedure, consult CPT code 44187.

Code 44310 cannot be reported with 44144, 44150-44151, 44155, 44156, 45113, 45119, 45136.

44312	Revision of ileostomy; simple (release of superficial scar) (separate procedure)	1 T 80 ◨

MED: 100-2,15,260; 100-4,12,90.3; 100-4,14,10

44314	complicated (reconstruction in-depth) (separate procedure)	C 80 ◨

---

26 Professional Component Only   80/80 Assist-at-Surgery Allowed/With Documentation   Unlisted   Not Covered

TC Technical Component Only   MED: Pub 100/NCD References   AMA: CPT Assistant References   1-9 ASC Group   ♂ Male Only   ♀ Female Only

166 — CPT Expert   CPT only © 2006 American Medical Association. All Rights Reserved. (Black Ink)   © 2006 Ingenix (Blue Ink)

44316	Continent ileostomy (Kock procedure) (separate procedure) C 80 ↻	

If a fiberoptic evaluation is performed, consult CPT code 44385.

44320	Colostomy or skin level cecostomy; C 80 ↻	

To report laparoscopic procedure, consult CPT code 44188.

Code 44320 cannot be reported with 44141, 44144, 44146, 44605, 45110, 45119, 45126, 45563, 45805, 45825, 50810, 51597, 57307, or 58240.

Mikulicz resection

44322	with multiple biopsies (eg, for congenital megacolon) (separate procedure) C 80 ↻	

Mikulicz resection

44340	Revision of colostomy; simple (release of superficial scar) (separate procedure) 3 T ↻	

MED: 100-2,15,260; 100-4,12,90.3; 100-4,14,10

44345	complicated (reconstruction in-depth) (separate procedure) C 80 ↻	

Skin

In 44346, the site of the colostomy may be moved. The bowel is mobilized and trimmed of any herniations. The former site is closed

Herniations that have formed around the site of a colostomy are repaired

The colon is mobilized, trimmed if necessary, and a new stoma is often created

44346	with repair of paracolostomy hernia (separate procedure) C 80 ↻	

ENDOSCOPY, SMALL INTESTINE AND STOMAL

Diagnostic endoscopy is always included in surgical endoscopy.

⊙ **44360** Small intestinal endoscopy, enteroscopy beyond second portion of duodenum, not including ileum; diagnostic, with or without collection of specimen(s) by brushing or washing (separate procedure)   2 T ↻

MED: 100-2,15,260; 100-3,100.2; 100-4,12,90.3; 100-4,14,10
AMA: 1994,Spring,7

⊙ **44361** with biopsy, single or multiple   2 T ↻
MED: 100-2,15,260; 100-3,100.2; 100-4,12,90.3; 100-4,14,10

⊙ **44363** with removal of foreign body   2 T 80 ↻
MED: 100-2,15,260; 100-3,100.2; 100-4,12,90.3; 100-4,14,10

⊙ **44364** with removal of tumor(s), polyp(s), or other lesion(s) by snare technique   2 T 80 ↻
MED: 100-2,15,260; 100-3,100.2; 100-4,12,90.3; 100-4,14,10

⊙ **44365** with removal of tumor(s), polyp(s), or other lesion(s) by hot biopsy forceps or bipolar cautery   2 T 80 ↻
MED: 100-2,15,260; 100-3,100.2; 100-4,12,90.3; 100-4,14,10

⊙ **44366** with control of bleeding (eg, injection, bipolar cautery, unipolar cautery, laser, heater probe, stapler, plasma coagulator)   2 T ↻
MED: 100-2,15,260; 100-3,100.2; 100-4,12,90.3; 100-4,14,10

⊙ **44369** with ablation of tumor(s), polyp(s), or other lesion(s) not amenable to removal by hot biopsy forceps, bipolar cautery or snare technique   2 T 80 ↻
MED: 100-2,15,260; 100-3,100.2; 100-4,12,90.3; 100-4,14,10

⊙ **44370** with transendoscopic stent placement (includes predilation)   9 T 80 ↻
MED: 100-2,15,260; 100-4,4,61.2; 100-4,12,90.3; 100-4,14,10
AMA: 2001,Nov,7

⊙ **44372** with placement of percutaneous jejunostomy tube   2 T ↻
MED: 100-2,15,260; 100-3,100.2; 100-4,12,90.3; 100-4,14,10
AMA: 1994,Spring,7

⊙ **44373** with conversion of percutaneous gastrostomy tube to percutaneous jejunostomy tube   2 T ↻
MED: 100-2,15,260; 100-3,100.2; 100-4,12,90.3; 100-4,14,10
AMA: 1994,Spring,7

⊙ **44376** Small intestinal endoscopy, enteroscopy beyond second portion of duodenum, including ileum; diagnostic, with or without collection of specimen(s) by brushing or washing (separate procedure)   2 T 80 ↻
MED: 100-2,15,260; 100-3,100.2; 100-4,12,90.3; 100-4,14,10
AMA: 1994,Spring,7

⊙ **44377** with biopsy, single or multiple   2 T 80 ↻
MED: 100-2,15,260; 100-3,100.2; 100-4,12,90.3; 100-4,14,10
AMA: 1994,Spring,7

⊙ **44378** with control of bleeding (eg, injection, bipolar cautery, unipolar cautery, laser, heater probe, stapler, plasma coagulator)   2 T 80 ↻
MED: 100-2,15,260; 100-3,100.2; 100-4,12,90.3; 100-4,14,10
AMA: 1994,Spring,7

⊙ **44379** with transendoscopic stent placement (includes predilation)   9 T 80 ↻
MED: 100-2,15,260; 100-4,4,61.2; 100-4,12,90.3; 100-4,14,10
AMA: 2001,Nov,7

⊙ **44380** Ileoscopy, through stoma; diagnostic, with or without collection of specimen(s) by brushing or washing (separate procedure)   1 T ↻
MED: 100-2,15,260; 100-3,100.2; 100-4,12,90.3; 100-4,14,10

⊙ **44382** with biopsy, single or multiple   1 T ↻
MED: 100-2,15,260; 100-3,100.2; 100-4,12,90.3; 100-4,14,10

⊙ **44383** with transendoscopic stent placement (includes predilation)   9 T ↻
MED: 100-2,15,260; 100-4,4,61.2; 100-4,12,90.3; 100-4,14,10
AMA: 2001,Nov,7

⊙ **44385** Endoscopic evaluation of small intestinal (abdominal or pelvic) pouch; diagnostic, with or without collection of specimen(s) by brushing or washing (separate procedure)   1 T ↻
MED: 100-2,15,260; 100-3,100.2; 100-4,12,90.3; 100-4,14,10

⊙ **44386** with biopsy, single or multiple   1 T 80 ↻
MED: 100-2,15,260; 100-3,100.2; 100-4,12,90.3; 100-4,14,10

⊙ **44388** Colonoscopy through stoma; diagnostic, with or without collection of specimen(s) by brushing or washing (separate procedure)   1 T ↻
MED: 100-2,15,260; 100-3,100.2; 100-4,12,90.3; 100-4,14,10

If colonoscopy is performed via rectum, consult CPT codes 45330-45385.

⊙ **44389** with biopsy, single or multiple   1 T ↻
MED: 100-2,15,260; 100-3,100.2; 100-4,12,90.3; 100-4,14,10

⊙ **44390** with removal of foreign body   1 T 80 ↻
MED: 100-2,15,260; 100-3,100.2; 100-4,12,90.3; 100-4,14,10

⊙ **44391** with control of bleeding (eg, injection, bipolar cautery, unipolar cautery, laser, heater probe, stapler, plasma coagulator)   1 T 80 ↻
MED: 100-2,15,260; 100-3,100.2; 100-4,12,90.3; 100-4,14,10

⊛ Modifier 63 Exempt Code	⊙ Conscious Sedation	+ CPT Add-on Code
Ⓜ Maternity Edit	Ⓐ Age Edit	A-Y APC Status Indicators

⊘ Modifier 51 Exempt Code	● New Code
↻ CCI Comprehensive Code	▲ Revised Code
	50 Bilateral Procedure

Digestive

44392 — 44899

⊙ **44392** with removal of tumor(s), polyp(s), or other lesion(s) by hot biopsy forceps or bipolar cautery 🔳 Ⓣ ▣

MED: 100-2,15,260; 100-3,100.2; 100-4,12,90.3; 100-4,14,10

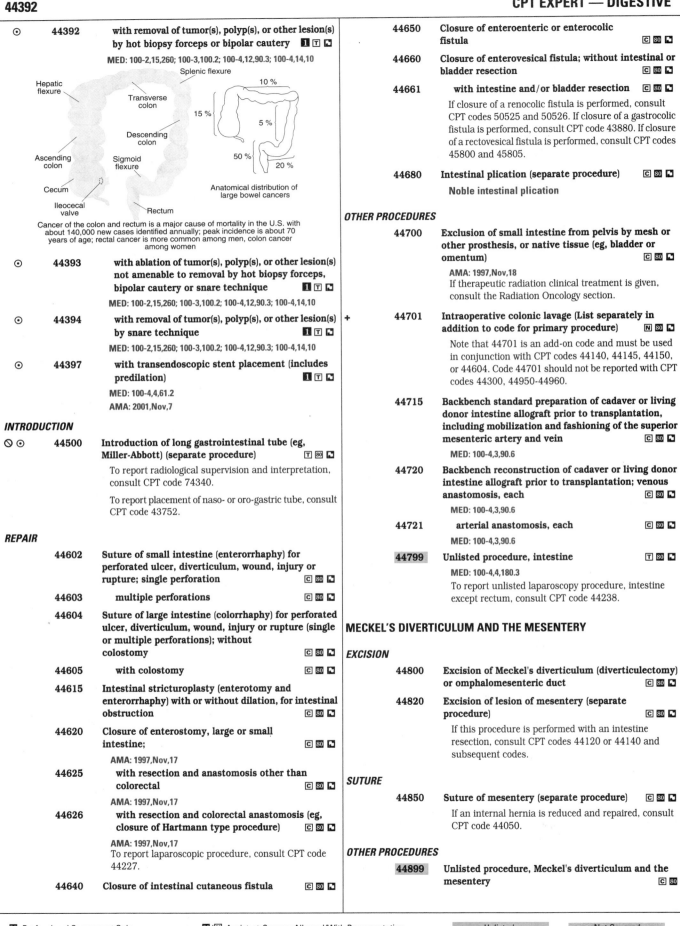

Hepatic flexure

Splenic flexure

Transverse colon

10 %

15 %

5 %

Descending colon

Ascending colon

Sigmoid flexure

50 %

20 %

Cecum

Ileocecal valve

Rectum

Anatomical distribution of large bowel cancers

Cancer of the colon and rectum is a major cause of mortality in the U.S. with about 140,000 new cases identified annually; peak incidence is about 70 years of age; rectal cancer is more common among men, colon cancer among women

⊙ **44393** with ablation of tumor(s), polyp(s), or other lesion(s) not amenable to removal by hot biopsy forceps, bipolar cautery or snare technique 🔳 Ⓣ ▣

MED: 100-2,15,260; 100-3,100.2; 100-4,12,90.3; 100-4,14,10

⊙ **44394** with removal of tumor(s), polyp(s), or other lesion(s) by snare technique 🔳 Ⓣ ▣

MED: 100-2,15,260; 100-3,100.2; 100-4,12,90.3; 100-4,14,10

⊙ **44397** with transendoscopic stent placement (includes predilation) 🔳 Ⓣ ▣

MED: 100-4,4,61.2

AMA: 2001,Nov,7

INTRODUCTION

⊘ ⊙ **44500** Introduction of long gastrointestinal tube (eg, Miller-Abbott) (separate procedure) Ⓣ 80 ▣

To report radiological supervision and interpretation, consult CPT code 74340.

To report placement of naso- or oro-gastric tube, consult CPT code 43752.

REPAIR

44602 Suture of small intestine (enterorrhaphy) for perforated ulcer, diverticulum, wound, injury or rupture; single perforation Ⓒ 80 ▣

44603 multiple perforations Ⓒ 80 ▣

44604 Suture of large intestine (colorrhaphy) for perforated ulcer, diverticulum, wound, injury or rupture (single or multiple perforations); without colostomy Ⓒ 80 ▣

44605 with colostomy Ⓒ 80 ▣

44615 Intestinal stricturoplasty (enterotomy and enterorrhaphy) with or without dilation, for intestinal obstruction Ⓒ 80 ▣

44620 Closure of enterostomy, large or small intestine; Ⓒ 80 ▣

AMA: 1997,Nov,17

44625 with resection and anastomosis other than colorectal Ⓒ 80 ▣

AMA: 1997,Nov,17

44626 with resection and colorectal anastomosis (eg, closure of Hartmann type procedure) Ⓒ 80 ▣

AMA: 1997,Nov,17
To report laparoscopic procedure, consult CPT code 44227.

44640 Closure of intestinal cutaneous fistula Ⓒ 80 ▣

44650 Closure of enteroenteric or enterocolic fistula Ⓒ 80 ▣

44660 Closure of enterovesical fistula; without intestinal or bladder resection Ⓒ 80 ▣

44661 with intestine and/or bladder resection Ⓒ 80 ▣

If closure of a renocolic fistula is performed, consult CPT codes 50525 and 50526. If closure of a gastrocolic fistula is performed, consult CPT code 43880. If closure of a rectovesical fistula is performed, consult CPT codes 45800 and 45805.

44680 Intestinal plication (separate procedure) Ⓒ 80 ▣

Noble intestinal plication

OTHER PROCEDURES

44700 Exclusion of small intestine from pelvis by mesh or other prosthesis, or native tissue (eg, bladder or omentum) Ⓒ 80 ▣

AMA: 1997,Nov,18
If therapeutic radiation clinical treatment is given, consult the Radiation Oncology section.

+ **44701** Intraoperative colonic lavage (List separately in addition to code for primary procedure) Ⓝ 80 ▣

Note that 44701 is an add-on code and must be used in conjunction with CPT codes 44140, 44145, 44150, or 44604. Code 44701 should not be reported with CPT codes 44300, 44950-44960.

44715 Backbench standard preparation of cadaver or living donor intestine allograft prior to transplantation, including mobilization and fashioning of the superior mesenteric artery and vein Ⓒ 80 ▣

MED: 100-4,3,90.6

44720 Backbench reconstruction of cadaver or living donor intestine allograft prior to transplantation; venous anastomosis, each Ⓒ 80 ▣

MED: 100-4,3,90.6

44721 arterial anastomosis, each Ⓒ 80 ▣

MED: 100-4,3,90.6

44799 Unlisted procedure, intestine Ⓣ 80 ▣

MED: 100-4,4,180.3
To report unlisted laparoscopy procedure, intestine except rectum, consult CPT code 44238.

MECKEL'S DIVERTICULUM AND THE MESENTERY

EXCISION

44800 Excision of Meckel's diverticulum (diverticulectomy) or omphalomesenteric duct Ⓒ 80 ▣

44820 Excision of lesion of mesentery (separate procedure) Ⓒ 80 ▣

If this procedure is performed with an intestine resection, consult CPT codes 44120 or 44140 and subsequent codes.

SUTURE

44850 Suture of mesentery (separate procedure) Ⓒ 80 ▣

If an internal hernia is reduced and repaired, consult CPT code 44050.

OTHER PROCEDURES

44899 Unlisted procedure, Meckel's diverticulum and the mesentery Ⓒ 80

CPT only © 2006 American Medical Association. All Rights Reserved. (Black Ink) © 2006 Ingenix (Blue Ink)

APPENDIX

INCISION

	44900	**Incision and drainage of appendiceal abscess; open** C 80
		AMA: 1997,Nov,18
⊙	**44901**	**percutaneous** T 80
		AMA: 1998,Mar,8; 1997,Nov,18

To report radiological supervision and interpretation, consult CPT code 75989.

EXCISION

Failure to treat appendicitis can lead to peritonitis

Ascending colon
Ileum
Cecum
Free tenia
Appendix and appendicular artery
Mesoappendix

Appendicitis, the inflammation and infection of the appendix, is most prevalent between the ages of 15 and 24

Peritonitis is the inflammation of the lining of the abdominal cavity

	44950	**Appendectomy;** C 80
		AMA: 1996,Sep,4

An incidental appendectomy during intra-abdominal surgery does not usually warrant a separate identification. However, if it is necessary to report, append modifier 52.

Battle's operation

+	**44955**	**when done for indicated purpose at time of other major procedure (not as separate procedure) (List separately in addition to code for primary procedure)** C 80
		AMA: 1996,Sep,4

Note that 44955 is an add-on code that must be used in conjunction with the appropriate code for the primary procedure. This code cannot be reported alone.

	44960	**for ruptured appendix with abscess or generalized peritonitis** C 80

Battle's operation

LAPAROSCOPY

Diagnostic laparoscopy is always include in surgical laparoscopy.

To report only diagnostic laparoscopy, consult CPT code 49320.

	44970	**Laparoscopy, surgical, appendectomy** T 80
		AMA: 2000,Mar,5; 1999,Nov,23
	44979	**Unlisted laparoscopy procedure, appendix** T 80 50
		AMA: 2000,Mar,5; 1999,Nov,23

RECTUM

INCISION

	45000	**Transrectal drainage of pelvic abscess** 1 T
		MED: 100-2,15,260; 100-4,12,90.3; 100-4,14,10
	45005	**Incision and drainage of submucosal abscess, rectum** 2 T
		MED: 100-2,15,260; 100-4,12,90.3; 100-4,14,10

	45020	**Incision and drainage of deep supralevator, pelvirectal, or retrorectal abscess** 2 T
		MED: 100-2,15,260; 100-4,12,90.3; 100-4,14,10

Consult also CPT codes 46050 and 46060.

EXCISION

	45100	**Biopsy of anorectal wall, anal approach (eg, congenital megacolon)** 1 T
		MED: 100-2,15,260; 100-4,12,90.3; 100-4,14,10

If an endoscopic biopsy is performed, consult CPT code 45305.

	45108	**Anorectal myomectomy** 2 T
		MED: 100-2,15,260; 100-4,12,90.3; 100-4,14,10
	45110	**Proctectomy; complete, combined abdominoperineal, with colostomy** C 80
	45111	**partial resection of rectum, transabdominal approach** C 80

Luschka proctectomy

	45112	**Proctectomy, combined abdominoperineal, pull-through procedure (eg, colo-anal anastomosis)** C 80
		AMA: 1997,Nov,18

If a colo-anal anastomosis is performed with the creation of a colonic reservoir or pouch, consult CPT code 45119.

	45113	**Proctectomy, partial, with rectal mucosectomy, ileoanal anastomosis, creation of ileal reservoir (S or J), with or without loop ileostomy** C 80
	45114	**Proctectomy, partial, with anastomosis; abdominal and transsacral approach** C 80
	45116	**transsacral approach only (Kraske type)** C 80
	45119	**Proctectomy, combined abdominoperineal pull-through procedure (eg, colo-anal anastomosis), with creation of colonic reservoir (eg, J-pouch), with diverting enterostomy when performed** C 80
		AMA: 1997,Nov,18

To report laparoscopic procedure, consult CPT code 45397.

	45120	**Proctectomy, complete (for congenital megacolon), abdominal and perineal approach; with pull-through procedure and anastomosis (eg, Swenson, Duhamel, or Soave type operation)** C 80
	45121	**with subtotal or total colectomy, with multiple biopsies** C 80
	45123	**Proctectomy, partial, without anastomosis, perineal approach** C 80
	45126	**Pelvic exenteration for colorectal malignancy, with proctectomy (with or without colostomy), with removal of bladder and ureteral transplantations, and/or hysterectomy, or cervicectomy, with or without removal of tube(s), with or without removal of ovary(s), or any combination thereof** C 80
		AMA: 1998,Nov,16
	45130	**Excision of rectal procidentia, with anastomosis; perineal approach** C 80

Altemeier procedure

	45135	**abdominal and perineal approach** C 80
	45136	**Excision of ileoanal reservoir with ileostomy** C 80

Code 45136 is not to be used with 44005, 44120, 44310.

45150   Division of stricture of rectum   2 T 80
         MED: 100-2,15,260; 100-4,12,90.3; 100-4,14,10

45160   Excision of rectal tumor by proctotomy, transsacral or transcoccygeal approach   2 T 80
         MED: 100-2,15,260; 100-4,12,90.3; 100-4,14,10

45170   Excision of rectal tumor, transanal approach   2 T 80
         MED: 100-2,15,260; 100-4,12,90.3; 100-4,14,10

DESTRUCTION

45190   Destruction of rectal tumor (eg, electrodesiccation, electrosurgery, laser ablation, laser resection, cryosurgery) transanal approach   9 T 80
         MED: 100-2,15,260; 100-4,12,90.3; 100-4,14,10

ENDOSCOPY

Diagnostic endoscopy is included in surgical endoscopy.

Transverse rectal fold
Transverse colon
Splenic flexure
Internal anal sphincter (involuntary)
Descending colon
Rectum
External anal sphincter (voluntary)
Pectinate line
Detail cutaway of lower rectum and anus
Sigmoid flexure
Anal canal
Rectum

The rectum is the section of colon below the sigmoid flexure and above the anal canal. The anal canal is the terminal part of the large intestine. The pectinate line marks the division in mucosal covering, innervation, and venous drainage

45300   Proctosigmoidoscopy, rigid; diagnostic, with or without collection of specimen(s) by brushing or washing (separate procedure)   T
         MED: 100-3,100.2
         AMA: 1997,Oct,6; 1994,Spring,8

⊙ 45303   with dilation (eg, balloon, guide wire, bougie)   T
         MED: 100-3,100.2
         AMA: 1997,Oct,6; 1994,Spring,8
         If radiological supervision and interpretation is performed, consult CPT code 74360.

⊙ 45305   with biopsy, single or multiple   1 T
         MED: 100-2,15,260; 100-3,100.2; 100-4,12,90.3; 100-4,14,10
         AMA: 1997,Oct,6

⊙ 45307   with removal of foreign body   1 T 80
         MED: 100-2,15,260; 100-3,100.2; 100-4,12,90.3; 100-4,14,10
         AMA: 1997,Oct,6; 1994,Spring,8

⊙ 45308   with removal of single tumor, polyp, or other lesion by hot biopsy forceps or bipolar cautery   1 T
         MED: 100-2,15,260; 100-3,100.2; 100-4,12,90.3; 100-4,14,10
         AMA: 1997,Oct,6; 1994,Spring,8

⊙ 45309   with removal of single tumor, polyp, or other lesion by snare technique   1 T
         MED: 100-2,15,260; 100-3,100.2; 100-4,12,90.3; 100-4,14,10
         AMA: 1997,Oct,6; 1994,Spring,8

⊙ 45315   with removal of multiple tumors, polyps, or other lesions by hot biopsy forceps, bipolar cautery or snare technique   1 T
         MED: 100-2,15,260; 100-3,100.2; 100-4,12,90.3; 100-4,14,10
         AMA: 1997,Oct,6; 1994,Spring,8

⊙ 45317   with control of bleeding (eg, injection, bipolar cautery, unipolar cautery, laser, heater probe, stapler, plasma coagulator)   1 T
         MED: 100-2,15,260; 100-3,100.2; 100-4,12,90.3; 100-4,14,10
         AMA: 1997,Oct,6; 1994,Spring,8

⊙ 45320   with ablation of tumor(s), polyp(s), or other lesion(s) not amenable to removal by hot biopsy forceps, bipolar cautery or snare technique (eg, laser)   1 T
         MED: 100-2,15,260; 100-3,100.2; 100-4,12,90.3; 100-4,14,10
         AMA: 1997,Oct,6; 1994,Spring,8

⊙ 45321   with decompression of volvulus   1 T
         MED: 100-2,15,260; 100-3,100.2; 100-4,12,90.3; 100-4,14,10
         AMA: 1997,Oct,6; 1994,Spring,8

⊙ 45327   with transendoscopic stent placement (includes predilation)   1 T
         MED: 100-4,4,61.2
         AMA: 2001,Nov,7

45330   Sigmoidoscopy, flexible; diagnostic, with or without collection of specimen(s) by brushing or washing (separate procedure)   T
         MED: 100-3,100.2; 100-4,12,30.1; 100-4,18,60.1
         AMA: 1994,Spring,9

45331   with biopsy, single or multiple   1 T
         MED: 100-2,15,260; 100-3,100.2; 100-4,12,90.3; 100-4,14,10
         AMA: 1996,Sep,6; 1994,Spring,9

⊙ 45332   with removal of foreign body   1 T
         MED: 100-2,15,260; 100-3,100.2; 100-4,12,90.3; 100-4,14,10
         AMA: 1994,Spring,9

⊙ 45333   with removal of tumor(s), polyp(s), or other lesion(s) by hot biopsy forceps or bipolar cautery   1 T
         MED: 100-2,15,260; 100-3,100.2; 100-4,12,90.3; 100-4,14,10
         AMA: 1994,Spring,9

⊙ 45334   with control of bleeding (eg, injection, bipolar cautery, unipolar cautery, laser, heater probe, stapler, plasma coagulator)   1 T
         MED: 100-2,15,260; 100-3,100.2; 100-4,12,90.3; 100-4,14,10
         AMA: 1996,Sep,6; 1994,Spring,9

⊙ 45335   with directed submucosal injection(s), any substance   1 T
         MED: 100-2,15,260; 100-3,100.2; 100-4,12,90.3; 100-4,14,10

⊙ 45337   with decompression of volvulus, any method   1 T
         MED: 100-2,15,260; 100-3,100.2; 100-4,12,90.3; 100-4,14,10
         AMA: 1994,Spring,9

⊙ 45338   with removal of tumor(s), polyp(s), or other lesion(s) by snare technique   1 T
         MED: 100-2,15,260; 100-3,100.2; 100-4,12,90.3; 100-4,14,10
         AMA: 1994,Spring,9

⊙ 45339   with ablation of tumor(s), polyp(s), or other lesion(s) not amenable to removal by hot biopsy forceps, bipolar cautery or snare technique   1 T
         MED: 100-2,15,260; 100-3,100.2; 100-4,12,90.3; 100-4,14,10
         AMA: 1994,Spring,9

⊙ 45340   with dilation by balloon, 1 or more strictures   1 T
         MED: 100-2,15,260; 100-3,100.2; 100-4,12,90.3; 100-4,14,10
         Do not report 45340 with CPT code 45345.

⊙ 45341   **with endoscopic ultrasound examination** 🔲 T 🔲
MED: 100-3,100.2; 100-3,220.5
AMA: 2001,Oct,4
To report transrectal ultrasound with rigid probe device, consult CPT code 76872.

Codes 76942 and 76975 cannot be reported with CPT code 45341.

⊙ 45342   **with transendoscopic ultrasound guided intramural or transmural fine needle aspiration/biopsy(s)** 🔲 T 🔲
MED: 100-3,100.2; 100-3,220.5
AMA: 2001,Oct,4
To report transrectal ultrasound with rigid probe device, consult CPT code 76872.

To report the interpretation of specimen, consult CPT codes 88172-88173.

Codes 76942 and 76975 cannot be reported with CPT code 45342.

⊙ 45345   **with transendoscopic stent placement (includes predilation)** 🔲 T 🔲
MED: 100-4,4,61.2
AMA: 2001,Nov,7

⊙ 45355   **Colonoscopy, rigid or flexible, transabdominal via colotomy, single or multiple** 🔲 T 🔲
MED: 100-2,15,260; 100-3,100.2; 100-4,12,40.6; 100-4,12,90.3; 100-4,14,10

⊙ 45378   **Colonoscopy, flexible, proximal to splenic flexure; diagnostic, with or without collection of specimen(s) by brushing or washing, with or without colon decompression (separate procedure)** 2 T 🔲
MED: 100-2,15,260; 100-3,100.2; 100-4,12,30.1; 100-4,12,40.6; 100-4,12,90.3; 100-4,14,10; 100-4,18,60.1
AMA: 1999,Aug,3; 1994,Spring,9

⊙ 45379   **with removal of foreign body** 2 T 🔲
MED: 100-2,15,260; 100-3,100.2; 100-4,12,90.3; 100-4,14,10
AMA: 1999,Aug,3; 1994,Spring,9

⊙ 45380   **with biopsy, single or multiple** 2 T 🔲
MED: 100-2,15,260; 100-3,100.2; 100-4,12,40.6; 100-4,12,90.3; 100-4,14,10
AMA: 1999,Feb,11; 1999,Aug,3; 1996,Jan,7; 1994,Spring,9

⊙ 45381   **with directed submucosal injection(s), any substance** 2 T 🔲
MED: 100-2,15,260; 100-3,100.2; 100-4,12,90.3; 100-4,14,10

⊙ 45382   **with control of bleeding (eg, injection, bipolar cautery, unipolar cautery, laser, heater probe, stapler, plasma coagulator)** 2 T 🔲
MED: 100-2,15,260; 100-3,100.2; 100-4,12,90.3; 100-4,14,10
AMA: 1999,Aug,3; 1994,Spring,9

⊙ 45383   **with ablation of tumor(s), polyp(s), or other lesion(s) not amenable to removal by hot biopsy forceps, bipolar cautery or snare technique** 2 T 🔲
MED: 100-2,15,260; 100-3,100.2; 100-4,12,90.3; 100-4,14,10
AMA: 1999,Aug,3; 1994,Spring,9

⊙ 45384   **with removal of tumor(s), polyp(s), or other lesion(s) by hot biopsy forceps or bipolar cautery** 2 T 🔲
MED: 100-2,15,260; 100-3,100.2; 100-4,12,90.3; 100-4,14,10
AMA: 1999,Feb,11; 1999,Aug,3; 1998,Jul,10; 1994,Spring,9

⊙ 45385   **with removal of tumor(s), polyp(s), or other lesion(s) by snare technique** 2 T 🔲
MED: 100-2,15,260; 100-3,100.2; 100-4,12,40.6; 100-4,12,90.3; 100-4,14,10
AMA: 1999,Aug,3; 1998,Jul,10; 1996,Jan,7; 1994,Spring,9
If a small intestine and stomal endoscopy is performed, consult CPT codes 44360-44393.

⊙ 45386   **with dilation by balloon, 1 or more strictures** 2 T 🔲
MED: 100-2,15,260; 100-3,100.2; 100-4,12,90.3; 100-4,14,10
Note that 45386 is not be used in conjunction with 45387.

⊙ 45387   **with transendoscopic stent placement (includes predilation)** 🔲 T 🔲
MED: 100-3,100.2; 100-4,4,61.2
AMA: 2001,Nov,7

⊙ 45391   **with endoscopic ultrasound examination** 2 T 🔲
Code 45391 cannot be reported with CPT codes 45330, 45341, 45342, 45378, 76872.

⊙ 45392   **with transendoscopic ultrasound guided intramural or transmural fine needle aspiration/biopsy(s)** 2 T 🔲
Code 45392 cannot be reported with CPT codes 45330, 45341, 45342, 45378, 76872.

LAPAROSCOPY

EXCISION

45395   **Laparoscopy, surgical; proctectomy, complete, combined abdominoperineal, with colostomy** C 80
To report open procedure, consult CPT code 45110.

45397   **proctectomy, combined abdominoperineal pull-through procedure (eg, colo-anal anastomosis), with creation of colonic reservoir (eg, J-pouch), with diverting enterostomy, when performed** C 80
To report open procedure, consult CPT code 45119.

REPAIR

45400   **Laparoscopy, surgical; proctopexy (for prolapse)** C 80
To report open procedure, consult CPT codes 45540, 45541.

45402   **proctopexy (for prolapse), with sigmoid resection** C 80
To report open procedure, consult CPT code 45550.

45499   **Unlisted laparoscopy procedure, rectum** T 80

REPAIR

45500   **Proctoplasty; for stenosis** 2 T 80 🔲
MED: 100-2,15,260; 100-4,12,90.3; 100-4,14,10

45505   **for prolapse of mucous membrane** 2 T 🔲
MED: 100-2,15,260; 100-4,12,90.3; 100-4,14,10

45520   **Perirectal injection of sclerosing solution for prolapse** T 🔲
AMA: 2001,Jul,11; 2001,Aug,10

45540   **Proctopexy (eg, for prolapse); abdominal approach** C 80 🔲
To report laparoscopic procedure, consult CPT code 45400.

45541   **perineal approach** T 80 🔲

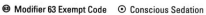

⑬ Modifier 63 Exempt Code   ⊙ Conscious Sedation   + CPT Add-on Code   ⊘ Modifier 51 Exempt Code   ● New Code   ▲ Revised Code

M Maternity Edit   A Age Edit   A-Y APC Status Indicators   🔲 CCI Comprehensive Code   50 Bilateral Procedure

Digestive

45550 — 46255

45550   **with sigmoid resection, abdominal approach**   C 80 ⬚

To report laparoscopic procedure, consult CPT code 45402.

Frickman proctopexy

45560   **Repair of rectocele (separate procedure)**   2 T 80 ⬚

MED: 100-2,15,260; 100-4,12,90.3; 100-4,14,10

If a rectocele is repaired with a posterior colporrhaphy, consult CPT code 57250.

45562   **Exploration, repair, and presacral drainage for rectal injury;**   C 80 ⬚

45563   **with colostomy**   C 80 ⬚

Maydl colostomy

Bladder | Pubic symphysis | Urethra

An anal fistula leading from the rectum to the skin near the anus contains a continual discharge that irritates the skin and causes discomfort or pain

Rectoperineal fistula

Fistulas are usually caused by a spreading abscess or an injury

Rectum

45800   **Closure of rectovesical fistula;**   C 80 ⬚

45805   **with colostomy**   C 80 ⬚

45820   **Closure of rectourethral fistula;**   C 80 ⬚

45825   **with colostomy**   C 80 ⬚

If a rectovaginal fistula is closed, consult CPT codes 57300-57308.

MANIPULATION

45900   **Reduction of procidentia (separate procedure) under anesthesia**   1 T 80 ⬚

MED: 100-2,15,260; 100-4,12,90.3; 100-4,14,10

45905   **Dilation of anal sphincter (separate procedure) under anesthesia other than local**   1 T ⬚

MED: 100-2,15,260; 100-4,12,90.3; 100-4,14,10

45910   **Dilation of rectal stricture (separate procedure) under anesthesia other than local**   1 T ⬚

MED: 100-2,15,260; 100-4,12,90.3; 100-4,14,10

45915   **Removal of fecal impaction or foreign body (separate procedure) under anesthesia**   1 T ⬚

MED: 100-2,15,260; 100-4,12,90.3; 100-4,14,10

OTHER PROCEDURES

45990   **Anorectal exam, surgical, requiring anesthesia (general, spinal, or epidural), diagnostic**   2 T 80

Code 45990 cannot be reported with 45300-45327, 46600, 57410, 99170.

45999   **Unlisted procedure, rectum**   T 80

MED: 100-4,4,180.3

To report unlisted laparoscopic procedure, rectum, consult CPT code 45499.

ANUS

INCISION

46020   **Placement of seton**   3 T ⬚

MED: 100-2,15,260; 100-4,14,90.3; 100-4,14,10

Code 46020 is not to be used in conjunction with 46060, 46280, 46600.

46030   **Removal of anal seton, other marker**   1 T 80 ⬚

MED: 100-2,15,260; 100-4,12,90.3; 100-4,14,10

46040   **Incision and drainage of ischiorectal and/or perirectal abscess (separate procedure)**   3 T ⬚

MED: 100-2,15,260; 100-4,12,90.3; 100-4,14,10

46045   **Incision and drainage of intramural, intramuscular, or submucosal abscess, transanal, under anesthesia**   2 T ⬚

MED: 100-2,15,260; 100-4,12,90.3; 100-4,14,10

46050   **Incision and drainage, perianal abscess, superficial**   1 T ⬚

MED: 100-2,15,260; 100-4,12,90.3; 100-4,14,10

Consult also CPT codes 45020 and 46060.

46060   **Incision and drainage of ischiorectal or intramural abscess, with fistulectomy or fistulotomy, submuscular, with or without placement of seton**   2 T ⬚

MED: 100-2,15,260; 100-4,12,90.3; 100-4,14,10

Consult also CPT code 45020.

Code 46060 is not to be used in conjunction with 46020.

46070   **Incision, anal septum (infant)**   A T 80 ⊛ ⬚

If anoplasty is performed, consult CPT codes 46700-46705.

46080   **Sphincterotomy, anal, division of sphincter (separate procedure)**   3 T ⬚

MED: 100-2,15,260; 100-4,12,90.3; 100-4,14,10

46083   **Incision of thrombosed hemorrhoid, external**   T ⬚

AMA: 1997,Jun,10

EXCISION

46200   **Fissurectomy, with or without sphincterotomy**   2 T ⬚

MED: 100-2,15,260; 100-4,12,90.3; 100-4,14,10

46210   **Cryptectomy; single**   2 T 80 ⬚

MED: 100-2,15,260; 100-4,12,90.3; 100-4,14,10

46211   **multiple (separate procedure)**   2 T 80 ⬚

MED: 100-2,15,260; 100-4,12,90.3; 100-4,14,10

46220   **Papillectomy or excision of single tag, anus (separate procedure)**   1 T ⬚

MED: 100-2,15,260; 100-4,12,90.3; 100-4,14,10

46221   **Hemorrhoidectomy, by simple ligature (eg, rubber band)**   T ⬚

AMA: 1997,Oct,6

46230   **Excision of external hemorrhoid tags and/or multiple papillae**   1 T ⬚

46250   **Hemorrhoidectomy, external, complete**   3 T ⬚

MED: 100-2,15,260; 100-4,12,90.3; 100-4,14,10

46255   **Hemorrhoidectomy, internal and external, simple;**   3 T ⬚

MED: 100-2,15,260; 100-4,12,90.3; 100-4,14,10

46257   with fissurectomy   ③ T ▣

MED: 100-2,15,260; 100-4,12,90.3; 100-4,14,10

46258   with fistulectomy, with or without fissurectomy   ③ T 80 ▣

MED: 100-2,15,260; 100-4,12,90.3; 100-4,14,10

46260   **Hemorrhoidectomy, internal and external, complex or extensive;**   ③ T ▣

MED: 100-2,15,260; 100-4,12,90.3; 100-4,14,10

Whitehead hemorrhoidectomy

46261   with fissurectomy   ④ T ▣

MED: 100-2,15,260; 100-4,12,90.3; 100-4,14,10

46262   with fistulectomy, with or without fissurectomy   ④ T ▣

MED: 100-2,15,260; 100-4,12,90.3; 100-4,14,10

To report injection of hemorrhoids, consult CPT code 46500; to report destruction, consult CPT codes 46934-46936; to report ligation, consult CPT codes 46945, 46946; to report hemorrhoidopexy consult, CPT code 46947.

46270   **Surgical treatment of anal fistula (fistulectomy/fistulotomy); subcutaneous**   ③ T ▣

MED: 100-2,15,260; 100-4,12,90.3; 100-4,14,10

46275   submuscular   ③ T ▣

MED: 100-2,15,260; 100-4,12,90.3; 100-4,14,10

46280   complex or multiple, with or without placement of seton   ④ T ▣

MED: 100-2,15,260; 100-4,12,90.3; 100-4,14,10

Do not report 46280 in conjunction with CPT code 46020.

46285   second stage   ① T ▣

MED: 100-2,15,260; 100-4,12,90.3; 100-4,14,10

46288   **Closure of anal fistula with rectal advancement flap**   ④ T ▣

MED: 100-2,15,260; 100-4,12,90.3; 100-4,14,10

46320   **Enucleation or excision of external thrombotic hemorrhoid**   T ▣

INTRODUCTION

Varicose veins commonly develop in the lower legs, particularly in the elderly, when impaired valves cause the vessels to swell and become inflamed; the risk of clot formation increases with inflamed veins; thrombophlebitis is the inflammation which may result in blood clots in veins

Rectum

Valve cusps become incompetent in the varicose vein causing blood to pool

Anal sphincter

Internal hemorrhoid

External hemorrhoid

Thrombus (blood clot)

Varicose veins and hemorrhoids (varicose rectal veins) are often associated; internal hemorrhoids (also called piles) are varicosities of the tributaries of the superior rectal veins and are covered by mucous membranes; external hemorrhoids are of the inferior rectal veins and are covered by skin

46500   **Injection of sclerosing solution, hemorrhoids**   T ▣

To report excision of hemorrhoids, consult CPT codes 46250-46262; to report destruction, consult CPT codes 46934-46936; to report ligation, consult CPT codes 46945, 46946; to report hemorrhoidopexy, consult CPT code 46947.

46505   **Chemodenervation of internal anal sphincter**   T 50

To report chemodenervation of other muscles, consult CPT codes 64612-64614, 64640.

Report the specific service in addition to the specific substance(s) or drug(s) provided.

ENDOSCOPY

Diagnostic endoscopy is always included in surgical endoscopy.

46600   **Anoscopy; diagnostic, with or without collection of specimen(s) by brushing or washing (separate procedure)**   ⊠ ▣

MED: 100-3,100.2

AMA: 1997,Oct,6; 1994,Spring,9

Do not report 46600 in conjunction with CPT code 46020.

46604   with dilation (eg, balloon, guide wire, bougie)   T ▣

MED: 100-3,100.2

AMA: 1997,Oct,6; 1994,Spring,9

46606   with biopsy, single or multiple   T ▣

MED: 100-3,100.2; 100-4,12,40.6

AMA: 1997,Oct,6; 1994,Spring,9

46608   with removal of foreign body   ① T 80 ▣

MED: 100-2,15,260; 100-3,100.2; 100-4,12,40.6; 100-4,12,90.3; 100-4,14,10

AMA: 1997,Oct,6; 1994,Spring,9

46610   with removal of single tumor, polyp, or other lesion by hot biopsy forceps or bipolar cautery   ① T ▣

MED: 100-2,15,260; 100-3,100.2; 100-4,12,90.3; 100-4,14,10

AMA: 1997,Oct,6; 1994,Spring,10

46611   with removal of single tumor, polyp, or other lesion by snare technique   ① T 80 ▣

MED: 100-2,15,260; 100-3,100.2; 100-4,12,90.3; 100-4,14,10

AMA: 1997,Oct,6; 1994,Spring,10

46612   with removal of multiple tumors, polyps, or other lesions by hot biopsy forceps, bipolar cautery or snare technique   ① T 80 ▣

MED: 100-2,15,260; 100-3,100.2; 100-4,12,90.3; 100-4,14,10

AMA: 1997,Oct,6; 1994,Spring,10

46614   with control of bleeding (eg, injection, bipolar cautery, unipolar cautery, laser, heater probe, stapler, plasma coagulator)   T ▣

MED: 100-3,100.2

AMA: 1997,Oct,6; 1994,Spring,10

46615   with ablation of tumor(s), polyp(s), or other lesion(s) not amenable to removal by hot biopsy forceps, bipolar cautery or snare technique   ② T 80 ▣

MED: 100-2,15,260; 100-3,100.2; 100-4,12,90.3; 100-4,14,10

AMA: 1997,Oct,6; 1994,Spring,10

REPAIR

46700   **Anoplasty, plastic operation for stricture; adult**   ③ T ▣

MED: 100-2,15,260; 100-4,12,90.3; 100-4,14,10

46705   infant   C 80 ⊛ ▣

If a simple incision of the anal septum is performed, consult CPT code 46070.

46706   **Repair of anal fistula with fibrin glue**   ① T ▣

46710   **Repair of ileoanal pouch fistula/sinus (eg, perineal or vaginal), pouch advancement; transperineal approach**   C 80

46712	combined transperineal and transabdominal approach	C 80
46715	Repair of low imperforate anus; with anoperineal fistula (cut-back procedure)	C 80 63 ⬚
46716	with transposition of anoperineal or anovestibular fistula	C 80 63 ⬚
46730	Repair of high imperforate anus without fistula; perineal or sacroperineal approach	C 80 63 ⬚
46735	combined transabdominal and sacroperineal approaches	C 80 63 ⬚
46740	Repair of high imperforate anus with rectourethral or rectovaginal fistula; perineal or sacroperineal approach	C 80 63 ⬚
46742	combined transabdominal and sacroperineal approaches	C 80 63 ⬚
46744	Repair of cloacal anomaly by anorectovaginoplasty and urethroplasty, sacroperineal approach	♀ C 80 63 ⬚
46746	Repair of cloacal anomaly by anorectovaginoplasty and urethroplasty, combined abdominal and sacroperineal approach;	♀ C 80 ⬚
46748	with vaginal lengthening by intestinal graft or pedicle flaps	♀ C 80 ⬚
46750	Sphincteroplasty, anal, for incontinence or prolapse; adult	3 T 80 ⬚

MED: 100-2,15,260; 100-3,230.10; 100-4,12,90.3; 100-4,14,10

| 46751 | child | A C 80 ⬚ |
| 46753 | Graft (Thiersch operation) for rectal incontinence and/or prolapse | 3 T ⬚ |

MED: 100-2,15,260; 100-3,230.10; 100-4,12,90.3; 100-4,14,10

| 46754 | Removal of Thiersch wire or suture, anal canal | 2 T 80 ⬚ |

MED: 100-2,15,260; 100-4,12,90.3; 100-4,14,10

| 46760 | Sphincteroplasty, anal, for incontinence, adult; muscle transplant | 2 T 80 ⬚ |

MED: 100-2,15,260; 100-3,230.10; 100-4,12,90.3; 100-4,14,10

| 46761 | levator muscle imbrication (Park posterior anal repair) | 3 T 80 ⬚ |

MED: 100-2,15,260; 100-4,12,90.3; 100-4,14,10

| 46762 | implantation artificial sphincter | 7 T 80 ⬚ |

MED: 100-2,15,260; 100-4,12,90.3; 100-4,14,10

DESTRUCTION

46900	Destruction of lesion(s), anus (eg, condyloma, papilloma, molluscum contagiosum, herpetic vesicle), simple; chemical	T ⬚
46910	electrodesiccation	T ⬚
46916	cryosurgery	T ⬚

MED: 100-3,140.5

| 46917 | laser surgery | 1 T ⬚ |

MED: 100-2,15,260; 100-3,140.5; 100-4,12,90.3; 100-4,14,10

| 46922 | surgical excision | 1 T ⬚ |

MED: 100-2,15,260; 100-4,12,90.3; 100-4,14,10

| 46924 | Destruction of lesion(s), anus (eg, condyloma, papilloma, molluscum contagiosum, herpetic vesicle), extensive (eg, laser surgery, electrosurgery, cryosurgery, chemosurgery) | 1 T ⬚ |

MED: 100-2,15,260; 100-4,12,90.3; 100-4,14,10

46934	Destruction of hemorrhoids, any method; internal	T ⬚
46935	external	T ⬚
46936	internal and external	T ⬚

To report excision of hemorrhoids, consult CPT codes 46250-46262; to report injection, consult CPT code 46500; to report ligation, consult CPT codes 46945, 46946; to report hemorrhoidopexy, consult CPT code 46947.

| 46937 | Cryosurgery of rectal tumor; benign | 2 T 80 ⬚ |

MED: 100-2,15,260; 100-4,12,90.3; 100-4,14,10

| 46938 | malignant | 2 T 80 ⬚ |

MED: 100-2,15,260; 100-4,12,90.3; 100-4,14,10

| 46940 | Curettage or cautery of anal fissure, including dilation of anal sphincter (separate procedure); initial | T ⬚ |
| 46942 | subsequent | T 80 ⬚ |

SUTURE

46945	Ligation of internal hemorrhoids; single procedure	T ⬚
46946	multiple procedures	1 T ⬚
46947	Hemorrhoidopexy (eg, for prolapsing internal hemorrhoids) by stapling	7 T ⬚

To report excision of hemorrhoids, consult CPT codes 46250-46262; to report injection, consult CPT code 46500; to report destruction, consult CPT codes 46934-46936.

OTHER PROCEDURES

| 46999 | Unlisted procedure, anus | T 80 |

MED: 100-4,4,180.3
AMA: 1997,Oct,6

LIVER

INCISION

The liver is divided into four lobes for descriptive purposes, although the left and right halves are functionally separate, each receiving its own arterial supply and venous drainage. The liver is the largest gland in the body and serves many metabolic purposes including secretion of bile. The gallbladder is located on the visceral side of the quadrate lobe and stores bile between active phases of digestion; positions of the sac and its structures varies

| 47000 | Biopsy of liver, needle; percutaneous | 1 T ⬚ |

MED: 100-2,15,260; 100-4,12,90.3; 100-4,14,10
AMA: 1993,Fall,12
To report imaging guidance, consult CPT codes 76942, 77002, 77012, and 77021.

26 Professional Component Only 80/80 Assist-at-Surgery Allowed/With Documentation   Unlisted   Not Covered

TC Technical Component Only **MED:** Pub 100/NCD References **AMA:** CPT Assistant References 1-9 ASC Group ♂ Male Only ♀ Female Only

174 — CPT Expert CPT only © 2006 American Medical Association. All Rights Reserved. *(Black Ink)* © *2006 Ingenix (Blue Ink)*

+ 47001   when done for indicated purpose at time of other major procedure (List separately in addition to code for primary procedure)   N ☐

To report imaging guidance, consult CPT codes 76942, 77002.

To report fine needle aspiration in conjunction with 47000, 47001, consult CPT codes 10021, 10022.

To report evaluation of fine needle aspirate consult CPT codes 88172, 88173.

Note that 47001 is an add-on code that must be used in conjunction with the appropriate code for the primary procedure. This code cannot be reported alone.

47010   Hepatotomy; for open drainage of abscess or cyst, one or two stages   C 80 ☐

AMA: 1997,Nov,18

⊙ **47011**   for percutaneous drainage of abscess or cyst, one or two stages   T 80 ☐

AMA: 1998,Mar,8; 1997,Nov,18

To report radiological supervision and interpretation, consult CPT code 75989.

Esophagus / Quadrate / Diaphragm / Right lobe / Left lobe / Caudate / Stomach

Quadrants are defined by H-shaped grooves on the visceral side

Steatosis (fatty liver) / Abstinence / Continued use / Cirrhosis / Normal / Continued use / Repeated attacks / Abstinence / Hepatitis

Interelationships among alcoholic steatosis, hepatitis, and cirrhosis

The liver is the largest gland in the body and serves many metabolic purposes including secretion of bile. Chronic alcohol use leads to three similar forms of alcoholic liver disease: steatosis (fatty liver), hepatitis, and cirrhosis. The conditions have many overlapping features and each may occur without involvement of alcohol. Alcoholic cirrhosis accounts for about 60 percent of all cirrhosis cases and the risk appears to rise with the amount of alcohol consumed daily. The liver tends to shrink and become fibrotic

47015   Laparotomy, with aspiration and/or injection of hepatic parasitic (eg, amoebic or echinococcal) cyst(s) or abscess(es)   C 80 ☐

EXCISION

47100   Biopsy of liver, wedge   C 80 ☐

MED: 100-4,3,20.2.1

47120   Hepatectomy, resection of liver; partial lobectomy   C 80 ☐

AMA: 1998,May,10

47122   trisegmentectomy   C 80 ☐

47125   total left lobectomy   C 80 ☐

47130   total right lobectomy   C 80 ☐

LIVER TRANSPLANTATION

Liver transplantation involves three different components:

- Cadaver or living donor hepatectomy which consists of harvesting and cold preparation of the graft prior to transplantation and care of the donor, in the case of living donor hepatectomy, (see 47133, 47140-47142).
- Backbench work consists of preparation of donor liver prior to transplantation. This includes preparation of whole liver graft including dissection and removal of surrounding tissue and soft tissue, preparation of the vena cava, portal vein, hepatic artery and common bile duct. Also included is preparation of the whole liver with splitting of the liver for partial grafts. Additional reconstruction of the liver graft including venous and arterial anastomosis(es) may also be performed. (See 47143-47147).
- Recipient transplantation which includes transplanting the liver into the patient and care of the recipient (see 47135-47136).

47133   Donor hepatectomy (including cold preservation), from cadaver donor   C ☐

MED: 100-4,3,90.4; 100-4,3,90.4.1; 100-4,3,90.4.2

47135   Liver allotransplantation; orthotopic, partial or whole, from cadaver or living donor, any age   C 80 ☐

MED: 100-2,15,50.5; 100-2,15,60.3; 100-3,260.1; 100-3,260.2; 100-4,3,90.4.1; 100-4,3,90.4.2; 100-4,3,90.6

47136   heterotopic, partial or whole, from cadaver or living donor, any age   C 80 ☐

MED: 100-2,15,50.5; 100-2,15,60.3; 100-3,260.1; 100-3,260.2; 100-4,3,90.4; 100-4,3,90.4.1; 100-4,3,90.4.2; 100-4,3,90.6

47140   Donor hepatectomy (including cold preservation), from living donor; left lateral segment only (segments II and III)   C 80 ☐

MED: 100-4,3,90.4.1; 100-4,3,90.4.2

47141   total left lobectomy (segments II, III and IV)   C 80 ☐

MED: 100-4,3,90.4.1; 100-4,3,90.4.2

47142   total right lobectomy (segments V, VI, VII and VIII)   C 80 ☐

MED: 100-4,3,90.4.1; 100-4,3,90.4.2

47143   Backbench standard preparation of cadaver donor whole liver graft prior to allotransplantation, including cholecystectomy, if necessary, and dissection and removal of surrounding soft tissues to prepare the vena cava, portal vein, hepatic artery, and common bile duct for implantation; without trisegment or lobe split   C 80 ☐

MED: 100-4,3,90.4.1; 100-4,3,90.4.2

47144   with trisegment split of whole liver graft into two partial liver grafts (ie, left lateral segment (segments II and III) and right trisegment (segments I and IV through VIII))   C 80 ☐

MED: 100-4,3,90.4.1; 100-4,3,90.4.2

47145   with lobe split of whole liver graft into two partial liver grafts (ie, left lobe (segments II, III, and IV) and right lobe (segments I and V through VIII))   C 80 ☐

MED: 100-4,3,90.4.1; 100-4,3,90.4.2

47146   Backbench reconstruction of cadaver or living donor liver graft prior to allotransplantation; venous anastomosis, each   C 80 ☐

MED: 100-4,3,90.4.1; 100-4,3,90.4.2

47147   arterial anastomosis, each   C 80 ☐

MED: 100-4,3,90.4.1; 100-4,3,90.4.2

Codes 47143-47147 cannot be reported with CPT codes 47120-47125, 47600, 47610.

REPAIR

47300   Marsupialization of cyst or abscess of liver   C 80 ☐

47350   Management of liver hemorrhage; simple suture of liver wound or injury   C 80 ☐

47360   complex suture of liver wound or injury, with or without hepatic artery ligation   C 80 ☐

47361   exploration of hepatic wound, extensive debridement, coagulation and/or suture, with or without packing of liver   C 80 ☐

47362   re-exploration of hepatic wound for removal of packing   C 80 ☐

LAPAROSCOPY

Diagnostic laparoscopy is included in surgical laparoscopy. To report only a diagnostic laparoscopy, consult CPT code 49320.

---

⑤ Modifier 63 Exempt Code   ⊙ Conscious Sedation   + CPT Add-on Code   ⊘ Modifier 51 Exempt Code   ● New Code   ▲ Revised Code

M Maternity Edit   A Age Edit   A-Y APC Status Indicators   ☐ CCI Comprehensive Code   50 Bilateral Procedure

47370 Laparoscopy, surgical, ablation of one or more liver tumor(s); radiofrequency T 80 ▣

AMA: 2002,Oct,1
To report imaging guidance, consult CPT code 76940.

47371 cryosurgical T 80 ▣

47379 Unlisted laparoscopic procedure, liver T 80

OTHER PROCEDURES

47380 Ablation, open, of one or more liver tumor(s); radiofrequency C 80 ▣

AMA: 2002,Oct,1
To report imaging guidance, consult CPT code 76940.

47381 cryosurgical C 80 ▣

47382 Ablation, one or more liver tumor(s), percutaneous, radiofrequency T 80 ▣

AMA: 2002,Oct,1
To report imaging guidance and monitoring, consult CPT codes 76940, 77013, or 77022.

47399 Unlisted procedure, liver T 80

MED: 100-4,4,180.3

BILIARY TRACT

INCISION

47400 Hepaticotomy or hepaticostomy with exploration, drainage, or removal of calculus C 80 ▣

47420 Choledochotomy or choledochostomy with exploration, drainage, or removal of calculus, with or without cholecystotomy; without transduodenal sphincterotomy or sphincteroplasty C 80 ▣

47425 with transduodenal sphincterotomy or sphincteroplasty C 80 ▣

47460 Transduodenal sphincterotomy or sphincteroplasty, with or without transduodenal extraction of calculus (separate procedure) C 80 ▣

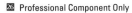

Gallbladder
R. hepatic duct
L. hepatic duct
Common hepatic duct
Cystic duct
Common bile duct (choledochus)
Drainage tube
Calculi (stones) are removed if present

The gallbladder is incised, explored, and possibly drained of infection or other fluids. Calculi, if present, are removed

Access is usually by a subcostal or upper midline incision. A drainage tube, if used, will be brought through the skin surface via a separate stab incision

47480 Cholecystotomy or cholecystostomy with exploration, drainage, or removal of calculus (separate procedure) C 80 ▣

47490 Percutaneous cholecystostomy T ▣

To report radiological supervision and interpretation, consult CPT code 75989.

INTRODUCTION

47500 Injection procedure for percutaneous transhepatic cholangiography N ▣

To report radiological supervision and interpretation, consult CPT code 74320.

47505 Injection procedure for cholangiography through an existing catheter (eg, percutaneous transhepatic or T-tube) N 80 ▣

To report radiological supervision and interpretation, consult CPT code 74305.

47510 Introduction of percutaneous transhepatic catheter for biliary drainage 2 T ▣

MED: 100-2,15,260; 100-4,12,90.3; 100-4,14,10
To report radiological supervision and interpretation, consult CPT code 75980.

47511 Introduction of percutaneous transhepatic stent for internal and external biliary drainage 9 T 50 ▣

MED: 100-2,15,260; 100-4,12,90.3; 100-4,14,10
To report radiological supervision and interpretation, consult CPT code 75982.

47525 Change of percutaneous biliary drainage catheter 1 T 50 ▣

MED: 100-2,15,260; 100-4,12,90.3; 100-4,14,10
To report radiological supervision and interpretation, consult CPT code 75984.

47530 Revision and/or reinsertion of transhepatic tube 1 T ▣

MED: 100-2,15,260; 100-4,12,90.3; 100-4,14,10
To report radiological supervision and interpretation, consult CPT code 75984.

ENDOSCOPY

Diagnostic endoscopy is always included in surgical endoscopy.

+ **47550** Biliary endoscopy, intraoperative (choledochoscopy) (List separately in addition to code for primary procedure) C 80

MED: 100-3,100.2
Note that 47550 is an add-on code that must be used in conjunction with the appropriate code for the primary procedure. This code cannot be reported alone.

47552 Biliary endoscopy, percutaneous via T-tube or other tract; diagnostic, with or without collection of specimen(s) by brushing and/or washing (separate procedure) 2 T ▣

MED: 100-2,15,260; 100-3,100.2; 100-4,12,90.3; 100-4,14,10

47553 with biopsy, single or multiple 3 T ▣

MED: 100-2,15,260; 100-3,100.2; 100-4,12,90.3; 100-4,14,10

47554 with removal of calculus/calculi 3 T ▣

MED: 100-2,15,260; 100-3,100.2; 100-4,12,90.3; 100-4,14,10

47555 with dilation of biliary duct stricture(s) without stent 3 T ▣

MED: 100-2,15,260; 100-3,100.2; 100-4,12,90.3; 100-4,14,10
If imaging guidance is provided, consult CPT codes 74363, 75982.

If an endoscopic retrograde cholangiopancreatography (ERCP) is performed, consult CPT codes 43260-43272 and 74363.

47556 with dilation of biliary duct stricture(s) with stent 9 T ▣

MED: 100-2,15,260; 100-3,100.2; 100-4,12,90.3; 100-4,14,10
If imaging guidance is provided, consult CPT codes 74363, 75982.

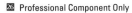
26 Professional Component Only   80/80 Assist-at-Surgery Allowed/With Documentation   Unlisted   Not Covered

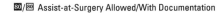
TC Technical Component Only   MED: Pub 100/NCD References   AMA: CPT Assistant References   1-9 ASC Group   ♂ Male Only   ♀ Female Only

176 — CPT Expert   CPT only © 2006 American Medical Association. All Rights Reserved. (Black Ink)   © 2006 Ingenix (Blue Ink)

LAPAROSCOPY

Diagnostic laparoscopy is always included in surgical laparoscopy. To report only a diagnostic laparoscopy, consult CPT code 49320.

47560 **Laparoscopy, surgical; with guided transhepatic cholangiography, without biopsy** ⓷ Ⓣ ⑧⓪ ◪

MED: 100-2,15,260; 100-4,12,90.3; 100-4,14,10
AMA: 2000,Mar,5; 1999,Nov,23

47561 **with guided transhepatic cholangiography with biopsy** ⓷ Ⓣ ⑧⓪ ◪

MED: 100-2,15,260; 100-3,100.13; 100-4,12,90.3; 100-4,14,10
AMA: 2000,Mar,5; 1999,Nov,23

47562 **cholecystectomy** Ⓣ ⑧⓪ ◪

MED: 100-3,100.13
AMA: 2000,Mar,5; 1999,Nov,23

47563 **cholecystectomy with cholangiography** Ⓣ ⑧⓪ ◪

MED: 100-3,100.13
AMA: 2000,Mar,5; 2000,Dec,14; 1999,Nov,23

47564 **cholecystectomy with exploration of common duct** Ⓣ ⑧⓪ ◪

MED: 100-3,100.13
AMA: 2000,Mar,5; 1999,Nov,23

47570 **cholecystoenterostomy** Ⓒ ⑧⓪ ◪

AMA: 2000,Mar,5; 1999,Nov,23

47579 Unlisted laparoscopy procedure, biliary tract Ⓣ ⑧⓪ ⑤⓪

AMA: 2000,Mar,5; 1999,Nov,23

EXCISION

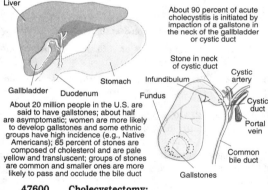

Liver

About 90 percent of acute cholecystitis is initiated by impaction of a gallstone in the neck of the gallbladder or cystic duct

Stone in neck of cystic duct

Cystic artery

Infundibulum

Gallbladder   Duodenum   Stomach   Fundus   Cystic duct

Portal vein

About 20 million people in the U.S. are said to have gallstones; about half are asymptomatic; women are more likely to develop gallstones and some ethnic groups have high incidence (e.g., Native Americans); 85 percent of stones are composed of cholesterol and are pale yellow and transluscent; groups of stones are common and smaller ones are more likely to pass and occlude the bile duct

Common bile duct

Gallstones

47600 **Cholecystectomy;** Ⓒ ⑧⓪ ◪

AMA: 1999,Nov,24
To report laparoscopic approach, consult CPT codes 47562-47564.

47605 **with cholangiography** Ⓒ ⑧⓪ ◪

AMA: 2002,Apr,19; 1999,Nov,24

47610 **Cholecystectomy with exploration of common duct;** Ⓒ ⑧⓪ ◪

AMA: 2002,Apr,19

47612 **with choledochoenterostomy** Ⓒ ⑧⓪ ◪

47620 **with transduodenal sphincterotomy or sphincteroplasty, with or without cholangiography** Ⓒ ⑧⓪ ◪

47630 **Biliary duct stone extraction, percutaneous via T-tube tract, basket, or snare (eg, Burhenne technique)** ⓷ Ⓣ ◪

MED: 100-2,15,260; 100-4,12,90.3; 100-4,14,10
AMA: 1998,Jun,10
To report radiological supervision and interpretation, consult CPT code 74327.

47700 **Exploration for congenital atresia of bile ducts, without repair, with or without liver biopsy, with or without cholangiography** Ⓒ ⑧⓪ ㊿ ◪

47701 **Portoenterostomy (eg, Kasai procedure)** Ⓒ ⑧⓪ ㊿ ◪

47711 **Excision of bile duct tumor, with or without primary repair of bile duct; extrahepatic** Ⓒ ⑧⓪ ◪

47712 **intrahepatic** Ⓒ ⑧⓪ ◪

If anastomosis is performed, consult CPT codes 47760-47800.

47715 **Excision of choledochal cyst** Ⓒ ⑧⓪ ◪

~~**47716**~~ ~~Anastomosis, choledochal cyst, without excision~~

Use 47719.

REPAIR

● **47719** Anastomosis, choledochal cyst, without excision Ⓒ

47720 **Cholecystoenterostomy; direct** Ⓒ ⑧⓪ ◪

AMA: 1999,Nov,24
If a laparoscopic approach is used, consult CPT code 47570.

47721 **with gastroenterostomy** Ⓒ ⑧⓪ ◪

47740 **Roux-en-Y** Ⓒ ⑧⓪ ◪

47741 **Roux-en-Y with gastroenterostomy** Ⓒ ⑧⓪ ◪

47760 **Anastomosis, of extrahepatic biliary ducts and gastrointestinal tract** Ⓒ ⑧⓪ ◪

47765 **Anastomosis, of intrahepatic ducts and gastrointestinal tract** Ⓒ ⑧⓪ ◪

Longmire anastomosis

47780 **Anastomosis, Roux-en-Y, of extrahepatic biliary ducts and gastrointestinal tract** Ⓒ ⑧⓪ ◪

47785 **Anastomosis, Roux-en-Y, of intrahepatic biliary ducts and gastrointestinal tract** Ⓒ ⑧⓪ ◪

47800 **Reconstruction, plastic, of extrahepatic biliary ducts with end-to-end anastomosis** Ⓒ ⑧⓪ ◪

47801 **Placement of choledochal stent** Ⓒ ⑧⓪ ◪

47802 **U-tube hepaticoenterostomy** Ⓒ ⑧⓪ ◪

47900 **Suture of extrahepatic biliary duct for pre-existing injury (separate procedure)** Ⓒ ⑧⓪ ◪

OTHER PROCEDURES

47999 Unlisted procedure, biliary tract Ⓣ ⑧⓪

MED: 100-4,4,180.3

PANCREAS

If peroral pancreatic endoscopic procedures are performed, consult CPT codes 43260-43272.

INCISION

48000 **Placement of drains, peripancreatic, for acute pancreatitis;** Ⓒ ⑧⓪ ◪

48001 **with cholecystostomy, gastrostomy, and jejunostomy** Ⓒ ⑧⓪ ◪

~~**48005**~~ ~~Resection or debridement of pancreas and peripancreatic tissue for acute necrotizing pancreatitis~~

Use 48105.

⊚ Modifier 63 Exempt Code   ⊙ Conscious Sedation   ＋ CPT Add-on Code   ⊘ Modifier 51 Exempt Code   ● New Code   ▲ Revised Code

Ⓜ Maternity Edit   Ⓐ Age Edit   Ⓐ-Ⓨ APC Status Indicators   ◪ CCI Comprehensive Code   ㊿ Bilateral Procedure

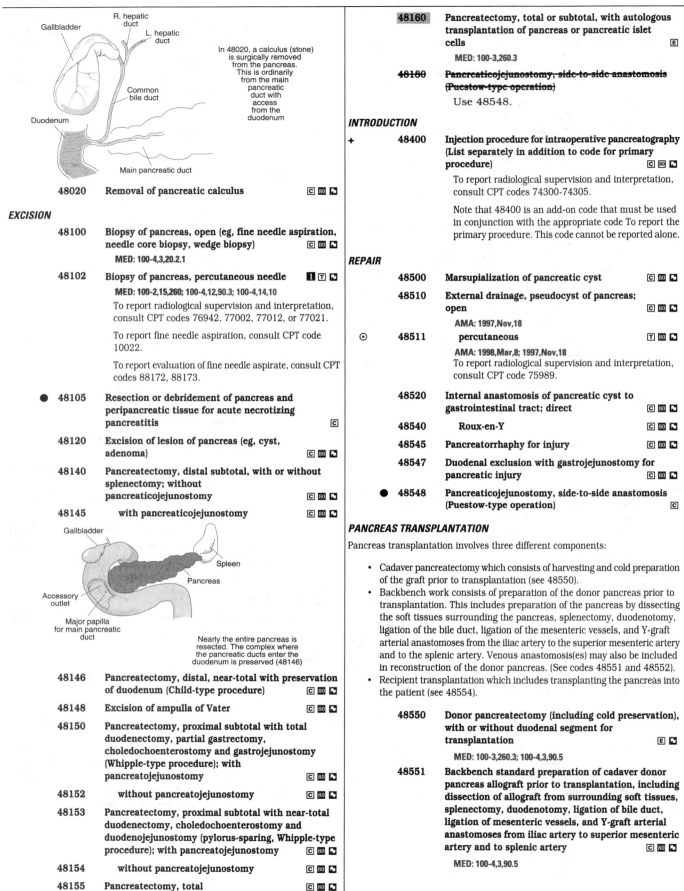

In 48020, a calculus (stone) is surgically removed from the pancreas. This is ordinarily from the main pancreatic duct with access from the duodenum

48020 Removal of pancreatic calculus 〔C〕〔80〕〔↺〕

EXCISION

48100 Biopsy of pancreas, open (eg, fine needle aspiration, needle core biopsy, wedge biopsy) 〔C〕〔80〕〔↺〕

MED: 100-4,3,20.2.1

48102 Biopsy of pancreas, percutaneous needle 〔1〕〔T〕〔↺〕

MED: 100-2,15,260; 100-4,12,90.3; 100-4,14,10

To report radiological supervision and interpretation, consult CPT codes 76942, 77002, 77012, or 77021.

To report fine needle aspiration, consult CPT code 10022.

To report evaluation of fine needle aspirate, consult CPT codes 88172, 88173.

● **48105** Resection or debridement of pancreas and peripancreatic tissue for acute necrotizing pancreatitis 〔C〕

48120 Excision of lesion of pancreas (eg, cyst, adenoma) 〔C〕〔80〕〔↺〕

48140 Pancreatectomy, distal subtotal, with or without splenectomy; without pancreaticojejunostomy 〔C〕〔80〕〔↺〕

48145 with pancreaticojejunostomy 〔C〕〔80〕〔↺〕

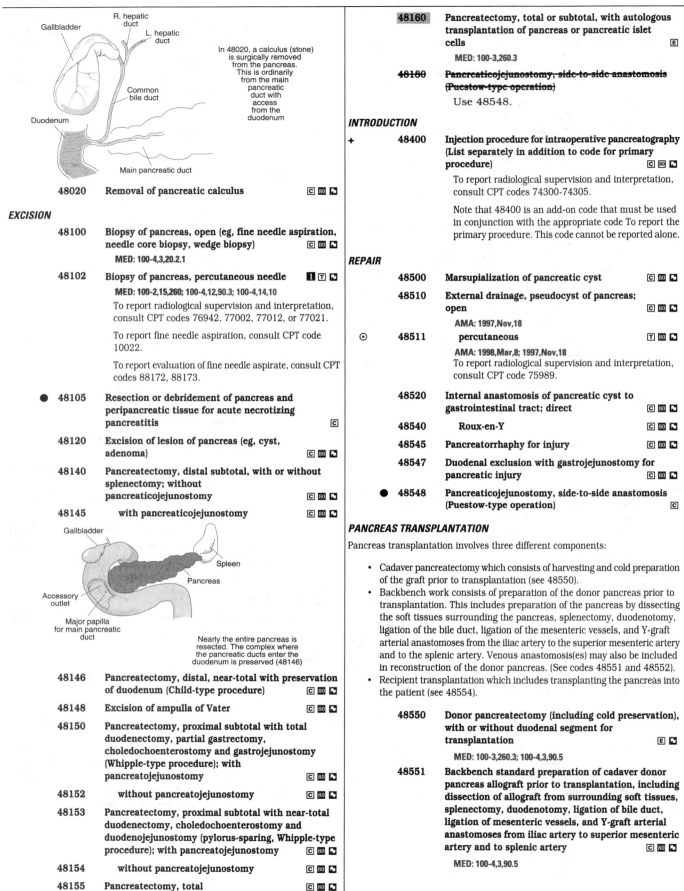

Nearly the entire pancreas is resected. The complex where the pancreatic ducts enter the duodenum is preserved (48146)

48146 Pancreatectomy, distal, near-total with preservation of duodenum (Child-type procedure) 〔C〕〔80〕〔↺〕

48148 Excision of ampulla of Vater 〔C〕〔80〕〔↺〕

48150 Pancreatectomy, proximal subtotal with total duodenectomy, partial gastrectomy, choledochoenterostomy and gastrojejunostomy (Whipple-type procedure); with pancreatojejunostomy 〔C〕〔80〕〔↺〕

48152 without pancreatojejunostomy 〔C〕〔80〕〔↺〕

48153 Pancreatectomy, proximal subtotal with near-total duodenectomy, choledochoenterostomy and duodenojejunostomy (pylorus-sparing, Whipple-type procedure); with pancreatojejunostomy 〔C〕〔80〕〔↺〕

48154 without pancreatojejunostomy 〔C〕〔80〕〔↺〕

48155 Pancreatectomy, total 〔C〕〔80〕〔↺〕

48160 Pancreatectomy, total or subtotal, with autologous transplantation of pancreas or pancreatic islet cells 〔E〕

MED: 100-3,260.3

~~**48180** Pancreaticojejunostomy, side-to-side anastomosis (Puestow-type operation)~~

Use 48548.

INTRODUCTION

+ **48400** Injection procedure for intraoperative pancreatography (List separately in addition to code for primary procedure) 〔C〕〔80〕〔↺〕

To report radiological supervision and interpretation, consult CPT codes 74300-74305.

Note that 48400 is an add-on code that must be used in conjunction with the appropriate code To report the primary procedure. This code cannot be reported alone.

REPAIR

48500 Marsupialization of pancreatic cyst 〔C〕〔80〕〔↺〕

48510 External drainage, pseudocyst of pancreas; open 〔C〕〔80〕〔↺〕

AMA: 1997,Nov,18

⊙ **48511** percutaneous 〔T〕〔80〕〔↺〕

AMA: 1998,Mar,8; 1997,Nov,18

To report radiological supervision and interpretation, consult CPT code 75989.

48520 Internal anastomosis of pancreatic cyst to gastrointestinal tract; direct 〔C〕〔80〕〔↺〕

48540 Roux-en-Y 〔C〕〔80〕〔↺〕

48545 Pancreatorrhaphy for injury 〔C〕〔80〕〔↺〕

48547 Duodenal exclusion with gastrojejunostomy for pancreatic injury 〔C〕〔80〕〔↺〕

● **48548** Pancreaticojejunostomy, side-to-side anastomosis (Puestow-type operation) 〔C〕

PANCREAS TRANSPLANTATION

Pancreas transplantation involves three different components:

- Cadaver pancreatectomy which consists of harvesting and cold preparation of the graft prior to transplantation (see 48550).
- Backbench work consists of preparation of the donor pancreas prior to transplantation. This includes preparation of the pancreas by dissecting the soft tissues surrounding the pancreas, splenectomy, duodenotomy, ligation of the bile duct, ligation of the mesenteric vessels, and Y-graft arterial anastomoses from the iliac artery to the superior mesenteric artery and to the splenic artery. Venous anastomosis(es) may also be included in reconstruction of the donor pancreas. (See codes 48551 and 48552).
- Recipient transplantation which includes transplanting the pancreas into the patient (see 48554).

48550 Donor pancreatectomy (including cold preservation), with or without duodenal segment for transplantation 〔E〕〔↺〕

MED: 100-3,260.3; 100-4,3,90.5

48551 Backbench standard preparation of cadaver donor pancreas allograft prior to transplantation, including dissection of allograft from surrounding soft tissues, splenectomy, duodenotomy, ligation of bile duct, ligation of mesenteric vessels, and Y-graft arterial anastomoses from iliac artery to superior mesenteric artery and to splenic artery 〔C〕〔80〕〔↺〕

MED: 100-4,3,90.5

48552	**Backbench reconstruction of cadaver donor pancreas allograft prior to transplantation, venous anastomosis, each**	C 80 ↻

MED: 100-4,3,90.5

Codes 48551 and 48552 cannot be reported with CPT codes 35531, 35563, 35685, 38100-38102, 44010, 44820, 44850, 47460, 47505-47525, 47550-47556, 48100-48120, 48545.

48554	**Transplantation of pancreatic allograft**	C 80 ↻

MED: 100-3,260.3; 100-4,3,90.5

48556	**Removal of transplanted pancreatic allograft**	C 80 ↻

MED: 100-3,260.3; 100-4,3,90.5

OTHER PROCEDURES

48999	Unlisted procedure, pancreas	T 80

MED: 100-4,4,180.3

ABDOMEN, PERITONEUM, AND OMENTUM

INCISION

49000	**Exploratory laparotomy, exploratory celiotomy with or without biopsy(s) (separate procedure)**	C 80 ↻

AMA; 2001,Mar,10

If wound exploration due to a penetrating trauma without laparotomy is performed, consult CPT code 20102.

49002	**Reopening of recent laparotomy**	C 80 ↻

If re-exploration is performed of a hepatic wound for removal of packing, consult CPT code 47362.

49010	**Exploration, retroperitoneal area with or without biopsy(s) (separate procedure)**	C 80 ↻

If wound exploration is performed due to a penetrating trauma without a laparotomy, consult CPT code 20102.

49020	**Drainage of peritoneal abscess or localized peritonitis, exclusive of appendiceal abscess; open**	C 80 ↻

If an appendiceal abscess is incised and drained, consult CPT code 44900.

⊙	49021	percutaneous	T ↻

To report radiological supervision and interpretation, consult CPT code 75989.

49040	**Drainage of subdiaphragmatic or subphrenic abscess; open**	C 80 ↻

AMA: 1997,Nov,18

⊙	49041	percutaneous	T 80 ↻

AMA: 1998,Mar,8; 1997,Nov,18
To report radiological supervision and interpretation, consult CPT code 75989.

49060	**Drainage of retroperitoneal abscess; open**	C ↻

AMA: 2001,Jul,11; 2001,Aug,10; 1999,Nov,24; 1997,Nov,18

⊙	49061	percutaneous	T 80 ↻

AMA: 2001,Jul,11; 2001,Aug,10; 1999,Nov,24; 1998,Mar,8; 1997,Nov,18
If laparoscopic drainage is performed, consult CPT code 49323.

For radiological supervision and interpretation, consult CPT code 75989.

49062	**Drainage of extraperitoneal lymphocele to peritoneal cavity, open**	C 80 ↻

AMA: 2001,Jul,11; 2001,Aug,10; 1997,Nov,19

49080	**Peritoneocentesis, abdominal paracentesis, or peritoneal lavage (diagnostic or therapeutic); initial**	2 T ↻

MED: 100-2,15,260; 100-4,12,90.3; 100-4,14,10

49081	subsequent	2 T ↻

MED: 100-2,15,260; 100-4,12,90.3; 100-4,14,10

To report imaging guidance, consult CPT codes 76942, 77012.

~~49085~~	~~Removal of peritoneal foreign body from peritoneal cavity~~	

Use 49402.

EXCISION, DESTRUCTION

49180	**Biopsy, abdominal or retroperitoneal mass, percutaneous needle**	1 T ↻

MED: 100-2,15,260; 100-4,12,90.3; 100-4,14,10
AMA: 1993,Fall,11
To report imaging guidance, consult CPT codes 76942, 77002, 77012, or 77021.

To report fine needle aspiration, consult CPT code 10021 or 10022.

To report evaluation of fine needle aspirate, consult CPT codes 88172, 88173.

49200	**Excision or destruction, open, intra-abdominal or retroperitoneal tumors or cysts or endometriomas;**	T 80 ↻
49201	extensive	C 80 ↻

See 58957 and 58958 for resection of recurrent ovarian, tubal, primary peritoneal, or uterine malignancy.

If open cryoablation of a renal tumor is performed, consult CPT code 50250.

If percutaneous cryotherapy ablation of renal tumors is performed, consult Category III code 0135T.

49215	**Excision of presacral or sacrococcygeal tumor**	C 80 ⊛ ↻
49220	**Staging laparotomy for Hodgkins disease or lymphoma (includes splenectomy, needle or open biopsies of both liver lobes, possibly also removal of abdominal nodes, abdominal node and/or bone marrow biopsies, ovarian repositioning)**	C 80 ↻

MED: 100-1,5,90.2; 100-2,15,80; 100-2,15,80.1; 100-4,16,10; 100-4,16,10.1; 100-4,16,110.4

49250	**Umbilectomy, omphalectomy, excision of umbilicus (separate procedure)**	4 T ↻

MED: 100-2,15,260; 100-4,12,90.3; 100-4,14,10

49255	**Omentectomy, epiploectomy, resection of omentum (separate procedure)**	C 80 ↻

AMA: 1999,Nov,24

LAPAROSCOPY

Surgical laparoscopy always includes diagnostic laparoscopy. To report only a diagnostic laparoscopy (peritoneoscopy), consult CPT code 49320. To report laparoscopic fulguration or excision of lesions of the ovary, pelvic viscera or peritoneal surface, consult CPT code 58662.

49320	**Laparoscopy, abdomen, peritoneum, and omentum, diagnostic, with or without collection of specimen(s) by brushing or washing (separate procedure)**	3 T 80 ↻

MED: 100-2,15,260; 100-4,12,90.3; 100-4,14,10
AMA: 2000,Mar,5; 1999,Nov,24

⊛ Modifier 63 Exempt Code ⊙ Conscious Sedation + CPT Add-on Code ⊘ Modifier 51 Exempt Code ● New Code ▲ Revised Code
M Maternity Edit A Age Edit A-Y APC Status Indicators ↻ CCI Comprehensive Code 80 Bilateral Procedure

49321	Laparoscopy, surgical; with biopsy (single or multiple) ⁴ T 80 ⌐

MED: 100-2,15,260; 100-4,12,90.3; 100-4,14,10
AMA: 2000,Mar,5; 1999,Nov,24

49322	with aspiration of cavity or cyst (eg, ovarian cyst) (single or multiple) ⁴ T 80 ⌐

MED: 100-2,15,260; 100-4,12,90.3; 100-4,14,10
AMA: 2000,Mar,5; 1999,Nov,24

49323	with drainage of lymphocele to peritoneal cavity T 80 ⌐

AMA: 2001,Jul,11; 2001,Aug,10; 2000,May,4; 2000,Mar,5; 1999,Nov,24

If percutaneous or open drainage is performed, consult CPT codes 49060 and 49061.

● 49324	with insertion of intraperitoneal cannula or catheter, permanent T

Use 49435 with 49324 for subcutaneous extension of iintraperitoneal catheter with remote chest exit site.

Use 49421 for open insertion of permanent intraperitoneal cannula or catheter.

● 49325	with revision of previously placed intraperitoneal cannula or catheter, with removal of intraluminal obstructive material if performed T

+ ● 49326	with omentopexy (omental tacking procedure) (List separately in addition to code for primary procedure) T

49329	Unlisted laparoscopy procedure, abdomen, peritoneum and omentum T 80 50

AMA: 2000,Mar,5; 1999,Nov,24

INTRODUCTION, REVISION, REMOVAL

49400	Injection of air or contrast into peritoneal cavity (separate procedure) N ⌐

To report radiological supervision and interpretation, consult CPT code 74190.

● 49402	Removal of peritoneal foreign body from peritoneal cavity ² T

For lysis of intestinal adhesions, use 44005.

49419	Insertion of intraperitoneal cannula or catheter, with subcutaneous reservoir, permanent (ie, totally implantable) ¹ T ⌐

To report removal, consult CPT code 49422.

49420	Insertion of intraperitoneal cannula or catheter for drainage or dialysis; temporary ¹ T ⌐

MED: 100-2,15,260; 100-4,12,90.3; 100-4,14,10
AMA: 1993,Fall,2

49421	permanent ¹ T ⌐

MED: 100-2,15,260; 100-4,12,90.3; 100-4,14,10
AMA: 1993,Fall,2

For laparoscopic insertion of intraperitoneal cannula or catheter, use 49324.

Use 49435 with 49421 for subcutanous extension of intraperitoneal catheter with remote chest exit site.

49422	Removal of permanent intraperitoneal cannula or catheter ¹ T ⌐

MED: 100-2,15,260; 100-4,12,90.3; 100-4,14,10
If a temporary catheter/cannula is removed, use the appropriate E/M code.

49423	Exchange of previously placed abscess or cyst drainage catheter under radiological guidance (separate procedure) T 80 ⌐

AMA: 1998,Mar,8; 1997,Nov,19
To report radiological supervision and interpretation, consult CPT code 75984.

49424	Contrast injection for assessment of abscess or cyst via previously placed drainage catheter or tube (separate procedure) N 80 ⌐

AMA: 1998,Mar,8; 1997,Nov,19
To report radiological supervision and interpretation, consult CPT code 76080.

49425	Insertion of peritoneal-venous shunt C 80 ⌐

49426	Revision of peritoneal-venous shunt ² T ⌐

MED: 100-2,15,260; 100-4,12,90.3; 100-4,14,10
If a shunt patency test is performed, consult CPT code 78291.

49427	Injection procedure (eg, contrast media) for evaluation of previously placed peritoneal-venous shunt N 80 ⌐

To report radiological supervision and interpretation, consult CPT code 75809, 78291.

49428	Ligation of peritoneal-venous shunt C ⌐

49429	Removal of peritoneal-venous shunt T ⌐

+ ● 49435	Insertion of subcutaneous extension to intraperitoneal cannula or catheter with remote chest exit site (List separately in addition to code for primary procedure) T

● 49436	Delayed creation of exit site from embedded subcutaneous segment of intraperitoneal cannula or catheter T

REPAIR

HERNIOPLASTY, HERNIORRHAPHY, HERNIOTOMY

Hernia repair codes are categorized primarily by type of hernia (inguinal, femoral, incisional/ventral, epigastric, umbilical, spigelian). Some hernias are further categorized based on whether there has been a previous hernia repair (initial, or recurrent). Additional variables include patient age and clinical presentation (reducible, strangulated/incarcerated).

Implantation of mesh or prosthesis may be performed with hernia repairs. However, the implantation should only be reported separately when used for repair of incisional and ventral hernias (49560-49566). When used for repair of other types of hernias, it is not considered a separately reportable procedure. For laparoscopic repair of inguinal and other hernias, see codes 49650-49659.

Repair of strangulated organs or structures should be reported in addition to the hernia repair. Structures most often involved include intestine (44120), testicles (54520), and ovaries (58940).

▲ 49491	Repair, initial inguinal hernia, preterm infant (younger than 37 weeks gestation at birth), performed from birth up to 50 weeks postconception age, with or without hydrocelectomy; reducible A T 80 50 ⊕ ⌐

▲ 49492	incarcerated or strangulated A T 80 50 ⊕ ⌐

Postconception age equals gestational age at birth plus age of infant in weeks at the time of the repair. To report initial inguinal hernia repairs that are performed on preterm infants who are over 50 weeks postconception age and under age 6 months at the time of surgery, consult CPT codes 49495, 49496.

---

26 Professional Component Only	80/80 Assist-at-Surgery Allowed/With Documentation	Unlisted	Not Covered
TC Technical Component Only	MED: Pub 100/NCD References AMA: CPT Assistant References	1-9 ASC Group ♂ Male Only	♀ Female Only

180 — CPT Expert   CPT only © 2006 American Medical Association. All Rights Reserved. *(Black Ink)*   © *2006 Ingenix (Blue Ink)*

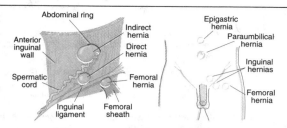

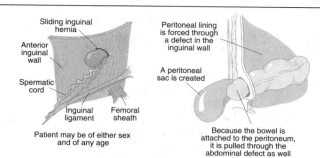

A hernia is a protrusion, usually through an abdominal wall containment. Often, hernias are congenital. Groin hernias are most common among both sexes and all age groups. In males, indirect hernias are often associated with incomplete closure of the path the testicle takes as it descends just prior to birth (the processus vaginalis). Direct hernias simply protrude through the wall. Femoral hernias occur below the inguinal ligament. Strangulation and necrosis of the protruding bowel section can occur. Umbilical hernias are often linked to incomplete closure of the umbilicus

In 49525, a sliding inguinal hernia (depicted above, right) is repaired in a patient of any age

▲ **49495** **Repair, initial inguinal hernia, full term infant younger than age 6 months, or preterm infant older than 50 weeks postconception age and younger than age 6 months at the time of surgery, with or without hydrocelectomy; reducible**   Ⓐ 4 T 80 50 ☺ ⌧
MED: 100-2,15,260; 100-4,12,90.3; 100-4,14,10
AMA: 1994,Winter,13; 1993,Winter,6
Halsted repair

▲ **49496** **incarcerated or strangulated**   Ⓐ 4 T 80 50 ☺ ⌧
MED: 100-2,15,260; 100-4,12,90.3; 100-4,14,10
AMA: 1994,Winter,13; 1993,Winter,6
Postconception age equals gestational age at birth plus age in weeks at the time of ther hernia repair. To report initial inguinal hernia repairs that are performed on preterm infants who are under or up to 50 weeks postconception age but under 6 months of age since birth, should be consult CPT codes 49491, 49492. For inguinal hernia repairs on infants age 6 months to under 5 years consult CPT codes 49500-49501.

▲ **49500** **Repair initial inguinal hernia, age 6 months to younger than 5 years, with or without hydrocelectomy; reducible**   Ⓐ 4 T 80 50 ⌧
MED: 100-2,15,260; 100-4,12,90.3; 100-4,14,10
AMA: 1994,Winter,13

▲ **49501** **incarcerated or strangulated**   Ⓐ 9 T 80 50 ⌧
MED: 100-2,15,260; 100-4,12,90.3; 100-4,14,10
AMA: 1994,Winter,13

▲ **49505** **Repair initial inguinal hernia, age 5 years or older; reducible**   4 T 80 50 ⌧
MED: 100-2,15,260; 100-4,12,90.3; 100-4,14,10
AMA: 2000,Sep,10; 1994,Winter,13
MacEwen hernia repair

▲ **49507** **incarcerated or strangulated**   Ⓐ 9 T 80 50 ⌧
MED: 100-2,15,260; 100-4,12,90.3; 100-4,14,10
AMA: 1994,Winter,13

49520 **Repair recurrent inguinal hernia, any age; reducible**   7 T 80 50 ⌧
MED: 100-2,15,260; 100-4,12,90.3; 100-4,14,10
AMA: 1994,Winter,13

49521 **incarcerated or strangulated**   9 T 80 50 ⌧
MED: 100-2,15,260; 100-4,12,90.3; 100-4,14,10
AMA: 1994,Winter,13

49525 **Repair inguinal hernia, sliding, any age**   4 T 80 50 ⌧
MED: 100-2,15,260; 100-4,12,90.3; 100-4,14,10
AMA: 1994,Winter,14

49540 **Repair lumbar hernia**   2 T 80 50 ⌧
MED: 100-2,15,260; 100-4,12,90.3; 100-4,14,10
AMA: 1994,Winter,14

49550 **Repair initial femoral hernia, any age; reducible**   5 T 80 50 ⌧
MED: 100-2,15,260; 100-4,12,90.3; 100-4,14,10
AMA: 1994,Winter,14

49553 **incarcerated or strangulated**   9 T 80 50 ⌧
MED: 100-2,15,260; 100-4,12,90.3; 100-4,14,10
AMA: 1994,Winter,14

49555 **Repair recurrent femoral hernia; reducible**   5 T 80 50 ⌧
MED: 100-2,15,260; 100-4,12,90.3; 100-4,14,10
AMA: 1994,Winter,14

49557 **incarcerated or strangulated**   9 T 80 50 ⌧
MED: 100-2,15,260; 100-4,12,90.3; 100-4,14,10
AMA: 1994,Winter,14

49560 **Repair initial incisional or ventral hernia; reducible**   4 T 80 50 ⌧
MED: 100-2,15,260; 100-4,12,90.3; 100-4,14,10
AMA: 1997,Nov,19; 1994,Winter,14; 1993,Winter,6

49561 **incarcerated or strangulated**   9 T 80 50 ⌧
MED: 100-2,15,260; 100-4,12,90.3; 100-4,14,10
AMA: 1994,Winter,14

49565 **Repair recurrent incisional or ventral hernia; reducible**   4 T 80 50 ⌧
MED: 100-2,15,260; 100-4,12,90.3; 100-4,14,10
AMA: 1997,Nov,19; 1994,Winter,14

49566 **incarcerated or strangulated**   9 T 80 50 ⌧
MED: 100-2,15,260; 100-4,12,90.3; 100-4,14,10
AMA: 1994,Winter,14

+ **49568** **Implantation of mesh or other prosthesis for incisional or ventral hernia repair (List separately in addition to code for the incisional or ventral hernia repair)**   7 T 80 ⌧
MED: 100-2,15,260; 100-4,12,90.3; 100-4,14,10
AMA: 2001,Sep,11; 1997,Nov,19; 1994,Winter,14
Note that 49568 is an add-on code that must be used in conjunction with the code for the incisional or ventral hernia repair . This code cannot be reported alone.

49570 **Repair epigastric hernia (eg, preperitoneal fat); reducible (separate procedure)**   4 T 80 50 ⌧
MED: 100-2,15,260; 100-4,12,90.3; 100-4,14,10
AMA: 1994,Winter,15

☺ Modifier 63 Exempt Code   ⊙ Conscious Sedation   + CPT Add-on Code   ⊘ Modifier 51 Exempt Code   ● New Code   ▲ Revised Code

Ⓜ Maternity Edit   Ⓐ Age Edit   Ⓐ-Ⓨ APC Status Indicators   ⌧ CCI Comprehensive Code   50 Bilateral Procedure

49572	incarcerated or strangulated	9 T 80 50

MED: 100-2,15,260; 100-4,12,90.3; 100-4,14,10
AMA: 1994,Winter,15

▲ 49580 Repair umbilical hernia, younger than age 5 years; reducible A 4 T 80 🔲
MED: 100-2,15,260; 100-4,12,90.3; 100-4,14,10
AMA: 1994,Winter,15

▲ 49582 incarcerated or strangulated A 9 T 80 🔲
MED: 100-2,15,260; 100-4,12,90.3; 100-4,14,10
AMA: 1994,Winter,15

▲ 49585 Repair umbilical hernia, age 5 years or older; reducible A 4 T 80 🔲
MED: 100-2,15,260; 100-4,12,90.3; 100-4,14,10
AMA: 1994,Winter,15
Mayo hernia repair

▲ 49587 incarcerated or strangulated A 9 T 80 🔲
MED: 100-2,15,260; 100-4,12,90.3; 100-4,14,10
AMA: 1994,Winter,15

49590 Repair spigelian hernia 3 T 80 50 🔲
MED: 100-2,15,260; 100-4,12,90.3; 100-4,14,10
AMA: 1994,Winter,15

49600 Repair of small omphalocele, with primary closure 4 T 80 63 🔲
MED: 100-2,15,260; 100-4,12,90.3; 100-4,14,10
AMA: 1994,Winter,15
If a diaphragmatic or hiatal hernia is repaired, consult CPT codes 39502-39541.

49605 Repair of large omphalocele or gastroschisis; with or without prosthesis C 80 63 🔲
AMA: 1994,Winter,15
If a diaphragmatic or hiatal hernia is repaired, consult CPT codes 39502-39541.

If an intra-abdominal hernia is reduced and repaired, consult CPT code 44050.

49606 with removal of prosthesis, final reduction and closure, in operating room C 80 63 🔲
AMA: 1994,Winter,15

49610 Repair of omphalocele (Gross type operation); first stage C 80 63 🔲
AMA: 1994,Winter,15

49611 second stage C 80 63 🔲
AMA: 1994,Winter,15

LAPAROSCOPY

Surgical laparoscopy always includes diagnostic laparoscopy. To report only diagnostic laparoscopy, consult CPT code 49320.

49650 Laparoscopy, surgical; repair initial inguinal hernia 4 T 80 50 🔲
MED: 100-2,15,260; 100-4,12,90.3; 100-4,14,10
AMA: 2000,Mar,5; 1999,Nov,24

49651 repair recurrent inguinal hernia 7 T 80 50 🔲
MED: 100-2,15,260; 100-4,12,90.3; 100-4,14,10
AMA: 2000,Mar,5; 1999,Nov,24

49659 Unlisted laparoscopy procedure, hernioplasty, herniorrhaphy, herniotomy T 80 50
AMA: 2001,Sep,11; 2000,Mar,5; 1999,Nov,25

SUTURE

49900 Suture, secondary, of abdominal wall for evisceration or dehiscence C 80 🔲
If a ruptured diaphragm is sutured, consult CPT codes 39540 and 39541. If debridement is performed on the abdominal wall, consult CPT codes 11042 and 11043.

OTHER PROCEDURES

49904 Omental flap, extra-abdominal (eg, for reconstruction of sternal and chest wall defects) C 🔲
Code 49904 includes both harvest and transplant. If a different surgeon harvests the flap, then both surgeons should report 49904 and append modifier 62.

+ 49905 Omental flap, intra-abdominal (List separately in addition to code for primary procedure) C 80 🔲
AMA: 2000,Nov,11
Note that code 49905 should not be reported in conjunction with CPT code 47700.

Note that 48400 is an add-on code that must be used in conjunction with the appropriate code for the primary procedure. This code cannot be reported alone.

49906 Free omental flap with microvascular anastomosis C 🔲
AMA: 1998,Nov,16; 1997,Apr,8
Do not report 69990 in addition to 49906 as the operating microscope is considered an inclusive component of the surgery.

49999 Unlisted procedure, abdomen, peritoneum and omentum T 80
MED: 100-4,4,180.3

26 Professional Component Only   80/80 Assist-at-Surgery Allowed/With Documentation   Unlisted   Not Covered

TC Technical Component Only   **MED:** Pub 100/NCD References **AMA:** CPT Assistant References   1-9 ASC Group   ♂ Male Only   ♀ Female Only

182 — CPT Expert   CPT only © 2006 American Medical Association. All Rights Reserved. *(Black Ink)*   © *2006 Ingenix (Blue Ink)*

URINARY SYSTEM

To report the provision of chemotherapeutic agents, report the code for the specific service as well as the specific substance(s) or drug(s) provided.

KIDNEY

If retroperitoneal exploration is performed on an abscess, tumor, or cyst, consult CPT codes 49101, 49060, 49200, and 49201.

INCISION

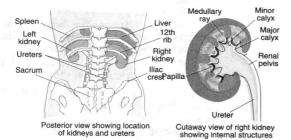

Spleen
Left kidney
Ureters
Sacrum

Liver
12th rib
Right kidney
Iliac crest
Papilla

Medullary ray
Minor calyx
Major calyx
Renal pelvis
Ureter

Posterior view showing location of kidneys and ureters

Cutaway view of right kidney showing internal structures

The kidneys remove waste products of protein metabolism and other excess materials and fluids from the blood. Variations in kidney anatomy are fairly common, though abnormalities can complicate procedures. "Pyelo" refers to the renal pelvis, an important access site to the inner kidney. Each kidney is imbedded in a mass of peritoneal fat that helps to enclose and position it

50010 **Renal exploration, not necessitating other specific procedures** Ⓒ 80 ↵

To report laparoscopic ablation of renal mass lesion(s), consult CPT code 50542.

50020 **Drainage of perirenal or renal abscess; open** Ⓣ ↵
AMA: 2001,Oct,8; 1997,Nov,19

⊙ **50021** **percutaneous** Ⓣ 80 ↵
AMA: 2001,Oct,8; 1998,Mar,8; 1997,Nov,19
To report radiological supervision and interpretation, consult CPT code 75989.

50040 **Nephrostomy, nephrotomy with drainage** Ⓒ ↵
AMA: 2001,Oct,8

50045 **Nephrotomy, with exploration** Ⓒ 80 ↵
AMA: 2001,Oct,8
If renal endoscopy is performed in conjunction with this procedure, consult CPT codes 50570-50580.

50060 **Nephrolithotomy; removal of calculus** Ⓒ 80 ↵
MED: 100-3,230.1
AMA: 2001,Oct,8

50065 **secondary surgical operation for calculus** Ⓒ 80 ↵
MED: 100-3,230.1
AMA: 2001,Oct,8

50070 **complicated by congenital kidney abnormality** Ⓒ 80 ↵
MED: 100-3,230.1
AMA: 2001,Oct,8

50075 **removal of large staghorn calculus filling renal pelvis and calyces (including anatrophic pyelolithotomy)** Ⓒ 80 ↵
MED: 100-3,230.1
AMA: 2001,Oct,8

50080 **Percutaneous nephrostolithotomy or pyelostolithotomy, with or without dilation, endoscopy, lithotripsy, stenting, or basket extraction; up to 2 cm** Ⓣ 50 ↵
MED: 100-3,100.2; 100-3,230.1
AMA: 2001,Oct,8
If nephrostomy is established without a nephrostolithotomy, consult CPT codes 50040, 50395, and 52334. If fluoroscopic guidance is used, consult CPT codes 76000 and 76001.

50081 **over 2 cm** Ⓣ 80 50 ↵
MED: 100-3,230.1
AMA: 2001,Oct,8
If nephrostomy is established without a nephrostolithotomy, consult CPT codes 50040, 50395, and 52334. If fluoroscopic guidance is used, consult CPT codes 76000 and 76001.

50100 **Transection or repositioning of aberrant renal vessels (separate procedure)** Ⓒ 80 ↵
AMA: 2001,Oct,8

50120 **Pyelotomy; with exploration** Ⓒ 80 50 ↵
AMA: 2001,Oct,8
If renal endoscopy is performed in conjunction with this procedure, consult CPT codes 50570-50580.

Gol-Vernet pyelotomy

50125 **with drainage, pyelostomy** Ⓒ 80 50 ↵
AMA: 2001,Oct,8
If retroperitoneal exploration is performed on an abscess, tumor, or cyst, consult CPT codes 49101, 49060, 49200, and 49201.

50130 **with removal of calculus (pyelolithotomy, pelviolithotomy, including coagulum pyelolithotomy)** Ⓒ 80 50 ↵
MED: 100-3,230.1
AMA: 2001,Oct,8

50135 **complicated (eg, secondary operation, congenital kidney abnormality)** Ⓒ 80 50 ↵
AMA: 2001,Oct,8
Report 99070 for supply of anticarcinogenic agents when used, in addition to primary procedure.

EXCISION

If a retroperitoneal tumor or cyst is excised, consult CPT codes 49200 and 49201.

To report laparoscopic ablation of renal mass lesion(s), consult CPT code 50542.

50200 **Renal biopsy; percutaneous, by trocar or needle** 1 Ⓣ 50 ↵
MED: 100-2,15,260; 100-3,190.4; 100-4,12,90.3; 100-4,14,10
AMA: 2001,Oct,8
To report radiological supervision and interpretation, consult CPT codes 76942, 77002, 77012, or 77021.
To report fine needle aspiration, consult CPT code 10022.
To report evaluation of fine needle aspirate, consult CPT codes 88172, 88173.

50205 **by surgical exposure of kidney** Ⓒ 80 50 ↵
MED: 100-4,3,20.2.1
AMA: 2001,Oct,8

50220 **Nephrectomy, including partial ureterectomy, any open approach including rib resection;** Ⓒ 80 50 ↵
AMA: 2002,Nov,1; 2001,Oct,8

Ⓢ Modifier 63 Exempt Code ⊙ Conscious Sedation ✚ CPT Add-on Code ⊘ Modifier 51 Exempt Code ● New Code ▲ Revised Code

Ⓜ Maternity Edit Ⓐ Age Edit Ⓐ-Ⓨ APC Status Indicators ↵ CCI Comprehensive Code 50 Bilateral Procedure

CPT only © 2006 American Medical Association. All Rights Reserved. (Black Ink)

50225   complicated because of previous surgery on same kidney   © 80 50 ▣
AMA: 2001,Oct,8

50230   radical, with regional lymphadenectomy and/or vena caval thrombectomy   © 80 50 ▣
AMA: 2001,Oct,8
If vena caval resection with reconstruction is necessary, consult CPT code 37799.

50234   Nephrectomy with total ureterectomy and bladder cuff; through same incision   © 80 ▣
AMA: 2001,Oct,8

50236   through separate incision   © 80 ▣
AMA: 2001,Oct,8

50240   Nephrectomy, partial   © 80 ▣
AMA: 2003,Jan,19; 2002,Nov,1; 2001,Oct,8
To report laparoscopic partial nephrectomy, consult CPT code 50543.

50250   Ablation, open, one or more renal mass lesion(s), cryosurgical, including intraoperative ultrasound, if performed   © 80
To report laparoscopic ablation of renal mass lesions, consult CPT code 50542.

To report percutaneous cryotherapy ablation of renal tumors, consult CPT Category III code 0135T.

50280   Excision or unroofing of cyst(s) of kidney   © 80 ▣
AMA: 2001,Oct,8; 1999,Nov,25
If laparoscopic ablation is performed on renal cysts, consult CPT code 50541.

50290   Excision of perinephric cyst   © 80 ▣
AMA: 2001,Oct,8

RENAL TRANSPLANTATION

Renal transplantation involves three different components:

- Cadaver or living donor nephrectomy which consists of harvesting and cold preparation of the graft prior to transplantation and care of the donor (see codes 50300, 50320, and 50547).
- Backbench work consists of preparation of the donor kidney prior to transplantation. This includes removal of perinephratic fat, diaphragmatic and retroperitoneal attachments, excision of adrenal gland; and preparation of ureter(s), renal vein(s), and renal artery(s), ligating branches as necessary. Other reconstruction procedures may involve venous, arterial, and/or ureteral anastomosis(es) necessary for the transplant (see codes 50323, 50325, 50327-50329).
- Recipient transplantation which includes transplanting the kidney into the patient (see 50360, 50365).

If dialysis is performed, consult CPT codes 90935-90999. If laparoscopic drainage of a lymphocele to peritoneal cavity is performed, consult CPT code 49323.

If a laparoscopic donor nephrectomy is performed, consult CPT code 50547.

50300   Donor nephrectomy (including cold preservation); from cadaver donor, unilateral or bilateral   © ▣
MED: 100-3,20.3; 100-3,110.16; 100-3,190.1; 100-3,230.12; 100-4,3,90.1; 100-4,3,90.1.1; 100-4,3,90.1.2
AMA: 1999,Nov,25

50320   open, from living donor   © 80 50 ▣
MED: 100-4,3,90.1; 100-4,3,90.1.1; 100-4,3,90.1.2
AMA: 2000,May,4; 1999,Nov,25

50323   Backbench standard preparation of cadaver donor renal allograft prior to transplantation, including dissection and removal of perinephric fat, diaphragmatic and retroperitoneal attachments, excision of adrenal gland, and preparation of ureter(s), renal vein(s), and renal artery(s), ligating branches, as necessary   © 80
MED: 100-4,3,90.1; 100-4,3,90.1.1; 100-4,3,90.1.2
Code 50323 cannot be reported with CPT codes 60540, 60545.

50325   Backbench standard preparation of living donor renal allograft (open or laparoscopic) prior to transplantation, including dissection and removal of perinephric fat and preparation of ureter(s), renal vein(s), and renal artery(s), ligating branches, as necessary   © 80 ▣
MED: 100-4,3,90.1; 100-4,3,90.1.1; 100-4,3,90.1.2

50327   Backbench reconstruction of cadaver or living donor renal allograft prior to transplantation; venous anastomosis, each   © 80 ▣
MED: 100-4,3,90.1; 100-4,3,90.1.1; 100-4,3,90.1.2

50328   arterial anastomosis, each   © 80 ▣
MED: 100-4,3,90.1; 100-4,3,90.1.1; 100-4,3,90.1.2

50329   ureteral anastomosis, each   © 80 ▣
MED: 100-4,3,90.1; 100-4,3,90.1.1; 100-4,3,90.1.2

50340   Recipient nephrectomy (separate procedure)   © 80 50 ▣
MED: 100-3,20.3; 100-3,110.16; 100-4,3,90.1; 100-4,3,90.1.1; 100-4,3,90.1.2

50360   Renal allotransplantation, implantation of graft; without recipient nephrectomy   © 80 ▣
MED: 100-3,190.1; 100-3,260.3; 100-3,260.7; 100-4,3,90.1; 100-4,3,90.1.1; 100-4,3,90.1.2

50365   with recipient nephrectomy   © 80 50 ▣
MED: 100-3,260.3; 100-3,260.7; 100-4,3,90.1; 100-4,3,90.1.1; 100-4,3,90.1.2

50370   Removal of transplanted renal allograft   © 80 ▣
MED: 100-3,190.1; 100-3,260.7; 100-4,3,90.1; 100-4,3,90.1.1; 100-4,3,90.1.2

50380   Renal autotransplantation, reimplantation of kidney   © 80 ▣
MED: 100-3,20.3; 100-3,110.16; 100-3,260.7; 100-4,3,90.1; 100-4,3,90.1.1; 100-4,3,90.1.2
If renal autotransplantation extra-corporeal (bench) surgery is performed, report autotransplantation as the primary procedure and then add the secondary procedure (e.g., partial nephrectomy, nephrolithotomy) and append modifier 51.

INTRODUCTION

RENAL PELVIS CATHETER PROCEDURES

INTERNALLY DWELLING

⊙   **50382**   Removal (via snare/capture) and replacement of internally dwelling ureteral stent via percutaneous approach, including radiological supervision and interpretation   Ⓣ 50
To report bilateral procedure, use modifier 50.

⊙   **50384**   Removal (via snare/capture) of internally dwelling ureteral stent via percutaneous approach, including radiological supervision and interpretation   Ⓣ 50
To report bilateral procedure, use modifier 50.
Codes 50382, 50384 cannot be reported with 50395.

EXTERNALLY ACCESSIBLE

⊙ **50387** **Removal and replacement of externally accessible transnephric ureteral stent (eg, external/internal stent) requiring fluoroscopic guidance, including radiological supervision and interpretation** T 80 50

MED: 100-4,4,61.2

To report bilateral procedure, use modifier 50.

To report removal and replacement of an externally accessible ureteral stent via ureterostomy or ilieal conduit, consult CPT code 50688.

To report removal without replacement of an externally accessible ureteral stent not requiring fluoroscopic guidance, consult E/M services codes.

50389 **Removal of nephrostomy tube, requiring fluoroscopic guidance (eg, with concurrent indwelling ureteral stent)** T 50

Removal of nephrostomy tube not requiring fluoroscopic guidance is included in the E/M services. Report the appropriate level of E/M service provided.

OTHER INTRODUCTION PROCEDURES

50390 **Aspiration and/or injection of renal cyst or pelvis by needle, percutaneous** 1 T 50

MED: 100-2,15,260; 100-4,12,90.3; 100-4,14,10

AMA: 2001,Oct,8; 1997,Dec,7; 1993,Fall,14

To report radiological supervision and interpretation, consult CPT codes 74425, 74470, 76942, 77002, 77012, or 77021.

To report evaluation of fine needle aspirate, consult CPT codes 88172, 88173.

50391 **Instillation(s) of therapeutic agent into renal pelvis and/or ureter through established nephrostomy, pyelostomy or ureterostomy tube (eg, anticarcinogenic or antifungal agent)** T

50392 **Introduction of intracatheter or catheter into renal pelvis for drainage and/or injection, percutaneous** 1 T 50

MED: 100-2,15,260; 100-4,12,90.3; 100-4,14,10

AMA: 2001,Oct,8; 1997,Dec,7

To report radiological supervision and interpretation, consult CPT codes 74475, 76942, or 77012.

50393 **Introduction of ureteral catheter or stent into ureter through renal pelvis for drainage and/or injection, percutaneous** 1 T 50

MED: 100-2,15,260; 100-4,12,90.3; 100-4,14,10

AMA: 2001,Oct,8; 1993,Fall,14

To report radiological supervision and interpretation, consult CPT codes 74480, 76942, 77002, or 77012.

50394 **Injection procedure for pyelography (as nephrostogram, pyelostogram, antegrade pyeloureterograms) through nephrostomy or pyelostomy tube, or indwelling ureteral catheter** N 50

AMA: 2001,Oct,8; 1997,Dec,7; 1993,Fall,15

To report radiological supervision and interpretation, consult CPT code 74425.

50395 **Introduction of guide into renal pelvis and/or ureter with dilation to establish nephrostomy tract, percutaneous** 1 T 50

MED: 100-2,15,260; 100-4,12,90.3; 100-4,14,10

AMA: 2001,Oct,8

If a nephrostolithotomy is performed, consult CPT codes 50080 and 50081. If a retrograde percutaneous nephrostomy is performed, consult CPT code 52334. If endoscopic surgery is performed, consult CPT codes 50551-50561.

For radiolgical supervision and interpretation, consult CPT codes 74475, 74480, 74485.

50396 **Manometric studies through nephrostomy or pyelostomy tube, or indwelling ureteral catheter** 1 T 80 50

MED: 100-2,15,260; 100-4,12,90.3; 100-4,14,10

AMA: 2001,Oct,8; 1997,Dec,7; 1993,Fall,16

To report radiological supervision and interpretation, consult CPT codes 74425, 74475, and 74480.

50398 **Change of nephrostomy or pyelostomy tube** 1 T 50

MED: 100-2,15,260; 100-4,12,90.3; 100-4,14,10

AMA: 2001,Oct,8

If radiological supervision and interpretation is performed, consult CPT code 75984.

REPAIR

50400 **Pyeloplasty (Foley Y-pyeloplasty), plastic operation on renal pelvis, with or without plastic operation on ureter, nephropexy, nephrostomy, pyelostomy, or ureteral splinting; simple** C 80

AMA: 2001,Oct,8; 2000,May,4; 1999,Nov,25

50405 **complicated (congenital kidney abnormality, secondary pyeloplasty, solitary kidney, calycoplasty)** C 80

AMA: 2001,Oct,8; 2000,May,4; 1999,Nov,25

If a laparoscopic approach is used, consult CPT code 50544.

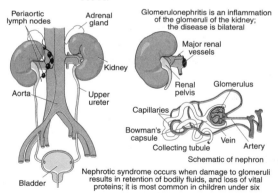

Periaortic lymph nodes — Adrenal gland — Kidney — Aorta — Upper ureter — Bladder

Glomerulonephritis is an inflammation of the glomeruli of the kidney; the disease is bilateral

Major renal vessels — Renal pelvis — Glomerulus — Capillaries — Bowman's capsule — Collecting tubule — Vein — Artery

Schematic of nephron

Nephrotic syndrome occurs when damage to glomeruli results in retention of bodily fluids, and loss of vital proteins; it is most common in children under six

50500 **Nephrorrhaphy, suture of kidney wound or injury** C 80

50520 **Closure of nephrocutaneous or pyelocutaneous fistula** C 80

50525 **Closure of nephrovisceral fistula (eg, renocolic), including visceral repair; abdominal approach** C 80

50526 **thoracic approach** C 80

50540 **Symphysiotomy for horseshoe kidney with or without pyeloplasty and/or other plastic procedure, unilateral or bilateral (one operation)** C 80

LAPAROSCOPY

Diagnostic laparoscopy is always included in surgical laparoscopy.

To report only a diagnostic laparoscopy (peritoneoscopy), consult CPT code 49320.

50541 Laparoscopy, surgical; ablation of renal cysts 〔T〕〔80〕▣
AMA: 2003,Jan,19; 2001,Oct,8; 2000,May,4; 1999,Nov,25

50542 ablation of renal mass lesion(s) 〔T〕〔80〕▣
AMA: 2003,Jan,19
To report open procedure, consult CPT codes 50220-50240.

If open cryoablation is performed, consult CPT code 50250.

If percutaneous cryotherapy ablation of renal tumors is performed, consult Category III code 0135T.

50543 partial nephrectomy 〔T〕〔80〕▣
AMA: 2003,Jan,19
To report open procedure, consult CPT code 50240.

50544 pyeloplasty 〔T〕〔80〕▣
AMA: 2001,Oct,8; 2000,May,4; 1999,Nov,25

50545 radical nephrectomy (includes removal of Gerota's fascia and surrounding fatty tissue, removal of regional lymph nodes, and adrenalectomy) 〔C〕〔80〕〔50〕▣
AMA: 2001,Oct,8
Consult CPT code 50230 for open procedure.

50546 nephrectomy, including partial ureterectomy 〔C〕〔80〕▣
AMA: 2001,Oct,8; 2000,May,4; 1999,Nov,25

50547 donor nephrectomy (including cold preservation), from living donor 〔C〕〔80〕〔50〕▣
MED: 100-4,3,90.1; 100-4,3,90.1.1; 100-4,3,90.1.2
AMA: 2001,Oct,8; 2000,May,4; 1999,Nov,25
Consult CPT code 50320 for open procedure.

For backbench renal allograft standard preparation before transplantation, consult CPT code 50325.

For backbench renal allograft reconstruction before transplantation, consult CPT code 50327-50329.

50548 nephrectomy with total ureterectomy 〔C〕〔80〕▣
AMA: 2001,Oct,8; 2000,May,4; 1999,Nov,25
Consult CPT codes 50234, 50236 for open procedure.

50549 Unlisted laparoscopy procedure, renal 〔T〕〔80〕〔50〕
AMA: 2000,May,4; 2000,Mar,5; 1999,Nov,25
If laparoscopic drainage is performed of a lymphocele to the peritoneal cavity, consult CPT code 49323.

ENDOSCOPY

To report supplies and material, consult CPT code 99070.

50551 Renal endoscopy through established nephrostomy or pyelostomy, with or without irrigation, instillation, or ureteropyelography, exclusive of radiologic service; 〔1〕〔T〕〔80〕〔50〕▣
MED: 100-2,15,260; 100-3,100.2; 100-4,12,90.3; 100-4,14,10
AMA: 2003,Jan,19; 2001,Oct,8

50553 with ureteral catheterization, with or without dilation of ureter 〔1〕〔T〕〔50〕▣
MED: 100-2,15,260; 100-3,100.2; 100-4,12,90.3; 100-4,14,10
AMA: 2001,Oct,8

50555 with biopsy 〔1〕〔T〕〔80〕〔50〕▣
MED: 100-2,15,260; 100-3,100.2; 100-4,12,90.3; 100-4,14,10
AMA: 2001,Oct,8

50557 with fulguration and/or incision, with or without biopsy 〔1〕〔T〕〔80〕〔50〕▣
MED: 100-2,15,260; 100-3,100.2; 100-4,12,90.3; 100-4,14,10
AMA: 2001,Oct,8

50561 with removal of foreign body or calculus 〔1〕〔T〕〔80〕〔50〕▣
MED: 100-2,15,260; 100-3,100.2; 100-3,230.1; 100-4,12,90.3; 100-4,14,10
AMA: 2003,Jan,19; 2001,Oct,8

50562 with resection of tumor 〔T〕〔80〕▣
AMA: 2003,Jan,19
If these procedures provide a significant identifiable service, they may be added to 50045 and 50120.

50570 Renal endoscopy through nephrotomy or pyelotomy, with or without irrigation, instillation, or ureteropyelography, exclusive of radiologic service; 〔T〕〔80〕〔50〕▣
MED: 100-3,100.2
AMA: 2001,Oct,8
If a nephrotomy is performed, consult CPT code 50045. If a pyelotomy is performed, consult CPT code 50120.

50572 with ureteral catheterization, with or without dilation of ureter 〔T〕〔80〕〔50〕▣
AMA: 2001,Oct,8

50574 with biopsy 〔T〕〔80〕〔50〕▣
AMA: 2001,Oct,8

50575 with endopyelotomy (includes cystoscopy, ureteroscopy, dilation of ureter and ureteral pelvic junction, incision of ureteral pelvic junction and insertion of endopyelotomy stent) 〔T〕〔50〕▣
AMA: 2002,Aug,11; 2001,Oct,8

50576 with fulguration and/or incision, with or without biopsy 〔T〕〔80〕〔50〕▣
AMA: 2001,Oct,8

50580 with removal of foreign body or calculus 〔C〕〔80〕〔50〕▣
MED: 100-3,100.2; 100-3,230.1
AMA: 2001,Oct,8

OTHER PROCEDURES

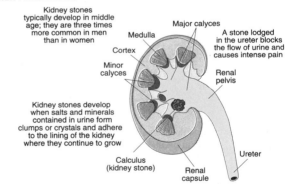

Kidney stones typically develop in middle age; they are three times more common in men than in women

Major calyces

Medulla

Cortex

A stone lodged in the ureter blocks the flow of urine and causes intense pain

Minor calyces

Renal pelvis

Kidney stones develop when salts and minerals contained in urine form clumps or crystals and adhere to the lining of the kidney where they continue to grow

Calculus (kidney stone)

Renal capsule

Ureter

50590 Lithotripsy, extracorporeal shock wave 〔T〕〔50〕▣
MED: 100-3,230.1
AMA: 2001,Oct,8; 2001,Jul,11; 2001,Aug,10

⊙ **50592** Ablation, one or more renal tumor(s), percutaneous, unilateral, radiofrequency 〔T〕〔80〕〔50〕
Code 50592 is a unilateral procedure. To report a bilateral service, report 50592 with modifier 50.

To report imaging guidance and monitoring, consult CPT codes 76940, 77013, 77022.

To report percutaneous cryotherapy ablation of renal tumors, consult Category III code 0135T.

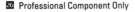

〔26〕 Professional Component Only 〔80〕/〔80〕 Assist-at-Surgery Allowed/With Documentation Unlisted Not Covered
〔TC〕 Technical Component Only MED: Pub 100/NCD References AMA: CPT Assistant References 〔1〕-〔9〕 ASC Group ♂ Male Only ♀ Female Only

186 — CPT Expert CPT only © 2006 American Medical Association. All Rights Reserved. (Black Ink) © 2006 Ingenix (Blue Ink)

URETER

INCISION

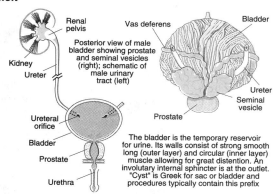

Renal pelvis

Vas deferens

Bladder

Kidney

Ureter

Posterior view of male bladder showing prostate and seminal vesicles (right); schematic of male urinary tract (left)

Ureter

Seminal vesicle

Ureteral orifice

Prostate

Bladder

Prostate

Urethra

The bladder is the temporary reservoir for urine. Its walls consist of strong smooth long (outer layer) and circular (inner layer) muscle allowing for great distention. An involutary internal sphincter is at the outlet. "Cyst" is Greek for sac or bladder and procedures typically contain this prefix

50600 **Ureterotomy with exploration or drainage (separate procedure)** C 80 50 ⟲

If ureteral endoscopy is performed in conjunction with this procedure, consult CPT codes 50970-50980.

50605 **Ureterotomy for insertion of indwelling stent, all types** C 80 50 ⟲
AMA: 2001,Oct,8

50610 **Ureterolithotomy; upper one-third of ureter** C 80 50 ⟲
AMA: 2001,Oct,8; 1999,Nov,26

50620 **middle one-third of ureter** C 80 50 ⟲
AMA: 2001,Oct,8; 1999,Nov,26

50630 **lower one-third of ureter** C 80 50 ⟲
AMA: 2001,Oct,8; 1999,Nov,26

If a laparoscopic approach is used, consult CPT code 50945. If a transvesical ureterolithotomy is performed, consult CPT code 51060. If a cystotomy is performed with stone basket extraction of the ureteral calculus, consult CPT code 51065. If an endoscopic extraction or manipulation of the ureteral calculus is performed, consult CPT codes 50080, 50081, 50561, 50961, 50980, 52320-52330, 52352, and 52353.

EXCISION

For ureterocele, consult CPT codes 51535, 52300.

50650 **Ureterectomy, with bladder cuff (separate procedure)** C 80 ⟲

50660 **Ureterectomy, total, ectopic ureter, combination abdominal, vaginal and/or perineal approach** C 80 ⟲

INTRODUCTION

50684 **Injection procedure for ureterography or ureteropyelography through ureterostomy or indwelling ureteral catheter** N 50 ⟲

To report radiological supervision and interpretation, consult CPT code 74425.

50686 **Manometric studies through ureterostomy or indwelling ureteral catheter** T 80 ⟲

50688 **Change of ureterostomy tube or externally accessible ureteral stent via ileal conduit** 1 T ⟲
MED: 100-2,15,260; 100-4,12,90.3; 100-4,14,10

To report imaging guidance, consult CPT code 75984

50690 **Injection procedure for visualization of ileal conduit and/or ureteropyelography, exclusive of radiologic service** N ⟲

To report radiological supervision and interpretation, consult CPT code 74425.

REPAIR

50700 **Ureteroplasty, plastic operation on ureter (eg, stricture)** C 80 ⟲

50715 **Ureterolysis, with or without repositioning of ureter for retroperitoneal fibrosis** C 80 50 ⟲

50722 **Ureterolysis for ovarian vein syndrome** ♀ C 80 ⟲

50725 **Ureterolysis for retrocaval ureter, with reanastomosis of upper urinary tract or vena cava** C 80 ⟲

50727 **Revision of urinary-cutaneous anastomosis (any type urostomy);** C 80 ⟲

50728 **with repair of fascial defect and hernia** C 80 ⟲

50740 **Ureteropyelostomy, anastomosis of ureter and renal pelvis** C 80 ⟲
AMA: 2001,Oct,8

50750 **Ureterocalycostomy, anastomosis of ureter to renal calyx** C 80 ⟲
AMA: 2001,Oct,8

50760 **Ureteroureterostomy** C 80 ⟲
AMA: 2001,Oct,8

50770 **Transureteroureterostomy, anastomosis of ureter to contralateral ureter** C 80 ⟲

Note that this procedure includes minor procedures to prevent vesicoureteral reflux.

50780 **Ureteroneocystostomy; anastomosis of single ureter to bladder** C 80 50 ⟲
AMA: 2001,Oct,8

If this procedure is combined with a cystourethroplasty or a vesical neck revision, consult CPT code 51820.

50782 **anastomosis of duplicated ureter to bladder** C 80 50 ⟲
AMA: 2001,Oct,8

50783 **with extensive ureteral tailoring** C 80 50 ⟲
AMA: 2001,Oct,8

Note that this procedure includes minor procedures to prevent vesicoureteral reflux.

50785 **with vesico-psoas hitch or bladder flap** C 80 50 ⟲
AMA: 2001,Oct,8

Note that this procedure includes minor procedures to prevent vesicoureteral reflux.

50800 **Ureteroenterostomy, direct anastomosis of ureter to intestine** C 80 50 ⟲
AMA: 2001,Oct,8

If procedures 50800-50820 are performed with a cystectomy, consult CPT codes 51580-51595.

50810 **Ureterosigmoidostomy, with creation of sigmoid bladder and establishment of abdominal or perineal colostomy, including intestine anastomosis** C 80 ⟲
AMA: 2001,Oct,8

50815 **Ureterocolon conduit, including intestine anastomosis** C 80 50 ⟲
AMA: 2001,Oct,8

50820 **Ureteroileal conduit (ileal bladder), including intestine anastomosis (Bricker operation)** C 80 50 ⟲
AMA: 2001,Oct,8

⊛ Modifier 63 Exempt Code ⊙ Conscious Sedation + CPT Add-on Code ⊘ Modifier 51 Exempt Code ● New Code ▲ Revised Code

M Maternity Edit A Age Edit A-Y APC Status Indicators ⟲ CCI Comprehensive Code 50 Bilateral Procedure

50825 Continent diversion, including intestine anastomosis using any segment of small and/or large intestine (Kock pouch or Camey enterocystoplasty) C 80 ⬀

AMA: 2001,Oct,8

50830 Urinary undiversion (eg, taking down of ureteroileal conduit, ureterosigmoidostomy or ureteroenterostomy with ureteroureterostomy or ureteroneocystostomy) C 80 ⬀

AMA: 2001,Oct,8

50840 Replacement of all or part of ureter by intestine segment, including intestine anastomosis C 80 50 ⬀

AMA: 2001,Oct,8

50845 Cutaneous appendico-vesicostomy C 80 ⬀

Mitrofanoff operation

50860 Ureterostomy, transplantation of ureter to skin C 80 50 ⬀

50900 Ureterorrhaphy, suture of ureter (separate procedure) C 80 ⬀

50920 Closure of ureterocutaneous fistula C 80 ⬀

50930 Closure of ureterovisceral fistula (including visceral repair) C 80 ⬀

50940 Deligation of ureter C 80 50 ⬀

If ureteroplasty or ureterolysis is performed, consult CPT codes 50700-50860.

LAPAROSCOPY

Diagnostic laparoscopy is always included with surgical laparoscopy

To report only a diagnostic laparoscopy (peritoneoscopy), consult CPT code 49320.

50945 Laparoscopy, surgical; ureterolithotomy T 80 50 ⬀

AMA: 2001,Oct,8; 2000,May,4; 1999,Nov,26

50947 ureteroneocystostomy with cystoscopy and ureteral stent placement 9 T 80 50 ⬀

MED: 100-2,15,260; 100-4,12,90.3; 100-4,14,10

AMA: 2001,Oct,8

50948 ureteroneocystostomy without cystoscopy and ureteral stent placement 9 T 80 50 ⬀

MED: 100-2,15,260; 100-4,12,90.3; 100-4,14,10

AMA: 2001,Oct,8

To report open ureterocystostomy, consult CPT codes 50780-50785.

50949 Unlisted laparoscopy procedure, ureter T 80 50

AMA: 2001,Oct,8

ENDOSCOPY

50951 Ureteral endoscopy through established ureterostomy, with or without irrigation, instillation, or ureteropyelography, exclusive of radiologic service; 1 T 80 50 ⬀

MED: 100-2,15,260; 100-3,100.2; 100-4,12,90.3; 100-4,14,10

AMA: 2001,Oct,8

50953 with ureteral catheterization, with or without dilation of ureter 1 T 80 50 ⬀

MED: 100-2,15,260; 100-4,12,90.3; 100-4,14,10

AMA: 2001,Oct,8

50955 with biopsy 1 T 80 50 ⬀

MED: 100-2,15,260; 100-4,12,90.3; 100-4,14,10

AMA: 2001,Oct,8

50957 with fulguration and/or incision, with or without biopsy 1 T 80 50 ⬀

MED: 100-2,15,260; 100-4,12,90.3; 100-4,14,10

AMA: 2001,Oct,8

50961 with removal of foreign body or calculus 1 T 80 50 ⬀

MED: 100-2,15,260; 100-4,12,90.3; 100-4,14,10

AMA: 2001,Oct,8

50970 Ureteral endoscopy through ureterotomy, with or without irrigation, instillation, or ureteropyelography, exclusive of radiologic service; 1 T 80 50 ⬀

MED: 100-2,15,260; 100-3,100.2; 100-4,12,90.3; 100-4,14,10

AMA: 2001,Oct,8

If a ureterotomy is performed, consult CPT code 50600.

If these procedures (50970-50980) provide a significant identifiable service, they may be added to 50600.

50972 with ureteral catheterization, with or without dilation of ureter 1 T 80 50 ⬀

MED: 100-2,15,260; 100-4,12,90.3; 100-4,14,10

AMA: 2001,Oct,8

50974 with biopsy 1 T 80 50 ⬀

MED: 100-2,15,260; 100-4,12,90.3; 100-4,14,10

AMA: 2001,Oct,8

50976 with fulguration and/or incision, with or without biopsy 1 T 80 50 ⬀

MED: 100-2,15,260; 100-4,12,90.3; 100-4,14,10

AMA: 2001,Oct,8

50980 with removal of foreign body or calculus 1 T 80 50 ⬀

MED: 100-2,15,260; 100-4,12,90.3; 100-4,14,10

AMA: 2001,Oct,8

BLADDER

INCISION

51000 Aspiration of bladder by needle T ⬀

51005 Aspiration of bladder; by trocar or intracatheter T ⬀

51010 with insertion of suprapubic catheter 1 T ⬀

MED: 100-2,15,260; 100-4,12,90.3; 100-4,14,10

To report imaging guidance, consult CPT codes 76942, 77002, or 77012.

51020 Cystotomy or cystostomy; with fulguration and/or insertion of radioactive material 4 T 80 ⬀

MED: 100-2,15,260; 100-4,12,90.3; 100-4,14,10

51030 with cryosurgical destruction of intravesical lesion 4 T 80 ⬀

MED: 100-2,15,260; 100-4,12,90.3; 100-4,14,10

51040 Cystostomy, cystotomy with drainage 4 T 80 ⬀

MED: 100-2,15,260; 100-4,12,90.3; 100-4,14,10

51045 Cystotomy, with insertion of ureteral catheter or stent (separate procedure) 4 T 80 ⬀

MED: 100-2,15,260; 100-4,12,90.3; 100-4,14,10

51050 Cystolithotomy, cystotomy with removal of calculus, without vesical neck resection 4 T 80 ⬀

MED: 100-2,15,260; 100-4,12,90.3; 100-4,14,10

51060 Transvesical ureterolithotomy C 80 ⬀

51065 Cystotomy, with calculus basket extraction and/or ultrasonic or electrohydraulic fragmentation of ureteral calculus 4 T 80 ⬀

MED: 100-2,15,260; 100-4,12,90.3; 100-4,14,10

51080 Drainage of perivesical or prevesical space abscess 1 T 80 ⬀

MED: 100-2,15,260; 100-4,12,90.3; 100-4,14,10

26 Professional Component Only   80/80 Assist-at-Surgery Allowed/With Documentation   Unlisted   Not Covered

TC Technical Component Only   MED: Pub 100/NCD References   AMA: CPT Assistant References   1-9 ASC Group   ♂ Male Only   ♀ Female Only

188 — CPT Expert   CPT only © 2006 American Medical Association. All Rights Reserved. (Black Ink)   © 2006 Ingenix (Blue Ink)

EXCISION

51500   Excision of urachal cyst or sinus, with or without umbilical hernia repair   4 T 80 ▣

     MED: 100-2,15,260; 100-4,12,90.3; 100-4,14,10

51520   Cystotomy; for simple excision of vesical neck (separate procedure)   4 T 80 ▣

     MED: 100-2,15,260; 100-4,12,90.3; 100-4,14,10

51525   for excision of bladder diverticulum, single or multiple (separate procedure)   C 80 ▣

51530   for excision of bladder tumor   C 80 ▣

     If transurethral resection is performed, consult CPT codes 52234-52240 and 52305.

51535   Cystotomy for excision, incision, or repair of ureterocele   C 80 50 ▣

     If a transurethral excision is performed, consult CPT code 52300.

51550   Cystectomy, partial; simple   C 80 ▣

51555   complicated (eg, postradiation, previous surgery, difficult location)   C 80 ▣

51565   Cystectomy, partial, with reimplantation of ureter(s) into bladder (ureteroneocystostomy)   C 80 ▣

51570   Cystectomy, complete; (separate procedure)   C 80 ▣

51575   with bilateral pelvic lymphadenectomy, including external iliac, hypogastric, and obturator nodes   C 80 ▣

51580   Cystectomy, complete, with ureterosigmoidostomy or ureterocutaneous transplantations;   C 80 ▣

51585   with bilateral pelvic lymphadenectomy, including external iliac, hypogastric, and obturator nodes   C 80 ▣

51590   Cystectomy, complete, with ureteroileal conduit or sigmoid bladder, including intestine anastomosis;   C 80 ▣

51595   with bilateral pelvic lymphadenectomy, including external iliac, hypogastric, and obturator nodes   C 80 ▣

51596   Cystectomy, complete, with continent diversion, any open technique, using any segment of small and/or large intestine to construct neobladder   C 80 ▣

51597   Pelvic exenteration, complete, for vesical, prostatic or urethral malignancy, with removal of bladder and ureteral transplantations, with or without hysterectomy and/or abdominoperineal resection of rectum and colon and colostomy, or any combination thereof   C 80 ▣

     If a pelvic exenteration is performed for gynecologic malignancy, consult CPT code 58240.

INTRODUCTION

If bladder catheterization is performed, consult CPT codes 53670 and 53675.

51600   Injection procedure for cystography or voiding urethrocystography   N ▣

     MED: 100-3,230.2

     To report radiological supervision and interpretation, consult CPT codes 74430 and 74455.

51605   Injection procedure and placement of chain for contrast and/or chain urethrocystography   N ▣

     To report radiological supervision and interpretation, consult CPT code 74430.

51610   Injection procedure for retrograde urethrocystography   N ▣

     To report radiological supervision and interpretation, consult CPT code 74450.

51700   Bladder irrigation, simple, lavage and/or instillation   T ▣

51701   Insertion of non-indwelling bladder catheter (eg, straight catheterization for residual urine)   X ▣

     When catheter insertion is a component of another procedure, do not report CPT codes 51701 or 51702 separately.

51702   Insertion of temporary indwelling bladder catheter; simple (eg, Foley)   X ▣

51703   complicated (eg, altered anatomy, fractured catheter/balloon)   T ▣

51705   Change of cystostomy tube; simple   T ▣

51710   complicated   1 T ▣

     MED: 100-2,15,260; 100-4,12,90.3; 100-4,14,10

     Consult CPT code 75984 for imaging guidance.

51715   Endoscopic injection of implant material into the submucosal tissues of the urethra and/or bladder neck   3 T 80 ▣

     MED: 100-2,15,260; 100-3,230.10; 100-4,12,90.3; 100-4,14,10

▲ **51720**   Bladder instillation of anticarcinogenic agent (including retention time)   T ▣

     AMA: 2002,Nov,11

URODYNAMICS

Urodynamics is a diagnostic service performed to evaluate the storage of urine and urine flow through the urinary tract. All procedures in this section represent complete procedures (both the professional and technical components). Physicians reporting these services as complete procedures are expected to supply all instruments/equipment, supplies, and technician services. A physician performing only the operation of the equipment and interpretation of the report should report only the professional component by appending modifier 26 Professional component, to the procedure codes.

When multiple procedures are performed at the same operative session, append modifier 51.

51725   Simple cystometrogram (CMG) (eg, spinal manometer)   T 80 ▣

     AMA: 2002,Sep,6

51726   Complex cystometrogram (eg, calibrated electronic equipment)   1 T ▣

     MED: 100-2,15,260; 100-4,12,90.3; 100-4,14,10

     AMA: 2002,Sep,6

51736   Simple uroflowmetry (UFR) (eg, stop-watch flow rate, mechanical uroflowmeter)   T 80 ▣

     MED: 100-3,230.2

     AMA: 2002,Sep,6

51741   Complex uroflowmetry (eg, calibrated electronic equipment)   T ▣

     MED: 100-3,230.2

     AMA: 2002,Sep,6

51772   Urethral pressure profile studies (UPP) (urethral closure pressure profile), any technique   1 T 80 ▣

     MED: 100-2,15,260; 100-4,12,90.3; 100-4,14,10

     AMA: 2002,Sep,6

     Keitzer test

51784   Electromyography studies (EMG) of anal or urethral sphincter, other than needle, any technique   T ▣

     AMA: 2002,Sep,6

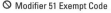

⊛ Modifier 63 Exempt Code   ☉ Conscious Sedation   + CPT Add-on Code   ⊘ Modifier 51 Exempt Code   ● New Code   ▲ Revised Code

M Maternity Edit   A Age Edit   A-Y APC Status Indicators   ▣ CCI Comprehensive Code   50 Bilateral Procedure

Urinary System

51785 — 52204

51785 Needle electromyography studies (EMG) of anal or
urethral sphincter, any technique   **1** T 80 ◩

MED: 100-2,15,260; 100-4,12,90.3; 100-4,14,10

AMA: 2002,Sep,6; 2002,Apr,1

51792 Stimulus evoked response (eg, measurement of
bulbocavernosus reflex latency time)   T 80 ◩

AMA: 2002,Sep,6; 2002,Apr,1

51795 Voiding pressure studies (VP); bladder voiding
pressure, any technique   T 80 ◩

MED: 100-3,230.2

AMA: 2002,Sep,6; 2001,Dec,7

51797 intra-abdominal voiding pressure (AP) (rectal,
gastric, intraperitoneal)   T 80 ◩

MED: 100-3,230.2

AMA: 2002,Sep,6; 2001,Dec,7

51798 Measurement of post-voiding residual urine and/or
bladder capacity by ultrasound,
non-imaging   X 80 ◩

REPAIR

51800 Cystoplasty or cystourethroplasty, plastic operation
on bladder and/or vesical neck (anterior Y-plasty,
vesical fundus resection), any procedure, with or
without wedge resection of posterior vesical
neck   C 80 ◩

51820 Cystourethroplasty with unilateral or bilateral
ureteroneocystostomy   C 80 ◩

51840 Anterior vesicourethropexy, or urethropexy (eg,
Marshall-Marchetti-Krantz, Burch); simple   C 80 ◩

AMA: 1998,Apr,15; 1997,Nov,19; 1997,Jan,1

51841 complicated (eg, secondary repair)   C 80 ◩

AMA: 1997,Jan,1

If urethropexy (Pereyra type) is performed, consult CPT
code 57289.

51845 Abdomino-vaginal vesical neck suspension, with or
without endoscopic control (eg, Stamey, Raz, modified
Pereyra)   ♀ C 80 ◩

AMA: 1997,Jan,3

51860 Cystorrhaphy, suture of bladder wound, injury or
rupture; simple   C 80 ◩

51865 complicated   C 80 ◩

51880 Closure of cystostomy (separate
procedure)   **1** T 80 ◩

MED: 100-2,15,260; 100-4,12,90.3; 100-4,14,10

51900 Closure of vesicovaginal fistula, abdominal
approach   ♀ C 80 ◩

If a vaginal approach is used, consult CPT codes
57320-57330.

51920 Closure of vesicouterine fistula;   ♀ C 80 ◩

51925 with hysterectomy   ♀ C 80 ◩

If a vesicoenteric fistula is closed, consult CPT codes
44660 and 44661. If a rectovesical fistula is closed,
consult CPT codes 45800-45805.

51940 Closure, exstrophy of bladder   C 80 ◩

Consult also CPT code 54390.

51960 Enterocystoplasty, including intestinal
anastomosis   C 80 ◩

51980 Cutaneous vesicostomy   C 80 ◩

LAPAROSCOPY

Diagnostic laparoscopy is always included in a surgical laparoscopy. For diagnostic
laparoscopy only (peritoneoscopy), consult CPT code 49320.

51990 Laparoscopy, surgical; urethral suspension for stress
incontinence   T 80 ◩

MED: 100-3,230.10

AMA: 2000,May,4; 1999,Nov,26

51992 sling operation for stress incontinence (eg, fascia
or synthetic)   ♀ **5** T 80 ◩

MED: 100-3,230.10

AMA: 2000,May,4; 1999,Nov,26

Consult CPT code 57288 for open sling operation for
stress incontinence. For removal or revision of sling
operation consult CPT code 57287.

51999 Unlisted laparoscopy procedure, bladder   T 80

ENDOSCOPY — CYSTOSCOPY, URETHROSCOPY, CYSTOURETHROSCOPY

Cystoscopy, urethroscopy, and cystourethroscopy are listed so that the main
procedure can be identified without listing all minor related procedures performed.
For example, a cystourethroscopy with dilation of a urethral stricture (52281)
includes calibration, meatotomy, and the injection procedure for cystography,
which are all explicitly described in the procedure.

Multiple procedures performed at the same operative session should be reported
and modifier 51 Multiple procedures should be appended.. Many procedures on
the ureter require placement of a temporary stent. Placement and removal of
temporary stents are not reported separately. However, placement of more
permanent, self-retaining, indwelling stents (52332) should be reported with the
code for the primary procedure.

52000 Cystourethroscopy (separate procedure)   **1** T ◩

MED: 100-4,15,260; 100-4,12,90.3; 100-4,14,10

AMA: 2001,May,5; 2000,Oct,7

52001 Cystourethroscopy with irrigation and evacuation of
multiple obstructing clots   **2** T ◩

MED: 100-2,15,260; 100-4,12,90.3; 100-4,14,10

Do not report 52001 in conjunction with 52000.

52005 Cystourethroscopy, with ureteral catheterization, with
or without irrigation, instillation, or
ureteropyelography, exclusive of radiologic
service;   **2** T ◩

MED: 100-2,15,260; 100-4,12,30.2; 100-4,12,90.3; 100-4,14,10

AMA: 2001,Oct,8; 2001,May,5; 2001,Jan,13; 2000,Sep,11
Howard test

52007 with brush biopsy of ureter and/or renal
pelvis   **2** T 50 ◩

MED: 100-2,15,260; 100-4,12,90.3; 100-4,14,10

AMA: 2001,Oct,8; 2001,May,5

52010 Cystourethroscopy, with ejaculatory duct
catheterization, with or without irrigation, instillation,
or duct radiography, exclusive of radiologic
service   ♂ **2** T ◩

MED: 100-2,15,260; 100-4,12,90.3; 100-4,14,10

AMA: 2001,May,5

To report radiological supervision and interpretation,
consult CPT code 74440.

TRANSURETHRAL SURGERY

URETHRA AND BLADDER

▲ **52204** Cystourethroscopy, with biopsy(s)   **2** T ◩

MED: 100-2,15,260; 100-4,12,90.3; 100-4,14,10

AMA: 2001,Sep,1; 2001,May,5

26 Professional Component Only   **80**/**80** Assist-at-Surgery Allowed/With Documentation   Unlisted   Not Covered

TC Technical Component Only   MED: Pub 100/NCD References   AMA: CPT Assistant References   **1**-**9** ASC Group   ♂ Male Only   ♀ Female Only

190 — CPT Expert   CPT only © 2006 American Medical Association. All Rights Reserved. (Black Ink)   © 2006 Ingenix (Blue Ink)

52214 Cystourethroscopy, with fulguration (including cryosurgery or laser surgery) of trigone, bladder neck, prostatic fossa, urethra, or periurethral glands 2 T 🗷

MED: 100-2,15,260; 100-4,12,90.3; 100-4,14,10
AMA: 2001,Sep,1; 2001,May,5

52224 Cystourethroscopy, with fulguration (including cryosurgery or laser surgery) or treatment of MINOR (less than 0.5 cm) lesion(s) with or without biopsy 2 T 🗷

MED: 100-2,15,260; 100-4,12,90.3; 100-4,14,10
AMA: 2001,Sep,1; 2001,May,5

52234 Cystourethroscopy, with fulguration (including cryosurgery or laser surgery) and/or resection of; SMALL bladder tumor(s) (0.5 up to 2.0 cm) 2 T 🗷

MED: 100-2,15,260; 100-4,12,30.2; 100-4,12,90.3; 100-4,14,10
AMA: 2003,Jan,19; 2002,Oct,12; 2001,Sep,1; 2001,May,5

52235 MEDIUM bladder tumor(s) (2.0 to 5.0 cm) 3 T 🗷

MED: 100-2,15,260; 100-4,12,30.2; 100-4,12,90.3; 100-4,14,10
AMA: 2003,Jan,19; 2002,Oct,12; 2001,Sep,1; 2001,May,5

52240 LARGE bladder tumor(s) 3 T 🗷

MED: 100-2,15,260; 100-4,12,30.2; 100-4,12,90.3; 100-4,14,10
AMA: 2001,Sep,1; 2001,May,5

52250 Cystourethroscopy with insertion of radioactive substance, with or without biopsy or fulguration 4 T 🗷

MED: 100-2,15,260; 100-3,230.12; 100-4,12,90.3; 100-4,14,10
AMA: 2001,Sep,1; 2001,May,5

52260 Cystourethroscopy, with dilation of bladder for interstitial cystitis; general or conduction (spinal) anesthesia 2 T 🗷

MED: 100-2,15,260; 100-3,230.12; 100-4,12,90.3; 100-4,14,10
AMA: 2001,Sep,1; 2001,May,5

52265 local anesthesia T 🗷

MED: 100-3,230.12
AMA: 2001,Sep,1; 2001,May,5

52270 Cystourethroscopy, with internal urethrotomy; female ♀ 2 T 🗷

MED: 100-2,15,260; 100-4,12,90.3; 100-4,14,10
AMA: 2001,Sep,1; 2001,May,5

52275 male ♂ 2 T 🗷

MED: 100-2,15,260; 100-4,12,90.3; 100-4,14,10
AMA: 2001,Sep,1; 2001,May,5

52276 Cystourethroscopy with direct vision internal urethrotomy 3 T 🗷

MED: 100-2,15,260; 100-4,12,90.3; 100-4,14,10
AMA: 2001,Sep,1; 2001,May,5

52277 Cystourethroscopy, with resection of external sphincter (sphincterotomy) 2 T 80 🗷

MED: 100-2,15,260; 100-4,12,90.3; 100-4,14,10
AMA: 2001,Sep,1; 2001,May,5

52281 Cystourethroscopy, with calibration and/or dilation of urethral stricture or stenosis, with or without meatotomy, with or without injection procedure for cystography, male or female 2 T 🗷

MED: 100-2,15,260; 100-4,12,90.3; 100-4,14,10
AMA: 2001,Sep,1; 2001,May,5; 1997,Nov,20

52282 Cystourethroscopy, with insertion of urethral stent 9 T 🗷

MED: 100-2,15,260; 100-4,12,90.3; 100-4,14,10
AMA: 2001,Sep,1; 2001,May,5; 1997,Nov,20

52283 Cystourethroscopy, with steroid injection into stricture 2 T 🗷

MED: 100-2,15,260; 100-4,12,90.3; 100-4,14,10
AMA: 2001,Sep,1; 2001,May,5

52285 Cystourethroscopy for treatment of the female urethral syndrome with any or all of the following: urethral meatotomy, urethral dilation, internal urethrotomy, lysis of urethrovaginal septal fibrosis, lateral incisions of the bladder neck, and fulguration of polyp(s) of urethra, bladder neck, and/or trigone ♀ 2 T 🗷

MED: 100-2,15,260; 100-4,12,90.3; 100-4,14,10
AMA: 2001,Sep,1; 2001,May,5

52290 Cystourethroscopy; with ureteral meatotomy, unilateral or bilateral 2 T 🗷

MED: 100-2,15,260; 100-4,12,40.7; 100-4,12,90.3; 100-4,14,10
AMA: 2001,Sep,1; 2001,May,5

52300 with resection or fulguration of orthotopic ureterocele(s), unilateral or bilateral 2 T 80 🗷

MED: 100-2,15,260; 100-4,12,40.7; 100-4,12,90.3; 100-4,14,10
AMA: 2001,Sep,1; 2001,May,5

52301 with resection or fulguration of ectopic ureterocele(s), unilateral or bilateral 3 T 80 🗷

MED: 100-4,12,40.7
AMA: 2001,Sep,1; 2001,May,5

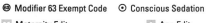

Diverticulum of bladder

Bladder

Rectum

Diverticula are pouches that push out through the wall of an organ; bladder diverticula may be acquired or congenital and may cause urinary incontinence or increased urgency to urinate

Pubic bone

This condition is most common in older men

Urethra

52305 with incision or resection of orifice of bladder diverticulum, single or multiple 2 T 🗷

MED: 100-2,15,260; 100-4,12,90.3; 100-4,14,10
AMA: 2001,Sep,1; 2001,May,5

52310 Cystourethroscopy, with removal of foreign body, calculus, or ureteral stent from urethra or bladder (separate procedure); simple 2 T 🗷

MED: 100-2,15,260; 100-4,12,90.3; 100-4,14,10
AMA: 2001,Sep,1; 2001,May,5
When reporting the removal of self-retaining, indwelling ureteral stent, append modifier 58 to code 52310 or 52315.

52315 complicated 2 T 🗷

MED: 100-2,15,260; 100-4,12,90.3; 100-4,14,10
AMA: 2001,Sep,1; 2001,May,5

52317 Litholapaxy: crushing or fragmentation of calculus by any means in bladder and removal of fragments; simple or small (less than 2.5 cm) 1 T 🗷

MED: 100-2,15,260; 100-4,12,90.3; 100-4,14,10
AMA: 2001,Sep,1; 2001,May,5

52318 complicated or large (over 2.5 cm) 2 T 🗷

MED: 100-2,15,260; 100-4,12,90.3; 100-4,14,10
AMA: 2001,Sep,1; 2001,May,5

 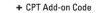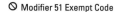

Urinary System

52320 — 52402

URETER AND PELVIS

CPT codes 52320-52355 include the insertion and removal of a temporary stent during a therapeutic or diagnostic cystourethroscopy and should not be separately reported.

For insertion of a self-retaining, indwelling stent performed during a cystourethroscopic diagnostic or therapeutic procedure(s) consult CPT code 52332 in addition to the primary procedure performed and add modifier 51. Code 52332 is used to report a unilateral procedure; add modifier 50 for insertion of a bilateral stent.

For the removal of a self-retaining indwelling ureteral stent, consult CPT codes 52310, 52315 and add modifier 58 if appropriate.

Diagnostic cystourethroscopy is always included in surgical cystourethroscopy. To report only a diagnostic cystourethroscopy, consult CPT code 52000. Therapeutic cystourethroscopy with ureteroscopy and/or pyeloscopy always includes diagnostic cystourethroscopy with ureteroscopy and/or pyeloscopy. Report code 52351 for a diagnostic cystourethroscopy with ureteroscopy and/or pyeloscopy.

52320 **Cystourethroscopy (including ureteral catheterization); with removal of ureteral calculus** 5 T 50

> MED: 100-2,15,260; 100-4,12,90.3; 100-4,14,10
> AMA: 2001,Sep,1; 2001,Oct,8; 2001,May,5; 2001,Jan,13; 1996,May,11; 1996,Mar,1

52325 **with fragmentation of ureteral calculus (eg, ultrasonic or electro-hydraulic technique)** 4 T 50

> MED: 100-2,15,260; 100-4,12,90.3; 100-4,14,10
> AMA: 2001,Sep,1; 2001,Oct,8; 2001,May,5; 1996,May,11; 1996,Mar,1

52327 **with subureteric injection of implant material** 2 T 50

> MED: 100-2,15,260; 100-3,230.10; 100-4,12,90.3; 100-4,14,10
> AMA: 2001,Sep,1; 2001,Oct,8; 2001,May,5; 1996,May,11; 1996,Mar,1

52330 **with manipulation, without removal of ureteral calculus** 2 T 50

> MED: 100-2,15,260; 100-4,12,90.3; 100-4,14,10
> AMA: 2001,Sep,1; 2001,Oct,8; 2001,May,5; 2000,Sep,11; 1996,May,11; 1996,Mar,1

52332 **Cystourethroscopy, with insertion of indwelling ureteral stent (eg, Gibbons or double-J type)** 2 T 50

> MED: 100-2,15,260; 100-4,12,90.3; 100-4,14,10
> AMA: 2001,Sep,1; 2001,Oct,8; 2001,May,5; 2001,Jan,13; 1996,May,11; 1996,Mar,1
> To report bilateral insertion, append modifier 50. If procedure is performed in addition to other diagnostic or therapeutic interventions, append modifier 51.

52334 **Cystourethroscopy with insertion of ureteral guide wire through kidney to establish a percutaneous nephrostomy, retrograde** 3 T 50

> MED: 100-2,15,260; 100-4,12,90.3; 100-4,14,10
> AMA: 2001,Sep,1; 2001,Oct,8; 2001,May,5; 1996,May,11; 1996,Mar,11
> If percutaneous nephrostolithotomy is performed, consult CPT codes 50080 and 50081. If establishment of the nephrostomy tract is performed by itself, consult CPT code 50395.

52341 **Cystourethroscopy; with treatment of ureteral stricture (eg, balloon dilation, laser, electrocautery, and incision)** 3 T 50

> MED: 100-2,15,260; 100-4,12,90.3; 100-4,14,10
> AMA: 2001,Sep,1; 2001,Oct,8; 2001,May,5; 2001,Apr,4

52342 **with treatment of ureteropelvic junction stricture (eg, balloon dilation, laser, electrocautery, and incision)** 3 T 50

> MED: 100-2,15,260; 100-4,12,90.3; 100-4,14,10
> AMA: 2001,Sep,1; 2001,Oct,8; 2001,May,5; 2001,Apr,4

52343 **with treatment of intra-renal stricture (eg, balloon dilation, laser, electrocautery, and incision)** 3 T 50

> MED: 100-2,15,260; 100-4,12,90.3; 100-4,14,10
> AMA: 2001,Sep,1; 2001,Oct,8; 2001,May,5; 2001,Apr,4

52344 **Cystourethroscopy with ureteroscopy; with treatment of ureteral stricture (eg, balloon dilation, laser, electrocautery, and incision)** 3 T 50

> MED: 100-2,15,260; 100-4,12,90.3; 100-4,14,10
> AMA: 2001,Sep,1; 2001,Oct,8; 2001,May,5; 2001,Apr,4

52345 **with treatment of ureteropelvic junction stricture (eg, balloon dilation, laser, electrocautery, and incision)** 3 T 80

> MED: 100-2,15,260; 100-4,12,90.3; 100-4,14,10
> AMA: 2001,Sep,1; 2001,Oct,8; 2001,May,5; 2001,Apr,4

52346 **with treatment of intra-renal stricture (eg, balloon dilation, laser, electrocautery, and incision)** 3 T 80

> MED: 100-2,15,260; 100-3,230.3; 100-4,12,90.3; 100-4,14,10
> AMA: 2001,Sep,1; 2001,Oct,8; 2001,May,5; 2001,Apr,4
> To report transurethral resection or incision of ejaculatory ducts, consult CPT code 52402.

52351 **Cystourethroscopy, with ureteroscopy and/or pyeloscopy; diagnostic** 3 T

> MED: 100-2,15,260; 100-4,12,90.3; 100-4,14,10
> AMA: 2001,Sep,1; 2001,Oct,8; 2001,May,5; 2001,Apr,4
> To report radiological supervision and interpretation, consult CPT code 74485.
>
> Do not report CPT code 52351 when reporting 52341-52346, or 52352-52355.

52352 **with removal or manipulation of calculus (ureteral catheterization is included)** 4 T 50

> MED: 100-2,15,260; 100-3,230.1; 100-4,12,90.3; 100-4,14,10
> AMA: 2001,Sep,1; 2001,Oct,8; 2001,May,5; 2001,Apr,4

52353 **with lithotripsy (ureteral catheterization is included)** 4 T 50

> MED: 100-2,15,260; 100-3,230.1; 100-4,12,90.3; 100-4,14,10
> AMA: 2001,Sep,1; 2001,Oct,8; 2001,May,5; 2001,Apr,4

52354 **with biopsy and/or fulguration of ureteral or renal pelvic lesion** 4 T 50

> MED: 100-2,15,260; 100-4,12,90.3; 100-4,14,10
> AMA: 2001,Sep,1; 2001,Oct,8; 2001,May,5; 2001,Apr,4

52355 **with resection of ureteral or renal pelvic tumor** 4 T 50

> MED: 100-2,15,260; 100-4,12,90.3; 100-4,14,10
> AMA: 2001,Sep,1; 2001,Oct,8; 2001,May,5; 2001,Apr,4

VESICAL NECK AND PROSTATE

To report abdominal and perineal gangrene debridement, consult CPT codes 11004-11006.

52400 **Cystourethroscopy with incision, fulguration, or resection of congenital posterior urethral valves, or congenital obstructive hypertrophic mucosal folds** 3 T

> MED: 100-2,15,260; 100-4,12,90.3; 100-4,14,10
> AMA: 2001,Apr,4

52402 **Cystourethroscopy with transurethral resection or incision of ejaculatory ducts** ♂ 3 T 80

26 Professional Component Only   80/80 Assist-at-Surgery Allowed/With Documentation   Unlisted   Not Covered

TC Technical Component Only   **MED:** Pub 100/NCD References   **AMA:** CPT Assistant References   1-9 ASC Group   ♂ Male Only   ♀ Female Only

192 — CPT Expert   **CPT only © 2006 American Medical Association. All Rights Reserved. (Black Ink)**   © 2006 Ingenix (Blue Ink)

52450 Transurethral incision of prostate ♂ 🔳 T 🔳

MED: 100-2,15,260; 100-4,12,90.3; 100-4,14,10

AMA: 2001,Apr,4

For abdominal and perineal gangrene debridement, consult CPT codes 11004-11006.

52500 Transurethral resection of bladder neck (separate procedure) ♂ 🔳 T 🔳

MED: 100-2,15,260; 100-4,12,90.3; 100-4,14,10

AMA: 2001,Apr,4

52510 Transurethral balloon dilation of the prostatic urethra ♂ 🔳 T 🔳

MED: 100-2,15,260; 100-4,12,90.3; 100-4,14,10

AMA: 2001,Apr,4

52601 Transurethral electrosurgical resection of prostate, including control of postoperative bleeding, complete (vasectomy, meatotomy, cystourethroscopy, urethral calibration and/or dilation, and internal urethrotomy are included) ♂ 🔳 T 🔳

MED: 100-2,15,260; 100-4,12,90.3; 100-4,14,10

AMA: 2001,Apr,4

If other approaches are used, consult CPT codes 55801-55845.

52606 Transurethral fulguration for postoperative bleeding occurring after the usual follow-up time ♂ 🔳 T 🔳

MED: 100-2,15,260; 100-4,12,90.3; 100-4,14,10

AMA: 2001,Apr,4

52612 Transurethral resection of prostate; first stage of two-stage resection (partial resection) ♂ 🔳 T 🔳

MED: 100-2,15,260; 100-4,12,90.3; 100-4,14,10

AMA: 2001,Apr,4

52614 second stage of two-stage resection (resection completed) ♂ 🔳 T 🔳

MED: 100-2,15,260; 100-4,12,90.3; 100-4,14,10

AMA: 2001,Apr,4

52620 Transurethral resection; of residual obstructive tissue after 90 days postoperative ♂ 🔳 T 🔳

MED: 100-2,15,260; 100-4,12,90.3; 100-4,14,10

AMA: 2001,Apr,4

52630 of regrowth of obstructive tissue longer than one year postoperative ♂ 🔳 T 🔳

MED: 100-2,15,260; 100-4,12,90.3; 100-4,14,10

AMA: 2001,Apr,4

52640 of postoperative bladder neck contracture ♂ 🔳 T 🔳

MED: 100-2,15,260; 100-4,12,90.3; 100-4,14,10

AMA: 2001,Apr,4

52647 Laser coagulation of prostate, including control of postoperative bleeding, complete (vasectomy, meatotomy, cystourethroscopy, urethral calibration and/or dilation, and internal urethrotomy are included if performed) ♂ 🔳 T 🔳

MED: 100-2,15,260; 100-4,12,90.3; 100-4,14,10

AMA: 2001,Apr,4; 1998,Mar,11

52648 Laser vaporization of prostate, including control of postoperative bleeding, complete (vasectomy, meatotomy, cystourethroscopy, urethral calibration and/or dilation, internal urethrotomy and transurethral resection of prostate are included if performed) ♂ 🔳 T 🔳

MED: 100-2,15,260; 100-4,12,90.3; 100-4,14,10

AMA: 2001,Apr,4; 1998,Mar,11

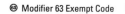

Bladder   Prostate   Urethra

In 52700, the physician drains abscess in and around prostate

52700 Transurethral drainage of prostatic abscess ♂ 🔳 T 🔳 🔳

MED: 100-2,15,260; 100-4,12,90.3; 100-4,14,10

AMA: 2001,Apr,4

URETHRA

If an endoscopy is performed, consult cystoscopy, urethroscopy, and cystourethroscopy procedures, 52000-52700. If an injection procedure is performed for urethrocystography, consult CPT codes 51600-51610.

INCISION

53000 Urethrotomy or urethrostomy, external (separate procedure); pendulous urethra 🔳 T 🔳

MED: 100-2,15,260; 100-4,12,90.3; 100-4,14,10

53010 perineal urethra, external 🔳 T 🔳

MED: 100-2,15,260; 100-4,12,90.3; 100-4,14,10

53020 Meatotomy, cutting of meatus (separate procedure); except infant 🔳 T 🔳

53025 infant 🔳 T 🔳 🔳

53040 Drainage of deep periurethral abscess 🔳 T 🔳 🔳

If a subcutaneous abscess is drained, consult CPT codes 10060 and 10061.

53060 Drainage of Skene's gland abscess or cyst ♀ T 🔳

53080 Drainage of perineal urinary extravasation; uncomplicated (separate procedure) 🔳 T 🔳

53085 complicated T 🔳 🔳

EXCISION

53200 Biopsy of urethra 🔳 T 🔳

53210 Urethrectomy, total, including cystostomy; female ♀ 🔳 T 🔳 🔳

53215 male ♂ 🔳 T 🔳 🔳

MED: 100-2,15,260; 100-4,12,90.3; 100-4,14,10

53220 Excision or fulguration of carcinoma of urethra 🔳 T 🔳

MED: 100-2,15,260; 100-4,12,90.3; 100-4,14,10

53230 Excision of urethral diverticulum (separate procedure); female ♀ 🔳 T 🔳 🔳

MED: 100-2,15,260; 100-4,12,90.3; 100-4,14,10

53235 male ♂ 🔳 T 🔳 🔳

MED: 100-2,15,260; 100-4,12,90.3; 100-4,14,10

53240 Marsupialization of urethral diverticulum, male or female 🔳 T 🔳

MED: 100-2,15,260; 100-4,12,90.3; 100-4,14,10

53250 Excision of bulbourethral gland (Cowper's gland) ♂ 2 T ▢
MED: 100-2,15,260; 100-4,12,90.3; 100-4,14,10

53260 Excision or fulguration; urethral polyp(s), distal urethra 2 T ▢
MED: 100-2,15,260; 100-4,12,90.3; 100-4,14,10
If an endoscopic approach is used, consult CPT codes 52214 and 52224.

53265 urethral caruncle 2 T ▢
MED: 100-2,15,260; 100-4,12,90.3; 100-4,14,10

53270 Skene's glands ♀ 2 T ▢
MED: 100-2,15,260; 100-4,12,90.3; 100-4,14,10

53275 urethral prolapse ♀ 2 T ▢
MED: 100-2,15,260; 100-4,12,90.3; 100-4,14,10

REPAIR

For hypospadias, consult CPT codes 54300-54352.

53400 Urethroplasty; first stage, for fistula, diverticulum, or stricture (eg, Johannsen type) 3 T 80 ▢
MED: 100-2,15,260; 100-4,12,90.3; 100-4,14,10

53405 second stage (formation of urethra), including urinary diversion 2 T 80 ▢
MED: 100-2,15,260; 100-4,12,90.3; 100-4,14,10

53410 Urethroplasty, one-stage reconstruction of male anterior urethra ♂ 2 T 80 ▢
MED: 100-2,15,260; 100-4,12,90.3; 100-4,14,10

53415 Urethroplasty, transpubic or perineal, one stage, for reconstruction or repair of prostatic or membranous urethra ♂ C 80 ▢
MED: 100-2,15,260; 100-4,12,90.3; 100-4,14,10

53420 Urethroplasty, two-stage reconstruction or repair of prostatic or membranous urethra; first stage ♂ 3 T 80 ▢
MED: 100-2,15,260; 100-4,12,90.3; 100-4,14,10

53425 second stage ♂ 2 T 80 ▢
MED: 100-2,15,260; 100-4,12,90.3; 100-4,14,10

53430 Urethroplasty, reconstruction of female urethra ♀ 2 T 80 ▢
MED: 100-2,15,260; 100-4,12,90.3; 100-4,14,10

53431 Urethroplasty with tubularization of posterior urethra and/or lower bladder for incontinence (eg, Tenago, Leadbetter procedure) 2 T 80 ▢
MED: 100-2,15,260; 100-3,230.10; 100-4,12,90.3; 100-4,14,10

53440 Sling operation for correction of male urinary incontinence (eg, fascia or synthetic) ♂ 2 S 80 ▢
MED: 100-2,15,260; 100-3,230.10; 100-4,12,90.3; 100-4,14,10

53442 Removal or revision of sling for male urinary incontinence (eg, fascia or synthetic) ♂ 1 T 80 ▢
MED: 100-2,15,260; 100-4,12,90.3; 100-4,14,10

53444 Insertion of tandem cuff (dual cuff) 2 S 80 ▢
MED: 100-2,15,260; 100-4,12,90.3; 100-4,14,10

53445 Insertion of inflatable urethral/bladder neck sphincter, including placement of pump, reservoir, and cuff 1 S 80 ▢
MED: 100-2,15,260; 100-3,230.10; 100-4,12,90.3; 100-4,14,10

53446 Removal of inflatable urethral/bladder neck sphincter, including pump, reservoir, and cuff 1 T 80 ▢
MED: 100-2,15,260; 100-4,12,90.3; 100-4,14,10

53447 Removal and replacement of inflatable urethral/bladder neck sphincter including pump, reservoir, and cuff at the same operative session 1 S 80 ▢
MED: 100-2,15,260; 100-3,230.10; 100-4,12,90.3; 100-4,14,10

53448 Removal and replacement of inflatable urethral/bladder neck sphincter including pump, reservoir, and cuff through an infected field at the same operative session including irrigation and debridement of infected tissue C 80 ▢
Do not report 11040-11043 in conjunction with CPT code 53448.

53449 Repair of inflatable urethral/bladder neck sphincter, including pump, reservoir, and cuff 1 T 80 ▢
MED: 100-2,15,260; 100-3,230.10; 100-4,12,90.3; 100-4,14,10

53450 Urethromeatoplasty, with mucosal advancement 1 T ▢
MED: 100-2,15,260; 100-4,12,90.3; 100-4,14,10
If a meatotomy is performed, consult CPT codes 53020 and 53025.

53460 Urethromeatoplasty, with partial excision of distal urethral segment (Richardson type procedure) 1 T 80 ▢
MED: 100-2,15,260; 100-4,12,90.3; 100-4,14,10

53500 Urethrolysis, transvaginal, secondary, open, including cystourethroscopy (eg, postsurgical obstruction, scarring) ♀ T 80 ▢
To report urethrolysis by retropubic approach, consult CPT code 53899.
Code 53500 cannot be reported with 52000.

53502 Urethrorrhaphy, suture of urethral wound or injury, female ♀ 2 T ▢
MED: 100-2,15,260; 100-4,12,90.3; 100-4,14,10

53505 Urethrorrhaphy, suture of urethral wound or injury; penile ♂ 2 T 80 ▢
MED: 100-2,15,260; 100-4,12,90.3; 100-4,14,10

53510 perineal 2 T 80 ▢
MED: 100-2,15,260; 100-4,12,90.3; 100-4,14,10

53515 prostatomembranous ♂ 2 T 80 ▢
MED: 100-2,15,260; 100-4,12,90.3; 100-4,14,10

53520 Closure of urethrostomy or urethrocutaneous fistula, male (separate procedure) ♂ 2 T ▢
MED: 100-2,15,260; 100-4,12,90.3; 100-4,14,10
If a urethrovaginal fistula is closed, consult CPT code 57310. If a urethrorectal fistula is closed, consult CPT codes 45820 and 45825.

MANIPULATION

For radiological supervision and interpretation, consult CPT code 74485.

53600 Dilation of urethral stricture by passage of sound or urethral dilator, male; initial ♂ T ▢

53601 subsequent ♂ T ▢

53605 Dilation of urethral stricture or vesical neck by passage of sound or urethral dilator, male, general or conduction (spinal) anesthesia ♂ 2 T ▢
MED: 100-2,15,260; 100-4,12,90.3; 100-4,14,10

53620 Dilation of urethral stricture by passage of filiform and follower, male; initial ♂ T ▢

53621 subsequent ♂ T ▢

53660	Dilation of female urethra including suppository and/or instillation; initial	♀ T ↩
53661	subsequent	♀ T ↩
53665	Dilation of female urethra, general or conduction (spinal) anesthesia	♀ 1 T ↩

MED: 100-2,15,260; 100-4,12,90.3; 100-4,14,10

OTHER PROCEDURES

53850	Transurethral destruction of prostate tissue; by microwave thermotherapy	♂ T ↩

MED: 100-2,15,260; 100-4,12,90.3; 100-4,14,10
AMA: 2001,Apr,4; 1997,Nov,20

53852	by radiofrequency thermotherapy	♂ T ↩

AMA: 2001,Apr,4; 1997,Nov,20

53853	by water-induced thermotherapy	♂ T ↩

Kidney
Ureter
Bladder
Prostate
Urethra
Testis

Bladder
Pubic bone
Corpus cavernosus
Corpus spongiosum
Glans penis
Foreskin (prepuce)
Urethra
Rectum
Prostate
Septa and lobules of testes

53899	Unlisted procedure, urinary system	T 80

MED: 100-4,4,180.3

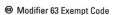

MALE GENITAL SYSTEM

PENIS

INCISION

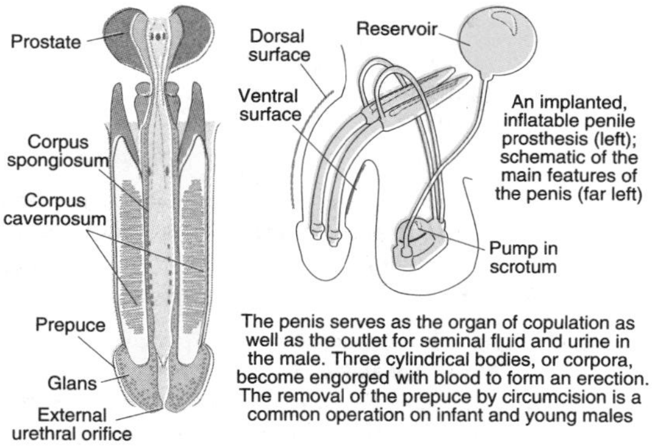
Prostate
Corpus spongiosum
Corpus cavernosum
Prepuce
Glans
External urethral orifice
Dorsal surface
Ventral surface
Reservoir
An implanted, inflatable penile prosthesis (left); schematic of the main features of the penis (far left)
Pump in scrotum

The penis serves as the organ of copulation as well as the outlet for seminal fluid and urine in the male. Three cylindrical bodies, or corpora, become engorged with blood to form an erection. The removal of the prepuce by circumcision is a common operation on infant and young males

54000 **Slitting of prepuce, dorsal or lateral (separate procedure); newborn** A ♂ 2 T 80 63 ⊡
MED: 100-2,15,260; 100-4,12,90.3; 100-4,14,10

54001 **except newborn** ♂ 2 T ⊡
MED: 100-2,15,260; 100-4,12,90.3; 100-4,14,10

54015 **Incision and drainage of penis, deep** ♂ 4 T 80 ⊡
MED: 100-2,15,260; 100-4,12,90.3; 100-4,14,10
If a subcutaneous abscess is incised and drained, consult CPT codes 10060-10160.

DESTRUCTION

54050 **Destruction of lesion(s), penis (eg, condyloma, papilloma, molluscum contagiosum, herpetic vesicle), simple; chemical** ♂ T ⊡

54055 **electrodesiccation** ♂ T ⊡

54056 **cryosurgery** ♂ T ⊡

54057 **laser surgery** ♂ 1 T ⊡
MED: 100-2,15,260; 100-3,140.5; 100-4,12,90.3; 100-4,14,10

54060 **surgical excision** ♂ 1 T ⊡
MED: 100-2,15,260; 100-4,12,90.3; 100-4,14,10

54065 **Destruction of lesion(s), penis (eg, condyloma, papilloma, molluscum contagiosum, herpetic vesicle), extensive (eg, laser surgery, electrosurgery, cryosurgery, chemosurgery)** ♂ 1 T ⊡
MED: 100-2,15,260; 100-3,140.5; 100-4,12,90.3; 100-4,14,10
If destruction or an excision is performed on other lesions, see the Integumentary System.

EXCISION

54100 **Biopsy of penis; (separate procedure)** ♂ 1 T ⊡
MED: 100-2,15,260; 100-4,12,90.3; 100-4,14,10
AMA: 1999,Nov,26

54105 **deep structures** ♂ 1 T ⊡
MED: 100-2,15,260; 100-4,12,90.3; 100-4,14,10

54110 **Excision of penile plaque (Peyronie disease);** ♂ 2 T 80 ⊡
MED: 100-2,15,260; 100-4,12,90.3; 100-4,14,10

54111 **with graft to 5 cm in length** ♂ 2 T 80 ⊡
MED: 100-2,15,260; 100-4,12,90.3; 100-4,14,10
AMA: 1999,Aug,5

54112 **with graft greater than 5 cm in length** ♂ 2 T 80 ⊡
MED: 100-2,15,260; 100-4,12,90.3; 100-4,14,10

54115 **Removal foreign body from deep penile tissue (eg, plastic implant)** ♂ 1 T 80 ⊡
MED: 100-2,15,260; 100-4,12,90.3; 100-4,14,10

54120 **Amputation of penis; partial** ♂ 2 T 80 ⊡
MED: 100-2,15,260; 100-4,12,90.3; 100-4,14,10

54125 **complete** ♂ C 80 ⊡

54130 **Amputation of penis, radical; with bilateral inguinofemoral lymphadenectomy** ♂ C 80 ⊡

54135 **in continuity with bilateral pelvic lymphadenectomy, including external iliac, hypogastric and obturator nodes** ♂ C 80 ⊡
If a lymphadenectomy (separate procedure) is performed, consult CPT codes 38760-38770.

▲ **54150** **Circumcision, using clamp or other device with regional dorsal penile or ring block** A ♂ 1 T 80 63 ⊡
MED: 100-2,15,260; 100-4,12,90.3; 100-4,14,10
AMA: 1998,May,11; 1996,Sep,11
Report modifier 52 with 54150 when perfomed without dorsal penile or ring block.

~~**54152**~~ ~~**except newborn**~~
Use 54150.

▲ **54160** **Circumcision, surgical excision other than clamp, device, or dorsal slit; neonate (28 days of age or less)** A ♂ 2 T 63 ⊡
MED: 100-2,15,260; 100-4,12,90.3; 100-4,14,10
AMA: 1998,May,11; 1996,Sep,11

▲ **54161** **older than 28 days of age** ♂ 2 T ⊡
MED: 100-2,15,260; 100-4,12,90.3; 100-4,14,10
AMA: 1998,May,11; 1996,Sep,11; 1996,Dec,10

54162 **Lysis or excision of penile post-circumcision adhesions** ♂ 2 T ⊡
MED: 100-2,15,260; 100-4,12,90.3; 100-4,14,10

54163 **Repair incomplete circumcision** ♂ 2 T ⊡
MED: 100-2,15,260; 100-4,12,90.3; 100-4,14,10

54164 **Frenulotomy of penis** ♂ 2 T ⊡
MED: 100-2,15,260; 100-4,12,90.3; 100-4,14,10
Do not use in conjunction with circumcision codes 54150-54161, 54162, 54163.

INTRODUCTION

54200 **Injection procedure for Peyronie disease;** ♂ T ⊡

54205 **with surgical exposure of plaque** ♂ 4 T 80 ⊡
MED: 100-2,15,260; 100-4,12,90.3; 100-4,14,10

54220 **Irrigation of corpora cavernosa for priapism** ♂ 1 T ⊡
MED: 100-2,15,260; 100-4,12,90.3; 100-4,14,10

54230 **Injection procedure for corpora cavernosography** ♂ N ⊡
To report radiological supervision and interpretation, consult CPT code 74445.

54231 **Dynamic cavernosometry, including intracavernosal injection of vasoactive drugs (eg, papaverine, phentolamine)** ♂ T ⊡

54235 **Injection of corpora cavernosa with pharmacologic agent(s) (eg, papaverine, phentolamine)** ♂ T ⊡
AMA: 1996,Sep,10

54240 Penile plethysmography ♂ T 80 ▢
MED: 100-3,20.14

If the physician only interprets the results and/or operates the equipment, modifier 26 should be appended to codes 54240 and 54250.

54250 Nocturnal penile tumescence and/or rigidity test ♂ T 80 ▢

If the physician only interprets the results and/or operates the equipment, modifier-26 should be appended to codes 54240 and 54250.

REPAIR

If other urethroplasties are performed, consult CPT codes 53400-53430. If penile revascularization is performed, consult CPT code 37788.

To report abdominal perineal gangrene debridement, consult 11004-11006.

54300 Plastic operation of penis for straightening of chordee (eg, hypospadias), with or without mobilization of urethra ♂ 3 T 80 ▢
MED: 100-2,15,260; 100-4,12,90.3; 100-4,14,10

54304 Plastic operation on penis for correction of chordee or for first stage hypospadias repair with or without transplantation of prepuce and/or skin flaps ♂ 3 T 80 ▢
MED: 100-2,15,260; 100-4,12,90.3; 100-4,14,10

54308 Urethroplasty for second stage hypospadias repair (including urinary diversion); less than 3 cm ♂ 3 T 80 ▢
MED: 100-2,15,260; 100-4,12,90.3; 100-4,14,10

54312 greater than 3 cm ♂ 3 T 80 ▢
MED: 100-2,15,260; 100-4,12,90.3; 100-4,14,10

54316 Urethroplasty for second stage hypospadias repair (including urinary diversion) with free skin graft obtained from site other than genitalia ♂ 3 T 80 ▢
MED: 100-2,15,260; 100-4,12,90.3; 100-4,14,10

54318 Urethroplasty for third stage hypospadias repair to release penis from scrotum (eg, third stage Cecil repair) ♂ 3 T 80 ▢
MED: 100-2,15,260; 100-4,12,90.3; 100-4,14,10

54322 One stage distal hypospadias repair (with or without chordee or circumcision); with simple meatal advancement (eg, Magpi, V-flap) ♂ 3 T 80 ▢
MED: 100-2,15,260; 100-4,12,90.3; 100-4,14,10

54324 with urethroplasty by local skin flaps (eg, flip-flap, prepucial flap) ♂ 3 T 80 ▢
MED: 100-2,15,260; 100-4,12,90.3; 100-4,14,10
Browne's operation

54326 with urethroplasty by local skin flaps and mobilization of urethra ♂ 3 T 80 ▢
MED: 100-2,15,260; 100-4,12,90.3; 100-4,14,10

54328 with extensive dissection to correct chordee and urethroplasty with local skin flaps, skin graft patch, and/or island flap ♂ 3 T 80 ▢
MED: 100-2,15,260; 100-4,12,90.3; 100-4,14,10

54332 One stage proximal penile or penoscrotal hypospadias repair requiring extensive dissection to correct chordee and urethroplasty by use of skin graft tube and/or island flap ♂ C 80 ▢

54336 One stage perineal hypospadias repair requiring extensive dissection to correct chordee and urethroplasty by use of skin graft tube and/or island flap ♂ C 80 ▢

54340 Repair of hypospadias complications (ie, fistula, stricture, diverticula); by closure, incision, or excision, simple ♂ 3 T 80 ▢
MED: 100-2,15,260; 100-4,12,90.3; 100-4,14,10

54344 requiring mobilization of skin flaps and urethroplasty with flap or patch graft ♂ 3 T 80 ▢
MED: 100-2,15,260; 100-4,12,90.3; 100-4,14,10

54348 requiring extensive dissection and urethroplasty with flap, patch or tubed graft (includes urinary diversion) ♂ 3 T 80 ▢
MED: 100-2,15,260; 100-4,12,90.3; 100-4,14,10

54352 Repair of hypospadias cripple requiring extensive dissection and excision of previously constructed structures including re-release of chordee and reconstruction of urethra and penis by use of local skin as grafts and island flaps and skin brought in as flaps or grafts ♂ 3 T 80 ▢
MED: 100-2,15,260; 100-4,12,90.3; 100-4,14,10

54360 Plastic operation on penis to correct angulation ♂ 3 T 80 ▢
MED: 100-2,15,260; 100-4,12,90.3; 100-4,14,10

54380 Plastic operation on penis for epispadias distal to external sphincter; ♂ 3 T 80 ▢
MED: 100-2,15,260; 100-4,12,90.3; 100-4,14,10
Lowsley's operation

54385 with incontinence ♂ 3 T 80 ▢
MED: 100-2,15,260; 100-3,230.10; 100-4,12,90.3; 100-4,14,10

54390 with exstrophy of bladder ♂ C 80 ▢

54400 Insertion of penile prosthesis; non-inflatable (semi-rigid) ♂ 3 S ▢
MED: 100-2,15,260; 100-3,230.4; 100-4,12,90.3; 100-4,14,10

54401 inflatable (self-contained) ♂ 3 S ▢
MED: 100-2,15,260; 100-3,230.4; 100-4,12,90.3; 100-4,14,10

54405 Insertion of multi-component, inflatable penile prosthesis, including placement of pump, cylinders, and reservoir ♂ 3 S 80 ▢
MED: 100-2,15,260; 100-3,230.4; 100-4,12,90.3; 100-4,14,10
If service is reduced, report 54405 with modifier 52.

54406 Removal of all components of a multi-component, inflatable penile prosthesis without replacement of prosthesis ♂ 3 T 80 ▢
MED: 100-2,15,260; 100-3,230.4; 100-4,12,90.3; 100-4,14,10
If service is reduced, report 54406 with modifier 52.

54408 Repair of component(s) of a multi-component, inflatable penile prosthesis ♂ 3 T 80 ▢
MED: 100-2,15,260; 100-3,230.4; 100-4,12,90.3; 100-4,14,10

54410 Removal and replacement of all component(s) of a multi-component, inflatable penile prosthesis at the same operative session ♂ 3 S 80 ▢
MED: 100-2,15,260; 100-3,230.4; 100-4,12,90.3; 100-4,14,10

---

26 Professional Component Only   80/80 Assist-at-Surgery Allowed/With Documentation   Unlisted   Not Covered

TC Technical Component Only   MED: Pub 100/NCD References   AMA: CPT Assistant References   1-9 ASC Group   ♂ Male Only   ♀ Female Only

198 — CPT Expert   CPT only © 2006 American Medical Association. All Rights Reserved. *(Black Ink)*   © 2006 Ingenix *(Blue Ink)*

54411 Removal and replacement of all components of a multi-component inflatable penile prosthesis through an infected field at the same operative session, including irrigation and debridement of infected tissue ♂ Ⓒ 80 ▢

MED: 100-3,230.4

If service is reduced, report 54411 with modifier 52.

Do not report 11040-11043 in conjunction with 54411.

54415 Removal of non-inflatable (semi-rigid) or inflatable (self-contained) penile prosthesis, without replacement of prosthesis ♂ ③ Ⓣ 80 ▢

MED: 100-2,15,260; 100-3,230.4; 100-4,12,90.3; 100-4,14,10

54416 Removal and replacement of non-inflatable (semi-rigid) or inflatable (self-contained) penile prosthesis at the same operative session ♂ ③ Ⓢ 80 ▢

MED: 100-2,15,260; 100-3,230.4; 100-4,12,90.3; 100-4,14,10

54417 Removal and replacement of non-inflatable (semi-rigid) or inflatable (self-contained) penile prosthesis through an infected field at the same operative session, including irrigation and debridement of infected tissue ♂ Ⓒ 80 ▢

MED: 100-3,230.4

Do not report 11040-11043 in conjunction with 54417.

54420 Corpora cavernosa-saphenous vein shunt (priapism operation), unilateral or bilateral ♂ ④ Ⓣ 80 ▢

MED: 100-2,15,260; 100-4,12,90.3; 100-4,14,10

54430 Corpora cavernosa-corpus spongiosum shunt (priapism operation), unilateral or bilateral ♂ Ⓒ 80 ▢

54435 Corpora cavernosa-glans penis fistulization (eg, biopsy needle, Winter procedure, rongeur, or punch) for priapism ♂ ④ Ⓣ ▢

MED: 100-2,15,260; 100-4,12,90.3; 100-4,14,10

54440 Plastic operation of penis for injury ♂ ④ Ⓣ 80 ▢

MED: 100-2,15,260; 100-4,12,90.3; 100-4,14,10

MANIPULATION

54450 Foreskin manipulation including lysis of preputial adhesions and stretching ♂ ① Ⓣ ▢

MED: 100-2,15,260; 100-4,12,90.3; 100-4,14,10

TESTIS

EXCISION

54500 Biopsy of testis, needle (separate procedure) ♂ ① Ⓣ 80 50 ▢

MED: 100-2,15,260; 100-4,12,90.3; 100-4,14,10

To report fine needle aspiration, consult CPT codes 10021, 10022.

To report evaluation of fine needle aspirate, consult CPT codes 88172, 88173.

54505 Biopsy of testis, incisional (separate procedure) ♂ ① Ⓣ 80 50 ▢

MED: 100-2,15,260; 100-4,12,90.3; 100-4,14,10

AMA: 2001,Oct,8

If this procedure is combined with a vasogram, a seminal vesiculogram, or a epididymogram, consult CPT code 55300.

54512 Excision of extraparenchymal lesion of testis ♂ ② Ⓣ 80 50 ▢

MED: 100-2,15,260; 100-4,12,90.3; 100-4,14,10

AMA: 2001,Oct,8

54520 Orchiectomy, simple (including subcapsular), with or without testicular prosthesis, scrotal or inguinal approach ♂ ③ Ⓣ 50 ▢

MED: 100-2,15,260; 100-3,230.3; 100-4,12,90.3; 100-4,14,10

AMA: 2001,Oct,8

Huggins'' orchiectomy

54522 Orchiectomy, partial ♂ ③ Ⓣ 80 50 ▢

MED: 100-2,15,260; 100-4,12,90.3; 100-4,14,10

AMA: 2001,Oct,8

54530 Orchiectomy, radical, for tumor; inguinal approach ♂ ④ Ⓣ 80 50 ▢

MED: 100-2,15,260; 100-3,230.3; 100-4,12,90.3; 100-4,14,10

AMA: 2001,Oct,8

54535 with abdominal exploration ♂ Ⓒ 80 50 ▢

MED: 100-3,230.3

AMA: 2001,Oct,8

If an orchiectomy is performed with repair of a hernia, consult CPT codes 49505 or 49507 and 54520. If a radical retroperitoneal lymphadenectomy is performed, consult CPT code 38780.

EXPLORATION

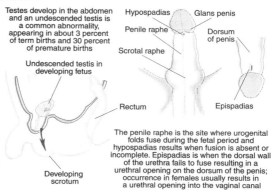

Testes develop in the abdomen and an undescended testis is a common abnormality, appearing in about 3 percent of term births and 30 percent of premature births

Undescended testis in developing fetus

Rectum

Developing scrotum

Hypospadias — Glans penis

Penile raphe — Dorsum of penis

Scrotal raphe

Epispadias

The penile raphe is the site where urogenital folds fuse during the fetal period and hypospadias results when fusion is absent or incomplete. Epispadias is when the dorsal wall of the urethra fails to fuse resulting in a urethral opening on the dorsum of the penis; occurrence in females usually results in a urethral opening into the vaginal canal

54550 Exploration for undescended testis (inguinal or scrotal area) ♂ ④ Ⓣ 80 50 ▢

MED: 100-2,15,260; 100-4,12,90.3; 100-4,14,10

AMA: 2001,Oct,8

54560 Exploration for undescended testis with abdominal exploration ♂ Ⓣ 80 50 ▢

AMA: 2001,Oct,8

REPAIR

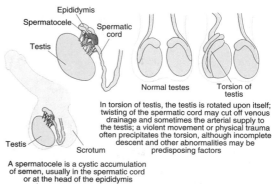

Spermatocele

Epididymis

Spermatic cord

Testis

Testis

Scrotum

Normal testes

Torsion of testis

In torsion of testis, the testis is rotated upon itself; twisting of the spermatic cord may cut off venous drainage and sometimes the arterial supply to the testis; a violent movement or physical trauma often precipitates the torsion, although incomplete descent and other abnormalities may be predisposing factors

A spermatocele is a cystic accumulation of semen, usually in the spermatic cord or at the head of the epididymis

54600 Reduction of torsion of testis, surgical, with or without fixation of contralateral testis ♂ ④ Ⓣ 50 ▢

MED: 100-2,15,260; 100-4,12,90.3; 100-4,14,10

54620 Fixation of contralateral testis (separate procedure) ♂ ③ Ⓣ 50 ▢

MED: 100-2,15,260; 100-4,12,90.3; 100-4,14,10

Male Genital System

54640 — 55120

54640 Orchiopexy, inguinal approach, with or without hernia repair ♂ 🔟 Ⓣ 🔟 🔟 🔟

MED: 100-2,15,260; 100-4,12,90.3; 100-4,14,10
AMA: 2001,Oct,8
To report inguinal hernia repair performed with inguinal orchiopexy, consult CPT codes 49495-49525.

Bevan's operation

54650 Orchiopexy, abdominal approach, for intra-abdominal testis (eg, Fowler-Stephens) ♂ Ⓒ 🔟 🔟 🔟

AMA: 2001,Oct,8; 2000,May,4; 1999,Nov,26
If a laparoscopic approach is used, consult CPT code 54692.

54660 Insertion of testicular prosthesis (separate procedure) ♂ 🔟 Ⓣ 🔟 🔟 🔟

MED: 100-2,15,260; 100-2,16,180; 100-4,12,90.3; 100-4,14,10
AMA: 2001,Oct,8

54670 Suture or repair of testicular injury ♂ 🔟 Ⓣ 🔟 🔟 🔟

MED: 100-2,15,260; 100-4,12,90.3; 100-4,14,10
AMA: 2001,Oct,8

54680 Transplantation of testis(es) to thigh (because of scrotal destruction) ♂ 🔟 Ⓣ 🔟 🔟 🔟

MED: 100-2,15,260; 100-4,12,90.3; 100-4,14,10
AMA: 2001,Oct,8

LAPAROSCOPY

Diagnostic laparoscopy is always included in surgical laparoscopy.

To report only a diagnostic laparoscopy (peritoneoscopy), consult CPT code 49320.

54690 Laparoscopy, surgical; orchiectomy ♂ 🔟 Ⓣ 🔟 🔟 🔟

MED: 100-2,15,260; 100-4,12,90.3; 100-4,14,10
AMA: 2001,Oct,8; 2000,Mar,5; 1999,Nov,26

54692 orchiopexy for intra-abdominal testis ♂ Ⓣ 🔟 🔟

AMA: 2001,Oct,8; 2000,May,4; 1999,Nov,27

54699 Unlisted laparoscopy procedure, testis Ⓣ 🔟 🔟

AMA: 2000,Mar,5; 1999,Nov,27

EPIDIDYMIS

INCISION

54700 Incision and drainage of epididymis, testis and/or scrotal space (eg, abscess or hematoma) ♂ 🔟 Ⓣ 🔟

MED: 100-2,15,260; 100-4,12,90.3; 100-4,14,10
AMA: 2001,Oct,8

EXCISION

54800 Biopsy of epididymis, needle ♂ 🔟 Ⓣ 🔟 🔟

MED: 100-2,15,260; 100-4,12,90.3; 100-4,14,10
AMA: 2001,Oct,8
To report fine needle aspiration, consult CPT codes 10021, 10022.

To report evaluation of fine needle aspirate, consult CPT codes 88172, 88173.

54820 ~~Exploration of epididymis, with or without biopsy~~
Use 54865.

54830 Excision of local lesion of epididymis ♂ 🔟 Ⓣ 🔟 🔟

MED: 100-2,15,260; 100-4,12,90.3; 100-4,14,10
AMA: 2001,Oct,8

54840 Excision of spermatocele, with or without epididymectomy ♂ 🔟 Ⓣ 🔟

MED: 100-2,15,260; 100-4,12,90.3; 100-4,14,10
AMA: 2001,Oct,8

54860 Epididymectomy; unilateral ♂ 🔟 Ⓣ 🔟

MED: 100-2,15,260; 100-4,12,90.3; 100-4,14,10

54861 bilateral ♂ 🔟 Ⓣ 🔟 🔟

MED: 100-2,15,260; 100-4,12,90.3; 100-4,14,10

EXPLORATION

● **54865** Exploration of epididymis, with or without biopsy 🔟 Ⓣ

REPAIR

54900 Epididymovasostomy, anastomosis of epididymis to vas deferens; unilateral ♂ 🔟 Ⓣ 🔟 🔟

MED: 100-2,15,260; 100-4,12,90.3; 100-4,14,10
AMA: 1998,Nov,16

54901 bilateral ♂ 🔟 Ⓣ 🔟 🔟

MED: 100-2,15,260; 100-4,12,90.3; 100-4,14,10
AMA: 1998,Nov,16
If an operating microscope is used, consult CPT code 69990.

TUNICA VAGINALIS

INCISION

Spermatic cord · Head of epididymis · Lobules · Open processus vaginalis · Testis · Abdominal cavity · Peritoneum · Hydrocele · Ductus deferens · Tail of epididymis · Tunica vaginalis

Schematic showing a communicating hydrocele flowing through unclosed processus vaginalis

The tunica vaginalis is a closed sac within the scrotum and is the lower remnant of the path taken by the testis as it descends from the abdomen just prior to birth. The presence of fluid in this pathway is called a hydrocele. The testes, or testicles, are the male reproductive organs. Each produces sperm and male sex hormones

55000 Puncture aspiration of hydrocele, tunica vaginalis, with or without injection of medication ♂ Ⓣ 🔟

EXCISION

55040 Excision of hydrocele; unilateral ♂ 🔟 Ⓣ 🔟

MED: 100-2,15,260; 100-4,12,90.3; 100-4,14,10

55041 bilateral ♂ 🔟 Ⓣ 🔟

MED: 100-2,15,260; 100-4,12,90.3; 100-4,14,10
If this procedure is performed with hernia repair, consult CPT codes 49495-49501.

REPAIR

55060 Repair of tunica vaginalis hydrocele (Bottle type) ♂ 🔟 Ⓣ 🔟 🔟 🔟

MED: 100-2,15,260; 100-4,12,90.3; 100-4,14,10

SCROTUM

INCISION

55100 Drainage of scrotal wall abscess ♂ 🔟 Ⓣ 🔟

MED: 100-2,15,260; 100-4,12,90.3; 100-4,14,10
Consult also CPT code 54700.

55110 Scrotal exploration ♂ 🔟 Ⓣ 🔟

MED: 100-2,15,260; 100-4,12,90.3; 100-4,14,10

55120 Removal of foreign body in scrotum ♂ 🔟 Ⓣ 🔟 🔟

MED: 100-2,15,260; 100-4,12,90.3; 100-4,14,10

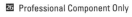
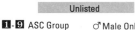

🄿🄲 Professional Component Only   🔟/🔟 Assist-at-Surgery Allowed/With Documentation   Unlisted   Not Covered

🅃🄲 Technical Component Only   **MED:** Pub 100/NCD References   **AMA:** CPT Assistant References   🔟-🔟 ASC Group   ♂ Male Only   ♀ Female Only

CPT only © 2006 American Medical Association. All Rights Reserved. *(Black Ink)*   © *2006 Ingenix (Blue Ink)*

EXCISION

55150   Resection of scrotum   ♂ **1** T 50 □
MED: 100-2,15,260; 100-4,12,90.3; 100-4,14,10
If a local lesion on the skin of the scrotum is excised, see the Integumentary System.

REPAIR

55175   Scrotoplasty; simple   ♂ **1** T 80 □
MED: 100-2,15,260; 100-4,12,90.3; 100-4,14,10

55180   complicated   ♂ **2** T 80 □
MED: 100-2,15,260; 100-4,12,90.3; 100-4,14,10

VAS DEFERENS

INCISION

55200   Vasotomy, cannulization with or without incision of vas, unilateral or bilateral (separate procedure)   ♂ **2** T 80 □
MED: 100-2,15,260; 100-4,12,90.3; 100-4,14,10

EXCISION

55250   Vasectomy, unilateral or bilateral (separate procedure), including postoperative semen examination(s)   ♂ **2** T □
MED: 100-2,15,260; 100-3,230.3; 100-4,12,90.3; 100-4,14,10
AMA: 1998,Jun,10; 1998,Jul,10

INTRODUCTION

55300   Vasotomy for vasograms, seminal vesiculograms, or epididymograms, unilateral or bilateral   ♂ **N** 80 □
To report radiological supervision and interpretation, consult CPT code 74440. If this procedure is combined with a biopsy of the testis, consult CPT code 54505 and append modifier 51.

REPAIR

55400   Vasovasostomy, vasovasorrhaphy   ♂ **1** T 80 50 □
MED: 100-2,15,260; 100-4,12,90.3; 100-4,14,10
AMA: 2001,Oct,8; 1998,Nov,16
If an operating microscope is used, consult CPT code 69990.

SUTURE

55450   Ligation (percutaneous) of vas deferens, unilateral or bilateral (separate procedure)   ♂ T 80 □

SPERMATIC CORD

EXCISION

Diagnostic laparosopy is always included in surgical laparoscopy.

55500   Excision of hydrocele of spermatic cord, unilateral (separate procedure)   ♂ **3** T 80 □
MED: 100-2,15,260; 100-4,12,90.3; 100-4,14,10
AMA: 2001,Oct,8

55520   Excision of lesion of spermatic cord (separate procedure)   ♂ **4** T 80 □
MED: 100-2,15,260; 100-4,12,90.3; 100-4,14,10
AMA: 2001,Oct,8; 2000,Sep,10

55530   Excision of varicocele or ligation of spermatic veins for varicocele; (separate procedure)   ♂ **4** T 50 □
MED: 100-2,15,260; 100-4,12,90.3; 100-4,14,10
AMA: 2001,Oct,8

55535   abdominal approach   ♂ **4** T 80 50 □
MED: 100-2,15,260; 100-4,12,90.3; 100-4,14,10
AMA: 2001,Oct,8

55540   with hernia repair   ♂ **5** T 80 50 □
MED: 100-2,15,260; 100-4,12,90.3; 100-4,14,10
AMA: 2001,Oct,8

LAPAROSCOPY

To report only a diagnostic laparoscopy (peritoneoscopy), consult CPT code 49320.

55550   Laparoscopy, surgical, with ligation of spermatic veins for varicocele   ♂ **9** T 80 50 □
MED: 100-2,15,260; 100-4,12,90.3; 100-4,14,10
AMA: 2001,Oct,8; 2000,Mar,5; 1999,Nov,27

55559   Unlisted laparoscopy procedure, spermatic cord   T 80 50
AMA: 2000,Mar,5; 1999,Nov,27

SEMINAL VESICLES

INCISION

55600   Vesiculotomy;   ♂ T 80 50 □

55605   complicated   ♂ C 80 50 □

EXCISION

55650   Vesiculectomy, any approach   ♂ C 80 50 □

55680   Excision of Mullerian duct cyst   ♂ **1** T 80 □
MED: 100-2,15,260; 100-4,12,90.3; 100-4,14,10
If an injection procedure is performed, consult CPT codes 52010 and 55300.

PROSTATE

INCISION

Perineal approach (retropubic) to prostate (above) and side view schematic of suprapubic approach

The walnut-sized prostate gland secretes a thin, milky fluid that mixes with spermatic fluids during ejaculation; its secretion constitutes about one-third of the volume of seminal fluid. The prostate is palpable via the rectum. Some procedures are via the urethra, which can be dilated to accommodate instruments. The seminal vesicles may also be palpated via the rectum. Each is a long, coiled tube which secretes a thick fluid that mixes with sperm as it passes along the ejaculatory ducts. The ejaculatory ducts are the union of the seminal vesicles and the sperm-carrying ductus deferens

55700   Biopsy, prostate; needle or punch, single or multiple, any approach   ♂ **2** T □
MED: 100-2,15,260; 100-4,12,90.3; 100-4,14,10
AMA: 1996,May,3
To report imaging guidance, consult CPT code 76942.

To report fine needle aspiration, consult CPT codes 10021, 10022.

To report evaluation of fine needle aspirate, consult CPT codes 88172, 88173.

55705   incisional, any approach   ♂ **2** T □
MED: 100-2,15,260; 100-4,12,90.3; 100-4,14,10

55720   Prostatotomy, external drainage of prostatic abscess, any approach; simple   ♂ **1** T 80 □
MED: 100-2,15,260; 100-4,12,90.3; 100-4,14,10

---

⑥³ Modifier 63 Exempt Code   ⊙ Conscious Sedation   + CPT Add-on Code   ⊘ Modifier 51 Exempt Code   ● New Code   ▲ Revised Code
M Maternity Edit   A Age Edit   A-Y APC Status Indicators   C CCI Comprehensive Code   50 Bilateral Procedure

| 55725 | complicated ♂ ☑ Ⓣ 80 ⧉ |

MED: 100-2,15,260; 100-4,12,90.3; 100-4,14,10

If transurethral drainage is performed, consult CPT code 52700.

EXCISION

If transurethral removal of the prostate is performed, consult CPT codes 52601-52640. If transurethral destruction of the prostate is performed, consult CPT codes 53850-53852. If a limited pelvic lymphadenectomy is performed for staging (separate procedure), consult CPT code 38562. If an independent node is dissected, consult CPT codes 38770-38780.

| 55801 | **Prostatectomy, perineal, subtotal (including control of postoperative bleeding, vasectomy, meatotomy, urethral calibration and/or dilation, and internal urethrotomy)** ♂ Ⓒ 80 ⧉ |

| 55810 | **Prostatectomy, perineal radical;** ♂ Ⓒ 80 ⧉ |
| | **Walsh modified radical prostatectomy** |

| 55812 | **with lymph node biopsy(s) (limited pelvic lymphadenectomy)** ♂ Ⓒ 80 ⧉ |

| 55815 | **with bilateral pelvic lymphadenectomy, including external iliac, hypogastric and obturator nodes** ♂ Ⓒ 80 ⧉ |

If this procedure is carried out on separate days, use CPT code 38770 and append modifier 50 and 55810.

| 55821 | **Prostatectomy (including control of postoperative bleeding, vasectomy, meatotomy, urethral calibration and/or dilation, and internal urethrotomy); suprapubic, subtotal, one or two stages** ♂ Ⓒ 80 ⧉ |

| 55831 | **retropubic, subtotal** ♂ Ⓒ 80 ⧉ |

| 55840 | **Prostatectomy, retropubic radical, with or without nerve sparing;** ♂ Ⓒ 80 ⧉ |

| 55842 | **with lymph node biopsy(s) (limited pelvic lymphadenectomy)** ♂ Ⓒ 80 ⧉ |

| 55845 | **with bilateral pelvic lymphadenectomy, including external iliac, hypogastric, and obturator nodes** ♂ Ⓒ 80 ⧉ |

If this procedure is carried out on separate days, use CPT code 38770 and append modifier 50 and 55840.

To report laparoscopic retropubic radical prostectomy, consult CPT code 55866.

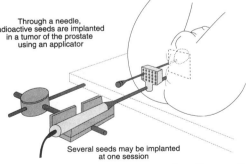

Through a needle, radioactive seeds are implanted in a tumor of the prostate using an applicator

Several seeds may be implanted at one session

| ~~55859~~ | ~~**Transperineal placement of needles or catheters into prostate for interstitial radioelement application, with or without cystoscopy**~~ |

Use 55875.

| 55860 | **Exposure of prostate, any approach, for insertion of radioactive substance;** ♂ Ⓣ ⧉ |
| | To report interstitial radioelement application, consult CPT codes 77776-77778. |

| 55862 | **with lymph node biopsy(s) (limited pelvic lymphadenectomy)** ♂ Ⓒ 80 ⧉ |

| 55865 | **with bilateral pelvic lymphadenectomy, including external iliac, hypogastric and obturator nodes** ♂ Ⓒ 80 ⧉ |

LAPAROSCOPY

Diagnostic laparoscopy is always included in surgical laparoscopy.

To report only a diagnostic laparoscopy (peritoneoscopy), consult CPT code 49320.

| 55866 | **Laparoscopy, surgical prostatectomy, retropubic radical, including nerve sparing** ♂ Ⓒ 80 ⧉ |
| | To report open procedure, consult CPT code 55840. |

OTHER PROCEDURES

To report artificial insemination, consult CPT codes 58321, 58322.

| 55870 | **Electroejaculation** ♂ Ⓣ ⧉ |

| 55873 | **Cryosurgical ablation of the prostate (includes ultrasonic guidance for interstitial cryosurgical probe placement)** ♂ ⑨ Ⓣ ⧉ |

MED: 100-3,230.9; 100-4,4,61.2
AMA: 2002,Sep,9; 2001,Apr,4

● | 55875 | **Transperineal placement of needles or catheters into prostate for interstitial radioelement application, with or without cystoscopy** ⑨ Ⓣ |
| | Consult codes 77776-77784 for interstitial radioelement application. |
| | Use 76965 for ultrasonic guidance for interstitial radioelement application. |

● | 55876 | **Placement of interstitial device(s) for radiation therapy guidance (eg, fiducial markers, dosimeter), prostate (via needle, any approach), single or multiple** Ⓣ |

| 55899 | **Unlisted procedure, male genital system** ♂ Ⓣ |

INTERSEX SURGERY

| 55970 | **Intersex surgery; male to female** Ⓔ |
| | MED: 13-3,140.3 |

| 55980 | **female to male** Ⓔ |
| | MED: 13-3,140.3 |

FEMALE GENITAL SYSTEM

VULVA, PERINEUM AND INTROITUS

INCISION

The following definitions would be employed when selecting a vulvectomy code:

- Simple: Removal of skin and superficial subcutaneous tissues
- Radical: Removal of skin and deep subcutaneous tissues
- Partial: Removal of less than 80 percent of the vulvar area
- Complete: Removal of more than 80 percent of the vulvar area

If a pelvic laparotomy is performed, consult CPT code 49000. If excision or destruction is performed of endometriomas, open method, consult CPT codes 49200 and 49201. If paracentesis is performed, consult CPT codes 49080 and 49081. If secondary closure of the abdominal wall evisceration or disruption is performed, consult CPT code 49900. If fulguration or excision of lesions is performed through a laparoscopic approach, consult CPT code 58662. If chemotherapy is needed, consult CPT codes 96401-96549.

If a sebaceous cyst, furuncle, or abscess is incised and drained, consult CPT codes 10040, 10060, and 10061.

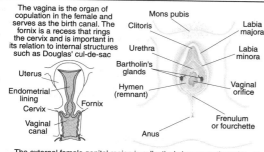

The vagina is the organ of copulation in the female and serves as the birth canal. The fornix is a recess that rings the cervix and is important in its relation to internal structures such as Douglas' cul-de-sac

The external female genital region is collectively known as the vulva, or sometimes, the pudendum. A Bartholin's gland is located on either side of the orifice. The perineum is the space between the anus and the vagina, but is often generally defined as the entire pelvic floor and its related structures. Introitus is a general term for the vaginal entrance

56405   Incision and drainage of vulva or perineal abscess   ♀ T C

56420   Incision and drainage of Bartholin's gland abscess   ♀ T C

To report incision and drainage of Skene's gland, consult CPT code 53060.

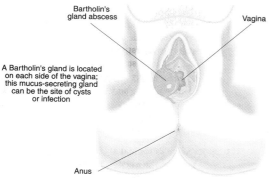

A Bartholin's gland is located on each side of the vagina; this mucus-secreting gland can be the site of cysts or infection

56440   Marsupialization of Bartholin's gland cyst   ♀ 2 T C

MED: 100-2,15,260; 100-4,12,90.3; 100-4,14,10

56441   Lysis of labial adhesions   ♀ 1 T 80 C

MED: 100-2,15,260; 100-4,12,90.3; 100-4,14,10

● **56442**   Hymenotomy, simple incision   1 T

DESTRUCTION

If destruction is performed on a Skene's gland cyst or abscess, consult CPT code 53270. If cautery destruction of a urethral caruncle is performed, consult CPT code 53265.

56501   Destruction of lesion(s), vulva; simple (eg, laser surgery, electrosurgery, cryosurgery, chemosurgery)   ♀ T C

MED: 100-3,140.5

56515   extensive (eg, laser surgery, electrosurgery, cryosurgery, chemosurgery)   ♀ 3 T C

MED: 100-2,15,260; 100-3,140.5; 100-4,12,90.3; 100-4,14,10

EXCISION

If a pelvic laparotomy is performed, consult CPT code 49000. If excision or destruction is performed of endometriomas, open method, consult CPT codes 49200 and 49201. If paracentesis is performed, consult CPT codes 49080 and 49081. If secondary closure of the abdominal wall evisceration or disruption is performed, consult CPT code 49900. If fulguration or excision of lesions is performed through a laparoscopic approach, consult CPT code 58662. If chemotherapy is needed, consult CPT codes 96401-96549.

56605   Biopsy of vulva or perineum (separate procedure); one lesion   ♀ T C

AMA: 2000,Sep,9

+   **56606**   each separate additional lesion (List separately in addition to code for primary procedure)   ♀ T C

Note that 56606 is an add-on code and must be used in conjunction with 56605.

If a local lesion is excised, consult CPT codes 11420-11426 and 11620-11626.

56620   Vulvectomy simple; partial   ♀ 5 T 80 C

MED: 100-2,15,260; 100-4,12,90.3; 100-4,14,10

56625   complete   ♀ 7 T 80 C

MED: 100-2,15,260; 100-4,12,90.3; 100-4,14,10

To report skin graft, consult CPT code 15002 and subsequent codes.

56630   Vulvectomy, radical, partial;   ♀ C 80 C

To report skin grafts, if necessary, consult CPT codes 15004, 15005, 15020, 15121, 15240, 15241.

Bassett's operation

56631   with unilateral inguinofemoral lymphadenectomy   ♀ C 80 C

Bassett's operation

56632   with bilateral inguinofemoral lymphadenectomy   ♀ C 80 C

Bassett's operation

56633   Vulvectomy, radical, complete;   ♀ C 80 C

Bassett's operation

56634   with unilateral inguinofemoral lymphadenectomy   ♀ C 80 C

Bassett's operation

56637   with bilateral inguinofemoral lymphadenectomy   ♀ C 80 C

Bassett's operation

56640   Vulvectomy, radical, complete, with inguinofemoral, iliac, and pelvic lymphadenectomy   ♀ C 80 50 C

If a lymphadenectomy is performed, consult CPT codes 38760-38780.

Bassett's operation

56700   Partial hymenectomy or revision of hymenal ring   ♀ 1 T 80 C

MED: 100-2,15,260; 100-4,12,90.3; 100-4,14,10

~~**56720**   Hymenotomy, simple incision~~
Use 56442.

56740   Excision of Bartholin's gland or cyst   ♀ 3 T C

MED: 100-2,15,260; 100-4,12,90.3; 100-4,14,10

If the Skene's gland is excised, consult CPT code 53270. If an excision is performed on the urethral caruncle, consult CPT code 53265. If excision or fulguration is performed on a urethral carcinoma, consult CPT code 53220. If excision or marsupialization is performed on the urethral diverticulum, consult CPT codes 53230 and 52340.

REPAIR

If a pelvic laparotomy is performed, consult CPT code 49000. If excision or destruction is performed of endometriomas, open method, consult CPT codes 49200 and 49201. If paracentesis is performed, consult CPT codes 49080 and 49081. If secondary closure of the abdominal wall evisceration or disruption is performed, consult CPT code 49900. If fulguration or excision of lesions is performed through a laparoscopic approach, consult CPT code 58662. If chemotherapy is needed, consult CPT codes 96401-96549.

Female Genital System

56800 — 57180

If a repair of the urethra is performed for mucosal prolapse, consult CPT code 53275.

56800 **Plastic repair of introitus** ♀ 3 T 80 ▢

MED: 100-2,15,260; 100-4,12,90.3; 100-4,14,10

Emmet's operation

56805 **Clitoroplasty for intersex state** ♀ T 80 ▢

56810 **Perineoplasty, repair of perineum, nonobstetrical (separate procedure)** ♀ 5 T 80 ▢

MED: 100-2,15,260; 100-4,12,90.3; 100-4,14,10

To report repair of nonobstetrical recent injury, consult CPT code 57210. Consult also CPT code 56800. To report anal sphincteroplasty, consult CPT codes 46750, 46751.

To report wound repair of genitalia, consult CPT codes 12001-12007, 12041-12047, and 13131-13133.

Emmet's operation

ENDOSCOPY

56820 **Colposcopy of the vulva;** ♀ T ▢

AMA: 2003,Feb,5

56821 **with biopsy(s)** ♀ T ▢

AMA: 2003,Feb,5

To report colposcopic services involving the vagina, consult CPT codes 57420-57421; cervix, consult CPT codes 57452-57461.

VAGINA

INCISION

If a pelvic laparotomy is performed, consult CPT code 49000. If excision or destruction is performed of endometriomas, open method, consult CPT codes 49200 and 49201. If paracentesis is performed, consult CPT codes 49080 and 49081. If secondary closure of the abdominal wall evisceration or disruption is performed, consult CPT code 49900. If fulguration or excision of lesions is performed through a laparoscopic approach, consult CPT code 58662. If chemotherapy is needed, consult CPT codes 96401-96549.

57000 **Colpotomy; with exploration** ♀ 1 T 80 ▢

MED: 100-2,15,260; 100-4,12,90.3; 100-4,14,10

57010 **with drainage of pelvic abscess** ♀ 2 T 80 ▢

MED: 100-2,15,260; 100-4,12,90.3; 100-4,14,10

Laroyenne operation

57020 **Colpocentesis (separate procedure)** ♀ 2 T 80 ▢

MED: 100-2,15,260; 100-4,12,90.3; 100-4,14,10

57022 **Incision and drainage of vaginal hematoma; obstetrical/postpartum** ♀ T 80 ▢

57023 **non-obstetrical (eg, post-trauma, spontaneous bleeding)** ♀ 1 T 80 ▢

MED: 100-2,15,260; 100-4,12,90.3; 100-4,14,10

DESTRUCTION

57061 **Destruction of vaginal lesion(s); simple (eg, laser surgery, electrosurgery, cryosurgery, chemosurgery)** ♀ T ▢

MED: 100-3,140.5

AMA: 1996,Apr,11

57065 **extensive (eg, laser surgery, electrosurgery, cryosurgery, chemosurgery)** ♀ 1 T ▢

MED: 100-2,15,260; 100-3,140.5; 100-4,12,90.3; 100-4,14,10

AMA: 1996,Apr,11

EXCISION

57100 **Biopsy of vaginal mucosa; simple (separate procedure)** ♀ T ▢

57105 **extensive, requiring suture (including cysts)** ♀ 2 T ▢

MED: 100-2,15,260; 100-4,12,90.3; 100-4,14,10

57106 **Vaginectomy, partial removal of vaginal wall;** ♀ T 80 ▢

AMA: 1999,Oct,4; 1998,Nov,17

57107 **with removal of paravaginal tissue (radical vaginectomy)** ♀ T 80 ▢

AMA: 1999,Oct,4; 1998,Nov,17

57109 **with removal of paravaginal tissue (radical vaginectomy) with bilateral total pelvic lymphadenectomy and para-aortic lymph node sampling (biopsy)** ♀ T 80 ▢

AMA: 1999,Oct,4; 1998,Nov,17

57110 **Vaginectomy, complete removal of vaginal wall;** ♀ C 80 ▢

AMA: 1999,Oct,4; 1998,Nov,17

57111 **with removal of paravaginal tissue (radical vaginectomy)** ♀ C 80 ▢

AMA: 1999,Oct,4; 1998,Nov,17

57112 **with removal of paravaginal tissue (radical vaginectomy) with bilateral total pelvic lymphadenectomy and para-aortic lymph node sampling (biopsy)** ♀ C 80 ▢

AMA: 1999,Oct,4; 1998,Nov,17

57120 **Colpocleisis (Le Fort type)** ♀ T 80 ▢

57130 **Excision of vaginal septum** ♀ 2 T 80 ▢

MED: 100-2,15,260; 100-4,12,90.3; 100-4,14,10

57135 **Excision of vaginal cyst or tumor** ♀ 2 T ▢

MED: 100-2,15,260; 100-4,12,90.3; 100-4,14,10

INTRODUCTION

57150 **Irrigation of vagina and/or application of medicament for treatment of bacterial, parasitic, or fungoid disease** ♀ T ▢

57155 **Insertion of uterine tandems and/or vaginal ovoids for clinical brachytherapy** ♀ 2 T ▢

AMA: 2002,Feb,7

To report insertion of radioelement sources of ribbons, consult CPT codes 77761-77763, 77781-77784.

57160 **Fitting and insertion of pessary or other intravaginal support device** ♀ T ▢

AMA: 2000,Jun,11; 1998,Oct,11

57170 **Diaphragm or cervical cap fitting with instructions** ♀ T 80 ▢

57180 **Introduction of any hemostatic agent or pack for spontaneous or traumatic nonobstetrical vaginal hemorrhage (separate procedure)** ♀ 1 T ▢

MED: 100-2,15,260; 100-4,12,90.3; 100-4,14,10

REPAIR

If an anterior vesicourethropexy or urethropexy is performed (e.g., Marshall-Marchetti-Krantz type), consult CPT codes 51840 and 51841. If laparoscopic suspension is performed on the ureter, consult CPT code 51990.

If a pelvic laparotomy is performed, consult CPT code 49000. If excision or destruction is performed of endometriomas, open method, consult CPT codes 49200 and 49201. If paracentesis is performed, consult CPT codes 49080 and 49081. If secondary closure of the abdominal wall evisceration or disruption is performed, consult CPT code 49900. If fulguration or excision of lesions is

26 Professional Component Only   80/80 Assist-at-Surgery Allowed/With Documentation   Unlisted   Not Covered

TC Technical Component Only   MED: Pub 100/NCD References   AMA: CPT Assistant References   1-9 ASC Group   ♂ Male Only   ♀ Female Only

204 — CPT Expert   CPT only © 2006 American Medical Association. All Rights Reserved. *(Black Ink)*   © 2006 Ingenix *(Blue Ink)*

performed through a laparoscopic approach, consult CPT code 58662. If chemotherapy is needed, consult CPT codes 96401-96549.

57200 Colporrhaphy, suture of injury of vagina (nonobstetrical) ♀ **1** T 80 ▣

MED: 100-2,15,260; 100-4,12,90.3; 100-4,14,10

57210 Colpoperineorrhaphy, suture of injury of vagina and/or perineum (nonobstetrical) ♀ **2** T 80 ▣

MED: 100-2,15,260; 100-4,12,90.3; 100-4,14,10

57220 Plastic operation on urethral sphincter, vaginal approach (eg, Kelly urethral plication) ♀ **3** T 80 ▣

MED: 100-2,15,260; 100-4,12,90.3; 100-4,14,10

57230 Plastic repair of urethrocele ♀ **3** T 80 ▣

MED: 100-2,15,260; 100-4,12,90.3; 100-4,14,10

57240 Anterior colporrhaphy, repair of cystocele with or without repair of urethrocele ♀ **5** T 80 ▣

MED: 100-2,15,260; 100-4,12,90.3; 100-4,14,10
AMA: 2002,Jun,4; 1997,Jan,3

57250 Posterior colporrhaphy, repair of rectocele with or without perineorrhaphy ♀ **5** T 80 ▣

MED: 100-2,15,260; 100-4,12,90.3; 100-4,14,10
AMA: 2002,Jun,4
If rectocele is repaired without posterior colporrhaphy, consult CPT code 45560.

57260 Combined anteroposterior colporrhaphy; ♀ **5** T 80 ▣

MED: 100-2,15,260; 100-4,12,90.3; 100-4,14,10
AMA: 2002,Jun,4

57265 with enterocele repair ♀ **7** T 80 ▣

MED: 100-2,15,260; 100-4,12,90.3; 100-4,14,10
AMA: 2002,Jun,4

+ **57267** Insertion of mesh or other prosthesis for repair of pelvic floor defect, each site (anterior, posterior compartment), vaginal approach (List separately in addition to code for primary procedure) ♀ **7** T 80

Note that 57267 must be used with 45560, 57240-57265.

57268 Repair of enterocele, vaginal approach (separate procedure) ♀ **3** T 80 ▣

MED: 100-2,15,260; 100-4,12,90.3; 100-4,14,10
AMA: 2002,Jun,4

57270 Repair of enterocele, abdominal approach (separate procedure) ♀ C 80 ▣

AMA: 2002,Jun,4

57280 Colpopexy, abdominal approach ♀ C 80 ▣

AMA: 2002,Jun,4; 1997,Jan,1

57282 Colpopexy, vaginal; extra-peritoneal approach (sacrospinous, iliococcygeus) ♀ T 80 ▣

AMA: 2002,Jun,4; 1997,Jan,1

57283 intra-peritoneal approach (uterosacral, levator myorrhaphy) ♀ T 80 ▣

57284 Paravaginal defect repair (including repair of cystocele, stress urinary incontinence, and/or incomplete vaginal prolapse) ♀ T 80 ▣

MED: 100-3,230.10
AMA: 2002,Jun,4; 1997,Jan,1

57287 Removal or revision of sling for stress incontinence (eg, fascia or synthetic) ♀ T 80 ▣

MED: 100-3,230.10
AMA: 2002,Jun,4

57288 Sling operation for stress incontinence (eg, fascia or synthetic) ♀ **5** T 80 ▣

AMA: 2002,Jun,4; 2002,Apr,18; 2000,Oct,7; 2000,May,4; 1999,Nov,28
If performed via laparoscope, consult CPT code 51992.

Millen-Read

57289 Pereyra procedure, including anterior colporrhaphy ♀ **5** T 80 ▣

MED: 100-2,15,260; 100-4,12,90.3; 100-4,14,10
AMA: 2002,Jun,4; 1997,Jan,3

57291 Construction of artificial vagina; without graft ♀ **5** T 80 ▣

MED: 100-2,15,260; 100-4,12,90.3; 100-4,14,10
McIndoe vaginal construction

57292 with graft ♀ T 80 ▣

57295 Revision (including removal) of prosthetic vaginal graft; vaginal approach T 80

● **57296** open abdominal approach C

57300 Closure of rectovaginal fistula; vaginal or transanal approach ♀ **3** T 80 ▣

MED: 100-2,15,260; 100-4,12,90.3; 100-4,14,10
AMA: 1997,Nov,21

57305 abdominal approach ♀ C 80 ▣

AMA: 1997,Nov,21

57307 abdominal approach, with concomitant colostomy ♀ C 80 ▣

AMA: 1997,Nov,21

57308 transperineal approach, with perineal body reconstruction, with or without levator plication ♀ C 80 ▣

AMA: 1997,Nov,21

57310 Closure of urethrovaginal fistula; ♀ T 80 ▣

57311 with bulbocavernosus transplant ♀ C 80 ▣

57320 Closure of vesicovaginal fistula; vaginal approach ♀ T 80 ▣

To report concomitant cystostomy, consult CPT codes 51005-51040.

57330 transvesical and vaginal approach ♀ T 80 ▣

If performed via abdominal approach, consult CPT code 51900.

57335 Vaginoplasty for intersex state ♀ T 80 ▣

MANIPULATION

57400 Dilation of vagina under anesthesia ♀ **2** T 80 ▣

MED: 100-2,15,260; 100-4,12,90.3; 100-4,14,10

57410 Pelvic examination under anesthesia ♀ **2** T ▣

MED: 100-2,15,260; 100-4,4,240; 100-4,12,90.3; 100-4,14,10
AMA: 1993,Spring,34

57415 Removal of impacted vaginal foreign body (separate procedure) under anesthesia ♀ **2** T 80 ▣

MED: 100-2,15,260; 100-4,12,90.3; 100-4,14,10
If removal of an impacted vaginal foreign body is performed without anesthesia, consult the appropriate E/M code.

ENDOSCOPY

To report speculoscopy, consult Category III codes 0031T and 0032T.

57420 Colposcopy of the entire vagina, with cervix if present; ♀ T ▣

AMA: 2003,Feb,5

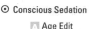

57421   with biopsy(s) of vagina/cervix   ♀ T ▯

AMA: 2003,Feb,5

To report colposcopic visualization of cervix and adjacent upper vagina, consult CPT code 57452.

To report colposcopies of multiple sites, append modifier 51 when appropriate.

To report colposcopic services of the vulva, consult CPT codes 56820, 56821; of the cervix, consult CPT codes 57452-57461.

To report endometrial sampling (biopsy) performed in conjunction with colposcopy, consult CPT code 58110.

57425   Laparoscopy, surgical, colpopexy (suspension of vaginal apex)   ♀ T 80 ▯

CERVIX UTERI

To report colposcopic services of the vulva, consult CPT codes 56820, 56821; of the vagina, consult CPT codes 57420, 57421.

ENDOSCOPY

57452   Colposcopy of the cervix including upper/adjacent vagina;   ♀ T ▯

AMA: 2003,Feb,5; 2000,Apr,5

Do not report 57452 in conjunction with CPT codes 57454-57461.

57454   with biopsy(s) of the cervix and endocervical curettage   ♀ T ▯

AMA: 2003,Feb,5; 2000,Apr,5

57455   with biopsy(s) of the cervix   ♀ T ▯

AMA: 2003,Feb,5

57456   with endocervical curettage   ♀ T ▯

AMA: 2003,Jan,23; 2003,Feb,5

57460   with loop electrode biopsy(s) of the cervix   ♀ T ▯

AMA: 2003,Jan,23; 2003,Feb,5; 2000,Apr,5

57461   with loop electrode conization of the cervix   ♀ T ▯

AMA: 2003,Jan,23; 2003,Feb,5

Do not report 57456 in conjunction with CPT code 57461.

To report endometrial sampling (biopsy) performed in conjunction with colposcopy, consult CPT code 58110.

EXCISION

If radical surgical procedures are performed, consult CPT codes 58200-58240. If an intrauterine device is inserted, consult CPT code 58300.

If a pelvic laparotomy is performed, consult CPT code 49000. If excision or destruction is performed of endometriomas, open method, consult CPT codes 49200 and 49201. If paracentesis is performed, consult CPT codes 49080 and 49081. If secondary closure of the abdominal wall evisceration or disruption is performed, consult CPT code 49900. If fulguration or excision of lesions is performed through a laparoscopic approach, consult CPT code 58662. If chemotherapy is needed, consult CPT codes 96401-96549.

To report insertion of hemostatic agent or pack for non-obstetrical hemorrhage control, consult CPT code 57180.

57500   Biopsy, single or multiple, or local excision of lesion, with or without fulguration (separate procedure)   ♀ T ▯

57505   Endocervical curettage (not done as part of a dilation and curettage)   ♀ T ▯

57510   Cautery of cervix; electro or thermal   ♀ T ▯

57511   cryocautery, initial or repeat   ♀ T ▯

57513   laser ablation   ♀ 2 T ▯

MED: 100-2,15,260; 100-4,12,90.3; 100-4,14,10

57520   Conization of cervix, with or without fulguration, with or without dilation and curettage, with or without repair; cold knife or laser   ♀ 2 T ▯

MED: 100-2,15,260; 100-4,12,90.3; 100-4,14,10

AMA: 2000,Apr,5

Consult also CPT code 58120.

57522   loop electrode excision   ♀ 2 T ▯

MED: 100-2,15,260; 100-4,12,90.3; 100-4,14,10

AMA: 2000,Apr,5

57530   Trachelectomy (cervicectomy), amputation of cervix (separate procedure)   ♀ 3 T 80 ▯

MED: 100-2,15,260; 100-4,12,90.3; 100-4,14,10

57531   Radical trachelectomy, with bilateral total pelvic lymphadenectomy and para-aortic lymph node sampling biopsy, with or without removal of tube(s), with or without removal of ovary(s)   ♀ C 80 ▯

AMA: 1997,Nov,21

If a radical abdominal hysterectomy is performed, consult CPT code 58210.

57540   Excision of cervical stump, abdominal approach;   ♀ C 80 ▯

57545   with pelvic floor repair   ♀ C 80 ▯

57550   Excision of cervical stump, vaginal approach;   ♀ 3 T 80 ▯

MED: 100-2,15,260; 100-4,12,90.3; 100-4,14,10

57555   with anterior and/or posterior repair   ♀ T 80 ▯

57556   with repair of enterocele   ♀ 5 T 80 ▯

MED: 100-2,15,260; 100-4,12,90.3; 100-4,14,10

● **57558**   Dilation and curettage of cervical stump   3 T

REPAIR

57700   Cerclage of uterine cervix, nonobstetrical   ♀ 1 T 80 ▯

MED: 100-2,15,260; 100-4,12,90.3; 100-4,14,10

McDonald cerclage

57720   Trachelorrhaphy, plastic repair of uterine cervix, vaginal approach   ♀ 3 T 80 ▯

MED: 100-2,15,260; 100-4,12,90.3; 100-4,14,10

MANIPULATION

57800   Dilation of cervical canal, instrumental (separate procedure)   ♀ T ▯

~~**57820**~~   ~~Dilation and curettage of cervical stump~~

Use 57558.

CORPUS UTERI

If an endocervical curettage is performed by itself, consult CPT code 57505.

If a pelvic laparotomy is performed, consult CPT code 49000. If excision or destruction is performed of endometriomas, open method, consult CPT codes 49200 and 49201. If paracentesis is performed, consult CPT codes 49080 and 49081. If secondary closure of the abdominal wall evisceration or disruption is performed, consult CPT code 49900. If fulguration or excision of lesions is performed through a laparoscopic approach, consult CPT code 58662. If chemotherapy is needed, consult CPT codes 96401-96549.

If a postpartum curettage is performed, consult CPT code 59160.

26 Professional Component Only   80/80 Assist-at-Surgery Allowed/With Documentation   Unlisted   Not Covered

TC Technical Component Only   MED: Pub 100/NCD References   AMA: CPT Assistant References   1-9 ASC Group   ♂ Male Only   ♀ Female Only

206 — CPT Expert   CPT only © 2006 American Medical Association. All Rights Reserved. (Black Ink)   © 2006 Ingenix (Blue Ink)

Female Genital System

EXCISION

58100 Endometrial sampling (biopsy) with or without endocervical sampling (biopsy), without cervical dilation, any method (separate procedure) ♀ T ▣

MED: 100-3,230.6

To report endometrial sampling (biopsy) performed in conjunction with colposcopy, consult CPT code 58110.

+ 58110 Endometrial sampling (biopsy) performed in conjunction with colposcopy (List separately in addition to code for primary procedure) T 80

Note that 58110 is an add-on code and must be used with 57420, 57421, 57452-57461.

58120 Dilation and curettage, diagnostic and/or therapeutic (nonobstetrical) ♀ 2 T ▣

MED: 100-2,15,260; 100-4,12,90.3; 100-4,14,10

AMA: 1997,Nov,21; 1995,Fall,16

▲ 58140 Myomectomy, excision of fibroid tumor(s) of uterus, 1 to 4 intramural myoma(s) with total weight of 250 g or less and/or removal of surface myomas; abdominal approach ♀ C 80 ▣

AMA: 2003,Feb,15

▲ 58145 Myomectomy, excision of fibroid tumor(s) of uterus, 1 to 4 intramural myoma(s) with total weight of 250 g or less and/or removal of surface myomas; vaginal approach ♀ 5 T 80 ▣

MED: 100-2,15,260; 100-4,12,90.3; 100-4,14,10

▲ 58146 Myomectomy, excision of fibroid tumor(s) of uterus, 5 or more intramural myomas and/or intramural myomas with total weight greater than 250 g, abdominal approach ♀ C 80 ▣

AMA: 2003,Feb,15

Do not report 58146 in conjunction with CPT codes 58140-58145, 58150-58240.

HYSTERECTOMY PROCEDURES

58150 Total abdominal hysterectomy (corpus and cervix), with or without removal of tube(s), with or without removal of ovary(s); ♀ C 80 ▣

MED: 100-3,230.3

AMA: 2001,Aug,11; 2000,Sep,9; 1997,Nov,21; 1997,Apr,3; 1996,Dec,10

58152 with colpo-urethrocystopexy (eg, Marshall-Marchetti-Krantz, Burch) ♀ C 80 ▣

MED: 100-3,230.3

AMA: 1997,Nov,22; 1997,Jan,1

If a urethrocystopexy is performed without a hysterectomy, consult CPT codes 51840 and 51841.

58180 Supracervical abdominal hysterectomy (subtotal hysterectomy), with or without removal of tube(s), with or without removal of ovary(s) ♀ C 80 ▣

MED: 100-3,230.3

58200 Total abdominal hysterectomy, including partial vaginectomy, with para-aortic and pelvic lymph node sampling, with or without removal of tube(s), with or without removal of ovary(s) ♀ C 80 ▣

MED: 100-3,230.3

To report hysterectomy with pelvic lymphadenectomy, consult CPT code 58210.

58210 Radical abdominal hysterectomy, with bilateral total pelvic lymphadenectomy and para-aortic lymph node sampling (biopsy), with or without removal of tube(s), with or without removal of ovary(s) ♀ C 80 ▣

MED: 100-3,230.3

If a radical hysterectomy is performed with an ovarian transposition, consult also CPT code 58825.

Wertheim hysterectomy

58240 Pelvic exenteration for gynecologic malignancy, with total abdominal hysterectomy or cervicectomy, with or without removal of tube(s), with or without removal of ovary(s), with removal of bladder and ureteral transplantations, and/or abdominoperineal resection of rectum and colon and colostomy, or any combination thereof ♀ C 80 ▣

MED: 100-3,230.3

If pelvic exenteration is performed for a lower urinary tract or a male genital malignancy, consult CPT code 51597.

▲ 58260 Vaginal hysterectomy, for uterus 250 g or less; ♀ T 80 ▣

MED: 100-3,230.3

▲ 58262 with removal of tube(s), and/or ovary(s) ♀ T 80 ▣

MED: 100-3,230.3

▲ 58263 with removal of tube(s), and/or ovary(s), with repair of enterocele ♀ T 80 ▣

MED: 100-3,230.3

Code 58263 cannot be reported with CPT code 57283.

▲ 58267 with colpo-urethrocystopexy (Marshall-Marchetti-Krantz type, Pereyra type) with or without endoscopic control ♀ C 80 ▣

MED: 100-3,230.3

▲ 58270 with repair of enterocele ♀ T 80 ▣

MED: 100-3,230.3

If an enterocele is repaired with removal of tubes and/or ovaries, consult CPT code 58263.

58275 Vaginal hysterectomy, with total or partial vaginectomy; ♀ C 80 ▣

MED: 100-3,230.3

58280 with repair of enterocele ♀ C 80 ▣

MED: 100-3,230.3

58285 Vaginal hysterectomy, radical (Schauta type operation) ♀ C 80 ▣

MED: 100-3,230.3

58290 Vaginal hysterectomy, for uterus greater than 250 g; ♀ T 80 ▣

58291 with removal of tube(s) and/or ovary(s) ♀ T 80 ▣

58292 with removal of tube(s) and/or ovary(s), with repair of enterocele ♀ T 80 ▣

58293 with colpo-urethrocystopexy (Marshall-Marchetti-Krantz type, Pereyra type) with or without endoscopic control ♀ C 80 ▣

58294 with repair of enterocele ♀ T 80 ▣

INTRODUCTION

If implantable contraceptive capsules are inserted or removed, consult CPT codes 11975, 11976, and 11977.

If a pelvic laparotomy is performed, consult CPT code 49000. If excision or destruction is performed of endometriomas, open method, consult CPT codes

---

◎ Modifier 63 Exempt Code · ⊙ Conscious Sedation · + CPT Add-on Code · ◯ Modifier 51 Exempt Code · ● New Code · ▲ Revised Code

Ⓜ Maternity Edit · Ⓐ Age Edit · Ⓐ-Ⓨ APC Status Indicators · ▣ CCI Comprehensive Code · 80 Bilateral Procedure

© 2006 Ingenix (Blue Ink) · CPT only © 2006 American Medical Association. All Rights Reserved. (Black Ink) · Female Genital System — 207

49200 and 49201. If paracentesis is performed, consult CPT codes 49080 and 49081. If secondary closure of the abdominal wall evisceration or disruption is performed, consult CPT code 49900. If fulguration or excision of lesions is performed through a laparoscopic approach, consult CPT code 58662. If chemotherapy is needed, consult CPT codes 96401-96549.

58300   **Insertion of intrauterine device (IUD)**   ♀ Ⓔ

AMA: 1998,Apr,14

58301   **Removal of intrauterine device (IUD)**   ♀ Ⓣ 80 🔲

AMA: 1998,Apr,14

58321   **Artificial insemination; intra-cervical**   ♀ Ⓣ 80 🔲

58322   **intra-uterine**   ♀ Ⓣ 80 🔲

58323   **Sperm washing for artificial insemination**   ♀ Ⓣ 80 🔲

AMA: 1998,Jan,6

58340   **Catheterization and introduction of saline or contrast material for saline infusion sonohysterography (SIS) or hysterosalpingography**   ♀ Ⓝ 🔲

AMA: 1999,Jul,8; 1997,Nov,22

To report radiological supervision and interpretation of a saline infusion hysterosonography, consult CPT code 76831. To report radiological supervision and interpretation of hysterosalpingography, consult CPT code 74740.

To report cryoablation of endometrium with ultrasonic guidance, consult CPT Category III code 0009T.

58345   **Transcervical introduction of fallopian tube catheter for diagnosis and/or re-establishing patency (any method), with or without hysterosalpingography**   ♀ Ⓣ 80 50 🔲

AMA: 1997,Nov,22

To report radiological supervision and interpretation, consult CPT code 74742.

58346   **Insertion of Heyman capsules for clinical brachytherapy**   ♀ ② Ⓣ 🔲

AMA: 2002,Feb,7

To report radioelement sources/ribbons insertion, consult CPT codes 77761-77763, 77781-77784.

58350   **Chromotubation of oviduct, including materials**   ♀ ③ Ⓣ 🔲

MED: 100-2,15,260; 100-4,12,90.3; 100-4,14,10

AMA: 2002,May,19

To report physician supplied materials, consult CPT code 99070.

58353   **Endometrial ablation, thermal, without hysteroscopic guidance**   ♀ ⑦ Ⓣ 80 50 🔲

MED: 100-2,15,260; 100-3,230.6; 100-4,12,90.3; 100-4,14,10

AMA: 2002,Mar,11; 2002,Apr,19

To report endometrial ablation with hysteroscopy consult CPT code 58563.

58356   **Endometrial cryoablation with ultrasonic guidance, including endometrial curettage, when performed**   ♀ Ⓣ 80 50 🔲

Code 58356 cannot be reported with CPT codes 58100, 58120, 58340, 76700, 76856.

REPAIR

If a pelvic laparotomy is performed, consult CPT code 49000. If excision or destruction is performed of endometriomas, open method, consult CPT codes 49200 and 49201. If paracentesis is performed, consult CPT codes 49080 and 49081. If secondary closure of the abdominal wall evisceration or disruption is performed, consult CPT code 49900. If fulguration or excision of lesions is performed through a laparoscopic approach, consult CPT code 58662. If chemotherapy is needed, consult CPT codes 96401-96549.

58400   **Uterine suspension, with or without shortening of round ligaments, with or without shortening of sacrouterine ligaments; (separate procedure)**   ♀ Ⓒ 80 🔲

Alexander's operation

58410   **with presacral sympathectomy**   ♀ Ⓒ 80 🔲

Alexander's operation

58520   **Hysterorrhaphy, repair of ruptured uterus (nonobstetrical)**   ♀ Ⓒ 80 🔲

58540   **Hysteroplasty, repair of uterine anomaly (Strassman type)**   ♀ Ⓒ 80 🔲

If a vesicouterine fistula is closed, consult CPT code 51920.

Tompkins metroplasty

LAPAROSCOPY/HYSTEROSCOPY

Diagnostic laparoscopy is always included in surgical laparoscopy. To report only a diagnostic laparoscopy, consult CPT code 49320.

For diagnostic hysteroscopy, consult CPT code 58555.

If a pelvic laparotomy is performed, consult CPT code 49000. If excision or destruction is performed of endometriomas, open method, consult CPT codes 49200 and 49201. If paracentesis is performed, consult CPT codes 49080 and 49081. If secondary closure of the abdominal wall evisceration or disruption is performed, consult CPT code 49900. If fulguration or excision of lesions is performed through a laparoscopic approach, consult CPT code 58662. If chemotherapy is needed, consult CPT codes 96400-96549.

● **58541**   **Laparoscopy, surgical, supracervical hysterectomy, for uterus 250 g or less;**   Ⓣ

● **58542**   **with removal of tube(s) and/or ovary(s)**   Ⓣ

Do not report 58541 or 58542 with 49320, 57410, 58140, 58150, 58661, 58670, or 58671.

● **58543**   **Laparoscopy, surgical, supracervical hysterectomy, for uterus greater than 250 g;**   Ⓣ

● **58544**   **with removal of tube(s) and/or ovary(s)**   Ⓣ

Do not report 58543 or 58544 with 49320, 57410, 58140, 58150, 58661, 58670, or 58671.

58545   **Laparoscopy, surgical, myomectomy, excision; 1 to 4 intramural myomas with total weight of 250 g or less and/or removal of surface myomas**   ♀ ⑨ Ⓣ 80 🔲

MED: 100-2,15,260; 100-4,12,90.3; 100-4,14,10

58546   **5 or more intramural myomas and/or intramural myomas with total weight greater than 250 grams**   ♀ ⑨ Ⓣ 80 🔲

MED: 100-2,15,260; 100-4,12,90.3; 100-4,14,10

● **58548**   **Laparoscopy, surgical, with radical hysterectomy, with bilateral total pelvic lymphadenectomy and para-aortic lymph node sampling (biopsy), with removal of tube(s) and ovary(s), if performed**   Ⓒ

Do not report 58548 with 38570-38572, 58210, 58285, or 58550-58554.

58550   **Laparoscopy, surgical, with vaginal hysterectomy, for uterus 250 g or less;**   ♀ ⑨ Ⓣ 80 🔲

MED: 100-2,15,260; 100-3,230.3; 100-4,12,90.3; 100-4,14,10

AMA: 2000,Mar,5; 1999,Nov,28

58552   **with removal of tube(s) and/or ovary(s)**   ♀ Ⓣ 80 🔲

58553   **Laparoscopy, surgical, with vaginal hysterectomy, for uterus greater than 250 g;**   ♀ Ⓣ 80 🔲

58554   **with removal of tube(s) and/or ovary(s)**   ♀ Ⓣ 80 🔲

26 Professional Component Only   80/80 Assist-at-Surgery Allowed/With Documentation   Unlisted   Not Covered

TC Technical Component Only   MED: Pub 100/NCD References   AMA: CPT Assistant References   1-9 ASC Group   ♂ Male Only   ♀ Female Only

208 — CPT Expert   CPT only © 2006 American Medical Association. All Rights Reserved. *(Black Ink)*   © *2006 Ingenix (Blue Ink)*

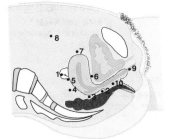

Some common sites
of endometriosis,
in descending order
of frequency:
(1) ovary,
(2) cul de sac,
(3) uterosacral ligaments,
(4) broad ligaments,
(5) fallopian tube,
(6) uterovesical fold,
(7) round ligament,
(8) vermiform appendix,
(9) vagina,
(10) rectovaginal septum

Endometriosis is a benign condition in which endometrial matter is present outside of the endometrial cavity; it is estimated that 15 percent of women have some degree of the disease; occurrence is most common in the ovaries and about 60 percent of patients will have ovarian involvement, many with cyst development

58555　　**Hysteroscopy, diagnostic (separate procedure)**　　♀ 🔳 T 80 🔲

MED: 100-2,15,260; 100-4,12,90.3; 100-4,14,10
AMA: 2000,Mar,5; 1999,Nov,28

58558　　**Hysteroscopy, surgical; with sampling (biopsy) of endometrium and/or polypectomy, with or without D & C**　　♀ 3 T 🔲

MED: 100-2,15,260; 100-4,12,90.3; 100-4,14,10
AMA: 2003,Jan,1; 2002,Sep,10; 2000,Mar,5; 1999,Nov,28

58559　　**with lysis of intrauterine adhesions (any method)**　　♀ 2 T 🔲

MED: 100-2,15,260; 100-4,12,90.3; 100-4,14,10
AMA: 2000,Mar,5; 1999,Nov,28

58560　　**with division or resection of intrauterine septum (any method)**　　♀ 3 T 80 🔲

MED: 100-2,15,260; 100-4,12,90.3; 100-4,14,10
AMA: 2000,Mar,5; 1999,Nov,28

58561　　**with removal of leiomyomata**　　♀ 3 T 80 🔲

MED: 100-2,15,260; 100-4,12,90.3; 100-4,14,10
AMA: 2003,Jan,1; 2000,Mar,5; 1999,Nov,28

58562　　**with removal of impacted foreign body**　　♀ 3 T 🔲

MED: 100-2,15,260; 100-4,12,90.3; 100-4,14,10
AMA: 2000,Mar,5; 1999,Nov,28

58563　　**with endometrial ablation (eg, endometrial resection, electrosurgical ablation, thermoablation)**　　♀ 9 T 80 🔲

MED: 100-2,15,260; 100-3,230.6; 100-4,12,90.3; 100-4,14,10
AMA: 2003,Jan,1; 2002,Mar,11; 2002,Apr,19; 2000,Mar,5; 1999,Nov,28

58565　　**with bilateral fallopian tube cannulation to induce occlusion by placement of permanent implants**　　♀ 9 T 🔲

Code 58565 cannot be reported with CPT code 58555 or 57800.

If this procedure is performed unilaterally, append modifier 52.

58578　　Unlisted laparoscopy procedure, uterus　　T 80 50

AMA: 2000,Mar,5; 1999,Nov,28

58579　　Unlisted hysteroscopy procedure, uterus　　T 80 50

AMA: 2000,Mar,5; 1999,Nov,28

OVIDUCT/OVARY

If a pelvic laparotomy is performed, consult CPT code 49000. If excision or destruction is performed of endometriomas, open method, consult CPT codes 49200 and 49201. If paracentesis is performed, consult CPT codes 49080 and 49081. If secondary closure of the abdominal wall evisceration or disruption is performed, consult CPT code 49900. If fulguration or excision of lesions is performed through a laparoscopic approach, consult CPT code 58662. If chemotherapy is needed, consult CPT codes 96400-96549.

INCISION

58600　　**Ligation or transection of fallopian tube(s), abdominal or vaginal approach, unilateral or bilateral**　　♀ T 80 🔲

MED: 100-3,230.3
AMA: 1999,Nov,28
Madlener operation

58605　　**Ligation or transection of fallopian tube(s), abdominal or vaginal approach, postpartum, unilateral or bilateral, during same hospitalization (separate procedure)**　　♀ C 80 🔲

MED: 100-3,230.3
AMA: 1999,Nov,28
If laparoscopic procedures are performed, consult CPT codes 58670 and 58371.

+　　**58611**　　**Ligation or transection of fallopian tube(s) when done at the time of cesarean delivery or intra-abdominal surgery (not a separate procedure) (List separately in addition to code for primary procedure)**　　♀ C 80 🔲

MED: 100-3,230.3
Note that 58611 is an add-on code that must be used in conjunction with the appropriate code for the primary procedure. This code cannot be reported alone.

58615　　**Occlusion of fallopian tube(s) by device (eg, band, clip, Falope ring) vaginal or suprapubic approach**　　♀ T 80 🔲

MED: 100-3,230.3
AMA: 1999,Nov,28
If a laparoscopic approach is used, consult CPT code 58671.

LAPAROSCOPY

If a laparoscopic biopsy is performed of the ovary or fallopian tube, consult CPT code 49321.

If a pelvic laparotomy is performed, consult CPT code 49000. If excision or destruction is performed of endometriomas, open method, consult CPT codes 49200 and 49201. If paracentesis is performed, consult CPT codes 49080 and 49081. If secondary closure of the abdominal wall evisceration or disruption is performed, consult CPT code 49900. If fulguration or excision of lesions is performed through a laparoscopic approach, consult CPT code 58662. If chemotherapy is needed, consult CPT codes 96401-96549.

Diagnostic laparoscopy is always included in surgical laparoscopy. To report only diagnostic laparoscopy, consult CT code 49320.

58660　　**Laparoscopy, surgical; with lysis of adhesions (salpingolysis, ovariolysis) (separate procedure)**　　♀ 5 T 80 🔲

MED: 100-2,15,260; 100-3,230.3; 100-4,12,90.3; 100-4,14,10
AMA: 2000,Mar,5; 1999,Nov,28

58661　　**with removal of adnexal structures (partial or total oophorectomy and/or salpingectomy)**　　♀ 5 T 80 🔲

MED: 100-2,15,260; 100-3,230.3; 100-4,12,90.3; 100-4,14,10
AMA: 2002,Jan,11; 2000,Mar,5; 1999,Nov,28

58662　　**with fulguration or excision of lesions of the ovary, pelvic viscera, or peritoneal surface by any method**　　♀ 5 T 80 🔲

MED: 100-2,15,260; 100-3,230.3; 100-4,12,90.3; 100-4,14,10
AMA: 2000,Mar,5; 1999,Nov,28

58670　　**with fulguration of oviducts (with or without transection)**　　♀ 3 T 🔲

MED: 100-2,15,260; 100-3,230.3; 100-4,12,90.3; 100-4,14,10
AMA: 2000,Mar,5; 1999,Nov,29

㊿ Modifier 63 Exempt Code　　⊙ Conscious Sedation　　+ CPT Add-on Code　　🚫 Modifier 51 Exempt Code　　● New Code　　▲ Revised Code

Ⓜ Maternity Edit　　🅰 Age Edit　　🅰-🆈 APC Status Indicators　　🔲 CCI Comprehensive Code　　50 Bilateral Procedure

58671　　with occlusion of oviducts by device (eg, band, clip, or Falope ring)　　♀ 🔳 🔲 🔲

MED: 100-2,15,260; 100-3,230.3; 100-4,12,90.3; 100-4,14,10
AMA: 2000,Mar,5; 1999,Nov,29

58672　　with fimbrioplasty　　♀ 🔳 🔲 🔲 🔲 🔲

MED: 100-2,15,260; 100-3,230.3; 100-4,12,90.3; 100-4,14,10
AMA: 2000,Mar,5; 1999,Nov,29

58673　　with salpingostomy (salpingoneostomy)　　♀ 🔳 🔲 🔲 🔲 🔲

MED: 100-2,15,260; 100-3,230.3; 100-4,12,90.3; 100-4,14,10
AMA: 2000,Mar,5; 1999,Nov,29
Codes 58672 and 58673 describe unilateral procedures. If performed bilaterally, append modifier 50.

58679　　Unlisted laparoscopy procedure, oviduct, ovary　　🔲 🔲 🔲

AMA: 2000,Mar,5; 1999,Nov,29
Use 49322 for laparoscopic aspiration of ovarian cyst.

Use 49321 for laparoscopic biopsy of ovary or fallopian tube.

EXCISION

58700　　Salpingectomy, complete or partial, unilateral or bilateral (separate procedure)　　♀ 🔲 🔲 🔲

58720　　Salpingo-oophorectomy, complete or partial, unilateral or bilateral (separate procedure)　　♀ 🔲 🔲 🔲

AMA: 2000,Sep,9

REPAIR

If a pelvic laparotomy is performed, consult CPT code 49000. If excision or destruction is performed of endometriomas, open method, consult CPT codes 49200 and 49201. If paracentesis is performed, consult CPT codes 49080 and 49081. If secondary closure of the abdominal wall evisceration or disruption is performed, consult CPT code 49900. If fulguration or excision of lesions is performed through a laparoscopic approach, consult CPT code 58662. If chemotherapy is needed, consult CPT codes 96401-96549.

58740　　Lysis of adhesions (salpingolysis, ovariolysis)　　♀ 🔲 🔲 🔲

AMA: 1999,Nov,29; 1996,Sep,9
If a laparoscopic approach is used, consult CPT code 58660. If excision or destruction is performed of endometriomas, open method, consult CPT codes 49200 and 49201. If fulguration or excision of lesions is performed, laparoscopic approach, consult CPT code 58662.

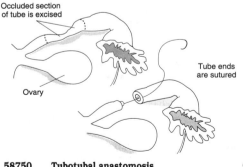

Occluded section of tube is excised

Tube ends are sutured

Ovary

58750　　Tubotubal anastomosis　　♀ 🔲 🔲 🔲

58752　　Tubouterine implantation　　♀ 🔲 🔲 🔲

58760　　Fimbrioplasty　　♀ 🔲 🔲 🔲 🔲

AMA: 1999,Nov,29
If a laparoscopic approach is used, consult CPT code 58672.

58770　　Salpingostomy (salpingoneostomy)　　♀ 🔲 🔲 🔲 🔲

AMA: 1999,Nov,29
If a laparoscopic approach is used, consult CPT code 58673.

OVARY

If a pelvic laparotomy is performed, consult CPT code 49000. If excision or destruction is performed of endometriomas, open method, consult CPT codes 49200 and 49201. If paracentesis is performed, consult CPT codes 49080 and 49081. If secondary closure of the abdominal wall evisceration or disruption is performed, consult CPT code 49900. If fulguration or excision of lesions is performed through a laparoscopic approach, consult CPT code 58662. If chemotherapy is needed, consult CPT codes 96401-96549.

INCISION

58800　　Drainage of ovarian cyst(s), unilateral or bilateral, (separate procedure); vaginal approach　　♀ 🔲 🔲 🔲

MED: 100-2,15,260; 100-4,12,90.3; 100-4,14,10

58805　　abdominal approach　　♀ 🔲 🔲 🔲

58820　　Drainage of ovarian abscess; vaginal approach, open　　♀ 🔲 🔲 🔲 🔲

MED: 100-2,15,260; 100-4,12,90.3; 100-4,14,10
AMA: 1997,Nov,22

58822　　abdominal approach　　♀ 🔲 🔲 🔲

AMA: 1997,Nov,22

⊙ **58823**　　Drainage of pelvic abscess, transvaginal or transrectal approach, percutaneous (eg, ovarian, pericolic)　　♀ 🔲 🔲 🔲

AMA: 1998,Mar,8; 1997,Nov,22
To report radiological supervision and interpretation, consult CPT code 75989.

58825　　Transposition, ovary(s)　　♀ 🔲 🔲 🔲

EXCISION

58900　　Biopsy of ovary, unilateral or bilateral (separate procedure)　　♀ 🔲 🔲 🔲 🔲

MED: 100-2,15,260; 100-4,3,20.2.1; 100-4,12,90.3; 100-4,14,10
AMA: 1999,Nov,29
If performed via laparoscope, consult CPT code 49321.

58920　　Wedge resection or bisection of ovary, unilateral or bilateral　　♀ 🔲 🔲 🔲

58925　　Ovarian cystectomy, unilateral or bilateral　　♀ 🔲 🔲 🔲

58940　　Oophorectomy, partial or total, unilateral or bilateral;　　♀ 🔲 🔲 🔲

MED: 100-3,230.3

58943　　for ovarian, tubal or primary peritoneal malignancy, with para-aortic and pelvic lymph node biopsies, peritoneal washings, peritoneal biopsies, diaphragmatic assessments, with or without salpingectomy(s), with or without omentectomy　　♀ 🔲 🔲 🔲

MED: 100-3,230.3

▲ **58950**　　Resection (initial) of ovarian, tubal or primary peritoneal malignancy with bilateral salpingo-oophorectomy and omentectomy;　　♀ 🔲 🔲 🔲

▲ **58951**　　with total abdominal hysterectomy, pelvic and limited para-aortic lymphadenectomy　　♀ 🔲 🔲 🔲

AMA: 2001,Aug,11

🔲 Professional Component Only　　　　🔲/🔲 Assist-at-Surgery Allowed/With Documentation　　　Unlisted　　　Not Covered

🔲 Technical Component Only　　**MED:** Pub 100/NCD References　　**AMA:** CPT Assistant References　　🔲-🔲 ASC Group　　♂ Male Only　　♀ Female Only

210 — CPT Expert　　　　**CPT only © 2006 American Medical Association. All Rights Reserved.** *(Black Ink)*　　　　**© 2006 Ingenix** *(Blue Ink)*

▲ 58952　with radical dissection for debulking (ie, radical excision or destruction, intra-abdominal or retroperitoneal tumors)　♀ C 80

AMA: 2001,Aug,11; 1996,Dec,10
Use 58957 and 58958 for resection of recurrent ovarian, tubal, primary peritoneal, or uterine malignancy.

58953　Bilateral salpingo-oophorectomy with omentectomy, total abdominal hysterectomy and radical dissection for debulking;　♀ C 80

AMA: 2002,Feb,7

58954　with pelvic lymphadenectomy and limited para-aortic lymphadenectomy　♀ C 80 ↻

AMA: 2002,Feb,7

58956　Bilateral salpingo-oophorectomy with total omentectomy, total abdominal hysterectomy for malignancy　♀ C 80 ↻

Code 58956 cannot be reported with CPT codes 49255, 58150, 58180, 58262, 58263, 58550, 58661, 58700, 58720, 58900, 58925, 58940, 58957, or 58958.

● 58957　Resection (tumor debulking) of recurrent ovarian, tubal, primary peritoneal, uterine malignancy (intra-abdominal, retroperitoneal tumors), with omentectomy, if performed;　C

● 58958　with pelvic lymphadenectomy and limited para-aortic lymphadenectomy　C

Do not report 58957 or 58958 with 38770, 38780, 44005, 49000, 49200-49215, 49255, or 58900-58960.

58960　Laparotomy, for staging or restaging of ovarian, tubal, or primary peritoneal malignancy (second look), with or without omentectomy, peritoneal washing, biopsy of abdominal and pelvic peritoneum, diaphragmatic assessment with pelvic and limited para-aortic lymphadenectomy　♀ C 80 ↻

Do not report 58960 with 58957 or 58958.

IN VITRO FERTILIZATION

58970　Follicle puncture for oocyte retrieval, any method　♀ 1 T 80 ↻

To report radiological supervision and interpretation, consult CPT code 76948.

58974　Embryo transfer, intrauterine　M ♀ 1 T 80 ↻

58976　Gamete, zygote, or embryo intrafallopian transfer, any method　M ♀ 1 T 80 ↻

AMA: 1999,Nov,29

OTHER PROCEDURES

58999　Unlisted procedure, female genital system (nonobstetrical)　♀ T 80

MED: 100-4,4,180.3

MATERNITY CARE AND DELIVERY

ANTEPARTUM SERVICES

Maternity care is outlined in the maternity care and delivery section. The codes for normal, uncomplicated care to the maternity patient (59400, 59510, 59610, 59618) include antepartum care, delivery, and postpartum care by the same physician.

Antepartum care includes the initial and routine subsequent history and physical exams, patient's weight, blood pressure, fetal heart tones, and routine urinalysis.

Delivery includes admission to the hospital, including the admitting history and exam, the management of uncomplicated labor, and either a vaginal or cesarean delivery.

Postpartum care includes the inpatient hospital care and any office visits following vaginal or cesarean delivery.

Codes for delivery following a previous cesarean delivery deserve some additional explanation. These codes report delivery after a previous cesarean delivery when an attempt is made to accomplish the delivery vaginally, also referred to as a VBAC.

When different physicians provide components of the total obstetric service, report the services separately using the codes designated for each component. Codes 59425 and 59426 identify a different physician providing four or more antepartum care visits. Use the appropriate E/M codes when a different physician provides one to three antepartum care visits. Use 59409, 59514, 59612, or 59620 when the physician performs vaginal or cesarean delivery only. Use 59410, 59515, 59614, or 59622 when the physician performs vaginal or cesarean delivery with postpartum care.

Services unrelated to the pregnancy should be reported with E/M codes or the procedure codes for the service. For example, a patient seen for a sore throat with a throat culture should have both the throat culture and E/M service reported separately. Clearly identify the reasons for the services as pharyngitis, not pregnancy.

Services directly related to the pregnancy, but not included in the global service, should be reported separately. Examples include ultrasound examination of pregnant uterus (76801-76817), glucose tolerance test (82951-82953), and Pap smear (88150). The neuraxial labor analgesia and anesthesia codes are reported in addition to the primary procedures.

Normal maternity care includes monthly visits up to 28 weeks gestation, biweekly visits to 36 weeks gestation, and weekly visits until delivery. For the patient at risk who is seen more frequently or for other medical/surgical intervention, report the additional services with a code representing the appropriate level of E/M service. The documentation must reflect the necessity of these visits as well as any additional laboratory or radiologic tests performed.

When the physician monitors the patient for a prolonged period, document the time spent in actual attendance and use prolonged services codes as appropriate. Codes 99356 and 99357 describe maternal-fetal monitoring, which is reported in addition to the delivery. Always include documentation to substantiate medical necessity.

59000　Amniocentesis; diagnostic　M ♀ T ↻

MED: 100-3,220.5
AMA: 2002,Feb,7; 1997,Apr,2
To report radiological supervision and interpretation, consult CPT code 76946.

59001　therapeutic amniotic fluid reduction (includes ultrasound guidance)　M ♀ T

AMA: 2002,Feb,7

59012　Cordocentesis (intrauterine), any method　M ♀ T 80

To report radiological supervision and interpretation, consult CPT code 76941.

59015　Chorionic villus sampling, any method　M ♀ T 80 ↻

AMA: 1997,Apr,2
To report radiological supervision and interpretation, consult CPT code 76945.

59020　Fetal contraction stress test　M ♀ T 80 ↻

AMA: 1997,Apr,2
If the physician only interprets the results and/or operates the equipment, modifier 26 should be appended to 59020.

59025　Fetal non-stress test　M ♀ T 80 ↻

AMA: 1998,May,10
If the physician only interprets the results and/or operates the equipment, modifier 26 should be appended to 59025.

| 59030 | Fetal scalp blood sampling | M ♀ T 80 ▢ |

| 59050 | Fetal monitoring during labor by consulting physician (ie, non-attending physician) with written report; supervision and interpretation | M ♀ M 80 ▢ |

AMA: 1997,Nov,22

| 59051 | interpretation only | M ♀ B 80 ▢ |

AMA: 1997,Nov,22

| 59070 | Transabdominal amnioinfusion, including ultrasound guidance | M ♀ T 80 ▢ |

| 59072 | Fetal umbilical cord occlusion, including ultrasound guidance | M ♀ T ▢ |

| 59074 | Fetal fluid drainage (eg, vesicocentesis, thoracocentesis, paracentesis), including ultrasound guidance | M ♀ T 80 ▢ |

| 59076 | Fetal shunt placement, including ultrasound guidance | M ♀ T 80 ▢ |

To report unlisted fetal invasive procedure, consult CPT code 59897.

EXCISION

| 59100 | Hysterotomy, abdominal (eg, for hydatidiform mole, abortion) | M ♀ T 80 ▢ |

If tubal ligation is performed at the same time as the hysterotomy, consult CPT code 58611 and report in addition to 59100.

| 59120 | Surgical treatment of ectopic pregnancy; tubal or ovarian, requiring salpingectomy and/or oophorectomy, abdominal or vaginal approach | M ♀ C 80 ▢ |

MED: 100-3,230.3

| 59121 | tubal or ovarian, without salpingectomy and/or oophorectomy | M ♀ C 80 ▢ |

| 59130 | abdominal pregnancy | M ♀ C 80 ▢ |

| 59135 | interstitial, uterine pregnancy requiring total hysterectomy | M ♀ C 80 ▢ |

MED: 100-3,230.3

| 59136 | interstitial, uterine pregnancy with partial resection of uterus | M ♀ C 80 ▢ |

MED: 100-3,230.3

| 59140 | cervical, with evacuation | M ♀ C 80 ▢ |

| 59150 | Laparoscopic treatment of ectopic pregnancy; without salpingectomy and/or oophorectomy | M ♀ T 80 ▢ |

AMA: 1996,Sep,9

Ectopic pregnancies are reported by site where abnormal attachment occurs; more than 95 percent occur in the fallopian tube

Ectopic pregnancy in tube

Abdominal pregnancy

Site of interstitial pregnancy

Cervix and cervical canal

Ectopic pregnancy in cervix

Ovarian pregnancy

Uterus

Broad ligament (mesometric)

Half of all ectopic pregnancies resolve spontaneously without rupture but surgical intervention is usually necessary for the remainder; rarely, an abdominal or mesometric pregnancy may continue until a viable fetus is delivered through an abdominal incision

| 59151 | with salpingectomy and/or oophorectomy | M ♀ T 80 ▢ |

MED: 100-3,230.3

| 59160 | Curettage, postpartum | M ♀ 3 T 80 ▢ |

MED: 100-2,15,260; 100-4,12,90.3; 100-4,14,10

AMA: 1997,Nov,22

INTRODUCTION

| 59200 | Insertion of cervical dilator (eg, laminaria, prostaglandin) (separate procedure) | M ♀ T ▢ |

AMA: 1997,Apr,3; 1993,Fall,9

If intrauterine fetal transfusion is conducted, consult CPT code 36460. If a hypertonic solution and/or prostaglandins are introduced to initiate labor, consult CPT codes 59850-59857.

REPAIR

If tracheloplasty is performed, consult CPT code 57700.

| 59300 | Episiotomy or vaginal repair, by other than attending physician | M ♀ T 80 ▢ |

| 59320 | Cerclage of cervix, during pregnancy; vaginal | M ♀ 1 T 80 ▢ |

MED: 100-2,15,260; 100-4,12,90.3; 100-4,14,10

| 59325 | abdominal | M ♀ C 80 ▢ |

| 59350 | Hysterorrhaphy of ruptured uterus | M ♀ C 80 ▢ |

VAGINAL DELIVERY, ANTEPARTUM AND POSTPARTUM CARE

This section addresses antepartum care, delivery, and postpartum care. Antepartum care includes monthly visits up to 28 weeks gestation, biweekly visits up to 36 weeks gestation and weekly visits until delivery. Services included are history, examinations, recording of weight, blood pressures, fetal health, urinalysis, and other examinations pertinent to the health of mother and child. Delivery services include admission, management of labor and vaginal delivery, or cesarean delivery. Postpartum care includes hospital and office visits following vaginal or cesarean section delivery.

If the physician provides all or part of the antepartum care, but does not perform the delivery, consult CPT codes 59425-59426. If only one to three visits are provided, consult the appropriate Evaluation and Management codes. For postpartum care only, consult CPT code 59430.

Breech presentation (left) and Simpson forceps delivery of aftercoming head (right)

Vacuum extractor attached to posterior fontanelle to flex head downward (below left)

Obstetric forceps provide traction, rotation, or both to the birthing head and designs vary to accomplish specific tasks (e.g., Kielland forceps to rotate the head). Low forceps is application when skull is at station plus 2 or lower; mid forceps is application above station plus 2; high forceps is application at point of engagement. Vacuum extraction holds certain advantages, especially when forced rotation is not wanted, but it is not used for breech presentations

| 59400 | Routine obstetric care including antepartum care, vaginal delivery (with or without episiotomy, and/or forceps) and postpartum care | M ♀ B ▢ |

MED: 100-2,15,20.1; 100-2,15,180

AMA: 2003,Feb,15; 2002,Aug,1; 1998,Jun,10; 1998,Apr,15; 1997,Feb,11; 1997,Apr,3; 1996,Mar,11

| 59409 | Vaginal delivery only (with or without episiotomy and/or forceps); | M ♀ T 80 ▢ |

MED: 100-2,15,20.1; 100-2,15,180

AMA: 2002,Aug,1; 1997,Feb,11; 1997,Apr,1; 1996,Sep,4; 1996,Mar,11; 1996,Jul,11

| 59410 | including postpartum care | M ♀ B ▢ |

MED: 100-2,15,20.1; 100-2,15,180

26 Professional Component Only

80/80 Assist-at-Surgery Allowed/With Documentation

Unlisted

Not Covered

TC Technical Component Only

MED: Pub 100/NCD References

AMA: CPT Assistant References

1-9 ASC Group

♂ Male Only

♀ Female Only

212 — CPT Expert

CPT only © 2006 American Medical Association. All Rights Reserved. (Black Ink)

© 2006 Ingenix (Blue Ink)

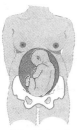
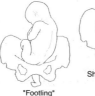

Shoulder presentation

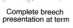

Complete breech presentation at term

"Footling"

Malposition and malpresentation occur when the fetus is in any presentation other than vertex; breech is most common at about 3 percent of deliveries; prematurity is a major predisposing factor

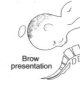

Brow presentation

59412 External cephalic version, with or without tocolysis Ⓜ ♀ Ⓣ 🔟 ☐

Report 59412 in conjunction with code(s) for delivery.

59414 Delivery of placenta (separate procedure) Ⓜ ♀ Ⓣ 🔟 ☐

AMA: 1998,Jun,10; 1996,Jun,10

59425 Antepartum care only; 4-6 visits Ⓜ ♀ Ⓑ 🔟 ☐

MED: 100-2,15,20.1; 100-2,15,180
AMA: 2002,Aug,1; 1997,Apr,11; 1994,Fall,21

If 1-3 visits for antepartum care are provided, consult the appropriate Evaluation and Management code(s).

59426 7 or more visits Ⓜ ♀ Ⓑ 🔟 ☐

MED: 100-2,15,20.1; 100-2,15,180
AMA: 2002,Aug,1; 1997,Apr,11; 1994,Fall,21

59430 Postpartum care only (separate procedure) Ⓜ ♀ Ⓑ ☐

MED: 100-2,15,20.1; 100-2,15,180
AMA: 2002,Aug,1; 1996,Jun,10

CESAREAN DELIVERY

If a standby physician is present for an infant, consult CPT code 99360.

To report low cervical Cesarean section, consult 59510, 59515, 59525.

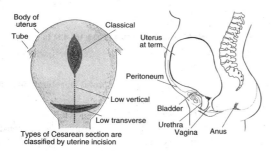

Types of Cesarean section are classified by uterine incision

Cesarean section is delivery through incisions in the anterior abdominal and uterine walls and is indicated for numerous conditions in both the fetus and the mother. Although other approaches may be warranted, low transverse is preferred to decrease chance of uterine rupture during future pregnancies

59510 Routine obstetric care including antepartum care, cesarean delivery, and postpartum care Ⓜ ♀ Ⓑ ☐

AMA: 2002,Aug,1; 1997,Feb,11; 1997,Apr,2; 1996,Sep,4; 1996,Oct,10; 1996,Jul,11

59514 Cesarean delivery only; Ⓜ ♀ Ⓒ 🔟 ☐

AMA: 1997,Feb,11; 1996,Oct,10

59515 including postpartum care Ⓜ ♀ Ⓑ ☐

+ **59525** Subtotal or total hysterectomy after cesarean delivery (List separately in addition to code for primary procedure) Ⓜ ♀ Ⓒ 🔟 ☐

Note that 59525 is an add-on code and must be used in conjunction with 59510, 59514, 59515, 59618, 59620, and 59622.

DELIVERY AFTER PREVIOUS CESAREAN DELIVERY

If a standby physician is present for an infant, consult CPT code 99360.

Codes 59610-59622 are used to report delivery services rendered to a patient who has had a previous cesarean delivery and now presents with the expectation of a vaginal delivery.

For a successful vaginal delivery after a previous cesarean section, consult CPT codes 59610-59614. If the attempt is unsuccessful and the patient has another cesarean section, consult codes 59618-59622. For elective cesarean deliveries, consult code 59510, 59514, or 59515.

59610 Routine obstetric care including antepartum care, vaginal delivery (with or without episiotomy, and/or forceps) and postpartum care, after previous cesarean delivery Ⓜ ♀ Ⓑ 🔟 ☐

MED: 100-2,15,20.1; 100-2,15,180
AMA: 2002,Aug,1; 1997,Apr,3; 1996,Feb,2

Codes 59610-59614 are reported for a successful vaginal delivery following a previous cesarean delivery.

59612 Vaginal delivery only, after previous cesarean delivery (with or without episiotomy and/or forceps); Ⓜ ♀ Ⓣ 🔟 ☐

MED: 100-2,15,20.1; 100-2,15,180
AMA: 2002,Aug,1; 1996,Feb,2

59614 including postpartum care Ⓜ ♀ Ⓑ ☐

MED: 100-2,15,20.1; 100-2,15,180
AMA: 1996,Feb,2

59618 Routine obstetric care including antepartum care, cesarean delivery, and postpartum care, following attempted vaginal delivery after previous cesarean delivery Ⓜ ♀ Ⓑ 🔟 ☐

AMA: 2002,Aug,1; 1996,Feb,2

Codes 59618-59622 are reported for an attempted vaginal delivery that is unsuccessful following a previous cesarean delivery which again must be performed via cesarean delivery.

59620 Cesarean delivery only, following attempted vaginal delivery after previous cesarean delivery; Ⓜ ♀ Ⓒ 🔟 ☐

AMA: 1996,Feb,2

59622 including postpartum care Ⓜ ♀ Ⓑ 🔟 ☐

AMA: 1996,Feb,2

ABORTION

If medical treatment is needed for a spontaneous complete abortion, any trimester, consult E/M codes 99201-99233.

59812 Treatment of incomplete abortion, any trimester, completed surgically Ⓜ ♀ 🟝 Ⓣ ☐

MED: 100-2,15,20.1; 100-2,15,260; 100-4,12,90.3; 100-4,14,10
AMA: 1995,Fall,16; 1993,Fall,9

59820 Treatment of missed abortion, completed surgically; first trimester Ⓜ ♀ 🟝 Ⓣ ☐

MED: 100-2,15,20.1; 100-2,15,260; 100-4,12,90.3; 100-4,14,10
AMA: 1999,Feb,10; 1995,Fall,16; 1993,Fall,9

59821 second trimester Ⓜ ♀ 🟝 Ⓣ 🔟 ☐

MED: 100-2,15,260; 100-4,12,90.3; 100-4,14,10
AMA: 1995,Fall,16; 1993,Fall,9

59830 Treatment of septic abortion, completed surgically Ⓜ ♀ Ⓒ 🔟 ☐

AMA: 1993,Fall,9

59840 Induced abortion, by dilation and curettage Ⓜ ♀ 🟝 Ⓣ 🔟 ☐

MED: 100-2,1,90; 100-2,15,260; 100-3,140.1; 100-4,3,100.1; 100-4,12,90.3; 100-4,14,10
AMA: 1993,Fall,9

⦾ Modifier 63 Exempt Code ⊙ Conscious Sedation + CPT Add-on Code ⊘ Modifier 51 Exempt Code ● New Code ▲ Revised Code

Ⓜ Maternity Edit Ⓐ Age Edit Ⓐ-Ⓨ APC Status Indicators ☐ CCI Comprehensive Code 🔟 Bilateral Procedure

59841 Induced abortion, by dilation and
evacuation   Ⓜ♀ 🖐 Ⓣ 🔲

MED: 100-2,1,90; 100-2,15,260; 100-3,140.1; 100-4,3,100.1;
100-4,12,90.3; 100-4,14,10

AMA: 1993,Fall,9

59850 Induced abortion, by one or more intra-amniotic
injections (amniocentesis-injections), including
hospital admission and visits, delivery of fetus and
secundines;   Ⓜ♀ Ⓒ 🔲

MED: 100-2,1,90; 100-3,140.1; 100-3,230.3; 100-4,3,100.1

AMA: 1993,Fall,10

59851 with dilation and curettage and/or
evacuation   Ⓜ♀ Ⓒ 🔲

MED: 100-2,1,90; 100-3,140.1; 100-4,3,100.1

AMA: 1993,Fall,10

59852 with hysterotomy (failed intra-amniotic
injection)   Ⓜ♀ Ⓒ 🔲

MED: 100-2,1,90; 100-3,140.1; 100-3,230.3; 100-4,3,100.1

AMA: 1993,Fall,10

If a cervical dilator is inserted, consult CPT code 59200.

59855 Induced abortion, by one or more vaginal suppositories
(eg, prostaglandin) with or without cervical dilation
(eg, laminaria), including hospital admission and visits,
delivery of fetus and secundines;   Ⓜ♀ Ⓒ 🔲

MED: 100-2,1,90; 100-3,140.1; 100-4,3,100.1

59856 with dilation and curettage and/or
evacuation   Ⓜ♀ Ⓒ 🔲

MED: 100-2,1,90; 100-3,140.1; 100-4,3,100.1

59857 with hysterotomy (failed medical
evacuation)   Ⓜ♀ Ⓒ 🔲

MED: 100-2,1,90; 100-3,140.1; 100-4,3,100.1

OTHER PROCEDURES

59866 Multifetal pregnancy reduction(s)
(MPR)   Ⓜ♀ Ⓣ 🔲

MED: 100-2,1,90; 100-3,140.1; 100-4,3,100.1

59870 Uterine evacuation and curettage for hydatidiform
mole   Ⓜ♀ 🖐 Ⓣ 🔲

MED: 100-2,15,260; 100-4,12,90.3; 100-4,14,10

AMA: 1999,Feb,10

59871 Removal of cerclage suture under anesthesia (other
than local)   Ⓜ♀ 🖐 Ⓣ 🔲

MED: 100-2,15,260; 100-4,12,90.3; 100-4,14,10

AMA: 1997,Nov,22

59897 Unlisted fetal invasive procedure, including ultrasound
guidance   Ⓣ 🔲

59898 Unlisted laparoscopy procedure, maternity care and
delivery   Ⓜ♀ Ⓣ 🔲

AMA: 2000,Mar,5; 1999,Nov,29

59899 Unlisted procedure, maternity care and
delivery   Ⓜ♀ Ⓣ 🔲

MED: 100-4,4,180.3

AMA: 1997,Jun,10

ENDOCRINE SYSTEM

If pituitary and pineal surgery is performed, consult the Nervous System section
of the CPT book.

THYROID GLAND

INCISION

60000 Incision and drainage of thyroglossal duct cyst,
infected   Ⓣ 🔲

MED: 100-2,15,260; 100-4,12,90.3; 100-4,14,10

EXCISION

60001 Aspiration and/or injection, thyroid cyst   Ⓣ 🔲

To report fine needle aspiration, consult CPT codes
10020, 10021.

To report imaging guidance, consult CPT codes 76942,
77012.

60100 Biopsy thyroid, percutaneous core needle   Ⓣ 🔲

AMA: 1997,Jun,5

To report imaging guidance, consult CPT codes 76942,
77002, 77012, and 77021.

To report needle aspiration, consult CPT codes 10021,
10022.

To report evaluation of fine needle aspirate, consult CPT
codes 88172, 88173.

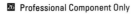

Epiglottis
Hyoid bone
Thyroglossal
duct (dotted line)
Cricothyroid
muscle
Hyoid
bone
Pyramid
lobe
Thyroid
cartilage
Cricoid
cartilage
Thyroid
cartilage
Thyroid
gland
Isthmus
Cricoid
cartilage
Thyroid
gland
Trachea
Esophagus

The thyroid is an important
endocrine gland and its size
and configuration can vary greatly.
A pyramid lobe occurs in about
40 percent of people and is a
remnant of the thyroglossal duct

60200 Excision of cyst or adenoma of thyroid, or transection
of isthmus   ② Ⓣ 🔲

MED: 100-2,15,260; 100-4,12,90.3; 100-4,14,10

60210 Partial thyroid lobectomy, unilateral; with or without
isthmusectomy   Ⓣ 🔲

60212 with contralateral subtotal lobectomy, including
isthmusectomy   Ⓣ 🔲

MED: 100-4,12,40.7

60220 Total thyroid lobectomy, unilateral; with or without
isthmusectomy   Ⓣ 🔲

60225 with contralateral subtotal lobectomy, including
isthmusectomy   Ⓣ 🔲

MED: 100-4,12,40.7

60240 Thyroidectomy, total or complete   Ⓣ 🔲

60252 Thyroidectomy, total or subtotal for malignancy; with
limited neck dissection   Ⓣ 🔲

AMA: 2000,Nov,10

60254 with radical neck dissection   Ⓒ 🔲

AMA: 2000,Nov,10

60260 Thyroidectomy, removal of all remaining thyroid
tissue following previous removal of a portion of
thyroid   Ⓣ 🔲

60270 Thyroidectomy, including substernal thyroid; sternal
split or transthoracic approach   Ⓒ 🔲

60271 cervical approach   Ⓒ 🔲

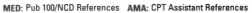

60280	Excision of thyroglossal duct cyst or sinus;	4 T 80 ⬚
	MED: 100-2,15,260; 100-4,12,90.3; 100-4,14,10	
60281	recurrent	4 T 80 ⬚
	MED: 100-2,15,260; 100-4,12,90.3; 100-4,14,10	

If a thyroid ultrasonography is performed, consult CPT code 76536.

PARATHYROID, THYMUS, ADRENAL GLANDS, PANCREAS, AND CAROTID BODY

If pituitary and pineal surgery is performed, consult the Nervous System section of CPT.

EXCISION

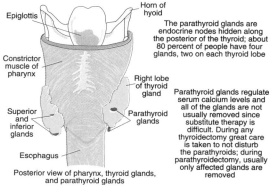

Epiglottis

Horn of hyoid

The parathyroid glands are endocrine nodes hidden along the posterior of the thyroid; about 80 percent of people have four glands, two on each thyroid lobe

Constrictor muscle of pharynx

Right lobe of thyroid gland

Parathyroid glands regulate serum calcium levels and all of the glands are not usually removed since substitute therapy is difficult. During any thyroidectomy great care is taken to not disturb the parathyroids; during parathyroidectomy, usually only affected glands are removed

Superior and inferior glands

Parathyroid glands

Esophagus

Posterior view of pharynx, thyroid glands, and parathyroid glands

60500	Parathyroidectomy or exploration of parathyroid(s);	T 80 ⬚
60502	re-exploration	T 80 ⬚
60505	with mediastinal exploration, sternal split or transthoracic approach	C 80 ⬚
+ 60512	Parathyroid autotransplantation (List separately in addition to code for primary procedure)	T 80

Note that 60512 is an add-on code and must be used in conjunction with 60500, 60502, 60505, 60212, 60225, 60240, 60252, 60254, 60260, 60270, and 60271.

60520	Thymectomy, partial or total; transcervical approach (separate procedure)	T 80 ⬚
60521	sternal split or transthoracic approach, without radical mediastinal dissection (separate procedure)	C 80 ⬚
60522	sternal split or transthoracic approach, with radical mediastinal dissection (separate procedure)	C 80 ⬚
60540	Adrenalectomy, partial or complete, or exploration of adrenal gland with or without biopsy, transabdominal, lumbar or dorsal (separate procedure);	C 80 50 ⬚
	AMA: 1998,Nov,17	
60545	with excision of adjacent retroperitoneal tumor	C 80 ⬚
	AMA: 1998,Nov,17	

Code 60540, 60545 cannot be reported with CPT code 50323.

If 60540 is performed bilaterally report with modifier 50.

If a remote or disseminated pheochromocytoma is excised, consult CPT codes 49200 and 49201. If a laparoscopic approach is used, consult CPT code 60650.

60600	Excision of carotid body tumor; without excision of carotid artery	C 80 ⬚
	MED: 100-3,20.18	
60605	with excision of carotid artery	C 80 ⬚
	MED: 100-3,20.18	

LAPAROSCOPY

Diagnostic laparoscopy is always included in surgical laparoscopy. To report diagnostic laparoscopy only, consult CPT code 49320.

60650	Laparoscopy, surgical, with adrenalectomy, partial or complete, or exploration of adrenal gland with or without biopsy, transabdominal, lumbar or dorsal	C 80 50 ⬚
	AMA: 2001,Nov,8; 2000,Mar,5; 1999,Nov,30	
60659	Unlisted laparoscopy procedure, endocrine system	T 80 50
	AMA: 2000,Mar,5; 1999,Nov,30	

OTHER PROCEDURES

60699	Unlisted procedure, endocrine system	T 80
	MED: 100-4,4,180.3	

⊕ Modifier 63 Exempt Code   ⊙ Conscious Sedation   + CPT Add-on Code   ⊘ Modifier 51 Exempt Code   ● New Code   ▲ Revised Code

Ⓜ Maternity Edit   Ⓐ Age Edit   Ⓐ-Ⓨ APC Status Indicators   ⬚ CCI Comprehensive Code   50 Bilateral Procedure

NERVOUS SYSTEM

SKULL, MENINGES, AND BRAIN

INJECTION, DRAINAGE, OR ASPIRATION

If an injection procedure is needed for cerebral angiography, consult CPT codes 36100-36218. If an injection procedure is needed for pneumoencephalography, consult CPT code 61055.

If an injection procedure is needed for ventriculography, consult CPT codes 61026, and 61120.

61000 Subdural tap through fontanelle, or suture, infant, unilateral or bilateral; initial

61001 subsequent taps

61020 Ventricular puncture through previous burr hole, fontanelle, suture, or implanted ventricular catheter/reservoir; without injection
MED: 100-2,15,260; 100-4,12,90.3; 100-4,14,10

61026 with injection of medication or other substance for diagnosis or treatment
MED: 100-2,15,260; 100-4,12,90.3; 100-4,14,10

61050 Cisternal or lateral cervical (C1-C2) puncture; without injection (separate procedure)
MED: 100-2,15,260; 100-4,12,90.3; 100-4,14,10

61055 with injection of medication or other substance for diagnosis or treatment (eg, C1-C2)
MED: 100-2,15,260; 100-4,12,90.3; 100-4,14,10
To report radiological supervision and interpretation, consult the Radiology section of the CPT book.

61070 Puncture of shunt tubing or reservoir for aspiration or injection procedure
MED: 100-2,15,260; 100-4,12,90.3; 100-4,14,10
To report radiological supervision and interpretation, consult CPT code 75809.

TWIST DRILL, BURR HOLE(S), OR TREPHINE

▲ **61105** Twist drill hole for subdural or ventricular puncture

⊘ ▲ **61107** Twist drill hole(s) for subdural, intracerebral, or ventricular puncture; for implanting ventricular catheter, pressure recording device, or other intracerebral monitoring device
To report intracranial neuroendoscopic ventricular catheter placement, consult CPT code 62160.

For twist drill or burr hole performed to place thermal perfusion probe, consult Category III code 0077T.

61108 for evacuation and/or drainage of subdural hematoma

61120 Burr hole(s) for ventricular puncture (including injection of gas, contrast media, dye, or radioactive material)

61140 Burr hole(s) or trephine; with biopsy of brain or intracranial lesion

61150 with drainage of brain abscess or cyst

61151 with subsequent tapping (aspiration) of intracranial abscess or cyst

61154 Burr hole(s) with evacuation and/or drainage of hematoma, extradural or subdural

61156 Burr hole(s); with aspiration of hematoma or cyst, intracerebral

⊘ ▲ **61210** for implanting ventricular catheter, reservoir, EEG electrode(s), pressure recording device, or other cerebral monitoring device (separate procedure)
To report intracranial neuroendoscopic ventricular catheter placement, consult CPT code 62160.

61215 Insertion of subcutaneous reservoir, pump or continuous infusion system for connection to ventricular catheter
MED: 100-2,15,260; 100-3,280.14; 100-4,12,90.3; 100-4,14,10
AMA: 1993,Spring,13
If chemotherapy is administered, consult CPT code 96450.

To report refilling and maintenance of implantable infusion pump for spinal or brain drug therapy, consult CPT code 95990.

61250 Burr hole(s) or trephine, supratentorial, exploratory, not followed by other surgery

61253 Burr hole(s) or trephine, infratentorial, unilateral or bilateral
AMA: 2002,Sep,10
If a burr hole(s) or trephine are followed by a craniotomy at the same operative session, consult CPT codes 61304-61321; do not use 61250 or 61253.

CRANIECTOMY OR CRANIOTOMY

61304 Craniectomy or craniotomy, exploratory; supratentorial

61305 infratentorial (posterior fossa)

61312 Craniectomy or craniotomy for evacuation of hematoma, supratentorial; extradural or subdural
AMA: 2002,Sep,10

61313 intracerebral

61314 Craniectomy or craniotomy for evacuation of hematoma, infratentorial; extradural or subdural

61315 intracerebellar

+ **61316** Incision and subcutaneous placement of cranial bone graft (List separately in addition to code for primary procedure)
Note that 61316 is an add-on code and must be used in conjunction with 61304, 61312, 61313, 61322, 61323, 61340, 61570, 61571, 61680-61705.

61320 Craniectomy or craniotomy, drainage of intracranial abscess; supratentorial

61321 infratentorial

61322 Craniectomy or craniotomy, decompressive, with or without duraplasty, for treatment of intracranial hypertension, without evacuation of associated intraparenchymal hematoma; without lobectomy
To report subtemporal decompression, consult CPT code 61340. Do not report 61313 in conjunction with CPT code 61322.

61323 with lobectomy
To report subtemporal decompression, consult CPT code 61340. Do not report 61313 in conjunction with CPT code 61323.

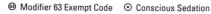 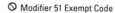 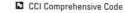

Nervous System

61330 — 61539

61330 Decompression of orbit only, transcranial approach [T] [80] [50] [↻]

Naffziger operation

61332 Exploration of orbit (transcranial approach); with biopsy [C] [80] [↻]

61333 with removal of lesion [C] [80] [↻]

61334 with removal of foreign body [T] [80] [↻]

61340 Subtemporal cranial decompression (pseudotumor cerebri, slit ventricle syndrome) [C] [80] [50] [↻]

To report decompression craniotomy or craniectomy for intracranial hypertension, without hematoma evauation, consult CPT codes 61322, 61323.

61343 Craniectomy, suboccipital with cervical laminectomy for decompression of medulla and spinal cord, with or without dural graft (eg, Arnold-Chiari malformation) [C] [80] [↻]

61345 Other cranial decompression, posterior fossa [C] [80] [↻]

If an orbital decompression is performed by a lateral wall approach, Kroenlein type, consult CPT code 67445.

61440 Craniotomy for section of tentorium cerebelli (separate procedure) [C] [80] [↻]

61450 Craniectomy, subtemporal, for section, compression, or decompression of sensory root of gasserian ganglion [C] [80] [↻]

Frazier-Spiller procedure

61458 Craniectomy, suboccipital; for exploration or decompression of cranial nerves [C] [80] [↻]

Jannetta decompression

61460 for section of one or more cranial nerves [C] [80] [↻]

61470 for medullary tractotomy [C] [80] [↻]

61480 for mesencephalic tractotomy or pedunculotomy [C] [80] [↻]

61490 Craniotomy for lobotomy, including cingulotomy [C] [80] [50] [↻]

61500 Craniectomy; with excision of tumor or other bone lesion of skull [C] [80] [↻]

61501 for osteomyelitis [C] [80] [↻]

61510 Craniectomy, trephination, bone flap craniotomy; for excision of brain tumor, supratentorial, except meningioma [C] [80] [↻]

61512 for excision of meningioma, supratentorial [C] [80] [↻]

61514 for excision of brain abscess, supratentorial [C] [80] [↻]

61516 for excision or fenestration of cyst, supratentorial [C] [80] [↻]

If an excision is performed of a pituitary tumor or a craniopharyngioma, consult CPT codes 61545, 61546, and 61548.

+ 61517 Implantation of brain intracavitary chemotherapy agent (List separately in addition to code for primary procedure) [C] [↻]

Note that 61517 is an add-on code and must be used in conjunction with 61510 or 61518. Do not use 61517 for brachytherapy insertion, consult CPT codes 77781-77784.

61518 Craniectomy for excision of brain tumor, infratentorial or posterior fossa; except meningioma, cerebellopontine angle tumor, or midline tumor at base of skull [C] [80] [↻]

61519 meningioma [C] [80] [↻]

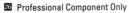

Cerebrum · Central sulcus · Corpus callosum · Left and right lateral ventricles · Third ventricle · White matter · Gray matter · Lateral sulcus (groove between ridges) · Cerebellum · Thalamus · Frontal section · Brain stem · Frontal lobe · Parietal lobe · Temporal lobe · Occipital lobe

Cancers of the central nervous system are grouped according to locations in the brain and spinal cord; many CNS tumors are grouped broadly as gliomas and rarely metastisize; secondary tumors are ones that have metastasized to the CNS and are often encountered with melanomas and lung cancers

61520 cerebellopontine angle tumor [C] [80] [↻]

61521 midline tumor at base of skull [C] [80] [↻]

61522 Craniectomy, infratentorial or posterior fossa; for excision of brain abscess [C] [80] [↻]

61524 for excision or fenestration of cyst [C] [80] [↻]

61526 Craniectomy, bone flap craniotomy, transtemporal (mastoid) for excision of cerebellopontine angle tumor; [C] [↻]

AMA: 1991,Summer,8

61530 combined with middle/posterior fossa craniotomy/craniectomy [C] [↻]

61531 Subdural implantation of strip electrodes through one or more burr or trephine hole(s) for long term seizure monitoring [C] [80] [↻]

MED: 100-3,160.5

If stereotactic implantation of electrodes is performed, consult CPT code 61760.

61533 Craniotomy with elevation of bone flap; for subdural implantation of an electrode array, for long term seizure monitoring [C] [80] [↻]

MED: 100-3,160.5

If continuous EEG monitoring is needed, consult CPT codes 95950-95954.

61534 for excision of epileptogenic focus without electrocorticography during surgery [C] [80] [↻]

61535 for removal of epidural or subdural electrode array, without excision of cerebral tissue (separate procedure) [C] [80] [↻]

MED: 100-3,160.5

61536 for excision of cerebral epileptogenic focus, with electrocorticography during surgery (includes removal of electrode array) [C] [80] [↻]

MED: 100-3,160.5

61537 for lobectomy, temporal lobe, without electrocorticography during surgery [C] [80] [↻]

61538 for lobectomy, temporal lobe, with electrocorticography during surgery [C] [80] [↻]

61539 for lobectomy, other than temporal lobe, partial or total, with electrocorticography during surgery [C] [80] [↻]

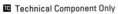

[2C] Professional Component Only · [TC] Technical Component Only · [80]/[80] Assist-at-Surgery Allowed/With Documentation · **MED:** Pub 100/NCD References · **AMA:** CPT Assistant References · [1]-[9] ASC Group · ♂ Male Only · ♀ Female Only · Unlisted · Not Covered

218 — CPT Expert · CPT only © 2006 American Medical Association. All Rights Reserved. *(Black Ink)* · © 2006 Ingenix *(Blue Ink)*

61540	for lobectomy, other than temporal lobe, partial or total, without electrocorticography during surgery	C 80 ↔
61541	for transection of corpus callosum	C 80 ↔
61542	for total hemispherectomy	C 80 ↔
61543	for partial or subtotal (functional) hemispherectomy	C 80 ↔
61544	for excision or coagulation of choroid plexus	C 80 ↔
61545	for excision of craniopharyngioma	C 80 ↔

To report craniotomy for selective amygdalohippocampectomy, consult CPT code 61566.

61546	**Craniotomy for hypophysectomy or excision of pituitary tumor, intracranial approach**	C 80 ↔
61548	**Hypophysectomy or excision of pituitary tumor, transnasal or transseptal approach, nonstereotactic**	C 80 ↔

AMA: 1998,Nov,17
Do not report 69990 in addition to code 61548 as the operating microscope is considered an inclusive component of the surgery.

61550	**Craniectomy for craniosynostosis; single cranial suture**	C 80 ↔
61552	**multiple cranial sutures**	C 80 ↔

If cranial reconstruction is performed for orbital hypertelorism, consult CPT codes 21260-21263.

61556	**Craniotomy for craniosynostosis; frontal or parietal bone flap**	C 80 ↔
61557	**bifrontal bone flap**	C 80 ↔
61558	**Extensive craniectomy for multiple cranial suture craniosynostosis (eg, cloverleaf skull); not requiring bone grafts**	C 80 ↔
61559	**recontouring with multiple osteotomies and bone autografts (eg, barrel-stave procedure) (includes obtaining grafts)**	C 80 ↔
61563	**Excision, intra and extracranial, benign tumor of cranial bone (eg, fibrous dysplasia); without optic nerve decompression**	C 80 ↔
61564	**with optic nerve decompression**	C 80 ↔

If reconstruction is required, consult CPT codes 21181-21183.

61566	**Craniotomy with elevation of bone flap; for selective amygdalohippocampectomy**	C 80 ↔
61567	**for multiple subpial transections, with electrocorticography during surgery**	C 80 ↔
61570	**Craniectomy or craniotomy; with excision of foreign body from brain**	C 80 ↔
61571	**with treatment of penetrating wound of brain**	C 80 ↔

If a sequestrectomy is performed for osteomyelitis, consult CPT code 61501.

61575	**Transoral approach to skull base, brain stem or upper spinal cord for biopsy, decompression or excision of lesion;**	C 80 ↔
61576	**requiring splitting of tongue and/or mandible (including tracheostomy)**	C 80 ↔

If arthrodesis is performed, consult CPT code 22548.

SURGERY OF SKULL BASE

Neurosurgical procedures of lesions involving the skull base often require the skills of several surgeons of different surgical specialties. These procedures have been broken into their component parts, categorized by the approach, definitive procedure, and repair/reconstruction of surgical defects following the definitive procedure.

The approach is defined as the portion of the procedure necessary to obtain adequate exposure of the lesion. It is described by anatomical area involved that includes anterior, middle, or posterior cranial fossa; brain stem; and upper spinal cord.

The definitive portion includes biopsy, excision, resection or repair of the lesion, and primary closure of the dura, mucous membrane and skin.

Repair/reconstruction is reported separately only when extensive dural grafting, cranioplasty, myocutaneous flaps, or extensive skin grafts are employed to close the surgical defect.

When different surgeons perform the component parts of skull base procedures, each reports only the code for the specific portion the physician has performed.

If one surgeon performs both the approach and definitive procedure, both codes should be reported, appending modifier 51 Multiple procedures to the secondary procedure.

Many physicians participate in the removal of lesions involving the skull base. Often working simultaneous, physicians from several specialties must work quickly to avoid infection. One physician may perform the approach procedure, another may perform the definitive procedure, and another may repair or reconstruct the dura, skull, and skin. Each must report the specific procedure performed.

APPROACH PROCEDURES

ANTERIOR CRANIAL FOSSA

61580	**Craniofacial approach to anterior cranial fossa; extradural, including lateral rhinotomy, ethmoidectomy, sphenoidectomy, without maxillectomy or orbital exenteration**	C 80 50 ↔

AMA: 1994,Spring,11

61581	**extradural, including lateral rhinotomy, orbital exenteration, ethmoidectomy, sphenoidectomy and/or maxillectomy**	C 50 ↔

AMA: 1994,Spring,11

61582	**extradural, including unilateral or bifrontal craniotomy, elevation of frontal lobe(s), osteotomy of base of anterior cranial fossa**	C 80 ↔

AMA: 1994,Spring,11

61583	**intradural, including unilateral or bifrontal craniotomy, elevation or resection of frontal lobe, osteotomy of base of anterior cranial fossa**	C 80 ↔

AMA: 1994,Spring,11

61584	**Orbitocranial approach to anterior cranial fossa, extradural, including supraorbital ridge osteotomy and elevation of frontal and/or temporal lobe(s); without orbital exenteration**	C 80 50 ↔
61585	**with orbital exenteration**	C 80 50 ↔
61586	**Bicoronal, transzygomatic and/or LeFort I osteotomy approach to anterior cranial fossa with or without internal fixation, without bone graft**	C 80 ↔

MIDDLE CRANIAL FOSSA

61590	**Infratemporal pre-auricular approach to middle cranial fossa (parapharyngeal space, infratemporal and midline skull base, nasopharynx), with or without disarticulation of the mandible, including parotidectomy, craniotomy, decompression and/or mobilization of the facial nerve and/or petrous carotid artery**	C 80 50 ↔

Nervous System

61591 — 61626

61591 Infratemporal post-auricular approach to middle cranial fossa (internal auditory meatus, petrous apex, tentorium, cavernous sinus, parasellar area, infratemporal fossa) including mastoidectomy, resection of sigmoid sinus, with or without decompression and/or mobilization of contents of auditory canal or petrous carotid artery   C 80 50 ◩

61592 Orbitocranial zygomatic approach to middle cranial fossa (cavernous sinus and carotid artery, clivus, basilar artery or petrous apex) including osteotomy of zygoma, craniotomy, extra- or intradural elevation of temporal lobe   C 80 50 ◩

POSTERIOR CRANIAL FOSSA

61595 Transtemporal approach to posterior cranial fossa, jugular foramen or midline skull base, including mastoidectomy, decompression of sigmoid sinus and/or facial nerve, with or without mobilization   C 80 50 ◩

61596 Transcochlear approach to posterior cranial fossa, jugular foramen or midline skull base, including labyrinthectomy, decompression, with or without mobilization of facial nerve and/or petrous carotid artery   C 80 50 ◩

61597 Transcondylar (far lateral) approach to posterior cranial fossa, jugular foramen or midline skull base, including occipital condylectomy, mastoidectomy, resection of C1-C3 vertebral body(s), decompression of vertebral artery, with or without mobilization   C 80 50 ◩

61598 Transpetrosal approach to posterior cranial fossa, clivus or foramen magnum, including ligation of superior petrosal sinus and/or sigmoid sinus   C 80 ◩

DEFINITIVE PROCEDURES

BASE OF ANTERIOR CRANIAL FOSSA

61600 Resection or excision of neoplastic, vascular or infectious lesion of base of anterior cranial fossa; extradural   C 80 ◩

AMA: 1994,Spring,12

61601 intradural, including dural repair, with or without graft   C 80 ◩

AMA: 1994,Spring,12

BASE OF MIDDLE CRANIAL FOSSA

61605 Resection or excision of neoplastic, vascular or infectious lesion of infratemporal fossa, parapharyngeal space, petrous apex; extradural   C 80 ◩

61606 intradural, including dural repair, with or without graft   C 80 ◩

61607 Resection or excision of neoplastic, vascular or infectious lesion of parasellar area, cavernous sinus, clivus or midline skull base; extradural   C 80 ◩

61608 intradural, including dural repair, with or without graft   C 80 ◩

+ 61609 Transection or ligation, carotid artery in cavernous sinus; without repair (List separately in addition to code for primary procedure)   C 80 ◩

Note that 61609-61612 are reported in addition to code(s) for primary procedure(s) 61605-61608. Only one transection or ligation of carotid artery code should be reported per operative session.

+ 61610 with repair by anastomosis or graft (List separately in addition to code for primary procedure)   C 80 ◩

+ 61611 Transection or ligation, carotid artery in petrous canal; without repair (List separately in addition to code for primary procedure)   C 80 ◩

+ 61612 with repair by anastomosis or graft (List separately in addition to code for primary procedure)   C 80 ◩

61613 Obliteration of carotid aneurysm, arteriovenous malformation, or carotid-cavernous fistula by dissection within cavernous sinus   C 80 50 ◩

BASE OF POSTERIOR CRANIAL FOSSA

61615 Resection or excision of neoplastic, vascular or infectious lesion of base of posterior cranial fossa, jugular foramen, foramen magnum, or C1-C3 vertebral bodies; extradural   C 80 ◩

61616 intradural, including dural repair, with or without graft   C 80 ◩

REPAIR AND/OR RECONSTRUCTION OF SURGICAL DEFECTS OF SKULL BASE

61618 Secondary repair of dura for cerebrospinal fluid leak, anterior, middle or posterior cranial fossa following surgery of the skull base; by free tissue graft (eg, pericranium, fascia, tensor fascia lata, adipose tissue, homologous or synthetic grafts)   C 80 ◩

AMA: 2000,Mar,11; 1994,Spring,19

61619 by local or regionalized vascularized pedicle flap or myocutaneous flap (including galea, temporalis, frontalis or occipitalis muscle)   C 80 ◩

AMA: 2000,Mar,11; 1994,Spring,19

ENDOVASCULAR THERAPY

Consult the glossary for terms and definitions and the front matter of this chapter for additional information.

61623 Endovascular temporary balloon arterial occlusion, head or neck (extracranial/intracranial) including selective catheterization of vessel to be occluded, positioning and inflation of occlusion balloon, concomitant neurological monitoring, and radiologic supervision and interpretation of all angiography required for balloon occlusion and to exclude vascular injury post occlusion   T ◩

MED: 100-4,4,61.2

If selective catheterization and angiography is performed on arteries other than the one being occluded, consult the appropriate CPT codes.

If complete angiography of artery to be occluded is performed immediately prior to temporary occlusion, consult the appropriate radiology supervision and interpretation CPT code only.

61624 Transcatheter permanent occlusion or embolization (eg, for tumor destruction, to achieve hemostasis, to occlude a vascular malformation), percutaneous, any method; central nervous system (intracranial, spinal cord)   C ◩

MED: 100-3,20.28
AMA: 1999,Jun,10
Consult also CPT code 37204. If radiological supervision and interpretation is needed, consult CPT code 75894.

61626 Transcatheter permanent occlusion or embolization (eg, for tumor destruction, to achieve hemostasis, to occlude a vascular malformation), percutaneous, any method; non-central nervous system, head or neck (extracranial, brachiocephalic branch)   T ◩

MED: 100-3,20.28; 100-4,4,61.2
Consult also CPT code 37204. If radiological supervision and interpretation is needed, consult CPT code 75894.

---

26 Professional Component Only   80/80 Assist-at-Surgery Allowed/With Documentation   Unlisted   Not Covered

TC Technical Component Only   MED: Pub 100/NCD References   AMA: CPT Assistant References   1-9 ASC Group   ♂ Male Only   ♀ Female Only

220 — CPT Expert   CPT only © 2006 American Medical Association. All Rights Reserved. (Black Ink)   © 2006 Ingenix (Blue Ink)

61630 Balloon angioplasty, intracranial (eg, atherosclerotic stenosis), percutaneous E

61635 Transcatheter placement of intravascular stent(s), intracranial (eg, atherosclerotic stenosis), including balloon angioplasty, if performed E

> Codes 61630 and 61635 include all selective vascular catheterization of the target vascular family, all diagnostic imaging for arteriography of the target vascular family, and all radiological supervision and interpretation services related to the procedure. When a diagnostic arteriogram (including imaging and selective catheterization) confirms the need for an angioplasty or stent placement, codes 61630 and 61635 include these services. When angioplasty or stenting is not indicated, the appropriate codes for selective catheterization and imaging should be reported instead of 61630 and 61635.

61640 Balloon dilatation of intracranial vasospasm, percutaneous; initial vessel E

+ **61641**   each additional vessel in same vascular family (List separately in addition to code for primary procedure) E

+ **61642**   each additional vessel in different vascular family (List separately in addition to code for primary procedure) E

> Note that 61641 and 61642 are add-on codes and must be used in conjunction with 61640.

> Codes 61640, 61641, and 61642 include all selective vascular catheterization of the target vessel, contrast injection(s), vessel measurement, roadmapping, postdilatation angiography, and fluoroscopic guidance for the balloon dilatation.

SURGERY FOR ANEURYSM, ARTERIOVENOUS MALFORMATION OR VASCULAR DISEASE

CPT codes 61680-61711 include craniotomy when it is appropriate for the procedure.

61680 Surgery of intracranial arteriovenous malformation; supratentorial, simple C 80 ▣

61682   supratentorial, complex C 80 ▣

61684   infratentorial, simple C 80 ▣

61686   infratentorial, complex C 80 ▣

61690   dural, simple C 80 ▣

61692   dural, complex C 80 ▣

61697 Surgery of complex intracranial aneurysm, intracranial approach; carotid circulation C 80 ▣

> CPT codes 61697, 61698 involve aneurysms that are larger than 15 mm or have calcification of the aneurysm neck, or if procedure requires temporary vessel occlusion, trapping or cardiopulmonary bypass to successfully treat the aneurysm.

61698   vertebrobasilar circulation C 80 ▣

61700 Surgery of simple intracranial aneurysm, intracranial approach; carotid circulation C 80 ▣

> AMA: 1999,Jun,11; 1999,Jul,10

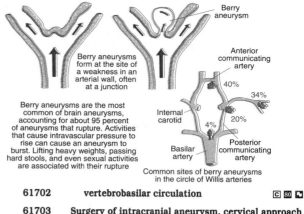

Berry aneurysms form at the site of a weakness in an arterial wall, often at a junction

Berry aneurysms are the most common of brain aneurysms, accounting for about 95 percent of aneurysms that rupture. Activities that cause intravascular pressure to rise can cause an aneurysm to burst. Lifting heavy weights, passing hard stools, and even sexual activities are associated with their rupture

Common sites of berry aneurysms in the circle of Willis arteries

61702   vertebrobasilar circulation C 80 ▣

61703 Surgery of intracranial aneurysm, cervical approach by application of occluding clamp to cervical carotid artery (Selverstone-Crutchfield type) C 80 ▣

> If direct ligation of the carotid artery is performed through a cervical approach, consult CPT codes 37600-37606.

61705 Surgery of aneurysm, vascular malformation or carotid-cavernous fistula; by intracranial and cervical occlusion of carotid artery C 80 ▣

61708   by intracranial electrothrombosis C 80 ▣

> If ligation or gradual occlusion is performed on an internal/common carotid artery, consult CPT codes 37605 and 37606.

61710   by intra-arterial embolization, injection procedure, or balloon catheter C 80 ▣

61711 Anastomosis, arterial, extracranial-intracranial (eg, middle cerebral/cortical) arteries C 80 ▣

> To report carotid or vertebral thomboendarterectomy, consult CPT code 35301.

STEREOTAXIS

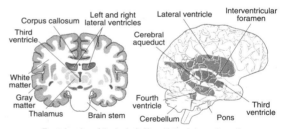

Frontal secion of the brain (left) and lateral view schematic showing the ventricular system in blue (right)

Cerebral spinal fluid (CSF) is secreted in the ventricles and flows generally from the laterals into the third ventricle via the interventricular foramina, and into the fourth ventricle via the cerebral aqueduct. Many brain disorders upset ventricular fluid pressures and shunts are employed to restore balance

61720 Creation of lesion by stereotactic method, including burr hole(s) and localizing and recording techniques, single or multiple stages; globus pallidus or thalamus T

61735   subcortical structure(s) other than globus pallidus or thalamus C ▣

> MED: 100-3,160.4

61750 Stereotactic biopsy, aspiration, or excision, including burr hole(s), for intracranial lesion; C ▣

> AMA: 1999,Nov,30

Nervous System

61751 — 62100

61751 with computed tomography and/or magnetic resonance guidance C ☒

MED: 100-3,220.1; 100-3,220.2; 100-3,220.3

AMA: 1999,Nov,30; 1996,Jun,10

If radiological supervision and interpretation of computerized tomography is needed, consult CPT codes 70450, 70460, and 70470 as appropriate. If radiological supervision and interpretation of magnetic resonance imaging is needed, consult CPT codes 70551, 70552, and 70553 as appropriate.

61760 Stereotactic implantation of depth electrodes into the cerebrum for long term seizure monitoring C ☒

MED: 100-3,160.5

61770 Stereotactic localization, including burr hole(s), with insertion of catheter(s) or probe(s) for placement of radiation source C ☒

61790 Creation of lesion by stereotactic method, percutaneous, by neurolytic agent (eg, alcohol, thermal, electrical, radiofrequency); gasserian ganglion 3 T ☒

MED: 100-2,15,260; 100-4,12,90.3; 100-4,14,10

61791 trigeminal medullary tract 3 T 80 ☒

MED: 100-2,15,260; 100-4,12,90.3; 100-4,14,10

61793 Stereotactic radiosurgery (particle beam, gamma ray or linear accelerator), one or more sessions B ☒

AMA: 1997,Nov,23

To report intensity modulated beam delivery plan and treatment, see 77301, 77418.

+ 61795 Stereotactic computer-assisted volumetric (navigational) procedure, intracranial, extracranial, or spinal (List separately in addition to code for primary procedure) 1 S ☒

AMA: 2001,Oct,10; 1999,Nov,30

Note that 61795 is an add-on code that must be used in conjunction with the appropriate code for the primary procedure. This code cannot be reported alone.

NEUROSTIMULATORS (INTRACRANIAL)

Consult the glossary for terms and definitions and the front matter of this chapter for additional information.

For programming or electronic analysis of neurostimulator pulse generators, initial or subsequent, consult CPT codes 95970-95975.

If microelectrode recording is performed by the operating surgeon it should not be reported separately. If another physician participates in neurophysiological mapping during deep brain stimulator implantation that physician may report 95961-95962.

61850 Twist drill or burr hole(s) for implantation of neurostimulator electrodes, cortical C 80 ☒

MED: 100-3,160.2; 100-3,160.7

AMA: 1999,Nov,30

61860 Craniectomy or craniotomy for implantation of neurostimulator electrodes, cerebral, cortical C 80 ☒

MED: 100-3,160.2; 100-3,160.7

AMA: 1999,Nov,30

61863 Twist drill, burr hole, craniotomy, or craniectomy with stereotactic implantation of neurostimulator electrode array in subcortical site (eg, thalamus, globus pallidus, subthalamic nucleus, periventricular, periaqueductal gray), without use of intraoperative microelectrode recording; first array C 80 50 ☒

+ 61864 each additional array (List separately in addition to primary procedure) C 80 ☒

Note that 61864 is an add-on code that must be used in conjunction with 61863.

61867 Twist drill, burr hole, craniotomy, or craniectomy with stereotactic implantation of neurostimulator electrode array in subcortical site (eg, thalamus, globus pallidus, subthalamic nucleus, periventricular, periaqueductal gray), with use of intraoperative microelectrode recording; first array C 80 50 ☒

MED: 100-4,32,50

+ 61868 each additional array (List separately in addition to primary procedure) C 80 ☒

MED: 100-4,32,50

Note that 61868 is an add-on code that must be used in conjunction with 61867.

61870 Craniectomy for implantation of neurostimulator electrodes, cerebellar; cortical C 80 ☒

MED: 100-3,160.2; 100-3,160.7

61875 subcortical C 80 ☒

MED: 100-3,160.2; 100-3,160.7

61880 Revision or removal of intracranial neurostimulator electrodes T 80 50 ☒

MED: 100-3,160.2; 100-3,160.7; 100-4,32,50

61885 Insertion or replacement of cranial neurostimulator pulse generator or receiver, direct or inductive coupling; with connection to a single electrode array 2 S 80 50 ☒

MED: 100-2,15,260; 100-3,160.2; 100-3,160.7; 100-3,230.1; 100-4,4,61.2; 100-4,12,90.3; 100-4,14,10; 100-4,32,50

AMA: 2001,Apr,8; 2000,Jun,3; 1999,Nov,30

61886 with connection to two or more electrode arrays 3 T 80 ☒

MED: 100-2,15,260; 100-3,160.2; 100-3,160.7; 100-4,4,61.2; 100-4,12,90.3; 100-4,14,10; 100-4,32,50

AMA: 2001,Apr,8; 2000,Jun,3; 1999,Nov,30

If open placement of a cranial nerve (e.g., vagal, trigeminal) neurostimulator electrode(s) is performed, consult CPT code 64573. If percutaneous placement of a cranial nerve (eg, vagal, trigeminal) neurostimulator electrode(s) is performed, consult CPT code 65443. If revision or removal of a cranial nerve (eg, vagal, trigeminal) neurostimulator electrode(s) is performed, consult CPT code 64585.

61888 Revision or removal of cranial neurostimulator pulse generator or receiver 1 T 50 ☒

MED: 100-2,15,260; 100-3,160.2; 100-3,160.7; 100-4,12,90.3; 100-4,14,10; 100-4,32,50

Code 61888 cannot be reported with CPT code 61885 or 61886 for the same pulse generator.

REPAIR

62000 Elevation of depressed skull fracture; simple, extradural T ☒

62005 compound or comminuted, extradural C 80 ☒

62010 with repair of dura and/or debridement of brain C 80 ☒

62100 Craniotomy for repair of dural/cerebrospinal fluid leak, including surgery for rhinorrhea/otorrhea C 80 ☒

If a spinal dural/CSF leak is repaired, consult CPT codes 63707 and 63709.

☒ Professional Component Only   80/80 Assist-at-Surgery Allowed/With Documentation   Unlisted   Not Covered

☒ Technical Component Only   **MED:** Pub 100/NCD References   **AMA:** CPT Assistant References   1-9 ASC Group   ♂ Male Only   ♀ Female Only

222 — CPT Expert   CPT only © 2006 American Medical Association. All Rights Reserved. (Black Ink)   © 2006 Ingenix (Blue Ink)

62115　Reduction of craniomegalic skull (eg, treated hydrocephalus); not requiring bone grafts or cranioplasty　C 80

62116　　with simple cranioplasty　C 80

62117　　requiring craniotomy and reconstruction with or without bone graft (includes obtaining grafts)　C 80

62120　Repair of encephalocele, skull vault, including cranioplasty　C 80

62121　Craniotomy for repair of encephalocele, skull base　C 80

62140　Cranioplasty for skull defect; up to 5 cm diameter　C 80

62141　　larger than 5 cm diameter　C 80

62142　Removal of bone flap or prosthetic plate of skull　C 80

62143　Replacement of bone flap or prosthetic plate of skull　C 80

62145　Cranioplasty for skull defect with reparative brain surgery　C 80

62146　Cranioplasty with autograft (includes obtaining bone grafts); up to 5 cm diameter　C 80

62147　　larger than 5 cm diameter　C 80

+　62148　Incision and retrieval of subcutaneous cranial bone graft for cranioplasty (List separately in addition to code for primary procedure)　C

> Note that 62148 is an add-on code and must be used in conjunction with 62140-62147.

NEUROENDOSCOPY

Diagnostic endoscopy is always included in surgical endoscopy.

+　62160　Neuroendoscopy, intracranial, for placement or replacement of ventricular catheter and attachment to shunt system or external drainage (List separately in addition to code for primary procedure)　T

> Note that 62160 is an add-on code and must be used in conjunction with 61107, 61210, 62220-62230 or 62258.

62161　Neuroendoscopy, intracranial; with dissection of adhesions, fenestration of septum pellucidum or intraventricular cysts (including placement, replacement, or removal of ventricular catheter)　C 80

62162　　with fenestration or excision of colloid cyst, including placement of external ventricular catheter for drainage　C 80

62163　　with retrieval of foreign body　C 80

62164　　with excision of brain tumor, including placement of external ventricular catheter for drainage　C 80

62165　　with excision of pituitary tumor, transnasal or trans-sphenoidal approach　C 80

CEREBROSPINAL FLUID (CSF) SHUNT

62180　Ventriculocisternostomy (Torkildsen type operation)　C 80

62190　Creation of shunt; subarachnoid/subdural-atrial, -jugular, -auricular　C

62192　　subarachnoid/subdural-peritoneal, -pleural, other terminus　C 80

62194　Replacement or irrigation, subarachnoid/subdural catheter　1 T 80

> MED: 100-2,15,260; 100-4,12,90.3; 100-4,14,10

62200　Ventriculocisternostomy, third ventricle;　C 80
　　　　Dandy ventriculocisternostomy

62201　　stereotactic, neuroendoscopic method　C

> To report intracranial neuroendoscopic procedures, consult CPT codes 62161-62165.

62220　Creation of shunt; ventriculo-atrial, -jugular, -auricular　C 80

> To report intracranial neuroendoscopic ventricular catheter placement, consult CPT code 62160.

62223　　ventriculo-peritoneal, -pleural, other terminus　C 80

> To report intracranial neuroendoscopic ventricular catheter placement, consult CPT code 62160.

62225　Replacement or irrigation, ventricular catheter　1 T

> MED: 100-2,15,260; 100-4,12,90.3; 100-4,14,10

> To report intracranial neuroendoscopic ventricular catheter placement, consult CPT code 62160.

62230　Replacement or revision of cerebrospinal fluid shunt, obstructed valve, or distal catheter in shunt system　2 T 80

> MED: 100-2,15,260; 100-4,12,90.3; 100-4,14,10

> To report intracranial neuroendoscopic ventricular catheter placement, consult CPT code 62160.

62252　Reprogramming of programmable cerebrospinal shunt　S 80

> If the physician interprets the results and/or operates the equipment, modifier 26 should be appended to 62252.

62256　Removal of complete cerebrospinal fluid shunt system; without replacement　C 80

62258　　with replacement by similar or other shunt at same operation　C 80

> If percutaneous irrigation or aspiration of a shunt reservoir is performed, consult CPT code 61070.

> For reprogramming of programmable CSF shunt, consult CPT code 62252.

> Use 62160 for intracranial neuroendoscopic ventricular catheter placement.

SPINE AND SPINAL CORD

If application of caliper or tongs is performed, consult CPT code 20660. If a fracture or dislocation of the spine is treated, consult CPT codes 22305-22327. CPT codes 62263, 62264, 62270-62273, 62280-62282, and 62310-62319 include the injection of contrast during fluoroscopic guidance and localization; do not report separately.

INJECTION, DRAINAGE, OR ASPIRATION

Note that injection of contrast during fluoroscopic guidance and localization should not be reported separately with codes 62263-62264, 62270-62273, 62280-62282, 62310-62319, and 0027T. For fluoroscopic guidance consult code 77003 unless a complete study such as myelography, eipdurography, or arthrography is performed. If this is the case, the fluoroscopy is included in the more extensive procedure. This includes the supervision and interpretation.

Report 62263 for a catheter-based treatment that involves targeted injections of various substances via an epidural catheter. This includes the insertion and removal of the catheter and the administration of one or more injections. This treatment may take more than one day. Adhesions or scarring may also be lysed during this treatment period. Do not report 62263 for each adhesiolysis treatment provided. This code should be reported only once for the entire series of treatment spanning two or more treatment days.

Report 62264 for multiple lysis of adhesions treatments performed on the same day. This may be performed by injection of neurolytic agent(s) or mechanically.

Both 62263 and 62264 include the injection of contrast material for fluoroscopy guidance and localization and epidurographyduring all treatment sessions.

To report endoscopic lysis of adhesions, consult Category III code 0027T. To report daily management of continuous epidural or subarachnoid drug administration performed with 62318-62319, consult CPT code 01996.

62263 Percutaneous lysis of epidural adhesions using solution injection (eg, hypertonic saline, enzyme) or mechanical means (eg, catheter) including radiologic localization (includes contrast when administered), multiple adhesiolysis sessions; 2 or more days ▪1▪ T ▪↩

MED: 100-2,15,260; 100-4,12,90.3; 100-4,14,10
AMA: 2002,Mar,11; 1999,Nov,33
62263 icludes 72275 and 77003.

62264 1 day ▪1▪ T ▪↩

Code 62264 includes 72275 and 77003.

Do not report 62264 in conjunction with code 62263.

62268 Percutaneous aspiration, spinal cord cyst or syrinx ▪1▪ T ▪↩

MED: 100-2,15,260; 100-4,12,90.3; 100-4,14,10
To report radiological supervision and interpretation, consult CPT codes 76942, 77002, and 77012.

62269 Biopsy of spinal cord, percutaneous needle ▪1▪ T ▪80▪ ▪↩

MED: 100-2,15,260; 100-4,12,90.3; 100-4,14,10
To report radiological supervision and interpretation, consult CPT codes 76942, 77002, and 77012.

To report fine needle aspiration, consult CPT codes 10021, 10022. To report evaluation of fine needle aspirate, consult CPT codes 88172, 88173.

Meninges

Most common agent in neonates is E. coli; Haemophilus influenzae b and streptococcus pneumoniae are common agents in adult cases

The brain and spinal cord are encased in a tough fibrous membrane known as the meninges and meningitis is an inflammation of that tissue and commonly affects the underlying central nervous system tissues and fluids; causes are numerous and classification is based on type of infection; purulent refers to forms usually caused by bacteria; chronic meningitis is usually caused by mycobacteria and fungi; aseptic or abacterial meningitis is commonly associated with a viral infection and is reported with the underlying disease. Encephalitis is inflammation of the brain and is also usually associated with a viral infection and also is reported with the underlying disease

62270 Spinal puncture, lumbar, diagnostic ▪1▪ T ▪↩

MED: 100-2,15,260; 100-4,12,90.3; 100-4,14,10
AMA: 1999,Nov,32-33

62272 Spinal puncture, therapeutic, for drainage of cerebrospinal fluid (by needle or catheter) ▪1▪ T ▪↩

MED: 100-2,15,260; 100-4,12,90.3; 100-4,14,10
AMA: 1999,Nov,32-33

62273 Injection, epidural, of blood or clot patch ▪1▪ T ▪↩

MED: 100-2,15,260; 100-3,10.5; 100-4,12,90.3; 100-4,14,10
AMA: 1999,Nov,32-34
To report injection of diagnostic or therapeutic substance(s), consult 62310, 62311, 62318, 62319.

62280 Injection/infusion of neurolytic substance (eg, alcohol, phenol, iced saline solutions), with or without other therapeutic substance; subarachnoid ▪1▪ T ▪↩

MED: 100-2,15,260; 100-4,12,90.3; 100-4,14,10
AMA: 2000,Jan,1; 1999,Nov,32-34

62281 epidural, cervical or thoracic ▪1▪ T ▪↩

MED: 100-2,15,260; 100-4,12,90.3; 100-4,14,10
AMA: 2000,Jan,1; 1999,Nov,32-34; 1996,Apr,10

62282 epidural, lumbar, sacral (caudal) ▪1▪ T ▪↩

MED: 100-2,15,260; 100-4,12,90.3; 100-4,14,10
AMA: 2000,Jan,1; 1999,Nov,32-34; 1996,Apr,10

62284 Injection procedure for myelography and/or computed tomography, spinal (other than C1-C2 and posterior fossa) ▪N▪ ▪↩

MED: 100-3,220.1
AMA: 1993,Fall,13
If an injection procedure is performed at C1-C2, consult CPT code 61055. For radiological supervision and interpretation, consult the Radiology section of the CPT book.

62287 Aspiration or decompression procedure, percutaneous, of nucleus pulposus of intervertebral disc, any method, single or multiple levels, lumbar (eg, manual or automated percutaneous discectomy, percutaneous laser discectomy) ▪9▪ T ▪↩

MED: 100-2,15,260; 100-4,12,90.3; 100-4,14,10
AMA: 2002,Mar,11; 1999,Nov,34
If fluoroscopic guidance is performed, consult CPT code 77002.

62290 Injection procedure for discography, each level; lumbar ▪N▪ ▪↩

AMA: 1999,Nov,35

62291 cervical or thoracic ▪N▪ ▪↩

AMA: 1999,Nov,35
To report radiological supervision and interpretation, consult CPT codes 72285 and 72295.

62292 Injection procedure for chemonucleolysis, including discography, intervertebral disc, single or multiple levels, lumbar ▪T▪ ▪80▪ ▪↩

AMA: 1999,Oct,10

62294 Injection procedure, arterial, for occlusion of arteriovenous malformation, spinal ▪3▪ T ▪↩

MED: 100-2,15,260; 100-4,12,90.3; 100-4,14,10

62310 Injection, single (not via indwelling catheter), not including neurolytic substances, with or without contrast (for either localization or epidurography), of diagnostic or therapeutic substance(s) (including anesthetic, antispasmodic, opioid, steroid, other solution), epidural or subarachnoid; cervical or thoracic ▪1▪ T ▪↩

MED: 100-2,15,260; 100-4,12,90.3; 100-4,14,10
AMA: 2000,Jan,1; 2000,Dec,15; 1999,Nov,32-35

62311 lumbar, sacral (caudal) ▪1▪ T ▪↩

MED: 100-2,15,260; 100-4,12,90.3; 100-4,14,10
AMA: 2000,Jan,1; 2000,Dec,15; 1999,Nov,32-35

▪26▪ Professional Component Only   ▪80/80▪ Assist-at-Surgery Allowed/With Documentation   Unlisted   Not Covered

▪TC▪ Technical Component Only   **MED:** Pub 100/NCD References   **AMA:** CPT Assistant References   ▪1-9▪ ASC Group   ♂ Male Only   ♀ Female Only

224 — CPT Expert   **CPT only © 2006 American Medical Association. All Rights Reserved.** *(Black Ink)*   © *2006 Ingenix (Blue Ink)*

62318 Injection, including catheter placement, continuous infusion or intermittent bolus, not including neurolytic substances, with or without contrast (for either localization or epidurography), of diagnostic or therapeutic substance(s) (including anesthetic, antispasmodic, opioid, steroid, other solution), epidural or subarachnoid; cervical or thoracic **1** **T** □

> MED: 100-2,15,260; 100-4,12,90.3; 100-4,14,10
>
> AMA: 2001,Oct,9; 2000,Jan,1; 2000,Dec,15; 1999,Nov,32-35

62319 lumbar, sacral (caudal) **1** **T** □

> MED: 100-2,15,260; 100-4,12,90.3; 100-4,14,10
>
> AMA: 2001,Oct,9; 2000,Jan,1; 2000,Dec,15; 1999,Nov,32-35
> To report transforaminal epidural injections, consult CPT codes 64479-64484.
>
> To report daily hospital management of continuous epidural or subarachnoid drug administration performed in conjunction with 62318-62319, consult CPT code 01996.

CATHETER IMPLANTATION

If an implantable infusion pump is refilled and maintained, consult CPT code 95990. If an intrathecal or epidural is place percutaneously, consult CPT codes 62270-62273, 62280-62284, and 62310-62319.

If application of caliper or tongs is performed, consult CPT code 20660. If a fracture or dislocation of the spine is treated, consult CPT codes 22305-22327.

62350 Implantation, revision or repositioning of tunneled intrathecal or epidural catheter, for long-term medication administration via an external pump or implantable reservoir/infusion pump; without laminectomy **2** **T** □

> MED: 100-2,15,260; 100-3,280.14; 100-4,12,90.3; 100-4,14,10
>
> AMA: 1999,Nov,36

62351 with laminectomy **T** **80** □

> MED: 100-3,280.14
>
> AMA: 1999,Nov,36
> If an implantable pump for spinal or brain drug therapy is refilled or maintained, consult CPT code 95990.

62355 Removal of previously implanted intrathecal or epidural catheter **2** **T** **80** □

> MED: 100-2,15,260; 100-4,12,90.3; 100-4,14,10

RESERVOIR/PUMP IMPLANTATION

62360 Implantation or replacement of device for intrathecal or epidural drug infusion; subcutaneous reservoir **2** **T** **80** □

> MED: 100-2,15,260; 100-3,280.14; 100-4,12,90.3; 100-4,14,10

62361 non-programmable pump **2** **T** **80** □

> MED: 100-2,15,260; 100-3,280.14; 100-4,12,90.3; 100-4,14,10

62362 programmable pump, including preparation of pump, with or without programming **2** **T** **80** □

> MED: 100-2,15,260; 100-4,12,90.3; 100-4,14,10
>
> AMA: 1997,Mar,11

62365 Removal of subcutaneous reservoir or pump, previously implanted for intrathecal or epidural infusion **2** **T** **80** □

> MED: 100-2,15,260; 100-3,280.14; 100-4,12,90.3; 100-4,14,10

62367 Electronic analysis of programmable, implanted pump for intrathecal or epidural drug infusion (includes evaluation of reservoir status, alarm status, drug prescription status); without reprogramming **S** **80** □

> MED: 100-3,280.14

62368 with reprogramming **S** **80** □

> MED: 100-3,280.14
>
> AMA: 2002,Nov,10
> If an implantable pump for spinal or brain drug therapy is refilled or maintained, consult CPT code 95990.

POSTERIOR EXTRADURAL LAMINOTOMY OR LAMINECTOMY FOR EXPLORATION/DECOMPRESSION OF NEURAL ELEMENTS OR EXCISION OF HERNIATED INTERVERTEBRAL DISKS

If application of caliper or tongs is performed, consult CPT code 20660. If a fracture or dislocation of the spine is treated, consult CPT codes 22305-22327.

If these procedures are followed by arthrodesis, consult CPT codes 22590-22614.

63001 Laminectomy with exploration and/or decompression of spinal cord and/or cauda equina, without facetectomy, foraminotomy or discectomy, (eg, spinal stenosis), one or two vertebral segments; cervical **T** **80** □

> AMA: 2001,Jan,12

63003 thoracic **T** **80** □

> AMA: 2001,Jan,12

63005 lumbar, except for spondylolisthesis **T** **80** □

> AMA: 2001,Jan,12

63011 sacral **T** **80** □

> AMA: 2001,Jan,12

63012 Laminectomy with removal of abnormal facets and/or pars inter-articularis with decompression of cauda equina and nerve roots for spondylolisthesis, lumbar (Gill type procedure) **T** **80** □

> AMA: 2001,Jan,12

63015 Laminectomy with exploration and/or decompression of spinal cord and/or cauda equina, without facetectomy, foraminotomy or discectomy, (eg, spinal stenosis), more than 2 vertebral segments; cervical **T** **80** □

> AMA: 2001,Jan,12

63016 thoracic **T** **80** □

> AMA: 2001,Jan,12

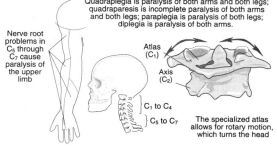

Quadraplegia is paralysis of both arms and both legs; quadraparesis is incomplete paralysis of both arms and both legs; paraplegia is paralysis of both legs; diplegia is paralysis of both arms.

Nerve root problems in C₅ through C₇ cause paralysis of the upper limb

Atlas (C₁)

Axis (C₂)

C₁ to C₄

C₅ to C₇

The specialized atlas allows for rotary motion, which turns the head

63017 lumbar **T** **80** □

> AMA: 2001,Jan,12

63020 Laminotomy (hemilaminectomy), with decompression of nerve root(s), including partial facetectomy, foraminotomy and/or excision of herniated intervertebral disc; one interspace, cervical **T** **80** **50** □

> AMA: 2001,Jan,12; 1999,Nov,36
> Codes 63020, 63030, and 63035 are unilateral procedures. To report these procedures performed bilaterally, append modifier 50.

63030 one interspace, lumbar (including open or endoscopically-assisted approach) **T** **80** **50** □

> AMA: 2002,Sep,10; 2001,Jan,12; 2001,Feb,10; 1999,Nov,36; 1996,Mar,7

---

⑥③ Modifier 63 Exempt Code ⊙ Conscious Sedation + CPT Add-on Code ⊘ Modifier 51 Exempt Code ● New Code ▲ Revised Code

M Maternity Edit **A** Age Edit **A-Y** APC Status Indicators □ CCI Comprehensive Code **50** Bilateral Procedure

Nervous System

63035 — 63081

+ **63035**   each additional interspace, cervical or lumbar (List separately in addition to code for primary procedure)   T 80 50

AMA: 2001,Jan,12; 2001,Feb,10; 1999,Nov,36; 1996,Mar,7

Note that 63035 is an add-on code and must be used in conjunction with 63020-63030.

63040   Laminotomy (hemilaminectomy), with decompression of nerve root(s), including partial facetectomy, foraminotomy and/or excision of herniated intervertebral disc, reexploration, single interspace; cervical   T 80 50

AMA: 2001,Jan,12; 1999,Jan,11

Codes 63040-63044 are unilateral procedures. To report these procedures performed bilaterally, append modifier 50.

63042   lumbar   T 80 50

AMA: 2001,Jan,12; 1999,Jan,11

+ **63043**   each additional cervical interspace (List separately in addition to code for primary procedure)   C 80 50

Note that CPT code 63043 is an add-on code and must be used in conjunction with 63040.

+ **63044**   each additional lumbar interspace (List separately in addition to code for primary procedure)   C 80 50

Note that CPT code 63044 is an add-on code and must be used in conjunction with 63042.

63045   Laminectomy, facetectomy and foraminotomy (unilateral or bilateral with decompression of spinal cord, cauda equina and/or nerve root(s), (eg, spinal or lateral recess stenosis)), single vertebral segment; cervical   T 80

AMA: 2001,Jan,12

63046   thoracic   T 80

AMA: 2001,Jan,12; 1999,Jan,11

63047   lumbar   T 80

AMA: 2002,Nov,11; 2001,Jan,12; 2001,Feb,10; 1999,Jan,11

+ **63048**   each additional segment, cervical, thoracic, or lumbar (List separately in addition to code for primary procedure)   T 80

AMA: 2001,Jan,12; 1999,Jan,11

Note that 63048 is an add-on code and must be used in conjunction with 63045-63047.

63050   Laminoplasty, cervical, with decompression of the spinal cord, two or more vertebral segments;   C 80

63051   with reconstruction of the posterior bony elements (including the application of bridging bone graft and non-segmental fixation devices (eg, wire, suture, mini-plates), when performed)   C 80

Code 63050 or 63051 cannot be reported with CPT codes 22600, 22614, 22840-22842, 63001, 63015, 63045, 63048, 63295 for the same vertebral segment(s).

TRANSPEDICULAR OR COSTOVERTEBRAL APPROACH FOR POSTEROLATERAL EXTRADURAL EXPLORATION/DECOMPRESSION

If application of caliper or tongs is performed, consult CPT code 20660. If a fracture or dislocation of the spine is treated, consult CPT codes 22305-22327.

63055   Transpedicular approach with decompression of spinal cord, equina and/or nerve root(s) (eg, herniated intervertebral disc), single segment; thoracic   T 80

AMA: 1999,Nov,36

63056   lumbar (including transfacet, or lateral extraforaminal approach) (eg, far lateral herniated intervertebral disk)   T 80

AMA: 1999,Nov,36

+ **63057**   each additional segment, thoracic or lumbar (List separately in addition to code for primary procedure)   T 80

AMA: 1999,Nov,36

Note that 63057 is an add-on code and must be used in conjunction with 63055, 63056.

63064   Costovertebral approach with decompression of spinal cord or nerve root(s), (eg, herniated intervertebral disc), thoracic; single segment   T 80

+ **63066**   each additional segment (List separately in addition to code for primary procedure)   T 80

Note that 63066 is an add-on code and must be used in conjunction with 63064.

To report excision of thoracic intraspinal lesions by laminectomy, consult CPT codes 63266, 63271, 63276, 63281, 63286.

ANTERIOR OR ANTEROLATERAL APPROACH FOR EXTRADURAL EXPLORATION/DECOMPRESSION

When two surgeons work together as primary surgeons performing distinct part(s) of spinal cord exploration/decompression surgery, each surgeon should assign one of the following codes and append modifier 62, Two surgeons. Modifier 62 can be reported with CPT code(s) 63075, 63077, 63081, 63085, 63087, 63090, and, as appropriate associated additional interspace codes 63076, 63078, or additional segment add-on code(s) 63082, 63086, 63088, 63091 provided that both surgeons continue to work together as primary surgeons.

Do not report 69990 in addition to codes 63075-63078 as the operating microscope is considered an inclusive component of these procedures.

If application of caliper or tongs is performed, consult CPT code 20660. If a fracture or dislocation of the spine is treated, consult CPT codes 22305-22327.

63075   Discectomy, anterior, with decompression of spinal cord and/or nerve root(s), including osteophytectomy; cervical, single interspace   T 80

AMA: 2001,Jan,12; 1998,Nov,18

+ **63076**   cervical, each additional interspace (List separately in addition to code for primary procedure)   C 80

AMA: 2001,Jan,12; 1998,Nov,18

Note that 63076 is an add-on code and must be used in conjunction with 63075.

63077   thoracic, single interspace   C 80

AMA: 2001,Jan,12; 1998,Nov,18

+ **63078**   thoracic, each additional interspace (List separately in addition to code for primary procedure)   C 80

AMA: 2001,Jan,12; 1998,Nov,18

Note that 63078 is an add-on code and must be used in conjunction with 63077.

63081   Vertebral corpectomy (vertebral body resection), partial or complete, anterior approach with decompression of spinal cord and/or nerve root(s); cervical, single segment   C 80

AMA: 1993,Spring,37

PC Professional Component Only   80/80 Assist-at-Surgery Allowed/With Documentation   Unlisted   Not Covered

TC Technical Component Only   MED: Pub 100/NCD References   AMA: CPT Assistant References   1-9 ASC Group   ♂ Male Only   ♀ Female Only

226 — CPT Expert   CPT only © 2006 American Medical Association. All Rights Reserved. (Black Ink)   © 2006 Ingenix (Blue Ink)

+ 63082 cervical, each additional segment (List separately in addition to code for primary procedure) C 80 🔳

AMA: 1993,Spring,37

Note that 63082 is an add-on code and must be used in conjunction with 63081.

If a transoral approach is used, consult CPT codes 61575 and 61576.

63085 Vertebral corpectomy (vertebral body resection), partial or complete, transthoracic approach with decompression of spinal cord and/or nerve root(s); thoracic, single segment C 80 🔳

AMA: 1993,Spring,37

+ 63086 thoracic, each additional segment (List separately in addition to code for primary procedure) C 80 🔳

AMA: 1993,Spring,37

Note that 63086 is an add-on code and must be used in conjunction with 63085.

63087 Vertebral corpectomy (vertebral body resection), partial or complete, combined thoracolumbar approach with decompression of spinal cord, cauda equina or nerve root(s), lower thoracic or lumbar; single segment C 80 🔳

AMA: 1993,Spring,37

+ 63088 each additional segment (List separately in addition to code for primary procedure) C 80 🔳

AMA: 1993,Spring,37

Note that 63088 is an add-on code and must be used in conjunction with 63087.

63090 Vertebral corpectomy (vertebral body resection), partial or complete, transperitoneal or retroperitoneal approach with decompression of spinal cord, cauda equina or nerve root(s), lower thoracic, lumbar, or sacral; single segment C 80 🔳

AMA: 1996,Mar,6; 1993,Spring,37

+ 63091 each additional segment (List separately in addition to code for primary procedure) C 80 🔳

AMA: 1996,Mar,6; 1993,Spring,37

Note that 63091 is an add-on code and must be used in conjunction with 63090.

LATERAL EXTRACAVITARY APPROACH FOR EXTRADURAL EXPLORATION/DECOMPRESSION

63101 Vertebral corpectomy (vertebral body resection), partial or complete, lateral extracavitary approach with decompression of spinal cord and/or nerve root(s) (eg, for tumor or retropulsed bone fragments); thoracic, single segment C 80 🔳

63102 lumbar, single segment C 80 🔳

+ 63103 thoracic or lumbar, each additional segment (List separately in addition to code for primary procedure) C 80 🔳

Note that 63103 is an add-on code that must be used in conjunction with 63101 and 63102.

INCISION

If application of caliper or tongs is performed, consult CPT code 20660. If a fracture or dislocation of the spine is treated, consult CPT codes 22305-22327.

63170 Laminectomy with myelotomy (eg, Bischof or DREZ type), cervical, thoracic, or thoracolumbar C 80 🔳

63172 Laminectomy with drainage of intramedullary cyst/syrinx; to subarachnoid space C 80 🔳

63173 to peritoneal or pleural space C 80 🔳

63180 Laminectomy and section of dentate ligaments, with or without dural graft, cervical; one or two segments C 80 🔳

63182 more than two segments C 80 🔳

63185 Laminectomy with rhizotomy; one or two segments C 80 🔳

Dana rhizotomy

63190 more than two segments C 80 🔳

63191 Laminectomy with section of spinal accessory nerve C 80 50 🔳

If resection of the sternocleidomastoid muscle is performed, consult CPT code 21720.

Code 63191 is a unilateral procedure. To report this procedure bilaterally, append modifier 50.

63194 Laminectomy with cordotomy, with section of one spinothalamic tract, one stage; cervical C 80 🔳

63195 thoracic C 80 🔳

63196 Laminectomy with cordotomy, with section of both spinothalamic tracts, one stage; cervical C 80 🔳

63197 thoracic C 80 🔳

63198 Laminectomy with cordotomy with section of both spinothalamic tracts, two stages within 14 days; cervical C 80 🔳

Keen laminectomy

63199 thoracic C 80 🔳

63200 Laminectomy, with release of tethered spinal cord, lumbar C 80 🔳

EXCISION BY LAMINECTOMY OF LESION OTHER THAN HERNIATED DISK

Cervical C_1 to C_7

Thoracic T_1 to T_{12}

Lumbar L_1 to L_5

Sacrum

Nerve roots

Pia mater

Dura mater (reflected)

Arachnoid

White matter

Gray matter

Schematic of spinal cord layers

The layers of the spinal cord are continuous with those of the brain; surgical access to the cord typically involves laminectomy or laminotomy. Delivery of a substance to the cord may be by injection or catheter and typically is to the epidural, subdural, or subarachnoid space

63250 Laminectomy for excision or occlusion of arteriovenous malformation of spinal cord; cervical C 80 🔳

63251 thoracic C 80 🔳

63252 thoracolumbar C 80 🔳

63265 Laminectomy for excision or evacuation of intraspinal lesion other than neoplasm, extradural; cervical C 80 🔳

63266 thoracic C 80 🔳

63267 lumbar C 80 🔳

63268 sacral C 80 🔳

63270 Laminectomy for excision of intraspinal lesion other than neoplasm, intradural; cervical C 80 🔳

63271 thoracic C 80 🔳

63272 lumbar C 80 🔳

Nervous System

63273 — 63688

63273	sacral	C 80 ▣
63275	Laminectomy for biopsy/excision of intraspinal neoplasm; extradural, cervical	C 80 ▣
63276	extradural, thoracic	C 80 ▣
63277	extradural, lumbar	C 80 ▣
63278	extradural, sacral	C 80 ▣
63280	intradural, extramedullary, cervical	C 80 ▣
63281	intradural, extramedullary, thoracic	C 80 ▣
63282	intradural, extramedullary, lumbar	C 80 ▣
63283	intradural, sacral	C 80 ▣
63285	intradural, intramedullary, cervical	C 80 ▣
63286	intradural, intramedullary, thoracic	C 80 ▣
63287	intradural, intramedullary, thoracolumbar	C 80 ▣
63290	combined extradural-intradural lesion, any level	C 80 ▣

If an intramedullary cyst syrinx is drained, consult CPT codes 63172 and 63173.

+ 63295 **Osteoplastic reconstruction of dorsal spinal elements, following primary intraspinal procedure (List separately in addition to code for primary procedure)** C 80

Note that 63295 is an add-on procedure and must be used in conjunction with 63172, 63173, 63185, 63190, 63200-63290. Code 63295 must not be used with 22590-22614, 22840-22844, 63050, 63051 for the same vertebral segment.

EXCISION, ANTERIOR OR ANTEROLATERAL APPROACH, INTRASPINAL LESION

Surgeons working together as primary surgeons, each performing distinct parts of an anterior approach for an intraspinal excision, should report the procedure with modifier 62.

If arthrodesis is performed, consult CPT codes 22548-22585. If the spine is reconstructed, consult CPT codes 20930-20938.

63300	Vertebral corpectomy (vertebral body resection), partial or complete, for excision of intraspinal lesion, single segment; extradural, cervical	C 80 ▣
63301	extradural, thoracic by transthoracic approach	C 80 ▣
63302	extradural, thoracic by thoracolumbar approach	C 80 ▣
63303	extradural, lumbar or sacral by transperitoneal or retroperitoneal approach	C 80 ▣
63304	intradural, cervical	C 80 ▣
63305	intradural, thoracic by transthoracic approach	C 80 ▣
63306	intradural, thoracic by thoracolumbar approach	C 80 ▣
63307	intradural, lumbar or sacral by transperitoneal or retroperitoneal approach	C 80 ▣
+ 63308	each additional segment (List separately in addition to codes for single segment)	C 80 ▣

Note that 63308 is an add-on code and must be used in conjunction with 63300-63307.

STEREOTAXIS

63600 **Creation of lesion of spinal cord by stereotactic method, percutaneous, any modality (including stimulation and/or recording)** 2 T 80 ▣

MED: 100-2,15,260; 100-4,12,90.3; 100-4,14,10

63610 **Stereotactic stimulation of spinal cord, percutaneous, separate procedure not followed by other surgery** 1 T 80 ▣

MED: 100-2,15,260; 100-4,12,90.3; 100-4,14,10

63615 **Stereotactic biopsy, aspiration, or excision of lesion, spinal cord** T ▣

NEUROSTIMULATORS (SPINAL)

Codes 63650-63688 apply to both simple and complex neurostimulators.

For programming or electronic analysis of neurostimulator pulse generators, initial or subsequent, consult CPT codes 95970-95975.

Report codes 63650, 63655, and 63660, as appropriate, for the placement, revision, or removal of the spinal neurostimulator system components to provide spinal electrical stimulation. The neurostimulator system includes a neurostimulator, external controller, extension, and collection of contacts.

For codes 63650, 63660 the contacts are on a catheter-like lead. An array defines the collection of contacts on one catheter.

Consult 63655, 63660 for systems placed by open surgical exposure. These contacts are on a plate or paddle-shaped surface.

63650 **Percutaneous implantation of neurostimulator electrode array, epidural** 2 S ▣

MED: 100-2,15,260; 100-3,160.2; 100-3,160.7; 100-4,12,90.3; 100-4,14,10

AMA: 1999,Nov,18; 1999,Mar,11; 1999,Apr,10; 1998,Jun,1

63655 **Laminectomy for implantation of neurostimulator electrodes, plate/paddle, epidural** S 80 ▣

MED: 100-3,160.2; 100-3,160.7

AMA: 1999,Sep,1; 1998,Nov,18; 1998,Jun,1

63660 **Revision or removal of spinal neurostimulator electrode percutaneous array(s) or plate/paddle(s)** 1 T ▣

MED: 100-2,15,260; 100-3,160.2; 100-3,160.7; 100-4,12,90.3; 100-4,14,10

AMA: 1998,Nov,18; 1998,Jun,1

63685 **Insertion or replacement of spinal neurostimulator pulse generator or receiver, direct or inductive coupling** 2 T 80 ▣

MED: 100-2,15,260; 100-3,160.7; 100-4,4,61.2; 100-4,12,90.3; 100-4,14,10

AMA: 1998,Jun,1

Code 63685 cannot be reported with CPT code 63688 for the same pulse generator or receiver.

63688 **Revision or removal of implanted spinal neurostimulator pulse generator or receiver** 1 T ▣

MED: 100-2,15,260; 100-3,160.7; 100-4,12,90.3; 100-4,14,10

AMA: 1998,Jun,1

26 Professional Component Only   80/80 Assist-at-Surgery Allowed/With Documentation   Unlisted   Not Covered

TC Technical Component Only   **MED:** Pub 100/NCD References   **AMA:** CPT Assistant References   1-9 ASC Group   ♂ Male Only   ♀ Female Only

228 — CPT Expert   CPT only © 2006 American Medical Association. All Rights Reserved. *(Black Ink)*   © 2006 Ingenix *(Blue Ink)*

REPAIR

Spina bifida results from the defective closure of the spinal column during early fetal development; classification is according to location along the spine

Degree of disability is related to location and type; mild spina bifida may include only a bony abnormality with no meningeal or nerve involvement

Cervical

Thoracic

Lumbar

A fluid-filled herniation that protrudes is spina bifida cystica, or meningocele

If nerves protrude into the defect, it is called rachischisis, or meningomyelocele

Dura mater

Spinal cord

Vertebra

Most children with severe spina bifida also have hydrocephalus, which is excessive fluid in the skull

63700 Repair of meningocele; less than 5 cm diameter 　ⓒ 80 ⊕ ↔

63702 　larger than 5 cm diameter 　ⓒ 80 ⊕ ↔

63704 Repair of myelomeningocele; less than 5 cm diameter 　ⓒ 80 ⊕ ↔

63706 　larger than 5 cm diameter 　ⓒ 80 ⊕ ↔

If this procedure involves complex skin closure, consult the Integumentary System section of the CPT book.

63707 Repair of dural/cerebrospinal fluid leak, not requiring laminectomy 　ⓒ 80 ↔

63709 Repair of dural/cerebrospinal fluid leak or pseudomeningocele, with laminectomy 　ⓒ 80 ↔

63710 Dural graft, spinal 　ⓒ 80 ↔

If a cervical laminectomy and section of dentate ligaments are performed, with or without a dural graft, consult CPT codes 63180 and 63182.

SHUNT, SPINAL CSF

63740 Creation of shunt, lumbar, subarachnoid-peritoneal, -pleural, or other; including laminectomy 　ⓒ 80 ↔

63741 　percutaneous, not requiring laminectomy 　T 80 ↔

63744 Replacement, irrigation or revision of lumbosubarachnoid shunt 　③ T 80 ↔

MED: 100-2,15,260; 100-4,12,90.3; 100-4,14,10

63746 Removal of entire lumbosubarachnoid shunt system without replacement 　② T 80 ↔

MED: 100-2,15,260; 100-4,12,90.3; 100-4,14,10

EXTRACRANIAL NERVES, PERIPHERAL NERVES, AND AUTONOMIC NERVOUS SYSTEM

To report intracranial surgery on cranial nerves, consult CPT codes 61450, 61460, 61790.

INTRODUCTION/INJECTION OF ANESTHETIC AGENT (NERVE BLOCK), DIAGNOSTIC, OR THERAPEUTIC

SOMATIC NERVES

64400 Injection, anesthetic agent; trigeminal nerve, any division or branch 　T ↔

AMA: 1999,Nov,36; 1999,May,8; 1998,Jul,10

64402 　facial nerve 　T ↔

AMA: 1998,Jul,10

64405 　greater occipital nerve 　T ↔

AMA: 1998,Jul,10

64408 　vagus nerve 　T 80 ↔

AMA: 1998,Jul,10

64410 　phrenic nerve 　① T 80 ↔

MED: 100-2,15,260; 100-4,12,90.3; 100-4,14,10

AMA: 1998,Jul,10

64412 　spinal accessory nerve 　T ↔

AMA: 1998,Jul,10

64413 　cervical plexus 　T ↔

AMA: 1998,Jul,10

64415 　brachial plexus, single 　① T ↔

MED: 100-2,15,260; 100-4,12,90.3; 100-4,14,10

AMA: 2001,Oct,9; 1999,May,8; 1998,Jul,10

64416 　brachial plexus, continuous infusion by catheter (including catheter placement) including daily management for anesthetic agent administration 　T ↔

Do not report 01996 in conjunction with CPT code 64416.

64417 　axillary nerve 　① T ↔

MED: 100-2,15,260; 100-4,12,90.3; 100-4,14,10

AMA: 1998,Jul,10

64418 　suprascapular nerve 　T ↔

AMA: 1998,Jul,10

64420 　intercostal nerve, single 　① T ↔

MED: 100-2,15,260; 100-4,12,90.3; 100-4,14,10

AMA: 1998,Jul,10

64421 　intercostal nerves, multiple, regional block 　① T ↔

MED: 100-2,15,260; 100-4,12,90.3; 100-4,14,10

AMA: 1998,Jul,10

64425 　ilioinguinal, iliohypogastric nerves 　T ↔

AMA: 1998,Jul,10

64430 　pudendal nerve 　① T ↔

MED: 100-2,15,260; 100-4,12,90.3; 100-4,14,10

AMA: 1998,Jul,10

64435 　paracervical (uterine) nerve 　♀ T ↔

AMA: 1998,Jul,10

64445 　sciatic nerve, single 　T ↔

AMA: 1999,May,8; 1998,Jul,10

64446 　sciatic nerve, continuous infusion by catheter, (including catheter placement) including daily management for anesthetic agent administration 　T ↔

Do not report 01996 in conjunction with CPT code 64446.

64447 　femoral nerve, single 　T ↔

Do not report 01996 in conjunction with CPT code 64447.

64448 　femoral nerve, continuous infusion by catheter (including catheter placement) including daily management for anesthetic agent administration 　T ↔

Do not report 01996 in conjunction with CPT code 64448.

64449 　lumbar plexus, posterior approach, continuous infusion by catheter (including catheter placement) including daily management for anesthetic agent administration 　T ↔

Do not report 01996 in conjunction with CPT code 64449.

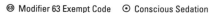 ⓢ Modifier 63 Exempt Code 　⊙ Conscious Sedation 　+ CPT Add-on Code 　 Ⓝ Modifier 51 Exempt Code 　 ● New Code 　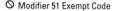 ▲ Revised Code

Ⓜ Maternity Edit 　Ⓐ Age Edit 　Ⓐ-Ⓨ APC Status Indicators 　 ↔ CCI Comprehensive Code 　50 Bilateral Procedure

Nervous System

64450 — 64575

64450 other peripheral nerve or branch ☐☐

AMA: 2001,Oct,9; 1999,Nov,37; 1999,Dec,7; 1998,Jul,10
If phenol destruction is performed, consult CPT codes 64622-64627.

If a subarachnoid or subdural injection is administered, consult CPT codes 62280, 62310-62319.

If an epidural or a caudal injection is administered, consult CPT codes 62273, 62281-62282, 62310-62319.

Use 77003 for fluoroscopic guidance and localization for needle placement and injection in conjunction with 64470-64484.

64470 Injection, anesthetic agent and/or steroid, paravertebral facet joint or facet joint nerve; cervical or thoracic, single level ☐☐☐☐

MED: 100-2,15,260; 100-4,12,90.3; 100-4,14,10
AMA: 2000,Feb,4; 1999,Nov,33, 37
If fluoroscopic guidance and localization for needle placement and injection is performed in conjunction with (64470-64484), consult CPT code 77003.

Codes 64470-64484 are unilateral procedures. To report these procedures performed bilaterally, append modifier 50.

+ **64472** cervical or thoracic, each additional level (List separately in addition to code for primary procedure) ☐☐☐☐

MED: 100-2,15,260; 100-4,12,90.3; 100-4,14,10
AMA: 2000,Feb,4; 1999,Nov,33, 37
Note that 64472 is an add-on code and must be used in conjunction with 64470.

64475 lumbar or sacral, single level ☐☐☐☐

MED: 100-2,15,260; 100-4,12,90.3; 100-4,14,10
AMA: 2000,Feb,4; 1999,Nov,33, 37

+ **64476** lumbar or sacral, each additional level (List separately in addition to code for primary procedure) ☐☐☐☐

MED: 100-2,15,260; 100-4,12,90.3; 100-4,14,10
AMA: 2000,Feb,4; 1999,Nov,33, 37
Note that 64476 is an add-on code and must be used in conjunction with 64475.

64479 Injection, anesthetic agent and/or steroid, transforaminal epidural; cervical or thoracic, single level ☐☐☐☐

MED: 100-2,15,260; 100-4,12,90.3; 100-4,14,10
AMA: 2000,Feb,4; 1999,Nov,33, 37

+ **64480** cervical or thoracic, each additional level (List separately in addition to code for primary procedure) ☐☐☐☐

MED: 100-2,15,260; 100-4,12,90.3; 100-4,14,10
AMA: 2000,Feb,4; 1999,Nov,33, 37
Note that 64480 is an add-on code and must be used in conjunction with 64479.

64483 lumbar or sacral, single level ☐☐☐☐

MED: 100-2,15,260; 100-4,12,90.3; 100-4,14,10
AMA: 2000,Feb,4; 1999,Nov,33, 37

+ **64484** lumbar or sacral, each additional level (List separately in addition to code for primary procedure) ☐☐☐☐

MED: 100-2,15,260; 100-4,12,90.3; 100-4,14,10
AMA: 2000,Feb,4; 1999,Nov,33, 37
Note that 64484 is an add-on code and must be used in conjunction with 64483.

SYMPATHETIC NERVES

64505 Injection, anesthetic agent; sphenopalatine ganglion ☐☐

AMA: 1998,Jul,10

64508 carotid sinus (separate procedure) ☐☐☐

AMA: 1998,Jul,10

64510 stellate ganglion (cervical sympathetic) ☐☐☐

MED: 100-2,15,260; 100-4,12,90.3; 100-4,14,10
AMA: 1998,Jul,10

64517 superior hypogastric plexus ☐☐☐

64520 lumbar or thoracic (paravertebral sympathetic) ☐☐☐

MED: 100-2,15,260; 100-4,12,90.3; 100-4,14,10
AMA: 1998,Jul,10

64530 celiac plexus, with or without radiologic monitoring ☐☐☐

MED: 100-2,15,260; 100-4,12,90.3; 100-4,14,10
AMA: 1998,Jul,10

NEUROSTIMULATORS (PERIPHERAL NERVE)

For programming or electronic analysis of neurostimulator pulse generators, initial or subsequent, consult CPT codes 95970-95975.

Consult the glossary for terms and definitions and the front matter of this chapter for additional information.

64550 Application of surface (transcutaneous) neurostimulator ☐☐

MED: 100-3,10.2; 100-3,130.5; 100-3,160.2; 100-3,160.7.1; 100-3,160.13; 100-3,280.13; 100-4,5,20
AMA: 2002,Apr,18

64553 Percutaneous implantation of neurostimulator electrodes; cranial nerve ☐☐☐☐

MED: 100-2,15,260; 100-3,160.2; 100-3,160.7; 100-4,12,90.3; 100-4,14,10
AMA: 2001,Apr,18; 1999,Nov,38
If this procedure involves open placement of a cranial nerve (e.g., vagal, trigeminal) neurostimulator pulse generator or receiver, consult CPT codes 61885 and 61886, as appropriate.

64555 peripheral nerve (excludes sacral nerve) ☐☐

MED: 100-3,30.1; 100-3,30.1.1; 100-3,160.2; 100-3,160.7.1

64560 autonomic nerve ☐☐☐

MED: 100-3,30.1; 100-3,30.1.1; 100-3,160.2

64561 sacral nerve (transforaminal placement) ☐☐☐

MED: 100-4,32,40

64565 neuromuscular ☐☐

MED: 100-3,30.1; 100-3,30.1.1; 100-3,160.2; 100-3,160.12; 100-3,160.13
AMA: 2000,Jul,11

64573 Incision for implantation of neurostimulator electrodes; cranial nerve ☐☐☐☐

MED: 100-2,15,260; 100-3,30.1; 100-3,160.2; 100-3,160.7; 100-3,160.18; 100-4,12,90.3; 100-4,14,10
AMA: 2001,Apr,8; 1999,Sep,1; 1999,Nov,38
If this procedure involves open placement of a cranial nerve neurostimulator pulse generator or receiver, consult CPT codes 61885, 61886.

To report revision or removal of cranial nerve neurostimulator pulse generator or receiver, consult CPT code 61888.

64575 peripheral nerve (excludes sacral nerve) ☐☐☐

MED: 100-2,15,260; 100-3,30.1; 100-3,30.1.1; 100-3,160.2; 100-3,160.7; 100-4,12,90.3; 100-4,14,10

☐ Professional Component Only   ☐/☐ Assist-at-Surgery Allowed/With Documentation   Unlisted   Not Covered

☐ Technical Component Only   **MED:** Pub 100/NCD References   **AMA:** CPT Assistant References   ☐-☐ ASC Group   ♂ Male Only   ♀ Female Only

230 — CPT Expert   CPT only © 2006 American Medical Association. All Rights Reserved. *(Black Ink)*   © 2006 Ingenix *(Blue Ink)*

64577	autonomic nerve	1 S 🔲

MED: 100-2,15,260; 100-3,30.1; 100-3,30.1.1; 100-3,160.2; 100-3,160.7; 100-4,12,90.3; 100-4,14,10

64580	neuromuscular	1 S 80 🔲

MED: 100-2,15,260; 100-3,30.1; 100-3,30.1.1; 100-3,160.2; 100-3,160.7; 100-3,160.12; 100-4,12,90.3; 100-4,14,10

64581	sacral nerve (transforaminal placement)	3 S 🔲

MED: 100-4,32,40

64585	Revision or removal of peripheral neurostimulator electrodes	1 T 80 🔲

MED: 100-2,15,260; 100-3,30.1; 100-3,160.2; 100-3,160.7; 100-3,160.7.1; 100-4,12,90.3; 100-4,14,10; 100-4,32,40

▲ **64590** Insertion or replacement of peripheral or gastric neurostimulator pulse generator or receiver, direct or inductive coupling 2 T 80 🔲

MED: 100-2,15,260; 100-3,30.1; 100-3,30.1.1; 100-3,160.2; 100-3,160.7; 100-3,160.7.1; 100-3,160.18; 100-4,4,61.2; 100-4,12,90.3; 100-4,14,10; 100-4,32,40

AMA: 2001,Apr,8; 1999,Sep,1
Code 64590 cannot be reported with CPT code 64595.

▲ **64595** Revision or removal of peripheral or gastric neurostimulator pulse generator or receiver 1 T 🔲

MED: 100-2,15,260; 100-3,30.1; 100-3,30.1.1; 100-3,160.2; 100-3,160.7; 100-3,160.7.1; 100-4,12,90.3; 100-4,14,10; 100-4,32,40

DESTRUCTION BY NEUROLYTIC AGENT (EG, CHEMICAL, THERMAL, ELECTRICAL, RADIOFREQUENCY) - SYMPATHETIC NERVES

The injection of other therapeutic agents (e.g., corticosteroids) is included in CPT codes 64680-64681. Do not report separately.

SOMATIC NERVES

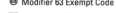

The main branches of the facial nerve (CN V2); Bell's palsy is paralysis of the facial nerve for no apparent reason and is marked for inability to close the eye and lip on the affected side

Trigeminal neuralgia, also known as tic douloureaux, is a severe facial pain brought on by mere touch in an area of one of the divisions of the trigeminal nerve, usually along the V2 branch

64600	Destruction by neurolytic agent, trigeminal nerve; supraorbital, infraorbital, mental, or inferior alveolar branch	1 T 🔲

MED: 100-2,15,260; 100-3,160.1; 100-4,12,90.3; 100-4,14,10

64605	second and third division branches at foramen ovale	1 T 80 🔲

MED: 100-2,15,260; 100-3,160.1; 100-4,12,90.3; 100-4,14,10

64610	second and third division branches at foramen ovale under radiologic monitoring	1 T 🔲

MED: 100-2,15,260; 100-3,160.1; 100-4,12,90.3; 100-4,14,10

64612	Chemodenervation of muscle(s); muscle(s) innervated by facial nerve (eg, for blepharospasm, hemifacial spasm)	T 50 🔲

MED: 100-3,160.1
AMA: 2001,Apr,1; 1998,Oct,10

64613	neck muscle(s) (eg, for spasmodic torticollis, spasmodic dysphonia)	T 🔲

MED: 100-3,160.1
AMA: 2001,Apr,1; 2000,Sep,10

64614	extremity(s) and/or trunk muscle(s) (eg, for dystonia, cerebral palsy, multiple sclerosis)	T 50 🔲

MED: 100-3,160.20
AMA: 2001,Apr,1
If chemodenervation is performed for strabismus involving the extraocular muscles, consult CPT code 67345.

To report chemodenervation that is guided by needle electromyography or muscle electrical stimulation, consult CPT codes 95873, 95874.

To report chemodenervation of the internal anal sphincter, consult CPT code 46505.

64620	Destruction by neurolytic agent, intercostal nerve	1 T 🔲

MED: 100-2,15,260; 100-3,160.1; 100-4,12,90.3; 100-4,14,10
AMA: 1999,Nov,38

Use 77003 for fluoroscopic guidance and loalization for needle placement and injection in conjunction with 64622-64627.

64622	Destruction by neurolytic agent, paravertebral facet joint nerve; lumbar or sacral, single level	1 T 50 🔲

MED: 100-2,15,260; 100-3,160.1; 100-4,12,90.3; 100-4,14,10
AMA: 2000,Mar,4; 1999,Nov,33, 39; 1999,Dec,7
To report fluoroscopic guidance and localization for needle placement and neurolysis with code 64622-64627, consult CPT code 77003.

Codes 64622-64627 are unilateral procedures. To report these procedures performed bilaterally, append modifier 50.

+ **64623** lumbar or sacral, each additional level (List separately in addition to code for primary procedure) 1 T 50 🔲

MED: 100-2,15,260; 100-3,160.1; 100-4,12,90.3; 100-4,14,10
AMA: 2000,Mar,4; 1999,Nov,33, 39
Note that 64623 is an add-on code and must be used in conjunction with 64622.

64626	cervical or thoracic, single level	1 T 50 🔲

MED: 100-2,15,260; 100-3,160.1; 100-4,12,90.3; 100-4,14,10
AMA: 2000,Mar,4; 1999,Nov,33, 39

+ **64627** cervical or thoracic, each additional level (List separately in addition to code for primary procedure) 1 T 50 🔲

MED: 100-2,15,260; 100-3,160.1; 100-4,12,90.3; 100-4,14,10
AMA: 2000,Mar,4; 1999,Nov,33, 39
Note that 64627 is an add-on code and must be used in conjunction with 64626.

64630	Destruction by neurolytic agent; pudendal nerve	2 T 80 🔲

MED: 100-2,15,260; 100-3,160.1; 100-4,12,90.3; 100-4,14,10

64640	other peripheral nerve or branch	T 50 🔲

MED: 100-3,160.1

SYMPATHETIC NERVES

64650	Chemodenervation of eccrine glands; both axillae	T 80

64653	other area(s) (eg, scalp, face, neck), per day	T 80

Report the specific service in addition to the code(s) for the specific substance(s) or drug(s) provided.

To report chemodenervation of extremities (eg, hands or feet), consult CPT code 64999.

Nervous System

64577 — 64653

Nervous System

64680 — 64771

64680   Destruction by neurolytic agent, with or without radiologic monitoring; celiac plexus   **2** T ▣
MED: 100-2,15,260; 100-3,160.1; 100-4,12,90.3; 100-4,14,10
AMA: 1999,Feb,10

64681   superior hypogastric plexus   **2** T ▣

NEUROPLASTY (EXPLORATION, NEUROLYSIS OR NERVE DECOMPRESSION)

If facial nerve decompression is performed, consult CPT code 69720.

If internal neurolysis is performed and requires the use of an operating microscope, consult CPT code 64727.

64702   Neuroplasty; digital, one or both, same digit   **1** T ▣
MED: 100-2,15,260; 100-4,12,90.3; 100-4,14,10
AMA: 2001,Jun,11

64704   nerve of hand or foot   **1** T 80 ▣
MED: 100-2,15,260; 100-4,12,90.3; 100-4,14,10
AMA: 2001,Jun,11

64708   Neuroplasty, major peripheral nerve, arm or leg; other than specified   **2** T 80 ▣
MED: 100-2,15,260; 100-4,12,90.3; 100-4,14,10
AMA: 2001,Jun,11

64712   sciatic nerve   **2** T 80 ▣
MED: 100-2,15,260; 100-4,12,90.3; 100-4,14,10
AMA: 2001,Jun,11

64713   brachial plexus   **2** T 80 ▣
MED: 100-2,15,260; 100-4,12,90.3; 100-4,14,10
AMA: 2001,Jun,11

64714   lumbar plexus   **2** T 80 ▣
MED: 100-2,15,260; 100-4,12,90.3; 100-4,14,10
AMA: 2001,Jun,11; 1997,Jun,11

64716   Neuroplasty and/or transposition; cranial nerve (specify)   **3** T 80 ▣
MED: 100-2,15,260; 100-4,12,90.3; 100-4,14,10
AMA: 2001,Jun,11

64718   ulnar nerve at elbow   **2** T 80 ▣
MED: 100-2,15,260; 100-4,12,90.3; 100-4,14,10
AMA: 2001,Jun,11

64719   ulnar nerve at wrist   **2** T ▣
MED: 100-2,15,260; 100-4,12,90.3; 100-4,14,10
AMA: 2001,Jun,11

64721   median nerve at carpal tunnel   **2** T 50 ▣
MED: 100-2,15,260; 100-4,12,90.3; 100-4,14,10
AMA: 2001,Jun,11; 1997,Sep,10
To report arthroscopic procedure, consult CPT code 29848.

64722   Decompression; unspecified nerve(s) (specify)   **1** T 80 ▣
MED: 100-2,15,260; 100-4,12,90.3; 100-4,14,10
AMA: 2001,Jun,11; 1999,May,11

64726   plantar digital nerve   **1** T ▣
MED: 100-2,15,260; 100-4,12,90.3; 100-4,14,10
AMA: 2001,Jun,11

+   64727   Internal neurolysis, requiring use of operating microscope (List separately in addition to code for neuroplasty) (Neuroplasty includes external neurolysis)   **1** T ▣
MED: 100-2,15,260; 100-4,12,90.3; 100-4,14,10
AMA: 2001,Jun,11; 1998,Nov,19
Do not report 69990 in addition to code 64727 as the operating microscope is considered an inclusive component of the surgery.

Note that 64727 is an add-on code that must be used in conjunction with the appropriate code for the primary procedure. This code cannot be reported alone.

TRANSECTION OR AVULSION

To report stereotactic lesion of gasserian ganglion, consult CPT code 61790.

64732   Transection or avulsion of; supraorbital nerve   **2** T 80 ▣
MED: 100-2,15,260; 100-4,12,90.3; 100-4,14,10
AMA: 1999,Nov,39

64734   infraorbital nerve   **2** T 80 ▣
MED: 100-2,15,260; 100-4,12,90.3; 100-4,14,10

64736   mental nerve   **2** T 80 ▣
MED: 100-2,15,260; 100-3,160.1; 100-4,12,90.3; 100-4,14,10

64738   inferior alveolar nerve by osteotomy   **2** T 80 ▣
MED: 100-2,15,260; 100-4,12,90.3; 100-4,14,10

64740   lingual nerve   **2** T 80 ▣
MED: 100-2,15,260; 100-4,12,90.3; 100-4,14,10

64742   facial nerve, differential or complete   **2** T 80 ▣
MED: 100-2,15,260; 100-4,12,90.3; 100-4,14,10

64744   greater occipital nerve   **2** T 80 50 ▣
MED: 100-2,15,260; 100-4,12,90.3; 100-4,14,10

64746   phrenic nerve   **2** T 80 ▣
MED: 100-2,15,260; 100-4,12,90.3; 100-4,14,10
To report section of a recurrent laryngeal nerve, consult CPT code 31595.

64752   vagus nerve (vagotomy), transthoracic   C 80 ▣

64755   vagus nerves limited to proximal stomach (selective proximal vagotomy, proximal gastric vagotomy, parietal cell vagotomy, supra- or highly selective vagotomy)   C 80 ▣
AMA: 1999,Nov,39
If a laparoscopic approach is used, consult CPT code 43652.

64760   vagus nerve (vagotomy), abdominal   C 80 ▣
AMA: 1999,Nov,39
If a laparoscopic approach is used, consult CPT code 43651.

64761   pudendal nerve   T 80 50 ▣

64763   Transection or avulsion of obturator nerve, extrapelvic, with or without adductor tenotomy   T 80 50 ▣

64766   Transection or avulsion of obturator nerve, intrapelvic, with or without adductor tenotomy   T 80 50 ▣
MED: 100-3,160.1

64771   Transection or avulsion of other cranial nerve, extradural   **2** T 80 ▣
MED: 100-2,15,260; 100-4,12,90.3; 100-4,14,10

64772 **Transection or avulsion of other spinal nerve, extradural** 2 T 80 ▣

MED: 100-2,15,260; 100-4,12,90.3; 100-4,14,10

If an excision is performed on a tender scar, skin, and subcutaneous tissue, with or without tiny neuroma, consult CPT codes 11400-11446 and 13100-13153.

EXCISION

SOMATIC NERVES

If a Morton Neurectomy is performed, consult CPT code 28080.

64774 **Excision of neuroma; cutaneous nerve, surgically identifiable** 2 T ▣

MED: 100-2,15,260; 100-4,12,90.3; 100-4,14,10

64776 **digital nerve, one or both, same digit** 3 T 80 ▣

MED: 100-2,15,260; 100-4,12,90.3; 100-4,14,10

+ **64778** **digital nerve, each additional digit (List separately in addition to code for primary procedure)** 2 T ▣

MED: 100-2,15,260; 100-4,12,90.3; 100-4,14,10

Note that 64778 is an add-on code and must be used in conjunction with 64776.

64782 **hand or foot, except digital nerve** 3 T ▣

MED: 100-2,15,260; 100-4,12,90.3; 100-4,14,10

+ **64783** **hand or foot, each additional nerve, except same digit (List separately in addition to code for primary procedure)** 2 T ▣

MED: 100-2,15,260; 100-4,12,90.3; 100-4,14,10

Note that 64783 is an add-on code and must be used in conjunction with 64782.

64784 **major peripheral nerve, except sciatic** 3 T 80 ▣

MED: 100-2,15,260; 100-4,12,90.3; 100-4,14,10

64786 **sciatic nerve** 3 T 80 ▣

MED: 100-2,15,260; 100-4,12,90.3; 100-4,14,10

+ **64787** **Implantation of nerve end into bone or muscle (List separately in addition to neuroma excision)** 2 T 80 ▣

MED: 100-2,15,260; 100-4,12,90.3; 100-4,14,10

Note that 64787 is an add-on code and must be used in conjunction with 64774-64786.

64788 **Excision of neurofibroma or neurolemmoma; cutaneous nerve** 3 T ▣

MED: 100-2,15,260; 100-4,12,90.3; 100-4,14,10

64790 **major peripheral nerve** 3 T 80 ▣

MED: 100-2,15,260; 100-4,12,90.3; 100-4,14,10

64792 **extensive (including malignant type)** 3 T 80 ▣

MED: 100-2,15,260; 100-4,12,90.3; 100-4,14,10

64795 **Biopsy of nerve** 2 T ▣

MED: 100-2,15,260; 100-4,12,90.3; 100-4,14,10

SYMPATHETIC NERVES

64802 **Sympathectomy, cervical** 2 T 80 50 ▣

MED: 100-2,15,260; 100-4,12,90.3; 100-4,14,10

64804 **Sympathectomy, cervicothoracic** T 80 50 ▣

64809 **Sympathectomy, thoracolumbar** C 80 50 ▣

   Leriche sympathectomy

64818 **Sympathectomy, lumbar** C 80 50 ▣

64820 **Sympathectomy; digital arteries, each digit** T ▣

   Code 69990 cannot be reported with 64820.

64821 **radial artery** 4 T 50 ▣

MED: 100-2,15,260; 100-4,12,90.3; 100-4,14,10

Code 69990 cannot be reported with 64821.

64822 **ulnar artery** T 50 ▣

Code 69990 cannot be reported with 64822.

64823 **superficial palmar arch** T 50 ▣

Code 69990 cannot be reported with 64823.

NEURORRHAPHY

64831 **Suture of digital nerve, hand or foot; one nerve** 4 T ▣

MED: 100-2,15,260; 100-4,12,90.3; 100-4,14,10

+ **64832** **each additional digital nerve (List separately in addition to code for primary procedure)** 1 T 80 ▣

MED: 100-2,15,260; 100-4,12,90.3; 100-4,14,10

AMA: 2000,Apr,6

Note that 64832 is an add-on code and must be used in conjunction with 64831.

64834 **Suture of one nerve, hand or foot; common sensory nerve** 2 T 80 ▣

MED: 100-2,15,260; 100-4,12,90.3; 100-4,14,10

64835 **median motor thenar** 3 T 80 ▣

MED: 100-2,15,260; 100-4,12,90.3; 100-4,14,10

64836 **ulnar motor** 3 T 80 ▣

MED: 100-2,15,260; 100-4,12,90.3; 100-4,14,10

+ **64837** **Suture of each additional nerve, hand or foot (List separately in addition to code for primary procedure)** 1 T 80 ▣

MED: 100-2,15,260; 100-4,12,90.3; 100-4,14,10

Note that 64837 is an add-on code and must be used in conjunction with 64834-64836.

64840 **Suture of posterior tibial nerve** 2 T 80 ▣

MED: 100-2,15,260; 100-4,12,90.3; 100-4,14,10

64856 **Suture of major peripheral nerve, arm or leg, except sciatic; including transposition** 2 T ▣

MED: 100-2,15,260; 100-4,12,90.3; 100-4,14,10

64857 **without transposition** 2 T 80 ▣

MED: 100-2,15,260; 100-4,12,90.3; 100-4,14,10

64858 **Suture of sciatic nerve** 2 T 80 ▣

MED: 100-2,15,260; 100-4,12,90.3; 100-4,14,10

+ **64859** **Suture of each additional major peripheral nerve (List separately in addition to code for primary procedure)** 1 T 80 ▣

MED: 100-2,15,260; 100-4,12,90.3; 100-4,14,10

Note that 64859 is an add-on code and must be used in conjunction with 64856 and 64857.

64861 **Suture of; brachial plexus** 3 T 80 ▣

MED: 100-2,15,260; 100-4,12,90.3; 100-4,14,10

64862 **lumbar plexus** 3 T 80 ▣

MED: 100-2,15,260; 100-4,12,90.3; 100-4,14,10

64864 **Suture of facial nerve; extracranial** 3 T 80 ▣

MED: 100-2,15,260; 100-4,12,90.3; 100-4,14,10

64865 **infratemporal, with or without grafting** 4 T 80 ▣

MED: 100-2,15,260; 100-4,12,90.3; 100-4,14,10

64866 **Anastomosis; facial-spinal accessory** C 80 ▣

Nervous System

64868 — 64999

64868	facial-hypoglossal	C 80
	Korte-Ballance anastomosis	

64870 facial-phrenic 4 T 80
MED: 100-2,15,260; 100-4,12,90.3; 100-4,14,10

+ **64872** Suture of nerve; requiring secondary or delayed suture (List separately in addition to code for primary neurorrhaphy) 2 T 80
MED: 100-2,15,260; 100-4,12,90.3; 100-4,14,10
Note that 64872 is an add-on code and must be used in conjunction with 64831-64865.

+ **64874** requiring extensive mobilization, or transposition of nerve (List separately in addition to code for nerve suture) 3 T 80
MED: 100-2,15,260; 100-4,12,90.3; 100-4,14,10
Note that 64874 is an add-on code and must be used in conjunction with 64831-64865.

+ **64876** requiring shortening of bone of extremity (List separately in addition to code for nerve suture) 3 T 80
MED: 100-2,15,260; 100-4,12,90.3; 100-4,14,10
Note that 64876 is an add-on code and must be used in conjunction with 64831-64865.

NEURORRHAPHY WITH NERVE GRAFT, VEIN GRAFT, OR CONDUIT

64885 Nerve graft (includes obtaining graft), head or neck; up to 4 cm in length 2 T 80
MED: 100-2,15,260; 100-4,12,90.3; 100-4,14,10
AMA: 2000,Nov,11

64886 more than 4 cm length 2 T 80
MED: 100-2,15,260; 100-4,12,90.3; 100-4,14,10
AMA: 2000,Nov,11

64890 Nerve graft (includes obtaining graft), single strand, hand or foot; up to 4 cm length 2 T 80
MED: 100-2,15,260; 100-4,12,90.3; 100-4,14,10

64891 more than 4 cm length 2 T 80
MED: 100-2,15,260; 100-4,12,90.3; 100-4,14,10

64892 Nerve graft (includes obtaining graft), single strand, arm or leg; up to 4 cm length 2 T 80
MED: 100-2,15,260; 100-4,12,90.3; 100-4,14,10

64893 more than 4 cm length 2 T 80
MED: 100-2,15,260; 100-4,12,90.3; 100-4,14,10

64895 Nerve graft (includes obtaining graft), multiple strands (cable), hand or foot; up to 4 cm length 3 T 80
MED: 100-2,15,260; 100-4,12,90.3; 100-4,14,10
AMA: 2000,Nov,11

64896 more than 4 cm length 3 T 80
MED: 100-2,15,260; 100-4,12,90.3; 100-4,14,10
AMA: 2000,Nov,11

64897 Nerve graft (includes obtaining graft), multiple strands (cable), arm or leg; up to 4 cm length 3 T 80
MED: 100-2,15,260; 100-4,12,90.3; 100-4,14,10
AMA: 2000,Nov,11

64898 more than 4 cm length 3 T 80
MED: 100-2,15,260; 100-4,12,90.3; 100-4,14,10
AMA: 2000,Nov,11

+ **64901** Nerve graft, each additional nerve; single strand (List separately in addition to code for primary procedure) 2 T 80
MED: 100-2,15,260; 100-4,12,90.3; 100-4,14,10
AMA: 2000,Nov,11
Note that 64901 is an add-on code and must be used in conjunction with 64885-64893.

+ **64902** multiple strands (cable) (List separately in addition to code for primary procedure) 2 T 80
MED: 100-2,15,260; 100-4,12,90.3; 100-4,14,10
AMA: 2000,Nov,11
Note that 64902 is an add-on code and must be used in conjunction with 64885, 64886, and 64895-64898.

64905 Nerve pedicle transfer; first stage 2 T 80
MED: 100-2,15,260; 100-4,12,90.3; 100-4,14,10

64907 second stage 1 T 80
MED: 100-2,15,260; 100-4,12,90.3; 100-4,14,10

● **64910** Nerve repair; with synthetic conduit or vein allograft (eg, nerve tube), each nerve T

● **64911** with autogenous vein graft (includes harvest of vein graft), each nerve T
Do not report 69990 in addition to 64910 and 64911.

OTHER PROCEDURES

64999 Unlisted procedure, nervous system T 80
AMA: 2000,Sep,10; 2000,Jan,10; 2000,Aug,7; 1998,Sep,16; 1998,Oct,10; 1996,Apr,10

26 Professional Component Only
TC Technical Component Only
80/80 Assist-at-Surgery Allowed/With Documentation
Unlisted   Not Covered
MED: Pub 100/NCD References AMA: CPT Assistant References   1-9 ASC Group   ♂ Male Only   ♀ Female Only
234 — CPT Expert
CPT only © 2006 American Medical Association. All Rights Reserved. *(Black Ink)*
© *2006 Ingenix (Blue Ink)*

EYE AND OCULAR ADNEXA

If a diagnostic and treatment program is initiated for ophthalmological services, consult the Medicine and Ophthalmology sections of CPT and CPT codes 92002. Do not report 69990 in addition to codes 65091-68850 as the operating microscope is considered an inclusive component of these procedures.

EYEBALL

REMOVAL OF EYE

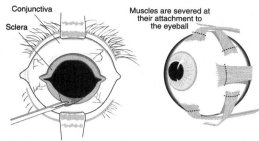

Conjunctiva
Sclera
Muscles are severed at their attachment to the eyeball

Evisceration involves removal of the contents of the eyeball: the vitreous; retina; choroid; lens; iris; and ciliary muscle. Only the scleral shell remains. A temporary or permanent implant is usually inserted

Enucleation involves severing the extraorbital muscles and optic nerve with removal of the eyeball. An implant is usually inserted and, if permanent, may involve attachment to the severed extraorbital muscles

65091   Evisceration of ocular contents; without implant   3 T 80 50 ⟲
MED: 100-2,15,260; 100-4,12,90.3; 100-4,14,10

65093   with implant   3 T 50 ⟲
MED: 100-2,15,260; 100-4,12,90.3; 100-4,14,10

65101   Enucleation of eye; without implant   3 T 50 ⟲
MED: 100-2,15,260; 100-4,12,90.3; 100-4,14,10

65103   with implant, muscles not attached to implant   3 T 50 ⟲
MED: 100-2,15,260; 100-4,12,90.3; 100-4,14,10

65105   with implant, muscles attached to implant   4 T 80 50 ⟲
MED: 100-2,15,260; 100-4,12,90.3; 100-4,14,10

If a conjunctivoplasty is performed after enucleation, consult CPT codes 68320 and subsequent codes.

65110   Exenteration of orbit (does not include skin graft), removal of orbital contents; only   5 T 80 50 ⟲
MED: 100-2,15,260; 100-4,12,90.3; 100-4,14,10

65112   with therapeutic removal of bone   7 T 80 50 ⟲
MED: 100-2,15,260; 100-4,12,90.3; 100-4,14,10

65114   with muscle or myocutaneous flap   7 T 80 50 ⟲
MED: 100-2,15,260; 100-4,12,90.3; 100-4,14,10

If a split skin graft is performed on the orbit, consult CPT codes 15120 and 15121. If a full thickness graft, free, is performed, consult CPT codes 15260 and 15261. If an eyelid, involving more than skin, is repaired, consult CPT codes 67930 and subsequent codes.

SECONDARY IMPLANT(S) PROCEDURES

Consult the glossary for terms and definitions and the front matter of this chapter for additional information.

If a diagnostic and treatment program is initiated for ophthalmological services, consult the Medicine and Ophthalmology sections of the CPT book and CPT codes 92002 and subsequent codes. Do not report 69990 in addition to codes 65091-68850 as the operating microscope is considered an inclusive component of these procedures.

65125   Modification of ocular implant with placement or replacement of pegs (eg, drilling receptacle for prosthesis appendage) (separate procedure)   T 50 ⟲

65130   Insertion of ocular implant secondary; after evisceration, in scleral shell   3 T 50 ⟲
MED: 100-2,15,260; 100-4,12,90.3; 100-4,14,10

65135   after enucleation, muscles not attached to implant   2 T 50 ⟲
MED: 100-2,15,260; 100-4,12,90.3; 100-4,14,10

65140   after enucleation, muscles attached to implant   3 T 50 ⟲
MED: 100-2,15,260; 100-4,12,90.3; 100-4,14,10

65150   Reinsertion of ocular implant; with or without conjunctival graft   2 T 80 50 ⟲
MED: 100-2,15,260; 100-4,12,90.3; 100-4,14,10

65155   with use of foreign material for reinforcement and/or attachment of muscles to implant   3 T 50 ⟲
MED: 100-2,15,260; 100-4,12,90.3; 100-4,14,10

65175   Removal of ocular implant   1 T 50 ⟲
MED: 100-2,15,260; 100-4,12,90.3; 100-4,14,10

If an orbital implant (implant outside muscle cone) is inserted, consult CPT code 67550. If the implant is removed, consult CPT code 67560.

REMOVAL OF FOREIGN BODY

If a diagnostic and treatment program is initiated for ophthalmological services, consult the Medicine and Ophthalmology sections of the CPT book and CPT codes 92002 and subsequent codes. Do not report 69990 in addition to codes 65091-68850 as the operating microscope is considered an inclusive component of these procedures.

If implanted material is removed, consult the following CPT codes: ocular implant, see 56175; anterior segment implant, see 65920; posterior segment implant, see 67120; and orbital implant, see 67560. If a diagnostic x-ray is taken for a foreign body, consult CPT code 70030. If a diagnostic echography is needed for a foreign body, consult CPT code 76529. If a foreign body is removed from the orbit, consult the following CPT codes: frontal approach, see 67413; lateral approach, see 67430; and transcranial approach, see 61334. If an embedded foreign body is removed from the eyelid, consult CPT code 67938. If a foreign body is removed from the lacrimal system, consult CPT code 68530.

65205   Removal of foreign body, external eye; conjunctival superficial   S 50 ⟲

65210   conjunctival embedded (includes concretions), subconjunctival, or scleral nonperforating   S 50 ⟲

65220   corneal, without slit lamp   S 50 ⟲

65222   corneal, with slit lamp   S 50 ⟲

To report repair of corneal laceration with foreign body, consult CPT code 65275.

65235   Removal of foreign body, intraocular; from anterior chamber of eye or lens   2 T 80 50 ⟲
MED: 100-2,15,260; 100-4,12,90.3; 100-4,14,10

To report removal of implant material from anterior segment, consult CPT code 65920.

65260   from posterior segment, magnetic extraction, anterior or posterior route   3 T 80 50 ⟲
MED: 100-2,15,260; 100-4,12,90.3; 100-4,14,10

⊗ Modifier 63 Exempt Code   ⊙ Conscious Sedation   + CPT Add-on Code   ⊘ Modifier 51 Exempt Code   ● New Code   ▲ Revised Code
M Maternity Edit   A Age Edit   A-Y APC Status Indicators   CCI Comprehensive Code   50 Bilateral Procedure

© 2006 Ingenix (Blue Ink)   CPT only © 2006 American Medical Association. All Rights Reserved. (Black Ink)   Eye and Ocular Adnexa — 235

65265   from posterior segment, nonmagnetic extraction   4 T 80 50 ⬛

MED: 100-2,15,260; 100-4,12,90.3; 100-4,14,10

To report removal of implant material from posterior segment, consult CPT code 67120.

REPAIR OF LACERATION

If a diagnostic and treatment program is initiated for ophthalmological services, consult the Medicine and Ophthalmology sections of the CPT book and CPT codes 92002 and subsequent codes. Do not report 69990 in addition to codes 65091-68850 as the operating microscope is considered an inclusive component of these procedures.

If the orbit is fractured, consult CPT codes 21385 and subsequent codes. If a wound on the skin of the eyelid is repaired, linear, simple, consult CPT codes 12011-12018; intermediate, layered closure, consult CPT codes 12051-12057; linear, complex, consult CPT codes 13150-13153; and other, consult CPT codes 67930 and 67935. If a wound of the lacrimal system is repaired, consult CPT code 68700. If an operative wound is repaired, consult CPT code 66250.

65270   Repair of laceration; conjunctiva, with or without nonperforating laceration sclera, direct closure   2 T 80 50 ⬛

MED: 100-2,15,260; 100-4,12,90.3; 100-4,14,10

65272   conjunctiva, by mobilization and rearrangement, without hospitalization   2 T 50 ⬛

MED: 100-2,15,260; 100-4,12,90.3; 100-4,14,10

65273   conjunctiva, by mobilization and rearrangement, with hospitalization   C 50 ⬛

65275   cornea, nonperforating, with or without removal foreign body   4 T 80 50 ⬛

MED: 100-2,15,260; 100-4,12,90.3; 100-4,14,10

65280   cornea and/or sclera, perforating, not involving uveal tissue   4 T 80 50 ⬛

MED: 100-2,15,260; 100-4,12,90.3; 100-4,14,10

65285   cornea and/or sclera, perforating, with reposition or resection of uveal tissue   4 T 80 50 ⬛

MED: 100-2,15,260; 100-4,12,90.3; 100-4,14,10

65286   application of tissue glue, wounds of cornea and/or sclera   T 50 ⬛

Note that this procedure includes use of a conjunctival flap and restoration of the anterior chamber, by air or saline injection when indicated. If the iris or ciliary body is repaired, consult CPT code 66680.

65290   Repair of wound, extraocular muscle, tendon and/or Tenon's capsule   3 T 50 ⬛

MED: 100-2,15,260; 100-4,12,90.3; 100-4,14,10

ANTERIOR SEGMENT

If a diagnostic and treatment program is initiated for ophthalmological services, consult the Medicine and Ophthalmology sections of the CPT book and CPT codes 92002 and subsequent codes. Do not report 69990 in addition to codes 65091-68850 as the operating microscope is considered an inclusive component of these procedures.

CORNEA

EXCISION

65400   Excision of lesion, cornea (keratectomy, lamellar, partial), except pterygium   1 T 50 ⬛

MED: 100-2,15,260; 100-4,12,90.3; 100-4,14,10

65410   Biopsy of cornea   2 T 80 50 ⬛

MED: 100-2,15,260; 100-4,12,90.3; 100-4,14,10

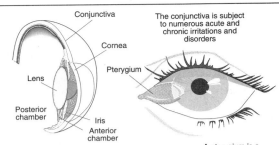

Conjunctiva

The conjunctiva is subject to numerous acute and chronic irritations and disorders

Cornea

Lens

Pterygium

Posterior chamber

Iris

Anterior chamber

Keratitis is an often painful inflammation of the cornea, the clear membrane covering the anterior segment of the eye

A pterygium is a wedge of excess tissue extending from the medial canthus toward the cornea

65420   Excision or transposition of pterygium; without graft   2 T 50 ⬛

MED: 100-2,15,260; 100-4,12,90.3; 100-4,14,10

65426   with graft   5 T 50 ⬛

MED: 100-2,15,260; 100-4,12,90.3; 100-4,14,10

REMOVAL OR DESTRUCTION

65430   Scraping of cornea, diagnostic, for smear and/or culture   S 50 ⬛

65435   Removal of corneal epithelium; with or without chemocauterization (abrasion, curettage)   T 50 ⬛

65436   with application of chelating agent (eg, EDTA)   T 50 ⬛

65450   Destruction of lesion of cornea by cryotherapy, photocoagulation or thermocauterization   S 50 ⬛

65600   Multiple punctures of anterior cornea (eg, for corneal erosion, tattoo)   T 50 ⬛

KERATOPLASTY

Corneal transplant procedures include the use of preserved or fresh grafts and the preparation of the donor material.

If refractive dermatoplasty procedures are performed in conjunction with this procedure, consult CPT codes 65760, 65765, and 65767.

If a diagnostic and treatment program is initiated for ophthalmological services, consult the Medicine and Ophthalmology sections of the CPT book and CPT codes 92002 and subsequent codes. Do not report 69990 in addition to codes 65091-68850 as the operating microscope is considered an inclusive component of these procedures.

65710   Keratoplasty (corneal transplant); lamellar   7 T 80 50 ⬛

MED: 100-2,15,260; 100-3,80.7; 100-4,12,90.3; 100-4,14,10

AMA: 2002,Oct,8

65730   penetrating (except in aphakia)   7 T 80 50 ⬛

MED: 100-2,15,260; 100-3,80.7; 100-4,12,90.3; 100-4,14,10

AMA: 2002,Oct,8

65750   penetrating (in aphakia)   7 T 80 50 ⬛

MED: 100-2,15,260; 100-3,80.7; 100-4,12,90.3; 100-4,14,10

AMA: 2002,Oct,8

65755   penetrating (in pseudophakia)   7 T 80 50 ⬛

MED: 100-2,15,260; 100-3,80.7; 100-4,12,90.3; 100-4,14,10

AMA: 2002,Oct,8

OTHER PROCEDURES

If a contact lens is fit for the treatment of a disease, consult CPT code 92070. If an unlisted procedure is performed on the cornea, consult CPT code 66999.

If a diagnostic and treatment program is initiated for ophthalmological services, consult the Medicine and Ophthalmology sections of the CPT book and CPT codes 92002 and subsequent codes. Do not report 69990 in addition to codes 65091-68850 as the operating microscope is considered an inclusive component of these procedures.

65760 Keratomileusis ⬜E

MED: 100-3,80.7

65765 Keratophakia ⬜E

MED: 100-3,80.7

65767 Epikeratoplasty ⬜E

MED: 100-3,80.7

65770 Keratoprosthesis ⑦ T 80 50 ⬜

MED: 100-2,15,260; 100-4,12,90.3; 100-4,14,10

65771 Radial keratotomy ⬜E

MED: 100-3,80.7

65772 Corneal relaxing incision for correction of surgically induced astigmatism ④ T 50 ⬜

MED: 100-2,15,260; 100-3,80.7; 100-4,12,90.3; 100-4,14,10

65775 Corneal wedge resection for correction of surgically induced astigmatism ④ T 50 ⬜

MED: 100-2,15,260; 100-3,80.7; 100-4,12,90.3; 100-4,14,10

65780 Ocular surface reconstruction; amniotic membrane transplantation ⑤ T 80 50 ⬜

65781 limbal stem cell allograft (eg, cadaveric or living donor) ⑤ T 80 50 ⬜

65782 limbal conjunctival autograft (includes obtaining graft) ⑤ T 80 50 ⬜

To report harvesting of conjunctival allograft, from a living donor, consult CPT 68371.

ANTERIOR CHAMBER

INCISION

If a diagnostic and treatment program is initiated for ophthalmological services, consult the Medicine and Ophthalmology sections of the CPT book and CPT codes 92002 and subsequent codes. Do not report 69990 in addition to codes 65091-68850 as the operating microscope is considered an inclusive component of these procedures.

65800 Paracentesis of anterior chamber of eye (separate procedure); with diagnostic aspiration of aqueous ① T 50 ⬜

MED: 100-2,15,260; 100-4,12,90.3; 100-4,14,10

65805 with therapeutic release of aqueous ① T 50 ⬜

MED: 100-2,15,260; 100-4,12,90.3; 100-4,14,10

65810 with removal of vitreous and/or discission of anterior hyaloid membrane, with or without air injection ③ T 50 ⬜

MED: 100-2,15,260; 100-4,12,90.3; 100-4,14,10

65815 with removal of blood, with or without irrigation and/or air injection ② T 50 ⬜

MED: 100-2,15,260; 100-4,12,90.3; 100-4,14,10

If an injection is needed, consult CPT codes 66020-66030.

To report removal of blood clot, consult CPT code 65930.

65820 Goniotomy ① T 80 50 ⑥③ ⬜

Barkan's operation

Use 66990 for use of ophthalmic endoscope with 65820.

65850 Trabeculotomy ab externo ④ T 50 ⬜

MED: 100-2,15,260; 100-4,12,90.3; 100-4,14,10

65855 Trabeculoplasty by laser surgery, one or more sessions (defined treatment series) T 50 ⬜

AMA: 1998,Mar,7

If re-treatment is necessary after several months because of disease progression, a new treatment or treatment series should be reported with a modifier to indicate lesser or greater complexity. If a trabeculectomy is performed, consult CPT code 66170.

65860 Severing adhesions of anterior segment, laser technique (separate procedure) T 80 50 ⬜

OTHER PROCEDURES

If a diagnostic and treatment program is initiated for ophthalmological services, consult the Medicine and Ophthalmology sections of the CPT book and CPT codes 92002 and subsequent codes. Do not report 69990 in addition to codes 65091-68850 as the operating microscope is considered an inclusive component of these procedures.

65865 Severing adhesions of anterior segment of eye, incisional technique (with or without injection of air or liquid) (separate procedure); goniosynechiae ① T 50 ⬜

MED: 100-2,15,260; 100-4,12,90.3; 100-4,14,10

If trabeculoplasty is performed by laser surgery, consult CPT code 65855.

65870 anterior synechiae, except goniosynechiae ④ T 50 ⬜

MED: 100-2,15,260; 100-4,12,90.3; 100-4,14,10

65875 posterior synechiae ④ T 50 ⬜

MED: 100-2,15,260; 100-4,12,90.3; 100-4,14,10

Use 66990 for use of ophthalmic endoscope with 65920.

65880 corneovitreal adhesions ④ T 50 ⬜

MED: 100-2,15,260; 100-4,12,90.3; 100-4,14,10

If laser surgery is performed, consult CPT code 66821.

65900 Removal of epithelial downgrowth, anterior chamber of eye ⑤ T 80 50 ⬜

MED: 100-2,15,260; 100-4,12,90.3; 100-4,14,10

65920 Removal of implanted material, anterior segment of eye ⑦ T 50 ⬜

MED: 100-2,15,260; 100-4,12,90.3; 100-4,14,10

Use code 66990 for use opthalmic endoscope with 65920.

65930 Removal of blood clot, anterior segment of eye ⑤ T 50 ⬜

MED: 100-2,15,260; 100-4,12,90.3; 100-4,14,10

66020 Injection, anterior chamber of eye (separate procedure); air or liquid ① T 50 ⬜

MED: 100-2,15,260; 100-4,12,90.3; 100-4,14,10

66030 medication ① T 50 ⬜

MED: 100-2,15,260; 100-4,12,90.3; 100-4,14,10

If the procedure performed on the anterior segment is unlisted, consult CPT code 66999.

ANTERIOR SCLERA

EXCISION

If a diagnostic and treatment program is initiated for ophthalmological services, consult the Medicine and Ophthalmology sections of the CPT book and CPT codes 92002 and subsequent codes. Do not report 69990 in addition to codes 65091-68850 as the operating microscope is considered an inclusive component of these procedures.

If an intraocular foreign body is removed, consult CPT code 65235. If an operation is performed on the posterior sclera, consult CPT codes 67250 and 67255.

66130   **Excision of lesion, sclera**   7 T 80 50

MED: 100-2,15,260; 100-4,12,90.3; 100-4,14,10

66150   **Fistulization of sclera for glaucoma; trephination with iridectomy**   4 T 50

MED: 100-2,15,260; 100-4,12,90.3; 100-4,14,10

66155   **thermocauterization with iridectomy**   4 T 50

MED: 100-2,15,260; 100-4,12,90.3; 100-4,14,10

66160   **sclerectomy with punch or scissors, with iridectomy**   2 T 50

MED: 100-2,15,260; 100-4,12,90.3; 100-4,14,10

Knapp's operation

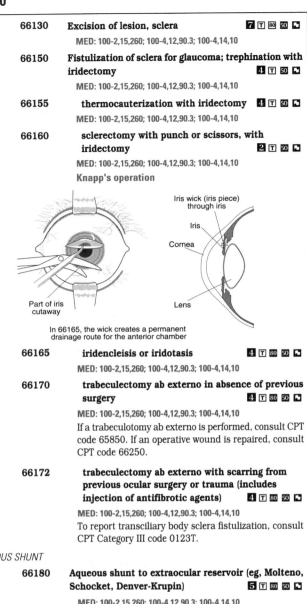

Iris wick (iris piece) through iris

Iris

Cornea

Lens

Part of iris cutaway

In 66165, the wick creates a permanent drainage route for the anterior chamber

66165   **iridencleisis or iridotasis**   4 T 80 50

MED: 100-2,15,260; 100-4,12,90.3; 100-4,14,10

66170   **trabeculectomy ab externo in absence of previous surgery**   4 T 80 50

MED: 100-2,15,260; 100-4,12,90.3; 100-4,14,10

If a trabeculotomy ab externo is performed, consult CPT code 65850. If an operative wound is repaired, consult CPT code 66250.

66172   **trabeculectomy ab externo with scarring from previous ocular surgery or trauma (includes injection of antifibrotic agents)**   4 T 80 50

MED: 100-2,15,260; 100-4,12,90.3; 100-4,14,10

To report transciliary body sclera fistulization, consult CPT Category III code 0123T.

AQUEOUS SHUNT

66180   **Aqueous shunt to extraocular reservoir (eg, Molteno, Schocket, Denver-Krupin)**   5 T 80 50

MED: 100-2,15,260; 100-4,12,90.3; 100-4,14,10

66185   **Revision of aqueous shunt to extraocular reservoir**   2 T 80 50

MED: 100-2,15,260; 100-4,12,90.3; 100-4,14,10

If an implanted shunt is removed, consult CPT code 67120.

REPAIR OR REVISION

If a diagnostic and treatment program is initiated for ophthalmological services, consult the Medicine and Ophthalmology sections of the CPT book and CPT codes 92002 and subsequent codes. Do not report 69990 in addition to codes 65091-68850 as the operating microscope is considered an inclusive component of these procedures.

If scleral procedures are performed in retinal surgery, consult CPT codes 67101 and subsequent codes.

66220   **Repair of scleral staphyloma; without graft**   3 T 80 50

MED: 100-2,15,260; 100-4,12,90.3; 100-4,14,10

66225   **with graft**   4 T 80 50

MED: 100-2,15,260; 100-4,12,90.3; 100-4,14,10

If scleral reinforcement is needed, consult CPT codes 67250 and 67255.

66250   **Revision or repair of operative wound of anterior segment, any type, early or late, major or minor procedure**   2 T 50

MED: 100-2,15,260; 100-4,12,90.3; 100-4,14,10

To report unlisted procedures on the anterior sclera, consult 66999.

IRIS, CILIARY BODY

INCISION

If a diagnostic and treatment program is initiated for ophthalmological services, consult the Medicine and Ophthalmology sections of the CPT book and CPT codes 92002 and subsequent codes. Do not report 69990 in addition to codes 65091-68850 as the operating microscope is considered an inclusive component of these procedures.

If an "iridotomy" is performed by photocoagulation, consult CPT code 66761.

66500   **Iridotomy by stab incision (separate procedure); except transfixion**   1 T 50

MED: 100-2,15,260; 100-4,12,90.3; 100-4,14,10

66505   **with transfixion as for iris bombe**   1 T 50

MED: 100-2,15,260; 100-4,12,90.3; 100-4,14,10

EXCISION

If a diagnostic and treatment program is initiated for ophthalmological services, consult the Medicine and Ophthalmology sections of the CPT book and CPT codes 92002 and subsequent codes. Do not report 69990 in addition to codes 65091-68850 as the operating microscope is considered an inclusive component of these procedures.

If "coreoplasty" is performed by photocoagulation, consult CPT code 66762.

66600   **Iridectomy, with corneoscleral or corneal section; for removal of lesion**   3 T 50

MED: 100-2,15,260; 100-4,12,90.3; 100-4,14,10

66605   **with cyclectomy**   3 T 50

MED: 100-2,15,260; 100-4,12,90.3; 100-4,14,10

66625   **peripheral for glaucoma (separate procedure)**   3 T 50

MED: 100-2,15,260; 100-4,12,90.3; 100-4,14,10

66630   **sector for glaucoma (separate procedure)**   3 T 50

MED: 100-2,15,260; 100-4,12,90.3; 100-4,14,10

66635   **optical (separate procedure)**   3 T 50

MED: 100-2,15,260; 100-4,12,90.3; 100-4,14,10

REPAIR

If a diagnostic and treatment program is initiated for ophthalmological services, consult the Medicine and Ophthalmology sections of the CPT book and CPT codes 92002 and subsequent codes. Do not report 69990 in addition to codes 65091-68850 as the operating microscope is considered an inclusive component of these procedures.

If uveal tissue is repositioned or resected because of a perforating wound of the cornea or the sclera, consult CPT code 65285.

66680   **Repair of iris, ciliary body (as for iridodialysis)**   3 T 50

MED: 100-2,15,260; 100-4,12,90.3; 100-4,14,10

66682   **Suture of iris, ciliary body (separate procedure) with retrieval of suture through small incision (eg, McCannel suture)**   2 T 50

MED: 100-2,15,260; 100-4,12,90.3; 100-4,14,10

DESTRUCTION

If an iridectomy is performed for removal of a lesion, with corneoscleral or corneal section, consult CPT codes 66600 and 66605. If an epithelial downgrowth is removed from the anterior chamber of the eye, consult CPT code 65900. If a procedure performed on the iris or ciliary body is unlisted, consult CPT code 66999.

26 Professional Component Only   80/80 Assist-at-Surgery Allowed/With Documentation   Unlisted   Not Covered

TC Technical Component Only   MED: Pub 100/NCD References AMA: CPT Assistant References   1 - 9 ASC Group   ♂ Male Only   ♀ Female Only

238 — CPT Expert   CPT only © 2006 American Medical Association. All Rights Reserved. *(Black Ink)*   © 2006 Ingenix *(Blue Ink)*

66700 Ciliary body destruction; diathermy ② T 80 50 🔲

   MED: 100-2,15,260; 100-4,12,90.3; 100-4,14,10

   Heine's operation

66710   cyclophotocoagulation, transscleral ② T 50 🔲

   MED: 100-2,15,260; 100-4,12,90.3; 100-4,14,10

66711   cyclophotocoagulation, endoscopic ② T 50 🔲

   Code 66711 cannot be reported with CPT code 66990.

⊙ 66720   cryotherapy ② T 50 🔲

   MED: 100-2,15,260; 100-4,12,90.3; 100-4,14,10

66740   cyclodialysis ② T 50 🔲

   MED: 100-2,15,260; 100-4,12,90.3; 100-4,14,10

66761 Iridotomy/iridectomy by laser surgery (eg, for glaucoma) (one or more sessions) T 50 🔲

   AMA: 1998,Mar,7

66762 Iridoplasty by photocoagulation (one or more sessions) (eg, for improvement of vision, for widening of anterior chamber angle) T 50 🔲

   AMA: 1998,Mar,7

66770 Destruction of cyst or lesion iris or ciliary body (nonexcisional procedure) T 50 🔲

LENS

INCISION

If a diagnostic and treatment program is initiated for ophthalmological services, consult the Medicine and Ophthalmology sections of the CPT book and CPT codes 92002 and subsequent codes. Do not report 69990 in addition to codes 65091-68850 as the operating microscope is considered an inclusive component of these procedures.

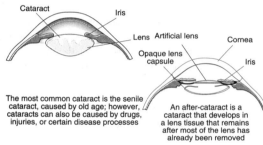

A cataract is a milky opacity on the normally clear lens of the eye; it obscures vision

Cataract   Iris

Lens   Artificial lens   Cornea

Opaque lens capsule   Iris

The most common cataract is the senile cataract, caused by old age; however, cataracts can also be caused by drugs, injuries, or certain disease processes

An after-cataract is a cataract that develops in a lens tissue that remains after most of the lens has already been removed

66820 Discission of secondary membranous cataract (opacified posterior lens capsule and/or anterior hyaloid); stab incision technique (Ziegler or Wheeler knife) T 50 🔲

66821   laser surgery (eg, YAG laser) (one or more stages) ② T 50 🔲

   MED: 100-2,15,260; 100-4,12,90.3; 100-4,14,10

66825 Repositioning of intraocular lens prosthesis, requiring an incision (separate procedure) ④ T 80 50 🔲

   MED: 100-2,15,260; 100-4,12,90.3; 100-4,14,10

REMOVAL CATARACT

If a diagnostic and treatment program is initiated for ophthalmological services, consult the Medicine and Ophthalmology sections of the CPT book and CPT codes 92002 and subsequent codes. Do not report 69990 in addition to codes 65091-68850 as the operating microscope is considered an inclusive component of these procedures.

Anterior and/or posterior capsulotomy, iridotomy, iridectomy, lateral canthotomy, use of viscoelastic agents, enzymatic zonulysis, or the use of other pharmacologic agents, subconjunctival or sub-tenon injections, are all included as part of the CPT code(s) for extraction of lens.

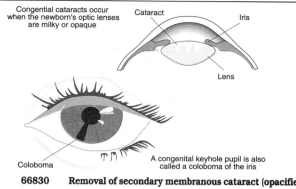

Congential cataracts occur when the newborn's optic lenses are milky or opaque

Cataract   Iris

Lens

Coloboma

A congenital keyhole pupil is also called a coloboma of the iris

66830 Removal of secondary membranous cataract (opacified posterior lens capsule and/or anterior hyaloid) with corneo-scleral section, with or without iridectomy (iridocapsulotomy, iridocapsulectomy) ④ T 50 🔲

   MED: 100-2,15,260; 100-3,80.10; 100-3,80.11; 100-4,12,90.3; 100-4,14,10

   If implanted material from the anterior segment is removed, consult CPT code 65920.

   Daviel's operation

66840 Removal of lens material; aspiration technique, one or more stages ④ T 50 🔲

   MED: 100-2,15,260; 100-3,80.10; 100-3,80.11; 100-4,12,90.3; 100-4,14,10

   AMA: 1992,Fall,4

   If implanted material from the anterior segment is removed, consult CPT code 65920.

   Fukala's operation

66850   phacofragmentation technique (mechanical or ultrasonic) (eg, phacoemulsification), with aspiration ⑦ T 50 🔲

   MED: 100-2,15,260; 100-3,80.10; 100-3,80.11; 100-4,12,90.3; 100-4,14,10

   AMA: 1992,Fall,6

66852   pars plana approach, with or without vitrectomy ④ T 80 50 🔲

   MED: 100-2,15,260; 100-3,80.10; 100-3,80.11; 100-4,12,90.3; 100-4,14,10

   AMA: 1992,Fall,8

66920   intracapsular ④ T 80 50 🔲

   MED: 100-2,15,260; 100-3,80.10; 100-3,80.11; 100-4,12,90.3; 100-4,14,10

   AMA: 1992,Fall,8

66930   intracapsular, for dislocated lens ⑤ T 80 50 🔲

   MED: 100-2,15,260; 100-3,80.10; 100-3,80.11; 100-4,12,90.3; 100-4,14,10

   AMA: 1992,Fall,8

66940   extracapsular (other than 66840, 66850, 66852) ⑤ T 80 50 🔲

   MED: 100-2,15,260; 100-3,80.10; 100-3,80.11; 100-4,12,90.3; 100-4,14,10

   AMA: 1992,Fall,4

   To report removal of intralenticular foreign body without lens extraction, consult CPT code 65235. To report repair of operative wound, consult CPT code 66250.

⊛ Modifier 63 Exempt Code   ⊙ Conscious Sedation   ＋ CPT Add-on Code   ⃠ Modifier 51 Exempt Code   ● New Code   ▲ Revised Code

Ⓜ Maternity Edit   Ⓐ Age Edit   Ⓐ-Ⓥ APC Status Indicators   🔲 CCI Comprehensive Code   50 Bilateral Procedure

66982 Extracapsular cataract removal with insertion of intraocular lens prosthesis (one stage procedure), manual or mechanical technique (eg, irrigation and aspiration or phacoemulsification), complex, requiring devices or techniques not generally used in routine cataract surgery (eg, iris expansion device, suture support for intraocular lens, or primary posterior capsulorrhexis) or performed on patients in the amblyogenic developmental stage **8** T 50 ▣

MED: 100-2,15,260; 100-3,80.10; 100-3,80.11; 100-4,12,90.3; 100-4,14,10
AMA: 2001,Feb,7

66983 Intracapsular cataract extraction with insertion of intraocular lens prosthesis (one stage procedure) **8** T 50 ▣

MED: 100-2,15,260; 100-3,80.10; 100-3,80.11; 100-4,12,90.3; 100-4,14,10
AMA: 1992,Fall,5, 8

66984 Extracapsular cataract removal with insertion of intraocular lens prosthesis (one stage procedure), manual or mechanical technique (eg, irrigation and aspiration or phacoemulsification) **8** T 50 ▣

MED: 100-2,15,260; 100-3,80.10; 100-3,80.11; 100-4,12,90.3; 100-4,14,10
AMA: 2001,Feb,7; 1992,Fall,5, 8
To report complex cataract removal, consult CPT code 66982.

66985 Insertion of intraocular lens prosthesis (secondary implant), not associated with concurrent cataract removal **6** T 50 ▣

MED: 100-2,15,260; 100-3,80.10; 100-3,80.11; 100-4,12,90.3; 100-4,14,10
If an implant is performed at the time of a concurrent cataract surgery, consult CPT code 66982, 66983 or 66984. If a secondary fixation (separate procedure) is performed, consult CPT code 66682.

To report intraocular lens prosthesis supplied by physician, consult CPT code 99070. To report removal of implant material from anterior segment, consult CPT code 65920. To report ultrasonic determination of intraocular lens power, consult CPT code 76519.

Use code 66990 for use of opthalmic endoscpe with 66985.

66986 Exchange of intraocular lens **6** T 50 ▣

MED: 100-2,15,260; 100-3,80.10; 100-3,80.11; 100-4,12,90.3; 100-4,14,10
Use code 66990 for use of opthalmic endoscope with 66986.

+ 66990 Use of ophthalmic endoscope (List separately in addition to code for primary procedure) N ▣

MED: 100-3,80.10; 100-3,80.11
Note that 66990 is an add-on code and must be used in conjunction with 65820, 65875, 65920, 66985, 66986, 67036, 67038, 67039, 67040, and 67112.

OTHER PROCEDURES

66999 Unlisted procedure, anterior segment of eye T 80 50

MED: 100-4,4,180.3

POSTERIOR SEGMENT

If a diagnostic and treatment program is initiated for ophthalmological services, consult the Medicine and Ophthalmology sections of the CPT book and CPT codes 92002 and subsequent codes. Do not report 69990 in addition to codes 65091-68850 as the operating microscope is considered an inclusive component of these procedures.

VITREOUS

67005 Removal of vitreous, anterior approach (open sky technique or limbal incision); partial removal **4** T 50 ▣

MED: 100-2,15,260; 100-3,80.11; 100-4,12,90.3; 100-4,14,10
AMA: 1992,Fall,4

67010 subtotal removal with mechanical vitrectomy **4** T 80 50 ▣

MED: 100-2,15,260; 100-3,80.11; 100-4,12,90.3; 100-4,14,10
AMA: 1992,Fall,4
If a procedure performed on the vitreous is unlisted, consult CPT code 67299.

If paracentesis is performed on the anterior chamber of the eye, with removal of the vitreous, consult CPT code 65810. If corneovitreal adhesions are removed, consult CPT code 65880.

67015 Aspiration or release of vitreous, subretinal or choroidal fluid, pars plana approach (posterior sclerotomy) **1** T 50 ▣

MED: 100-2,15,260; 100-4,12,90.3; 100-4,14,10

67025 Injection of vitreous substitute, pars plana or limbal approach, (fluid-gas exchange), with or without aspiration (separate procedure) **1** T 50 ▣

MED: 100-2,15,260; 100-4,12,90.3; 100-4,14,10

67027 Implantation of intravitreal drug delivery system (eg, ganciclovir implant), includes concomitant removal of vitreous **4** T 80 50 ▣

MED: 100-2,15,260; 100-3,80.11; 100-4,12,90.3; 100-4,14,10
AMA: 1998,Nov,1; 1997,Nov,23
If the implant is removed, consult CPT code 67121.

67028 Intravitreal injection of a pharmacologic agent (separate procedure) T 50 ▣

67030 Discission of vitreous strands (without removal), pars plana approach **1** T 80 50 ▣

MED: 100-2,15,260; 100-4,12,90.3; 100-4,14,10

67031 Severing of vitreous strands, vitreous face adhesions, sheets, membranes or opacities, laser surgery (one or more stages) **2** T 50 ▣

MED: 100-2,15,260; 100-4,12,90.3; 100-4,14,10

67036 Vitrectomy, mechanical, pars plana approach; **4** T 80 50 ▣

MED: 100-2,15,260; 100-3,80.11; 100-4,12,90.3; 100-4,14,10
AMA: 1992,Fall,6

67038 with epiretinal membrane stripping **5** T 80 50 ▣

MED: 100-2,15,260; 100-3,80.11; 100-4,12,90.3; 100-4,14,10

67039 with focal endolaser photocoagulation **7** T 80 50 ▣

MED: 100-2,15,260; 100-3,80.11; 100-4,12,90.3; 100-4,14,10

67040 with endolaser panretinal photocoagulation **7** T 80 50 ▣

MED: 100-2,15,260; 100-3,80.11; 100-4,12,90.3; 100-4,14,10
If an associated lensectomy is performed, consult CPT code 66850. If the retinal detachment surgery includes a vitrectomy, consult CPT code 67108. If a foreign body is removed, consult CPT codes 65260 and 65265.

To report use of ophthalmic endoscope in conjunction with codes 67036, 67038, 67039 or 67040, consult CPT code 66990.

26 Professional Component Only
TC Technical Component Only
80/80 Assist-at-Surgery Allowed/With Documentation
MED: Pub 100/NCD References AMA: CPT Assistant References
Unlisted
1-9 ASC Group ♂ Male Only
Not Covered
♀ Female Only

240 — CPT Expert   CPT only © 2006 American Medical Association. All Rights Reserved. *(Black Ink)*   © 2006 Ingenix *(Blue Ink)*

RETINA OR CHOROID

REPAIR

If a diagnostic and treatment program is initiated for ophthalmological services, consult the Medicine and Ophthalmology sections of CPT and CPT code 92002 and subsequent codes. Do not report 69990 in addition to codes 65091-68850 as the operating microscope is considered an inclusive component of these procedures.

If diathermy, cryotherapy, and/or photocoagulation are combined, report the procedure under the principal modality used.

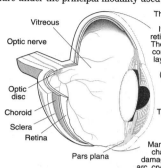

Vitreous
Optic nerve
Optic disc
Choroid
Sclera
Retina
Pars plana
Posterior chamber

The choroid is the vascular layer of the posterior chamber. It provides nourishment to the retina, to which it is firmly attached. The retina is a delicate membrane containing a light-sensitive neural layer fed by the optic nerve. This neural layer can delaminate (known as a detached retina). The optic nerve enters the chamber at the optic disc where the fibers spread throughout the retina. The vitreous is the transparent gel filling the interior of the posterior chamber.

Many surgeries to the posterior chamber center on repairing damage to the retina. Laser, zenon arc, cryoprobe, and diathermal probe are common techniques. Access to the retina is often via the pars plana.

67101 **Repair of retinal detachment, one or more sessions; cryotherapy or diathermy, with or without drainage of subretinal fluid** T 50

    AMA: 1998,Mar,7

67105 **photocoagulation, with or without drainage of subretinal fluid** T 50

    AMA: 1998,Mar,7

67107 **Repair of retinal detachment; scleral buckling (such as lamellar scleral dissection, imbrication or encircling procedure), with or without implant, with or without cryotherapy, photocoagulation, and drainage of subretinal fluid** 5 T 80 50

    MED: 100-2,15,260; 100-3,140.5; 100-4,12,90.3; 100-4,14,10
    Gonin's operation

67108 **with vitrectomy, any method, with or without air or gas tamponade, focal endolaser photocoagulation, cryotherapy, drainage of subretinal fluid, scleral buckling, and/or removal of lens by same technique** 7 T 80 50

    MED: 100-2,15,260; 100-3,80.11; 100-3,140.5; 100-4,12,90.3; 100-4,14,10

67110 **by injection of air or other gas (eg, pneumatic retinopexy)** T 50

The retina may detach due to injury, shrinkage of the vitreous, or as a result of a hole in the retina caused by another disorder

Lens
Vitreous
Iris
Choroid
Area of detachment
Cornea
Retina
Sclera

Nearsighted people are more susceptible to retinal detachment

In retinal detachment, the photo-sensitive retinal layer of the eye separates from the blood-rich choroid layer; this can damage the retina and lead to blindness if not repaired

67112 **by scleral buckling or vitrectomy, on patient having previous ipsilateral retinal detachment repair(s) using scleral buckling or vitrectomy techniques** 7 T 80 50

    MED: 100-2,15,260; 100-4,12,90.3; 100-4,14,10
    If subretinal or subchoroidal fluid is aspirated or drained, consult CPT code 67015.

    Use code 66990 for use of opthalmic endoscope with 67112.

67115 **Release of encircling material (posterior segment)** 2 T 50

    MED: 100-2,15,260; 100-4,12,90.3; 100-4,14,10

67120 **Removal of implanted material, posterior segment; extraocular** 2 T 50

    MED: 100-2,15,260; 100-4,12,90.3; 100-4,14,10

67121 **intraocular** 2 T 80 50

    MED: 100-2,15,260; 100-4,12,90.3; 100-4,14,10
    AMA: 1998,Nov,19; 1997,Nov,23
    To report removal from anterior segment, consult CPT code 65920.

    To report removal of foreign body, consult CPT codes 65260, 65265.

PROPHYLAXIS

If a diagnostic and treatment program is initiated for ophthalmological services, consult the Medicine and Ophthalmology sections of the CPT book and CPT codes 92002 and subsequent codes. Do not report 69990 in addition to codes 65091-68850 as the operating microscope is considered an inclusive component of these procedures.

Codes 67141-67145 are usually provided in multiple sessions or groups of sessions. These codes include all sessions in a defined treatment period.

67141 **Prophylaxis of retinal detachment (eg, retinal break, lattice degeneration) without drainage, one or more sessions; cryotherapy, diathermy** 2 T 50

    MED: 100-2,15,260; 100-4,12,90.3; 100-4,14,10
    AMA: 1998,Mar,7

67145 **photocoagulation (laser or xenon arc)** T 50

    MED: 100-3,140.5
    AMA: 1998,Mar,7; 1992,Fall,4

DESTRUCTION

If a diagnostic and treatment program is initiated for ophthalmological services, consult the Medicine and Ophthalmology sections of the CPT book and CPT codes 92002 and subsequent codes. Do not report 69990 in addition to codes 65091-68850 as the operating microscope is considered an inclusive component of these procedures.

If a procedure performed on the retina is unlisted, consult CPT code 67299.

67208 **Destruction of localized lesion of retina (eg, macular edema, tumors), one or more sessions; cryotherapy, diathermy** T 50

    AMA: 1998,Nov,19; 1998,Mar,7

67210 **photocoagulation** T 50

    MED: 100-3,140.5
    AMA: 1998,Nov,19; 1998,Mar,7

67218 **radiation by implantation of source (includes removal of source)** 5 T 50

    MED: 100-2,15,260; 100-4,12,90.3; 100-4,14,10
    AMA: 1998,Mar,7

67220 Destruction of localized lesion of choroid (eg, choroidal neovascularization); photocoagulation (eg, laser), one or more sessions   T 50 ⬛

MED: 100-3,140.5

AMA: 2001,Feb,7; 1999,Nov,39; 1998,Nov,19

To report destruction of macular drusen, photocoagulation, consult CPT Category III code 0017T.

For destruction of localized lesion of choroid by transpupillary thermotherapy, consult CPT Category III code 0016T.

67221 photodynamic therapy (includes intravenous infusion)   T ⬛

MED: 100-3,80.2; 100-3,80.3

AMA: 2002,Jun,10; 2001,Sep,10; 2001,Feb,7

+ 67225 photodynamic therapy, second eye, at single session (List separately in addition to code for primary eye treatment)   T ⬛

MED: 100-3,80.3

AMA: 2002,Jun,10

Note that 67225 is an add-on code and must be used in conjunction with 67221.

67227 Destruction of extensive or progressive retinopathy (eg, diabetic retinopathy), one or more sessions; cryotherapy, diathermy   1 T 50 ⬛

MED: 100-2,15,260; 100-4,12,90.3; 100-4,14,10

AMA: 1998,Mar,7

67228 photocoagulation (laser or xenon arc)   T 50 ⬛

MED: 100-3,140.5

AMA: 1998,Mar,7

POSTERIOR SCLERA

REPAIR

If a diagnostic and treatment program is initiated for ophthalmological services, consult the Medicine and Ophthalmology sections of the CPT book and CPT codes 92002 and subsequent codes. Do not report 69990 in addition to codes 65091-68850 as the operating microscope is considered an inclusive component of these procedures.

If a procedure performed on the retina is unlisted, consult CPT code 67299.

To report excision of a lesion of the sclera, consult CPT code 66130.

67250 Scleral reinforcement (separate procedure); without graft   3 T 50 ⬛

MED: 100-2,15,260; 100-4,12,90.3; 100-4,14,10

67255 with graft   3 T 80 50 ⬛

MED: 100-2,15,260; 100-4,12,90.3; 100-4,14,10

If a scleral staphyloma is repaired, consult CPT codes 66220 and 66225.

OTHER PROCEDURES

67299 Unlisted procedure, posterior segment   T 80 50

MED: 100-4,4,180.3

OCULAR ADNEXA

EXTRAOCULAR MUSCLES

If a diagnostic and treatment program is initiated for ophthalmological services, consult the Medicine and Ophthalmology sections of the CPT book and CPT codes 92002 and subsequent codes. Do not report 69990 in addition to codes 65091-68850 as the operating microscope is considered an inclusive component of these procedures.

If adjustable sutures are used, consult CPT code 67335 in addition to primary procedure (67311-67334) used that reflects the number of muscles operated on.

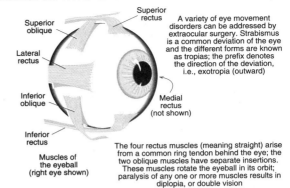

Superior oblique

Superior rectus

Superior oblique

Lateral rectus

Inferior oblique

Inferior rectus

Medial rectus (not shown)

Muscles of the eyeball (right eye shown)

A variety of eye movement disorders can be addressed by extraocular surgery. Strabismus is a common deviation of the eye and the different forms are known as tropias; the prefix denotes the direction of the deviation, i.e., exotropia (outward)

The four rectus muscles (meaning straight) arise from a common ring tendon behind the eye; the two oblique muscles have separate insertions. These muscles rotate the eyeball in its orbit; paralysis of any one or more muscles results in diplopia, or double vision

67311 Strabismus surgery, recession or resection procedure; one horizontal muscle   3 T 50 ⬛

MED: 100-2,15,260; 100-4,12,90.3; 100-4,14,10

AMA: 2002,Sep,10; 1998,Nov,1; 1997,Mar,5; 1993,Summer,20

67312 two horizontal muscles   4 T 50 ⬛

MED: 100-2,15,260; 100-4,12,90.3; 100-4,14,10

AMA: 1997,Mar,5; 1993,Summer,20

67314 one vertical muscle (excluding superior oblique)   4 T 50 ⬛

MED: 100-2,15,260; 100-4,12,90.3; 100-4,14,10

AMA: 1997,Mar,5; 1993,Summer,20

67316 two or more vertical muscles (excluding superior oblique)   4 T 80 50 ⬛

MED: 100-2,15,260; 100-4,12,90.3; 100-4,14,10

AMA: 1997,Mar,5; 1993,Summer,20

67318 Strabismus surgery, any procedure, superior oblique muscle   4 T 50 ⬛

MED: 100-2,15,260; 100-4,12,90.3; 100-4,14,10

AMA: 1998,Nov,19; 1997,Mar,5; 1993,Summer,20

+ 67320 Transposition procedure (eg, for paretic extraocular muscle), any extraocular muscle (specify) (List separately in addition to code for primary procedure)   4 T ⬛

MED: 100-2,15,260; 100-4,12,90.3; 100-4,14,10

AMA: 1997,Mar,5; 1993,Summer,20

Note that 67320 is an add-on code and must be used in conjunction with 67311-67318.

+ 67331 Strabismus surgery on patient with previous eye surgery or injury that did not involve the extraocular muscles (List separately in addition to code for primary procedure)   4 T ⬛

MED: 100-2,15,260; 100-4,12,90.3; 100-4,14,10

AMA: 1997,Mar,5; 1993,Summer,20

Note that 67331 is an add-on code and must be used in conjunction with 67311-67318.

+ 67332 Strabismus surgery on patient with scarring of extraocular muscles (eg, prior ocular injury, strabismus or retinal detachment surgery) or restrictive myopathy (eg, dysthyroid ophthalmopathy) (List separately in addition to code for primary procedure)   4 T 80 ⬛

MED: 100-2,15,260; 100-4,12,90.3; 100-4,14,10

AMA: 1997,Mar,5; 1993,Summer,20

Note that 67332 is an add-on code and must be used in conjunction with 67311-67318.

26 Professional Component Only   80/80 Assist-at-Surgery Allowed/With Documentation   Unlisted   Not Covered

TC Technical Component Only   **MED:** Pub 100/NCD References   **AMA:** CPT Assistant References   1-9 ASC Group   ♂ Male Only   ♀ Female Only

242 — CPT Expert   CPT only © 2006 American Medical Association. All Rights Reserved. *(Black Ink)*   © *2006 Ingenix (Blue Ink)*

+ **67334** Strabismus surgery by posterior fixation suture technique, with or without muscle recession (List separately in addition to code for primary procedure) `4` `T` `□`

MED: 100-2,15,260; 100-4,12,90.3; 100-4,14,10

AMA: 1997,Mar,5; 1993,Summer,20

Note that 67334 is an add-on code and must be used in conjunction with 67311-67318.

+ **67335** Placement of adjustable suture(s) during strabismus surgery, including postoperative adjustment(s) of suture(s) (List separately in addition to code for specific strabismus surgery) `4` `T` `□`

MED: 100-2,15,260; 100-4,12,90.3; 100-4,14,10

AMA: 1997,Mar,5; 1993,Summer,20

Note that 67335 is an add-on code and must be used in conjunction with codes 67311-67334.

+ **67340** Strabismus surgery involving exploration and/or repair of detached extraocular muscle(s) (List separately in addition to code for primary procedure) `4` `T` `80` `□`

MED: 100-2,15,260; 100-4,12,90.3; 100-4,14,10

AMA: 1997,Mar,5; 1993,Summer,20

Note that 67340 is an add-on code and must be used in conjunction with 67311-67334.

Hummelshein operation

67343 Release of extensive scar tissue without detaching extraocular muscle (separate procedure) `7` `T` `80` `50` `□`

AMA: 1997,Mar,5; 1993,Summer,20

Report 67343 in conjunction with 67311-67340, when performed other than on the affected muscle.

67345 Chemodenervation of extraocular muscle `T` `50` `□`

AMA: 1997,Mar,5; 1993,Summer,20

If chemodenervation is performed for blepharospasm and other neurological disorders, consult CPT codes 64612 and 64613.

● **67346** Biopsy of extraocular muscle `1` `T`

Use code 65290 for repair of wound, extraocular muscle, tendon or Tenon's capsule.

OTHER PROCEDURES

~~67350~~ ~~Biopsy of extraocular muscle~~

Use 67346.

67399 Unlisted procedure, ocular muscle `T` `80` `50`

MED: 100-4,4,180.3

ORBIT

EXPLORATION, EXCISION, DECOMPRESSION

If a diagnostic and treatment program is initiated for ophthalmological services, consult the Medicine and Ophthalmology sections of the CPT book and CPT codes 92002 and subsequent codes. Do not report 69990 in addition to codes 65091-68850 as the operating microscope is considered an inclusive component of these procedures.

If an orbitotomy is performed through a transcranial approach, consult CPT codes 61330-61334. If an orbital implant is inserted, consult CPT codes 67550 and 67560. If an eyeball is removed or repaired after removal, consult CPT codes 65091-65175.

67400 Orbitotomy without bone flap (frontal or transconjunctival approach); for exploration, with or without biopsy `3` `T` `80` `50` `□`

MED: 100-2,15,260; 100-4,12,90.3; 100-4,14,10

67405 with drainage only `4` `T` `80` `50` `□`

MED: 100-2,15,260; 100-4,12,90.3; 100-4,14,10

67412 with removal of lesion `5` `T` `80` `50` `□`

MED: 100-2,15,260; 100-4,12,90.3; 100-4,14,10

67413 with removal of foreign body `5` `T` `80` `50` `□`

MED: 100-2,15,260; 100-4,12,90.3; 100-4,14,10

67414 with removal of bone for decompression `T` `80` `50` `□`

AMA: 1999,Jul,10

67415 Fine needle aspiration of orbital contents `1` `T` `80` `50` `□`

MED: 100-2,15,260; 100-4,12,90.3; 100-4,14,10

If exenteration, enucleation, and repair are performed, consult CPT codes 65101 and subsequent codes. If optic nerve decompression is performed, consult CPT code 67570.

67420 Orbitotomy with bone flap or window, lateral approach (eg, Kroenlein); with removal of lesion `5` `T` `80` `50` `□`

MED: 100-2,15,260; 100-4,12,90.3; 100-4,14,10

67430 with removal of foreign body `5` `T` `80` `50` `□`

MED: 100-2,15,260; 100-4,12,90.3; 100-4,14,10

67440 with drainage `5` `T` `80` `50` `□`

MED: 100-2,15,260; 100-4,12,90.3; 100-4,14,10

67445 with removal of bone for decompression `5` `T` `80` `50` `□`

If optic nerve sheath decompression is performed, consult CPT codes 67570.

67450 for exploration, with or without biopsy `5` `T` `80` `50` `□`

MED: 100-2,15,260; 100-4,12,90.3; 100-4,14,10

OTHER PROCEDURES

If a diagnostic and treatment program is initiated for ophthalmological services, consult the Medicine and Ophthalmology sections of the CPT book and CPT codes 92002 and subsequent codes. Do not report 69990 in addition to codes 65091-68850 as the operating microscope is considered an inclusive component of these procedures.

67500 Retrobulbar injection; medication (separate procedure, does not include supply of medication) `S` `50` `□`

67505 alcohol `T` `50` `□`

67515 Injection of medication or other substance into Tenon's capsule `T` `50` `□`

If a subconjunctival injection is needed, consult CPT code 68200.

67550 Orbital implant (implant outside muscle cone); insertion `4` `T` `50` `□`

MED: 100-2,15,260; 100-4,12,90.3; 100-4,14,10

If an ocular implant is needed (implant inside muscle cone), consult CPT codes 65093-65105 and 65130-65175. If treatment is needed for fractures of the malar area or orbit, consult CPT codes 21355 et seq.

67560 removal or revision `2` `T` `80` `50` `□`

MED: 100-2,15,260; 100-4,12,90.3; 100-4,14,10

If an ocular implant is needed (implant inside muscle cone), consult CPT codes 65093-65105 and 65130-65175. If treatment is needed for fractures of the malar area or orbit, consult CPT codes 21355 et seq.

67570 Optic nerve decompression (eg, incision or fenestration of optic nerve sheath) `4` `T` `80` `50` `□`

67599 Unlisted procedure, orbit `T` `80` `50`

MED: 100-4,4,180.3

⊕ Modifier 63 Exempt Code	⊙ Conscious Sedation	+ CPT Add-on Code	⊘ Modifier 51 Exempt Code	● New Code	▲ Revised Code

`M` Maternity Edit 　`A` Age Edit 　`A`-`Y` APC Status Indicators 　`□` CCI Comprehensive Code 　`50` Bilateral Procedure

EYELIDS

INCISION

67700	Blepharotomy, drainage of abscess, eyelid	T 50 ⟲
67710	Severing of tarsorrhaphy	T 50 ⟲
67715	Canthotomy (separate procedure)	❶ T 50 ⟲

MED: 100-2,15,260; 100-4,12,90.3; 100-4,14,10

If canthoplasty is performed, consult CPT code 67950. If a division of the symblepharon is performed, consult CPT code 68340.

EXCISION, DESTRUCTION

These codes include the lid margin, palpebral conjunctiva, and tarsus.

If a diagnostic and treatment program is initiated for ophthalmological services, consult the Medicine and Ophthalmology sections of the CPT book and CPT codes 92002 and subsequent codes. Do not report 69990 in addition to codes 65091-68850 as the operating microscope is considered an inclusive component of these procedures.

If a lesion involving mainly the skin of the eyelid is removed, consult CPT codes 11310-11313, 11400-11446, 11640-11646, and 17000-17004.

To report repair of wounds, blepharoplasty, grafts and reconstructive surgery, consult CPT codes 67930-67975.

67800	Excision of chalazion; single	T ⟲

AMA: 1999,Sep,10

67801	multiple, same lid	T ⟲
67805	multiple, different lids	T ⟲

AMA: 1999,Sep,10

67808	under general anesthesia and/or requiring hospitalization, single or multiple	❷ T ⟲

MED: 100-2,15,260; 100-4,12,90.3; 100-4,14,10

67810	Biopsy of eyelid	T 50 ⟲
67820	Correction of trichiasis; epilation, by forceps only	S 50 ⟲

AMA: 1998,Jul,1

67825	epilation by other than forceps (eg, by electrosurgery, cryotherapy, laser surgery)	T 50 ⟲

AMA: 1998,Jul,10

67830	incision of lid margin	❷ T 50 ⟲

MED: 100-2,15,260; 100-4,12,90.3; 100-4,14,10

67835	incision of lid margin, with free mucous membrane graft	❷ T 80 50 ⟲

MED: 100-2,15,260; 100-4,12,90.3; 100-4,14,10

67840	Excision of lesion of eyelid (except chalazion) without closure or with simple direct closure	T 50 ⟲

If an eyelid is excised and repaired by reconstructive surgery, consult CPT codes 67961 and 67966.

67850	Destruction of lesion of lid margin (up to 1 cm)	T 50 ⟲

If Mohs micrographic surgery is performed, consult CPT codes 17311-17315.

Report the appropriate E/M office visit codes for initiation or follow-up care of topical chemotherapy administration.

TARSORRHAPHY

If a diagnostic and treatment program is initiated for ophthalmological services, consult the Medicine and Ophthalmology sections of the CPT book and CPT codes 92002 and subsequent codes. Do not report 69990 in addition to codes 65091-68850 as the operating microscope is considered an inclusive component of these procedures.

67875	Temporary closure of eyelids by suture (eg, Frost suture)	T 50 ⟲
67880	Construction of intermarginal adhesions, median tarsorrhaphy, or canthorrhaphy;	❸ T 50 ⟲

MED: 100-2,15,260; 100-4,12,90.3; 100-4,14,10

67882	with transposition of tarsal plate	❸ T 50 ⟲

MED: 100-2,15,260; 100-4,12,90.3; 100-4,14,10

If severing of the tarsorrhaphy occurs, consult CPT codes 67710. If canthoplasty is performed for reconstruction of the canthus, consult CPTcode 67950. If a canthotomy is performed, consult CPT code 67715.

REPAIR (BROW PTOSIS, BLEPHAROPTOSIS, LID RETRACTION, ECTROPION, ENTROPION)

If a diagnostic and treatment program is initiated for ophthalmological services, consult the Medicine and Ophthalmology sections of the CPT book and CPT codes 92002 and subsequent codes. Do not report 69990 in addition to codes 65091-68850 as the operating microscope is considered an inclusive component of these procedures.

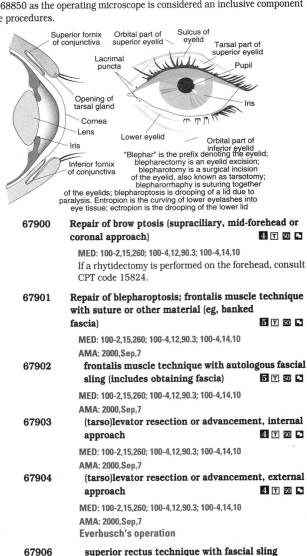

"Blephar" is the prefix denoting the eyelid; blepharectomy is an eyelid excision; blepharotomy is a surgical incision of the eyelid, also known as tarsotomy; blepharorrhaphy is suturing together of the eyelids; blepharoptosis is drooping of a lid due to paralysis. Entropion is the curving of lower eyelashes into eye tissue; ectropion is the drooping of the lower lid

67900	Repair of brow ptosis (supraciliary, mid-forehead or coronal approach)	❹ T 50 ⟲

MED: 100-2,15,260; 100-4,12,90.3; 100-4,14,10

If a rhytidectomy is performed on the forehead, consult CPT code 15824.

67901	Repair of blepharoptosis; frontalis muscle technique with suture or other material (eg, banked fascia)	❺ T 50 ⟲

MED: 100-2,15,260; 100-4,12,90.3; 100-4,14,10
AMA: 2000,Sep,7

67902	frontalis muscle technique with autologous fascial sling (includes obtaining fascia)	❺ T 50 ⟲

MED: 100-2,15,260; 100-4,12,90.3; 100-4,14,10
AMA: 2000,Sep,7

67903	(tarso)levator resection or advancement, internal approach	❹ T 50 ⟲

MED: 100-2,15,260; 100-4,12,90.3; 100-4,14,10
AMA: 2000,Sep,7

67904	(tarso)levator resection or advancement, external approach	❹ T 50 ⟲

MED: 100-2,15,260; 100-4,12,90.3; 100-4,14,10
AMA: 2000,Sep,7
Everbusch's operation

67906	superior rectus technique with fascial sling (includes obtaining fascia)	❺ T 50 ⟲

MED: 100-2,15,260; 100-4,12,90.3; 100-4,14,10
AMA: 2000,Sep,7

67908	conjunctivo-tarso-Muller's muscle-levator resection (eg, Fasanella-Servat type)	❹ T 50 ⟲

MED: 100-2,15,260; 100-4,12,90.3; 100-4,14,10
AMA: 2000,Sep,7

2️⃣6️⃣ Professional Component Only   8️⃣0️⃣/8️⃣0️⃣ Assist-at-Surgery Allowed/With Documentation   Unlisted   Not Covered

🆃�🅲 Technical Component Only   **MED:** Pub 100/NCD References   **AMA:** CPT Assistant References   ❶-❾ ASC Group   ♂ Male Only   ♀ Female Only

244 — CPT Expert   CPT only © 2006 American Medical Association. All Rights Reserved. *(Black Ink)*   © 2006 Ingenix *(Blue Ink)*

67909	Reduction of overcorrection of ptosis	4 T 50 ⬛
	MED: 100-2,15,260; 100-4,12,90.3; 100-4,14,10	
67911	Correction of lid retraction	3 T 50 ⬛
	MED: 100-2,15,260; 100-4,12,90.3; 100-4,14,10	
67912	Correction of lagophthalmos, with implantation of upper eyelid lid load (eg, gold weight)	3 T 50 ⬛
67914	Repair of ectropion; suture	3 T 50 ⬛
	MED: 100-2,15,260; 100-4,12,90.3; 100-4,14,10	
67915	thermocauterization	T 50 ⬛
67916	excision tarsal wedge	4 T 50 ⬛
	MED: 100-2,15,260; 100-4,12,90.3; 100-4,14,10	
67917	extensive (eg, tarsal strip operations)	4 T 50 ⬛
	MED: 100-2,15,260; 100-4,12,90.3; 100-4,14,10	

To report correction of everted punctum, consult CPT code 68705.

67921	Repair of entropion; suture	3 T 50 ⬛
	MED: 100-2,15,260; 100-4,12,90.3; 100-4,14,10	
67922	thermocauterization	T 50 ⬛
67923	excision tarsal wedge	4 T 50 ⬛
	MED: 100-2,15,260; 100-4,12,90.3; 100-4,14,10	
67924	extensive (eg, tarsal strip or capsulopalpebral fascia repairs operation)	4 T 50 ⬛
	MED: 100-2,15,260; 100-4,12,90.3; 100-4,14,10	

If a cicatricial ectropion or an entropion requiring scar excision or skin graft is repaired, consult also CPT codes 67961 and subsequent codes.

RECONSTRUCTION

These codes include the lid margin, palpebral conjunctiva, and tarsus.

If a diagnostic and treatment program is initiated for ophthalmological services, consult the Medicine and Ophthalmology sections of the CPT book and CPT codes 92002 and subsequent codes. Do not report 69990 in addition to codes 65091-68850 as the operating microscope is considered an inclusive component of these procedures.

If the skin of the eyelid is repaired, consult CPT codes 12011-12018, 12051-12057, 13150, and 13153. If tarsorrhaphy or canthorrhaphy is performed, consult CPT codes 67880 and 67882. If blepharoptosis and lid retraction is repaired, consult CPT codes 67901-67911.

To report blepharoplasty for entropion/ectropion, consult CPT codes 67916, 67917, 67923 and 67924. To report correction of blepharochalasis, consult CPT codes 15820-15823. To repair skin of eyelid with adjacent tissue transfer, consult CPT codes 14060, 14061; preparation of graft, see 15002-15005; free graft, see 15120, 15121, 15260, and 15261.

To report excision of lesion of eyelid, consult CPT code 67800 and subsequent codes. To report repair of lacrimal canaliculi, consult CPT code 68700.

67930	Suture of recent wound, eyelid, involving lid margin, tarsus, and/or palpebral conjunctiva direct closure; partial thickness	T 50 ⬛
67935	full thickness	2 T 50 ⬛
	MED: 100-2,15,260; 100-4,12,90.3; 100-4,14,10	
67938	Removal of embedded foreign body, eyelid	S 50 ⬛

See codes 14060,14061 for repair of skin of eyelid, adjacent tissue transfers. Use code 15004 for preparation of graft. See codes 15120, 15121, 15260, and 15261 for free graft.

| 67950 | Canthoplasty (reconstruction of canthus) | 2 T 50 ⬛ |
| | MED: 100-2,15,260; 100-4,12,90.3; 100-4,14,10 | |

67961	Excision and repair of eyelid, involving lid margin, tarsus, conjunctiva, canthus, or full thickness, may include preparation for skin graft or pedicle flap with adjacent tissue transfer or rearrangement; up to one-fourth of lid margin	3 T 80 50 ⬛
	MED: 100-2,15,260; 100-4,12,90.3; 100-4,14,10	
67966	over one-fourth of lid margin	3 T 50 ⬛
	MED: 100-2,15,260; 100-4,12,90.3; 100-4,14,10	
67971	Reconstruction of eyelid, full thickness by transfer of tarsoconjunctival flap from opposing eyelid; up to two-thirds of eyelid, one stage or first stage	3 T 80 50 ⬛
	MED: 100-2,15,260; 100-4,12,90.3; 100-4,14,10	
	Dupuy-Dutemp reconstruction	
67973	total eyelid, lower, one stage or first stage	3 T 80 50 ⬛
	MED: 100-2,15,260; 100-4,12,90.3; 100-4,14,10	
67974	total eyelid, upper, one stage or first stage	3 T 80 50 ⬛
	MED: 100-2,15,260; 100-4,12,90.3; 100-4,14,10	
	Landboldt's operation	
67975	second stage	3 T 50 ⬛
	MED: 100-2,15,260; 100-4,12,90.3; 100-4,14,10	
	Landboldt's operation	

OTHER PROCEDURES

| 67999 | Unlisted procedure, eyelids | T 80 50 |
| | MED: 100-4,4,180.3 | |

CONJUNCTIVA

INCISION AND DRAINAGE

If a foreign body is removed, consult CPT codes 65205 and subsequent codes.

If a diagnostic and treatment program is initiated for ophthalmological services, consult the Medicine and Ophthalmology sections of the CPT book and CPT codes 92002 and subsequent codes. Do not report 69990 in addition to codes 65091-68850 as the operating microscope is considered an inclusive component of these procedures.

| 68020 | Incision of conjunctiva, drainage of cyst | T 50 ⬛ |
| 68040 | Expression of conjunctival follicles (eg, for trachoma) | S 50 ⬛ |

EXCISION AND/OR DESTRUCTION

If a diagnostic and treatment program is initiated for ophthalmological services, consult the Medicine and Ophthalmology sections of the CPT book and CPT codes 92002 and subsequent codes. Do not report 69990 in addition to codes 65091-68850 as the operating microscope is considered an inclusive component of these procedures.

68100	Biopsy of conjunctiva	T 50 ⬛
68110	Excision of lesion, conjunctiva; up to 1 cm	T 50 ⬛
68115	over 1 cm	2 T 50 ⬛
	MED: 100-2,15,260; 100-4,12,90.3; 100-4,14,10	
68130	with adjacent sclera	2 T 50 ⬛
	MED: 100-2,15,260; 100-4,12,90.3; 100-4,14,10	
68135	Destruction of lesion, conjunctiva	T 50 ⬛

INJECTION

| 68200 | Subconjunctival injection | S 50 ⬛ |

If an injection is made into the Tenon's capsule or if a retrobulbar injection is needed, consult CPT codes 67500-67515.

⊛ Modifier 63 Exempt Code   ⊙ Conscious Sedation   + CPT Add-on Code   ⊘ Modifier 51 Exempt Code   ● New Code   ▲ Revised Code

M Maternity Edit   A Age Edit   A-Y APC Status Indicators   ⬛ CCI Comprehensive Code   50 Bilateral Procedure

Eye and Ocular Adnexa

68320 — 68760

CONJUNCTIVOPLASTY

If a diagnostic and treatment program is initiated for ophthalmological services, consult the Medicine and Ophthalmology sections of the CPT book and CPT codes 92002 and subsequent codes. Do not report 69990 in addition to codes 65091-68850 as the operating microscope is considered an inclusive component of these procedures.

If a wound is repaired, consult CPT codes 65270-65273.

68320 Conjunctivoplasty; with conjunctival graft or extensive rearrangement [4] [T] [50]
MED: 100-2,15,260; 100-4,12,90.3; 100-4,14,10

68325 with buccal mucous membrane graft (includes obtaining graft) [4] [T] [50]
MED: 100-2,15,260; 100-4,12,90.3; 100-4,14,10

68326 Conjunctivoplasty, reconstruction cul-de-sac; with conjunctival graft or extensive rearrangement [4] [T] [50]
MED: 100-2,15,260; 100-4,12,90.3; 100-4,14,10

68328 with buccal mucous membrane graft (includes obtaining graft) [4] [T] [80] [50]
MED: 100-2,15,260; 100-4,12,90.3; 100-4,14,10

68330 Repair of symblepharon; conjunctivoplasty, without graft [4] [T] [80] [50]
MED: 100-2,15,260; 100-4,12,90.3; 100-4,14,10

68335 with free graft conjunctiva or buccal mucous membrane (includes obtaining graft) [4] [T] [50]
MED: 100-2,15,260; 100-4,12,90.3; 100-4,14,10

68340 division of symblepharon, with or without insertion of conformer or contact lens [4] [T] [80] [50]
MED: 100-2,15,260; 100-4,12,90.3; 100-4,14,10

OTHER PROCEDURES

68360 Conjunctival flap; bridge or partial (separate procedure) [2] [T] [50]
MED: 100-2,15,260; 100-4,12,90.3; 100-4,14,10

68362 total (such as Gunderson thin flap or purse string flap) [2] [T] [50]
MED: 100-2,15,260; 100-4,12,90.3; 100-4,14,10
If a conjunctival flap is used for a perforating injury, consult CPT codes 65280 and 65285. If an operative wound is repaired, consult CPT code 66250. If a conjunctival foreign body is removed, consult CPT codes 65205 and 65210.

68371 Harvesting conjunctival allograft, living donor [2] [T] [50]

68399 Unlisted procedure, conjunctiva [T] [80] [50]
MED: 100-4,4,180.3

LACRIMAL SYSTEM

INCISION

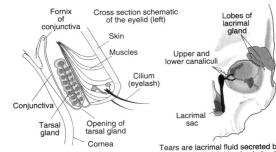

Fornix of conjunctiva — Cross section schematic of the eyelid (left) — Lobes of lacrimal gland — Skin — Muscles — Upper and lower canaliculi — Cilium (eyelash) — Conjunctiva — Tarsal gland — Opening of tarsal gland — Cornea — Lacrimal sac

The eyelid is a moveable fold covered by skin externally and highly vascularized conjunctiva internally. The tarsal glands secrete lubricant to the edges of the eyelid

Tears are lacrimal fluid secreted by the almond-sized lacrimal gland through ducts into the fornix of the conjunctiva; fluid is drained through the puncta and into the lacrimal sac and into the nose

68400 Incision, drainage of lacrimal gland [T] [50]

68420 Incision, drainage of lacrimal sac (dacryocystotomy or dacryocystostomy) [T] [50]

68440 Snip incision of lacrimal punctum [T] [50]

EXCISION

68500 Excision of lacrimal gland (dacryoadenectomy), except for tumor; total [3] [T] [50]
MED: 100-2,15,260; 100-4,12,90.3; 100-4,14,10

68505 partial [3] [T] [50]
MED: 100-2,15,260; 100-4,12,90.3; 100-4,14,10

68510 Biopsy of lacrimal gland [1] [T] [80] [50]
MED: 100-2,15,260; 100-4,12,90.3; 100-4,14,10

68520 Excision of lacrimal sac (dacryocystectomy) [3] [T] [80] [50]
MED: 100-2,15,260; 100-4,12,90.3; 100-4,14,10

68525 Biopsy of lacrimal sac [1] [T] [50]
MED: 100-2,15,260; 100-4,12,90.3; 100-4,14,10

68530 Removal of foreign body or dacryolith, lacrimal passages [T] [50]
Meller's excision

68540 Excision of lacrimal gland tumor; frontal approach [3] [T] [50]
MED: 100-2,15,260; 100-4,12,90.3; 100-4,14,10

68550 involving osteotomy [3] [T] [50]
MED: 100-2,15,260; 100-4,12,90.3; 100-4,14,10

REPAIR

68700 Plastic repair of canaliculi [2] [T] [50]
MED: 100-2,15,260; 100-4,12,90.3; 100-4,14,10

68705 Correction of everted punctum, cautery [T] [50]

68720 Dacryocystorhinostomy (fistulization of lacrimal sac to nasal cavity) [4] [T] [80] [50]
MED: 100-2,15,260; 100-4,12,90.3; 100-4,14,10
AMA: 2001,Sep,10

68745 Conjunctivorhinostomy (fistulization of conjunctiva to nasal cavity); without tube [4] [T] [80] [50]
MED: 100-2,15,260; 100-4,12,90.3; 100-4,14,10

68750 with insertion of tube or stent [4] [T] [80] [50]
MED: 100-2,15,260; 100-4,12,90.3; 100-4,14,10

68760 Closure of the lacrimal punctum; by thermocauterization, ligation, or laser surgery [S] [50]

68761	by plug, each	S 80 50 ↺
	AMA: 1996,Jun,1	
68770	Closure of lacrimal fistula (separate procedure)	4 T 80 50 ↺
	MED: 100-2,15,260; 100-4,12,90.3; 100-4,14,10	

PROBING AND/OR RELATED PROCEDURES

68801	Dilation of lacrimal punctum, with or without irrigation	S 50 ↺
68810	Probing of nasolacrimal duct, with or without irrigation;	1 S 50 ↺
	MED: 100-2,15,260; 100-4,12,90.3; 100-4,14,10	
	AMA: 2002,Nov,11	
68811	requiring general anesthesia	2 T 50 ↺
	MED: 100-2,15,260; 100-4,12,90.3; 100-4,14,10	
	AMA: 2002,Nov,11	
68815	with insertion of tube or stent	2 T 50 ↺
	MED: 100-2,15,260; 100-4,12,90.3; 100-4,14,10	
	AMA: 2002,Nov,11	
	Consult also CPT code 92018.	
68840	Probing of lacrimal canaliculi, with or without irrigation	S 50 ↺
68850	Injection of contrast medium for dacryocystography	N 50 ↺
	AMA: 2001,Feb,7	
	If radiological supervision and interpretation is needed, consult CPT codes 70170, 78660.	

OTHER PROCEDURES

| 68899 | Unlisted procedure, lacrimal system | T 80 50 |
| | MED: 100-4,4,180.3 | |

AUDITORY SYSTEM

EXTERNAL EAR

INCISION

If diagnostic services are performed (e.g., audiometry, vestibular tests), consult CPT codes 92502 and subsequent codes.

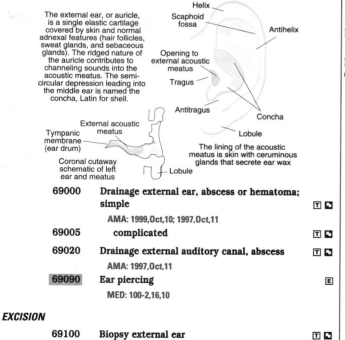

The external ear, or auricle, is a single elastic cartilage covered by skin and normal adnexal features (hair follicles, sweat glands, and sebaceous glands). The ridged nature of the auricle contributes to channeling sounds into the acoustic meatus. The semi-circular depression leading into the middle ear is named the concha, Latin for shell.

Helix
Scaphoid fossa
Antihelix
Opening to external acoustic meatus
Tragus
Antitragus
Concha
Lobule
External acoustic meatus
Tympanic membrane (ear drum)
Coronal cutaway schematic of left ear and meatus
Lobule
The lining of the acoustic meatus is skin with ceruminous glands that secrete ear wax

69000	Drainage external ear, abscess or hematoma; simple	T ↺
	AMA: 1999,Oct,10; 1997,Oct,11	
69005	complicated	T ↺
69020	Drainage external auditory canal, abscess	T ↺
	AMA: 1997,Oct,11	
69090	Ear piercing	E
	MED: 100-2,16,10	

EXCISION

| 69100 | Biopsy external ear | T ↺ |

69105	Biopsy external auditory canal	T ↺
69110	Excision external ear; partial, simple repair	1 T ↺
	MED: 100-2,15,260; 100-4,12,90.3; 100-4,14,10	
69120	complete amputation	2 T ↺
	MED: 100-2,15,260; 100-4,12,90.3; 100-4,14,10	
	If the ear is reconstructed, consult CPT codes 15120 and subsequent codes.	
69140	Excision exostosis(es), external auditory canal	2 T 80 ↺
	MED: 100-2,15,260; 100-4,12,90.3; 100-4,14,10	
69145	Excision soft tissue lesion, external auditory canal	2 T ↺
	MED: 100-2,15,260; 100-4,12,90.3; 100-4,14,10	
69150	Radical excision external auditory canal lesion; without neck dissection	3 T ↺
	MED: 100-2,15,260; 100-4,12,90.3; 100-4,14,10	
69155	with neck dissection	C 80 ↺
	If skin grafting is necessary, consult CPT codes 15004-15261.	
	If the temporal bone is resected, consult CPT code 69535.	

REMOVAL

If diagnostic services are performed (e.g., audiometry, vestibular tests), consult CPT codes 92502 and subsequent codes.

69200	Removal foreign body from external auditory canal; without general anesthesia	X ↺
69205	with general anesthesia	1 T ↺
	MED: 100-2,15,260; 100-4,12,90.3; 100-4,14,10	
69210	Removal impacted cerumen (separate procedure), one or both ears	X ↺
69220	Debridement, mastoidectomy cavity, simple (eg, routine cleaning)	T 50 ↺
69222	Debridement, mastoidectomy cavity, complex (eg, with anesthesia or more than routine cleaning)	T 50 ↺

REPAIR

If a wound or injury of the external ear is sutured, consult CPT codes 12011-14300.

If diagnostic services are performed (e.g., audiometry, vestibular tests), consult CPT codes 92502 and subsequent codes.

⊙	69300	Otoplasty, protruding ear, with or without size reduction	3 T 80 50 ↺
		MED: 100-2,15,260; 100-4,12,90.3; 100-4,14,10	
	69310	Reconstruction of external auditory canal (meatoplasty) (eg, for stenosis due to injury, infection) (separate procedure)	3 T ↺
		MED: 100-2,15,260; 100-4,12,90.3; 100-4,14,10	
	69320	Reconstruction external auditory canal for congenital atresia, single stage	7 T 80 ↺
		MED: 100-2,15,260; 100-4,12,90.3; 100-4,14,10	
		To report procedure performed in conjunction with middle ear reconstruction, consult CPT codes 69631 and 69641. To report other reconstruction procedures with grafts, consult CPT codes 13150-15760 and 21230-21235.	

Auditory System

69399 — 69631

OTHER PROCEDURES

If diagnostic services are performed (e.g., audiometry, vestibular tests), consult CPT codes 92502 and subsequent codes.

If otoscopy is performed under general anesthesia, consult CPT code 92502.

69399   Unlisted procedure, external ear   [T] [80]
        MED: 100-4,4,180.3

MIDDLE EAR

INTRODUCTION

69400   Eustachian tube inflation, transnasal; with catheterization   [T] [⤴]

69401   without catheterization   [T] [⤴]

69405   Eustachian tube catheterization, transtympanic   [T] [80] [⤴]

INCISION

69420   Myringotomy including aspiration and/or eustachian tube inflation   [T] [50] [⤴]

69421   Myringotomy including aspiration and/or eustachian tube inflation requiring general anesthesia   [3] [T] [50] [⤴]
        MED: 100-2,15,260; 100-4,12,90.3; 100-4,14,10

69424   Ventilating tube removal requiring general anesthesia   [T] [50] [⤴]

Do not report 69424 in addition to CPT codes 69205, 69210, 69420, 69421, 69433-69676, 69710-69745, 69801-69930.

This is a unilateral procedure. To report this procedure performed bilaterally, append modifier 50.

69433   Tympanostomy (requiring insertion of ventilating tube), local or topical anesthesia   [T] [50] [⤴]

69436   Tympanostomy (requiring insertion of ventilating tube), general anesthesia   [3] [T] [50] [⤴]
        MED: 100-2,15,260; 100-4,12,90.3; 100-4,14,10

69440   Middle ear exploration through postauricular or ear canal incision   [3] [T] [50] [⤴]
        MED: 100-2,15,260; 100-4,12,90.3; 100-4,14,10

If an atticotomy is performed, consult CPT codes 69601 and subsequent codes.

69450   Tympanolysis, transcanal   [1] [T] [80] [50] [⤴]
        MED: 100-2,15,260; 100-4,12,90.3; 100-4,14,10

EXCISION

69501   Transmastoid antrotomy (simple mastoidectomy)   [7] [T] [50] [⤴]
        MED: 100-2,15,260; 100-4,12,90.3; 100-4,14,10

69502   Mastoidectomy; complete   [7] [T] [80] [50] [⤴]
        MED: 100-2,15,260; 100-4,12,90.3; 100-4,14,10

69505   modified radical   [7] [T] [80] [50] [⤴]
        MED: 100-2,15,260; 100-4,12,90.3; 100-4,14,10

69511   radical   [7] [T] [80] [50] [⤴]
        MED: 100-2,15,260; 100-4,12,90.3; 100-4,14,10

If a skin graft is needed, consult CPT codes 15004 and subsequent codes.

If debridement is performed on the mastoidectomy cavity, consult CPT codes 69220 and 69222.

69530   Petrous apicectomy including radical mastoidectomy   [7] [T] [80] [50] [⤴]
        MED: 100-2,15,260; 100-4,12,90.3; 100-4,14,10

69535   Resection temporal bone, external approach   [C] [50] [⤴]

If a middle fossa approach is used, consult CPT codes 69950-69970.

69540   Excision aural polyp   [T] [50] [⤴]

69550   Excision aural glomus tumor; transcanal   [5] [T] [80] [50] [⤴]
        MED: 100-2,15,260; 100-4,12,90.3; 100-4,14,10

69552   transmastoid   [7] [T] [80] [50] [⤴]
        MED: 100-2,15,260; 100-4,12,90.3; 100-4,14,10

69554   extended (extratemporal)   [C] [80] [50] [⤴]

REPAIR

Squamous part of temporal bone — Petrous part of temporal bone — Mastoid process — Petrous part of temporal bone — Internal acoustic canal — Petrous apex — Mastoid — Cutaway of mastoid process — Oval window — Plane of view above — Mastoid air cells — Facial nerve canal — The internal structure of the mastoid process resembles a honeycomb; infections of the middle ear sometimes spread to the mastoid cells

69601   Revision mastoidectomy; resulting in complete mastoidectomy   [7] [T] [80] [50] [⤴]
        MED: 100-2,15,260; 100-4,12,90.3; 100-4,14,10

69602   resulting in modified radical mastoidectomy   [7] [T] [80] [50] [⤴]
        MED: 100-2,15,260; 100-4,12,90.3; 100-4,14,10

69603   resulting in radical mastoidectomy   [7] [T] [80] [50] [⤴]
        MED: 100-2,15,260; 100-4,12,90.3; 100-4,14,10

69604   resulting in tympanoplasty   [7] [T] [50] [⤴]
        MED: 100-2,15,260; 100-4,12,90.3; 100-4,14,10

If a secondary tympanoplasty is planned after mastoidectomy, consult CPT codes 69631 and 69632.

69605   with apicectomy   [7] [T] [80] [50] [⤴]
        MED: 100-2,15,260; 100-4,12,90.3; 100-4,14,10

If a skin graft is performed, consult CPT codes 15120, 15121, 15260, and 15261.

69610   Tympanic membrane repair, with or without site preparation of perforation for closure, with or without patch   [T] [50] [⤴]
        AMA: 2001,Mar,10

69620   Myringoplasty (surgery confined to drumhead and donor area)   [2] [T] [50] [⤴]
        MED: 100-2,15,260; 100-4,12,90.3; 100-4,14,10
        AMA: 2001,Mar,10

69631   Tympanoplasty without mastoidectomy (including canalplasty, atticotomy and/or middle ear surgery), initial or revision; without ossicular chain reconstruction   [5] [T] [50] [⤴]
        MED: 100-2,15,260; 100-4,12,90.3; 100-4,14,10
        AMA: 2001,Mar,10; 1998,Jul,11

69632	with ossicular chain reconstruction (eg, postfenestration) 🔲5 T 50 🔲

MED: 100-2,15,260; 100-4,12,90.3; 100-4,14,10

▲ 69633 with ossicular chain reconstruction and synthetic prosthesis (eg, partial ossicular replacement prosthesis (PORP), total ossicular replacement prosthesis (TORP)) 🔲5 T 50 🔲

MED: 100-2,15,260; 100-4,12,90.3; 100-4,14,10

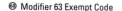

The tympanic membrane is a thin, sensitive tissue and is the gateway to the middle ear; the membrane vibrates in response to sound waves and the movement is transmitted via the ossicular chain to the internal ear. Many surgeries to the middle ear involve repair to the tympanic membrane and reconstruction to the various components of the ossicular chain

69635 Tympanoplasty with antrotomy or mastoidotomy (including canalplasty, atticotomy, middle ear surgery, and/or tympanic membrane repair); without ossicular chain reconstruction 🔲7 T 50 🔲

MED: 100-2,15,260; 100-4,12,90.3; 100-4,14,10

69636 with ossicular chain reconstruction 🔲7 T 80 50 🔲

MED: 100-2,15,260; 100-4,12,90.3; 100-4,14,10

▲ 69637 with ossicular chain reconstruction and synthetic prosthesis (eg, partial ossicular replacement prosthesis (PORP), total ossicular replacement prosthesis (TORP)) 🔲7 T 80 50 🔲

MED: 100-2,15,260; 100-4,12,90.3; 100-4,14,10

69641 Tympanoplasty with mastoidectomy (including canalplasty, middle ear surgery, tympanic membrane repair); without ossicular chain reconstruction 🔲7 T 50 🔲

MED: 100-2,15,260; 100-4,12,90.3; 100-4,14,10

69642 with ossicular chain reconstruction 🔲7 T 50 🔲

MED: 100-2,15,260; 100-4,12,90.3; 100-4,14,10

69643 with intact or reconstructed wall, without ossicular chain reconstruction 🔲7 T 50 🔲

MED: 100-2,15,260; 100-4,12,90.3; 100-4,14,10

69644 with intact or reconstructed canal wall, with ossicular chain reconstruction 🔲7 T 50 🔲

MED: 100-2,15,260; 100-4,12,90.3; 100-4,14,10

69645 radical or complete, without ossicular chain reconstruction 🔲7 T 50 🔲

MED: 100-2,15,260; 100-4,12,90.3; 100-4,14,10

69646 radical or complete, with ossicular chain reconstruction 🔲7 T 80 50 🔲

MED: 100-2,15,260; 100-4,12,90.3; 100-4,14,10

69650 Stapes mobilization 🔲7 T 50 🔲

MED: 100-2,15,260; 100-4,12,90.3; 100-4,14,10

69660 Stapedectomy or stapedotomy with reestablishment of ossicular continuity, with or without use of foreign material; 🔲5 T 50 🔲

MED: 100-2,15,260; 100-4,12,90.3; 100-4,14,10

69661 with footplate drill out 🔲5 T 80 50 🔲

MED: 100-2,15,260; 100-4,12,90.3; 100-4,14,10

69662 Revision of stapedectomy or stapedotomy 🔲5 T 50 🔲

MED: 100-2,15,260; 100-4,12,90.3; 100-4,14,10

69666 Repair oval window fistula 🔲4 T 80 50 🔲

MED: 100-2,15,260; 100-4,12,90.3; 100-4,14,10

69667 Repair round window fistula 🔲4 T 80 50 🔲

MED: 100-2,15,260; 100-4,12,90.3; 100-4,14,10

69670 Mastoid obliteration (separate procedure) 🔲3 T 80 50 🔲

MED: 100-2,15,260; 100-4,12,90.3; 100-4,14,10

69676 Tympanic neurectomy 🔲3 T 50 🔲

MED: 100-2,15,260; 100-4,12,90.3; 100-4,14,10

OTHER PROCEDURES

69700 Closure postauricular fistula, mastoid (separate procedure) 🔲3 T 50 🔲

MED: 100-2,15,260; 100-4,12,90.3; 100-4,14,10

69710 Implantation or replacement of electromagnetic bone conduction hearing device in temporal bone E

The replacement procedure includes the removal of the old device.

69711 Removal or repair of electromagnetic bone conduction hearing device in temporal bone 🔲1 T 80 50 🔲

MED: 100-2,15,260; 100-4,12,90.3; 100-4,14,10

69714 Implantation, osseointegrated implant, temporal bone, with percutaneous attachment to external speech processor/cochlear stimulator; without mastoidectomy 🔲9 T 50 🔲

MED: 100-2,15,260; 100-4,12,90.3; 100-4,14,10

69715 with mastoidectomy 🔲9 T 50 🔲

MED: 100-2,15,260; 100-4,12,90.3; 100-4,14,10

69717 Replacement (including removal of existing device), osseointegrated implant, temporal bone, with percutaneous attachment to external speech processor/cochlear stimulator; without mastoidectomy 🔲9 T 50 🔲

MED: 100-2,15,260; 100-4,12,90.3; 100-4,14,10

69718 with mastoidectomy 🔲9 T 50 🔲

MED: 100-2,15,260; 100-4,12,90.3; 100-4,14,10

69720 Decompression facial nerve, intratemporal; lateral to geniculate ganglion 🔲5 T 80 50 🔲

MED: 100-2,15,260; 100-4,12,90.3; 100-4,14,10

69725 including medial to geniculate ganglion 🔲T 80 50 🔲

MED: 100-2,15,260; 100-4,12,90.3; 100-4,14,10

69740 Suture facial nerve, intratemporal, with or without graft or decompression; lateral to geniculate ganglion 🔲5 T 80 50 🔲

MED: 100-2,15,260; 100-4,12,90.3; 100-4,14,10

If an extracranial suture of facial nerve is performed, consult CPT code 64864.

69745 including medial to geniculate ganglion 🔲5 T 80 50 🔲

MED: 100-2,15,260; 100-4,12,90.3; 100-4,14,10

69799 Unlisted procedure, middle ear T 80 50

MED: 100-4,4,180.3
AMA: 1999,Oct,10

⊛ Modifier 63 Exempt Code   ⊙ Conscious Sedation   + CPT Add-on Code   ⊘ Modifier 51 Exempt Code   ● New Code   ▲ Revised Code

M Maternity Edit   A Age Edit   A-Y APC Status Indicators   C CCI Comprehensive Code   50 Bilateral Procedure

Operating Microscope

69801 — 69990

INNER EAR

INCISION AND/OR DESTRUCTION

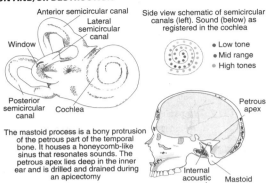

Anterior semicircular canal
Lateral semicircular canal
Side view schematic of semicircular canals (left). Sound (below) as registered in the cochlea
Window
● Low tone
● Mid range
● High tones
Posterior semicircular canal
Cochlea
Petrous apex

The mastoid process is a bony protrusion of the petrous part of the temporal bone. It houses a honeycomb-like sinus that resonates sounds. The petrous apex lies deep in the inner ear and is drilled and drained during an apicectomy

Internal acoustic canal
Mastoid

| 69801 | Labyrinthotomy, with or without cryosurgery including other nonexcisional destructive procedures or perfusion of vestibuloactive drugs (single or multiple perfusions); transcanal | 5 T 80 50 |

MED: 100-2,15,260; 100-4,12,90.3; 100-4,14,10
This procedure includes all of the required infusions performed on initial and subsequent days of treatment.

| 69802 | with mastoidectomy | 7 T 80 50 |

MED: 100-2,15,260; 100-4,12,90.3; 100-4,14,10

| 69805 | Endolymphatic sac operation; without shunt | 7 T 80 50 |

MED: 100-2,15,260; 100-4,12,90.3; 100-4,14,10

| 69806 | with shunt | 7 T 50 |

MED: 100-2,15,260; 100-4,12,90.3; 100-4,14,10

| 69820 | Fenestration semicircular canal | 5 T 80 50 |

MED: 100-2,15,260; 100-4,12,90.3; 100-4,14,10
Lempert's fenestration

| 69840 | Revision fenestration operation | 5 T 80 50 |

MED: 100-2,15,260; 100-4,12,90.3; 100-4,14,10

EXCISION

| 69905 | Labyrinthectomy; transcanal | 7 T 50 |

MED: 100-2,15,260; 100-4,12,90.3; 100-4,14,10

| 69910 | with mastoidectomy | 7 T 80 50 |

MED: 100-2,15,260; 100-4,12,90.3; 100-4,14,10

| 69915 | Vestibular nerve section, translabyrinthine approach | 7 T 80 50 |

MED: 100-2,15,260; 100-4,12,90.3; 100-4,14,10
If a transcranial approach is used, consult CPT code 69950.

INTRODUCTION

| 69930 | Cochlear device implantation, with or without mastoidectomy | 7 T 80 50 |

MED: 100-2,15,260; 100-3,50.3; 100-4,12,90.3; 100-4,14,10; 100-4,32,100

OTHER PROCEDURES

| 69949 | Unlisted procedure, inner ear | T 80 50 |

MED: 100-4,4,180.3

TEMPORAL BONE, MIDDLE FOSSA APPROACH
If an external approach is used, consult CPT code 69535.

| 69950 | Vestibular nerve section, transcranial approach | C 80 50 |

| 69955 | Total facial nerve decompression and/or repair (may include graft) | T 80 50 |

| 69960 | Decompression internal auditory canal | T 80 50 |

| 69970 | Removal of tumor, temporal bone | C 80 50 |

OTHER PROCEDURES

| 69979 | Unlisted procedure, temporal bone, middle fossa approach | T 80 50 |

MED: 100-4,4,180.3

OPERATING MICROSCOPE

+ | 69990 | Microsurgical techniques, requiring use of operating microscope (List separately in addition to code for primary procedure) | N 80 |

AMA: 2002,Oct,8; 1999,Oct,10; 1999,Jun,11; 1999,Jul,11; 1999,Apr,11; 1998,Nov,20
Note that 69990 is an add-on code that must be used in conjunction with the appropriate code for the primary procedure. This code cannot be reported alone.

Do not report 69990 with the following CPT codes 15756-15758, 15842, 19364, 19368, 20955-20962, 20969-20973, 26551-26554, 26556, 31526, 31531, 31536, 31541, 31545, 31546, 31561, 31571, 43116, 43496, 49906, 61548, 63075-63078, 64727, 64820-64823, 65091-68850.

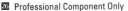

26 Professional Component Only
80/80 Assist-at-Surgery Allowed/With Documentation
Unlisted
Not Covered

TC Technical Component Only
MED: Pub 100/NCD References
AMA: CPT Assistant References
1-9 ASC Group
♂ Male Only
♀ Female Only

250 — CPT Expert
CPT only © 2006 American Medical Association. All Rights Reserved. (Black Ink)
© 2006 Ingenix (Blue Ink)

Radiology

CODING INFORMATION

Radiology services regularly employ imaging, diagnostic, and therapeutic technologies developed only a few decades ago. Consequently, the radiology section (70010–79999) is under constant review to reflect current standards of service.

Radiological procedures are divided into four subsections in the CPT book: diagnostic radiology, including computed tomography (CT), magnetic resonance imaging (MRI), and interventional radiology procedures; diagnostic ultrasound; radiation oncology; and diagnostic and therapeutic nuclear medicine. Codes are ordered according to anatomic site (head, chest, abdomen), and body system (gastrointestinal, aorta, and arteries). The subject listings in the radiology section may be reported when a physician either performs or supervises the services.

Procedures are described by type of service (modality), specific body site, and are followed by additional information regarding the use of contrast material and the complexity of the procedure.

Procedures frequently performed by radiologists may be found outside the radiology section, such as noninvasive vascular diagnostic studies (93875–93990), which are found in the medicine section. Services involving the invasive or interventional component of interventional radiology services are found in the surgery section. These include percutaneous biopsies, injection procedures, and transcatheter procedures.

TECHNICAL AND PROFESSIONAL COMPONENTS

Radiology procedures are made up of two components: technical and professional. The technical component includes the provision of the equipment, supplies, technical personnel, and costs attendant to the performance of the procedure other than the professional services. The professional component encompasses the physician's work in providing the service, including supervision, interpretation, and report of the procedure. Education, malpractice insurance, and other expenses incident to maintaining a practice are also part of the professional component.

A common division for reimbursement of routine diagnostic procedures is 60 percent for the technical component and 40 percent for the professional component.

Coding radiology services has been difficult due to the technical component inherent to this area of medicine. The advent of freestanding medical facilities including physician offices capable of offering imaging services, catheterizations, and other diagnostic and therapeutic radiology services poses a challenge in securing reimbursement for both components. The CPT book reports the physician component of services rather than the technical. Coders will not find a modifier in the CPT book to reflect technical services. HCPCS Level II provides the modifier TC specifically for reporting the technical component. Unless instructed otherwise by payers, the professional component should be reported with modifier 26, the technical component with modifier TC.

RESULTS/TESTING/REPORTS

Results indicate the technical component of a procedure or service. Testing is the service that leads to the report and interpretation. Reports provide interpretation of the tests.

GLOBAL SERVICE

A global service may be reported when one physician provides both components of the radiology procedure, such as owning the equipment, employing the technologist, and providing a written interpretation of the examination.

SUBSECTIONS

The radiology section of the CPT book is divided into four subsections. These are:

- Functional MRI
- Aorta and Arteries
- Veins and Lymphatics
- Transcatheter Procedures
- Diagnostic Ultrasound
- Abdomen and Retroperitoneum
- Obstetrical
- Non-Obstetrical
- Radiation Oncology
- Clinical Treatment Planning
- Radiation Treatment Management
- Proton Beam Treatment Delivery
- Hyperthermia
- Clinical Brachytherapy
- Nuclear Medicine
- Musculoskeletal System
- Cardiovascular System
- Therapeutic
- Nuclear Medicine

DIAGNOSTIC RADIOLOGY

Procedures in diagnostic radiology subsection establish a diagnosis or follow the progression or remission of a disease process. However, also included in this section are procedures that are therapeutic. These therapeutic procedures are often referred to as interventional or invasive radiology services. Codes in this chapter of the CPT book report the radiological supervision and interpretation of these interventional and invasive procedures.

Diagnostic radiology uses different modalities, including x-rays, fluoroscopy, computed tomography (CT), and magnetic resonance imaging (MRI). Procedures in the diagnostic radiology section are ordered by anatomic site and described by type of service (modality), specific body site, number of views, and use of contrast materials.

Terms and Instructions

A radiological examination refers to plain films of specific sites. Other terms used to describe plain films include standard or conventional films. Services employing other modalities and additional techniques are described as such (i.e., radiography with fluoroscopy, computerized axial tomography, or magnetic resonance imaging).

Computed axial tomography (CT scan) is a type of imaging that employs basic tomographic technique enhanced by computer imaging. Computer enhancement synthesizes the images obtained from different directions in a given plane, effectively reconstructing a cross-sectional plane of the body.

Computed tomography angiography (CTA) provides multiple rapid thin section CT scans, a series of x-ray beams taken from different angles to create cross-sectional images of organs, bones, and tissues.

Magnetic resonance imaging (MRI) involves the application of an external magnetic field that forces a uniform alignment of hydrogen atom nuclei in the soft tissue. The nuclei emit radiofrequency signals that are converted into sets of tomographic images and displayed on a computer screen for three-dimensional visualization of the soft tissue structure.

Views describe the patient's position in relation to the camera. A code may specify a position, as in 71010 that describes a single frontal view of the chest. Other codes do not specify a position, but designate the number of views, as in 73610 that specifies a minimum of three views of the ankle.

Procedures performed with contrast material often do not specify the type of contrast, as in 74160 that reports computed axial tomography of the abdomen with contrast. However, other codes are more specific. Radiologic examination of the colon using barium enema contrast is reported with code 74270. An air contrast with specific high-density barium is reported with code 74280.

The radiological supervision and interpretation of many interventional and invasive procedures are reported with codes from diagnostic radiology. Interventional/invasive codes may be used to report procedures that are diagnostic in nature, such as fluoroscopic localization code 77002. Or, the codes may be used to report therapeutic procedures, such as radiologic supervision and interpretation of transcatheter embolization 75894.

Administration of Contrast Material(s)

The phrases "with contrast" or "without contrast followed by contrast" appears within the code narrative of some radiology services codes. This represents contrast material administered intravascularly, intrathecally, or intra-articularly.

DIAGNOSTIC ULTRASOUND

Permanent records of ultrasound examinations such as description of anatomic region, measurements, obstructed view and site to be localized for a guided surgical procedure must be kept. A written report of the exam should be included in the patient's medical record. Ultrasound should not be reported unless there is image documentation and a final written report.

Procedures in the diagnostic ultrasound subsection are organized by anatomic site. However, when the ultrasound is part of an interventional radiology procedure for localization purposes, the procedure is listed under "Ultrasonic Guidance Procedures."

Codes for ultrasounds performed for diagnostic purposes are selected based on the technique or type of study (A-mode, B-scan), the extent of the study (limited, complete, follow-up), and additional services performed with certain ultrasounds (intraocular lens power calculation).

Technique

A-mode (a-scan) is an ultrasonic scanning procedure providing one-dimensional measurement.

M-mode is an ultrasonic scanning procedure that measures the amplitude and velocity of moving echo-producing structures to allow one-dimensional viewing.

B-scan is a two-dimensional ultrasonic scanning procedure providing a two-dimensional display.

Real-time is a two-dimensional scanning procedure that displays both structure and movement in time.

Doppler is an ultrasonic scanning procedure that measures the velocity of moving objects and often applied in the study of blood flow.

Extent

"Complete" defines a complete procedure that implies a scan of the entire body area.

"Limited" defines a limited procedure that involves scanning a single organ, quadrant, or completing a partial examination.

"Follow-up/repeat" implies performing a limited study on an area previously scanned.

Ultrasound procedures may be found in other sections of the CPT book. For example, echocardiography procedures are in the medicine section under "Cardiovascular Services." Color mapping in conjunction with fetal echocardiography (76825–76826) is reported with 93325 in the medicine section. Duplex scans and Doppler studies of the vascular system are found in the medicine section under the heading "Noninvasive Vascular Diagnostic Studies."

RADIATION ONCOLOGY

Radiation oncology is a therapeutic method as opposed to a diagnostic service. The radiologist manages and prescribes treatment for patients who have malignant neoplasms responsive to radiation therapy.

Radiation oncology involves the following services: consultation, clinical treatment, planning, medical radiation physics, and treatment delivery and management.

Consultation codes from the evaluation and management (E/M) section of the CPT book report consultations conducted by radiation oncologists and the E/M guidelines must be followed when applying these codes. Office/outpatient consultations are reported with codes 99241–99245; codes 99251–99255 are reported for inpatient consultations.

Clinical treatment planning consists of two services, planning and simulation to determine the best course of treatment. Planning is reported with codes 77261–77263, depending on the extent or complexity of the process. Simulation is reported with codes 77280–77295, depending on the extent or complexity of the service.

- Report 77261 for simple planning that requires assessment of a single treatment area. No interpretation of special tests is required. The treatment site can be in a single port or simple parallel opposed ports with simple or no blocking.

- Report 77262 for an intermediate level of planning that requires interpretation of tests performed for tumor localization. The radiation oncologist may need to assess two separate treatment areas or protect sensitive organs.

- Report 77263 for the interpretation of complex testing procedures, including CT and MR localization and/or special laboratory tests. Planning requires complex blocks and/or custom shielding blocks for the protection of sensitive normal structures. Tangential ports may be required. Three or more areas may require treatment. In addition, complex treatment planning often involves a combination of modalities such as brachytherapy, hyperthermia, chemotherapy and surgery.

- Simulation sets the treatment portals to specific treatment volumes. Simulation should be reported only once per time of set-up procedure.

- Simple simulation (77280) involves a single port or single pair of parallel ports on a single treatment area.

- Intermediate simulation (77285) involves three or more ports directed at a single treatment area. It also is required when two separate treatment areas are involved.

- Complex simulation (77290) involves a combination of multiple treatment areas, complex blocking rotation or arc therapy, multiple modalities, and use of contrast materials.

- Three-dimensional simulation (77295) involves computer-generated three-dimensional reconstruction of the tumor and surrounding critical structures.

- Medical radiation physics involves dosimetry calculation, the design and construction of treatment devices, and special services as defined below:

- Dosimetry calculation is the process a facility-based physicist uses to select the proper energy and modality to be used for each portal.

- Design and construction involves fabricating devices for the blocks. The physician must be involved in the design, selection, and placement of the devices and must document the involvement.

- Special services include hyperthermia or brachytherapy.

Treatment delivery and management (77401–77499) involves the delivery of radiation therapy and care of the patient during the course of therapy. While a nonphysician may deliver the treatment, the physician is responsible for checking and documenting the accuracy of the treatment. In addition, the physician responds to any adverse reactions to treatment and monitors the effects of the treatment on the tumor and surrounding tissues. Ongoing patient examinations are part of this service and not reported separately.

NUCLEAR MEDICINE

Nuclear medicine relies on radium or other radioelements for either diagnostic imaging or radiopharmaceutical therapy. Radiopharmaceutical therapy destroys diseased tissues, usually malignant neoplasms, using radioelements. This subsection is organized first by the nature of the procedure, diagnostic or therapeutic. The diagnostic codes are organized by body system and defined by the extent or complexity of the service.

Procedures in nuclear medicine are independent services. Diagnostic work-up or follow-up care is reported separately, except when specifically noted as included in the service. These services do not include the provision of radium or other radioelements.

SPECIAL CODING SITUATIONS

INTERVENTIONAL RADIOLOGY

Interventional radiology services involve both an invasive component (such as a biopsy or injection) and a radiological component (radiological supervision and interpretation of the procedure). The invasive component, which may be either a diagnostic or therapeutic service, is reported with codes from the surgery section. Examples of the invasive component include injection procedure for shoulder arthrography (23350), percutaneous renal biopsy (50200), and transcatheter occlusion of a vascular malformation (61624–61626). The radiology component for supervision and interpretation is reported with codes from the diagnostic radiology and diagnostic ultrasound subsections.

Component coding was developed for services that can be performed by a single physician, usually an interventional radiologist or by two physicians, a surgeon and a radiologist. Whether performed by one or two physicians, an interventional radiology procedure must be documented as thoroughly as a surgical procedure. When two physicians perform an invasive procedure, each physician documents the portion of the service provided and references the other's involvement in the written report. Each physician reports only the CPT code for the portion of the service the respective physician provided.

The following diagnostic angiography procedures include the work provided in the interventional procedure and should not be reported separately:

- Contrast injections, angiography, roadmapping, and/or fluoroscopy

- Vessel measurement

- Post angiography or stent angiography

Diagnostic procedure codes may be used in addition to the interventional procedure only if the following criteria are met:

- No prior catheter-based angiographic study is available and a full diagnostic study is performed and the decision to intervene is based on the diagnostic study.

- A diagnostic study is documented in the medical records but the patient's condition has changed, there is not adequate visualization or there is a clinical change during the procedure that requires reevaluation.

- The diagnostic study is performed in a different area from the interventional surgery.

- Do not separately report a diagnostic angiography performed at the same time as an interventional procedure if it is specifically included in the interventional code procedure description.

The following venography diagnostic procedures include the work provided in the interventional procedure and should not be reported separately:

- Contrast injections, venography, roadmapping, and/or fluoroscopy

- Vessel measurement

- Post venography or stent venography

Diagnostic procedure codes may only be used in addition to the interventional procedure if the following are met:

- A full diagnostic study was done but is not available and a full diagnostic study and the basis for an interventional procedure was based on the diagnostic study.

- A diagnostic study is documented in the medical records but the patient's condition has changed, there is not adequate visualization, or there is a clinical change during the procedure that requires re-evaluation.

- The diagnostic study is performed in a different area from the interventional surgery.

- Do not separately report a diagnostic venography performed at the same time as an interventional procedure if it is specifically included in the interventional code procedure description.

The following procedures are included in a therapeutic transcatheter interventional procedure:

- Contrast injections, venography, roadmapping, and/or fluoroscopy

- Vessel measurement

- Except for services allowed by 75898, completion of angiography/venography

Noninvasive Vascular Diagnostic Studies
A description of noninvasive vascular diagnostic services (93875–93990) are mentioned here since radiologists frequently perform them also. Vascular study procedures are comprised of the following services: patient care required during performance of the study, supervision of the study, written interpretation of study results, a hard copy of output, and analysis of all data.

MODIFIERS
As in other specialties, modifiers in radiology denote circumstances that affect the performance of services and procedures. Radiologists most frequently apply modifier 26 Professional component which reports the physician (professional) component of a service separately from the technical portion. Other modifiers for radiology include, but are not limited to:

22 Unusual procedural services

52 Reduced services

59 Distinct procedural service

76 Repeat procedure by same physician

77 Repeat procedure by another physician

X-RAY CONSULTATIONS
Code 76140 Consultation on x-ray examination made elsewhere, written report is used by a physician providing a second interpretation and report on a radiologic procedure. The previous interpretation is usually from a source outside of the physician's practice and is provided at the request of another physician. Both written reports must be maintained as part of the patient's medical record. The initial report and the consultation must document the specific procedure reviewed and the complexity of the procedure, such as the number of views. Do not report 76140 for outside films that are reviewed in conjunction with evaluation and management services. The medical decision making component of E/M codes includes "amount and/or complexity of data to be reviewed."

DOCUMENTING RADIOLOGY SERVICES
Diagnostic coding is critical in establishing medical necessity, even though the radiologist may not have the information necessary to assign a definitive diagnosis. For example, many radiological services are performed to rule out a particular problem. Tests that are normal effectively rule out the suspected condition; however, the radiologist must be given sufficient information about the patient's clinical history to justify medical necessity. In instances of a rule-out diagnosis, the physician must provide the radiologist with information, regarding the patient's symptoms, signs, or complaints.

PHYSICIAN REQUIREMENTS
In general, the patient's physician orders the study and a radiologist performs and/or interprets the procedure. The radiologist sends a report to the referring physician who includes it in the overall assessment of the patient. For coding and reimbursement purposes, the radiologist's portion of the service is reported as a complete procedure or as the professional component of the study. The ordering physician evaluates the results of the study for consideration in the medical decision making but does not file a claim for any portion of the radiological study.

Requesting Physician Responsibilities
The physician should sign or initial the radiologist's report as evidence the information was reviewed and considered in medical decision making. While the actual film may be stored elsewhere, a written report should be incorporated into the patient's medical record to prove the study was medically necessary.

Radiologist Responsibilities
Radiologists must complete a written report for every service claimed. The specific name or title of the study must appear on the report; for example, "Chest x-ray, PA and lateral." In addition to reporting the number and type of views taken, reports also must indicate any other circumstances that may affect the exam such as, a patient's state of fasting for a bowel study. Documentation should also include:

- Quality of the study (clear or blurry)

- Pertinent positive findings (abnormal)

- Pertinent negative findings (normal)

- Other aspects of the film such as incidental findings in other areas

- Radiologist's impression and diagnosis

- Recommendations for further studies or treatment

- Signature

Although the ordering physician must indicate the medical necessity, the radiologist must indicate the reason in the report. The complexity of the study dictates the depth of the radiology statement. Results from radiological studies done for urgent, acute problems must be communicated verbally by the radiologist to the physician as soon as they are available (and, also, documented later in the patient record).

REPORTS
Radiology reports are almost universally transcribed. For that reason, precautions must be taken to keep the patient's record current. Whenever possible, apply the rules for dictated operative reports to radiology reports. For example, a handwritten summary of the study should be placed in the chart until the transcription is available. The radiologist should read the transcription for accuracy and sign it before it is sent to the ordering physician or placed permanently in the patient's record.

Dictated reports should include the number and type of views taken, whether the study required a contrast medium, and the type and amount of contrast medium or radionuclide. This information plus other pertinent documentation is necessary to support CPT code selection and eliminate any extra time that could be necessary for verification.

Document all additional views beyond the usual number. Report with modifier 22 Unusual procedural services added to the CPT code that may qualify the service for higher reimbursement. This does not apply to codes that specify "minimum number of views" in their descriptions.

Second Readings
The requesting physician may interpret a radiological study following the radiologist's interpretation. A second interpretation cannot be billed since it is part of the overall patient assessment. If the physician disagrees with the radiologist's findings, it should not be recorded in the patient chart. The physician should discuss any differences of opinion with the radiologist and if a change in interpretation is made, a final corrected statement should be made in the chart. A brief note stating the reason for the change should be included. This clarifies the final diagnostic interpretation of the service that simplifies the process of assigning accurate codes.

ADDITIONAL STUDIES

Findings from a routine x-ray exam may warrant further studies. For example, a radiologist may elect to do tomograms on a patient whose chest x-ray revealed a mass. The documentation must indicate that the existence of the mass establishes the medical necessity for further studies. In such a situation, the radiologist usually is not required to check with the ordering physician before proceeding with additional studies.

STEPS FOR ACCURATE CODING AND DOCUMENTATION

The following procedures should be followed for complete and accurate coding and documentation:

1. Obtain sufficient history from the ordering physician to assign an accurate diagnosis code.

2. Document the exam in sufficient detail to allow complete and accurate procedure coding.

3. If the report is dictated, review the transcribed report for accuracy. Correct any error on the transcribed report and return to the transcriptionist to generate new and corrected hard copy.

DIAGNOSTIC RADIOLOGY (DIAGNOSTIC IMAGING)

HEAD AND NECK

70010 Myelography, posterior fossa, radiological supervision and interpretation ⑤ 80 ▣

MED: 100-2,6,10; 100-2,15,80; 100-4,3,10.4; 100-4,13,10; 100-4,13,100

To report procedure, consult CPT codes 61055, 62284.

70015 Cisternography, positive contrast, radiological supervision and interpretation ⑤ 80 ▣

MED: 100-2,6,10; 100-2,15,80; 100-4,3,10.4; 100-4,13,10; 100-4,13,100

To report procedure, consult, CPT codes 61055, 62284.

70030 Radiologic examination, eye, for detection of foreign body ⓧ 80

MED: 100-2,6,10; 100-2,15,80; 100-4,3,10.4; 100-4,13,10; 100-4,13,100

70100 Radiologic examination, mandible; partial, less than four views ⓧ 80

MED: 100-2,6,10; 100-2,15,80; 100-4,3,10.4; 100-4,13,10; 100-4,13,100

70110 complete, minimum of four views ⓧ 80 ▣

MED: 100-2,6,10; 100-2,15,80; 100-4,3,10.4; 100-4,13,10; 100-4,13,100

70120 Radiologic examination, mastoids; less than three views per side ⓧ 80

MED: 100-2,6,10; 100-2,15,80; 100-4,3,10.4; 100-4,13,10; 100-4,13,100

70130 complete, minimum of three views per side ⓧ 80 ▣

MED: 100-2,6,10; 100-2,15,80; 100-4,3,10.4; 100-4,13,10; 100-4,13,100

70134 Radiologic examination, internal auditory meati, complete ⓧ 80

MED: 100-2,6,10; 100-2,15,80; 100-4,3,10.4; 100-4,13,10; 100-4,13,100

70140 Radiologic examination, facial bones; less than three views ⓧ 80

MED: 100-2,6,10; 100-2,15,80; 100-4,3,10.4; 100-4,13,10; 100-4,13,100

70150 complete, minimum of three views ⓧ 80 ▣

MED: 100-2,6,10; 100-2,15,80; 100-4,3,10.4; 100-4,13,10; 100-4,13,100

70160 Radiologic examination, nasal bones, complete, minimum of three views ⓧ 80

MED: 100-2,6,10; 100-2,15,80; 100-4,3,10.4; 100-4,13,10; 100-4,13,100

70170 Dacryocystography, nasolacrimal duct, radiological supervision and interpretation ⓧ 80 ▣

MED: 100-2,6,10; 100-2,15,80; 100-4,3,10.4; 100-4,13,10; 100-4,13,100

To report procedure, consult CPT code 68850.

70190 Radiologic examination; optic foramina ⓧ 80

MED: 100-2,6,10; 100-2,15,80; 100-4,3,10.4; 100-4,13,10; 100-4,13,100

70200 orbits, complete, minimum of four views ⓧ 80

MED: 100-2,6,10; 100-2,15,80; 100-4,3,10.4; 100-4,13,10; 100-4,13,100

70210 Radiologic examination, sinuses, paranasal, less than three views ⓧ 80

MED: 100-2,6,10; 100-2,15,80; 100-4,3,10.4; 100-4,13,10; 100-4,13,100

70220 Radiologic examination, sinuses, paranasal, complete, minimum of three views ⓧ 80 ▣

MED: 100-2,6,10; 100-2,15,80; 100-4,3,10.4; 100-4,13,10; 100-4,13,100

70240 Radiologic examination, sella turcica ⓧ 80

MED: 100-2,6,10; 100-2,15,80; 100-4,3,10.4; 100-4,13,10; 100-4,13,100

70250 Radiologic examination, skull; less than four views ⓧ 80

MED: 100-2,6,10; 100-2,15,80; 100-4,3,10.4; 100-4,13,10; 100-4,13,100

70260 complete, minimum of four views ⓧ 80 ▣

MED: 100-2,6,10; 100-2,15,80; 100-4,3,10.4; 100-4,13,10; 100-4,13,100

Crown, Neck, Root, Mandible — Enamel, Dentin, Pulp cavity, Root cavity, Apical foramen — Section of incisor

Dentine, Gingiva (gum), Cementum — Enamel, Root canal — Section of molar

Normal dentition numbers 16 teeth in each jaw: two incisors, two canines, four premolars, and six molars. A common tooth eruption problem occurs with the third molars (wisdom teeth) which may be malposed and become impacted. Caries means "rotten" and is a decalcification of tooth enamel and sometimes penetration into the dentin and pulp. Disease processes may cause resorption of the dentin and cementum

70300 Radiologic examination, teeth; single view ⓧ 80

MED: 100-2,6,10; 100-2,15,80; 100-4,3,10.4; 100-4,13,10; 100-4,13,100

70310 partial examination, less than full mouth ⓧ 80 ▣

MED: 100-2,6,10; 100-2,15,80; 100-4,3,10.4; 100-4,13,10; 100-4,13,100

70320 complete, full mouth ⓧ 80 ▣

MED: 100-2,6,10; 100-2,15,80; 100-4,3,10.4; 100-4,13,10; 100-4,13,100

70328 Radiologic examination, temporomandibular joint, open and closed mouth; unilateral ⓧ 80

MED: 100-2,6,10; 100-2,15,80; 100-4,3,10.4; 100-4,13,10; 100-4,13,100

70330 bilateral ⓧ 80 ▣

MED: 100-2,6,10; 100-2,15,80; 100-4,3,10.4; 100-4,13,10; 100-4,13,100

70332 Temporomandibular joint arthrography, radiological supervision and interpretation ⑤ 80 ▣

MED: 100-2,6,10; 100-2,15,80; 100-4,3,10.4; 100-4,13,10; 100-4,13,100

Code 77002 cannot be used with 70332.

70336 Magnetic resonance (eg, proton) imaging, temporomandibular joint(s) ⑤ 80 ▣

MED: 100-2,6,10; 100-2,15,80; 100-3,220.2; 100-4,3,10.4; 100-4,13,10; 100-4,13,40; 100-4,13,100

AMA: 2001,Jul,3; 1999,Jul,11

70350 Cephalogram, orthodontic ⓧ 80

MED: 100-2,6,10; 100-2,15,80; 100-4,3,10.4; 100-4,13,10; 100-4,13,100

70355 Orthopantogram ⊠ 80 ◰

MED: 100-2,6,10; 100-2,15,80; 100-4,3,10.4; 100-4,13,10;
100-4,13,100

70360 Radiologic examination; neck, soft tissue ⊠ 80

MED: 100-2,6,10; 100-2,15,80; 100-4,3,10.4; 100-4,13,10;
100-4,13,100

70370 pharynx or larynx, including fluoroscopy and/or magnification technique ⊠ 80 ◰

MED: 100-2,6,10; 100-2,15,80; 100-4,3,10.4; 100-4,13,10;
100-4,13,100

70371 Complex dynamic pharyngeal and speech evaluation by cine or video recording ⊠ 80 ◰

MED: 100-2,6,10; 100-2,15,80; 100-4,3,10.4; 100-4,13,10;
100-4,13,100

70373 Laryngography, contrast, radiological supervision and interpretation ⊠ 80 ◰

MED: 100-2,6,10; 100-2,15,80; 100-4,3,10.4; 100-4,13,10;
100-4,13,100

70380 Radiologic examination, salivary gland for calculus ⊠ 80

MED: 100-2,6,10; 100-2,15,80; 100-4,3,10.4; 100-4,13,10;
100-4,13,100

70390 Sialography, radiological supervision and interpretation ⊠ 80 ◰

MED: 100-2,6,10; 100-2,15,80; 100-4,3,10.4; 100-4,13,10;
100-4,13,100

To report procedure, consult CPT code 42550.

70450 Computed tomography, head or brain; without contrast material S 80 ◰

MED: 100-2,6,10; 100-2,15,80; 100-3,220.1; 100-4,3,10.4;
100-4,13,10; 100-4,13,30; 100-4,13,100

AMA: 1996,Apr,11

70460 with contrast material(s) S 80 ◰

MED: 100-2,6,10; 100-2,15,80; 100-3,220.1; 100-4,3,10.4;
100-4,13,10; 100-4,13,30; 100-4,13,100

AMA: 1996,Apr,11

70470 without contrast material, followed by contrast material(s) and further sections S 80 ◰

MED: 100-2,6,10; 100-2,15,80; 100-3,220.1; 100-4,3,10.4;
100-4,13,10; 100-4,13,30; 100-4,13,100

AMA: 1996,Apr,11

If 3D rendering is performed, consult CPT codes 76376, 76377.

70480 Computed tomography, orbit, sella, or posterior fossa or outer, middle, or inner ear; without contrast material S 80 ◰

MED: 100-2,6,10; 100-2,15,80; 100-3,220.1; 100-4,3,10.4;
100-4,13,10; 100-4,13,30; 100-4,13,100

70481 with contrast material(s) S 80 ◰

MED: 100-2,6,10; 100-2,15,80; 100-3,220.1; 100-4,3,10.4;
100-4,13,10; 100-4,13,30; 100-4,13,100

70482 without contrast material, followed by contrast material(s) and further sections S 80 ◰

MED: 100-2,6,10; 100-2,15,80; 100-3,220.1; 100-4,3,10.4;
100-4,13,10; 100-4,13,30; 100-4,13,100

If 3D rendering is performed, consult CPT codes 76376, 76377.

70486 Computed tomography, maxillofacial area; without contrast material S 80 ◰

MED: 100-2,6,10; 100-2,15,80; 100-3,220.1; 100-4,3,10.4;
100-4,13,10; 100-4,13,30; 100-4,13,100

AMA: 2002,Mar,11

70487 with contrast material(s) S 80 ◰

MED: 100-2,6,10; 100-2,15,80; 100-3,220.1; 100-4,3,10.4;
100-4,13,10; 100-4,13,30; 100-4,13,100

70488 without contrast material, followed by contrast material(s) and further sections S 80 ◰

MED: 100-2,6,10; 100-2,15,80; 100-3,220.1; 100-4,3,10.4;
100-4,13,10; 100-4,13,30; 100-4,13,100

If 3D rendering is performed, consult CPT codes 76376, 76377.

70490 Computed tomography, soft tissue neck; without contrast material S 80 ◰

MED: 100-2,6,10; 100-2,15,80; 100-3,220.1; 100-4,3,10.4;
100-4,13,10; 100-4,13,30; 100-4,13,100

70491 with contrast material(s) S 80 ◰

MED: 100-2,6,10; 100-2,15,80; 100-3,220.1; 100-4,3,10.4;
100-4,13,10; 100-4,13,30; 100-4,13,100

70492 without contrast material followed by contrast material(s) and further sections S 80 ◰

MED: 100-2,6,10; 100-2,15,80; 100-3,220.1; 100-4,3,10.4;
100-4,13,10; 100-4,13,30; 100-4,13,100

If 3D rendering is performed, consult CPT codes 76376, 76377.

If computed axial axial tomography is performed on the cervical spine, consult CPT codes 72125 and 72126.

70496 Computed tomographic angiography, head, without contrast material(s), followed by contrast material(s) and further sections, including image post-processing S 80 ◰

MED: 100-2,6,10; 100-2,15,80; 100-3,220.1; 100-4,3,10.4;
100-4,13,10; 100-4,13,30; 100-4,13,100

AMA: 2001,Jul,3

70498 Computed tomographic angiography, neck, without contrast material(s), followed by contrast material(s) and further sections, including image post-processing S 80 ◰

MED: 100-2,6,10; 100-2,15,80; 100-3,220.1; 100-4,3,10.4;
100-4,13,10; 100-4,13,30; 100-4,13,100

AMA: 2001,Jul,3

▲ **70540 Magnetic resonance (eg, proton) imaging, orbit, face, and/or neck; without contrast material(s)** S 80 ◰

MED: 100-2,6,10; 100-2,15,80; 100-3,220.2; 100-4,3,10.4;
100-4,13,10; 100-4,13,40; 100-4,13,100

AMA: 2001,Jul,3

▲ **70542 with contrast material(s)** S 80 ◰

MED: 100-2,6,10; 100-2,15,80; 100-3,220.2; 100-4,3,10.4;
100-4,13,10; 100-4,13,40; 100-4,13,100

AMA: 2001,Jul,3

▲ **70543 without contrast material(s), followed by contrast material(s) and further sequences** S 80 ◰

MED: 100-2,6,10; 100-2,15,80; 100-3,220.2; 100-4,3,10.4;
100-4,13,10; 100-4,13,40; 100-4,13,100

AMA: 2001,Jul,3

Rport codes 70540-70543 once per imaging session.

70544 Magnetic resonance angiography, head; without contrast material(s) S 80 ◰

MED: 100-2,6,10; 100-2,15,80; 100-3,220.3; 100-4,3,10.4;
100-4,13,10; 100-4,13,40.1; 100-4,13,40.1.1; 100-4,13,100

AMA: 2001,Sep,4

70545 with contrast material(s) S 80 ◰

MED: 100-2,6,10; 100-2,15,80; 100-3,220.3; 100-4,3,10.4;
100-4,13,10; 100-4,13,40.1; 100-4,13,40.1.1; 100-4,13,100

AMA: 2001,Sep,4

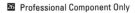 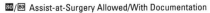

70546 **without contrast material(s), followed by contrast material(s) and further sequences** 〔S〕〔80〕〔◻〕

MED: 100-2,6,10; 100-2,15,80; 100-3,220.3; 100-4,3,10.4; 100-4,13,10; 100-4,13,40.1; 100-4,13,40.1.1; 100-4,13,100

AMA: 2001,Sep,4

70547 **Magnetic resonance angiography, neck; without contrast material(s)** 〔S〕〔80〕〔◻〕

MED: 100-2,6,10; 100-2,15,80; 100-3,220.3; 100-4,3,10.4; 100-4,13,10; 100-4,13,40.1; 100-4,13,40.1.1; 100-4,13,100

AMA: 2001,Sep,4

70548 **with contrast material(s)** 〔S〕〔80〕〔◻〕

MED: 100-2,6,10; 100-2,15,80; 100-3,220.3; 100-4,3,10.4; 100-4,13,10; 100-4,13,40.1; 100-4,13,40.1.1; 100-4,13,100

AMA: 2001,Sep,4

70549 **without contrast material(s), followed by contrast material(s) and further sequences** 〔S〕〔80〕〔◻〕

MED: 100-2,6,10; 100-2,15,80; 100-3,220.3; 100-4,3,10.4; 100-4,13,10; 100-4,13,40.1; 100-4,13,40.1.1; 100-4,13,100

AMA: 2001,Sep,4

70551 **Magnetic resonance (eg, proton) imaging, brain (including brain stem); without contrast material** 〔S〕〔80〕〔◻〕

MED: 100-2,6,10; 100-2,15,80; 100-3,220.2; 100-4,3,10.4; 100-4,12,70; 100-4,13,10; 100-4,13,20; 100-4,13,40; 100-4,13,90; 100-4,13,100

AMA: 1998,May,10

70552 **with contrast material(s)** 〔S〕〔80〕〔◻〕

MED: 100-2,6,10; 100-2,15,80; 100-3,220.2; 100-4,3,10.4; 100-4,13,10; 100-4,13,40; 100-4,13,100

AMA: 2001,Jul,3

70553 **without contrast material, followed by contrast material(s) and further sequences** 〔S〕〔80〕〔◻〕

MED: 100-2,6,10; 100-2,15,80; 100-3,220.2; 100-4,3,10.4; 100-4,12,70; 100-4,13,10; 100-4,13,20; 100-4,13,40; 100-4,13,90; 100-4,13,100

AMA: 2001,Jul,3; 1997,Nov,24

If magnetic spectroscopy is performed, consult CPT code 76390.

Identification and mapping of stimulation of brain functions is reported with codes 70554-70555. If the neurofunctional tests are performed by a technologist or nonphysician or nonpsychologist, consult 70554. When the service is provided entirely by a physician or psychologist, consult 70555.

● **70554** **Magnetic resonance imaging, brain, functional MRI; including test selection and administration of repetitive body part movement and/or visual stimulation, not requiring physician or psychologist administration** 〔S〕

Do not report 70554 with 96020.

● **70555** **requiring physician or psychologist administration of entire neurofunctional testing** 〔S〕

Do not report 70555 unless 96020 is performed.

Do not report 70554 or 70555 with 70551-70553 unless a separate diagnostic MRI is performed.

70557 **Magnetic resonance (eg, proton) imaging, brain (including brain stem and skull base), during open intracranial procedure (eg, to assess for residual tumor or residual vascular malformation); without contrast material** 〔S〕〔80〕〔◻〕

To report stereotactic biopsy of intracranial lesion with magnetic resonance guidance, use 61751.

Codes 70557, 70558 or 70559 can be reported only if a separate report is generated. Report only one of these codes once per operative session.

Do not report these codes in conjunction with 61751, 77021 or 77022.

70558 **with contrast material(s)** 〔S〕〔80〕〔◻〕

70559 **without contrast material(s), followed by contrast material(s) and further sequences** 〔S〕〔80〕〔◻〕

Use 61751 for stereotactic biopsy of intracranial lesion with magnetic resonance guidance.

Codes 70557, 70558, or 70559 may be reported only if a separate report is generated. Report only one of these codes once per operative session. Do not use these codes in conjunction with 61751, 77021, or 77022.

CHEST

To report fluoroscopic or ultrasonic guidance for needle placement procedure such as a biopsy, aspiration, injection, or localization device of the thorax, consult 76942, 77002.

71010 **Radiologic examination, chest; single view, frontal** 〔X〕〔80〕〔◻〕

MED: 100-2,6,10; 100-2,15,80; 100-4,3,10.4; 100-4,12,30.6.12; 100-4,13,10; 100-4,13,90; 100-4,13,100

If chest x-ray, single view, frontal is performed as part of critical care services do not report separately.

71015 **stereo, frontal** 〔X〕〔80〕〔◻〕

MED: 100-2,15,80; 100-4,3,10.4; 100-4,12,30.6.12; 100-4,13,10; 100-4,13,100

71020 **Radiologic examination, chest, two views, frontal and lateral;** 〔X〕〔80〕〔◻〕

MED: 100-2,6,10; 100-2,15,80; 100-4,3,10.4; 100-4,12,30.6.12; 100-4,13,10; 100-4,13,90; 100-4,13,100

If chest x-ray, two views, frontal and lateral is performed as part of critical care services do not report separately.

71021 **with apical lordotic procedure** 〔X〕〔80〕〔◻〕

MED: 100-2,15,80; 100-4,3,10.4; 100-4,13,10; 100-4,13,90; 100-4,13,100

71022 **with oblique projections** 〔X〕〔80〕〔◻〕

MED: 100-2,6,10; 100-2,15,80; 100-4,3,10.4; 100-4,13,10; 100-4,13,100

71023 **with fluoroscopy** 〔X〕〔80〕〔◻〕

MED: 100-2,15,80; 100-4,3,10.4; 100-4,13,10; 100-4,13,100

71030 **Radiologic examination, chest, complete, minimum of four views;** 〔X〕〔80〕〔◻〕

MED: 100-2,6,10; 100-2,15,80; 100-4,3,10.4; 100-4,13,10; 100-4,13,90; 100-4,13,100

71034 **with fluoroscopy** 〔X〕〔80〕〔◻〕

MED: 100-2,15,80; 100-4,3,10.4; 100-4,13,10; 100-4,13,100

If a separate chest fluoroscopy is performed, consult CPT code 76000.

71035 **Radiologic examination, chest, special views (eg, lateral decubitus, Bucky studies)** 〔X〕〔80〕

MED: 100-2,6,10; 100-2,15,80; 100-4,3,10.4; 100-4,13,10; 100-4,13,100

71040 **Bronchography, unilateral, radiological supervision and interpretation** 〔X〕〔80〕〔◻〕

MED: 100-2,15,80; 100-4,3,10.4; 100-4,13,10; 100-4,13,100

To report procedure, consult CPT codes 31656, 31715.

71060 **Bronchography, bilateral, radiological supervision and interpretation** 〔X〕〔80〕〔◻〕

MED: 100-2,15,80; 100-4,3,10.4; 100-4,13,10; 100-4,13,100

To report procedure, consult CPT codes 31656, 31715.

71090 **Insertion pacemaker, fluoroscopy and radiography, radiological supervision and interpretation** 〔X〕〔80〕〔◻〕

MED: 100-2,15,80; 100-4,3,10.4; 100-4,13,10; 100-4,13,100

To report procedure, consult CPT for appropriate code.

⊛ Modifier 63 Exempt Code   ⊙ Conscious Sedation   ✚ CPT Add-on Code   ⊘ Modifier 51 Exempt Code   ● New Code   ▲ Revised Code

Ⓜ Maternity Edit   Ⓐ Age Edit   Ⓐ-Ⓨ APC Status Indicators   ◻ CCI Comprehensive Code   〔50〕 Bilateral Procedure

71100	Radiologic examination, ribs, unilateral; two views	X 80 ▣

MED: 100-2,6,10; 100-2,15,80; 100-4,3,10.4; 100-4,13,10; 100-4,13,100

71101	including posteroanterior chest, minimum of three views	X 80 ▣

MED: 100-2,15,80; 100-4,3,10.4; 100-4,13,10; 100-4,13,100

71110	Radiologic examination, ribs, bilateral; three views	X 80 ▣

MED: 100-2,6,10; 100-2,15,80; 100-4,3,10.4; 100-4,13,10; 100-4,13,100

71111	including posteroanterior chest, minimum of four views	X 80 ▣

MED: 100-2,15,80; 100-4,3,10.4; 100-4,13,10; 100-4,13,100

71120	Radiologic examination; sternum, minimum of two views	X 80

MED: 100-2,15,80; 100-4,3,10.4; 100-4,13,10; 100-4,13,100

71130	sternoclavicular joint or joints, minimum of three views	X 80

MED: 100-2,15,80; 100-4,3,10.4; 100-4,13,10; 100-4,13,100

71250	Computed tomography, thorax; without contrast material	S 80 ▣

MED: 100-2,6,10; 100-2,15,80; 100-3,220.1; 100-4,3,10.4; 100-4,13,10; 100-4,13,30; 100-4,13,100

71260	with contrast material(s)	S 80 ▣

MED: 100-2,15,80; 100-3,220.1; 100-4,3,10.4; 100-4,13,10; 100-4,13,30; 100-4,13,100

AMA: 2001,Jul,3

71270	without contrast material, followed by contrast material(s) and further sections	S 80 ▣

MED: 100-2,15,80; 100-3,220.1; 100-4,3,10.4; 100-4,13,10; 100-4,13,30; 100-4,13,100

AMA: 2001,Jun,10

If 3D rendering is performed, consult CPT codes 76376, 76377.

See codes 0144T-0151T for cardiac computed tomography of the heart.

▲ **71275**	Computed tomographic angiography, chest (noncoronary), without contrast material(s), followed by contrast material(s) and further sections, including image postprocessing	S 80 ▣

MED: 100-2,6,10; 100-2,15,80; 100-3,220.1; 100-4,3,10.4; 100-4,13,10; 100-4,13,30; 100-4,13,100

Consult codes 0146T-0149T for coronary artery computed tomographic angiography including calcification score and/or cardiac morphology.

71550	Magnetic resonance (eg, proton) imaging, chest (eg, for evaluation of hilar and mediastinal lymphadenopathy); without contrast material(s)	S 80 ▣

MED: 100-2,6,10; 100-2,15,80; 100-3,220.2; 100-4,3,10.4; 100-4,13,10; 100-4,13,40; 100-4,13,100

AMA: 2001,Jul,3

71551	with contrast material(s)	S 80 ▣

MED: 100-2,15,80; 100-3,220.2; 100-4,3,10.4; 100-4,13,10; 100-4,13,40; 100-4,13,100

AMA: 2001,Jul,3

71552	without contrast material(s), followed by contrast material(s) and further sequences	S 80 ▣

MED: 100-2,15,80; 100-3,220.2; 100-4,3,10.4; 100-4,13,10; 100-4,13,40; 100-4,13,100

AMA: 2001,Jul,3

If a breast MRI is performed, consult CPT codes 77058 and 77059.

71555	Magnetic resonance angiography, chest (excluding myocardium), with or without contrast material(s)	B 80 ▣

MED: 100-2,6,10; 100-2,15,80; 100-3,220.3; 100-4,3,10.4; 100-4,13,10; 100-4,13,40.1; 100-4,13,40.1.1; 100-4,13,100

AMA: 1995,Fall,2

SPINE AND PELVIS

72010	Radiologic examination, spine, entire, survey study, anteroposterior and lateral	X 80 ▣

MED: 100-2,6,10; 100-2,15,80; 100-4,3,10.4; 100-4,13,10; 100-4,13,100

AMA: 2002,May,18

72020	Radiologic examination, spine, single view, specify level	X 80

MED: 100-2,15,80; 100-4,3,10.4; 100-4,13,10; 100-4,13,100

72040	Radiologic examination, spine, cervical; two or three views	X 80

MED: 100-2,6,10; 100-2,15,80; 100-4,3,10.4; 100-4,13,10; 100-4,13,90; 100-4,13,100

AMA: 2001,Sep,4

72050	minimum of four views	X 80 ▣

MED: 100-2,15,80; 100-4,3,10.4; 100-4,13,10; 100-4,13,90; 100-4,13,100

72052	complete, including oblique and flexion and/or extension studies	X 80 ▣

MED: 100-2,15,80; 100-4,3,10.4; 100-4,13,10; 100-4,13,90; 100-4,13,100

72069	Radiologic examination, spine, thoracolumbar, standing (scoliosis)	X 80 ▣

MED: 100-2,15,80; 100-4,3,10.4; 100-4,13,10; 100-4,13,90; 100-4,13,100

72070	Radiologic examination, spine; thoracic, two views	X 80 ▣

MED: 100-2,6,10; 100-2,15,80; 100-4,3,10.4; 100-4,13,10; 100-4,13,90; 100-4,13,100

AMA: 2001,Sep,4

72072	thoracic, three views	X 80 ▣

MED: 100-2,15,80; 100-4,3,10.4; 100-4,13,10; 100-4,13,90; 100-4,13,100

AMA: 2001,Sep,4

72074	thoracic, minimum of four views	X 80 ▣

MED: 100-2,15,80; 100-4,3,10.4; 100-4,13,10; 100-4,13,90; 100-4,13,100

AMA: 2001,Sep,4

72080	thoracolumbar, two views	X 80 ▣

MED: 100-2,15,80; 100-4,3,10.4; 100-4,13,10; 100-4,13,90; 100-4,13,100

AMA: 2001,Sep,4

72090	scoliosis study, including supine and erect studies	X 80 ▣

MED: 100-2,15,80; 100-4,3,10.4; 100-4,13,10; 100-4,13,100

72100	Radiologic examination, spine, lumbosacral; two or three views	X 80 ▣

MED: 100-2,6,10; 100-2,15,80; 100-4,3,10.4; 100-4,13,10; 100-4,13,100

AMA: 2001,Sep,4

72110	minimum of four views	X 80 ▣

MED: 100-2,15,80; 100-4,3,10.4; 100-4,13,10; 100-4,13,100

AMA: 2001,Sep,4

72114	complete, including bending views	X 80 ▣

MED: 100-2,15,80; 100-4,3,10.4; 100-4,13,10; 100-4,13,90; 100-4,13,100

72120 Radiologic examination, spine, lumbosacral, bending views only, minimum of four views 🅇 80 ▮
MED: 100-2,15,80; 100-4,3,10.4; 100-4,13,10; 100-4,13,100

72125 Computed tomography, cervical spine; without contrast material 🅂 80 ▮
MED: 100-2,6,10; 100-2,15,80; 100-3,220.1; 100-4,3,10.4; 100-4,13,10; 100-4,13,30; 100-4,13,100

72126 with contrast material 🅂 80 ▮
MED: 100-2,15,80; 100-3,220.1; 100-4,3,10.4; 100-4,13,10; 100-4,13,30; 100-4,13,100

72127 without contrast material, followed by contrast material(s) and further sections 🅂 80 ▮
MED: 100-2,15,80; 100-3,220.1; 100-4,3,10.4; 100-4,13,10; 100-4,13,30; 100-4,13,100

72128 Computed tomography, thoracic spine; without contrast material 🅂 80 ▮
MED: 100-2,6,10; 100-2,15,80; 100-3,220.1; 100-4,3,10.4; 100-4,13,10; 100-4,13,30; 100-4,13,100

72129 with contrast material 🅂 80 ▮
MED: 100-2,15,80; 100-3,220.1; 100-4,3,10.4; 100-4,13,10; 100-4,13,30; 100-4,13,100

72130 without contrast material, followed by contrast material(s) and further sections 🅂 80 ▮
MED: 100-2,15,80; 100-3,220.1; 100-4,3,10.4; 100-4,13,10; 100-4,13,30; 100-4,13,100

72131 Computed tomography, lumbar spine; without contrast material 🅂 80 ▮
MED: 100-2,6,10; 100-2,15,80; 100-3,220.1; 100-4,3,10.4; 100-4,13,10; 100-4,13,30; 100-4,13,100

72132 with contrast material 🅂 80 ▮
MED: 100-2,15,80; 100-3,220.1; 100-4,3,10.4; 100-4,13,10; 100-4,13,30; 100-4,13,100
AMA: 1993,Fall,13

72133 without contrast material, followed by contrast material(s) and further sections 🅂 80 ▮
MED: 100-2,15,80; 100-3,220.1; 100-4,3,10.4; 100-4,13,10; 100-4,13,30; 100-4,13,100
If 3D rendering is performed, consult CPT codes 76376, 76377.

To report intrathecal injections, consult CPT codes 61055, 62284.

72141 Magnetic resonance (eg, proton) imaging, spinal canal and contents, cervical; without contrast material 🅂 80 ▮
MED: 100-2,6,10; 100-2,15,80; 100-3,220.2; 100-4,3,10.4; 100-4,13,10; 100-4,13,40; 100-4,13,100

72142 with contrast material(s) 🅂 80 ▮
MED: 100-2,15,80; 100-3,220.2; 100-4,3,10.4; 100-4,13,10; 100-4,13,40; 100-4,13,100
If cervical spine canal imaging is performed first without contrast material followed by contrast material, consult CPT code 72156.

72146 Magnetic resonance (eg, proton) imaging, spinal canal and contents, thoracic; without contrast material 🅂 80 ▮
MED: 100-2,6,10; 100-2,15,80; 100-3,220.2; 100-4,3,10.4; 100-4,13,10; 100-4,13,40; 100-4,13,100
AMA: 1999,May,10

72147 with contrast material(s) 🅂 80 ▮
MED: 100-2,15,80; 100-3,220.2; 100-4,3,10.4; 100-4,13,10; 100-4,13,40; 100-4,13,100
AMA: 1999,May,10
If thoracic spinal canal imaging is performed first without contrast material followed by contrast material, consult CPT code 72157.

72148 Magnetic resonance (eg, proton) imaging, spinal canal and contents, lumbar; without contrast material 🅂 80 ▮
MED: 100-2,6,10; 100-2,15,80; 100-3,220.2; 100-4,3,10.4; 100-4,13,10; 100-4,13,40; 100-4,13,100

72149 with contrast material(s) 🅂 80 ▮
MED: 100-2,15,80; 100-3,220.2; 100-4,3,10.4; 100-4,13,10; 100-4,13,40; 100-4,13,100
If lumbar spinal canal imaging is performed first without contrast material followed by contrast material, consult CPT code 72158.

72156 Magnetic resonance (eg, proton) imaging, spinal canal and contents, without contrast material, followed by contrast material(s) and further sequences; cervical 🅂 80 ▮
MED: 100-2,6,10; 100-2,15,80; 100-3,220.2; 100-4,3,10.4; 100-4,12,70; 100-4,13,10; 100-4,13,20; 100-4,13,40; 100-4,13,90; 100-4,13,100

72157 thoracic 🅂 80 ▮
MED: 100-2,15,80; 100-3,220.2; 100-4,3,10.4; 100-4,12,70; 100-4,13,10; 100-4,13,20; 100-4,13,40; 100-4,13,90; 100-4,13,100

72158 lumbar 🅂 80 ▮
MED: 100-2,15,80; 100-3,220.2; 100-4,3,10.4; 100-4,12,70; 100-4,13,10; 100-4,13,20; 100-4,13,40; 100-4,13,90; 100-4,13,100

72159 Magnetic resonance angiography, spinal canal and contents, with or without contrast material(s) 🅔
MED: 100-2,6,10; 100-2,15,80; 100-3,220.3; 100-4,3,10.4; 100-4,13,10; 100-4,13,40.1; 100-4,13,40.1.1; 100-4,13,100

72170 Radiologic examination, pelvis; one or two views 🅇 80
MED: 100-2,15,80; 100-4,3,10.4; 100-4,13,10; 100-4,13,100
AMA: 2001,Sep,4

72190 complete, minimum of three views 🅇 80 ▮
MED: 100-2,6,10; 100-2,15,80; 100-4,3,10.4; 100-4,13,10; 100-4,13,90; 100-4,13,100
If pelvimetry is performed, consult CPT code 74710.

72191 Computed tomographic angiography, pelvis, without contrast material(s), followed by contrast material(s) and further sections, including image post-processing 🅂 80 ▮
MED: 100-2,6,10; 100-2,15,80; 100-3,220.1; 100-4,3,10.4; 100-4,13,10; 100-4,13,30; 100-4,13,100
AMA: 2001,Jul,3
To report CTA aorto-iliofemoral runoff, consult CPT code 75635.

72192 Computed tomography, pelvis; without contrast material 🅂 80 ▮
MED: 100-2,6,10; 100-2,15,80; 100-3,220.1; 100-4,3,10.4; 100-4,13,10; 100-4,13,30; 100-4,13,100

72193 with contrast material(s) 🅂 80 ▮
MED: 100-2,15,80; 100-3,220.1; 100-4,3,10.4; 100-4,13,10; 100-4,13,30; 100-4,13,100

 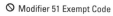

Radiology

72194   without contrast material, followed by contrast material(s) and further sections   [S] [80] [▣]

MED: 100-2,15,80; 100-3,220.1; 100-4,3,10.4; 100-4,13,10; 100-4,13,30; 100-4,13,100

If 3D rendering is performed, consult CPT codes 76376, 76377.

For computed tomographic colonography, consult Category III codes 0066T, 0067T.

Codes 72192-72194 cannot be reported with Category III codes 0066T, 0067T.

72195   **Magnetic resonance (eg, proton) imaging, pelvis; without contrast material(s)**   [S] [80] [▣]

MED: 100-2,6,10; 100-2,15,80; 100-3,220.1; 100-3,220.2; 100-4,3,10.4; 100-4,13,10; 100-4,13,40; 100-4,13,100

AMA: 2001,Jul,3

72196   **with contrast material(s)**   [S] [80] [▣]

MED: 100-2,15,80; 100-3,220.1; 100-3,220.2; 100-4,3,10.4; 100-4,13,10; 100-4,13,40; 100-4,13,100

AMA: 2001,Jul,3

72197   **without contrast material(s), followed by contrast material(s) and further sequences**   [S] [80] [▣]

MED: 100-2,15,80; 100-3,220.1; 100-3,220.2; 100-4,3,10.4; 100-4,13,10; 100-4,13,40; 100-4,13,100

AMA: 2001,Jul,3

72198   **Magnetic resonance angiography, pelvis, with or without contrast material(s)**   [B] [80] [▣]

MED: 100-2,6,10; 100-2,15,80; 100-3,220.3; 100-4,3,10.4; 100-4,13,10; 100-4,13,40.1; 100-4,13,40.1.1; 100-4,13,100

72200   **Radiologic examination, sacroiliac joints; less than three views**   [X] [80]

MED: 100-2,15,80; 100-4,3,10.4; 100-4,13,10; 100-4,13,100

72202   **three or more views**   [X] [80]

MED: 100-2,15,80; 100-4,3,10.4; 100-4,13,10; 100-4,13,100

72220   **Radiologic examination, sacrum and coccyx, minimum of two views**   [X] [80]

MED: 100-2,6,10; 100-2,15,80; 100-4,3,10.4; 100-4,13,10; 100-4,13,90; 100-4,13,100

72240   **Myelography, cervical, radiological supervision and interpretation**   [S] [80] [▣]

MED: 100-2,6,10; 100-2,15,80; 100-4,3,10.4; 100-4,13,10; 100-4,13,100

AMA: 1993,Fall,13

To report procedure, consult CPT codes 61055, 62284.

72255   **Myelography, thoracic, radiological supervision and interpretation**   [S] [80] [▣]

MED: 100-2,6,10; 100-2,15,80; 100-4,3,10.4; 100-4,13,10; 100-4,13,100

To report procedure, consult CPT codes 61055, 62284.

72265   **Myelography, lumbosacral, radiological supervision and interpretation**   [S] [80] [▣]

MED: 100-2,6,10; 100-2,15,80; 100-4,3,10.4; 100-4,13,10; 100-4,13,100

AMA: 2000,Aug,7; 1993,Fall,13

To report procedure, consult CPT codes 61055, 62284.

72270   **Myelography, two or more regions (eg, lumbar/thoracic, cervical/thoracic, lumbar/cervical, lumbar/thoracic/cervical), radiological supervision and interpretation**   [S] [80] [▣]

MED: 100-2,6,10; 100-2,15,80; 100-4,3,10.4; 100-4,13,10; 100-4,13,100

To report procedure, consult CPT codes 61055, 62284.

72275   **Epidurography, radiological supervision and interpretation**   [S] [▣]

MED: 100-2,15,80; 100-4,3,10.4; 100-4,13,10; 100-4,13,100

AMA: 2000,Jan,1; 2000,Aug,7; 1999,Nov,40

To report the injection procedure consult CPT codes 62280-62282, 62310-62319, 64479-64484, and 0027T.

Code 72275 includes code 77003.

Report 72275 only when an epidurogram is performed, images documented, and a formal radiology report is written.

▲ **72285**   **Discography, cervical or thoracic, radiological supervision and interpretation**   [S] [80] [▣]

MED: 100-2,6,10; 100-2,15,80; 100-4,3,10.4; 100-4,13,10; 100-4,13,100

AMA: 1999,Nov,35, 40

To report procedure, consult CPT code 62291.

● **72291**   **Radiological supervision and interpretation, percutaneous vertebroplasty or vertebral augmentation including cavity creation, per vertebral body; under fluoroscopic guidance**   [S]

See codes 22520-22525 for procedure.

● **72292**   **under CT guidance**   [S]

See codes 22520-22525 for procedure.

▲ **72295**   **Discography, lumbar, radiological supervision and interpretation**   [S] [80] [▣]

MED: 100-2,6,10; 100-2,15,80; 100-4,3,10.4; 100-4,13,10; 100-4,13,100

To report procedure, consult CPT code 62290.

UPPER EXTREMITIES

If a radiological examination of stress views is performed, any joint, consult CPT code 77071.

Gold wedding band absorbs all x-rays (white)

Air allows all rays to reach film (black)

Calcium in bone absorbs most of rays and is nearly white

Radiograph (left)

Film

X-ray beam

Soft tissues absorb part of rays and will vary in gray intensity

Posterioranterior (PA) chest study; lateral views also common

Traditional diagnostic radiography is defined by the x-ray. Radiographs, or x-rays, are "shadowgrams" of body structures and tissues and show radiopaque matter, such as bone, to be whiter and radiolucent substances, such as air, to be blacker. Each study is oriented by the direction path of the x-ray beam: e.g., PA, the most common, means the beam travels from posterior to anterior. Contrast agents are commonly used to highlight particular areas or structures

73000   **Radiologic examination; clavicle, complete**   [X] [80]

MED: 100-2,15,80; 100-4,3,10.4; 100-4,13,10; 100-4,13,100

73010   **scapula, complete**   [X] [80]

MED: 100-2,15,80; 100-4,3,10.4; 100-4,13,10; 100-4,13,100

73020   **Radiologic examination, shoulder; one view**   [X] [80]

MED: 100-2,15,80; 100-4,3,10.4; 100-4,13,10; 100-4,13,100

73030   **complete, minimum of two views**   [X] [80] [▣]

MED: 100-2,6,10; 100-2,15,80; 100-4,3,10.4; 100-4,13,10; 100-4,13,100

73040   **Radiologic examination, shoulder, arthrography, radiological supervision and interpretation**   [S] [80] [▣]

MED: 100-2,15,80; 100-4,3,10.4; 100-4,13,10; 100-4,13,100

AMA: 2001,Jul,3

Code 77002 cannot be reported with 73040.

To report injection procedure, consult CPT code 23350.

72194 — 73040

---

[26] Professional Component Only

[80]/[80] Assist-at-Surgery Allowed/With Documentation

Unlisted

Not Covered

[TC] Technical Component Only   **MED:** Pub 100/NCD References   **AMA:** CPT Assistant References   [1]-[9] ASC Group   ♂ Male Only   ♀ Female Only

73050 Radiologic examination; acromioclavicular joints, bilateral, with or without weighted distraction ⊠ 80

MED: 100-2,15,80; 100-4,3,10.4; 100-4,13,10; 100-4,13,100

73060 humerus, minimum of two views ⊠ 80

MED: 100-2,15,80; 100-4,3,10.4; 100-4,13,10; 100-4,13,100

73070 Radiologic examination, elbow; two views ⊠ 80

MED: 100-2,15,80; 100-4,3,10.4; 100-4,13,10; 100-4,13,100
AMA: 2001,Sep,4

73080 complete, minimum of three views ⊠ 80 ◪

MED: 100-2,6,10; 100-2,15,80; 100-4,3,10.4; 100-4,13,10; 100-4,13,100

73085 Radiologic examination, elbow, arthrography, radiological supervision and interpretation ⑤ 80 ◪

MED: 100-2,15,80; 100-4,3,10.4; 100-4,13,10; 100-4,13,100
Code 77002 cannot be reported with 73085.

To report injection procedure, consult CPT code 24220.

73090 Radiologic examination; forearm, two views ⊠ 80

MED: 100-2,6,10; 100-2,15,80; 100-4,3,10.4; 100-4,13,10; 100-4,13,100
AMA: 2001,Sep,4

73092 upper extremity, infant, minimum of two views Ⓐ ⊠ 80 ◪

MED: 100-2,15,80; 100-4,3,10.4; 100-4,13,10; 100-4,13,100

73100 Radiologic examination, wrist; two views ⊠ 80

MED: 100-2,6,10; 100-2,15,80; 100-4,3,10.4; 100-4,13,10; 100-4,13,100
AMA: 2001,Sep,4

73110 complete, minimum of three views ⊠ 80 ◪

MED: 100-2,15,80; 100-4,3,10.4; 100-4,13,10; 100-4,13,100
AMA: 1997,Mar,10

73115 Radiologic examination, wrist, arthrography, radiological supervision and interpretation ⑤ 80 ◪

MED: 100-2,15,80; 100-4,3,10.4; 100-4,13,10; 100-4,13,100
Code 77002 cannot be reported with 73115.

To report injection procedure, consult CPT code 25246.

73120 Radiologic examination, hand; two views ⊠ 80 ◪

MED: 100-2,6,10; 100-2,15,80; 100-4,3,10.4; 100-4,13,10; 100-4,13,100

73130 minimum of three views ⊠ 80 ◪

MED: 100-2,15,80; 100-4,3,10.4; 100-4,13,10; 100-4,13,100

73140 Radiologic examination, finger(s), minimum of two views ⊠ 80

MED: 100-2,15,80; 100-4,3,10.4; 100-4,13,10; 100-4,13,100

73200 Computed tomography, upper extremity; without contrast material ⑤ 80 ◪

MED: 100-2,6,10; 100-2,15,80; 100-3,220.1; 100-4,3,10.4; 100-4,13,10; 100-4,13,30; 100-4,13,100

73201 with contrast material(s) ⑤ 80 ◪

MED: 100-2,15,80; 100-3,220.1; 100-4,3,10.4; 100-4,13,10; 100-4,13,30; 100-4,13,100

73202 without contrast material, followed by contrast material(s) and further sections ⑤ 80 ◪

MED: 100-2,15,80; 100-3,220.1; 100-4,3,10.4; 100-4,13,10; 100-4,13,30; 100-4,13,100

73206 Computed tomographic angiography, upper extremity, without contrast material(s), followed by contrast material(s) and further sections, including image post-processing ⑤ 80 ◪

MED: 100-2,6,10; 100-2,15,80; 100-3,220.1; 100-4,3,10.4; 100-4,13,10; 100-4,13,30; 100-4,13,100
AMA: 2001,Jul,3

73218 Magnetic resonance (eg, proton) imaging, upper extremity, other than joint; without contrast material(s) ⑤ 80 ◪

MED: 100-2,6,10; 100-2,15,80; 100-4,3,10.4; 100-4,13,10; 100-4,13,30; 100-4,13,100
AMA: 2001,Jul,3

73219 with contrast material(s) ⑤ 80 ◪

MED: 100-2,15,80; 100-3,220.2; 100-4,3,10.4; 100-4,13,10; 100-4,13,40; 100-4,13,100
AMA: 2001,Jul,3

73220 without contrast material(s), followed by contrast material(s) and further sequences ⑤ 80 ◪

MED: 100-2,15,80; 100-3,220.2; 100-4,3,10.4; 100-4,13,10; 100-4,13,40; 100-4,13,100
AMA: 2001,Jul,3

73221 Magnetic resonance (eg, proton) imaging, any joint of upper extremity; without contrast material(s) ⑤ 80 ◪

MED: 100-2,6,10; 100-2,15,80; 100-3,220.2; 100-4,3,10.4; 100-4,13,10; 100-4,13,40; 100-4,13,100
AMA: 2001,Jul,3

73222 with contrast material(s) ⑤ 80 ◪

MED: 100-2,15,80; 100-3,220.2; 100-4,3,10.4; 100-4,13,10; 100-4,13,40; 100-4,13,100
AMA: 2001,Jul,3

73223 without contrast material(s), followed by contrast material(s) and further sequences ⑤ 80 ◪

MED: 100-2,15,80; 100-3,220.2; 100-4,3,10.4; 100-4,13,10; 100-4,13,40; 100-4,13,100
AMA: 2001,Jul,3

73225 Magnetic resonance angiography, upper extremity, with or without contrast material(s) Ⓔ

MED: 100-2,6,10; 100-2,15,80; 100-3,220.3; 100-4,3,10.4; 100-4,13,10; 100-4,13,40.1; 100-4,13,40.1.1; 100-4,13,100

LOWER EXTREMITIES

If a radiological examination of stress views is performed, any joint, consult CPT code 77071.

73500 Radiologic examination, hip, unilateral; one view ⊠ 80

MED: 100-2,6,10; 100-2,15,80; 100-4,3,10.4; 100-4,13,10; 100-4,13,100

73510 complete, minimum of two views ⊠ 80 ◪

MED: 100-2,15,80; 100-4,3,10.4; 100-4,13,10; 100-4,13,100
AMA: 2002,Apr,19; 1999,May,10; 1992,Spring,9

73520 Radiologic examination, hips, bilateral, minimum of two views of each hip, including anteroposterior view of pelvis ⊠ 80 ◪

MED: 100-2,6,10; 100-2,15,80; 100-4,3,10.4; 100-4,13,10; 100-4,13,100
AMA: 2002,Apr,19

73525 Radiologic examination, hip, arthrography, radiological supervision and interpretation ⑤ 80 ◪

MED: 100-2,15,80; 100-4,3,10.4; 100-4,13,10; 100-4,13,100
Code 77002 cannot be reported with 73525.

To report injection procedure, consult CPT codes 27093, 27095.

73530 Radiologic examination, hip, during operative procedure ⊠ 80

MED: 100-2,15,80; 100-4,3,10.4; 100-4,13,10; 100-4,13,100

73540 Radiologic examination, pelvis and hips, infant or child, minimum of two views Ⓐ ⊠ 80 ◪

MED: 100-2,15,80; 100-4,3,10.4; 100-4,13,10; 100-4,13,100

73542 — 74010

73542 Radiological examination, sacroiliac joint arthrography, radiological supervision and interpretation ⑤ ☒

MED: 100-2,6,10; 100-2,15,80; 100-4,3,10.4; 100-4,13,10; 100-4,13,100
AMA: 1999,Nov,40-41
Code 77002 cannot be reported with 73542.

For injection procedure, use 27096. If formal arthrography is not performed, recorded, and a formal radiologic report is not issued, use 77003 for fluoroscopic guidance for sacroiliac joint injections.

73550 Radiologic examination, femur, two views ☒ ⑧⓪

MED: 100-2,15,80; 100-4,3,10.4; 100-4,13,10; 100-4,13,100
AMA: 2001,Sep,4

73560 Radiologic examination, knee; one or two views ☒ ⑧⓪ ☒

MED: 100-2,6,10; 100-2,15,80; 100-4,3,10.4; 100-4,13,10; 100-4,13,100

73562 three views ☒ ⑧⓪ ☒

MED: 100-2,15,80; 100-4,3,10.4; 100-4,13,10; 100-4,13,100

73564 complete, four or more views ☒ ⑧⓪ ☒

MED: 100-2,15,80; 100-4,3,10.4; 100-4,13,10; 100-4,13,100
AMA: 1998,Nov,21; 1998,Jun,11

73565 both knees, standing, anteroposterior ☒ ⑧⓪ ☒

MED: 100-2,15,80; 100-4,3,10.4; 100-4,13,10; 100-4,13,100

73580 Radiologic examination, knee, arthrography, radiological supervision and interpretation ⑤ ⑧⓪ ☒

MED: 100-2,15,80; 100-4,3,10.4; 100-4,13,10; 100-4,13,100
Code 77002 cannot be reported with 73580.

To report injection procedure, consult CPT code 27370.

73590 Radiologic examination; tibia and fibula, two views ☒ ⑧⓪ ☒

MED: 100-2,6,10; 100-2,15,80; 100-4,3,10.4; 100-4,13,10; 100-4,13,100
AMA: 2001,Sep,4

73592 lower extremity, infant, minimum of two views Ⓐ☒ ⑧⓪ ☒

MED: 100-2,6,10; 100-2,15,80; 100-4,3,10.4; 100-4,13,10; 100-4,13,100

73600 Radiologic examination, ankle; two views ☒ ⑧⓪ ☒

MED: 100-2,15,80; 100-4,3,10.4; 100-4,13,10; 100-4,13,100
AMA: 2001,Sep,4

73610 complete, minimum of three views ☒ ⑧⓪ ☒

MED: 100-2,15,80; 100-4,3,10.4; 100-4,13,10; 100-4,13,100

73615 Radiologic examination, ankle, arthrography, radiological supervision and interpretation ⑤ ⑧⓪ ☒

MED: 100-2,15,80; 100-4,3,10.4; 100-4,13,10; 100-4,13,100
Code 77002 cannot be reported with 73615.

To report injection procedure, consult CPT code 27648.

73620 Radiologic examination, foot; two views ☒ ⑧⓪ ☒

MED: 100-2,15,80; 100-4,3,10.4; 100-4,13,10; 100-4,13,100
AMA: 2001,Sep,4

73630 complete, minimum of three views ☒ ⑧⓪ ☒

MED: 100-2,15,80; 100-4,3,10.4; 100-4,13,10; 100-4,13,100

73650 Radiologic examination; calcaneus, minimum of two views ☒ ⑧⓪

MED: 100-2,15,80; 100-4,3,10.4; 100-4,13,10; 100-4,13,100

73660 toe(s), minimum of two views ☒ ⑧⓪

MED: 100-2,15,80; 100-4,3,10.4; 100-4,13,10; 100-4,13,100

73700 Computed tomography, lower extremity; without contrast material ⑤ ⑧⓪ ☒

MED: 100-2,6,10; 100-2,13,30; 100-2,15,80; 100-3,220.1; 100-4,3,10.4; 100-4,13,10; 100-4,13,100

73701 with contrast material(s) ⑤ ⑧⓪ ☒

MED: 100-2,13,30; 100-2,15,80; 100-3,220.1; 100-4,3,10.4; 100-4,13,10; 100-4,13,100

73702 without contrast material, followed by contrast material(s) and further sections ⑤ ⑧⓪ ☒

MED: 100-2,13,30; 100-2,15,80; 100-3,220.1; 100-4,3,10.4; 100-4,13,10; 100-4,13,100
If 3D rendering is performed, consult CPT codes 76376, 76377.

73706 Computed tomographic angiography, lower extremity, without contrast material(s), followed by contrast material(s) and further sections, including image post-processing ⑤ ⑧⓪ ☒

MED: 100-2,6,10; 100-2,15,80; 100-4,3,10.4; 100-4,13,10; 100-4,13,100
AMA: 2001,Jul,3
To report CTA aorto-iliofemoral runoff, consult CPT code 75635.

73718 Magnetic resonance (eg, proton) imaging, lower extremity other than joint; without contrast material(s) ⑤ ⑧⓪ ☒

MED: 100-2,6,10; 100-2,15,80; 100-3,220.2; 100-4,3,10.4; 100-4,13,10; 100-4,13,40; 100-4,13,100
AMA: 2001,Jul,3

73719 with contrast material(s) ⑤ ⑧⓪ ☒

MED: 100-2,15,80; 100-3,220.2; 100-4,3,10.4; 100-4,13,10; 100-4,13,40; 100-4,13,100
AMA: 2001,Jul,3

73720 without contrast material(s), followed by contrast material(s) and further sequences ⑤ ⑧⓪ ☒

MED: 100-2,15,80; 100-3,220.2; 100-4,3,10.4; 100-4,13,10; 100-4,13,40; 100-4,13,100
AMA: 2001,Jul,3

73721 Magnetic resonance (eg, proton) imaging, any joint of lower extremity; without contrast material ⑤ ⑧⓪ ☒

MED: 100-2,6,10; 100-2,15,80; 100-3,220.2; 100-4,3,10.4; 100-4,13,10; 100-4,13,40; 100-4,13,100
AMA: 2001,Jul,3

73722 with contrast material(s) ⑤ ⑧⓪ ☒

MED: 100-2,15,80; 100-3,220.2; 100-4,3,10.4; 100-4,13,10; 100-4,13,40; 100-4,13,100
AMA: 2001,Jul,3

73723 without contrast material(s), followed by contrast material(s) and further sequences ⑤ ⑧⓪ ☒

MED: 100-2,15,80; 100-3,220.2; 100-4,3,10.4; 100-4,13,10; 100-4,13,40; 100-4,13,100
AMA: 2001,Jul,3

73725 Magnetic resonance angiography, lower extremity, with or without contrast material(s) Ⓑ ⑧⓪ ☒

MED: 100-2,6,10; 100-2,15,80; 100-3,220.3; 100-4,3,10.4; 100-4,13,10; 100-4,13,40.1; 100-4,13,40.1.1; 100-4,13,100

ABDOMEN

74000 Radiologic examination, abdomen; single anteroposterior view ☒ ⑧⓪

MED: 100-2,15,80; 100-4,3,10.4; 100-4,13,10; 100-4,13,90; 100-4,13,100
AMA: 1998,Nov,21

74010 anteroposterior and additional oblique and cone views ☒ ⑧⓪ ☒

MED: 100-2,15,80; 100-4,3,10.4; 100-4,13,10; 100-4,13,100

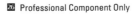

74020 complete, including decubitus and/or erect views ⊠ 80 ▣

MED: 100-2,15,80; 100-4,3,10.4; 100-4,13,10; 100-4,13,100

74022 complete acute abdomen series, including supine, erect, and/or decubitus views, single view chest ⊠ 80 ▣

MED: 100-2,6,10; 100-2,15,80; 100-4,3,10.4; 100-4,13,10; 100-4,13,100

74150 Computed tomography, abdomen; without contrast material Ⓢ 80 ▣

MED: 100-2,6,10; 100-2,15,80; 100-3,220.1; 100-4,3,10.4; 100-4,13,10; 100-4,13,30; 100-4,13,100

AMA: 2002,Oct,12

74160 with contrast material(s) Ⓢ 80 ▣

MED: 100-2,15,80; 100-3,220.1; 100-4,3,10.4; 100-4,13,10; 100-4,13,30; 100-4,13,100

74170 without contrast material, followed by contrast material(s) and further sections Ⓢ 80 ▣

MED: 100-2,15,80; 100-3,220.1; 100-4,3,10.4; 100-4,13,10; 100-4,13,30; 100-4,13,100

For computed tomographic colonography, consult Category III codes 0066T, 0067T.

Codes 72192-72194 cannot be reported with Category III codes 0066T, 0067T.

74175 Computed tomographic angiography, abdomen, without contrast material(s), followed by contrast material(s) and further sections, including image post-processing Ⓢ 80 ▣

MED: 100-2,6,10; 100-2,15,80; 100-3,220.1; 100-4,3,10.4; 100-4,13,10; 100-4,13,30; 100-4,13,100

AMA: 2001,Jul,3

To report CTA aorto-iliofemoral runoff, consult CPT code 75635.

74181 Magnetic resonance (eg, proton) imaging, abdomen; without contrast material(s) Ⓢ 80 ▣

MED: 100-2,6,10; 100-2,15,80; 100-3,220.2; 100-4,3,10.4; 100-4,13,10; 100-4,13,40; 100-4,13,100

AMA: 2001,Jul,3

74182 with contrast material(s) Ⓢ 80 ▣

MED: 100-2,15,80; 100-3,220.2; 100-4,3,10.4; 100-4,13,10; 100-4,13,40; 100-4,13,100

AMA: 2001,Jul,3

74183 without contrast material(s), followed by with contrast material(s) and further sequences Ⓢ 80 ▣

MED: 100-2,15,80; 100-3,220.2; 100-4,3,10.4; 100-4,13,10; 100-4,13,40; 100-4,13,100

AMA: 2001,Jul,3

74185 Magnetic resonance angiography, abdomen, with or without contrast material(s) Ⓑ 80 ▣

MED: 100-2,6,10; 100-3,220.3; 100-4,3,10.4; 100-4,13,40.1; 100-4,13,40.1.1

74190 Peritoneogram (eg, after injection of air or contrast), radiological supervision and interpretation ⊠ 80 ▣

MED: 100-2,15,80; 100-4,3,10.4; 100-4,13,10; 100-4,13,100

If air or contrast is injected into the peritoneal cavity, consult CPT code 49400. If computed tomography is performed on the pelvis, consult CPT code 72192 or 74150.

GASTROINTESTINAL TRACT

If the gastrostomy tube is placed percutaneously, consult CPT code 43750.

74210 Radiologic examination; pharynx and/or cervical esophagus Ⓢ 80

MED: 100-2,15,80; 100-4,3,10.4; 100-4,13,10; 100-4,13,100

74220 esophagus Ⓢ 80 ▣

MED: 100-2,15,80; 100-4,3,10.4; 100-4,13,10; 100-4,13,100

74230 Swallowing function, with cineradiography/videoradiography Ⓢ 80 ▣

MED: 100-2,15,80; 100-4,3,10.4; 100-4,13,10; 100-4,13,100

74235 Removal of foreign body(s), esophageal, with use of balloon catheter, radiological supervision and interpretation Ⓢ 80 ▣

MED: 100-2,15,80; 100-4,3,10.4; 100-4,13,10; 100-4,13,100

To report esophagoscopy or upper gastrointestinal endoscopy procedure with removal of a foreign body, consult CPT codes 43215 and 43247.

74240 Radiologic examination, gastrointestinal tract, upper; with or without delayed films, without KUB Ⓢ 80 ▣

MED: 100-2,6,10; 100-2,15,80; 100-4,3,10.4; 100-4,13,10; 100-4,13,100

74241 with or without delayed films, with KUB Ⓢ 80 ▣

MED: 100-2,15,80; 100-4,3,10.4; 100-4,13,10; 100-4,13,100

74245 with small intestine, includes multiple serial films Ⓢ 80 ▣

MED: 100-2,15,80; 100-4,3,10.4; 100-4,13,10; 100-4,13,100

74246 Radiological examination, gastrointestinal tract, upper, air contrast, with specific high density barium, effervescent agent, with or without glucagon; with or without delayed films, without KUB Ⓢ 80 ▣

MED: 100-2,15,80; 100-4,3,10.4; 100-4,13,10; 100-4,13,100

Moynihan test

74247 with or without delayed films, with KUB Ⓢ 80 ▣

MED: 100-2,15,80; 100-4,3,10.4; 100-4,13,10; 100-4,13,100

74249 with small intestine follow-through Ⓢ 80 ▣

MED: 100-2,15,80; 100-4,3,10.4; 100-4,13,10; 100-4,13,100

74250 Radiologic examination, small intestine, includes multiple serial films; Ⓢ 80 ▣

MED: 100-2,6,10; 100-2,15,80; 100-4,3,10.4; 100-4,13,10; 100-4,13,100

74251 via enteroclysis tube Ⓢ 80 ▣

MED: 100-2,15,80; 100-4,3,10.4; 100-4,13,10; 100-4,13,100

74260 Duodenography, hypotonic Ⓢ 80 ▣

MED: 100-2,15,80; 100-4,3,10.4; 100-4,13,10; 100-4,13,100

74270 Radiologic examination, colon; barium enema, with or without KUB Ⓢ 80 ▣

MED: 100-2,15,80; 100-4,3,10.4; 100-4,13,10; 100-4,13,100

74280 air contrast with specific high density barium, with or without glucagon Ⓢ 80 ▣

MED: 100-2,15,80; 100-4,3,10.4; 100-4,13,10; 100-4,13,100; 100-4,18,60.1

74283 Therapeutic enema, contrast or air, for reduction of intussusception or other intraluminal obstruction (eg, meconium ileus) Ⓢ 80

MED: 100-2,15,80; 100-4,3,10.4; 100-4,13,10; 100-4,13,100

AMA: 1997,Nov,24

74290 Cholecystography, oral contrast; Ⓢ 80

MED: 100-2,15,80; 100-4,3,10.4; 100-4,13,10; 100-4,13,100

74291 additional or repeat examination or multiple day examination Ⓢ 80

MED: 100-2,15,80; 100-4,3,10.4; 100-4,13,10; 100-4,13,100

Radiology

74300 — 74450

74300 Cholangiography and/or pancreatography; intraoperative, radiological supervision and interpretation ☒ 80 ◪

MED: 100-2,15,80; 100-4,3,10.4; 100-4,13,10; 100-4,13,100
AMA: 2000,Dec,14; 1999,Nov,41

+ **74301** additional set intraoperative, radiological supervision and interpretation (List separately in addition to code for primary procedure) ☒ 80 ◪

MED: 100-2,15,80; 100-4,3,10.4; 100-4,13,10; 100-4,13,100

Note that 74301 is an add-on code and must be used in conjunction with 74300.

74305 through existing catheter, radiological supervision and interpretation ☒ 80 ◪

MED: 100-2,15,80; 100-4,3,10.4; 100-4,13,10; 100-4,13,100
AMA: 1999,Nov,41
To report procedure performed, consult CPT codes 47505, 47560-47561, 47563, and 48400. If a biliary duct stone extraction is performed percutaneously, consult CPT codes 47630 and 74327.

74320 Cholangiography, percutaneous, transhepatic, radiological supervision and interpretation ☒ 80 ◪

MED: 100-2,15,80; 100-4,3,10.4; 100-4,13,10; 100-4,13,100
To report procedure, consult CPT code 47500.

74327 Postoperative biliary duct calculus removal, percutaneous via T-tube tract, basket, or snare (eg, Burhenne technique), radiological supervision and interpretation ⑤ 80 ◪

MED: 100-2,6,10; 100-2,15,80; 100-4,3,10.4; 100-4,13,10; 100-4,13,100

If a biliary duct stone extraction is performed percutaneously, consult CPT code 47630.

74328 Endoscopic catheterization of the biliary ductal system, radiological supervision and interpretation Ⓝ 80 ◪

MED: 100-2,15,80; 100-4,3,10.4; 100-4,13,10; 100-4,13,100
To report endoscopic retrograde cholangiopancreatography (ECRP) procedure, consult CPT codes 43260-43272 as appropriate.

74329 Endoscopic catheterization of the pancreatic ductal system, radiological supervision and interpretation Ⓝ 80 ◪

MED: 100-2,15,80; 100-4,3,10.4; 100-4,13,10; 100-4,13,100
To report endoscopic retrograde cholangiopancreatography (ECRP) procedure, consult CPT codes 43260-43272 as appropriate.

74330 Combined endoscopic catheterization of the biliary and pancreatic ductal systems, radiological supervision and interpretation Ⓝ 80 ◪

MED: 100-2,15,80; 100-4,3,10.4; 100-4,13,10; 100-4,13,100
To report endoscopic retrograde cholangiopancreatography (ECRP) procedure, consult CPT codes 43260-43272 as appropriate.

74340 Introduction of long gastrointestinal tube (eg, Miller-Abbott), including multiple fluoroscopies and films, radiological supervision and interpretation ☒ 80 ◪

MED: 100-2,15,80; 100-4,3,10.4; 100-4,13,10; 100-4,13,100
If tube is placed, consult CPT code 44500.

74350 Percutaneous placement of gastrostomy tube, radiological supervision and interpretation ☒ 80 ◪

MED: 100-2,15,80; 100-4,3,10.4; 100-4,13,10; 100-4,13,100

74355 Percutaneous placement of enteroclysis tube, radiological supervision and interpretation ☒ 80 ◪

MED: 100-2,15,80; 100-4,3,10.4; 100-4,13,10; 100-4,13,100
To report procedure, consult CPT code 44015.

74360 Intraluminal dilation of strictures and/or obstructions (eg, esophagus), radiological supervision and interpretation ⑤ 80 ◪

MED: 100-2,15,80; 100-4,3,10.4; 100-4,13,10; 100-4,13,100
AMA: 1994,Spring,3
To report procedure, consult CPT codes 43220 or 43458.

74363 Percutaneous transhepatic dilation of biliary duct stricture with or without placement of stent, radiological supervision and interpretation ⑤ 80 ◪

MED: 100-2,15,80; 100-4,3,10.4; 100-4,13,10; 100-4,13,100
If a transhepatic catheter/stent is introduced percutaneously, consult CPT codes 47510 and 47511. If a biliary endoscopy is performed percutaneously via a T-tube or other tract with dilation of the biliary duct stricture(s), consult CPT codes 47555 and 47556.

URINARY TRACT

74400 Urography (pyelography), intravenous, with or without KUB, with or without tomography ⑤ 80 ◪

MED: 100-2,15,80; 100-4,3,10.4; 100-4,13,10; 100-4,13,100

74410 Urography, infusion, drip technique and/or bolus technique; ⑤ 80 ◪

MED: 100-2,15,80; 100-4,3,10.4; 100-4,13,10; 100-4,13,100

74415 with nephrotomography ⑤ 80 ◪

MED: 100-2,15,80; 100-4,3,10.4; 100-4,13,10; 100-4,13,100

74420 Urography, retrograde, with or without KUB ⑤ 80 ◪

MED: 100-2,15,80; 100-4,3,10.4; 100-4,13,10; 100-4,13,100
AMA: 2000,Sep,11

74425 Urography, antegrade, (pyelostogram, nephrostogram, loopogram), radiological supervision and interpretation ⑤ 80 ◪

MED: 100-2,15,80; 100-4,3,10.4; 100-4,13,10; 100-4,13,100
AMA: 1997,Dec,7; 1993,Fall,14
To report procedure, consult CPT codes 50394, 50684, and 50690.

74430 Cystography, minimum of three views, radiological supervision and interpretation ⑤ 80 ◪

MED: 100-2,15,80; 100-4,3,10.4; 100-4,13,10; 100-4,13,100
To report procedure, consult CPT codes 51600 and 51605.

74440 Vasography, vesiculography, or epididymography, radiological supervision and interpretation ♂ ⑤ 80 ◪

MED: 100-2,15,80; 100-4,3,10.4; 100-4,13,10; 100-4,13,100
To report procedure, consult CPT codes 52010 and 55300.

74445 Corpora cavernosography, radiological supervision and interpretation ♂ ⑤ 80 ◪

MED: 100-2,15,80; 100-4,3,10.4; 100-4,13,10; 100-4,13,100
To report procedure, consult CPT code 54230.

74450 Urethrocystography, retrograde, radiological supervision and interpretation ⑤ 80 ◪

MED: 100-2,15,80; 100-3,230.2; 100-4,3,10.4; 100-4,13,10; 100-4,13,100
To report procedure, consult CPT code 51610.

74455   **Urethrocystography, voiding, radiological supervision and interpretation** ⑤ 80 ☐

MED: 100-2,15,80; 100-3,230.2; 100-4,3,10.4; 100-4,13,10; 100-4,13,100

To report procedure, consult CPT code 51600.

74470   **Radiologic examination, renal cyst study, translumbar, contrast visualization, radiological supervision and interpretation** 区 80 ☐

MED: 100-2,15,80; 100-4,3,10.4; 100-4,13,10; 100-4,13,100

To report procedure, consult CPT code 50390.

74475   **Introduction of intracatheter or catheter into renal pelvis for drainage and/or injection, percutaneous, radiological supervision and interpretation** ⑤ 80 ☐

MED: 100-2,15,80; 100-4,3,10.4; 100-4,13,10; 100-4,13,100

AMA: 1997,Dec,7

To report procedure, consult CPT codes 50392 and 50396.

74480   **Introduction of ureteral catheter or stent into ureter through renal pelvis for drainage and/or injection, percutaneous, radiological supervision and interpretation** ⑤ 80 ☐

MED: 100-2,15,80; 100-4,3,10.4; 100-4,13,10; 100-4,13,100

AMA: 1993,Fall,14

To report surgical procedure performed consult CPT codes 50393, 50395, and 50396 as appropriate. If transurethral surgery (ureter and pelvis) is performed, consult CPT codes 52320-52355.

74485   **Dilation of nephrostomy, ureters, or urethra, radiological supervision and interpretation** ⑤ 80 ☐

MED: 100-2,15,80; 100-4,3,10.4; 100-4,13,10; 100-4,13,100

If the ureter is dilated without radiological guidance, consult CPT codes 52341, 52344. If a nephrostomy or pyelostomy tube is changed, consult CPT code 50395.

To report procedure, consult CPT codes 50395 and 53600-53621.

GYNECOLOGICAL AND OBSTETRICAL

If radiological examination is performed on the abdomen and pelvis, consult CPT codes 72170-72190, 74000-74170.

74710   **Pelvimetry, with or without placental localization** ♀ 区 80

MED: 100-2,15,80; 100-4,3,10.4; 100-4,13,10; 100-4,13,100

74740   **Hysterosalpingography, radiological supervision and interpretation** ♀ 区 80 ☐

MED: 100-2,15,80; 100-4,3,10.4; 100-4,13,10; 100-4,13,100

AMA: 1999,Jul,8; 1997,Nov,24

If saline or contrast is introduced for hysterosalpingography, see 58340.

74742   **Transcervical catheterization of fallopian tube, radiological supervision and interpretation** ♀ 区 80 ☐

MED: 100-2,15,80; 100-4,3,10.4; 100-4,13,10; 100-4,13,100

To report the transcervical introduction of a fallopian tube catheter with or without hysterosalpingography, consult CPT code 58345.

74775   **Perineogram (eg, vaginogram, for sex determination or extent of anomalies)** Ⓜ ♀ ⑤ 80 ☐

MED: 100-2,15,80; 100-4,3,10.4; 100-4,13,10; 100-4,13,100

HEART

To report cardiac catheterization procedures, consult CPT codes 93501-93556.

75552   **Cardiac magnetic resonance imaging for morphology; without contrast material** ⑤ 80 ☐

MED: 100-2,6,10; 100-2,15,80; 100-3,220.2; 100-4,3,10.4; 100-4,13,10; 100-4,13,40; 100-4,13,100

AMA: 1995,Fall,1

75553   **with contrast material** ⑤ 80 ☐

MED: 100-2,15,80; 100-3,220.2; 100-4,3,10.4; 100-4,13,10; 100-4,13,40; 100-4,13,100

AMA: 1995,Fall,1

75554   **Cardiac magnetic resonance imaging for function, with or without morphology; complete study** ⑤ 80 ☐

MED: 100-2,6,10; 100-2,15,80; 100-3,220.2; 100-4,3,10.4; 100-4,13,10; 100-4,13,40; 100-4,13,100

AMA: 1995,Fall,2

75555   **limited study** ⑤ 80 ☐

MED: 100-2,15,80; 100-3,220.2; 100-4,3,10.4; 100-4,13,10; 100-4,13,40; 100-4,13,100

AMA: 1995,Fall,2

75556   **Cardiac magnetic resonance imaging for velocity flow mapping** Ⓔ

MED: 100-2,6,10; 100-2,15,80; 100-3,220.2; 100-4,3,10.4; 100-4,13,10; 100-4,13,40; 100-4,13,100

AMA: 1995,Fall,2

To report intravenous procedures, consult CPT codes 36000-36013, 36400-36425 and 36100-36248 for intra-arterial procedures. To report radiological supervision and interpretation, consult CPT codes 75600-75978.

VASCULAR PROCEDURES

AORTA AND ARTERIES

Include introduction and all lesser order catheterization used in the approach. Additional order catheterization within the same family of arteries should be reported using codes in the 36000 range The following diagnostic angiography procedures include the work provided in the interventional procedure and should not be reported separately:

- Contrast injections, angiography, roadmapping, and/or fluoroscopy
- Vessel measurement
- Post angiography or stent angiography

Diagnostic codes may only be used in addition to the interventional procedure if the following are met:

- No previous angiographic study is available, and a full diagnostic study is performed that is the basis for the interventional procedure.
- A diagnostic study is documented in the medical records but the patient's condition has changed, there is not adequate visualization, or there is a clinical change during the procedure that requires reevaluation.
- The diagnostic study is performed in a different area from the interventional surgery

Do not separately report a diagnostic angiography performed at the same time as an interventional procedure if it specifically included in the interventional code procedure description.

75600   **Aortography, thoracic, without serialography, radiological supervision and interpretation** ⑤ 80 ☐

MED: 100-2,15,80; 100-4,3,10.4; 100-4,13,10; 100-4,13,100

To report the injection procedure, consult CPT code 93544.

75605   **Aortography, thoracic, by serialography, radiological supervision and interpretation** ⑤ 80 ☐

MED: 100-2,15,80; 100-4,3,10.4; 100-4,13,10; 100-4,13,100

AMA: 1998,Dec,9; 1994,Spring,29

To report the injection procedure, consult CPT code 93544.

⊗ Modifier 63 Exempt Code   ⊙ Conscious Sedation   + CPT Add-on Code   ⊘ Modifier 51 Exempt Code   ● New Code   ▲ Revised Code

Ⓜ Maternity Edit   Ⓐ Age Edit   Ⓐ-Ⓨ APC Status Indicators   ☐ CCI Comprehensive Code   80 Bilateral Procedure

75625 Aortography, abdominal, by serialography, radiological supervision and interpretation [S] [80] [ ]

    MED: 100-2,15,80; 100-4,3,10.4; 100-4,13,10; 100-4,13,100

    AMA: 2001,Jan,14; 1993,Fall,16

    To report the injection procedure, consult CPT code 93544.

75630 Aortography, abdominal plus bilateral iliofemoral lower extremity, catheter, by serialography, radiological supervision and interpretation [S] [80] [ ]

    MED: 100-2,15,80; 100-4,3,10.4; 100-4,13,10; 100-4,13,100

    AMA: 2001,Jan,14; 1993,Fall,16

    Include introduction and all lesser order catheterization used in the approach. Additional order catheterization within the same family of arteries should be reported using codes in the 36000s.

75635 Computed tomographic angiography, abdominal aorta and bilateral iliofemoral lower extremity runoff, radiological supervision and interpretation, without contrast material(s), followed by contrast material(s) and further sections, including image post-processing [S] [80] [ ]

    MED: 100-2,15,80; 100-4,3,10.4; 100-4,13,10; 100-4,13,100

    AMA: 2001,Jul,3

75650 Angiography, cervicocerebral, catheter, including vessel origin, radiological supervision and interpretation [S] [80] [ ]

    MED: 100-2,15,80; 100-4,3,10.4; 100-4,13,10; 100-4,13,100

    AMA: 2000,Oct,4; 1998,Apr,3; 1994,Spring,29

75658 Angiography, brachial, retrograde, radiological supervision and interpretation [S] [80] [ ]

    MED: 100-2,15,80; 100-4,3,10.4; 100-4,13,10; 100-4,13,100

75660 Angiography, external carotid, unilateral, selective, radiological supervision and interpretation [S] [80] [ ]

    MED: 100-2,15,80; 100-4,3,10.4; 100-4,13,10; 100-4,13,100

75662 Angiography, external carotid, bilateral, selective, radiological supervision and interpretation [S] [80] [ ]

    MED: 100-2,15,80; 100-4,3,10.4; 100-4,13,10; 100-4,13,100

75665 Angiography, carotid, cerebral, unilateral, radiological supervision and interpretation [S] [80] [ ]

    MED: 100-2,15,80; 100-4,3,10.4; 100-4,13,10; 100-4,13,100

75671 Angiography, carotid, cerebral, bilateral, radiological supervision and interpretation [S] [80] [ ]

    MED: 100-2,15,80; 100-4,3,10.4; 100-4,13,10; 100-4,13,100

    AMA: 2000,Oct,4

75676 Angiography, carotid, cervical, unilateral, radiological supervision and interpretation [S] [80] [ ]

    MED: 100-2,15,80; 100-4,3,10.4; 100-4,13,10; 100-4,13,100

75680 Angiography, carotid, cervical, bilateral, radiological supervision and interpretation [S] [80] [ ]

    MED: 100-2,15,80; 100-4,3,10.4; 100-4,13,10; 100-4,13,100

    AMA: 2000,Oct,4

75685 Angiography, vertebral, cervical, and/or intracranial, radiological supervision and interpretation [S] [80] [ ]

    MED: 100-2,15,80; 100-4,3,10.4; 100-4,13,10; 100-4,13,100

    AMA: 2000,Oct,4

75705 Angiography, spinal, selective, radiological supervision and interpretation [S] [80] [ ]

    MED: 100-2,15,80; 100-4,3,10.4; 100-4,13,10; 100-4,13,100

75710 Angiography, extremity, unilateral, radiological supervision and interpretation [S] [80] [ ]

    MED: 100-2,15,80; 100-4,3,10.4; 100-4,13,10; 100-4,13,100

    AMA: 2001,Jan,14; 1999,Apr,11

75716 Angiography, extremity, bilateral, radiological supervision and interpretation [S] [80] [ ]

    MED: 100-2,15,80; 100-4,3,10.4; 100-4,13,10; 100-4,13,100

    AMA: 2001,Jan,14; 1993,Fall,16

75722 Angiography, renal, unilateral, selective (including flush aortogram), radiological supervision and interpretation [S] [80] [ ]

    MED: 100-2,15,80; 100-4,3,10.4; 100-4,13,10; 100-4,13,100

75724 Angiography, renal, bilateral, selective (including flush aortogram), radiological supervision and interpretation [S] [80] [ ]

    MED: 100-2,15,80; 100-4,3,10.4; 100-4,13,10; 100-4,13,100

75726 Angiography, visceral, selective or supraselective, (with or without flush aortogram), radiological supervision and interpretation [S] [80] [ ]

    MED: 100-2,15,80; 100-4,3,10.4; 100-4,13,10; 100-4,13,100

    If selective angiography is performed, each additional visceral vessel studied after basic examination, consult CPT code 75774.

75731 Angiography, adrenal, unilateral, selective, radiological supervision and interpretation [S] [80] [ ]

    MED: 100-2,15,80; 100-4,3,10.4; 100-4,13,10; 100-4,13,100

75733 Angiography, adrenal, bilateral, selective, radiological supervision and interpretation [S] [80] [ ]

    MED: 100-2,15,80; 100-4,3,10.4; 100-4,13,10; 100-4,13,100

75736 Angiography, pelvic, selective or supraselective, radiological supervision and interpretation [S] [80] [ ]

    MED: 100-2,15,80; 100-4,3,10.4; 100-4,13,10; 100-4,13,100

75741 Angiography, pulmonary, unilateral, selective, radiological supervision and interpretation [S] [80] [ ]

    MED: 100-2,15,80; 100-4,3,10.4; 100-4,13,10; 100-4,13,100

    To report an injection procedure during pulmonary angiography, consult CPT code 93541.

75743 Angiography, pulmonary, bilateral, selective, radiological supervision and interpretation [S] [80] [ ]

    MED: 100-2,15,80; 100-4,3,10.4; 100-4,13,10; 100-4,13,100

    AMA: 1998,Apr,3; 1994,Spring,29

    For an injection procedure during pulmonary angiography, consult CPT code 93541.

75746 Angiography, pulmonary, by nonselective catheter or venous injection, radiological supervision and interpretation [S] [80] [ ]

    MED: 100-2,15,80; 100-4,3,10.4; 100-4,13,10; 100-4,13,100

    To report an injection procedure during cardiac catheterization To report pulmonary angiography, consult CPT code 93541. To report catheter introduction, injection procedure, consult CPT codes 93501-93533, 93539, 93540, 93545, and 93556.

    If an intravenous procedure is reported, consult CPT codes 36000-36013, 36400-36425, and 36100-36248 To report an intra-arterial procedure.

75756 Angiography, internal mammary, radiological supervision and interpretation [S] [80] [ ]

    MED: 100-2,15,80; 100-4,3,10.4; 100-4,13,10; 100-4,13,100

    To report catheter introduction, injection procedure, consult CPT codes 93501-93533, 93545, and 93556.

---

[26] Professional Component Only   [80]/[80] Assist-at-Surgery Allowed/With Documentation   Unlisted   Not Covered

[TC] Technical Component Only   **MED:** Pub 100/NCD References   **AMA:** CPT Assistant References   [1]-[9] ASC Group   ♂ Male Only   ♀ Female Only

266 — CPT Expert   CPT only © 2006 American Medical Association. All Rights Reserved. *(Black Ink)*   © *2006 Ingenix (Blue Ink)*

+ **75774** **Angiography, selective, each additional vessel studied after basic examination, radiological supervision and interpretation (List separately in addition to code for primary procedure)** S 80 ▣

MED: 100-2,15,80; 100-4,3,10.4; 100-4,13,10; 100-4,13,100
AMA: 1994,Spring,29; 1993,Fall,17
To report angiography, consult CPT code 75600-75790.

To report catheterizations, consult CPT codes 36215-36248.

To report introduction of catheter, injection procedure, consult CPT codes 93501-93533, 93545, 93555, 93556.

Note that 75774 is an add-on code that must be used in conjunction with the appropriate code To report the specific initial vessel studied. This code cannot be reported alone.

75790 **Angiography, arteriovenous shunt (eg, dialysis patient), radiological supervision and interpretation** S 80 ▣

MED: 100-2,15,80; 100-4,3,10.4; 100-4,13,10; 100-4,13,100
AMA: 2001,May,1
To report catheter introduction, consult CPT codes 36140, 36145, 36215-36217, and 36245-36247.

VEINS AND LYMPHATICS

The following venography diagnostic procedures include the work provided in the interventional procedure and should not be reported separately:

- Contrast injections, venography, roadmapping, and/or fluoroscopy
- Vessel measurement
- Post venography or stent venography

Diagnostic procedure codes may only be used in addition to the interventional procedure if the following are met:

- No prior catheter-based venographic study is available and a full diagnostic study is performed, and the decision to intervene is based on that diagnostic study.
- A diagnostic study is documented in the medical records but the patient's condition has changed, there is not adequate visualization or there is a clinical change during the procedure that requires reevaluation.
- The diagnostic study is performed in a different area from the interventional surgery

Do not separately report a diagnostic venography performed at the same time as an interventional procedure if it specifically included in the interventional code procedure description.

The following procedures are included in a therapeutic transcatheter interventional procedure:

- Contrast injections, venography, roadmapping, and/or fluoroscopy
- Vessel measurement
- Except for services allowed by 75898, completion of angiography/venography

If an injection procedure is performed for the lymphatic system, consult CPT code 38790. If an injection procedure is performed for the venous system, consult CPT codes 36000-36015 and 36400-36510.

75801 **Lymphangiography, extremity only, unilateral, radiological supervision and interpretation** X 80 ▣

MED: 100-2,15,80; 100-4,3,10.4; 100-4,13,10; 100-4,13,100

75803 **Lymphangiography, extremity only, bilateral, radiological supervision and interpretation** X 80 ▣

MED: 100-2,15,80; 100-4,3,10.4; 100-4,13,10; 100-4,13,100

75805 **Lymphangiography, pelvic/abdominal, unilateral, radiological supervision and interpretation** X 80 ▣

MED: 100-2,15,80; 100-4,3,10.4; 100-4,13,10; 100-4,13,100

75807 **Lymphangiography, pelvic/abdominal, bilateral, radiological supervision and interpretation** X 80 ▣

MED: 100-2,15,80; 100-4,3,10.4; 100-4,13,10; 100-4,13,100

75809 **Shuntogram for investigation of previously placed indwelling nonvascular shunt (eg, LeVeen shunt, ventriculoperitoneal shunt, indwelling infusion pump), radiological supervision and interpretation** X 80 ▣

MED: 100-2,15,80; 100-4,3,10.4; 100-4,13,10; 100-4,13,100
If an injection procedure is performed for the evaluation of a previously placed peritoneovenous shunt, consult CPT code 49427. For puncture of shunt tubing or reservoir for aspiration or injection procedure, consult CPT code 61070.

75810 **Splenoportography, radiological supervision and interpretation** S 80 ▣

MED: 100-2,15,80; 100-4,3,10.4; 100-4,13,10; 100-4,13,100

75820 **Venography, extremity, unilateral, radiological supervision and interpretation** S 80 ▣

MED: 100-2,15,80; 100-4,3,10.4; 100-4,13,10; 100-4,13,100
AMA: 1997,Oct,10

75822 **Venography, extremity, bilateral, radiological supervision and interpretation** S 80 ▣

MED: 100-2,15,80; 100-4,3,10.4; 100-4,13,10; 100-4,13,100

75825 **Venography, caval, inferior, with serialography, radiological supervision and interpretation** S 80 ▣

MED: 100-2,15,80; 100-4,3,10.4; 100-4,13,10; 100-4,13,100

75827 **Venography, caval, superior, with serialography, radiological supervision and interpretation** S 80 ▣

MED: 100-2,15,80; 100-4,3,10.4; 100-4,13,10; 100-4,13,100
AMA: 1998,Apr,3

75831 **Venography, renal, unilateral, selective, radiological supervision and interpretation** S 80 ▣

MED: 100-2,15,80; 100-4,3,10.4; 100-4,13,10; 100-4,13,100

75833 **Venography, renal, bilateral, selective, radiological supervision and interpretation** S 80 ▣

MED: 100-2,15,80; 100-4,3,10.4; 100-4,13,10; 100-4,13,100

75840 **Venography, adrenal, unilateral, selective, radiological supervision and interpretation** S 80 ▣

MED: 100-2,15,80; 100-4,3,10.4; 100-4,13,10; 100-4,13,100

75842 **Venography, adrenal, bilateral, selective, radiological supervision and interpretation** S 80 ▣

MED: 100-2,15,80; 100-4,3,10.4; 100-4,13,10; 100-4,13,100

75860 **Venography, venous sinus (eg, petrosal and inferior sagittal) or jugular, catheter, radiological supervision and interpretation** S 80 ▣

MED: 100-2,15,80; 100-4,3,10.4; 100-4,13,10; 100-4,13,100

75870 **Venography, superior sagittal sinus, radiological supervision and interpretation** S 80 ▣

MED: 100-2,15,80; 100-4,3,10.4; 100-4,13,10; 100-4,13,100

75872 **Venography, epidural, radiological supervision and interpretation** S 80 ▣

MED: 100-2,15,80; 100-4,3,10.4; 100-4,13,10; 100-4,13,100

75880 **Venography, orbital, radiological supervision and interpretation** S 80 ▣

MED: 100-2,15,80; 100-4,3,10.4; 100-4,13,10; 100-4,13,100

75885 **Percutaneous transhepatic portography with hemodynamic evaluation, radiological supervision and interpretation** S 80 ▣

MED: 100-2,15,80; 100-4,3,10.4; 100-4,13,10; 100-4,13,100
AMA: 2002,Mar,10; 1996,Oct,4

75887 **Percutaneous transhepatic portography without hemodynamic evaluation, radiological supervision and interpretation** S 80 ▢

MED: 100-2,15,80; 100-4,3,10.4; 100-4,13,10; 100-4,13,100
AMA: 2002,Mar,10

75889 **Hepatic venography, wedged or free, with hemodynamic evaluation, radiological supervision and interpretation** S 80 ▢

MED: 100-2,15,80; 100-4,3,10.4; 100-4,13,10; 100-4,13,100

75891 **Hepatic venography, wedged or free, without hemodynamic evaluation, radiological supervision and interpretation** S 80 ▢

MED: 100-2,15,80; 100-4,3,10.4; 100-4,13,10; 100-4,13,100

75893 **Venous sampling through catheter, with or without angiography (eg, for parathyroid hormone, renin), radiological supervision and interpretation** Q 80 ▢

MED: 100-2,15,80; 100-4,3,10.4; 100-4,13,10; 100-4,13,100

If venous catheterization is performed for selective organ blood sampling, consult CPT code 36500.

TRANSCATHETER PROCEDURES

The following transcatheter procedures include the work provided in the interventional procedure and should not be reported separately:

- Contrast injections, venography, roadmapping, and/or fluoroscopy
- Vessel measurement
- Post venography or stent venography (except for those uses permitted by 75898).

Diagnostic angiography/venography performed at the same time as a transcatheter procedure is separately reportable unless it is specifically included in the descriptor. This includes instances when no prior catheter-based diagnostic angiography/venography study of the target vessel is available, prior diagnostic study is not adequate, or the patient's condition has changed since the previous study or during the intervention (see 75600-75893).

Codes 75956 and 75956 include all angiography of the thoracic aorta and its branches for diagnostic imaging prior to deployment of the primary endovascular devices, fluoroscopic guidance in the delivery of the endovascular components, and arterial angiography during the procedure.

CPT code 75958 includes the analogous services for placement of each proximal thoracic endovascular extension, and code 75959 includes the analogous services for placement of a distal thoracic endovascular extension(s) placed during a procedure after the primary repair.

75894 **Transcatheter therapy, embolization, any method, radiological supervision and interpretation** S 80 ▢

MED: 100-2,15,80; 100-3,20.28; 100-4,3,10.4; 100-4,13,10; 100-4,13,100
AMA: 1998,Sep,7
Use code 37210 for uterine fibroid embolization. Use code 37204 for obstetrical or gynecologic embolization procedures for other than uterine fibroids, e.g. embolization to treat postpartum hemorrhage.

75896 **Transcatheter therapy, infusion, any method (eg, thrombolysis other than coronary), radiological supervision and interpretation** S 80 ▢

MED: 100-2,15,80; 100-4,3,10.4; 100-4,13,10; 100-4,13,100
AMA: 2001,May,1
To report injection procedure performed, consult CPT codes 37201, 37202. If coronary thrombolysis is performed, consult CPT codes 92975 and 92977.

75898 **Angiography through existing catheter for follow-up study for transcatheter therapy, embolization or infusion** X 80 ▢

MED: 100-2,15,80; 100-4,3,10.4; 100-4,13,10; 100-4,13,100

75900 **Exchange of a previously placed intravascular catheter during thrombolytic therapy with contrast monitoring, radiological supervision and interpretation** C 80 ▢

MED: 100-2,15,80; 100-4,3,10.4; 100-4,13,10; 100-4,13,100
If a previously placed arterial catheter is exchanged during thrombolytic therapy, consult CPT code 37209.

75901 **Mechanical removal of pericatheter obstructive material (eg, fibrin sheath) from central venous device via separate venous access, radiologic supervision and interpretation** X 80 ▢

MED: 100-2,15,80; 100-4,3,10.4; 100-4,13,10; 100-4,13,100
To report procedure, consult CPT code 36595.

To report venous catheterization, consult CPT codes 36010-36012.

75902 **Mechanical removal of intraluminal (intracatheter) obstructive material from central venous device through device lumen, radiologic supervision and interpretation** X 80 ▢

MED: 100-2,15,80; 100-4,3,10.4; 100-4,13,10; 100-4,13,100
To report procedure, consult CPT code 36596.

To report venous catheterization, consult CPT codes 36010-36012.

75940 **Percutaneous placement of IVC filter, radiological supervision and interpretation** S 80 ▢

MED: 100-2,15,80; 100-4,3,10.4; 100-4,13,10; 100-4,13,100
AMA: 2000,Nov,11
To report procedure, consult CPT code 37620.

75945 **Intravascular ultrasound (non-coronary vessel), radiological supervision and interpretation; initial vessel** S 80 ▢

MED: 100-3,220.5; 100-4,3,10.4; 100-4,13,10; 100-4,13,100

+ **75946** **each additional non-coronary vessel (List separately in addition to code for primary procedure)** S 80 ▢

MED: 100-2,15,80; 100-3,220.5; 100-4,3,10.4; 100-4,13,10; 100-4,13,100
To report placement of catheter, consult CPT codes 36215-36248. If transcatheter therapies are performed, consult CPT codes 37200-37208, 61624, and 61626. If an intravascular ultrasound is performed during a diagnostic evaluation and/or a therapeutic intervention, consult CPT codes 37250 and 37251.

Note that 75946 is an add-on code and must be used in conjunction with 75945.

75952 **Endovascular repair of infrarenal abdominal aortic aneurysm or dissection, radiological supervision and interpretation** C 80 ▢

MED: 100-2,15,80; 100-4,3,10.4; 100-4,13,10; 100-4,13,100
To report implantation of endovascular grafts, consult CPT codes 38400-38408.

To report radiologic supervision and interpretation of endovascular repair of abdominal aortic aneurysm involving visceral vessels, consult Category III codes 0078T-0081T.

75953 **Placement of proximal or distal extension prosthesis for endovascular repair of infrarenal aortic or iliac artery aneurysm, pseudoaneurysm, or dissection, radiological supervision and interpretation** C 80 ▢

MED: 100-2,15,80; 100-4,3,10.4; 100-4,13,10; 100-4,13,100
AMA: 2003,Feb,1
To report implantation of endovascular extension prostheses, consult CPT codes 34825 and 34826.

26 Professional Component Only   80/80 Assist-at-Surgery Allowed/With Documentation   Unlisted   Not Covered

TC Technical Component Only   MED: Pub 100/NCD References   AMA: CPT Assistant References   1-9 ASC Group   ♂ Male Only   ♀ Female Only

268 — CPT Expert   CPT only © 2006 American Medical Association. All Rights Reserved. (Black Ink)   © 2006 Ingenix (Blue Ink)

75954 Endovascular repair of iliac artery aneurysm, pseudoaneurysm, arteriovenous malformation, or trauma, radiological supervision and interpretation [C] [80] [■]

MED: 100-2,15,80; 100-4,3,10.4; 100-4,13,10; 100-4,13,100
AMA: 2003,Feb,1
To report procedure, consult CPT code 34900.

75956 Endovascular repair of descending thoracic aorta (eg, aneurysm, pseudoaneurysm, dissection, penetrating ulcer, intramural hematoma, or traumatic disruption); involving coverage of left subclavian artery origin, initial endoprosthesis plus descending thoracic aortic extension(s), if required, to level of celiac artery origin, radiological supervision and interpretation [C] [80]

MED: 100-4,3,10.4
To report implantation of endovascular graft, consult CPT code 33880.

75957 not involving coverage of left subclavian artery origin, initial endoprosthesis plus descending thoracic aortic extension(s), if required, to level of celiac artery origin, radiological supervision and interpretation [C] [80]

MED: 100-4,3,10.4
To report implantation of endovascular graft, consult CPT code 33881.

75958 Placement of proximal extension prosthesis for endovascular repair of descending thoracic aorta (eg, aneurysm, pseudoaneurysm, dissection, penetrating ulcer, intramural hematoma, or traumatic disruption), radiological supervision and interpretation [C] [80]

MED: 100-4,3,10.4
Code 75958 should be reported for each proximal extension.

To report implantation of proximal endovascular extension, consult CPT codes 33883, 33884.

75959 Placement of distal extension prosthesis(s) (delayed) after endovascular repair of descending thoracic aorta, as needed, to level of celiac origin, radiological supervision and interpretation [C] [80]

MED: 100-4,3,10.4
Code 75959 cannot be reported with 75956, 57957.

Code 75959 should be reported only once, regardless of the number of modules deployed.

To report implantation of a distal endovascular extension, consult CPT code 33886.

75960 Transcatheter introduction of intravascular stent(s), (except coronary, carotid, and vertebral vessel), percutaneous and/or open, radiological supervision and interpretation, each vessel [S] [80] [■]

MED: 100-2,15,80; 100-4,3,10.4; 100-4,13,10; 100-4,13,100
AMA: 2001,May,1; 1996,Oct,2; 1993,Fall,18
To report procedure, consult CPT codes 37205-37208.

To report radiologic supervision and interpretation of transcatheter placement of extracranial vertebral or intrathoracic carotid artery stent(s), consult CPT Category III code 0075T, 0076T.

75961 Transcatheter retrieval, percutaneous, of intravascular foreign body (eg, fractured venous or arterial catheter), radiological supervision and interpretation [S] [80] [■]

MED: 100-2,15,80; 100-4,3,10.4; 100-4,13,10; 100-4,13,100
To report procedure consult CPT code 37203.

75962 Transluminal balloon angioplasty, peripheral artery, radiological supervision and interpretation [S] [80] [■]

MED: 100-2,15,80; 100-4,3,10.4; 100-4,13,10; 100-4,13,100
AMA: 2001,May,1; 1993,Fall,18
To report transluminal balloon angioplasty procedure consult CPT codes 35450-35460 or 35470-35476.

+ **75964** Transluminal balloon angioplasty, each additional peripheral artery, radiological supervision and interpretation (List separately in addition to code for primary procedure) [S] [80] [■]

MED: 100-3,20.7; 100-4,3,10.4; 100-4,13,10; 100-4,13,100
Note that 75964 is an add-on code and must be used in conjunction with 75962.

For transluminal balloon angioplasty procedure consult CPT codes 35450-35460 or 35470-35476.

75966 Transluminal balloon angioplasty, renal or other visceral artery, radiological supervision and interpretation [S] [80] [■]

MED: 100-3,20.7; 100-4,3,10.4; 100-4,13,10; 100-4,13,100
To report transluminal balloon angioplasty procedure consult CPT codes 35450-35460 or 35470-35476.

+ **75968** Transluminal balloon angioplasty, each additional visceral artery, radiological supervision and interpretation (List separately in addition to code for primary procedure) [S] [80] [■]

MED: 100-3,20.7; 100-4,3,10.4; 100-4,13,10; 100-4,13,100
Note that 75968 is an add-on code and must be used in conjunction with 75966. If a percutaneous transluminal coronary angioplasty is performed, consult CPT codes 92982-92984.

75970 Transcatheter biopsy, radiological supervision and interpretation [S] [80] [■]

MED: 100-2,15,80; 100-4,3,10.4; 100-4,13,10; 100-4,13,100
If an injection procedure is performed for transcatheter therapy or for a biopsy, consult CPT codes 36100-36299. If a transcatheter renal and ureteral biopsy is performed, consult CPT code 52007. If a biopsy of the pancreas is performed through a percutaneous needle, consult CPT code 48102. If a biopsy of the abdominal or retroperitoneal mass is performed, consult CPT code 49180.

75978 Transluminal balloon angioplasty, venous (eg, subclavian stenosis), radiological supervision and interpretation [S] [80] [■]

MED: 100-2,15,80; 100-3,20.7; 100-4,3,10.4; 100-4,13,10; 100-4,13,100
AMA: 2001,May,1; 1996,Oct,4
To report procedures performed, consult CPT codes 35460 and 35476.

75980 Percutaneous transhepatic biliary drainage with contrast monitoring, radiological supervision and interpretation [S] [80] [■]

MED: 100-2,15,80; 100-4,3,10.4; 100-4,13,10; 100-4,13,100
To report introduction procedure of percutaneous transhepatic catheter for bilary drainage, consult CPT code 47510.

⊛ Modifier 63 Exempt Code   ⊙ Conscious Sedation   + CPT Add-on Code   ⊘ Modifier 51 Exempt Code   ● New Code   ▲ Revised Code
[M] Maternity Edit   [A] Age Edit   [A]-[Y] APC Status Indicators   [■] CCI Comprehensive Code   [50] Bilateral Procedure

Radiology

75982 — 76040

75982 Percutaneous placement of drainage catheter for combined internal and external biliary drainage or of a drainage stent for internal biliary drainage in patients with an inoperable mechanical biliary obstruction, radiological supervision and interpretation ⑤ ⑧⓪ ▣

MED: 100-2,15,80; 100-4,3,10.4; 100-4,13,10; 100-4,13,100

To report procedures performed, consult CPT codes 47511 or 47556.

75984 Change of percutaneous tube or drainage catheter with contrast monitoring (eg, gastrointestinal system, genitourinary system, abscess), radiological supervision and interpretation ⓧ ⑧⓪ ▣

MED: 100-2,15,80; 100-4,3,10.4; 100-4,13,10; 100-4,13,100

To report procedure performed consult CPT codes 43760, 47525, 47530, 50398, 50688, 51705, 51710.

If a nephrostomy or pyelostomy tube is changed, consult CPT code 50398. If a percutaneous nephrostolithotomy or pyelostolithotomy is performed, consult CPT codes 50080 and 50081. To report percutaneous cholecystostomy, consult CPT code 47490.

To report introduction procedure only for percutaneous biliary drainage, consult CPT codes 47510 and 47511. To report change of percutaneous biliary drainage catheter only, consult CPT code 47525.

75989 Radiological guidance (ie, fluoroscopy, ultrasound, or computed tomography), for percutaneous drainage (eg, abscess, specimen collection), with placement of catheter, radiological supervision and interpretation ⓝ ⑧⓪ ▣

MED: 100-2,15,80; 100-3,220.1; 100-3,220.5; 100-4,3,10.4; 100-4,13,10; 100-4,13,30; 100-4,13,100
AMA: 1998,Mar,8; 1997,Nov,24

TRANSLUMINAL ATHERECTOMY

75992 Transluminal atherectomy, peripheral artery, radiological supervision and interpretation ⑤ ⑧⓪ ▣

MED: 100-2,15,80; 100-4,3,10.4; 100-4,13,10; 100-4,13,100

To report procedure performed, consult CPT codes 35481-35485, 35491-35495.

+ **75993** Transluminal atherectomy, each additional peripheral artery, radiological supervision and interpretation (List separately in addition to code for primary procedure) ⑤ ⑧⓪ ▣

MED: 100-2,15,80; 100-4,3,10.4; 100-4,13,10; 100-4,13,100

Note that 75993 is an add-on code and must be used in conjunction with 75992. If an open or a percutaneous transluminal peripheral atherectomy is performed, consult CPT codes 35481-35485 and 35491-35495.

75994 Transluminal atherectomy, renal, radiological supervision and interpretation ⑤ ⑧⓪ ▣

MED: 100-2,15,80; 100-4,3,10.4; 100-4,13,10; 100-4,13,100

To report an open transluminal peripheral artherectomy consult CPT code 35480. To report a percutaneous transluminal peripheral atherectomy, consult CPT code 35490.

75995 Transluminal atherectomy, visceral, radiological supervision and interpretation ⑤ ⑧⓪ ▣

MED: 100-2,15,80; 100-4,3,10.4; 100-4,13,10; 100-4,13,100

+ **75996** Transluminal atherectomy, each additional visceral artery, radiological supervision and interpretation (List separately in addition to code for primary procedure) ⑤ ⑧⓪ ▣

MED: 100-2,15,80; 100-4,3,10.4; 100-4,13,10; 100-4,13,100

Note that 75996 is an add-on code and must be used in conjunction with 75995.

OTHER PROCEDURES

If an arthrography is performed, of shoulder, consult CPT code 73040; elbow, consult CPT code 73085; wrist, consult CPT code 73115; hip, consult CPT code 73525; knee, consult CPT 73580; and ankle, consult CPT code 73615. To report computed tomography cerebral perfusion analysis, consult Category III code 0042T.

75998 ~~Fluoroscopic guidance for central venous access device placement, replacement (catheter only or complete), or removal (includes fluoroscopic guidance for vascular access and catheter manipulation, any necessary contrast injections through access site or catheter with related venography radiologic supervision and interpretation, and radiographic documentation of final catheter position) (List separately in addition to code for primary procedure)~~

Use 77001.

76000 Fluoroscopy (separate procedure), up to 1 hour physician time, other than 71023 or 71034 (eg, cardiac fluoroscopy) ⓧ ⑧⓪ ▣

MED: 100-2,15,80; 100-4,3,10.4; 100-4,13,10; 100-4,13,100
AMA: 2000,Dec,14; 1999,Nov,32; 1996,Apr,10

76001 Fluoroscopy, physician time more than 1 hour, assisting a nonradiologic physician (eg, nephrostolithotomy, ERCP, bronchoscopy, transbronchial biopsy) ⓝ ⑧⓪ ▣

MED: 100-2,15,80; 100-4,3,10.4; 100-4,13,10; 100-4,13,100

76003 ~~Fluoroscopic guidance for needle placement (eg, biopsy, aspiration, injection, localization device)~~

Use 77002.

76005 ~~Fluoroscopic guidance and localization of needle or catheter tip for spine or paraspinous diagnostic or therapeutic injection procedures (epidural, transforaminal epidural, subarachnoid, paravertebral facet joint, paravertebral facet joint nerve or sacroiliac joint), including neurolytic agent destruction~~

Use 77003.

76006 ~~Manual application of stress performed by physician for joint radiography, including contralateral joint if indicated~~

Use 77071.

76010 Radiologic examination from nose to rectum for foreign body, single view, child Ⓐ ⓧ ⑧⓪ ▣

MED: 100-2,15,80; 100-4,3,10.4; 100-4,13,10; 100-4,13,100

76012 ~~Radiological supervision and interpretation, percutaneous vertebroplasty or vertebral augmentation including cavity creation, per vertebral body; under fluoroscopic guidance~~

Use 72291.

76013 ~~under CT guidance~~

Use 72292.

76020 ~~Bone age studies~~

Use 77072.

76040 ~~Bone length studies (orthoroentgenogram, scanogram)~~

Use 77073.

~~76061~~	~~Radiologic examination, osseous survey; limited (eg, for metastases)~~
	Use 77074.
~~76062~~	~~complete (axial and appendicular skeleton)~~
	Use 77075.
~~76065~~	~~Radiologic examination, osseous survey, infant~~
	Use 77076.
~~76066~~	~~Joint survey, single view, two or more joints (specify)~~
	Use 77077.
~~76070~~	~~Computed tomography, bone mineral density study, one or more sites; axial skeleton (eg, hips, pelvis, spine)~~
	MED: 100-3,150.3; 100-3,220.1
	Use 77078.
~~76071~~	~~appendicular skeleton (peripheral) (eg, radius, wrist, heel)~~
	MED: 100-3,150.3; 100-3,220.1
	Use 77079.
~~76075~~	~~Dual energy X-ray absorptiometry (DXA), bone density study, one or more sites; axial skeleton (eg, hips, pelvis, spine)~~
	MED: 100-3,150.3
	Use 77080.
~~76076~~	~~appendicular skeleton (peripheral) (eg, radius, wrist, heel)~~
	MED: 100-3,150.3
	Use 77079.
~~76077~~	~~vertebral fracture assessment~~
	Use 77080-77082.
~~76078~~	~~Radiographic absorptiometry (eg, photodensitometry, radiogrammetry), one or more sites~~
	MED: 100-3,150.3
	Use 77083.

76080 Radiologic examination, abscess, fistula or sinus tract study, radiological supervision and interpretation   X 80 🖸

    MED: 100-2,15,80; 100-4,3,10.4; 100-4,13,10; 100-4,13,100
    AMA: 1998,Mar,8; 1997,Nov,24
    To report procedure, consult CPT code 20501, 49424.

~~76082~~	~~Computer aided detection (computer algorithm analysis of digital image data for lesion detection) with further physician review for interpretation, with or without digitization of film radiographic images; diagnostic mammography (List separately in addition to code for primary procedure)~~
	MED: 100-3,220.4
	Use 77051.
~~76083~~	~~screening mammography (List separately in addition to code for primary procedure)~~
	MED: 100-3,220.4
	Use 77052.
~~76086~~	~~Mammary ductogram or galactogram; single duct, radiological supervision and interpretation~~
	Use 77053.
~~76088~~	~~Mammary ductogram or galactogram, multiple ducts, radiological supervision and interpretation~~
	Use 77054.
~~76090~~	~~Mammography; unilateral~~
	MED: 100-3,220.4
	Use 77055.

~~76091~~	~~bilateral~~
	MED: 100-3,220.4
	Use 77056.
~~76092~~	~~Screening mammography, bilateral (two view film study of each breast)~~
	MED: 100-3,220.4
	Use 77057.
~~76093~~	~~Magnetic resonance imaging, breast, without and/or with contrast material(s); unilateral~~
	MED: 100-3,220.2
	Use 77058.
~~76094~~	~~bilateral~~
	MED: 100-3,220.2
	Use 77059.
~~76095~~	~~Stereotactic localization guidance for breast biopsy or needle placement (eg, for wire localization or for injection), each lesion, radiological supervision and interpretation~~
	MED: 100-3,220.13
	Use 77031.
~~76096~~	~~Mammographic guidance for needle placement, breast (eg, for wire localization or for injection), each lesion, radiological supervision and interpretation~~
	MED: 100-3,220.4
	Use 77032.

76098 Radiological examination, surgical specimen   X 80

    MED: 100-2,15,80; 100-4,3,10.4; 100-4,13,10; 100-4,13,100

76100 Radiologic examination, single plane body section (eg, tomography), other than with urography   X 80 🖸

    MED: 100-2,15,80; 100-4,3,10.4; 100-4,13,10; 100-4,13,100

76101 Radiologic examination, complex motion (ie, hypercycloidal) body section (eg, mastoid polytomography), other than with urography; unilateral   X 80

    MED: 100-2,15,80; 100-4,3,10.4; 100-4,13,10; 100-4,13,100

76102 bilateral   X 80 🖸

    MED: 100-2,15,80; 100-4,3,10.4; 100-4,13,10; 100-4,13,100
    If a nephrotomography is performed, consult CPT code 74415.

76120 Cineradiography/videoradiography, except where specifically included   X 80 🖸

    MED: 100-2,15,80; 100-4,3,10.4; 100-4,13,10; 100-4,13,100
    AMA: 2000,Sep,4

+ **76125** Cineradiography/videoradiography to complement routine examination (List separately in addition to code for primary procedure)   X 80 🖸

    MED: 100-2,15,80; 100-4,3,10.4; 100-4,13,10; 100-4,13,100
    AMA: 2000,Sep,4
    Note that 76125 is an add-on code that must be used in conjunction with the appropriate code for the primary procedure. This code cannot be reported alone.

76140 Consultation on X-ray examination made elsewhere, written report   E

    MED: 100-2,15,80; 100-4,3,10.4; 100-4,13,10; 100-4,13,100
    AMA: 1991,Summer,13

76150 Xeroradiography   X TC 80

    MED: 100-2,15,80; 100-4,3,10.4; 100-4,13,10; 100-4,13,100
    Note that 76150 is to be used only for non-mammographic studies.

76350 Subtraction in conjunction with contrast studies   N TC 80

    MED: 100-2,15,80; 100-3,220.1; 100-3,220.9; 100-4,3,10.4; 100-4,13,10; 100-4,13,100

⑥⑨ Modifier 63 Exempt Code   ☉ Conscious Sedation   + CPT Add-on Code   ⊘ Modifier 51 Exempt Code   ● New Code   ▲ Revised Code
M Maternity Edit   A Age Edit   A-Y APC Status Indicators   🖸 CCI Comprehensive Code   50 Bilateral Procedure

© 2006 Ingenix (Blue Ink)   CPT only © 2006 American Medical Association. All Rights Reserved. (Black Ink)   Radiology — 271

Radiology

76355 — 76519

~~76355~~ ~~Computed tomography guidance for stereotactic localization~~

    MED: 100-3,220.1

    Use 77011.

~~76360~~ ~~Computed tomography guidance for needle placement (eg, biopsy, aspiration, injection, localization device), radiological supervision and interpretation~~

    MED: 100-3,20.7; 100-3,220.1; 100-3,220.13

    Use 77012.

~~76362~~ ~~Computed tomography guidance for, and monitoring of, visceral tissue ablation~~

    MED: 100-3,220.1

    Use 77013.

~~76370~~ ~~Computed tomography guidance for placement of radiation therapy fields~~

    MED: 100-3,220.1

    Use 77014.

76376 **3D rendering with interpretation and reporting of computed tomography, magnetic resonance imaging, ultrasound, or other tomographic modality; not requiring image postprocessing on an independent workstation** [X] [80]

    MED: 100-4,3,10.4

    Report code 76376 in conjunction with code(s) for base imaging procedure(s).

    Code 76376 cannot be reported with 70496, 70498, 70544-70549, 71275, 71555, 72159, 72191, 72198, 73206, 73225, 73706, 73725, 74175, 74185, 75635, 76377, 78000-78999, 0066T, 0067T, and 0144T-0151T.

76377 **requiring image postprocessing on an independent workstation** [S] [80]

    MED: 100-4,3,10.4

    Report code 76377 in conjunction with code(s) for base imaging procedure(s).

    Code 76377 cannot be used with 70496, 70498, 70544-70549, 71275, 71555, 72159, 72191, 72198, 73206, 73225, 73706, 73725, 74175, 74185, 75635, 76376, 78000-78999, 0066T, 0067T, and 0144T-0151T.

76380 **Computed tomography, limited or localized follow-up study** [S] [80]

    MED: 100-2,15,80; 100-3,220.1; 100-4,3,10.4; 100-4,13,10; 100-4,13,30; 100-4,13,100

76390 **Magnetic resonance spectroscopy** [E]

    MED: 100-2,15,80; 100-4,3,10.4; 100-4,13,10; 100-4,13,100

    AMA: 1997,Nov,25

    If magnetic resonance imaging is performed, consult the appropriate MRI body site code.

~~76393~~ ~~Magnetic resonance guidance for needle placement (eg, for biopsy, needle aspiration, injection, or placement of localization device) radiological supervision and interpretation~~

    MED: 100-3,220.2; 100-3,220.13

    Use 77021.

~~76394~~ ~~Magnetic resonance guidance for, and monitoring of, visceral tissue ablation~~

    MED: 100-3,220.2

    Use 77022.

~~76400~~ ~~Magnetic resonance (eg, proton) imaging, bone marrow blood supply~~

    MED: 100-3,220.2

    Use 77084.

76496 **Unlisted fluoroscopic procedure (eg, diagnostic, interventional)** [X] [80]

    MED: 100-2,15,80; 100-4,3,10.4; 100-4,13,10; 100-4,13,100

76497 **Unlisted computed tomography procedure (eg, diagnostic, interventional)** [S] [80]

    MED: 100-2,15,80; 100-3,220.2; 100-4,3,10.4; 100-4,13,10; 100-4,13,40; 100-4,13,40.1; 100-4,13,100

76498 **Unlisted magnetic resonance procedure (eg, diagnostic, interventional)** [S] [80]

    MED: 100-2,15,80; 100-3,220.2; 100-3,220.3; 100-4,3,10.4; 100-4,13,10; 100-4,13,40; 100-4,13,40.1; 100-4,13,100

76499 **Unlisted diagnostic radiographic procedure** [X] [80]

    MED: 100-2,15,80; 100-4,3,10.4; 100-4,13,10; 100-4,13,100

    AMA: 2000,Sep,4; 1999,Jul,10

    To report diagnostic vascular ultrasound studies, consult 93875-93990. To report focused ultrasound ablation treatment of uterine leiomyomata, consult Category III codes 0071T, 0072T.

DIAGNOSTIC ULTRASOUND

Permanent records of ultrasound examinations such as description of anatomic region, measurements, obstructed view, and site to be localized for a guided surgical procedure are required. A written report of the exam should be included in the patient's medical record. Do not report an ultrasound without a thorough examination of the organ(s) or anatomic region, documentation of the image, and a final written report

HEAD AND NECK

▲ 76506 **Echoencephalography, real time with image documentation (gray scale) (for determination of ventricular size, delineation of cerebral contents, and detection of fluid masses or other intracranial abnormalities), including A-mode encephalography as secondary component where indicated** [S] [80] [▣]

    MED: 100-2,15,80; 100-3,220.5; 100-4,3,10.4

76510 **Ophthalmic ultrasound, diagnostic; B-scan and quantitative A-scan performed during the same patient encounter** [S] [80] [▣]

    MED: 100-4,3,10.4

76511 **quantitative A-scan only** [S] [80] [▣]

    MED: 100-2,15,80; 100-3,10.1; 100-3,220.5; 100-4,3,10.4

    AMA: 1999,Nov,42; 1996,Oct,9

76512 **B-scan (with or without superimposed non-quantitative A-scan)** [S] [80] [▣]

    MED: 100-2,15,80; 100-3,10.1; 100-3,220.5; 100-4,3,10.4

    AMA: 1996,Oct,9

76513 **anterior segment ultrasound, immersion (water bath) B-scan or high resolution biomicroscopy** [S] [80] [▣]

    MED: 100-2,15,80; 100-3,10.1; 100-3,220.5; 100-4,3,10.4

    AMA: 1999,Nov,42

76514 **corneal pachymetry, unilateral or bilateral (determination of corneal thickness)** [X] [80]

    MED: 100-3,80.7; 100-4,3,10.4

76516 **Ophthalmic biometry by ultrasound echography, A-scan;** [S] [80] [▣]

    MED: 100-2,15,80; 100-3,10.1; 100-3,220.5; 100-4,3,10.4

76519 **with intraocular lens power calculation** [S] [80] [▣]

    MED: 100-2,15,80; 100-3,10.1; 100-3,220.5; 100-4,3,10.4

    To report partial coherence interferometry, consult CPT code 92136.

[26] Professional Component Only   [80]/[80] Assist-at-Surgery Allowed/With Documentation   Unlisted   Not Covered

[TC] Technical Component Only   **MED:** Pub 100/NCD References   **AMA:** CPT Assistant References   [1]-[9] ASC Group   ♂ Male Only   ♀ Female Only

272 — CPT Expert   CPT only © 2006 American Medical Association. All Rights Reserved. *(Black Ink)*   © *2006 Ingenix (Blue Ink)*

	76529	Ophthalmic ultrasonic foreign body localization [S][80][↻]

MED: 100-2,15,80; 100-3,220.5; 100-4,3,10.4

▲ 76536 Ultrasound, soft tissues of head and neck (eg, thyroid, parathyroid, parotid), real time with image documentation [S][80][↻]

MED: 100-2,15,80; 100-3,220.5; 100-4,3,10.4

CHEST

▲ 76604 Ultrasound, chest (includes mediastinum), real time with image documentation [S][80][↻]

MED: 100-2,15,80; 100-3,220.5; 100-4,3,10.4

▲ 76645 Ultrasound, breast(s) (unilateral or bilateral), real time with image documentation [S][80][↻]

MED: 100-2,15,80; 100-3,220.5; 100-4,3,10.4

ABDOMEN AND RETROPERITONEUM

A complete ultrasound of the abdomen (76700) consists of real time scans of: liver, gall bladder, common bile duct, pancreas, spleen, kidneys, upper abdominal aorta, and inferior vena cava including any demonstrated abdominal abnormality.

A complete ultrasound examination of the retroperitoneum (76770) includes real time scans of the kidneys, abdominal aorta, common iliac artery origins, and inferior vena cava, including any demonstrated retroperitoneal abnormality. If clinical history points to urinary tract pathology, complete evaluation of the kidneys and urinary bladder also comprises a complete retroperitoneal ultrasound.

Do not report an ultrasound without a thorough examination of the organ(s) or anatomic region, documentation of the image, and a final written report.

▲ 76700 Ultrasound, abdominal, real time with image documentation; complete [S][80][↻]

MED: 100-2,15,80; 100-3,220.5; 100-4,3,10.4
AMA: 2001,Oct,1; 1993,Fall,13

▲ 76705 limited (eg, single organ, quadrant, follow-up) [S][80][↻]

MED: 100-2,15,80; 100-3,220.5; 100-4,3,10.4
AMA: 2001,Oct,1; 1993,Fall,13

▲ 76770 Ultrasound, retroperitoneal (eg, renal, aorta, nodes), real time with image documentation; complete [S][80][↻]

MED: 100-2,15,80; 100-3,220.5; 100-4,3,10.4
AMA: 1999,May,10; 1999,Jun,10

▲ 76775 limited [S][80][↻]

MED: 100-2,15,80; 100-3,220.5; 100-4,3,10.4
AMA: 1999,May,10; 1999,Jun,10

● 76776 Ultrasound, transplanted kidney, real time and duplex Doppler with image documentation [S]

Do not report code 76776 with 93975 or 93976.

Use code 76775 for ultrasound of transplanted kidney without duplex Doppler.

~~76778~~ ~~Ultrasound, transplanted kidney, B-scan and/or real time with image documentation, with or without duplex Doppler study~~

MED: 100-3,220.5
Use 76775, 76776.

SPINAL CANAL

76800 Ultrasound, spinal canal and contents [S][80][↻]

MED: 100-2,15,80; 100-3,220.5; 100-4,3,10.4
AMA: 1998,Apr,15

PELVIS

OBSTETRICAL

76801 Ultrasound, pregnant uterus, real time with image documentation, fetal and maternal evaluation, first trimester (<14 weeks 0 days), transabdominal approach; single or first gestation [M][♀][S][80][↻]

MED: 100-3,220.5; 100-4,3,10.4

Use 76813 to report first trimester fetal nuchal translucency measurement.

+ 76802 each additional gestation (List separately in addition to code for primary procedure) [M][♀][S][80][↻]

MED: 100-3,220.5; 100-4,3,10.4

Note that 76802 is an add-on code and must be used in conjunction with code 76801.

Use 76814 to report first trimester fetal nuchal translucency measurement.

76805 Ultrasound, pregnant uterus, real time with image documentation, fetal and maternal evaluation, after first trimester (> or = 14 weeks 0 days), transabdominal approach; single or first gestation [M][♀][S][80][↻]

MED: 100-2,15,80; 100-3,220.5; 100-4,3,10.4
AMA: 2001,Oct,1; 1997,Nov,25; 1997,Apr,2

+ 76810 each additional gestation (List separately in addition to code for primary procedure) [M][♀][S][80][↻]

MED: 100-2,15,80; 100-3,220.5; 100-4,3,10.4
AMA: 2001,Oct,1; 1997,Apr,2

Note that 76810 is an add-on code and must be used in conjunction with CPT code 76805.

76811 Ultrasound, pregnant uterus, real time with image documentation, fetal and maternal evaluation plus detailed fetal anatomic examination, transabdominal approach; single or first gestation [M][♀][S][80][↻]

MED: 100-3,220.5; 100-4,3,10.4

+ 76812 each additional gestation (List separately in addition to code for primary procedure) [M][♀][S][80][↻]

MED: 100-3,220.5; 100-4,3,10.4

Note that 76812 is an add-on code and must be used in conjunction with CPT code 76811.

● 76813 Ultrasound, pregnant uterus, real time with image documentation, first trimester fetal nuchal translucency measurement, transabdominal or transvaginal approach; single or first gestation [S]

+ ● 76814 each additional gestation (List separately in addition to code for primary procedure) [S]

Note that 76814 is an add-on code and must be reported with 76813.

76815 Ultrasound, pregnant uterus, real time with image documentation, limited (eg, fetal heart beat, placental location, fetal position and/or qualitative amniotic fluid volume), one or more fetuses [M][♀][S][80][↻]

MED: 100-2,15,80; 100-3,220.5; 100-4,3,10.4
AMA: 2001,Oct,1; 2001,Dec,6; 1997,Nov,25; 1997,Apr,2
Report 76815 only once per exam.

Use 76813 and 76814 to report first trimester fetal nuchal translucency measurement.

---

⑥³ Modifier 63 Exempt Code ⊙ Conscious Sedation + CPT Add-on Code ⊘ Modifier 51 Exempt Code ● New Code ▲ Revised Code
[M] Maternity Edit [A] Age Edit [A]-[Y] APC Status Indicators [↻] CCI Comprehensive Code [50] Bilateral Procedure

76816 Ultrasound, pregnant uterus, real time with image documentation, follow-up (eg, re-evaluation of fetal size by measuring standard growth parameters and amniotic fluid volume, re-evaluation of organ system(s) suspected or confirmed to be abnormal on a previous scan), transabdominal approach, per fetus Ⓜ♀ Ⓢ 80 🔲

MED: 100-2,15,80; 100-3,220.5; 100-4,3,10.4

AMA: 2001,Oct,1; 1997,Apr,2

To report each fetus examined in a multiple pregnancy, append modifier 59 to code 76816.

76817 Ultrasound, pregnant uterus, real time with image documentation, transvaginal Ⓜ♀ Ⓢ 80 🔲

MED: 100-3,220.5; 100-4,3,10.4

To report non-obstetrical transvaginal ultrasound, consult CPT code 76830.

To report transvaginal exam done at time of transabdominal obstetrical exam, report 76817 in addition to appropriate transabdominal obstetric ultrasound code.

76818 Fetal biophysical profile; with non-stress testing Ⓜ♀ Ⓢ 80 🔲

MED: 100-2,15,80; 100-3,220.5; 100-4,3,10.4

AMA: 2001,Sep,4; 2001,Dec,6; 1998,May,10; 1997,Apr,2

76819 without non-stress testing Ⓜ♀ Ⓢ 80 🔲

MED: 100-2,15,80; 100-3,220.5; 100-4,3,10.4

AMA: 2001,Sep,4; 2001,Dec,6

To report fetal biophysical profile assessments for any additional fetuses, modifier 59 should be appended.

To report amniotic fluid index without non-stress test, consult CPT code 76815.

76820 Doppler velocimetry, fetal; umbilical artery ♀ Ⓢ 80

MED: 100-4,3,10.4

76821 middle cerebral artery ♀ Ⓢ 80

MED: 100-4,3,10.4

76825 Echocardiography, fetal, cardiovascular system, real time with image documentation (2D), with or without M-mode recording; Ⓜ♀ Ⓢ 80 🔲

MED: 100-2,15,80; 100-3,220.5; 100-4,3,10.4

AMA: 1997,Apr,2

76826 follow-up or repeat study Ⓜ♀ Ⓢ 80 🔲

MED: 100-2,15,80; 100-3,220.5; 100-4,3,10.4

AMA: 1997,Apr,2

76827 Doppler echocardiography, fetal, pulsed wave and/or continuous wave with spectral display; complete Ⓜ♀ Ⓢ 80 🔲

MED: 100-2,15,80; 100-3,220.5; 100-4,3,10.4

AMA: 1997,Apr,2

76828 follow-up or repeat study Ⓜ♀ Ⓢ 80 🔲

MED: 100-2,15,80; 100-3,220.5; 100-4,3,10.4

AMA: 1997,Apr,2

If color mapping is performed, consult CPT code 93325.

NON-OBSTETRICAL

Code 76856 includes the complete evaluation of the female pelvis. Included in this exam is a description and measurement of the uterus and adnexal structures, measurement of the endometrium, measurement of the bladder (when applicable), and a description of any pelvic problems. This includes ovarian cysts, uterine leiomyomata, and free pelvic fluid.

Report 76856 for a complete evaluation of the male pelvis. This exam includes evaluation and measurement (when applicable) of the urinary bladder, evaluation of the prostate and seminal vesicles to the extent that they are visualized transabdominally, and any pelvic pathology. This includes bladder tumor, enlarged prostate, free pelvic fluid, and pelvic abscess.

Report 76857 for a focused limited examination of one or more pelvic abnormalities previously seen on ultrasound. Report 76857 rather than 76770 when for an examination of the urinary bladder alone (i.e., not including kidneys). Report 51798 for a bladder volume or post-void residual measurement is obtained without imaging the bladder.

Do not report an ultrasound without a thorough examination of the organ(s) or anatomic region, documentation of the image, and a final written report.

76830 Ultrasound, transvaginal ♀ Ⓢ 80 🔲

MED: 100-2,15,80; 100-3,220.5; 100-4,3,10.4

AMA: 1999,Jul,8; 1996,Aug,10

To report obstetrical transvaginal ultrasound, consult CPT code 76817.

To report non-obstetrical transvaginal exam performed at time of transabdominal non-obstetrical exam, report both 76830 and appropriate transabdominal code.

76831 Saline infusion sonohysterography (SIS), including color flow Doppler, when performed ♀ Ⓢ 80 🔲

MED: 100-2,15,80; 100-3,220.5; 100-4,3,10.4

AMA: 1999,Jul,8; 1997,Nov,25

To report the introduction of saline, consult CPT code 58340.

▲ **76856** Ultrasound, pelvic (nonobstetric), real time with image documentation; complete Ⓢ 80 🔲

MED: 100-2,15,80; 100-3,220.5; 100-4,3,10.4

AMA: 2001,Oct,1

▲ **76857** limited or follow-up (eg, for follicles) Ⓢ 80 🔲

MED: 100-2,15,80; 100-3,220.5; 100-4,3,10.4

AMA: 2001,Oct,1; 1997,Jun,10

GENITALIA

76870 Ultrasound, scrotum and contents ♂ Ⓢ 80 🔲

MED: 100-2,15,80; 100-3,220.5; 100-4,3,10.4

76872 Ultrasound, transrectal; Ⓢ 80 🔲

MED: 100-2,15,80; 100-3,220.5; 100-4,3,10.4

AMA: 1999,Nov,42; 1996,May,3

76873 prostate volume study for brachytherapy treatment planning (separate procedure) ♂ Ⓢ 80

MED: 100-2,15,80; 100-3,220.5; 100-4,3,10.4

AMA: 1999,Nov,42

EXTREMITIES

▲ **76880** Ultrasound, extremity, nonvascular, real time with image documentation Ⓢ 80 🔲

MED: 100-2,15,80; 100-3,220.5; 100-4,3,10.4

76885 Ultrasound, infant hips, real time with imaging documentation; dynamic (requiring physician manipulation) Ⓐ Ⓢ 80 🔲

MED: 100-2,15,80; 100-3,220.5; 100-4,3,10.4

AMA: 1997,Nov,25

76886 limited, static (not requiring physician manipulation) Ⓐ Ⓢ 80 🔲

MED: 100-2,15,80; 100-3,220.5; 100-4,3,10.4

AMA: 1997,Nov,25

ULTRASONIC GUIDANCE PROCEDURES

76930 Ultrasonic guidance for pericardiocentesis, imaging supervision and interpretation Ⓢ 80 🔲

MED: 100-3,220.5; 100-4,3,10.4

To report procedure, consult CPT codes 33010 and 33011.

---

26 Professional Component Only

TC Technical Component Only

80/80 Assist-at-Surgery Allowed/With Documentation

MED: Pub 100/NCD References AMA: CPT Assistant References

Unlisted

🔢-🔢 ASC Group ♂ Male Only

Not Covered

♀ Female Only

76932 Ultrasonic guidance for endomyocardial biopsy, imaging supervision and interpretation ⓢ 80 ◪

MED: 100-3,220.5; 100-4,3,10.4

To report procedure, consult CPT code 93505.

76936 Ultrasound guided compression repair of arterial pseudoaneurysm or arteriovenous fistulae (includes diagnostic ultrasound evaluation, compression of lesion and imaging) ⓢ 80 ◪

MED: 100-3,220.5; 100-4,3,10.4

+ **76937** Ultrasound guidance for vascular access requiring ultrasound evaluation of potential access sites, documentation of selected vessel patency, concurrent realtime ultrasound visualization of vascular needle entry, with permanent recording and reporting (List separately in addition to code for primary procedure) Ⓝ 80 ◪

MED: 100-4,3,10.4

Code 76937 cannot be reported in conjunction with 76942.

To report a non-invasive extremity venous vascular diagnostic study performed separate from venous access guidance, consult CPT codes 93965, 93970 or 93971.

▲ **76940** Ultrasound guidance for, and monitoring of, parenchymal tissue ablation ⓢ 80 ◪

MED: 100-4,3,10.4

Code 76940 cannot be reported in conjunction with 76998.

See codes 32998, 47340-47382, and 50592 for ablation.

76941 Ultrasonic guidance for intrauterine fetal transfusion or cordocentesis, imaging supervision and interpretation Ⓜ ♀ ⓢ 80 ◪

MED: 100-3,220.5; 100-4,3,10.4

To report fetal intrauterine transfusion procedure, consult CPT code 36460. If cordocentesis is performed, consult CPT code 59012.

76942 Ultrasonic guidance for needle placement (eg, biopsy, aspiration, injection, localization device), imaging supervision and interpretation ⓢ 80 ◪

MED: 100-3,20.7; 100-3,220.5; 100-3,220.13; 100-4,3,10.4
AMA: 2001,Oct,1; 1997,Jun,5; 1996,May,3; 1993,Fall,12
Code 76942 cannot be reported in conjunction with 43232, 43237, 43242, 45341, 45342, or 76975.

To report microwave thermotherapy of the breast, consult CPT Category III code 0061T.

76945 Ultrasonic guidance for chorionic villus sampling, imaging supervision and interpretation Ⓜ ♀ ⓢ 80 ◪

MED: 100-3,220.5; 100-4,3,10.4

To report chorionic villus sampling, consult CPT code 59015.

76946 Ultrasonic guidance for amniocentesis, imaging supervision and interpretation Ⓜ ♀ ⓢ 80 ◪

MED: 100-3,220.5; 100-4,3,10.4

To report procedure, consult CPT code 59000.

76948 Ultrasonic guidance for aspiration of ova, imaging supervision and interpretation ♀ ⓢ 80 ◪

MED: 100-3,220.5; 100-4,3,10.4

To report procedure, consult CPT code 58970.

76950 Ultrasonic guidance for placement of radiation therapy fields ⓢ 80 ◪

MED: 100-3,220.5; 100-4,3,10.4

76965 Ultrasonic guidance for interstitial radioelement application ⓢ 80 ◪

MED: 100-3,220.5; 100-4,3,10.4

OTHER PROCEDURES

76970 Ultrasound study follow-up (specify) ⓢ 80 ◪

MED: 100-3,220.5; 100-4,3,10.4

76975 Gastrointestinal endoscopic ultrasound, supervision and interpretation ⓢ 80 ◪

MED: 100-3,220.5; 100-4,3,10.4; 100-4,12,30.1
AMA: 1994,Spring,5
Code 76975 cannot be reported in conjunction with 43231, 43232, 43237, 43238, 43242, 43259, 45341, 45342, or 76942.

76977 Ultrasound bone density measurement and interpretation, peripheral site(s), any method Ⓧ 80 ◪

MED: 100-3,220.5; 100-4,3,10.4; 100-4,4,240; 100-4,13,140.2; 100-4,13,140.3
AMA: 1998,Nov,21

~~**76986** Ultrasonic guidance, intraoperative~~

MED: 100-3,220.5

Use 76998.

● **76998** Ultrasonic guidance, intraoperative ⓢ

Do not report 76998 with codes 47370-47382.

Use code 76940 for ultrasound guidance for open and laparoscopic radiofrequency tissue ablation.

76999 Unlisted ultrasound procedure (eg, diagnostic, interventional) ⓢ 80

MED: 100-3,220.5

RADIOLOGIC GUIDANCE

FLUOROSCOPIC GUIDANCE

+ ● **77001** Fluoroscopic guidance for central venous access device placement, replacement (catheter only or complete), or removal (includes fluoroscopic guidance for vascular access and catheter manipulation, any necessary contrast injections through access site or catheter with related venography radiologic supervision and interpretation, and radiographic documentation of final catheter position) (List separately in addition to code for primary procedure) Ⓝ

Do not use code 77001 with code 77002.

If formal extremity venography is performed from separate venous access and separately interpreted, use codes 36005 and 75820, 75822, 75825, or 75827.

● **77002** Fluoroscopic guidance for needle placement (eg, biopsy, aspiration, injection, localization device) Ⓝ

Also report appropriate surgical code for procedure and anatomical location.

77002 includes all radiographic arthroscopy with the exception of supervision and interpretation for CT and MR arthrography.

Do not report code 77002 in addition to codes 70332, 73040, 73085, 73115, 73525, 73580, or 73615.

Code 77002 is included in and should not be separately reported for the organ/anatomical specific radiological supervision and interpretation procedures 74320, 74350, 74355, 74445, 74470, 74475, 75809, 75810, 75885, 75887, 75980, 75982, and 75989.

---

⑥³ Radiology 63 Exempt Code   ☉ Conscious Sedation   + CPT Add-on Code   ⊘ Modifier 51 Exempt Code   ● New Code   ▲ Revised Code

Ⓜ Maternity Edit   Ⓐ Age Edit   Ⓐ-Ⓨ APC Status Indicators   ◪ CCI Comprehensive Code   50 Bilateral Procedure

● **77003** Fluoroscopic guidance and localization of needle or catheter tip for spine or paraspinous diagnostic or therapeutic injection procedures (epidural, transforaminal epidural, subarachnoid, paravertebral facet joint, paravertebral facet joint nerve, or sacroiliac joint), including neurolytic agent destruction [N]

Injection of contrast during fluoroscopic guidance and localization, code 77003, is included in codes 22526, 22527, 62263, 62264, 62270-62282, 62310-62319, and 0027T.

Fluoroscopic guidance for subarachnoid puncture for diagnostic radiograhpic myelography is included in the supervision and interpretation codes 72240-72270.

See codes 62270-62282 and 62310-62319 for epidural and subarachnoid needle or catheter placement and injection.

See codes 27096 and 73542 for sacroiliac joint arthrography. If formal arthrography is not performed, recorded, and a formal radiographic report is not issued, use code 77003 for the fluoroscopic guidance of sacroliliac injections.

See codes 64470-64475 for paravertebral facet joint injection. See codes 64479-64484 for transforaminal epidural needle placement and injection.

See codes 64600-64680 for destruction by neurolytic agent.

Codes 62263, 62264, and 0027T for percutaneous or endoscopic lysis of adhesions include fluoroscopic guidance and localization.

COMPUTED TOMOGRAPHY GUIDANCE

● **77011** Computed tomography guidance for stereotactic localization [S]

● **77012** Computed tomography guidance for needle placement (eg, biopsy, aspiration, injection, localization device), radiological supervision and interpretation [S]

● **77013** Computerized tomography guidance for, and monitoring of, parenchymal tissue ablation [S]

Do not report code 77013 with code 20982.

Use code 0135T for percutaneous cryotherapy ablation of renal tumorrs. See codes 32998, 47382 and 50592 for percutaneous radiofrequency ablation.

● **77014** Computed tomography guidance for placement of radiation therapy fields [S]

MAGNETIC RESONANCE GUIDANCE

● **77021** Magnetic resonance guidance for needle placement (eg, for biopsy, needle aspiration, injection, or placement of localization device) radiological supervision and interpretation [S]

See the appropiate organ or site for procedure.

● **77022** Magnetic resonance guidance for, and monitoring of, parenchymal tissue ablation [S]

See codes 32998, 47382, and 50592 for percutaneous radiofrequency ablation.

Use code 0135T for percutaneous cryotherapy ablation of renal tumors.

See codes 0071T and 0072T for focused ultrasound ablation treatment of uterine leiomyomata.

OTHER RADIOLOGIC GUIDANCE

● **77031** Stereotactic localization guidance for breast biopsy or needle placement (eg, for wire localization or for injection), each lesion, radiological supervision and interpretation [X]

See codes 10022, 19000-19103, 19290 and 19291 for procedure.

Use code 38792 for injection for sentinel node localization without lymphoscintigraphy.

● **77032** Mammographic guidance for needle placement, breast (eg, for wire localization or for injection), each lesion, radiological supervision and interpretation [X]

See codes 10022, 19000, 19102, 19103, 19290, and 19291 for procedure.

Use code 38792 for injection for sentinel node localization without lymphoscintigraphy.

BREAST, MAMMOGRAPHY

+ ● **77051** Computer-aided detection (computer algorithm analysis of digital image data for lesion detection) with further physician review for interpretation, with or without digitization of film radiographic images; diagnostic mammography (List separately in addition to code for primary procedure) [A]

Note that code 77051 is an add-on code and must be reproted with code 77055 or 77056.

+ ● **77052** screening mammography (List separately in addition to code for primary procedure) [A]

Note that code 77052 is an add-on code and must be reproted with code 77057.

● **77053** Mammary ductogram or galactogram, single duct, radiological supervision and interpretation [X]

Use code 19030 for mammary ductogram or galactogram injection.

● **77054** Mammary ductogram or galactogram, multiple ducts, radiological supervision and interpretation [X]

● **77055** Mammography; unilateral [A]

● **77056** bilateral [A]

Use codes 77055 or 77056 with code 77051 for computer-aided detection applied to a diagnostic mammogram.

● **77057** Screening mammography, bilateral (2-view film study of each breast) [A]

Use code 77052 with code 77057 for computer-aided detection applied to a screening mmmogram.

Use code 0060T for bilateral eletrical impedance scan of the breast.

● **77058** Magnetic resonance imaging, breast, without and/or with contrast material(s); unilateral [B]

● **77059** bilateral [B]

BONE/JOINT STUDIES

● **77071** Manual application of stress performed by physician for joint radiography, including contralateral joint if indicated [X]

See the appropriate anatomic site and number of views for radiographic interpretation of stressed images.

● **77072** Bone age studies [X]

26 Professional Component Only

80/80 Assist-at-Surgery Allowed/With Documentation

Unlisted

Not Covered

TC Technical Component Only

MED: Pub 100/NCD References   **AMA:** CPT Assistant References

1-9 ASC Group

♂ Male Only

♀ Female Only

276 — CPT Expert

CPT only © 2006 American Medical Association. All Rights Reserved. *(Black Ink)*

© 2006 Ingenix *(Blue Ink)*

● 77073　Bone length studies (orthoroentgenogram, scanogram)　⊠

● 77074　Radiologic examination, osseous survey; limited (eg, for metastases)　⊠

● 77075　complete (axial and appendicular skeleton)　⊠

● 77076　Radiologic examination, osseous survey, infant　⊠

● 77077　Joint survey, single view, 2 or more joints (specify)　⊠

● 77078　Computed tomography, bone mineral density study, 1 or more sites; axial skeleton (eg, hips, pelvis, spine)　Ⓢ

● 77079　appendicular skeleton (peripheral) (eg, radius, wrist, heel)　Ⓢ

● 77080　Dual-energy X-ray absorptiometry (DXA), bone density study, 1 or more sites; axial skeleton (eg, hips, pelvis, spine)　Ⓢ

● 77081　appendicular skeleton (peripheral) (eg, radius, wrist, heel)　Ⓢ

● 77082　vertebral fracture assessment　⊠

Use code 0028T to report dual-energy X-ray absorptiometry (DXA) body composition study, one or more sites.

● 77083　Radiographic absorptiometry (eg, photodensitometry, radiogrammetry), 1 or more sites　⊠

● 77084　Magnetic resonance (eg, proton) imaging, bone marrow blood supply　Ⓢ

RADIATION ONCOLOGY

CLINICAL TREATMENT PLANNING (EXTERNAL AND INTERNAL SOURCES)

The codes in this section provide for brachytherapy and teletherapy to include the initial consultation, clinical treatment planning, dosimetry, radiation physics, treatment devices and treatment management services. These codes also include follow-up care for up to three months following completion. Identify preliminary consultation and patient evaluation performed by the therapeutic radiologist by the evaluation and management code. Consult the glossary for terms and definitions and the front matter of this chapter for additional information.

77261　Therapeutic radiology treatment planning; simple　Ⓑ 26 80 🞖

MED: 100-2,6,10; 100-4,3,10.4; 100-4,4,240; 100-4,12,70; 100-4,13,90
AMA: 1997,Oct,1

77262　intermediate　Ⓑ 26 80 🞖

MED: 100-2,6,10; 100-4,3,10.4; 100-4,4,240; 100-4,13,20; 100-4,13,90
AMA: 1997,Oct,1

77263　complex　Ⓑ 26 80 🞖

MED: 100-2,6,10; 100-4,3,10.4; 100-4,4,240; 100-4,12,70; 100-4,13,20; 100-4,13,90
AMA: 1997,Oct,1; 1991,Fall,12

77280　Therapeutic radiology simulation-aided field setting; simple　⊠ 80 🞖

MED: 100-2,6,10; 100-4,3,10.4; 100-4,4,220.4; 100-4,4,240; 100-4,12,70; 100-4,13,20; 100-4,13,90
AMA: 1997,Oct,1; 1997,Nov,26

77285　intermediate　⊠ 80 🞖

MED: 100-2,6,10; 100-4,3,10.4; 100-4,4,220.4; 100-4,4,240; 100-4,12,70; 100-4,13,20; 100-4,13,90
AMA: 1997,Oct,1

77290　complex　⊠ 80 🞖

MED: 100-2,6,10; 100-4,3,10.4; 100-4,4,220.4; 100-4,4,240; 100-4,12,70; 100-4,13,20; 100-4,13,90
AMA: 1997,Oct,1; 1991,Fall,12

77295　3-dimensional　⊠ 80 🞖

MED: 100-2,6,10; 100-4,3,10.4; 100-4,4,220.4; 100-4,4,240; 100-4,12,70; 100-4,13,20; 100-4,13,90
AMA: 1997,Oct,1; 1997,Nov,26

77299　Unlisted procedure, therapeutic radiology clinical treatment planning　⊠ 80

MED: 100-2,6,10; 100-4,3,10.4; 100-4,4,240; 100-4,12,70; 100-4,13,20; 100-4,13,90

MEDICAL RADIATION PHYSICS, DOSIMETRY, TREATMENT DEVICES, AND SPECIAL SERVICES

77300　Basic radiation dosimetry calculation, central axis depth dose calculation, TDF, NSD, gap calculation, off axis factor, tissue inhomogeneity factors, calculation of non-ionizing radiation surface and depth dose, as required during course of treatment, only when prescribed by the treating physician　⊠ 80 🞖

MED: 100-4,3,10.4; 100-4,4,220.4; 100-4,4,240; 100-4,12,70; 100-4,13,20; 100-4,13,90
AMA: 1997,Oct,1; 1991,Fall,13

77301　Intensity modulated radiotherapy plan, including dose-volume histograms for target and critical structure partial tolerance specifications　⊠ 80 🞖

MED: 100-4,3,10.4; 100-4,4,220.1; 100-4,4,220.4; 100-4,4,240; 100-4,12,70; 100-4,13,20; 100-4,13,90

Dose plan is optimized using inverse or forward planning technique for modulated beam delivery (eg, binary, dynamic MLC) to create highly conformal dose distribution. Computer plan distribution must be verified for positional accuracy based on dosimetric verification of the intensity map with verification of treatment set up and interpretation of verification methodology.

77305　Teletherapy, isodose plan (whether hand or computer calculated); simple (one or two parallel opposed unmodified ports directed to a single area of interest)　⊠ 80 🞖

MED: 100-4,3,10.4; 100-4,4,220.4; 100-4,4,240; 100-4,12,70; 100-4,13,20; 100-4,13,90
AMA: 1997,Oct,1

77310　intermediate (three or more treatment ports directed to a single area of interest)　⊠ 80 🞖

MED: 100-4,3,10.4; 100-4,4,220.4; 100-4,4,240; 100-4,12,70; 100-4,13,20; 100-4,13,90
AMA: 1997,Oct,1

77315　complex (mantle or inverted Y, tangential ports, the use of wedges, compensators, complex blocking, rotational beam, or special beam considerations)　⊠ 80 🞖

MED: 100-4,3,10.4; 100-4,4,220.4; 100-4,4,240; 100-4,12,70; 100-4,13,20; 100-4,13,90
AMA: 1997,Oct,1; 1991,Fall,13

Note that only one teletherapy isodose plan may be reported for a given course of therapy to a specific treatment area.

77321　Special teletherapy port plan, particles, hemibody, total body　⊠ 80 🞖

MED: 100-4,3,10.4; 100-4,4,220.4; 100-4,4,240; 100-4,12,70; 100-4,13,20; 100-4,13,90
AMA: 1997,Oct,1; 1991,Fall,14

⊛ Modifier 63 Exempt Code　　⊙ Conscious Sedation　　+ CPT Add-on Code　　⊘ Modifier 51 Exempt Code　　● New Code　　▲ Revised Code
Ⓜ Maternity Edit　　Ⓐ Age Edit　　Ⓐ-Ⓨ APC Status Indicators　　🞖 CCI Comprehensive Code　　50 Bilateral Procedure

Radiology

77326 — 77413

77326 Brachytherapy isodose plan; simple (calculation made from single plane, one to four sources/ribbon application, remote afterloading brachytherapy, 1 to 8 sources) ☒ 80 ▣

MED: 100-4,3,10.4; 100-4,4,240; 100-4,12,70; 100-4,13,20; 100-4,13,90

AMA: 1991,Winter,17

77327 intermediate (multiplane dosage calculations, application involving 5 to 10 sources/ribbons, remote afterloading brachytherapy, 9 to 12 sources) ☒ 80 ▣

MED: 100-4,3,10.4; 100-4,4,240

AMA: 1991,Winter,17

77328 complex (multiplane isodose plan, volume implant calculations, over 10 sources/ribbons used, special spatial reconstruction, remote afterloading brachytherapy, over 12 sources) ☒ 80 ▣

MED: 100-4,3,10.4; 100-4,4,240

AMA: 1991,Winter,17

77331 Special dosimetry (eg, TLD, microdosimetry) (specify), only when prescribed by the treating physician ☒ 80 ▣

MED: 100-4,3,10.4; 100-4,4,240; 100-4,12,70; 100-4,13,20; 100-4,13,90

AMA: 1997,Oct,1; 1991,Fall,13

77332 Treatment devices, design and construction; simple (simple block, simple bolus) ☒ 80 ▣

MED: 100-4,3,10.4; 100-4,4,220.4; 100-4,4,240; 100-4,12,70; 100-4,13,20; 100-4,13,90

AMA: 1997,Oct,1

77333 intermediate (multiple blocks, stents, bite blocks, special bolus) ☒ 80 ▣

MED: 100-4,3,10.4; 100-4,4,220.4; 100-4,4,240; 100-4,12,70; 100-4,13,20; 100-4,13,90

AMA: 1997,Oct,1

77334 complex (irregular blocks, special shields, compensators, wedges, molds or casts) ☒ 80 ▣

MED: 100-4,3,10.4; 100-4,4,220.4; 100-4,4,240; 100-4,12,70; 100-4,13,20; 100-4,13,90

AMA: 1997,Oct,1; 1991,Fall,13

77336 Continuing medical physics consultation, including assessment of treatment parameters, quality assurance of dose delivery, and review of patient treatment documentation in support of the radiation oncologist, reported per week of therapy ☒ TC 80 ▣

MED: 100-4,3,10.4; 100-4,4,220.4; 100-4,4,240; 100-4,12,70; 100-4,13,20; 100-4,13,90

AMA: 1998,Nov,21; 1997,Oct,1; 1991,Fall,15

77370 Special medical radiation physics consultation ☒ TC 80 ▣

MED: 100-4,3,10.4; 100-4,4,220.4; 100-4,4,240; 100-4,12,70; 100-4,13,20; 100-4,13,90

AMA: 1997,Oct,1; 1991,Fall,14

STEREOTACTIC RADIATION TREATMENT DELIVERY

● **77371** Radiation treatment delivery, stereotactic radiosurgery (SRS), complete course of treatment of cerebral lesion(s) consisting of 1 session; multi-source Cobalt 60 based ⓢ

● **77372** linear accelerator based Ⓑ

Use 77432 for radiation treatment management.

● **77373** Stereotactic body radiation therapy, treatment delivery, per fraction to 1 or more lesions, including image guidance, entire course not to exceed 5 fractions Ⓑ

Do not report code 77373 with codes 77401-77416 or 77418.

See codes 77371 and 77372 for single fraction cranial lesion(s).

OTHER PROCEDURES

77399 Unlisted procedure, medical radiation physics, dosimetry and treatment devices, and special services ☒ 80

MED: 100-4,3,10.4; 100-4,4,240

AMA: 1998,Nov,21

RADIATION TREATMENT DELIVERY

Radiation treatment delivery codes 77401-77416 recognize the technical component and the assorted energy levels.

For stereotactic body radiation therapy treatment delivery, consult 77371-77373.

77401 Radiation treatment delivery, superficial and/or ortho voltage ⓢ TC 80 ▣

MED: 100-2,6,10; 100-4,3,10.4; 100-4,4,220.1; 100-4,4,240; 100-4,12,70; 100-4,13,20; 100-4,13,70.3; 100-4,13,90

77402 Radiation treatment delivery, single treatment area, single port or parallel opposed ports, simple blocks or no blocks; up to 5 MeV ⓢ TC 80 ▣

MED: 100-2,6,10; 100-4,3,10.4; 100-4,4,220.1; 100-4,4,240; 100-4,12,70; 100-4,13,20; 100-4,13,70.3; 100-4,13,90

77403 6-10 MeV ⓢ TC 80 ▣

MED: 100-4,3,10.4; 100-4,4,220.1; 100-4,4,240; 100-4,12,70; 100-4,13,20; 100-4,13,70.3; 100-4,13,90

77404 11-19 MeV ⓢ TC 80 ▣

MED: 100-4,3,10.4; 100-4,4,220.1; 100-4,4,240; 100-4,12,70; 100-4,13,20; 100-4,13,70.3; 100-4,13,90

77406 20 MeV or greater ⓢ TC 80 ▣

MED: 100-4,3,10.4; 100-4,4,220.1; 100-4,4,240; 100-4,12,70; 100-4,13,20; 100-4,13,70.3; 100-4,13,90

77407 Radiation treatment delivery, two separate treatment areas, three or more ports on a single treatment area, use of multiple blocks; up to 5 MeV ⓢ TC 80 ▣

MED: 100-2,6,10; 100-4,3,10.4; 100-4,4,220.1; 100-4,4,240; 100-4,12,70; 100-4,13,20; 100-4,13,70.3; 100-4,13,90

77408 6-10 MeV ⓢ TC 80 ▣

MED: 100-4,3,10.4; 100-4,4,220.1; 100-4,4,240; 100-4,12,70; 100-4,13,20; 100-4,13,70.3; 100-4,13,90

77409 11-19 MeV ⓢ TC 80 ▣

MED: 100-4,3,10.4; 100-4,4,220.1; 100-4,4,240; 100-4,12,70; 100-4,13,20; 100-4,13,70.3; 100-4,13,90

77411 20 MeV or greater ⓢ TC 80 ▣

MED: 100-4,3,10.4; 100-4,4,220.1; 100-4,4,240; 100-4,12,70; 100-4,13,20; 100-4,13,70.3; 100-4,13,90

77412 Radiation treatment delivery, three or more separate treatment areas, custom blocking, tangential ports, wedges, rotational beam, compensators, electron beam; up to 5 MeV ⓢ TC 80 ▣

MED: 100-2,6,10; 100-4,3,10.4; 100-4,4,220.1; 100-4,4,240; 100-4,12,70; 100-4,13,20; 100-4,13,70.3; 100-4,13,90

77413 6-10 MeV ⓢ TC 80 ▣

MED: 100-4,3,10.4; 100-4,4,220.1; 100-4,4,240; 100-4,12,70; 100-4,13,20; 100-4,13,70.3; 100-4,13,90

AMA: 1991,Fall,14

26 Professional Component Only   80/80 Assist-at-Surgery Allowed/With Documentation   Unlisted   Not Covered

TC Technical Component Only   MED: Pub 100/NCD References   AMA: CPT Assistant References   1-9 ASC Group   ♂ Male Only   ♀ Female Only

278 — CPT Expert   CPT only © 2006 American Medical Association. All Rights Reserved. (Black Ink)   © 2006 Ingenix (Blue Ink)

77414   11-19 MeV   `S` `TC` `80` `◻`

MED: 100-4,3,10.4; 100-4,4,220.1; 100-4,4,240; 100-4,12,70; 100-4,13,20; 100-4,13,70.3; 100-4,13,90

77416   20 MeV or greater   `S` `TC` `80` `◻`

MED: 100-4,3,10.4; 100-4,4,220.1; 100-4,4,240; 100-4,12,70; 100-4,13,20; 100-4,13,70.3; 100-4,13,90

77417   Therapeutic radiology port film(s)   `X` `TC` `80` `◻`

MED: 100-4,3,10.4; 100-4,4,240; 100-4,12,70; 100-4,13,20; 100-4,13,70.3; 100-4,13,90

AMA: 1997,Dec,11; 1991,Fall,14

77418   Intensity modulated treatment delivery, single or multiple fields/arcs, via narrow spatially and temporally modulated beams, binary, dynamic MLC, per treatment session   `S` `TC` `80` `◻`

MED: 100-2,6,10; 100-4,3,10.4; 100-4,4,220.1; 100-4,4,240; 100-4,12,70; 100-4,13,20; 100-4,13,90

To report intensity modulated treatment planning, consult CPT code 77301.

To report compensator based beam modulation treatment delivery, consult Category III code 0073T.

77421   Stereoscopic X-ray guidance for localization of target volume for the delivery of radiation therapy   `S` `80`

MED: 100-4,3,10.4; 100-4,4,240

Code 77421 cannot be reported with 77432, or 77435.

See code 55876 for placement of interstitial device(s) for radiation therapy guidance for prostate.

NEUTRON BEAM TREATMENT DELIVERY

77422   High energy neutron radiation treatment delivery; single treatment area using a single port or parallel-opposed ports with no blocks or simple blocking   `S` `TC` `80`

MED: 100-2,6,10; 100-4,3,10.4; 100-4,4,240

77423   1 or more isocenter(s) with coplanar or non-coplanar geometry with blocking and/or wedge, and/or compensator(s)   `S` `TC` `80`

MED: 100-2,6,10; 100-4,3,10.4; 100-4,4,240

RADIATION TREATMENT MANAGEMENT

The codes in this section provide for brachytherapy and teletherapy to include the initial consultation, clinical treatment planning, dosimetry, radiation physics, treatment devices and treatment management services. These codes also include follow-up care for up to three months following completion. Identify preliminary consultation and patient evaluation performed by the therapeutic radiologist by the evaluation and management code. Consult the glossary for terms and definitions and the front matter of this chapter for additional information.

For radiation treatment management, the professional services usually furnished consist of review of patient treatment setup, port films, dosimetry, dose delivery and treatment parameters, and medical evaluation and management services.

Report radiation treatment management in units of five treatment sessions; this is not reflective of the actual time period in which the treatment are furnished. Treatment management consists of review of dosimetry, dose delivery, and treatment parameters; review of port films; review of treatment set-up; and examination of patient for medical evaluation and management.

77427   Radiation treatment management, five treatments   `B` `26` `◻`

AMA: 2000,Feb,7; 1999,Nov,42

77431   Radiation therapy management with complete course of therapy consisting of one or two fractions only   `B` `26` `80` `◻`

MED: 100-4,3,10.4; 100-4,4,240; 100-4,12,70; 100-4,13,20; 100-4,13,90

AMA: 1997,Oct,1

Note that 77431 is not to be used to fill in the last week of a long course of therapy.

77432   Stereotactic radiation treatment management of cerebral lesion(s) (complete course of treatment consisting of one session)   `B` `26` `80` `◻`

MED: 100-4,3,10.4; 100-4,4,240; 100-4,12,70; 100-4,13,20; 100-4,13,90

AMA: 1997,Oct,1

To report stereotactic body radiation treatment management, consult code 77371-77373.

● **77435**   Stereotactic body radiation therapy, treatment management, per treatment course, to one or more lesions, including image guidance, entire course not to exceed 5 fractions   `N`

Do not report code 77435 with codes 77427-77432.

When stereotactic radiation therapy is performed jointly by a surgeon and radiation oncologist (e.g. spinal or cranial), the surgeon reports radiosurgery with code 61793.

77470   Special treatment procedure (eg, total body irradiation, hemibody radiation, per oral, endocavitary or intraoperative cone irradiation)   `S` `80` `◻`

MED: 100-4,3,10.4; 100-4,4,240; 100-4,12,70; 100-4,13,20; 100-4,13,90

AMA: 1997,Oct,1; 1991,Winter,22

Note that 77470 assumes that this procedure is performed one or more times during the course of therapy, in addition to daily or weekly patient management.

77499   Unlisted procedure, therapeutic radiology treatment management   `B` `80`

MED: 100-4,3,10.4; 100-4,4,240; 100-4,12,70; 100-4,13,20; 100-4,13,90

AMA: 2000,Feb,7; 1999,Nov,42

PROTON BEAM TREATMENT DELIVERY

The codes in this section provide for brachytherapy and teletherapy to include the initial consultation, clinical treatment planning, dosimetry, radiation physics, treatment devices and treatment management services. These codes also include follow-up care for up to three months following completion. Identify preliminary consultation and patient evaluation performed by the therapeutic radiologist by the evaluation and management code. Consult the glossary for terms and definitions and the front matter of this chapter for additional information.

77520   Proton treatment delivery; simple, without compensation   `S` `TC` `80`

MED: 100-2,6,10; 100-4,3,10.4; 100-4,4,240; 100-4,12,70; 100-4,13,20; 100-4,13,90

AMA: 1999,Nov,43

77522   simple, with compensation   `S` `TC` `80` `◻`

MED: 100-2,6,10; 100-4,3,10.4; 100-4,4,240; 100-4,12,70; 100-4,13,20; 100-4,13,90

77523   intermediate   `S` `TC` `80` `◻`

MED: 100-2,6,10; 100-4,3,10.4; 100-4,4,240; 100-4,12,70; 100-4,13,20; 100-4,13,90

AMA: 1999,Nov,43

77525   complex   `S` `TC` `80` `◻`

MED: 100-2,6,10; 100-4,3,10.4; 100-4,4,240; 100-4,12,70; 100-4,13,20; 100-4,13,90

HYPERTHERMIA

The codes in this section provide for brachytherapy and teletherapy to include the initial consultation, clinical treatment planning, dosimetry, radiation physics, treatment devices and treatment management services. These codes also include follow-up care for up to three months following completion. Identify preliminary consultation and patient evaluation performed by the therapeutic radiologist by the evaluation and management code. Consult the glossary for terms and definitions and the front matter of this chapter for additional information.

Microwaves, ultrasound, probes, and radio frequencies may be used in concert with radiation therapy to provide external, interstitial, and intracavitary hyperthermia. Include the management and follow-up care in the following codes; physics planning and insertion of the sources are also included.

⊙ **77600** **Hyperthermia, externally generated; superficial (ie, heating to a depth of 4 cm or less)** S 80 ▣

MED: 100-3,110.1; 100-4,3,10.4; 100-4,4,240; 100-4,12,70; 100-4,13,20; 100-4,13,90

AMA: 1991,Winter,22

⊙ **77605** **deep (ie, heating to depths greater than 4 cm)** S 80 ▣

MED: 100-3,110.1; 100-4,3,10.4; 100-4,4,240; 100-4,12,70; 100-4,13,20; 100-4,13,90

AMA: 1991,Winter,22

⊙ **77610** **Hyperthermia generated by interstitial probe(s); 5 or fewer interstitial applicators** S 80 ▣

MED: 100-3,110.1; 100-4,3,10.4; 100-4,4,240; 100-4,12,70; 100-4,13,20; 100-4,13,90

AMA: 1991,Winter,22

⊙ **77615** **more than 5 interstitial applicators** S 80 ▣

MED: 100-3,110.1; 100-4,3,10.4; 100-4,4,240; 100-4,12,70; 100-4,13,20; 100-4,13,90

AMA: 1991,Winter,22

CLINICAL INTRACAVITARY HYPERTHERMIA

77620 **Hyperthermia generated by intracavitary probe(s)** S 80 ▣

MED: 100-3,110.1; 100-4,3,10.4; 100-4,4,240; 100-4,12,70; 100-4,13,20; 100-4,13,90

AMA: 1991,Winter,22

CLINICAL BRACHYTHERAPY

The codes in this section provide for brachytherapy and teletherapy to include the initial consultation, clinical treatment planning, dosimetry, radiation physics, treatment devices and treatment management services. These codes also include follow-up care for up to three months following completion. Identify preliminary consultation and patient evaluation performed by the therapeutic radiologist by the evaluation and management code. Consult the glossary for terms and definitions and the front matter of this chapter for additional information.

Man-made or natural radioactive elements are placed in or around the treatment field by a radiotherapist. CPT codes 77750-77799 include hospital admission and daily visits.

77750 **Infusion or instillation of radioelement solution (includes 3 months follow-up care)** S 80 ▣

MED: 100-4,3,10.4; 100-4,4,240; 100-4,12,70; 100-4,13,20; 100-4,13,70.4; 100-4,13,90

To report the administration of radiolabeled monoclonal antibodies, consult CPT code 79403.

To report non-antibody radiopharmaceutical therapy by IV administration, not including the three-month follow-up care, consult CPT code 79101.

77761 **Intracavitary radiation source application; simple** S 80 ▣

MED: 100-4,3,10.4; 100-4,4,240; 100-4,12,70; 100-4,13,20; 100-4,13,70.4; 100-4,13,90

AMA: 1999,Mar,3; 1996,Jan,7; 1991,Winter,23

77762 **intermediate** S 80 ▣

MED: 100-4,3,10.4; 100-4,4,240; 100-4,12,70; 100-4,13,20; 100-4,13,70.4; 100-4,13,90

AMA: 1991,Winter,23

77763 **complex** S 80 ▣

MED: 100-4,3,10.4; 100-4,4,240; 100-4,12,70; 100-4,13,20; 100-4,13,70.4; 100-4,13,90

AMA: 1999,Mar,3; 1991,Winter,23

77776 **Interstitial radiation source application; simple** S 80 ▣

MED: 100-4,3,10.4; 100-4,4,240; 100-4,12,70; 100-4,13,20; 100-4,13,70.4; 100-4,13,90

AMA: 1991,Winter,23

77777 **intermediate** S 80 ▣

MED: 100-4,3,10.4; 100-4,4,240; 100-4,12,70; 100-4,13,20; 100-4,13,70.4; 100-4,13,90

AMA: 1991,Winter,23

77778 **complex** S 80 ▣

MED: 100-4,3,10.4; 100-4,4,240; 100-4,12,70; 100-4,13,20; 100-4,13,70.4; 100-4,13,90

AMA: 1991,Winter,23

77781 **Remote afterloading high intensity brachytherapy; 1-4 source positions or catheters** S 80 ▣

MED: 100-4,3,10.4; 100-4,4,240; 100-4,12,70; 100-4,13,20; 100-4,13,70.4; 100-4,13,90

AMA: 1999,Mar,3; 1991,Winter,23

77782 **5-8 source positions or catheters** S 80 ▣

MED: 100-4,3,10.4; 100-4,4,240; 100-4,12,70; 100-4,13,20; 100-4,13,70.4; 100-4,13,90

AMA: 1999,Mar,3; 1991,Winter,23

77783 **9-12 source positions or catheters** S 80 ▣

MED: 100-4,3,10.4; 100-4,4,240; 100-4,12,70; 100-4,13,20; 100-4,13,70.4; 100-4,13,90

AMA: 1999,Mar,3; 1991,Winter,23

77784 **over 12 source positions or catheters** S 80 ▣

MED: 100-4,3,10.4; 100-4,4,240; 100-4,12,70; 100-4,13,20; 100-4,13,70.4; 100-4,13,90

AMA: 1999,Mar,3; 1991,Winter,23

77789 **Surface application of radiation source** S 80 ▣

MED: 100-4,3,10.4; 100-4,4,240; 100-4,12,70; 100-4,13,20; 100-4,13,70.4; 100-4,13,90

77790 **Supervision, handling, loading of radiation source** N 80 ▣

MED: 100-4,3,10.4; 100-4,4,240; 100-4,12,70; 100-4,13,20; 100-4,13,70.4; 100-4,13,90

77799 **Unlisted procedure, clinical brachytherapy** S 80

MED: 100-4,3,10.4; 100-4,4,240; 100-4,12,70; 100-4,13,20; 100-4,13,70.4; 100-4,13,90

NUCLEAR MEDICINE

DIAGNOSTIC

ENDOCRINE SYSTEM

In Nuclear Medicine, the procedures can be listed separately or as part of the overall medical care of the patient. The provision of radium or other radioelements is not included in CPT codes 78000-79999. Report diagnostic and therapeutic radiopharmaceuticals supplied by the physician separately.

78000 **Thyroid uptake; single determination** S 80 ▣

MED: 100-2,6,10; 100-2,15,80; 100-3,220.8; 100-4,3,10.4

78001 **multiple determinations** S 80 ▣

MED: 100-2,15,80; 100-3,220.8; 100-4,3,10.4

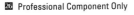
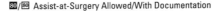

26 Professional Component Only   80/80 Assist-at-Surgery Allowed/With Documentation   Unlisted   Not Covered

TC Technical Component Only   MED: Pub 100/NCD References   AMA: CPT Assistant References   1 - 9 ASC Group   ♂ Male Only   ♀ Female Only

280 — CPT Expert   CPT only © 2006 American Medical Association. All Rights Reserved. *(Black Ink)*   © 2006 *Ingenix (Blue Ink)*

78003   stimulation, suppression or discharge (not including initial uptake studies) [S] [80] [CCI]

MED: 100-2,15,80; 100-3,220.8; 100-4,3,10.4

78006   Thyroid imaging, with uptake; single determination [S] [80] [CCI]

MED: 100-2,6,10; 100-2,15,80; 100-3,220.8; 100-4,3,10.4

78007   multiple determinations [S] [80] [CCI]

MED: 100-2,15,80; 100-3,220.8; 100-4,3,10.4

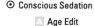

Thyroid cartilage
Cricoid cartilage
Thyroid gland
First four tracheal rings
Trachea
Thyroid gland
Cross-section view
Vocal folds
Jugular vein
Esophagus
Spine
Common carotid artery and vein

Hypothyroidism is the syndrome caused by a deficiency of thyroid hormone; the condition may be congenital, acquired, or iatrogenic (resulting from medical treatment)

The thyroid gland secretes hormones governing the body's metabolic rate; excess levels result in hyperthyroidism; abnormal enlargement of the gland is called goiter and there are numerous forms

78010   Thyroid imaging; only [S] [80] [CCI]

MED: 100-2,6,10; 100-2,15,80; 100-3,220.8; 100-4,3,10.4

78011   with vascular flow [S] [80] [CCI]

MED: 100-2,15,80; 100-3,220.8; 100-4,3,10.4

78015   Thyroid carcinoma metastases imaging; limited area (eg, neck and chest only) [S] [80] [CCI]

MED: 100-2,6,10; 100-2,15,80; 100-3,220.8; 100-4,3,10.4
AMA: 1998,Nov,21

78016   with additional studies (eg, urinary recovery) [S] [80] [CCI]

MED: 100-2,15,80; 100-3,220.8; 100-4,3,10.4

78018   whole body [S] [80] [CCI]

MED: 100-2,15,80; 100-3,220.8; 100-4,3,10.4
AMA: 1999,Apr,4

+   **78020**   Thyroid carcinoma metastases uptake (List separately in addition to code for primary procedure) [S] [80] [CCI]

MED: 100-2,15,80; 100-3,220.8; 100-4,3,10.4
AMA: 1999,Apr,4; 1998,Nov,21
Note that 78020 is an add-on code and must be used in conjunction with 78018.

78070   Parathyroid imaging [S] [80] [CCI]

MED: 100-2,15,80; 100-3,220.8; 100-4,3,10.4

78075   Adrenal imaging, cortex and/or medulla [S] [80] [CCI]

MED: 100-2,15,80; 100-3,220.8; 100-4,3,10.4

Epiglottis
Hyoid bone
Thyroid cartilage
Cricoid cartilage
Thyroid gland
Pyramid lobe
Thyroglossal duct (dotted line)
Hyoid bone
Cricothyroid muscle
Thyroid cartilage
Cricoid cartilage
Thyroid gland
Trachea
Esophagus
Isthmus

The thyroid is an important endocrine gland and its size and configuration can vary greatly. A pyramid lobe occurs in about 40 percent of people and is a remnant of the thyroglossal duct

78099   Unlisted endocrine procedure, diagnostic nuclear medicine [S] [80]

MED: 100-2,15,80; 100-3,220.8; 100-4,3,10.4
If a chemical analysis is needed, consult the Chemistry section of the CPT book.

HEMATOPOIETIC, RETICULOENDOTHELIAL AND LYMPHATIC SYSTEM

78102   Bone marrow imaging; limited area [S] [80] [CCI]

MED: 100-2,15,80; 100-3,220.8; 100-4,3,10.4

78103   multiple areas [S] [80] [CCI]

MED: 100-2,15,80; 100-3,220.8; 100-4,3,10.4

78104   whole body [S] [80] [CCI]

MED: 100-2,15,80; 100-3,220.8; 100-4,3,10.4

78110   Plasma volume, radiopharmaceutical volume-dilution technique (separate procedure); single sampling [S] [80] [CCI]

MED: 100-2,15,80; 100-3,220.8; 100-4,3,10.4

78111   multiple samplings [S] [80] [CCI]

MED: 100-2,15,80; 100-3,220.8; 100-4,3,10.4

78120   Red cell volume determination (separate procedure); single sampling [S] [80] [CCI]

MED: 100-2,15,80; 100-3,220.8; 100-4,3,10.4

78121   multiple samplings [S] [80] [CCI]

MED: 100-2,15,80; 100-3,220.8; 100-4,3,10.4

78122   Whole blood volume determination, including separate measurement of plasma volume and red cell volume (radiopharmaceutical volume-dilution technique) [S] [80] [CCI]

MED: 100-2,15,80; 100-3,220.8; 100-4,3,10.4

78130   Red cell survival study; [S] [80] [CCI]

MED: 100-2,15,80; 100-3,220.8; 100-4,3,10.4

78135   differential organ/tissue kinetics, (eg, splenic and/or hepatic sequestration) [S] [80] [CCI]

MED: 100-2,15,80; 100-3,220.8; 100-4,3,10.4

78140   Labeled red cell sequestration, differential organ/tissue, (eg, splenic and/or hepatic) [S] [80] [CCI]

MED: 100-2,15,80; 100-3,220.8; 100-4,3,10.4

78185   Spleen imaging only, with or without vascular flow [S] [80] [CCI]

MED: 100-2,15,80; 100-3,220.8; 100-4,3,10.4
If this procedure is combined with a liver study, consult CPT codes 78215 and 78216.

78190   Kinetics, study of platelet survival, with or without differential organ/tissue localization [S] [80] [CCI]

MED: 100-2,15,80; 100-3,220.8; 100-4,3,10.4

78191   Platelet survival study [S] [80] [CCI]

MED: 100-2,15,80; 100-3,220.8; 100-4,3,10.4

78195   Lymphatics and lymph nodes imaging [S] [80] [CCI]

MED: 100-2,15,80; 100-3,220.8; 100-4,3,10.4
AMA: 1999,Nov,43; 1999,Dec,8; 1998,Nov,22
If sentinel node identification is performed without scintigraphy imaging, consult CPT code 38792. If the sentinel node is excised, consult CPT codes 38500-38542.

78199   Unlisted hematopoietic, reticuloendothelial and lymphatic procedure, diagnostic nuclear medicine [S] [80]

MED: 100-2,15,80; 100-3,220.8; 100-4,3,10.4
If chemical analysis is needed, consult the Chemistry section of CPT.

GASTROINTESTINAL SYSTEM

78201 Liver imaging; static only ⓈⒺ 80 🔄
MED: 100-2,15,80; 100-3,220.8; 100-4,3,10.4

78202 with vascular flow Ⓢ 80 🔄
MED: 100-2,15,80; 100-3,220.8; 100-4,3,10.4

If spleen imaging is performed by itself, consult CPT code 78185.

78205 Liver imaging (SPECT); Ⓢ 80 🔄
MED: 100-2,15,80; 100-3,220.8; 100-3,220.12; 100-4,3,10.4
AMA: 1998,Nov,22

78206 with vascular flow Ⓢ 80 🔄
MED: 100-2,15,80; 100-3,220.8; 100-4,3,10.4
AMA: 1998,Nov,22

78215 Liver and spleen imaging; static only Ⓢ 80 🔄
MED: 100-2,15,80; 100-3,220.8; 100-4,3,10.4

78216 with vascular flow Ⓢ 80 🔄
MED: 100-2,15,80; 100-3,220.8; 100-4,3,10.4

78220 Liver function study with hepatobiliary agents, with serial images Ⓢ 80 🔄
MED: 100-2,15,80; 100-3,220.8; 100-4,3,10.4

78223 Hepatobiliary ductal system imaging, including gallbladder, with or without pharmacologic intervention, with or without quantitative measurement of gallbladder function Ⓢ 80 🔄
MED: 100-2,15,80; 100-3,220.8; 100-4,3,10.4

78230 Salivary gland imaging; Ⓢ 80 🔄
MED: 100-2,15,80; 100-3,220.8; 100-4,3,10.4

78231 with serial images Ⓢ 80 🔄
MED: 100-2,15,80; 100-3,220.8; 100-4,3,10.4

78232 Salivary gland function study Ⓢ 80 🔄
MED: 100-2,15,80; 100-3,220.8; 100-4,3,10.4

78258 Esophageal motility Ⓢ 80 🔄
MED: 100-2,15,80; 100-3,220.8; 100-4,3,10.4

78261 Gastric mucosa imaging Ⓢ 80 🔄
MED: 100-2,15,80; 100-3,220.8; 100-4,3,10.4

78262 Gastroesophageal reflux study Ⓢ 80 🔄
MED: 100-2,15,80; 100-3,220.8; 100-4,3,10.4

78264 Gastric emptying study Ⓢ 80 🔄
MED: 100-2,15,80; 100-3,220.8; 100-4,3,10.4

78267 Urea breath test, C-14 (isotopic); acquisition for analysis Ⓐ 🔄
MED: 100-2,15,80; 100-3,220.8; 100-4,3,10.4
AMA: 1999,Nov,43

78268 analysis Ⓐ 🔄
MED: 100-2,15,80; 100-3,220.8; 100-4,3,10.4
AMA: 1999,Nov,43

78270 Vitamin B-12 absorption study (eg, Schilling test); without intrinsic factor Ⓢ 80 🔄
MED: 100-2,15,80; 100-3,220.8; 100-4,3,10.4

78271 with intrinsic factor Ⓢ 80 🔄
MED: 100-2,15,80; 100-3,220.8; 100-4,3,10.4

78272 Vitamin B-12 absorption studies combined, with and without intrinsic factor Ⓢ 80 🔄
MED: 100-2,15,80; 100-3,220.8; 100-4,3,10.4

78278 Acute gastrointestinal blood loss imaging Ⓢ 80 🔄
MED: 100-2,15,80; 100-3,220.8; 100-4,3,10.4

78282 Gastrointestinal protein loss Ⓢ 80 🔄
MED: 100-2,15,80; 100-3,220.8; 100-4,3,10.4

78290 Intestine imaging (eg, ectopic gastric mucosa, Meckel's localization, volvulus) Ⓢ 80 🔄
MED: 100-2,15,80; 100-3,220.8; 100-4,3,10.4

78291 Peritoneal-venous shunt patency test (eg, for LeVeen, Denver shunt) Ⓢ 80 🔄
MED: 100-2,15,80; 100-3,220.8; 100-4,3,10.4

To report injection procedure, consult CPT code 49427.

78299 Unlisted gastrointestinal procedure, diagnostic nuclear medicine Ⓢ 80
MED: 100-2,15,80; 100-3,220.8; 100-4,3,10.4

If chemical analysis is needed, consult the Chemistry section of the CPT book.

MUSCULOSKELETAL SYSTEM

78300 Bone and/or joint imaging; limited area Ⓢ 80 🔄
MED: 100-2,15,80; 100-3,220.8; 100-4,3,10.4
AMA: 1997,Mar,11

78305 multiple areas Ⓢ 80 🔄
MED: 100-2,15,80; 100-3,220.8; 100-4,3,10.4
AMA: 1997,Mar,11

78306 whole body Ⓢ 80 🔄
MED: 100-2,15,80; 100-3,220.8; 100-4,3,10.4; 100-4,12,70; 100-4,13,20; 100-4,13,90
AMA: 2002,Jan,10; 1997,Mar,11

78315 three phase study Ⓢ 80 🔄
MED: 100-2,15,80; 100-3,220.8; 100-4,3,10.4
AMA: 2002,Jan,10

78320 tomographic (SPECT) Ⓢ 80 🔄
MED: 100-2,15,80; 100-3,220.8; 100-3,220.12; 100-4,3,10.4; 100-4,12,70; 100-4,13,20; 100-4,13,90
AMA: 1997,Mar,11

78350 Bone density (bone mineral content) study, one or more sites; single photon absorptiometry Ⓧ 80 🔄
MED: 100-2,6,10; 100-2,15,80; 100-3,150.3; 100-3,220.8; 100-4,3,10.4; 100-4,4,240; 100-4,13,140.2; 100-4,13,140.3
AMA: 1997,Nov,26

78351 dual photon absorptiometry, one or more sites Ⓔ
MED: 100-2,6,10; 100-2,15,80; 100-3,150.3; 100-3,220.8; 100-4,3,10.4; 100-4,4,240
AMA: 1997,Nov,26

If radiographic bone density (photodensitometry) is performed, consult CPT code 77083.

78399 Unlisted musculoskeletal procedure, diagnostic nuclear medicine Ⓢ 80
MED: 100-2,15,80; 100-3,220.8; 100-4,3,10.4

CARDIOVASCULAR SYSTEM

In Nuclear Medicine, the procedures can be listed separately or as part of the overall medical care of the patient. The provision of radium or other radioelements is not included in CPT codes 78000-79999. These materials should be reported separately.

Use stress testing codes from 93015-93018 series when the following procedures are performed during exercise or medication-induced stress. Infusion and blood pool imaging can be performed at rest or during stress.

78414 Determination of central c-v hemodynamics (non-imaging) (eg, ejection fraction with probe technique) with or without pharmacologic intervention or exercise, single or multiple determinations Ⓢ 80 🔄
MED: 100-2,15,80; 100-3,220.8; 100-4,3,10.4

78428 Cardiac shunt detection Ⓢ 80 🔄
MED: 100-2,15,80; 100-3,220.8; 100-4,3,10.4

🄯 Professional Component Only   80/80 Assist-at-Surgery Allowed/With Documentation   Unlisted   Not Covered
🆃🅲 Technical Component Only   MED: Pub 100/NCD References   AMA: CPT Assistant References   🅰-🅰 ASC Group   ♂ Male Only   ♀ Female Only

282 — CPT Expert

78445   Non-cardiac vascular flow imaging (ie, angiography, venography)   S 80 ⟲
    MED: 100-2,15,80; 100-3,220.8; 100-4,3,10.4

78456   Acute venous thrombosis imaging, peptide   S ⟲
    MED: 100-2,15,80; 100-3,220.8; 100-4,3,10.4
    AMA: 1999,Nov,43

78457   Venous thrombosis imaging, venogram; unilateral   S 80 ⟲
    MED: 100-2,15,80; 100-3,220.8; 100-4,3,10.4
    AMA: 1999,Nov,43

78458   bilateral   S 80 ⟲
    MED: 100-2,15,80; 100-3,220.8; 100-4,3,10.4
    AMA: 1999,Nov,43

78459   Myocardial imaging, positron emission tomography (PET), metabolic evaluation   S 80 ⟲
    MED: 100-2,6,10; 100-2,15,80; 100-3,220.6; 100-3,220.8; 100-4,3,10.4; 100-4,13,60; 100-4,13,60.1; 100-4,13,60.2; 100-4,13,60.3; 100-4,13,60.3.1; 100-4,13,60.4; 100-4,13,60.9; 100-4,13,60.11
    AMA: 1997,Nov,26; 1996,Jun,5
    If a myocardial perfusion study is performed, consult CPT codes 78491-78492.

78460   Myocardial perfusion imaging; (planar) single study, at rest or stress (exercise and/or pharmacologic), with or without quantification   S 80 ⟲
    MED: 100-2,6,10; 100-2,15,80; 100-3,220.8; 100-4,3,10.4
    AMA: 2000,Apr,1; 1999,Mar,10

78461   multiple studies, (planar) at rest and/or stress (exercise and/or pharmacologic), and redistribution and/or rest injection, with or without quantification   S 80 ⟲
    MED: 100-2,15,80; 100-3,220.8; 100-4,3,10.4
    AMA: 1999,Mar,10

78464   tomographic (SPECT), single study (including attenuation correction when performed), at rest or stress (exercise and/or pharmacologic), with or without quantification   S 80 ⟲
    MED: 100-3,220.8; 100-4,3,10.4
    AMA: 1999,Mar,10

78465   tomographic (SPECT), multiple studies (including attenuation correction when performed), at rest and/or stress (exercise and/or pharmacologic) and redistribution and/or rest injection, with or without quantification   S 80 ⟲
    MED: 100-2,15,80; 100-3,220.8; 100-3,220.12; 100-4,3,10.4
    AMA: 1999,Mar,10; 1998,Aug,11

78466   Myocardial imaging, infarct avid, planar; qualitative or quantitative   S 80 ⟲
    MED: 100-2,6,10; 100-2,15,80; 100-3,220.8; 100-4,3,10.4

78468   with ejection fraction by first pass technique   S 80 ⟲
    MED: 100-2,15,80; 100-3,220.8; 100-4,3,10.4

78469   tomographic SPECT with or without quantification   S 80 ⟲
    MED: 100-2,15,80; 100-3,220.8; 100-4,3,10.4

78472   Cardiac blood pool imaging, gated equilibrium; planar, single study at rest or stress (exercise and/or pharmacologic), wall motion study plus ejection fraction, with or without additional quantitative processing   S 80 ⟲
    MED: 100-2,15,80; 100-3,220.8; 100-4,3,10.4
    AMA: 1999,Nov,44; 1999,Jun,8; 1998,Nov,22

78473   multiple studies, wall motion study plus ejection fraction, at rest and stress (exercise and/or pharmacologic), with or without additional quantification   S 80 ⟲
    MED: 100-2,15,80; 100-3,220.8; 100-4,3,10.4
    AMA: 1999,Jun,11

+ **78478**   Myocardial perfusion study with wall motion, qualitative or quantitative study (List separately in addition to code for primary procedure)   S 80 ⟲
    MED: 100-2,15,80; 100-3,220.8; 100-4,3,10.4
    AMA: 1999,Mar,10
    Note that 78478 is an add-on code and must be used in conjunction with 78460, 78461, 78464, and 78465.

+ **78480**   Myocardial perfusion study with ejection fraction (List separately in addition to code for primary procedure)   S 80 ⟲
    MED: 100-2,15,80; 100-3,220.8; 100-4,3,10.4
    AMA: 1997,Mar,10
    Note that 78480 is an add-on code and must be used in conjunction with 78460, 78461, 78464, and 78465.

78481   Cardiac blood pool imaging, (planar), first pass technique; single study, at rest or with stress (exercise and/or pharmacologic), wall motion study plus ejection fraction, with or without quantification   S 80 ⟲
    MED: 100-2,15,80; 100-3,220.8; 100-4,3,10.4

78483   multiple studies, at rest and with stress (exercise and/or pharmacologic), wall motion study plus ejection fraction, with or without quantification   S 80 ⟲
    MED: 100-2,15,80; 100-3,220.8; 100-4,3,10.4
    If a cerebral blood flow study is conducted, consult CPT code 78615.

78491   Myocardial imaging, positron emission tomography (PET), perfusion; single study at rest or stress   S 80 ⟲
    MED: 100-2,15,80; 100-3,220.6; 100-3,220.8; 100-4,3,10.4; 100-4,13,60; 100-4,13,60.2; 100-4,13,60.3; 100-4,13,60.3.1; 100-4,13,60.4; 100-4,13,60.9; 100-4,13,60.11
    AMA: 1997,Nov,27

78492   multiple studies at rest and/or stress   S 80 ⟲
    MED: 100-2,15,80; 100-3,220.6; 100-3,220.8; 100-4,3,10.4; 100-4,13,60; 100-4,13,60.1; 100-4,13,60.2; 100-4,13,60.3; 100-4,13,60.4; 100-4,13,60.9; 100-4,13,60.11
    AMA: 1997,Nov,27

78494   Cardiac blood pool imaging, gated equilibrium, SPECT, at rest, wall motion study plus ejection fraction, with or without quantitative processing   S 80 ⟲
    MED: 100-2,15,80; 100-3,220.8; 100-4,3,10.4
    AMA: 1999,Jun,3; 1998,Nov,22

+ **78496**   Cardiac blood pool imaging, gated equilibrium, single study, at rest, with right ventricular ejection fraction by first pass technique (List separately in addition to code for primary procedure)   S 80 ⟲
    MED: 100-2,15,80; 100-3,220.8; 100-4,3,10.4
    AMA: 1999,Jun,3, 11; 1998,Nov,22
    Note that 78496 is an add-on code and must be used in conjunction with 78472.

78499   Unlisted cardiovascular procedure, diagnostic nuclear medicine   S 80
    MED: 100-2,15,80; 100-3,220.8; 100-4,3,10.4
    If chemical analysis is needed, consult the Chemistry section of the CPT book.

⊛ Modifier 63 Exempt Code   ⊙ Conscious Sedation   + CPT Add-on Code   ⊘ Modifier 51 Exempt Code   ● New Code   ▲ Revised Code

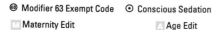 Maternity Edit   A Age Edit   A-Y APC Status Indicators   ⟲ CCI Comprehensive Code   50 Bilateral Procedure

Radiology

RESPIRATORY SYSTEM

78580   Pulmonary perfusion imaging, particulate   [S] [80] [⟲]

MED: 100-2,15,80; 100-3,220.7; 100-3,220.8; 100-4,3,10.4

AMA: 1999,Mar,4

78584   Pulmonary perfusion imaging, particulate, with ventilation; single breath   [S] [80] [⟲]

MED: 100-2,15,80; 100-3,220.7; 100-3,220.8; 100-4,3,10.4

AMA: 1999,Mar,4

78585   rebreathing and washout, with or without single breath   [S] [80] [⟲]

MED: 100-2,15,80; 100-3,220.8; 100-4,3,10.4

AMA: 1999,Mar,4

78586   Pulmonary ventilation imaging, aerosol; single projection   [S] [80] [⟲]

MED: 100-2,15,80; 100-3,220.8; 100-4,3,10.4

AMA: 1999,Mar,4

78587   multiple projections (eg, anterior, posterior, lateral views)   [S] [80] [⟲]

MED: 100-2,15,80; 100-3,220.8; 100-4,3,10.4

AMA: 1999,Mar,4

78588   Pulmonary perfusion imaging, particulate, with ventilation imaging, aerosol, one or multiple projections   [S] [80] [⟲]

MED: 100-2,15,80; 100-3,220.7; 100-3,220.8; 100-4,3,10.4

AMA: 1999,Mar,4; 1998,Nov,22

78591   Pulmonary ventilation imaging, gaseous, single breath, single projection   [S] [80] [⟲]

MED: 100-2,15,80; 100-3,220.8; 100-4,3,10.4

AMA: 1999,Mar,4

78593   Pulmonary ventilation imaging, gaseous, with rebreathing and washout with or without single breath; single projection   [S] [80] [⟲]

MED: 100-2,15,80; 100-3,220.8; 100-4,3,10.4

AMA: 1999,Mar,4

78594   multiple projections (eg, anterior, posterior, lateral views)   [S] [80] [⟲]

MED: 100-2,15,80; 100-3,220.8; 100-4,3,10.4

78596   Pulmonary quantitative differential function (ventilation/perfusion) study   [S] [80] [⟲]

MED: 100-2,15,80; 100-3,220.8; 100-4,3,10.4

78599   Unlisted respiratory procedure, diagnostic nuclear medicine   [S] [80]

MED: 100-2,15,80; 100-3,220.8; 100-4,3,10.4

NERVOUS SYSTEM

Diagram of tomography principal (left)

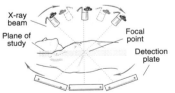

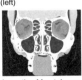

Schematic of frontal coronal CT section of skull

Tomogram is a general term for radiographic studies that focus on a single body plane, unimpeded by shadows cast by surrounding tissues and structures. The x-ray tube and the film are rotated around the patient during exposure of the focal point. Computed tomography (CT) offers a "slice" view of the study area and information is typically digitized and viewed on monitors. Magnetic resonance imaging (MRI) places a patient within the field of a powerful magnet while radio waves pass through the body; as with CT studies, views are usually of a "slice" of tissue. Ultrasound and nuclear imaging are other common radiological approaches

78600   Brain imaging, limited procedure; static   [S] [80] [⟲]

MED: 100-2,15,80; 100-3,220.8; 100-4,3,10.4

78601   with vascular flow   [S] [80] [⟲]

MED: 100-2,15,80; 100-3,220.8; 100-4,3,10.4

78605   Brain imaging, complete study; static   [S] [80] [⟲]

MED: 100-2,15,80; 100-3,220.8; 100-4,3,10.4

78606   with vascular flow   [S] [80] [⟲]

MED: 100-2,15,80; 100-3,220.8; 100-4,3,10.4

78607   tomographic (SPECT)   [S] [80] [⟲]

MED: 100-2,15,80; 100-3,220.8; 100-4,3,10.4

78608   Brain imaging, positron emission tomography (PET); metabolic evaluation   [S] [80] [⟲]

MED: 100-2,15,80; 100-3,220.6; 100-3,220.8; 100-4,3,10.4; 100-4,13,60.3; 100-4,13,60.3.1; 100-4,13,60.12

78609   perfusion evaluation   [E] [80] [⟲]

MED: 100-2,15,80; 100-3,220.6; 100-3,220.7; 100-3,220.8; 100-4,3,10.4; 100-4,13,60.3; 100-4,13,60.12

78610   Brain imaging, vascular flow only   [S] [80] [⟲]

MED: 100-2,15,80; 100-3,220.8; 100-4,3,10.4

78615   Cerebral vascular flow   [S] [80] [⟲]

MED: 100-2,15,80; 100-3,220.8; 100-4,3,10.4

78630   Cerebrospinal fluid flow, imaging (not including introduction of material); cisternography   [S] [80] [⟲]

MED: 100-2,15,80; 100-3,220.8; 100-4,3,10.4

If an injection procedure is performed, consult CPT codes 61000-61070 and 62270-62319.

78635   ventriculography   [S] [80] [⟲]

MED: 100-2,15,80; 100-3,220.8; 100-4,3,10.4

If an injection procedure is performed, consult CPT codes 61000-61070 and 62270-62294.

78645   shunt evaluation   [S] [80] [⟲]

MED: 100-2,15,80; 100-3,220.8; 100-4,3,10.4

If an injection procedure is performed, consult CPT codes 61000-61070 and 62270-62294.

78647   tomographic (SPECT)   [S] [80] [⟲]

MED: 100-2,15,80; 100-3,220.8; 100-3,220.12; 100-4,3,10.4

78650   Cerebrospinal fluid leakage detection and localization   [S] [80] [⟲]

MED: 100-2,15,80; 100-3,220.8; 100-4,3,10.4

If an injection procedure is performed, consult CPT codes 61000-61070 and 62270-62294.

78660   Radiopharmaceutical dacryocystography   [S] [80] [⟲]

MED: 100-2,15,80; 100-3,220.8; 100-4,3,10.4

78699   Unlisted nervous system procedure, diagnostic nuclear medicine   [S] [80]

MED: 100-2,15,80; 100-3,220.8; 100-4,3,10.4

GENITOURINARY SYSTEM

▲ **78700**   Kidney imaging morphology;   [S] [80] [⟲]

MED: 100-2,15,80; 100-3,220.8; 100-4,3,10.4

▲ **78701**   with vascular flow   [S] [80] [⟲]

MED: 100-2,15,80; 100-3,220.8; 100-4,3,10.4

~~**78704**~~   ~~with function study (ie, imaging renogram)~~

MED: 100-3,220.8

Use 78707-78709.

▲ **78707**   Kidney imaging morphology; with vascular flow and function, single study without pharmacological intervention   [S] [80] [⟲]

MED: 100-2,15,80; 100-3,220.8; 100-4,3,10.4

AMA: 1997,Nov,27

[26] Professional Component Only

[TC] Technical Component Only

[80]/[80] Assist-at-Surgery Allowed/With Documentation

MED: Pub 100/NCD References   AMA: CPT Assistant References

Unlisted

Not Covered

[1]-[9] ASC Group   ♂ Male Only   ♀ Female Only

284 — CPT Expert   CPT only © 2006 American Medical Association. All Rights Reserved. (*Black Ink*)   © 2006 *Ingenix* (*Blue Ink*)

▲ **78708** with vascular flow and function, single study, with pharmacological intervention (eg, angiotensin converting enzyme inhibitor and/or diuretic) [S] [80] [CCI]

MED: 100-2,15,80; 100-3,220.8; 100-4,3,10.4
AMA: 1997,Nov,27

▲ **78709** with vascular flow and function, multiple studies, with and without pharmacological intervention (eg, angiotensin converting enzyme inhibitor and/or diuretic) [S] [80] [CCI]

MED: 100-2,15,80; 100-3,220.8; 100-4,3,10.4
AMA: 1997,Nov,27

If a radioactive substance is introduced in association with renal endoscopy, consult CPT codes 77776-77778.

▲ **78710** Kidney imaging morphology; tomographic (SPECT) [S] [80] [CCI]

MED: 100-2,15,80; 100-3,220.8; 100-3,220.12; 100-4,3,10.4
AMA: 1997,Nov,27

~~**78715**~~ ~~Kidney vascular flow only~~

MED: 100-3,220.8

Use 78701-78709.

78725 Kidney function study, non-imaging radioisotopic study [S] [80] [CCI]

MED: 100-2,15,80; 100-3,220.8; 100-4,3,10.4
AMA: 1998,Nov,22

+ ▲ **78730** Urinary bladder residual study (List separately in addition to code for primary procedure) [X] [80] [CCI]

MED: 100-2,15,80; 100-3,220.8; 100-4,3,10.4

Note that code 78730 is an add-on code and must be reported with code 78740.

Use code 51798 for measurement of postvoid residual urine and/or lbadder capacity by ultrasound, nonimaging.

Use code 76857 for ultrasound imaging of bladder only, with measurement of postvoid urine, when performed.

78740 Ureteral reflux study (radiopharmaceutical voiding cystogram) [S] [80] [CCI]

MED: 100-2,15,80; 100-3,220.8; 100-3,230.2; 100-4,3,10.4

Use code 78730 with code 78740 for urinary bladder residual study.

To report catheterization, consult CPT codes 51701, 51702, 51703.

~~**78760**~~ ~~Testicular imaging;~~

MED: 100-3,220.8

Use 78761.

▲ **78761** Testicular imaging with vascular flow ♂ [S] [80] [CCI]

MED: 100-2,15,80; 100-3,220.8; 100-4,3,10.4

To report introduction of radioactive substance with ureteral endoscopy, consult CPT codes 50959, 50978.

78799 Unlisted genitourinary procedure, diagnostic nuclear medicine [S] [80]

MED: 100-2,15,80; 100-3,220.8; 100-4,3,10.4

If chemistry analysis is needed, consult the Chemistry section of the CPT book.

OTHER PROCEDURES

See appropriate heading for specific organ sites.

78800 Radiopharmaceutical localization of tumor or distribution of radiopharmaceutical agent(s); limited area [S] [80] [CCI]

MED: 100-2,15,80; 100-3,220.8; 100-4,3,10.4

Use 78800 to report radiophosphorus ocular tumor identification.

78801 multiple areas [S] [80] [CCI]

MED: 100-2,15,80; 100-3,220.8; 100-4,3,10.4

78802 whole body, single day imaging [S] [80] [CCI]

MED: 100-2,15,80; 100-3,220.8; 100-4,3,10.4; 100-4,12,70; 100-4,13,20; 100-4,13,90

78803 tomographic (SPECT) [S] [80] [CCI]

MED: 100-2,15,80; 100-3,220.8; 100-3,220.12; 100-4,3,10.4; 100-4,12,70; 100-4,13,20; 100-4,13,90

78804 whole body, requiring two or more days imaging [S] [80] [CCI]

MED: 100-4,3,10.4

78805 Radiopharmaceutical localization of inflammatory process; limited area [S] [80] [CCI]

MED: 100-2,15,80; 100-3,220.8; 100-4,3,10.4
AMA: 1999,Nov,44

To report bone and/or joint imaging, consult CPT codes 78300, 78305, and 78306.

78806 whole body [S] [80] [CCI]

MED: 100-2,15,80; 100-3,220.8; 100-4,3,10.4; 100-4,12,70; 100-4,13,20; 100-4,13,90
AMA: 1999,Nov,44

78807 tomographic (SPECT) [S] [80] [CCI]

MED: 100-2,15,80; 100-3,220.8; 100-3,220.12; 100-4,3,10.4; 100-4,12,70; 100-4,13,20; 100-4,13,90

To report imaging bone infectious or inflammatory disease with a bone imaging radiopharmaceutical, consult 78300, 78305, 78306.

To report PET of brain, consult 78608, 78609. To report PET myocardial imaging, see 78491, 784992.

78811 Tumor imaging, positron emission tomography (PET); limited area (eg, chest, head/neck) [S] [80] [CCI]

MED: 100-4,3,10.4; 100-4,13,60.3; 100-4,13,60.3.1

78812 skull base to mid-thigh [S] [80] [CCI]

MED: 100-4,3,10.4; 100-4,13,60.3; 100-4,13,60.3.1

78813 whole body [S] [80] [CCI]

MED: 100-4,3,10.4; 100-4,13,60.3; 100-4,13,60.3.1

78814 Tumor imaging, positron emission tomography (PET) with concurrently acquired computed tomography (CT) for attenuation correction and anatomical localization; limited area (eg, chest, head/neck) [S] [80] [CCI]

MED: 100-4,3,10.4; 100-4,13,60.3; 100-4,13,60.3.1

78815 skull base to mid-thigh [S] [80] [CCI]

MED: 100-4,3,10.4; 100-4,13,60.3; 100-4,13,60.3.1

78816 whole body [S] [80] [CCI]

MED: 100-4,3,10.4; 100-4,13,60.3; 100-4,13,60.3.1

Codes 78811-78816 should be reported only once per session.

Report the CT scan code for other than attenuation correction and anatomical localization with the code for the specific site and append modifier 59.

---

⑥³ Modifier 63 Exempt Code   ⊙ Conscious Sedation   + CPT Add-on Code   ∅ Modifier 51 Exempt Code   ● New Code   ▲ Revised Code
[M] Maternity Edit   [A] Age Edit   [A]-[Y] APC Status Indicators   [CCI] CCI Comprehensive Code   [50] Bilateral Procedure

78890 Generation of automated data: interactive process involving nuclear physician and/or allied health professional personnel; simple manipulations and interpretation, not to exceed 30 minutes N

MED: 100-3,220.8; 100-4,3,10.4; 100-4,12,70; 100-4,13,20; 100-4,13,90

Report 78890 and 78891 in addition to primary procedure.

78891 complex manipulations and interpretation, exceeding 30 minutes N

MED: 100-3,220.8; 100-4,3,10.4; 100-4,12,70; 100-4,13,20; 100-4,13,90

Note that 78890 and 78891 should be used in addition to the primary procedure.

78999 Unlisted miscellaneous procedure, diagnostic nuclear medicine S 80

MED: 100-3,220.8

THERAPEUTIC

The oral and intravenous administration codes in this section include the method of administration. For intra-arterial, intra-cavitary, and intra-articular administration, also report the appropriate injection and/or procedure codes, as well as imaging guidance and radiological supervision and interpretation codes, when applicable. .

79005 Radiopharmaceutical therapy, by oral administration S 80

MED: 100-4,4,240

To report monoclonal antibody therrapy, consult 79403.

79101 Radiopharmaceutical therapy, by intravenous administration S 80 ▢

MED: 100-4,4,240

Code 79101 cannot be reported with CPT codes 36400, 36410, 79403, 90780, 96408.

To report radiolabeled monochlonal antibody by IV infusion, consult 79403.

To report infusion or instillation of non-antibody radioelement solution including three months after follow-up consult CPT code 77750.

79200 Radiopharmaceutical therapy, by intracavitary administration S 80 ▢

MED: 100-3,220.8; 100-4,4,240

79300 Radiopharmaceutical therapy, by interstitial radioactive colloid administration S 80 ▢

MED: 100-3,220.8; 100-4,4,240

79403 Radiopharmaceutical therapy, radiolabeled monoclonal antibody by intravenous infusion S 80 ▢

MED: 100-3,220.8; 100-4,4,240

To report pre-treatment imaging, consult CPT codes 78802, 78804.

Code 79403 cannot be reported in conjunction with 79101.

79440 Radiopharmaceutical therapy, by intra-articular administration S 80 ▢

MED: 100-3,220.8; 100-4,4,240

79445 Radiopharmaceutical therapy, by intra-arterial particulate administration S 80 ▢

MED: 100-4,4,240

Code 79445 cannot be reported with 90773, 96420.

If angiography and interventional procedures are done, report the radiologic procedural codes for supervision and interpretation and the procedure before the intra-arterial radiopharmaceutical therapy.

79999 Radiopharmaceutical therapy, unlisted procedure S 80

MED: 100-3,220.8; 100-4,3,10.4; 100-4,4,240; 100-4,12,70; 100-4,13,20; 100-4,13,90

2C Professional Component Only

TC Technical Component Only

80/**80** Assist-at-Surgery Allowed/With Documentation

MED: Pub 100/NCD References **AMA:** CPT Assistant References

Unlisted   Not Covered

1-**9** ASC Group   ♂ Male Only   ♀ Female Only

286 — CPT Expert   CPT only © 2006 American Medical Association. All Rights Reserved. *(Black Ink)*   © *2006 Ingenix (Blue Ink)*

Pathology and Laboratory

CODING INFORMATION

ORGANIZATION
The pathology and laboratory section of CPT is divided into the following subsections:

- Organ or Disease Oriented Panels
- Drug Testing
- Therapeutic Drug Assays
- Evocative/Suppression Testing
- Consultations (Clinical Pathology)
- Urinalysis
- Chemistry
- Molecular Diagnostics
- Infectious Agents: Detection of Antibodies
- Hematology and Coagulation
- Microbiology
- Anatomic Pathology
- Cytopathology
- Cytogenetic Studies
- Surgical Pathology

RESULTS/TESTING/REPORTS

Results indicate the technical component of a procedure or service. Testing is the service that leads to the report and interpretation. Reports provide interpretation of the tests.

GUIDELINES

Inpatient coders are not required to code pathology or laboratory tests since they are not necessary in the assignment of diagnosis-related groups (DRGs). However, pathology and laboratory codes are itemized on chargemasters for reporting services and supplies to patients.

Outpatient coders frequently code pathology and laboratory tests. Coding instructions include listing each laboratory procedure separately, unless it is part of a panel. Never use modifier 51 Multiple procedures in pathology or laboratory coding.

Many lab tests can be performed by different methods. To choose the correct code, carefully review code descriptions as well as any notes. When in doubt, request information from the physician or laboratory for clarification, or consult an authoritative reference.

Pathology and laboratory services are provided by the physician or by technologists under the supervision of a physician. The majority of the codes represent a technical component only, but certain codes represent a global service-a combination of professional and technical components. If the pathologist reviews a test result or renders an opinion of a test that is represented by a global code, the code selected should be identified with modifier 26 to indicate that only the professional component was provided.

SUBSECTIONS

ORGAN OR DISEASE-ORIENTED PANELS
Nine codes (80048–80076) report panels listing definitive test components: basic metabolic; general health; electrolyte; comprehensive metabolic; obstetric; lipid; renal function; acute hepatitis; and hepatic function. These panels neither specify clinical parameters nor do they preclude performance of other tests. Tests performed in addition to the procedures defined in a panel can be reported separately. However, panel tests should not be reported separately on the same day as single test codes listed as part of the panel. For example, a hepatic function panel code 80076 includes codes 82040

(albumin), 82247 (bilirubin, total), 82248 (bilirubin, direct), 84075 (phosphatase, alkaline), 84155 (protein, total), 84460 (transferase, alanine amino (ALT) (SGBT), and 84450 (transferase, aspartate amino (AST) (SGOT).

DRUG TESTING
The drug testing subsection lists codes (80100–80103) for qualitative screens that are usually confirmed by a second technique. Thirteen drugs or classes of drugs are listed as examples of commonly assayed qualitative screens: alcohols; amphetamines; barbiturates; opiates; benzodiazepines; cocaine and metabolites; methadones; methaqualones; phencyclidines; phenothiazines; propoxyphenes; tetrahydrocannabinoids; and tricyclic antidepressants.

Reporting Drug Screens
Qualitative screens should be reported when a provider is testing for the presence of a particular substance or substances. Coding for qualitative screening tests is based on procedure, not method or analyte. For example, if confirmation of five drugs requires three procedures, 80102 Drug confirmation, each procedure is identified three times. Drugs that have been confirmed through qualitative testing may also be quantitated. Use codes from the chemistry section (82000–84999) or therapeutic drug assay section (80150–80299) to report quantitative testing.

THERAPEUTIC DRUG ASSAYS
The therapeutic drug assays subsection (80150–80299) lists codes for quantitative assays. Several of these codes were found in the chemistry and toxicology subsection in past editions of the CPT book and reported as either qualitative or quantitative tests.

Coding for Drug Assays
Codes listed under therapeutic drug assays or under chemistry are used when a drug is quantitated, or measured. Screening may be used to detect a substance, but it is not a prerequisite for quantitation. For example, screening is not necessary when a known drug has been overdosed. Coding for quantitative assays is based on the substance tested. Unless the code description notes otherwise, the examination material may be from any source.

EVOCATIVE/SUPPRESSION TESTING
These procedures (80400–80440) measure the effects of administered evocative (stimulating) or suppressive agents upon the patient and represent the technical component of the service. These panels measure levels of multiple constituents or the same constituent multiple times after administering the stimulating or suppressing agent. Most of these tests are performed to evaluate specific conditions stated in the code narrative. For example, 80400 ACTH stimulation panel (adrenocorticotropic hormone) is performed for adrenal insufficiency. Supplies and drugs are reported separately, (99070 or HCPCS Level II codes). To report physician attendance and monitoring during the tests, refer to the appropriate evaluation and management codes. Prolonged physician care codes may be reported separately, except when testing is performed by prolonged infusion (90780–90781).

CONSULTATION (CLINICAL PATHOLOGY)
Two consultation codes (80500 and 80502) are reserved for the pathologist to indicate a service, not a test. The pathology consultation is performed at the request of an attending physician and requires a written report. Code 80500 is a limited service without review of the patient's history and medical records. Code 80502 is a comprehensive service for a complex diagnostic problem, with review of the patient's history and medical records.

URINALYSIS
Codes 81000–81099 are used for specific analysis of one or more components of the urine. Select the appropriate code based on method (e.g., dip stick, tablet reagent, qualitative, semiquantitative) purpose (e.g., pregnancy test, timed-volume, bacteriuria screen) and specific constituents evaluated (e.g., bilirubin, glucose, pH). Not all urine analyses are listed in this section. For other tests, see appropriate section. For example, urine chloride can be found in the chemistry section.

CHEMISTRY
Chemistry codes (82000–84999) report only quantitative tests unless the description specifies otherwise, as is the case with the chromatography codes (82486–82492). Qualitative screens are reported by the four drug testing codes (80100–80103).

An individual code or a series of codes may be required for appropriate reporting. Glucose testing is an example:

82947	Glucose; quantitative, blood (except reagent strip)
82948	blood, reagent strip
82950	post glucose dose (includes glucose)
82951	tolerance test (GTT), three specimens (includes glucose)
82952	tolerance test, each additional beyond three specimens

Code 82951 reports a three–specimen glucose tolerance test (GTT). This code includes obtaining the fasting blood sample, supplying and administering the oral glucose dose, and obtaining the next two samples (e.g., at one-half hour and one hour). Code 82952 reports additional samples beyond the first three. Report 82951 once and 82952 twice for a three-hour GTT in which specimens are obtained at zero, one-half, one, two, and three hours.

Multiple specimens from different sources as well as specimens obtained at different times should be reported separately. For example, total bilirubin levels (82247) obtained in the morning and afternoon would be reported twice on that date of service.

MOLECULAR DIAGNOSTICS
Tests in these series (83890–83913) are reported by procedure rather than analyte and should be coded separately for each procedure used in an analysis.

HEMATOLOGY AND COAGULATION
The infectious agent antibodies subsection (85002–85999) lists those laboratory procedures specific to blood and blood-forming organs, including complete blood counts (CBC), clotting factors, clotting inhibitors, prothrombin and thrombin time, platelets, and sickling.

Code 85097 for bone marrow and smear interpretation is found in this subsection. However, when reporting interpretation services read procedure descriptions carefully as cell block interpretations and bone marrow biopsy interpretations should be reported with 88305.

IMMUNOLOGY
The immunology subsection (86000–86849) identifies codes for antigen and antibody studies. Detection of antibodies to infectious agents using multiple step qualitative or semiquantitative immunoassays should be reported with codes 86602–86804.

Specific tissue typing procedures are also found in the immunology subsection, see 86805–86822.

High-volume procedures include cardiolipin antibody; antigen complement; deoxyribonucleic acid antibody; hepatitis C antibody; delta agent hepatitis; heterophile antibodies; and streptococcus screening.

TRANSFUSION MEDICINE
Once listed in immunology, most blood bank codes are now grouped together under the transfusion medicine subsection (86850–86999). Since more blood bank procedures are likely to be performed on an outpatient basis, this subsection may expand in the future.

Be aware that the present codes do not report the supply of blood or blood products, and their cost may not be covered by insurance. Payers usually cover antibody screening, autologous blood or component collection, processing and storage, blood typing, and blood praeparata. Some payers require blood to be replaced (when the unit given is replaceable) instead of paid. Some payers will not cover the cost of blood components, such as albumin, plasma, or plasmanate. There may also be restrictions on procedures involving pheresis.

MICROBIOLOGY
These microbiology codes (87001–87999) identify services related to cultures, organism identification, and sensitivity studies. Many of the narratives are similar to those in the immunology section, so it is important to pay close attention to technique. Infectious agents identified by antigen detection, nucleic acid probe, or fluorescence microscopy is reported with codes 87260–87999 from microbiology. Infectious agents identified by antibody detection are reported with codes 86602–86804 from immunology. For example, cytomegalovirus (CMV) identified by infectious agent antigen detection by enzyme immunoassay technique, qualitative or semiquantitative, multiple step method is reported with 87332 from microbiology. However, CMV antibody detection by qualitative or semiquantitative immunoassay, multiple step method is reported with 86644.

ANATOMIC PATHOLOGY
Anatomic pathology (88000–88099) includes postmortem examinations (e.g., necropsy, autopsy), cytopathology (e.g., fluids, washing or brushing, Pap smears, fine needle aspirations, flow cytometry, etc.) and cytogenetic studies (e.g., tissue cultures for chromosome studies, etc.). Postmortem examination procedures report only the physician portion of the service. To report outside laboratory services, append modifier 90.

CYTOPATHOLOGY
Codes for reporting cervical and vaginal screening (Pap smears) (88141–88155, 88164–88167, 88174–88175) have undergone considerable revision and expansion in recent years. Codes 88142–88143 report cervical or vaginal specimens collected in a preservative fluid using automated thin layer preparation, with manual screening. Codes 88174–88175 report cervical or vaginal specimens collected in a preservative fluid using automated thin layer preparation, with automated screening. These specimens may then be examined by either Bethesda or non-Bethesda reporting systems. Codes 88150–88154 report cervical or vaginal specimens (Pap smears) prepared on slides and examined using non-Bethesda reporting systems. Codes 88164–88167 report cervical or vaginal specimens (Pap smears) prepared on slides and examined using Bethesda reporting systems. All of the above codes report manual screening and rescreening using various techniques under physician supervision. Cervical or vaginal cytopathology services requiring physician interpretation are reported separately with code 88141. Definitive hormonal evaluation is also reported separately with code 88155.

CYTOGENETIC STUDIES
Codes in this section (88230–88299) are related to the branch of genetics that studies cellular (cyto) structure and function as it relates to heredity (genetics). White blood cells, specifically T-lymphocytes, are the most commonly used specimen for chromosome analysis (88245–88289). Chromosome analysis for breakage syndromes (88245–88248) may be requested by the name of the specific syndrome being investigated, such as Fragile X, Xeroderma pigmentosum (XP), Ataxia-telangiectasia (A-T), and Fanconi anemia (FA), while 88249 reports a specific technique for the analysis of breakage syndromes involving clastogen stress. Other codes in this section include chromosome analysis for the presence of mosaicism (88263), malignant neoplasms (88264), and possible genetic abnormalities detectable within the cells of amniotic fluid (88269). Tissue and skin biopsies are reported separately using codes from the CPT surgery section. Physician interpretation and report are also reported separately, with 88291 from the cytogenetic studies section.

SURGICAL PATHOLOGY
The primary surgical pathology codes (88300–88309) describe gross and microscopic examination of specimens submitted for pathologic evaluation.

The specimen is the unit of service to report for surgical pathology. A specimen is defined as each tissue or tissues submitted for individual and separate evaluation. Each separate specimen requires individual examination and pathologic diagnosis. When two or more individual specimens are submitted from the same patient, each specimen is assigned an individual CPT code that should reflect the proper level of service.

The type of exam and the type of tissue define the level of service. CPT code 88300 should be reported for specimens requiring only gross examination. All other surgical pathology services require both gross and microscopic examination of the tissue and are defined by the type of specimen. The type of specimen included in each level is listed in the code description. For example, tissue submitted labeled "synovium knee" is examined by the pathologist and determined to be a synovial cyst. The surgical pathology code reported is 88304 because "bursa/synovial cyst" is listed under CPT code 88304.

Codes listed in 88300–88309 do not include any of the special services described by procedures 88311–88399. Procedures 88311–88399 describe additional services which may be reported separately and include the following: special stains, histochemistry, immunocytochemistry, immunofluorescent studies, electron microscopy, nerve teasing preparations, protein analysis by the Western Blot method, and pathology consultations during surgery.

TRANSCUTANEOUS PROCEDURES
This section (code 88400) describes the procedure to test bilirubin using a transdermal approach such as in a patch form applied to the skin.

OTHER PROCEDURES
Codes in this subsection (89050–89240) describe such procedures as crystal identification by light microscopy, duodenal intubation and aspiration, gastric intubation and aspiration, and nasal smear for eosinophils.

REPRODUCTIVE MEDICINE PROCEDURES
Reproductive laboratory services in this subsection include culture and co-culture of oocytes with coding options for extended culture and the use of microtechniques. There are codes for oocyte biopsies for pre-implantation genetic diagnoses, as well as coding options for storage and thawing of cryopreserved specimens.

LABORATORY CODING

Verify that all services performed have a signed physician order, are medically necessary and each is coded correctly, and supported by documentation in the medical record. Maintaining a current chargemaster or fee schedule is critical. Laboratories, (physician/clinic-based, hospital-based, or freestanding) must update their chargemasters and fee schedule annually and verify that the codes and descriptors match the services performed. Never report a service with a code that appears to be "close enough" to the actual service performed. If the descriptor does not match the service performed, review the CPT book to identify a more specific code. If a code cannot be identified, assign an unlisted procedure code and supply supporting documentation with the claim.

To avoid unbundling become familiar with the following subsections: Organ and Disease Oriented Panels (80048–80076), and Evocative/Suppression Testing (80400–80440). Do not report individual codes when the individual laboratory procedures are included in a panel.

ORGAN OR DISEASE ORIENTED PANELS

80048   Basic metabolic panel   Ⓐ ◪

MED: 100-2,6,10; 100-2,15,80; 100-4,3,10.4

AMA: 2000,Jan,7; 1999,Nov,44; 1998,Jan,6

This panel must include the following: Calcium (82310) Carbon dioxide (82374) Chloride (82435) Creatinine (82565) Glucose (82947) Potassium (84132) Sodium (84295) Urea nitrogen (BUN) (84520)

Code 80048 cannot be reported in conjunction with 80053.

80050   General health panel   Ⓔ

MED: 100-2,6,10; 100-2,15,80; 100-4,3,10.4

AMA: 1998,Jan,6; 1997,Nov,28; 1997,Jun,10; 1993,Summer,14; 1992,Winter,14

This panel must include the following: Comprehensive metabolic panel (80053) Blood count, complete (CBC), automated and automated differential WBC count (85025 or 85027 and 85004) OR Blood count, complete (CBC), automated (85027) and appropriate manual differential WBC count (85007 or 85009) Thyroid stimulating hormone (TSH) (84443)

80051   Electrolyte panel   Ⓐ ◪

MED: 100-2,6,10; 100-2,15,80; 100-4,3,10.4

AMA: 1998,Jan,6; 1997,Nov,28

This panel must include the following: carbon dioxide (82374), chloride (82435), potassium (84132), sodium (84295)

80053   Comprehensive metabolic panel   Ⓐ ◪

MED: 100-2,6,10; 100-2,15,80; 100-4,3,10.4

AMA: 2000,May,11; 2000,Jan,7; 1999,Nov,44; 1999,Dec,1; 1998,Nov,23; 1998,Jan,6

This panel must include the following: Albumin (82040) Bilirubin, total (82247) Calcium (82310) Carbon dioxide (bicarbonate) (82374) Chloride (82435) Creatinine (82565) Glucose (82947) Phosphatase, alkaline (84075) Potassium (84132) Protein, total (84155) Sodium (84295) Transferase, alanine amino (ALT) (SGPT) (84460) Transferase, aspartate amino (AST) (SGOT) (84450) Urea nitrogen (BUN) (84520)

Note that 80053 cannot be used in addition to CPT codes 80048 and 80076.

80055   Obstetric panel   Ⓜ ♀ Ⓔ

MED: 100-2,6,10; 100-2,15,80; 100-4,3,10.4

AMA: 1997,Jun,10; 1993,Summer,14; 1992,Winter,14

This panel must include the following: Blood count, complete (CBC), automated and automated differential WBC count (85025 or 85027 and 85004) OR Blood count, complete (CBC), automated (85027) and appropriate manual differential WBC count (85007 or 85009) Hepatitis B surface antigen (HBsAg) (87340) Antibody, rubella (86762) Syphilis test, qualitative (eg, VDRL, RPR, ART) (86592) Antibody screen, RBC, each serum technique (86850) Blood typing, ABO (86900) AND Blood typing, Rh (D) (86901)

80061   Lipid panel   Ⓐ ◪ ☒

MED: 100-2,6,10; 100-2,15,80; 100-3,190.23; 100-4,3,10.4

AMA: 2000,Mar,11; 1997,Jun,10; 1993,Summer,14; 1992,Winter,14

This panel must include the following: Cholesterol, serum, total (82465) Lipoprotein, direct measurement, high density cholesterol (HDL cholesterol) (83718) Triglycerides (84478)

80069   Renal function panel   Ⓐ ◪

MED: 100-2,6,10; 100-2,15,80; 100-3,190.10; 100-4,3,10.4

AMA: 2000,Jan,7; 1999,Nov,44

This panel must include the following: Albumin (82040) Calcium (82310) Carbon dioxide (bicarbonate) (82374) Chloride (82435) Creatinine (82565) Glucose (82947) Phosphorus inorganic (phosphate) (84100) Potassium (84132) Sodium (84295) Urea nitrogen (BUN) (84520)

80074   Acute hepatitis panel   Ⓐ ◪

MED: 100-2,6,10; 100-2,15,80; 100-3,190.33; 100-4,3,10.4

AMA: 2000,Jan,7; 1999,Nov,45

This panel must include the following: Hepatitis A antibody (HAAb), IgM antibody (86709) Hepatitis B core antibody (HBcAb), IgM antibody (86705) Hepatitis B surface antigen (HBsAg) (87340) Hepatitis C antibody (86803)

80076   Hepatic function panel   Ⓐ ◪

MED: 100-2,6,10; 100-2,15,80; 100-4,3,10.4

AMA: 2000,Jan,7; 1999,Nov,45; 1999,Apr,6; 1998,Jan,6; 1997,Jun,10; 1993,Summer,14; 1992,Winter,14

This panel must include the following: Albumin (82040) Bilirubin, total (82247) Bilirubin, direct (82248) Phosphatase, alkaline (84075) Protein, total (84155) Transferase, alanine amino (ALT) (SGPT) (84460) Transferase, aspartate amino (AST) (SGOT) (84450)

Note that 80076 cannot be used in addition to CPT code 80053.

DRUG TESTING

Consult CPT codes 82000-84999 (Chemistry) or 80150-80299 (Therapeutic drug assay) for quantitation of drugs screened.

80100   Drug screen, qualitative; multiple drug classes chromatographic method, each procedure   Ⓐ ◪

MED: 100-2,6,10; 100-2,15,80; 100-4,3,10.4

AMA: 2000,Mar,1; 1993,Fall,26

80101   single drug class method (eg, immunoassay, enzyme assay), each drug class   Ⓐ ◪ ☒

MED: 100-2,6,10; 100-2,15,80; 100-3,190.8; 100-4,3,10.4

AMA: 2000,Mar,1; 1993,Fall,26

80102   Drug confirmation, each procedure   Ⓐ ◪

MED: 100-2,6,10; 100-2,15,80; 100-4,3,10.4

AMA: 2000,Mar,1; 1993,Fall,26

80103   Tissue preparation for drug analysis   Ⓝ

MED: 100-2,15,80; 100-4,3,10.4

AMA: 2000,Mar,1

THERAPEUTIC DRUG ASSAYS

For nonquantitative testing, consult CPT codes 80100-80103.

The specimen used for analysis may be from any source.

80150   Amikacin   Ⓐ

MED: 100-2,15,80; 100-4,3,10.4

AMA: 2000,Mar,1; 1993,Fall,26; 1992,Winter,14

80152   Amitriptyline   Ⓐ

MED: 100-2,15,80; 100-4,3,10.4

AMA: 2000,Mar,1; 1993,Fall,26; 1992,Winter,14

80154   Benzodiazepines   Ⓐ

MED: 100-2,15,80; 100-4,3,10.4

AMA: 2000,Mar,1; 1993,Fall,26; 1992,Winter,14

80156   Carbamazepine; total   Ⓐ

MED: 100-2,15,80; 100-4,3,10.4

AMA: 2000,Mar,1; 1993,Fall,26; 1992,Winter,14

Pathology and Laboratory

80157 — 80410

80157	free	Ⓐ

MED: 100-2,15,80; 100-4,3,10.4
AMA: 2000,Mar,1; 1993,Fall,26; 1992,Winter,14

80158 Cyclosporine Ⓐ

MED: 100-2,15,80; 100-4,3,10.4
AMA: 2000,Mar,1; 1993,Fall,26; 1992,Winter,14

80160 Desipramine Ⓐ

MED: 100-2,15,80; 100-4,3,10.4
AMA: 2000,Mar,1; 1993,Fall,26; 1992,Winter,14

80162 Digoxin Ⓐ

MED: 100-2,15,80; 100-3,190.24; 100-4,3,10.4
AMA: 2000,Mar,1; 1993,Fall,26; 1992,Winter,14

80164 Dipropylacetic acid (valproic acid) Ⓐ

MED: 100-2,15,80; 100-4,3,10.4
AMA: 2000,Mar,1; 1993,Fall,26; 1992,Winter,14

80166 Doxepin Ⓐ

MED: 100-2,15,80; 100-4,3,10.4
AMA: 2000,Mar,1; 1993,Fall,26; 1992,Winter,14

80168 Ethosuximide Ⓐ

MED: 100-2,15,80; 100-4,3,10.4
AMA: 2000,Mar,1; 1993,Fall,26; 1992,Winter,14

80170 Gentamicin Ⓐ

MED: 100-2,15,80; 100-4,3,10.4
AMA: 2000,Mar,1; 1993,Fall,26; 1992,Winter,14

80172 Gold Ⓐ

MED: 100-2,15,80; 100-4,3,10.4
AMA: 2000,Mar,1; 1993,Fall,26; 1992,Winter,14

80173 Haloperidol Ⓐ

MED: 100-2,15,80; 100-4,3,10.4
AMA: 2000,Mar,1; 1993,Fall,26; 1992,Winter,14

80174 Imipramine Ⓐ

MED: 100-2,15,80; 100-4,3,10.4
AMA: 2000,Mar,1; 1993,Fall,26; 1992,Winter,14

80176 Lidocaine Ⓐ

MED: 100-2,15,80; 100-4,3,10.4
AMA: 2000,Mar,1; 1993,Fall,26; 1992,Winter,14

80178 Lithium Ⓐ

MED: 100-2,15,80; 100-4,3,10.4
AMA: 2000,Mar,1; 1993,Fall,26; 1992,Winter,14

80182 Nortriptyline Ⓐ

MED: 100-2,15,80; 100-4,3,10.4
AMA: 2000,Mar,1; 1993,Fall,26; 1992,Winter,14

80184 Phenobarbital Ⓐ

MED: 100-2,15,80; 100-4,3,10.4
AMA: 2000,Mar,1; 1993,Fall,26; 1992,Winter,14

80185 Phenytoin; total Ⓐ

MED: 100-2,15,80; 100-4,3,10.4
AMA: 2000,Mar,1; 1993,Fall,26; 1992,Winter,14

80186 free Ⓐ

MED: 100-2,15,80; 100-4,3,10.4
AMA: 2000,Mar,1; 1993,Fall,26; 1992,Winter,14

80188 Primidone Ⓐ

MED: 100-2,15,80; 100-4,3,10.4
AMA: 2000,Mar,1; 1993,Fall,26; 1992,Winter,14

80190 Procainamide; Ⓐ

MED: 100-2,15,80; 100-4,3,10.4
AMA: 2000,Mar,1; 1993,Fall,26; 1992,Winter,14

80192 with metabolites (eg, n-acetyl procainamide) Ⓐ ▣

MED: 100-2,15,80; 100-4,3,10.4
AMA: 2000,Mar,1; 1993,Fall,26; 1992,Winter,14

80194 Quinidine Ⓐ

MED: 100-2,15,80; 100-4,3,10.4
AMA: 2000,Mar,1; 1993,Fall,26; 1992,Winter,14

80195 Sirolimus Ⓐ

MED: 100-4,3,10.4

80196 Salicylate Ⓐ

MED: 100-2,15,80; 100-4,3,10.4
AMA: 2000,Mar,1; 1993,Fall,26; 1992,Winter,14

80197 Tacrolimus Ⓐ

MED: 100-2,15,80; 100-4,3,10.4
AMA: 2000,Mar,1; 1993,Fall,26; 1992,Winter,14

80198 Theophylline Ⓐ

MED: 100-2,15,80; 100-4,3,10.4
AMA: 2000,Mar,1; 1993,Fall,26; 1992,Winter,14

80200 Tobramycin Ⓐ

MED: 100-2,15,80; 100-4,3,10.4
AMA: 2000,Mar,1; 1993,Fall,26; 1992,Winter,14

80201 Topiramate Ⓐ

MED: 100-2,15,80; 100-4,3,10.4
AMA: 2000,Mar,1; 1993,Fall,26; 1992,Winter,14

80202 Vancomycin Ⓐ

MED: 100-2,15,80; 100-4,3,10.4
AMA: 2000,Mar,1; 1993,Fall,26; 1992,Winter,14

80299 Quantitation of drug, not elsewhere specified Ⓐ

MED: 100-2,15,80; 100-4,3,10.4
AMA: 2000,Mar,"1, 3"; 1993,Fall,26; 1992,Winter,14

EVOCATIVE/SUPPRESSION TESTING

80400 ACTH stimulation panel; for adrenal insufficiency Ⓐ ▣

MED: 100-2,15,80; 100-4,3,10.4
AMA: 1994,Summer,1
This panel must include the following: Cortisol (82533 x 2)

80402 for 21 hydroxylase deficiency Ⓐ ▣

MED: 100-2,15,80; 100-4,3,10.4
AMA: 1994,Summer,1
This panel must include the following: Cortisol (82533 x 2) 17 hydroxyprogesterone (83498 x 2)

80406 for 3 beta-hydroxydehydrogenase deficiency Ⓐ ▣

MED: 100-2,15,80; 100-4,3,10.4
AMA: 1994,Summer,1
This panel must include the following: Cortisol (82533 x 2) 17 hydroxypregnenolone (84143 x 2)

80408 Aldosterone suppression evaluation panel (eg, saline infusion) Ⓐ ▣

MED: 100-2,15,80; 100-4,3,10.4
AMA: 1994,Summer,1
This panel must include the following: Aldosterone (82088 x 2) Renin (84244 x 2)

80410 Calcitonin stimulation panel (eg, calcium, pentagastrin) Ⓐ ▣

MED: 100-2,15,80; 100-4,3,10.4
AMA: 1994,Summer,1
This panel must include the following: Calcitonin (82308 x 3)

---

26 Professional Component Only   80/ 80 Assist-at-Surgery Allowed/With Documentation   Unlisted   Not Covered
TC Technical Component Only   MED: Pub 100/NCD References   AMA: CPT Assistant References   1-9 ASC Group   ♂ Male Only   ♀ Female Only

292 — CPT Expert   CPT only © 2006 American Medical Association. All Rights Reserved. (Black Ink)   © 2006 Ingenix (Blue Ink)

80412 Corticotropic releasing hormone (CRH) stimulation panel Ⓐ 🗎

MED: 100-2,15,80; 100-4,3,10.4
AMA: 1994,Summer,1
This panel must include the following: Cortisol (82533 x 6) Adrenocorticotropic hormone (ACTH) (82024 x 6)

80414 Chorionic gonadotropin stimulation panel; testosterone response ♀ Ⓐ 🗎

MED: 100-2,15,80; 100-4,3,10.4
AMA: 1994,Summer,1
This panel must include the following: Testosterone (84403 x 2 on three pooled blood samples)

80415 estradiol response Ⓐ 🗎

MED: 100-2,15,80; 100-4,3,10.4
AMA: 1994,Summer,1
This panel must include the following: Estradiol (82670 x 2 on three pooled blood samples)

80416 Renal vein renin stimulation panel (eg, captopril) Ⓐ 🗎

MED: 100-2,15,80; 100-4,3,10.4
AMA: 1994,Summer,1
This panel must include the following: Renin (84244 x 6)

80417 Peripheral vein renin stimulation panel (eg, captopril) Ⓐ 🗎

MED: 100-2,15,80; 100-4,3,10.4
This panel must include the following: Renin (84244 x 2)

80418 Combined rapid anterior pituitary evaluation panel Ⓐ 🗎

MED: 100-2,15,80; 100-4,3,10.4
AMA: 1994,Summer,1
This panel must include the following: Adrenocorticotropic hormone (ACTH) (82024 x 4) Luteinizing hormone (LH) (83002 x 4) Follicle stimulating hormone (FSH) (83001 x 4) Prolactin (84146 x 4) Human growth hormone (HGH) (83003 x 4) Cortisol (82533 x 4) Thyroid stimulating hormone (TSH) (84443 x 4)

80420 Dexamethasone suppression panel, 48 hour Ⓐ 🗎

MED: 100-2,15,80; 100-4,3,10.4
AMA: 1994,Summer,1
This panel must include the following: Free cortisol, urine (82530 x 2) Cortisol (82533 x 2) Volume measurement for timed collection (81050 x 2) (For single dose dexamethasone, use 82533)

If a single dose of dexamethasone is given, consult CPT code 82533.

80422 Glucagon tolerance panel; for insulinoma Ⓐ 🗎

MED: 100-2,15,80; 100-4,3,10.4
AMA: 1994,Summer,1
This panel must include the following: Glucose (82947 x 3) Insulin (83525 x 3)

80424 for pheochromocytoma Ⓐ 🗎

MED: 100-2,15,80; 100-4,3,10.4
AMA: 1994,Summer,1
This panel must include the following: Catecholamines, fractionated (82384 x 2)

80426 Gonadotropin releasing hormone stimulation panel Ⓐ 🗎

MED: 100-2,15,80; 100-4,3,10.4
AMA: 1994,Summer,1
This panel must include the following: Follicle stimulating hormone (FSH) (83001 x 4) Luteinizing hormone (LH) (83002 x 4)

80428 Growth hormone stimulation panel (eg, arginine infusion, l-dopa administration) Ⓐ 🗎

MED: 100-2,15,80; 100-4,3,10.4
AMA: 1994,Summer,1
This panel must include the following: Human growth hormone (HGH) (83003 x 4)

80430 Growth hormone suppression panel (glucose administration) Ⓐ 🗎

MED: 100-2,15,80; 100-4,3,10.4
AMA: 1994,Summer,1
This panel must include the following: Glucose (82947 x 3) Human growth hormone (HGH) (83003 x 4)

80432 Insulin-induced C-peptide suppression panel Ⓐ 🗎

MED: 100-2,15,80; 100-4,3,10.4
AMA: 1994,Summer,1
This panel must include the following: Insulin (83525) C-peptide (84681 x 5) Glucose (82947 x 5)

80434 Insulin tolerance panel; for ACTH insufficiency Ⓐ 🗎

MED: 100-2,15,80; 100-4,3,10.4
AMA: 1994,Summer,1
This panel must include the following: Cortisol (82533 x 5) Glucose (82947 x 5)

80435 for growth hormone deficiency Ⓐ 🗎

MED: 100-2,15,80; 100-4,3,10.4
AMA: 1994,Summer,1
This panel must include the following: Glucose (82947 x 5) Human growth hormone (HGH) (83003 x 5)

80436 Metyrapone panel Ⓐ 🗎

MED: 100-2,15,80; 100-4,3,10.4
AMA: 1994,Summer,1
This panel must include the following: Cortisol (82533 x 2) 11 deoxycortisol (82634 x 2)

80438 Thyrotropin releasing hormone (TRH) stimulation panel; one hour Ⓐ 🗎

MED: 100-2,15,80; 100-4,3,10.4
AMA: 1994,Summer,1
This panel must include the following: Thyroid stimulating hormone (TSH) (84443 x 3)

80439 two hour Ⓐ 🗎

MED: 100-2,15,80; 100-4,3,10.4
AMA: 1994,Summer,1
This panel must include the following: Thyroid stimulating hormone (TSH) (84443 x 4)

80440 for hyperprolactinemia Ⓐ 🗎

MED: 100-2,15,80; 100-4,3,10.4
AMA: 1994,Summer,1
This panel must include the following: Prolactin (84146 x 3)

Pathology and Laboratory

CONSULTATIONS (CLINICAL PATHOLOGY)

80500 Clinical pathology consultation; limited, without review of patient's history and medical records ⊠ 80 ↻

MED: 100-2,15,80; 100-4,3,10.4; 100-4,4,20.5; 100-4,12,60

AMA: 2002,Nov,9; 1997,Apr,9

80502 comprehensive, for a complex diagnostic problem, with review of patient's history and medical records ⊠ 80 ↻

MED: 100-2,15,80; 100-4,3,10.4; 100-4,4,20.5; 100-4,12,60

AMA: 2002,Nov,9; 1997,Apr,9

Note that 80502 may also be used for pharmacokinetic consultations. If a patient must be examined and evaluated, consult CPT codes 99241-99275.

URINALYSIS

To report urinalysis, infectious agent detection, semi-quantitative analysis of volatile compounds, consult Category III code 0041T.

81000 Urinalysis, by dip stick or tablet reagent for bilirubin, glucose, hemoglobin, ketones, leukocytes, nitrite, pH, protein, specific gravity, urobilinogen, any number of these constituents; non-automated, with microscopy A ↻

MED: 100-2,6,10; 100-2,15,80; 100-4,3,10.4

AMA: 1993,Fall,25; 1990-1991,Winter,10

81001 automated, with microscopy A ↻

MED: 100-2,15,80; 100-4,3,10.4

81002 non-automated, without microscopy A ↻

MED: 100-2,15,80; 100-4,3,10.4

AMA: 1998,Mar,3

Mosenthal test

81003 automated, without microscopy A ↻ ⊠

MED: 100-2,15,80; 100-4,3,10.4

81005 Urinalysis; qualitative or semiquantitative, except immunoassays A ↻

MED: 100-2,6,10; 100-2,15,80; 100-4,3,10.4

AMA: 1993,Fall,25; 1990-1991,Winter,10

If urinalysis is performed of a non-immunoassay reagent strip, consult CPT codes 81000 and 81002. For qualitative or semiquantitative immunoassay, consult CPT code 83518.

To report microalbumin, consult CPT codes 82043, 82044.

Benedict test for dextrose

81007 bacteriuria screen, except by culture or dipstick A ↻ ⊠

MED: 100-2,15,80; 100-4,3,10.4

To report dipstick urinalysis consult CPT codes 81000 or 81002. To report urine culture, consult CPT codes 87086-87088.

81015 microscopic only A

MED: 100-2,15,80; 100-4,3,10.4

81020 two or three glass test A ↻

MED: 100-2,15,80; 100-4,3,10.4

AMA: 1990-1991,Winter,10

Valentine's test

81025 Urine pregnancy test, by visual color comparison methods ♀ A

MED: 100-2,15,80; 100-4,3,10.4

AMA: 1998,Mar,3

81050 Volume measurement for timed collection, each A

MED: 100-2,15,80; 100-4,3,10.4

81099 Unlisted urinalysis procedure ⊠

MED: 100-2,15,80; 100-4,3,10.4

CHEMISTRY

Report codes 83890-83914 for use with molecular diagnostic techniques for analysis of nucleic acids.

Report codes 83890-83914 by procedure rather than analyte.

Report each procedure used in an analysis separately. For example, a procedure requiring isolation of DNA, restriction endonuclease digestion, electrophoresis, and nucleic acid probe amplification would be reported with codes 83890, 83892, 83894, and 83898.

Report the appropriate modifier when diagnostic procedures are performed to test for oncology, hematology, neurology, or inherited disorders.

82000 Acetaldehyde, blood A

MED: 100-2,15,80; 100-4,3,10.4

AMA: 2000,Mar,1

82003 Acetaminophen A

MED: 100-2,15,80; 100-4,3,10.4

82009 Acetone or other ketone bodies, serum; qualitative A

MED: 100-2,15,80; 100-4,3,10.4

82010 quantitative A ⊠

MED: 100-2,15,80; 100-4,3,10.4

82013 Acetylcholinesterase A

MED: 100-2,15,80; 100-4,3,10.4

To report gastric acid, free and/or total, consult CPT codes 82926 and 82928. To report acid phosphatase, consult CPT codes 84060-84066.

82016 Acylcarnitines; qualitative, each specimen A

MED: 100-2,15,80; 100-4,3,10.4

AMA: 1998,Nov,23

Report quantitative carnitine (total and free) separately, consult CPT code 82379.

82017 quantitative, each specimen A ↻

MED: 100-2,15,80; 100-4,3,10.4

AMA: 1998,Nov,23

82024 Adrenocorticotropic hormone (ACTH) A ↻

MED: 100-2,15,80; 100-3,300.1; 100-4,3,10.4

82030 Adenosine, 5-monophosphate, cyclic (cyclic AMP) A

MED: 100-2,15,80; 100-4,3,10.4

82040 Albumin; serum A

MED: 100-2,15,80; 100-3,190.10; 100-4,3,10.4

AMA: 1999,Dec,2

82042 urine or other source, quantitative, each specimen A

MED: 100-2,15,80; 100-4,3,10.4

82043 urine, microalbumin, quantitative A ↻

MED: 100-2,15,80; 100-3,190.10; 100-4,3,10.4

AMA: 1994,Summer,2

82044 urine, microalbumin, semiquantitative (eg, reagent strip assay) A ⊠

MED: 100-2,15,80; 100-3,190.10; 100-4,3,10.4

AMA: 2002,Sep,10; 1998,Mar,3; 1994,Summer,2

To report prealbumin, consult CPT code 84134.

82045 ischemia modified A

MED: 100-4,3,10.4

---

26 Professional Component Only   80/ 80 Assist-at-Surgery Allowed/With Documentation   Unlisted   Not Covered

TC Technical Component Only   **MED:** Pub 100/NCD References   **AMA:** CPT Assistant References   1 - 9 ASC Group   ♂ Male Only   ♀ Female Only

82055   Alcohol (ethanol); any specimen except breath   Ⓐ 🅧

MED: 100-2,15,80; 100-4,3,10.4

To report other volatiles including isopropyl alcohol and methanol, consult CPT code 84600.

82075   breath   Ⓐ

MED: 100-2,15,80; 100-4,3,10.4

82085   Aldolase   Ⓐ

82088   Aldosterone   Ⓐ 🔁

MED: 100-2,15,80; 100-4,3,10.4

To report alkaline phosphatase, consult CPT codes 84075 and 84080.

82101   Alkaloids, urine, quantitative   Ⓐ

MED: 100-2,15,80; 100-4,3,10.4

To report quantitative or qualitative acetone or other ketone bodies, serum, consult CPT codes 82009 and 82010. To report alpha tocopherol (Vitamin E), consult CPT code 84446.

82103   Alpha-1-antitrypsin; total   Ⓐ

MED: 100-2,15,80; 100-4,3,10.4

82104   phenotype   Ⓐ

MED: 100-2,15,80; 100-4,3,10.4

▲ 82105   Alpha-fetoprotein (AFP); serum   Ⓐ 🔁

MED: 100-2,15,80; 100-3,190.25; 100-4,3,10.4

▲ 82106   amniotic fluid   Ⓜ ♀ Ⓐ 🔁

MED: 100-2,15,80; 100-4,3,10.4

● 82107   AFP-L3 fraction isoform and total AFP (including ratio)   Ⓐ

82108   Aluminum   Ⓐ

MED: 100-2,15,80; 100-3,190.10; 100-4,3,10.4

82120   Amines, vaginal fluid, qualitative   ♀ Ⓐ 🅧

MED: 100-2,15,80; 100-4,3,10.4

AMA: 1999,Nov,45

If a combined pH and amines test is performed for vaginitis, use 83986 in addition to 82120.

82127   Amino acids; single, qualitative, each specimen   Ⓐ

MED: 100-2,15,80; 100-4,3,10.4

AMA: 1998,Nov,24

82128   multiple, qualitative, each specimen   Ⓐ 🔁

MED: 100-2,15,80; 100-4,3,10.4

AMA: 1998,Nov,24

82131   single, quantitative, each specimen   Ⓐ 🔁

MED: 100-2,15,80; 100-4,3,10.4

AMA: 1998,Nov,24; 1998,May,11

Van Slyke method

82135   Aminolevulinic acid, delta (ALA)   Ⓐ

MED: 100-2,15,80; 100-4,3,10.4

82136   Amino acids, 2 to 5 amino acids, quantitative, each specimen   Ⓐ 🔁

MED: 100-2,15,80; 100-4,3,10.4

AMA: 1998,Nov,24

82139   Amino acids, 6 or more amino acids, quantitative, each specimen   Ⓐ 🔁

MED: 100-2,15,80; 100-4,3,10.4

AMA: 1998,Nov,24

82140   Ammonia   Ⓐ

MED: 100-2,15,80; 100-4,3,10.4

82143   Amniotic fluid scan (spectrophotometric)   Ⓜ ♀ Ⓐ

MED: 100-2,15,80; 100-4,3,10.4

To report amniotic fluid L/S ratio, consult CPT code 83611. To report amobarbital, consult CPT codes 80100-80103 to report qualitative analysis and 82205 to report quantitative analysis.

82145   Amphetamine or methamphetamine   Ⓐ

MED: 100-2,15,80; 100-4,3,10.4

Prior to obtaining a quantitative analysis for amphetamine/methamphetamine, a qualitative drug screen (80100-80101) and drug confirmation test (80102) are normally performed.

82150   Amylase   Ⓐ

MED: 100-2,15,80; 100-4,3,10.4

82154   Androstanediol glucuronide   Ⓐ

MED: 100-2,15,80; 100-4,3,10.4

AMA: 1994,Summer,5

82157   Androstenedione   Ⓐ

MED: 100-2,15,80; 100-4,3,10.4

82160   Androsterone   Ⓐ

MED: 100-2,15,80; 100-4,3,10.4

82163   Angiotensin II   Ⓐ

MED: 100-2,15,80; 100-4,3,10.4

82164   Angiotensin I - converting enzyme (ACE)   Ⓐ

MED: 100-2,15,80; 100-4,3,10.4

To report vasopressin (antidiuretic hormone, ADH), consult CPT code 84588. To report heavy metal screening (arsenic, barium, beryllium, bismuth, antimony, mercury), consult CPT code 83015. To report alpha-1-antitrypsin, consult CPT codes 82103 and 82104.

82172   Apolipoprotein, each   Ⓐ

MED: 100-2,15,80; 100-4,3,10.4

82175   Arsenic   Ⓐ

MED: 100-2,15,80; 100-4,3,10.4

To report heavy metal screening (arsenic, barium, beryllium, bismuth, antimony, mercury), consult CPT code 83015.

82180   Ascorbic acid (Vitamin C), blood   Ⓐ 🔁

MED: 100-2,15,80; 100-4,3,10.4

To report salicylate, consult CPT code 80196.

To report atherogenic index, blood, ultracentrifugation, quantitative, consult CPT code 83716.

82190   Atomic absorption spectroscopy, each analyte   Ⓐ

MED: 100-2,15,80; 100-4,3,10.4

82205   Barbiturates, not elsewhere specified   Ⓐ

MED: 100-2,15,80; 100-4,3,10.4

Prior to obtaining a quantitative analysis for amphetamine/methamphetamine, a qualitative drug screen (80100-80101) and drug confirmation test (80102) are normally performed.

To report B-Natriuretic peptide, consult CPT code 83880.

82232   Beta-2 microglobulin   Ⓐ

MED: 100-2,15,80; 100-4,3,10.4

To report carbon dioxide (bicarbonate), consult CPT code 82374.

82239   Bile acids; total   Ⓐ

MED: 100-4,3,10.4

⊗ Modifier 63 Exempt Code   ⊙ Conscious Sedation   + CPT Add-on Code   ⊘ Modifier 51 Exempt Code   ● New Code   ▲ Revised Code

Ⓜ Maternity Edit   Ⓐ Age Edit   🅧 CLIA Waived Test   Ⓐ-Ⓨ APC Status Indicators   🔁 CCI Comprehensive Code   🔟 Bilateral Procedure

82240   **cholylglycine**   Ⓐ

MED: 100-2,15,80; 100-4,3,10.4

To report urine bile pigments, consult CPT codes 81000-81005.

82247   **Bilirubin; total**   Ⓐ

MED: 100-2,15,80; 100-4,3,10.4

AMA: 2000,Jan,7; 1999,Dec,1; 1999,Apr,6; 1998,Nov,24

Van Den Bergh test

82248   **direct**   Ⓐ

MED: 100-2,15,80; 100-4,3,10.4

AMA: 1999,Dec,1; 1999,Apr,6; 1998,Nov,24

82252   **feces, qualitative**   Ⓐ

MED: 100-2,15,80; 100-4,3,10.4

82261   **Biotinidase, each specimen**   Ⓐ

MED: 100-2,15,80; 100-4,3,10.4

AMA: 1998,Nov,24

82270   **Blood, occult, by peroxidase activity (eg, guaiac), qualitative; feces, consecutive collected specimens with single determination, for colorectal neoplasm screening (ie, patient was provided three cards or single triple card for consecutive collection)**   Ⓐ

MED: 100-2,15,80; 100-3,190.34; 100-4,3,10.4; 100-4,18,60.1; 100-4,18,60.2; 100-4,18,60.2.1; 100-4,18,60.6

Day test

82271   **other sources**   Ⓐ

MED: 100-4,3,10.4

82272   **Blood, occult, by peroxidase activity (eg, guaiac), qualitative, feces, single specimen (eg, from digital rectal exam)**   Ⓐ

MED: 100-4,3,10.4

82274   **Blood, occult, by fecal hemoglobin determination by immunoassay, qualitative, feces, 1-3 simultaneous determinations**   Ⓐ ◨ ☒

MED: 100-2,15,80; 100-4,3,10.4

82286   **Bradykinin**   Ⓐ

MED: 100-2,15,80; 100-4,3,10.4

82300   **Cadmium**   Ⓐ

MED: 100-2,15,80; 100-4,3,10.4

82306   **Calcifediol (25-OH Vitamin D-3)**   Ⓐ ◨

MED: 100-2,15,80; 100-4,3,10.4

82307   **Calciferol (Vitamin D)**   Ⓐ ◨

MED: 100-2,15,80; 100-4,3,10.4

To report 1, 25-Dihydroxyvitamin D, consult CPT code 82652.

82308   **Calcitonin**   Ⓐ ◨

MED: 100-2,15,80; 100-4,3,10.4

82310   **Calcium; total**   Ⓐ ◨

MED: 100-2,15,80; 100-3,190.10; 100-4,3,10.4

AMA: 1999,Dec,1

82330   **ionized**   Ⓐ

MED: 100-2,15,80; 100-4,3,10.4

82331   **after calcium infusion test**   Ⓐ ◨

MED: 100-2,15,80; 100-4,3,10.4

82340   **urine quantitative, timed specimen**   Ⓐ

MED: 100-2,15,80; 100-4,3,10.4

82355   **Calculus; qualitative analysis**   Ⓐ ◨

MED: 100-2,15,80; 100-4,3,10.4

82360   **quantitative analysis, chemical**   Ⓐ ◨

MED: 100-2,15,80; 100-4,3,10.4

82365   **infrared spectroscopy**   Ⓐ ◨

MED: 100-2,15,80; 100-4,3,10.4

82370   **x-ray diffraction**   Ⓐ ◨

MED: 100-2,15,80; 100-4,3,10.4

To report carbamates, see individual listings.

82373   **Carbohydrate deficient transferrin**   Ⓐ

MED: 100-2,15,80; 100-4,3,10.4

82374   **Carbon dioxide (bicarbonate)**   Ⓐ

MED: 100-2,15,80; 100-3,190.10; 100-4,3,10.4

AMA: 1999,Dec,1

Consult also CPT code 82803.

82375   **Carbon monoxide, (carboxyhemoglobin); quantitative**   Ⓐ

MED: 100-2,15,80; 100-4,3,10.4

82376   **qualitative**   Ⓐ

MED: 100-2,15,80; 100-4,3,10.4

To report end-tidal carbon monoxide, consult CPT Category III code 0043T.

82378   **Carcinoembryonic antigen (CEA)**   Ⓐ

MED: 100-2,15,80; 100-3,190.26; 100-4,3,10.4

AMA: 1996,Aug,11; 1993,Fall,25

82379   **Carnitine (total and free), quantitative, each specimen**   Ⓐ

MED: 100-2,15,80; 100-4,3,10.4

AMA: 1998,Nov,24

To report acylcarnitine, qualitative, consult CPT code 82016; quantitative, consult CPT code 82017.

82380   **Carotene**   Ⓐ

MED: 100-2,15,80; 100-4,3,10.4

82382   **Catecholamines; total urine**   Ⓐ

MED: 100-2,15,80; 100-4,3,10.4

82383   **blood**   Ⓐ

MED: 100-2,15,80; 100-4,3,10.4

82384   **fractionated**   Ⓐ ◨

MED: 100-2,15,80; 100-4,3,10.4

To report metanephrine, consult CPT code 83835. To report vanillylmandelic acid (VMA), consult CPT code 84585.

82387   **Cathepsin-D**   Ⓐ

MED: 100-2,15,80; 100-4,3,10.4

82390   **Ceruloplasmin**   Ⓐ

MED: 100-2,15,80; 100-4,3,10.4

82397   **Chemiluminescent assay**   Ⓐ

MED: 100-2,15,80; 100-4,3,10.4

AMA: 1993,Fall,25

82415   **Chloramphenicol**   Ⓐ

MED: 100-2,15,80; 100-4,3,10.4

82435   **Chloride; blood**   Ⓐ

MED: 100-2,15,80; 100-3,190.10; 100-4,3,10.4

AMA: 1999,Dec,1

82436   **urine**   Ⓐ

MED: 100-2,15,80; 100-4,3,10.4

82438   **other source**   Ⓐ

MED: 100-2,15,80; 100-4,3,10.4

To report sweat collection by iontophoresis, consult CPT code 89230.

82441	Chlorinated hydrocarbons, screen	Ⓐ

MED: 100-2,15,80; 100-4,3,10.4

To report phenothiazine, consult CPT code 84022. To report calciferol (Vitamin D), consult CPT code 82307.

82465	Cholesterol, serum or whole blood, total	Ⓐ ▣ Ⓧ

MED: 100-2,15,80; 100-3,190.23; 100-4,3,10.4

AMA: 2000,Mar,11; 1999,Dec,1

To report high density lipoprotein (HDL) cholesterol, consult CPT code 83718.

82480	Cholinesterase; serum	Ⓐ

MED: 100-2,15,80; 100-4,3,10.4

82482	RBC	Ⓐ

MED: 100-2,15,80; 100-4,3,10.4

82485	Chondroitin B sulfate, quantitative	Ⓐ

MED: 100-2,15,80; 100-4,3,10.4

To report quantitative or qualitative chorionic gonadotropin (hCG), consult CPT codes 84702 and 84703.

82486	Chromatography, qualitative; column (eg, gas liquid or HPLC), analyte not elsewhere specified	Ⓐ

MED: 100-2,15,80; 100-4,3,10.4

AMA: 1998,Nov,24-25

82487	paper, 1-dimensional, analyte not elsewhere specified	Ⓐ

MED: 100-2,15,80; 100-4,3,10.4

82488	paper, 2-dimensional, analyte not elsewhere specified	Ⓐ

MED: 100-2,15,80; 100-4,3,10.4

82489	thin layer, analyte not elsewhere specified	Ⓐ

MED: 100-2,15,80; 100-4,3,10.4

82491	Chromatography, quantitative, column (eg, gas liquid or HPLC); single analyte not elsewhere specified, single stationary and mobile phase	Ⓐ

MED: 100-2,15,80; 100-4,3,10.4

AMA: 2000,Mar,1; 1998,Nov,24-25; 1993,Fall,25

82492	multiple analytes, single stationary and mobile phase	Ⓐ ▣

MED: 100-2,15,80; 100-4,3,10.4

AMA: 2000,Mar,1; 1998,Nov,24-25

82495	Chromium	Ⓐ

MED: 100-2,15,80; 100-3,300.1; 100-4,3,10.4

82507	Citrate	Ⓐ

MED: 100-2,15,80; 100-4,3,10.4

82520	Cocaine or metabolite	Ⓐ

MED: 100-2,15,80; 100-4,3,10.4

Prior to quantification, a drug screen is normally performed and is reported separately. For drug screen, consult CPT codes 80100-80103. For quantitative urine alkaloids, consult CPT code 82101. For complement, consult CPT codes 86160-86162.

82523	Collagen cross links, any method	Ⓐ Ⓧ

MED: 100-2,15,80; 100-3,190.19; 100-4,3,10.4

82525	Copper	Ⓐ

MED: 100-2,15,80; 100-4,3,10.4

To report urine porphyrins, consult CPT codes 84119 and 84120. To report hydroxycorticosteroids, 17-(17-OHCS), consult CPT code 83491.

82528	Corticosterone	Ⓐ

MED: 100-2,15,80; 100-4,3,10.4

Porter-Silber test

82530	Cortisol; free	Ⓐ ▣

MED: 100-2,15,80; 100-4,3,10.4

AMA: 1994,Summer,3

82533	total	Ⓐ ▣

MED: 100-2,15,80; 100-4,3,10.4

AMA: 1994,Summer,3

To report C-peptide, consult CPT code 84681.

82540	Creatine	Ⓐ

MED: 100-2,15,80; 100-4,3,10.4

82541	Column chromatography/mass spectrometry (eg, GC/MS, or HPLC/MS), analyte not elsewhere specified; qualitative, single stationary and mobile phase	Ⓐ

MED: 100-2,15,80; 100-4,3,10.4

AMA: 1998,Nov,24-25

82542	quantitative, single stationary and mobile phase	Ⓐ

MED: 100-2,15,80; 100-4,3,10.4

AMA: 1998,Nov,24-25

82543	stable isotope dilution, single analyte, quantitative, single stationary and mobile phase	Ⓐ

MED: 100-2,15,80; 100-4,3,10.4

AMA: 1998,Nov,24-25

82544	stable isotope dilution, multiple analytes, quantitative, single stationary and mobile phase	Ⓐ ▣

MED: 100-2,15,80; 100-4,3,10.4

AMA: 1999,Dec,7; 1998,Nov,24-25

82550	Creatine kinase (CK), (CPK); total	Ⓐ ▣

MED: 100-2,15,80; 100-4,3,10.4

AMA: 1999,Dec,1; 1998,Feb,1

82552	isoenzymes	Ⓐ ▣

MED: 100-2,15,80; 100-4,3,10.4

AMA: 1998,Feb,1

82553	MB fraction only	Ⓐ ▣

MED: 100-2,15,80; 100-4,3,10.4

AMA: 1998,Feb,1

82554	isoforms	Ⓐ ▣

MED: 100-2,15,80; 100-4,3,10.4

AMA: 1998,Feb,1

82565	Creatinine; blood	Ⓐ

MED: 100-2,15,80; 100-3,190.10; 100-4,3,10.4

AMA: 1999,Dec,1

82570	other source	Ⓐ Ⓧ

MED: 100-2,15,80; 100-4,3,10.4

82575	clearance	Ⓐ ▣

MED: 100-2,15,80; 100-4,3,10.4

Holten test

82585	Cryofibrinogen	Ⓐ

MED: 100-2,15,80; 100-4,3,10.4

82595	Cryoglobulin, qualitative or semi-quantitative (eg, cryocrit)	Ⓐ

MED: 100-2,15,80; 100-4,3,10.4

If quantitative cryoglobulin is performed consult CPT codes 82784, 82785.

If crystal is identified by light microscopy with or without polarizing lens analysis, any body fluid except urine, consult CPT code 89060.

82600	Cyanide	Ⓐ

MED: 100-2,15,80; 100-4,3,10.4

82607	Cyanocobalamin (Vitamin B-12);	Ⓐ ▣

MED: 100-2,15,80; 100-4,3,10.4

---

⑬ Modifier 63 Exempt Code   ⊙ Conscious Sedation   + CPT Add-on Code   ⊘ Modifier 51 Exempt Code   ● New Code   ▲ Revised Code

Ⓜ Maternity Edit   Ⓐ Age Edit   Ⓧ CLIA Waived Test   Ⓐ-Ⓨ APC Status Indicators   ▣ CCI Comprehensive Code   ㊿ Bilateral Procedure

 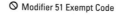

82608   **unsaturated binding capacity**   Ⓐ

MED: 100-2,15,80; 100-4,3,10.4
To report adenosine, 5-monophosphate, cyclic (cyclic AMP), consult CPT code 82030. To report guanosine monophosphate (GMP), cyclic, consult CPT code 83008. To report cyclosporine, consult CPT code 80158.

82615   **Cystine and homocystine, urine, qualitative**   Ⓐ

MED: 100-2,15,80; 100-4,3,10.4

82626   **Dehydroepiandrosterone (DHEA)**   Ⓐ

MED: 100-2,15,80; 100-4,3,10.4
AMA: 1994,Summer,4

82627   **Dehydroepiandrosterone-sulfate (DHEA-S)**   Ⓐ

MED: 100-2,15,80; 100-4,3,10.4
AMA: 1994,Summer,4
To report delta-aminolevulinic acid (ALA), consult CPT code 82135.

82633   **Desoxycorticosterone, 11-**   Ⓐ

MED: 100-2,15,80; 100-4,3,10.4

82634   **Deoxycortisol, 11-**   Ⓐ ↻

MED: 100-2,15,80; 100-4,3,10.4
To report a dexamethasone suppression test, consult CPT code 80420. For amylase, consult CPT code 82150.

82638   **Dibucaine number**   Ⓐ

MED: 100-2,15,80; 100-4,3,10.4
To report volatiles (e.g., acetic anhydride, carbon tetrachloride, dichloroethane, dichloromethane, diethylether, isopropyl alcohol, methanol), consult CPT code 84600.

82646   **Dihydrocodeinone**   Ⓐ

MED: 100-2,15,80; 100-4,3,10.4
A drug screen (qualitative analysis) is normally performed prior to quantitative analysis. For drug screen, consult CPT codes 80100-80103.

82649   **Dihydromorphinone**   Ⓐ

MED: 100-2,15,80; 100-4,3,10.4
A drug screen (qualitative analysis) is normally performed prior to quantitative analysis. For drug screen, consult CPT codes 80100-80103.

82651   **Dihydrotestosterone (DHT)**   Ⓐ

MED: 100-2,15,80; 100-4,3,10.4

▲ **82652**   **Dihydroxyvitamin D, 1,25-**   Ⓐ ↻

MED: 100-2,15,80; 100-4,3,10.4

82654   **Dimethadione**   Ⓐ

MED: 100-2,15,80; 100-4,3,10.4
A drug screen (qualitative analysis) is normally performed prior to quantitative analysis. For drug screen, consult CPT codes 80100-80103. For total phenytoin, consult CPT code 80185. For dipropylacetic acid, consult CPT code 80164. For catecholamines, consult CPT codes 82382-82384. For duodenal intubation and aspiration, consult CPT code 89100. For endocrine receptor assays, consult CPT codes 84233-84235.

82656   **Elastase, pancreatic (EL-1), fecal, qualitative or semi-quantitative**   Ⓐ

MED: 100-4,3,10.4

82657   **Enzyme activity in blood cells, cultured cells, or tissue, not elsewhere specified; nonradioactive substrate, each specimen**   Ⓐ

MED: 100-2,15,80; 100-4,3,10.4
AMA: 1998,Nov,25

82658   **radioactive substrate, each specimen**   Ⓐ

MED: 100-2,15,80; 100-4,3,10.4
AMA: 1998,Nov,25

82664   **Electrophoretic technique, not elsewhere specified**   Ⓐ

MED: 100-2,15,80; 100-4,3,10.4

82666   **Epiandrosterone**   Ⓐ

MED: 100-2,15,80; 100-4,3,10.4
To report catecholamines, consult CPT codes 82382-82384.

82668   **Erythropoietin**   Ⓐ

MED: 100-2,15,80; 100-4,3,10.4

82670   **Estradiol**   Ⓐ ↻

MED: 100-2,15,80; 100-4,3,10.4

82671   **Estrogens; fractionated**   Ⓐ

MED: 100-2,15,80; 100-4,3,10.4

82672   **total**   Ⓐ

MED: 100-2,15,80; 100-4,3,10.4
To report estrogen receptor assay, consult CPT code 84233.

82677   **Estriol**   Ⓐ

MED: 100-2,15,80; 100-4,3,10.4

82679   **Estrone**   Ⓐ ✖

MED: 100-2,15,80; 100-4,3,10.4
To report alcohol (ethanol), consult CPT codes 82055 and 82075.

82690   **Ethchlorvynol**   Ⓐ

MED: 100-2,15,80; 100-4,3,10.4
To report alcohol (ethanol), consult CPT codes 82055 and 82075.

82693   **Ethylene glycol**   Ⓐ

MED: 100-2,15,80; 100-4,3,10.4

82696   **Etiocholanolone**   Ⓐ

MED: 100-2,15,80; 100-4,3,10.4
To report fractionation of ketosteroids, consult CPT code 83593.

82705   **Fat or lipids, feces; qualitative**   Ⓐ

MED: 100-2,15,80; 100-4,3,10.4

82710   **quantitative**   Ⓐ

MED: 100-2,15,80; 100-4,3,10.4

82715   **Fat differential, feces, quantitative**   Ⓐ

MED: 100-2,15,80; 100-4,3,10.4

82725   **Fatty acids, nonesterified**   Ⓐ

MED: 100-2,15,80; 100-4,3,10.4

82726   **Very long chain fatty acids**   Ⓐ

MED: 100-2,15,80; 100-4,3,10.4
AMA: 1998,Nov,25

82728   **Ferritin**   Ⓐ

To report fetal hemoglobin, consult CPT codes 83030, 83033, and 85460. To report alpha-1 fetoprotein, consult CPT codes 82105 and 82106.

82731   **Fetal fibronectin, cervicovaginal secretions, semi-quantitative**   Ⓜ ♀

MED: 100-2,15,80; 100-4,3,10.4
AMA: 1998,Nov,25

82735   **Fluoride**   Ⓐ

MED: 100-2,15,80; 100-4,3,10.4

---

② Professional Component Only   ⑧⁰/⑧⁰ Assist-at-Surgery Allowed/With Documentation   Unlisted   Not Covered

ⓣⓒ Technical Component Only   MED: Pub 100/NCD References   AMA: CPT Assistant References   ❶-❾ ASC Group   ♂ Male Only   ♀ Female Only

298 — CPT Expert   CPT only © 2006 American Medical Association. All Rights Reserved. *(Black Ink)*   © 2006 Ingenix *(Blue Ink)*

82742	**Flurazepam**	A

MED: 100-2,15,80; 100-4,3,10.4

A drug screen (qualitative analysis) is normally performed prior to quantitative analysis. For drug screen, consult CPT codes 80100-80103. If a foam stability test is performed, consult CPT code 83662.

82746	**Folic acid; serum**	A

MED: 100-2,15,80; 100-4,3,10.4

82747	**RBC**	A

MED: 100-2,15,80; 100-4,3,10.4

To report gonadotropin; follicle stimulating hormone (FSH), consult CPT code 83001.

82757	**Fructose, semen**	♂ A

MED: 100-2,15,80; 100-4,3,10.4

To report fructosamine, consult CPT code 82985. To report sugars, chromatographic, TLC or paper chromatography, consult CPT code 84375.

82759	**Galactokinase, RBC**	A

MED: 100-2,15,80; 100-4,3,10.4

82760	**Galactose**	A

MED: 100-2,15,80; 100-4,3,10.4

82775	**Galactose-1-phosphate uridyl transferase; quantitative**	A

MED: 100-2,15,80; 100-4,3,10.4

82776	**screen**	A

MED: 100-2,15,80; 100-4,3,10.4

82784	**Gammaglobulin; IgA, IgD, IgG, IgM, each**	A

MED: 100-2,15,80; 100-4,3,10.4
AMA: 2000,Aug,11; 1994,Spring,31
Farr test

82785	**IgE**	A

MED: 100-2,15,80; 100-4,3,10.4
AMA: 1994,Spring,31

To report allergen specific IgE, consult CPT code 86003 and 86005.

Farr test

82787	**immunoglobulin subclasses, (IgG1, 2, 3, or 4), each**	A

MED: 100-2,15,80; 100-4,3,10.4

To report Gamma-glutamyltransferase (GGT), consult CPT code 82977.

82800	**Gases, blood, pH only**	A

MED: 100-2,15,80; 100-4,3,10.4

82803	**Gases, blood, any combination of pH, pCO2, pO2, CO2, HCO3 (including calculated O2 saturation);**	A

MED: 100-2,15,80; 100-4,3,10.4

Note that 82803 is to be used for two or more of the following analytes: Gases, blood, any combination of pH, Carbon Dioxide, Hydrochloric acid, including calculated oxygen saturation.

82805	**with O2 saturation, by direct measurement, except pulse oximetry**	A

MED: 100-2,15,80; 100-4,3,10.4

82810	**Gases, blood, O2 saturation only, by direct measurement, except pulse oximetry**	A

MED: 100-2,15,80; 100-4,3,10.4

To report pulse oximetry, consult CPT code 94760.

82820	**Hemoglobin-oxygen affinity (pO2 for 50% hemoglobin saturation with oxygen)**	A

MED: 100-2,15,80; 100-4,3,10.4

82926	**Gastric acid, free and total, each specimen**	A

MED: 100-2,15,80; 100-4,3,10.4

82928	**Gastric acid, free or total, each specimen**	A

MED: 100-2,15,80; 100-4,3,10.4

82938	**Gastrin after secretin stimulation**	A

MED: 100-2,15,80; 100-4,3,10.4

82941	**Gastrin**	A

MED: 100-2,15,80; 100-4,3,10.4

To report gentamicin, consult CPT code 80170. To report glutamyltransferase, gamma (GGT), consult CPT code 82977. To report gas liquid or HPLA chromatography, consult CPT code 82486.

82943	**Glucagon**	A

MED: 100-2,15,80; 100-4,3,10.4

82945	**Glucose, body fluid, other than blood**	A

MED: 100-2,15,80; 100-4,3,10.4

82946	**Glucagon tolerance test**	A

MED: 100-2,15,80; 100-4,3,10.4

82947	**Glucose; quantitative, blood (except reagent strip)**	A

MED: 100-3,160.17; 100-3,190.10; 100-3,190.20; 100-4,3,10.4
AMA: 2002,Jun,1; 1999,Sep,10; 1999,Dec,1; 1994,Summer,5; 1993,Summer,14

82948	**blood, reagent strip**	A

MED: 100-2,15,80; 100-3,160.17; 100-3,190.20; 100-4,3,10.4
AMA: 1999,Jan,10; 1994,Summer,5

82950	**post glucose dose (includes glucose)**	A

MED: 100-2,15,80; 100-3,160.17; 100-4,3,10.4
AMA: 2002,Jun,1; 1999,Sep,10

82951	**tolerance test (GTT), three specimens (includes glucose)**	A

MED: 100-2,15,80; 100-4,3,10.4
AMA: 2001,Feb,10

82952	**tolerance test, each additional beyond three specimens**	A

MED: 100-2,15,80; 100-4,3,10.4
AMA: 2001,Feb,10

82953	**tolbutamide tolerance test**	A

MED: 100-2,15,80; 100-4,3,10.4

If an insulin tolerance test is performed, consult CPT codes 80434 and 80435. If a leucine tolerance test is performed, consult CPT code 80428. For semiquantitative urine glucose, consult CPT codes 81000, 81002, 81005, and 81099.

82955	**Glucose-6-phosphate dehydrogenase (G6PD); quantitative**	A

MED: 100-2,15,80; 100-4,3,10.4

82960	**screen**	A

MED: 100-2,15,80; 100-4,3,10.4

If a glucose tolerance test is performed with medication, consult CPT code 90774 in addition.

82962	**Glucose, blood by glucose monitoring device(s) cleared by the FDA specifically for home use**	A

MED: 100-2,15,80; 100-3,160.17; 100-3,190.20; 100-4,3,10.4
AMA: 1999,Jan,10; 1994,Summer,4

82963	**Glucosidase, beta**	A

MED: 100-2,15,80; 100-4,3,10.4

⊛ Modifier 63 Exempt Code	⊙ Conscious Sedation	+ CPT Add-on Code	⊘ Modifier 51 Exempt Code	● New Code	▲ Revised Code

M Maternity Edit	A Age Edit	X CLIA Waived Test	A-Y APC Status Indicators	C CCI Comprehensive Code	50 Bilateral Procedure

 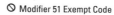

82965 Glutamate dehydrogenase [A]

MED: 100-2,15,80; 100-4,3,10.4

82975 Glutamine (glutamic acid amide) [A]

MED: 100-2,15,80; 100-4,3,10.4

82977 Glutamyltransferase, gamma (GGT) [A]

MED: 100-2,15,80; 100-3,190.32; 100-4,3,10.4
AMA: 1999,Dec,1

82978 Glutathione [A]

MED: 100-2,15,80; 100-4,3,10.4

82979 Glutathione reductase, RBC [A]

MED: 100-2,15,80; 100-4,3,10.4

82980 Glutethimide [A]

MED: 100-2,15,80; 100-4,3,10.4
To report glycohemoglobin, consult CPT code 83036.

82985 Glycated protein [A] [⟳] [✗]

MED: 100-2,15,80; 100-3,190.21; 100-4,3,10.4
AMA: 1994,Summer,2
To report chorionic gonadotropin, consult CPT codes 84702 and 84703.

83001 Gonadotropin; follicle stimulating hormone (FSH) [A] [⟳] [✗]

MED: 100-2,15,80; 100-4,3,10.4

83002 luteinizing hormone (LH) [A] [⟳] [✗]

MED: 100-2,15,80; 100-4,3,10.4
To report luteinizing releasing factor (LRH), consult CPT code 83727.

83003 Growth hormone, human (HGH) (somatotropin) [A] [⟳]

MED: 100-2,15,80; 100-4,3,10.4
To report antibody to human growth hormone, consult CPT code 86277.

83008 Guanosine monophosphate (GMP), cyclic [A]

MED: 100-2,15,80; 100-4,3,10.4

83009 Helicobacter pylori, blood test analysis for urease activity, non-radioactive isotope (eg, C-13) [A]

MED: 100-4,3,10.4
To report H. pylori breath test analysis for urease activity, consult 83013, 83014.

83010 Haptoglobin; quantitative [A]

MED: 100-2,15,80; 100-4,3,10.4

83012 phenotypes [A]

MED: 100-2,15,80; 100-4,3,10.4

83013 Helicobacter pylori; breath test analysis for urease activity, non-radioactive isotope (eg, C-13) [A] [⟳]

MED: 100-2,15,80; 100-4,3,10.4
AMA: 1999,Nov,45; 1999,Feb,8; 1998,Nov,25
To report H. pylori, stool, consult CPT code 87338. To report H. pylori, liquid scintillation counter, consult CPT codes 78267, 78268. To report H. pylori, enzyme immunoassay, consult CPT code 87339.

83014 drug administration [A] [⟳]

MED: 100-2,15,80; 100-4,3,10.4
AMA: 1999,Nov,45; 1999,Feb,8; 1998,Nov,25
To report H. pylori, stool, consult CPT code 87338. To report H. pylori, liquid scintillation counter, consult CPT codes 78267, 78268. To report H. pylori, enzyme immunoassay, consult CPT code 87339.

To report H pylori, blood test analysis for urease activity, consult CPT code 83009.

83015 Heavy metal (eg, arsenic, barium, beryllium, bismuth, antimony, mercury); screen [A]

MED: 100-2,15,80; 100-4,3,10.4
Reinsch test

83018 quantitative, each [A]

MED: 100-2,15,80; 100-4,3,10.4

83020 Hemoglobin fractionation and quantitation; electrophoresis (eg, A2, S, C, and/or F) [A] [80] [⟳]

MED: 100-2,15,80; 100-4,3,10.4; 100-4,12,60
AMA: 1998,Nov,25

83021 chromatography (eg, A2, S, C, and/or F) [A] [⟳]

MED: 100-2,15,80; 100-4,3,10.4
AMA: 1999,Dec,7; 1998,Nov,25

83026 Hemoglobin; by copper sulfate method, non-automated [A] [✗]

MED: 100-2,15,80; 100-4,3,10.4

83030 F (fetal), chemical [A] [⟳]

MED: 100-2,15,80; 100-4,3,10.4

83033 F (fetal), qualitative [A] [⟳]

MED: 100-2,15,80; 100-4,3,10.4

83036 glycosylated (A1C) [A] [✗]

MED: 100-2,15,80; 100-3,190.21; 100-4,3,10.4
AMA: 1994,Summer,2
To report fecal hemoglobin detection by immunoassay, consult CPT code 82274.

83037 glycosylated (A1C) by device cleared by FDA for home use [A]

83045 methemoglobin, qualitative [A]

MED: 100-2,15,80; 100-4,3,10.4

83050 methemoglobin, quantitative [A]

MED: 100-2,15,80; 100-4,3,10.4

83051 plasma [A]

MED: 100-2,15,80; 100-4,3,10.4

83055 sulfhemoglobin, qualitative [A]

MED: 100-2,15,80; 100-4,3,10.4

83060 sulfhemoglobin, quantitative [A]

MED: 100-2,15,80; 100-4,3,10.4

83065 thermolabile [A]

MED: 100-2,15,80; 100-4,3,10.4

83068 unstable, screen [A] [⟳]

MED: 100-2,15,80; 100-4,3,10.4

83069 urine [A]

MED: 100-2,15,80; 100-4,3,10.4

83070 Hemosiderin; qualitative [A]

MED: 100-2,15,80; 100-4,3,10.4

83071 quantitative [A]

MED: 100-2,15,80; 100-4,3,10.4
A drug screen (qualitative analysis) is normally performed prior to quantitative analysis. For drug screen, consult CPT codes 80100-80103. For hydroxyindoleacetic acid, 5- (HIAA), consult CPT code 83497. For high performance liquid chromatography HPLC, consult CPT code 82486.

83080 b-Hexosaminidase, each assay [A]

MED: 100-2,15,80; 100-4,3,10.4
AMA: 1998,Nov,25

[26] Professional Component Only   [80]/[80] Assist-at-Surgery Allowed/With Documentation   Unlisted   Not Covered

[TC] Technical Component Only   MED: Pub 100/NCD References   AMA: CPT Assistant References   [1]-[9] ASC Group   ♂ Male Only   ♀ Female Only

300 — CPT Expert   CPT only © 2006 American Medical Association. All Rights Reserved. *(Black Ink)*   © 2006 Ingenix *(Blue Ink)*

83088 **Histamine**
MED: 100-2,15,80; 100-3,30.6; 100-4,3,10.4
If a Hollander test is performed, consult CPT code 91052.

83090 **Homocysteine**
MED: 100-2,15,80; 100-4,3,10.4
AMA: 2001,Jan,13

83150 **Homovanillic acid (HVA)**
MED: 100-2,15,80; 100-4,3,10.4
If a hydrogen breath test is performed, consult CPT code 91065.

83491 **Hydroxycorticosteroids, 17- (17-OHCS)**
MED: 100-2,15,80; 100-4,3,10.4
To report cortisol, consult CPT code 82530, 82533. To report deoxycortisol, 11- consult CPT code 82634.

83497 **Hydroxyindolacetic acid, 5-(HIAA)**
MED: 100-2,15,80; 100-4,3,10.4
If a urine qualitative test is performed, consult CPT code 81005. For 5-Hydroxytryptamine, consult CPT code 84260.

83498 **Hydroxyprogesterone, 17-d**
MED: 100-2,15,80; 100-4,3,10.4

83499 **Hydroxyprogesterone, 20-**
MED: 100-2,15,80; 100-4,3,10.4

83500 **Hydroxyproline; free**
MED: 100-2,15,80; 100-4,3,10.4

83505 **total**
MED: 100-2,15,80; 100-4,3,10.4

83516 **Immunoassay for analyte other than infectious agent antibody or infectious agent antigen, qualitative or semiquantitative; multiple step method**
MED: 100-2,15,80; 100-4,3,10.4
AMA: 1998,Nov,25

83518 **single step method (eg, reagent strip)**
MED: 100-2,15,80; 100-4,3,10.4
AMA: 1993,Fall,26

83519 **Immunoassay, analyte, quantitative; by radiopharmaceutical technique (eg, RIA)**
MED: 100-2,15,80; 100-4,3,10.4
AMA: 1994,Summer,2; 1993,Fall,26

83520 **not otherwise specified**
MED: 100-2,15,80; 100-4,3,10.4
AMA: 1993,Fall,26
To report qualitative or semi-quantitative immunoassay excluding infectious agent antibody or infectious agent antigen, multiple step method, consult CPT code 83516; single step method, consult CPT code 83518. For quantitative immunoassay by radiopharmaceutical immunoassay or radioimmunoassay (RIA), consult CPT code 83519. To report immunoassay for infectious agent antibody, qualitative or semi-quantitative, single step method (e.g., reagent strip), consult CPT code 86318. To report immunoassays for infectious agent antibody, qualitative or semi-quantitative multiple step method, consult CPT codes 86602-86804. To report infectious agent antigen detection by enzyme immunoassay, qualitative or semi-quantitative, consult CPT codes 87301-87899. For immunoassay for tumor antigen, consult CPT code 86316. To report immunoassay for infectious agent antibody not elsewhere specified, quantitative, consult CPT code 86317.

83525 **Insulin; total**
MED: 100-2,15,80; 100-4,3,10.4
To report proinsulin, consult CPT code 84206.

83527 **free**
MED: 100-2,15,80; 100-4,3,10.4
AMA: 1994,Summer,5

83528 **Intrinsic factor**
MED: 100-2,15,80; 100-4,3,10.4
To report intrinsic factor antibodies, consult CPT code 86340.

83540 **Iron**
AMA: 1993,Fall,25

83550 **Iron binding capacity**

83570 **Isocitric dehydrogenase (IDH)**
MED: 100-2,15,80; 100-4,3,10.4
To report isopropyl alcohol, consult CPT code 84600.

83582 **Ketogenic steroids, fractionation**
MED: 100-2,15,80; 100-4,3,10.4
To report ketone bodies for serum, consult CPT codes 82009 and 82010. To report ketone bodies for urine, consult CPT codes 81000-81003.

83586 **Ketosteroids, 17- (17-KS); total**
MED: 100-2,15,80; 100-4,3,10.4

83593 **fractionation**
MED: 100-2,15,80; 100-4,3,10.4

83605 **Lactate (lactic acid)**
MED: 100-2,15,80; 100-4,3,10.4

83615 **Lactate dehydrogenase (LD), (LDH);**
MED: 100-2,15,80; 100-3,190.10; 100-4,3,10.4
AMA: 1999,Dec,1; 1998,Feb,1; 1993,Fall,25

83625 **isoenzymes, separation and quantitation**
MED: 100-2,15,80; 100-3,190.10; 100-4,3,10.4
AMA: 1998,Feb,1; 1993,Fall,25

83630 **Lactoferrin, fecal; qualitative**
MED: 100-4,3,10.4

83631 **quantitative**
MED: 100-4,3,10.4

83632 **Lactogen, human placental (HPL) human chorionic somatomammotropin**
MED: 100-2,15,80; 100-4,3,10.4

83633 **Lactose, urine; qualitative**
MED: 100-2,15,80; 100-4,3,10.4

83634 **quantitative**
MED: 100-2,15,80; 100-4,3,10.4
To report tolerance, consult CPT codes 82951 and 82952. If a breath hydrogen test is performed to report lactase deficiency, consult CPT code 91065.

83655 **Lead**
MED: 100-2,15,80; 100-4,3,10.4

83661 **Fetal lung maturity assessment; lecithin sphingomyelin (L/S) ratio**
MED: 100-2,15,80; 100-4,3,10.4

83662 **foam stability test**
MED: 100-2,15,80; 100-4,3,10.4

83663 **fluorescence polarization**
MED: 100-2,15,80; 100-4,3,10.4

83664   **lamellar body density**

MED: 100-2,15,80; 100-4,3,10.4

To report phosphatidylglycerol, consult CPT code 84081.

83670   **Leucine aminopeptidase (LAP)**

MED: 100-2,15,80; 100-4,3,10.4

83690   **Lipase**

MED: 100-2,15,80; 100-4,3,10.4

83695   **Lipoprotein (a)**

MED: 100-4,3,10.4

● **83698**   **Lipoprotein-associated phospholipase A2, (Lp-PLA2)**

83700   **Lipoprotein, blood; electrophoretic separation and quantitation**

MED: 100-4,3,10.4

83701   **high resolution fractionation and quantitation of lipoproteins including lipoprotein subclasses when performed (eg, electrophoresis, ultracentrifugation)**

MED: 100-4,3,10.4

83704   **quantitation of lipoprotein particle numbers and lipoprotein particle subclasses (eg, by nuclear magnetic resonance spectroscopy)**

MED: 100-4,3,10.4

83718   **Lipoprotein, direct measurement; high density cholesterol (HDL cholesterol)**

MED: 100-2,15,80; 100-3,190.23; 100-4,3,10.4

AMA: 1999,Oct,11

83719   **VLDL cholesterol**

MED: 100-2,15,80; 100-4,3,10.4

AMA: 1999,Oct,11

83721   **LDL cholesterol**

MED: 100-2,15,80; 100-3,190.23; 100-4,3,10.4

AMA: 1999,Oct,11; 1998,Nov,25

To report fractionation by high resolution electrophoresis or ultracentrifugation, consult CPT code 83701.

To report lipoprotein paricle numbers and subclasses analysis by nuclear magnetic resonance spectroscopy, consult CPT code 83695.

For direct meaasurement, intermediate density lipoproteins (remnant lipoproteins), consult CPT Category III code 0026T.

83727   **Luteinizing releasing factor (LRH)**

MED: 100-2,15,80; 100-4,3,10.4

If qualitative analysis is performed, consult CPT codes 80100-80103. For macroglobulins, alpha-2, consult CPT code 86329.

83735   **Magnesium**

MED: 100-2,15,80; 100-4,3,10.4

83775   **Malate dehydrogenase**

MED: 100-2,15,80; 100-4,3,10.4

To report maltose tolerance, consult CPT codes 82951 and 82952. To report mammotropin, consult CPT code 84146.

83785   **Manganese**

MED: 100-2,15,80; 100-4,3,10.4

To report marijuana, consult CPT codes 80100-80103.

83788   **Mass spectrometry and tandem mass spectrometry (MS, MS/MS), analyte not elsewhere specified; qualitative, each specimen**

MED: 100-2,15,80; 100-4,3,10.4

AMA: 1998,Nov,26

83789   **quantitative, each specimen**

MED: 100-2,15,80; 100-4,3,10.4

AMA: 1998,Nov,26

83805   **Meprobamate**

MED: 100-2,15,80; 100-4,3,10.4

A drug screen (qualitative analysis) is normally performed prior to quantitative analysis. For drug screen, consult CPT codes 80100-80103.

83825   **Mercury, quantitative**

MED: 100-2,15,80; 100-4,3,10.4

To report mercury screen, consult CPT code 83015.

83835   **Metanephrines**

MED: 100-2,15,80; 100-4,3,10.4

To report catecholamines, consult CPT codes 82382-82384.

83840   **Methadone**

MED: 100-2,15,80; 100-4,3,10.4

A drug screen (qualitative analysis) is normally performed prior to quantitative analysis. For drug screen, consult CPT codes 80100-80103 and 82145. For methanol, consult CPT code 84600.

83857   **Methemalbumin**

MED: 100-2,15,80; 100-4,3,10.4

To report methemoglobin, see hemoglobin CPT codes 83045 and 83050.

83858   **Methsuximide**

MED: 100-2,15,80; 100-4,3,10.4

To report methyl alcohol, consult CPT code 84600. To report microalbumin, quantitative, consult CPT code 82043; semiquantitative, consult CPT code 82044. To report microglobulin, beta-2, consult CPT code 82232.

83864   **Mucopolysaccharides, acid; quantitative**

MED: 100-2,15,80; 100-4,3,10.4

83866   **screen**

MED: 100-2,15,80; 100-4,3,10.4

83872   **Mucin, synovial fluid (Ropes test)**

MED: 100-2,15,80; 100-4,3,10.4

83873   **Myelin basic protein, cerebrospinal fluid**

MED: 100-2,15,80; 100-4,3,10.4

To report oligoclonal bands, consult CPT code 83916.

83874   **Myoglobin**

MED: 100-2,15,80; 100-4,3,10.4

AMA: 1998,Feb,1

To report Nalorphine, consult CPT code 83925.

83880   **Natriuretic peptide**

MED: 100-4,3,10.4

83883   **Nephelometry, each analyte not elsewhere specified**

MED: 100-2,15,80; 100-4,3,10.4

83885   **Nickel**

MED: 100-2,15,80; 100-4,3,10.4

83887   **Nicotine**

MED: 100-2,15,80; 100-4,3,10.4

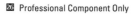 Professional Component Only   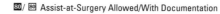 Assist-at-Surgery Allowed/With Documentation   Unlisted   Not Covered

Technical Component Only   **MED:** Pub 100/NCD References   **AMA:** CPT Assistant References   **1-9** ASC Group   ♂ Male Only   ♀ Female Only

302 — CPT Expert   CPT only © 2006 American Medical Association. All Rights Reserved. *(Black Ink)*   © *2006 Ingenix (Blue Ink)*

83890 Molecular diagnostics; molecular isolation or extraction 🅐 🄲
MED: 100-2,15,80; 100-4,3,10.4
AMA: 1998,Nov,26; 1993,Fall,26
To report microbial identification, consult CPT codes 87797 and 87798.

Code 83890-83912 separately for each procedure used in analysis rather than by analyte.

83891 isolation or extraction of highly purified nucleic acid 🅐 🄲
MED: 100-2,15,80; 100-4,3,10.4
AMA: 1998,Nov,26

83892 enzymatic digestion 🅐 🄲
MED: 100-2,15,80; 100-4,3,10.4
AMA: 1993,Fall,26

83893 dot/slot blot production 🅐 🄲
MED: 100-2,15,80; 100-4,3,10.4
AMA: 1998,Nov,26

83894 separation by gel electrophoresis (eg, agarose, polyacrylamide) 🅐 🄲
MED: 100-2,15,80; 100-4,3,10.4
AMA: 1998,Nov,26; 1993,Fall,25

83896 nucleic acid probe, each 🅐 🄲
MED: 100-2,15,80; 100-4,3,10.4
AMA: 2002,Aug,10; 1993,Fall,26

83897 nucleic acid transfer (eg, Southern, Northern) 🅐 🄲
MED: 100-2,15,80; 100-4,3,10.4
AMA: 1998,Nov,26

83898 amplification of patient nucleic acid, each nucleic acid sequence 🅐 🄲
MED: 100-2,15,80; 100-4,3,10.4
AMA: 1998,Nov,26; 1993,Fall,26

83900 amplification of patient nucleic acid, multiplex, first two nucleic acid sequences 🅐
MED: 100-4,3,10.4

+ 83901 amplification of patient nucleic acid, multiplex, each additional nucleic acid sequence (List separately in addition to code for primary procedure) 🅐 🄲
MED: 100-2,15,80; 100-4,3,10.4
AMA: 1998,Nov,26
Note that 83901 is an add-on code and should be reported in conjunction with 83900.

83902 reverse transcription 🅐 🄲
MED: 100-2,15,80; 100-4,3,10.4

83903 mutation scanning, by physical properties (eg, single strand conformational polymorphisms (SSCP), heteroduplex, denaturing gradient gel electrophoresis (DGGE), RNA'ase A), single segment, each 🅐 🄲
MED: 100-2,15,80; 100-4,3,10.4
AMA: 1998,Nov,26

83904 mutation identification by sequencing, single segment, each segment 🅐 🄲
MED: 100-2,15,80; 100-4,3,10.4
AMA: 1998,Nov,26

83905 mutation identification by allele specific transcription, single segment, each segment 🅐 🄲
MED: 100-2,15,80; 100-4,3,10.4
AMA: 1998,Nov,26

83906 mutation identification by allele specific translation, single segment, each segment 🅐 🄲
MED: 100-2,15,80; 100-4,3,10.4
AMA: 1998,Nov,26

83907 lysis of cells prior to nucleic acid extraction (eg, stool specimens, paraffin embedded tissue) 🅐
MED: 100-4,3,10.4

83908 signal amplification of patient nucleic acid, each nucleic acid sequence 🅐
MED: 100-4,3,10.4
To report multiplex amplification, consult CPT codes 83900, 83901.

83909 separation and identification by high resolution technique (eg, capillary electrophoresis) 🅐
MED: 100-4,3,10.4

83912 interpretation and report 🅐 80 🄲
MED: 100-2,15,80; 100-4,3,10.4; 100-4,12,60

83913 RNA stabilization 🅐

● **83913** RNA stabilization

83914 Mutation identification by enzymatic ligation or primer extension, single segment, each segment (eg, oligonucleotide ligation assay (OLA), single base chain extension (SBCE), or allele-specific primer extension (ASPE)) 🅐
MED: 100-4,3,10.4

83915 Nucleotidase 5'- 🅐
MED: 100-2,15,80; 100-4,3,10.4

83916 Oligoclonal immune (oligoclonal bands) 🅐 🄲
MED: 100-2,15,80; 100-4,3,10.4

83918 Organic acids; total, quantitative, each specimen 🅐 🄲
MED: 100-2,15,80; 100-4,3,10.4
AMA: 1998,Nov,26; 1996,Mar,11

83919 qualitative, each specimen 🅐
MED: 100-2,15,80; 100-4,3,10.4
AMA: 1998,Nov,26

83921 Organic acid, single, quantitative 🅐 🄲
MED: 100-2,15,80; 100-4,3,10.4

83925 Opiates, (eg, morphine, meperidine) 🅐
MED: 100-2,15,80; 100-4,3,10.4

83930 Osmolality; blood 🅐
MED: 100-2,15,80; 100-4,3,10.4

83935 urine 🅐
MED: 100-2,15,80; 100-4,3,10.4

83937 Osteocalcin (bone g1a protein) 🅐
MED: 100-2,15,80; 100-4,3,10.4
AMA: 1994,Summer,5

83945 Oxalate 🅐
MED: 100-2,15,80; 100-4,3,10.4

83950 Oncoprotein, HER-2/neu 🅐 🄲
MED: 100-2,15,80; 100-4,3,10.4
To report tissue analysis, consult CPT codes 88342, 88365.

83970 Parathormone (parathyroid hormone) 🅐
MED: 100-2,15,80; 100-4,3,10.4
To report screening for chlorinated hydrocarbons, consult CPT code 82441.

 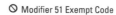
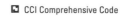

83986 pH, body fluid, except blood [A] [X]
MED: 100-2,15,80; 100-4,3,10.4
To report blood pH, consult CPT codes 82800 and 82803.

83992 Phencyclidine (PCP) [A]
MED: 100-2,15,80; 100-4,3,10.4
A drug screen (qualitative analysis) is normally performed prior to quantitative analysis. For drug screen, consult CPT codes 80100-80103. For phenobarbital, consult CPT code 80184.

84022 Phenothiazine [A]
MED: 100-2,15,80; 100-4,3,10.4
A drug screen (qualitative analysis) is normally performed prior to quantitative analysis. For drug screen, consult CPT codes 80100-80101.

84030 Phenylalanine (PKU), blood [A]
MED: 100-2,15,80; 100-4,3,10.4
To report phenylalanine-tyrosine ratio, consult CPT codes 84030 and 84510.

Guthrie test

84035 Phenylketones, qualitative [A]
MED: 100-2,15,80; 100-4,3,10.4

84060 Phosphatase, acid; total [A]
MED: 100-2,15,80; 100-4,3,10.4

84061 forensic examination [A]
MED: 100-2,15,80; 100-4,3,10.4

84066 prostatic ♂ [A]
MED: 100-2,15,80; 100-4,3,10.4

84075 Phosphatase, alkaline; [A]
MED: 100-2,15,80; 100-3,160.17; 100-3,190.10; 100-4,3,10.4
AMA: 1999,Dec,1

84078 heat stable (total not included) [A]
MED: 100-2,15,80; 100-3,160.17; 100-4,3,10.4

84080 isoenzymes [A] [□]
MED: 100-2,15,80; 100-3,160.17; 100-4,3,10.4

84081 Phosphatidylglycerol [A]
MED: 100-2,15,80; 100-4,3,10.4
To report inorganic phosphates, consult CPT code 84100. To report organic phosphates, see code for specific method. For cholinesterase, consult CPT codes 82480 and 82482.

84085 Phosphogluconate, 6-, dehydrogenase, RBC [A]
MED: 100-2,15,80; 100-4,3,10.4

84087 Phosphohexose isomerase [A]
MED: 100-2,15,80; 100-4,3,10.4

84100 Phosphorus inorganic (phosphate); [A]
MED: 100-2,15,80; 100-3,190.10; 100-4,3,10.4
AMA: 1999,Dec,1

84105 urine [A]
MED: 100-2,15,80; 100-4,3,10.4
To report pituitary gonadotropins, consult CPT codes 83001-83002. To report PKU, consult CPT codes 84030 and 84035.

84106 Porphobilinogen, urine; qualitative [A]
MED: 100-2,15,80; 100-4,3,10.4

84110 quantitative [A]
MED: 100-2,15,80; 100-4,3,10.4

84119 Porphyrins, urine; qualitative [A]
MED: 100-2,15,80; 100-4,3,10.4

84120 quantitation and fractionation [A]
MED: 100-2,15,80; 100-4,3,10.4

84126 Porphyrins, feces; quantitative [A]
MED: 100-2,15,80; 100-4,3,10.4

84127 qualitative [A]
MED: 100-2,15,80; 100-4,3,10.4
To report porphyrin precursors, consult CPT codes 82135, 84106, and 84110. To report protoporphyrin, RBC, consult CPT codes 84202 and 84203.

84132 Potassium; serum [A]
MED: 100-2,15,80; 100-3,190.10; 100-4,3,10.4
AMA: 2002,Jun,1; 1999,Dec,1

84133 urine [A]
MED: 100-2,15,80; 100-4,3,10.4

84134 Prealbumin [A]
MED: 100-2,15,80; 100-4,3,10.4
To report microalbumin, consult CPT codes 82043 and 82044.

84135 Pregnanediol [A]
MED: 100-2,15,80; 100-4,3,10.4

84138 Pregnanetriol [A]
MED: 100-2,15,80; 100-4,3,10.4

84140 Pregnenolone [A]
MED: 100-2,15,80; 100-4,3,10.4
AMA: 1994,Summer,6

84143 17-hydroxypregnenolone [A]
MED: 100-2,15,80; 100-4,3,10.4
AMA: 1994,Summer,6

84144 Progesterone [A]
MED: 100-2,15,80; 100-4,3,10.4
To report progesterone receptor assay, consult CPT code 84234. To report proinsulin, consult CPT code 84206.

84146 Prolactin [A] [□]
MED: 100-2,15,80; 100-4,3,10.4

84150 Prostaglandin, each [A]
MED: 100-2,15,80; 100-4,3,10.4

84152 Prostate specific antigen (PSA); complexed (direct measurement) ♂ [A]
MED: 100-2,15,80; 100-3,210.1; 100-4,3,10.4

84153 total ♂ [A]
MED: 100-2,15,80; 100-3,190.31; 100-3,210.1; 100-4,3,10.4
AMA: 1999,Dec,10; 1999,Aug,5; 1998,Nov,26; 1997,Jan,10; 1996,May,10; 1996,Aug,10; 1993,Fall,26

84154 free ♂ [A]
MED: 100-3,210.1; 100-4,3,10.4
AMA: 1999,Dec,10; 1999,Aug,5; 1998,Nov,26

84155 Protein, total, except by refractometry; serum [A] [□]
MED: 100-2,15,80; 100-3,190.10; 100-4,3,10.4
AMA: 2000,Jan,7; 1999,Dec,1

84156 urine [A]
MED: 100-4,3,10.4

84157 other source (eg, synovial fluid, cerebrospinal fluid) [A]
MED: 100-4,3,10.4

84160	Protein, total, by refractometry, any source ⒶⒸ

MED: 100-2,15,80; 100-4,3,10.4

To report urine total protein by dipstick method, consult CPT codes 81000-81003.

84163	Pregnancy-associated plasma protein-A (PAPP-A) ♀ Ⓐ

MED: 100-4,3,10.4

84165	Protein; electrophoretic fractionation and quantitation, serum Ⓐ ⑧⓪ Ⓒ

MED: 100-2,15,80; 100-4,3,10.4; 100-4,12,60

84166	electrophoretic fractionation and quantitation, other fluids with concentration (eg, urine, CSF) Ⓐ ⑧⓪ Ⓒ

MED: 100-4,3,10.4

84181	Western Blot, with interpretation and report, blood or other body fluid Ⓐ ⑧⓪ Ⓒ

MED: 100-2,15,80; 100-3,190.9; 100-4,3,10.4; 100-4,12,60

84182	Western Blot, with interpretation and report, blood or other body fluid, immunological probe for band identification, each Ⓐ ⑧⓪ Ⓒ

MED: 100-2,15,80; 100-3,190.9; 100-4,3,10.4; 100-4,12,60

If a Western Blot tissue analysis is performed, consult CPT code 88371.

84202	Protoporphyrin, RBC; quantitative Ⓐ

MED: 100-2,15,80; 100-4,3,10.4

84203	screen Ⓐ

MED: 100-2,15,80; 100-4,3,10.4

84206	Proinsulin Ⓐ

MED: 100-2,15,80; 100-4,3,10.4

To report pseudocholinesterase, consult CPT code 82480.

84207	Pyridoxal phosphate (Vitamin B-6) Ⓐ Ⓒ

MED: 100-2,15,80; 100-4,3,10.4

84210	Pyruvate Ⓐ

MED: 100-2,15,80; 100-4,3,10.4

84220	Pyruvate kinase Ⓐ

MED: 100-2,15,80; 100-4,3,10.4

84228	Quinine Ⓐ

MED: 100-2,15,80; 100-4,3,10.4

84233	Receptor assay; estrogen Ⓐ Ⓒ

MED: 100-2,15,80; 100-4,3,10.4

84234	progesterone Ⓐ Ⓒ

MED: 100-2,15,80; 100-4,3,10.4

84235	endocrine, other than estrogen or progesterone (specify hormone) Ⓐ Ⓒ

MED: 100-2,15,80; 100-4,3,10.4

84238	non-endocrine (specify receptor) Ⓐ Ⓒ

MED: 100-2,15,80; 100-4,3,10.4

84244	Renin Ⓐ Ⓒ

MED: 100-2,15,80; 100-4,3,10.4

84252	Riboflavin (Vitamin B-2) Ⓐ Ⓒ

MED: 100-2,15,80; 100-4,3,10.4

To report salicylates, consult CPT code 80196. If a secretin test is performed, consult CPT codes 99070, 89100 and appropriate analyses.

84255	Selenium Ⓐ

MED: 100-2,15,80; 100-4,3,10.4

84260	Serotonin Ⓐ

MED: 100-2,15,80; 100-4,3,10.4

To report urine metabolites (HIAA), consult CPT code 83497.

84270	Sex hormone binding globulin (SHBG) Ⓐ

MED: 100-2,15,80; 100-4,3,10.4

AMA: 1994,Summer,4

84275	Sialic acid Ⓐ

MED: 100-2,15,80; 100-4,3,10.4

To report sickle hemoglobin, consult CPT code 85660.

84285	Silica Ⓐ

MED: 100-2,15,80; 100-4,3,10.4

84295	Sodium; serum Ⓐ

MED: 100-2,15,80; 100-3,190.10; 100-4,3,10.4

AMA: 1999,Dec,1

84300	urine Ⓐ

MED: 100-2,15,80; 100-4,3,10.4

84302	other source Ⓐ

MED: 100-4,3,10.4

To report somatomammotropin, consult CPT code 83632. To report somatotropin, consult CPT code 83003.

84305	Somatomedin Ⓐ

MED: 100-2,15,80; 100-4,3,10.4

AMA: 1994,Summer,4

84307	Somatostatin Ⓐ

MED: 100-2,15,80; 100-4,3,10.4

AMA: 1994,Summer,4

84311	Spectrophotometry, analyte not elsewhere specified Ⓐ

MED: 100-2,15,80; 100-4,3,10.4

84315	Specific gravity (except urine) Ⓐ

MED: 100-2,15,80; 100-4,3,10.4

To report specific gravity, urine, consult CPT codes 81000-81003. If stone analysis is performed, consult CPT codes 82355-82370.

84375	Sugars, chromatographic, TLC or paper chromatography Ⓐ

MED: 100-2,15,80; 100-4,3,10.4

84376	Sugars (mono-, di-, and oligosaccharides); single qualitative, each specimen Ⓐ

MED: 100-2,15,80; 100-4,3,10.4

AMA: 1999,Dec,7; 1998,Nov,26-27

84377	multiple qualitative, each specimen Ⓐ Ⓒ

MED: 100-2,15,80; 100-4,3,10.4

AMA: 1998,Nov,26-27

84378	single quantitative, each specimen Ⓐ Ⓒ

MED: 100-2,15,80; 100-4,3,10.4

AMA: 1998,Nov,26-27

84379	multiple quantitative, each specimen Ⓐ Ⓒ

MED: 100-2,15,80; 100-4,3,10.4

AMA: 1999,Dec,7; 1998,Nov,26-27

84392	Sulfate, urine Ⓐ

MED: 100-2,15,80; 100-4,3,10.4

To report T-3, consult CPT codes 84479-84481. To report T-4, consult CPT codes 84436-84439. To report sulfhemoglobin, see hemoglobin CPT codes 83055 and 83060.

84402	Testosterone; free Ⓐ

MED: 100-2,15,80; 100-4,3,10.4

 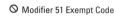

Pathology and Laboratory

84403 — 84588

84403	total	A ↴

MED: 100-2,15,80; 100-4,3,10.4

84425	Thiamine (Vitamin B-1)	A ↴

MED: 100-2,15,80; 100-4,3,10.4

84430	Thiocyanate	A

MED: 100-2,15,80; 100-4,3,10.4

84432	Thyroglobulin	A

MED: 100-2,15,80; 100-4,3,10.4
AMA: 1994,Summer,2

Thyroglobulin, antibody, see 86800. If a thyrotropin releasing hormone (TRH) test is performed, consult CPT codes 80438 and 80439.

84436	Thyroxine; total	A ↴

MED: 100-2,15,80; 100-3,190.22; 100-4,3,10.4
AMA: 1994,Summer,3; 1993,Fall,25

84437	requiring elution (eg, neonatal)	A

MED: 100-2,15,80; 100-4,3,10.4

84439	free	A ↴

MED: 100-2,15,80; 100-3,190.22; 100-4,3,10.4

84442	Thyroxine binding globulin (TBG)	A

MED: 100-2,15,80; 100-4,3,10.4

84443	Thyroid stimulating hormone (TSH)	A ↴

MED: 100-2,15,80; 100-3,190.22; 100-4,3,10.4
AMA: 1994,Summer,3

84445	Thyroid stimulating immune globulins (TSI)	A ↴

MED: 100-2,15,80; 100-4,3,10.4
AMA: 1994,Summer,3

To report tobramycin, consult CPT code 80200.

84446	Tocopherol alpha (Vitamin E)	A ↴

MED: 100-2,15,80; 100-4,3,10.4

To report tolbutamide tolerance, consult CPT code 82953.

84449	Transcortin (cortisol binding globulin)	A

MED: 100-2,15,80; 100-4,3,10.4
AMA: 1994,Summer,6

84450	Transferase; aspartate amino (AST) (SGOT)	A ✕

MED: 100-2,15,80; 100-3,160.17; 100-3,190.10; 100-4,3,10.4
AMA: 1999,Dec,1

84460	alanine amino (ALT) (SGPT)	A ✕

MED: 100-2,15,80; 100-3,160.17; 100-4,3,10.4
AMA: 1999,Dec,1

84466	Transferrin	A ↴

AMA: 1994,Summer,4
To report iron binding capacity, consult CPT code 83550.

84478	Triglycerides	A ↴ ✕

MED: 100-2,15,80; 100-3,190.23; 100-4,3,10.4
AMA: 2000,Mar,11; 1999,Dec,1

84479	Thyroid hormone (T3 or T4) uptake or thyroid hormone binding ratio (THBR)	A ↴

MED: 100-2,15,80; 100-3,190.22; 100-4,3,10.4
AMA: 1994,Summer,3; 1993,Fall,25

84480	Triiodothyronine T3; total (TT-3)	A ↴

MED: 100-2,15,80; 100-4,3,10.4

84481	free	A ↴

MED: 100-2,15,80; 100-4,3,10.4

84482	reverse	A ↴

MED: 100-2,15,80; 100-4,3,10.4
AMA: 1994,Summer,2

84484	Troponin, quantitative	A

MED: 100-2,15,80; 100-4,3,10.4
AMA: 1998,Jan,6; 1998,Feb,1; 1997,Nov,29
To report Troponin, qualitative assay, consult CPT code 84512.

84485	Trypsin; duodenal fluid	A

MED: 100-2,15,80; 100-4,3,10.4

84488	feces, qualitative	A

MED: 100-2,15,80; 100-4,3,10.4

84490	feces, quantitative, 24-hour collection	A

MED: 100-2,15,80; 100-4,3,10.4

84510	Tyrosine	A

MED: 100-2,15,80; 100-4,3,10.4

To report urate crystal identification, consult CPT code 89060.

84512	Troponin, qualitative	A

MED: 100-2,15,80; 100-4,3,10.4
AMA: 1998,Jan,6; 1998,Feb,1; 1997,Nov,29
To report Troponin, quantitative assay, consult CPT code 84484.

84520	Urea nitrogen; quantitative	A

MED: 100-2,15,80; 100-3,160.17; 100-3,190.10; 100-4,3,10.4
AMA: 1999,Dec,1

84525	semiquantitative (eg, reagent strip test)	A

MED: 100-2,15,80; 100-3,160.17; 100-4,3,10.4
AMA: 1998,Mar,3
Patterson's test

84540	Urea nitrogen, urine	A

MED: 100-2,15,80; 100-4,3,10.4

84545	Urea nitrogen, clearance	A

MED: 100-2,15,80; 100-4,3,10.4

84550	Uric acid; blood	A

MED: 100-2,15,80; 100-4,3,10.4
AMA: 1999,Dec,1

84560	other source	A

MED: 100-2,15,80; 100-4,3,10.4

84577	Urobilinogen, feces, quantitative	A

MED: 100-2,15,80; 100-4,3,10.4

84578	Urobilinogen, urine; qualitative	A

MED: 100-2,15,80; 100-4,3,10.4

84580	quantitative, timed specimen	A ↴

MED: 100-2,15,80; 100-4,3,10.4

84583	semiquantitative	A

MED: 100-2,15,80; 100-4,3,10.4

To report uroporphyrins, consult CPT Code 84120. To report dipropylacetic acid (valproic acid), consult CPT code 80164.

84585	Vanillylmandelic acid (VMA), urine	A

MED: 100-2,15,80; 100-4,3,10.4

84586	Vasoactive intestinal peptide (VIP)	A

MED: 100-2,15,80; 100-4,3,10.4
AMA: 1994,Summer,6

84588	Vasopressin (antidiuretic hormone, ADH)	A

MED: 100-2,15,80; 100-4,3,10.4

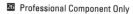

26 Professional Component Only
TC Technical Component Only
80/80 Assist-at-Surgery Allowed/With Documentation
MED: Pub 100/NCD References   AMA: CPT Assistant References
Unlisted
Not Covered
1-9 ASC Group   ♂ Male Only   ♀ Female Only

306 — CPT Expert   CPT only © 2006 American Medical Association. All Rights Reserved. (Black Ink)   © 2006 Ingenix (Blue Ink)

84590 | Vitamin A [A] [C]
MED: 100-2,15,80; 100-4,3,10.4

To report thiamine (Vitamin B-1), consult CPT code 84425. To report Riboflavin (Vitamin B-2), consult CPT code 84252. To report pyridoxal phosphate (Vitamin B-6), consult CPT code 84207. To report cyanocobalamin (Vitamin B-12), consult CPT code 82607. If a Vitamin B-12 absorption study is performed, (e.g., Schilling test), consult CPT codes 78270 and 78271. To report ascorbic acid (Vitamin C), consult CPT code 82180. To report Vitamin D, consult CPT codes 82306, 82307, and 82652. To report tocopherol alpha (Vitamin E), consult CPT code 84446.

84591 | Vitamin, not otherwise specified [A]
MED: 100-2,15,80; 100-4,3,10.4

84597 | Vitamin K [A] [C]
MED: 100-2,15,80; 100-4,3,10.4

To report vanillylmandelic acid (VMA), consult CPT code 84585.

84600 | Volatiles (eg, acetic anhydride, carbon tetrachloride, dichloroethane, dichloromethane, diethylether, isopropyl alcohol, methanol) [A]
MED: 100-2,15,80; 100-4,3,10.4

To report acetaldehyde, consult CPT code 82000. To report plasma volume, radiopharmaceutical volume-dilution technique, consult CPT codes 78110 and 78111.

84620 | Xylose absorption test, blood and/or urine [A] [C]
MED: 100-2,15,80; 100-4,3,10.4

Administration of d-xylose is reported separately, consult CPT code 99070.

84630 | Zinc [A]
MED: 100-2,15,80; 100-4,3,10.4

84681 | C-peptide [A] [C]
MED: 100-2,15,80; 100-4,3,10.4

84702 | Gonadotropin, chorionic (hCG); quantitative [A] [C]
MED: 100-2,15,80; 100-3,190.27; 100-4,3,10.4

If a urine pregnancy test is conducted by visual color comparison, consult CPT code 81025.

84703 | qualitative [A] [X]
MED: 100-2,15,80; 100-4,3,10.4

If a urine pregnancy test is conducted by visual color comparison, consult CPT code 81025.

84830 | Ovulation tests, by visual color comparison methods for human luteinizing hormone ♀ [A] [X]
MED: 100-2,15,80; 100-4,3,10.4

84999 | Unlisted chemistry procedure [X]
MED: 100-2,15,80; 100-4,3,10.4
AMA: 2000,Oct,7

HEMATOLOGY AND COAGULATION

For agglutinins, see the Immunology section of the CPT book. For antiplasmin, consult CPT code 85410. For antithrombin III, consult CPT codes 85300 and 85301.

For blood banking procedures, see the Transfusion Medicine section.

85002 | Bleeding time [A]
MED: 100-2,15,80; 100-4,3,10.4

85004 | Blood count; automated differential WBC count [A] [C]
MED: 100-3,190.15; 100-4,3,10.4

85007 | blood smear, microscopic examination with manual differential WBC count [A] [C]
MED: 100-2,15,80; 100-3,190.15; 100-4,3,10.4

85008 | blood smear, microscopic examination without manual differential WBC count [A] [C]
MED: 100-2,15,80; 100-3,190.15; 100-4,3,10.4

To report other fluids (e.g., CSF), consult CPT codes 89050 and 89051.

85009 | manual differential WBC count, buffy coat [A] [C]
MED: 100-2,15,80; 100-4,3,10.4

To report eosinophils, nasal smear, consult CPT code 89190.

85013 | spun microhematocrit [A] [X]
MED: 100-2,15,80; 100-3,190.10; 100-3,190.15; 100-4,3,10.4

85014 | hematocrit (Hct) [A] [C] [X]
MED: 100-2,15,80; 100-3,190.15; 100-4,3,10.4

85018 | hemoglobin (Hgb) [A] [C] [X]
MED: 100-2,15,80; 100-3,190.10; 100-3,190.15; 100-4,3,10.4

To report fecal hemoglobin detection by immunoassay, consult CPT code 82274.

To report other hemoglobin determinations, consult CPT codes 83020-83069.

85025 | complete (CBC), automated (Hgb, Hct, RBC, WBC and platelet count) and automated differential WBC count [A] [C]
MED: 100-2,15,80; 100-3,160.17; 100-3,190.10; 100-3,190.15; 100-4,3,10.4
AMA: 2000,Jul,11

85027 | complete (CBC), automated (Hgb, Hct, RBC, WBC and platelet count) [A] [C]
MED: 100-2,15,80; 100-3,160.17; 100-3,190.15; 100-4,3,10.4

85032 | manual cell count (erythrocyte, leukocyte, or platelet) each [A] [C]
MED: 100-3,190.15; 100-4,3,10.4

85041 | red blood cell (RBC), automated [A] [C]
MED: 100-2,15,80; 100-4,3,10.4

Do not report 85041 with CPT codes 85025 or 85027.

85044 | reticulocyte, manual [A]
MED: 100-2,15,80; 100-4,3,10.4

85045 | reticulocyte, automated [A] [C]
MED: 100-2,15,80; 100-4,3,10.4

85046 | reticulocytes, automated, including one or more cellular parameters (eg, reticulocyte hemoglobin content (CHr), immature reticulocyte fraction (IRF), reticulocyte volume (MRV), RNA content), direct measurement [A] [C]
MED: 100-2,15,80; 100-4,3,10.4
AMA: 1998,Nov,27

85048 | leukocyte (WBC), automated [A] [C]
MED: 100-2,15,80; 100-3,190.15; 100-4,3,10.4

85049 | platelet, automated [A] [C]
MED: 100-3,190.15; 100-4,3,10.4

85055 | Reticulated platelet assay [A]
MED: 100-4,3,10.4

85060 | Blood smear, peripheral, interpretation by physician with written report [B] [50]
MED: 100-2,15,80; 100-4,3,10.4; 100-4,4,20.5; 100-4,12,60

⑥ Modifier 63 Exempt Code   ⊙ Conscious Sedation   + CPT Add-on Code   ⊘ Modifier 51 Exempt Code   ● New Code   ▲ Revised Code

[M] Maternity Edit   [A] Age Edit   [X] CLIA Waived Test   [A]-[Y] APC Status Indicators   [C] CCI Comprehensive Code   [50] Bilateral Procedure

© 2006 Ingenix (Blue Ink)   CPT only © 2006 American Medical Association. All Rights Reserved. (Black Ink)   Path/Lab — 307

85097	**Bone marrow, smear interpretation**	X 80

MED: 100-2,15,80; 100-4,3,10.4; 100-4,4,20.5; 100-4,12,60
AMA: 1998,Jul,4; 1992,Winter,17
To report special stains, consult CPT codes 85540, 88312, and 88313.

To report bone biopsy, consult CPT codes 20220, 20225, 20240, 20245, 20250, 20251.

85130	**Chromogenic substrate assay**	A C

MED: 100-2,15,80; 100-4,3,10.4
To report circulating anti-coagulant screen (mixing studies), consult CPT codes 85611 and 85732.

85170	**Clot retraction**	A C

MED: 100-2,15,80; 100-4,3,10.4

85175	**Clot lysis time, whole blood dilution**	A C

MED: 100-2,15,80; 100-4,3,10.4
To report clotting factor I (fibrinogen), consult CPT codes 85384 and 85385.

85210	**Clotting; factor II, prothrombin, specific**	A C

MED: 100-2,15,80; 100-4,3,10.4; 100-4,3,20.7.3
Consult also CPT codes 85610-85613.

85220	**factor V (AcG or proaccelerin), labile factor**	A C

MED: 100-2,15,80; 100-4,3,10.4; 100-4,3,20.7.3

85230	**factor VII (proconvertin, stable factor)**	A C

MED: 100-2,15,80; 100-4,3,10.4; 100-4,3,20.7.3

85240	**factor VIII (AHG), one stage**	A C

MED: 100-2,15,80; 100-4,3,10.4; 100-4,3,20.7.3

85244	**factor VIII related antigen**	A C

MED: 100-2,15,80; 100-4,3,10.4; 100-4,3,20.7.3

85245	**factor VIII, VW factor, ristocetin cofactor**	A C

MED: 100-2,15,80; 100-4,3,10.4; 100-4,3,20.7.3

85246	**factor VIII, VW factor antigen**	A C

MED: 100-2,15,80; 100-4,3,10.4; 100-4,3,20.7.3

85247	**factor VIII, von Willebrand factor, multimetric analysis**	A C

MED: 100-2,15,80; 100-4,3,10.4; 100-4,3,20.7.3

85250	**factor IX (PTC or Christmas)**	A C

MED: 100-2,15,80; 100-4,3,10.4; 100-4,3,20.7.3

85260	**factor X (Stuart-Prower)**	A C

MED: 100-2,15,80; 100-4,3,10.4; 100-4,3,20.7.3

85270	**factor XI (PTA)**	A C

MED: 100-2,15,80; 100-4,3,10.4; 100-4,3,20.7.3

85280	**factor XII (Hageman)**	A C

MED: 100-2,15,80; 100-4,3,10.4; 100-4,3,20.7.3

85290	**factor XIII (fibrin stabilizing)**	A C

MED: 100-2,15,80; 100-4,3,10.4; 100-4,3,20.7.3

85291	**factor XIII (fibrin stabilizing), screen solubility**	A C

MED: 100-2,15,80; 100-4,3,10.4; 100-4,3,20.7.3

85292	**prekallikrein assay (Fletcher factor assay)**	A C

MED: 100-2,15,80; 100-4,3,10.4; 100-4,3,20.7.3

85293	**high molecular weight kininogen assay (Fitzgerald factor assay)**	A C

MED: 100-2,15,80; 100-4,3,10.4; 100-4,3,20.7.3

85300	**Clotting inhibitors or anticoagulants; antithrombin III, activity**	A C

85301	**antithrombin III, antigen assay**	A C

MED: 100-2,15,80; 100-4,3,10.4

85302	**protein C, antigen**	A C

MED: 100-2,15,80; 100-4,3,10.4

85303	**protein C, activity**	A C

MED: 100-2,15,80; 100-4,3,10.4

85305	**protein S, total**	A C

MED: 100-2,15,80; 100-4,3,10.4

85306	**protein S, free**	A C

MED: 100-2,15,80; 100-4,3,10.4

85307	**Activated Protein C (APC) resistance assay**	A C

MED: 100-2,15,80; 100-4,3,10.4

85335	**Factor inhibitor test**	A C

85337	**Thrombomodulin**	A C

MED: 100-2,15,80; 100-4,3,10.4
To report mixing studies for inhibitors, consult CPT code 85732.

85345	**Coagulation time; Lee and White**	A C

MED: 100-2,15,80; 100-4,3,10.4

85347	**activated**	A C

MED: 100-2,15,80; 100-4,3,10.4

85348	**other methods**	A C

MED: 100-2,15,80; 100-4,3,10.4
To report a differential count, consult CPT codes 85007 and subsequent codes. For duke bleeding time, consult CPT code 85002. For eosinophils, nasal smear, consult CPT code 89190.

85360	**Euglobulin lysis**	A C

MED: 100-2,15,80; 100-4,3,10.4
To report fetal hemoglobin, consult CPT codes 83030, 83033, and 85460.

85362	**Fibrin(ogen) degradation (split) products (FDP)(FSP); agglutination slide, semiquantitative**	A C

MED: 100-2,15,80; 100-4,3,10.4
To report immunoelectrophoresis, consult CPT code 86320.

85366	**paracoagulation**	A C

MED: 100-2,15,80; 100-4,3,10.4

85370	**quantitative**	A C

MED: 100-2,15,80; 100-4,3,10.4

85378	**Fibrin degradation products, D-dimer; qualitative or semiquantitative**	A C

MED: 100-2,15,80; 100-4,3,10.4

85379	**quantitative**	A C

MED: 100-2,15,80; 100-4,3,10.4
To report ultrasensitive and standard sensitivity quantitative D-dimer, consult CPT code 85379.

85380	**ultrasensitive (eg, for evaluation for venous thromboembolism), qualitative or semiquantitative**	A C

MED: 100-4,3,10.4

85384	**Fibrinogen; activity**	A C

MED: 100-2,15,80; 100-4,3,10.4; 100-4,3,20.7.3

85385	**antigen**	A C

MED: 100-2,15,80; 100-4,3,10.4; 100-4,3,20.7.3

85390	**Fibrinolysins or coagulopathy screen, interpretation and report**	A 80 C

MED: 100-2,15,80; 100-4,3,10.4; 100-4,12,60

85396	Coagulation/fibrinolysis assay, whole blood (eg, viscoelastic clot assessment), including use of any pharmacologic additive(s), as indicated, including interpretation and written report, per day [N] [80]
	MED: 100-4,3,10.4
85400	Fibrinolytic factors and inhibitors; plasmin [A] [C]
	MED: 100-2,15,80; 100-4,3,10.4
85410	alpha-2 antiplasmin [A] [C]
	MED: 100-2,15,80; 100-4,3,10.4
85415	plasminogen activator [A] [C]
	MED: 100-2,15,80; 100-4,3,10.4
85420	plasminogen, except antigenic assay [A] [C]
	MED: 100-2,15,80; 100-4,3,10.4
85421	plasminogen, antigenic assay [A] [C]
	MED: 100-2,15,80; 100-4,3,10.4
	To report fragility, red blood cell, consult CPT codes 85547 and 85555-85557.
85441	Heinz bodies; direct [A] [C]
	MED: 100-2,15,80; 100-4,3,10.4
85445	induced, acetyl phenylhydrazine [A] [C]
	MED: 100-2,15,80; 100-4,3,10.4
	To report hematocrit (PCV), consult CPT codes 85014 and 85025, 85027. To report hemoglobin, consult CPT codes 83020-83068 and 85018, 85025, 85027.
85460	Hemoglobin or RBCs, fetal, for fetomaternal hemorrhage; differential lysis (Kleihauer-Betke) [M] ♀ [A] [C]
	MED: 100-2,15,80; 100-4,3,10.4
	AMA: 1993,Fall,25
	Consult also CPT codes 83030 and 83033. For hemolysins, consult CPT codes 86940 and 86941.
85461	rosette [M] ♀ [A] [C]
	MED: 100-2,15,80; 100-4,3,10.4
85475	Hemolysin, acid [A] [C]
	MED: 100-2,15,80; 100-4,3,10.4
	Consult also CPT codes 86940 and 86941.
	Ham test
85520	Heparin assay [A] [C]
	MED: 100-2,15,80; 100-4,3,10.4
85525	Heparin neutralization [A] [C]
	MED: 100-2,15,80; 100-4,3,10.4
85530	Heparin-protamine tolerance test [A] [C]
	MED: 100-2,15,80; 100-4,3,10.4
85536	Iron stain, peripheral blood [A] [C]
	MED: 100-2,15,80; 100-4,3,10.4
	To report iron stains on bone marrow or other tissues with physician evaluation, consult CPT code 88313.
85540	Leukocyte alkaline phosphatase with count [A] [C]
	MED: 100-2,15,80; 100-4,3,10.4
85547	Mechanical fragility, RBC [A] [C]
	MED: 100-2,15,80; 100-4,3,10.4
85549	Muramidase [A] [C]
	MED: 100-2,15,80; 100-4,3,10.4
	To report nitroblue tetrazolium dye test, consult CPT code 86384.
85555	Osmotic fragility, RBC; unincubated [A] [C]
	MED: 100-2,15,80; 100-4,3,10.4
85557	incubated [A] [C]
	MED: 100-2,15,80; 100-4,3,10.4
	To report packed cell volume, consult CPT code 85013. To report partial throboplastin time, consult CPT codes 85730 and 85732. To report parasites, blood (e.g., malaria smears), consult CPT code 87207. To report plasmin, consult CPT code 85400. To report plasminogen, consult CPT code 85420. To report plasminogen factor, consult CPT code 85415.
85576	Platelet, aggregation (in vitro), each agent [A] [80] [C]
	MED: 100-2,15,80; 100-4,3,10.4; 100-4,12,60
	AMA: 1996,Jul,10
85597	Platelet neutralization [A] [C]
	MED: 100-2,15,80; 100-4,3,10.4
85610	Prothrombin time; [A] [C] [X]
	MED: 100-2,15,80; 100-3,190.10; 100-3,190.17; 100-4,3,10.4; 100-4,3,20.7.3
85611	substitution, plasma fractions, each [A] [C]
	MED: 100-2,15,80; 100-4,3,10.4; 100-4,3,20.7.3
85612	Russell viper venom time (includes venom); undiluted [A] [C]
	MED: 100-2,15,80; 100-4,3,10.4
85613	diluted [A] [C]
	MED: 100-2,15,80; 100-4,3,10.4
	To report red blood cell count, consult CPT codes 85025, 85027, and 85041.
85635	Reptilase test [A] [C]
	MED: 100-2,15,80; 100-4,3,10.4
	To report reticulocyte count, consult CPT codes 85044 and 85045.
85651	Sedimentation rate, erythrocyte; non-automated [A] [X]
	MED: 100-2,15,80; 100-4,3,10.4
85652	automated [A] [C]
	MED: 100-2,15,80; 100-4,3,10.4
	Westergren test
85660	Sickling of RBC, reduction [A] [C]
	MED: 100-2,15,80; 100-4,3,10.4
	If hemoglobin electophoresis is performed, consult CPT codes 83020. For smears (e.g., for parasites, malaria), consult CPT code 87207.
85670	Thrombin time; plasma [A] [C]
	MED: 100-2,15,80; 100-4,3,10.4
85675	titer [A] [C]
	MED: 100-2,15,80; 100-4,3,10.4
85705	Thromboplastin inhibition, tissue [A] [C]
	MED: 100-2,15,80; 100-4,3,10.4
	To report individual clotting factors, consult CPT codes 85245-85247.
85730	Thromboplastin time, partial (PTT); plasma or whole blood [A] [C]
	MED: 100-2,15,80; 100-3,190.16; 100-4,3,10.4
	Hicks-Pitney test
85732	substitution, plasma fractions, each [A] [C]
	MED: 100-2,15,80; 100-4,3,10.4

 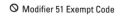

Pathology and Laboratory

85810 — 86156

85810   Viscosity   [A]

MED: 100-2,15,80; 100-4,3,10.4

To report Von Willebrand factor assay, consult CPT codes 85245-85247. To report a white blood cell (WBC) count, consult CPT codes 85025, 85027, 85048, and 89050.

85999   Unlisted hematology and coagulation procedure   [X]

MED: 100-2,15,80; 100-4,3,10.4

IMMUNOLOGY

Acetylcholine receptor antibody, consult CPT codes 86255, 86256. Actinomyces to antibodies, consult CPT codes 86602. Adrenal cortex antibodies, consult CPT codes 86255, 86256. To report tuberculosis test, cell mediated immunity measurement of gamma interferon antigen response, consult CPT Category III code 0010T.

CPT codes 86602-86804 are qualitative or semiquantitative immunoassays performed by multiple step methods for the detection of antibodies to infectious agents. To report immunoassays by single step method such as reagent strips, consult code 86318. Report procedure codes for identification of antibodies as precisely as possible. When multiple tests are performed to detect antibodies to organisms classified more precisely than the specificity allowed by available codes, it is appropriate to code each as a separate service. To report assays that are performed for antibodies to Coxsackie A and B species, each assay should be reported separately. If multiple assays are performed for antibodies of different immunoglobulin classes, each assay should be reported separately.

To report the detection of antibodies other than those to infectious agents, consult specific antibody (e.g., 86021, 86022, 86023, 86376, 86800, 86850-86870) or specific method (e.g., 83516, 86255, 86256). To report infectious agent/antigen detection, consult 87260-87899.

To report infectious agent/antigen detection, consult CPT codes 87620-87899.

86000   Agglutinins, febrile (eg, Brucella, Francisella, Murine typhus, Q fever, Rocky Mountain spotted fever, scrub typhus), each antigen   [A]

MED: 100-2,15,80; 100-4,3,10.4

To report antibodies to infectious agents, consult CPT codes 86602-86804.

86001   Allergen specific IgG quantitative or semiquantitative, each allergen   [A] [TC]

MED: 100-2,15,80; 100-4,3,10.4

To report agglutinins and autohemolysins, consult CPT codes 86940 and 86941.

86003   Allergen specific IgE; quantitative or semiquantitative, each allergen   [A] [TC]

MED: 100-2,15,80; 100-4,3,10.4

AMA: 1994,Spring,31

To report total quantitative IgE, consult CPT code 82785.

86005   qualitative, multiallergen screen (dipstick, paddle or disk)   [A]

MED: 100-2,15,80; 100-4,3,10.4

AMA: 1994,Spring,31

To report total qualitative IgE, consult CPT code 83518. To report alpha-1 antitrypsin, consult CPT codes 82103 and 82104. To report alpha-1 feto-protein, consult CPT codes 82105 and 82106. To report anti-AChR (acetylcholine receptor) antibody titer, consult CPT codes 86255 and 86256. To report anticardiolipin antibody, consult CPT code 86147. To report anti-DNA, consult CPT code 86225. To report anti-deoxyribonuclease titer, consult CPT code 86215.

86021   Antibody identification; leukocyte antibodies   [A] [TC]

MED: 100-2,15,80; 100-4,3,10.4

86022   platelet antibodies   [A] [TC]

MED: 100-2,15,80; 100-4,3,10.4

86023   platelet associated immunoglobulin assay   [A] [TC]

MED: 100-2,15,80; 100-4,3,10.4

86038   Antinuclear antibodies (ANA);   [A] [TC]

MED: 100-2,15,80; 100-4,3,10.4

86039   titer   [A] [TC]

MED: 100-2,15,80; 100-4,3,10.4

To report antistreptococcal antibody (e.g., anti-DNAse), consult CPT code 86215. To report antistreptokinase titer, consult CPT code 86590.

86060   Antistreptolysin 0; titer   [A] [TC]

MED: 100-2,15,80; 100-4,3,10.4

To report antibodies to infectious agents, consult CPT codes 86602-86804.

86063   screen   [A]

MED: 100-2,15,80; 100-4,3,10.4

To report antibodies to infectious agents, consult CPT codes 86602-86804. To report antibodies to Blastomyces, consult CPT code 86612.

86077   Blood bank physician services; difficult cross match and/or evaluation of irregular antibody(s), interpretation and written report   [X] [80]

MED: 100-2,15,80; 100-4,3,10.4; 100-4,4,20.5; 100-4,12,60

86078   investigation of transfusion reaction including suspicion of transmissible disease, interpretation and written report   [X] [80]

MED: 100-2,15,80; 100-4,3,10.4; 100-4,4,20.5; 100-4,12,60

86079   authorization for deviation from standard blood banking procedures (eg, use of outdated blood, transfusion of Rh incompatible units), with written report   [X] [80]

MED: 100-2,15,80; 100-4,3,10.4; 100-4,4,20.5; 100-4,12,60

To report antibodies to candida, consult CPT code 86628. To report skin testing, consult CPT code 86485. To report antibodies to brucella, consult CPT code 86622.

86140   C-reactive protein;   [A]

MED: 100-2,15,80; 100-4,3,10.4

To report candidiasis, consult CPT code 86628.

86141   high sensitivity (hsCRP)   [A] [TC]

MED: 100-2,15,80; 100-4,3,10.4

86146   Beta 2 Glycoprotein I antibody, each   [A]

MED: 100-2,15,80; 100-4,3,10.4

86147   Cardiolipin (phospholipid) antibody, each Ig class   [A]

MED: 100-2,15,80; 100-4,3,10.4

86148   Anti-phosphatidylserine (phospholipid) antibody   [A]

MED: 100-2,15,80; 100-4,3,10.4

AMA: 1997,Nov,30

To report antiprothrombin (phopholipid cofactor) antibody, consult CPT Category III code 0030T.

86155   Chemotaxis assay, specify method   [A]

MED: 100-2,15,80; 100-4,3,10.4

To report antibodies to coccidioides, consult CPT code 86635. To report skin testing, consult CPT code 86490.

To report clostridium difficile toxin, consult CPT code 87230.

86156   Cold agglutinin; screen   [A]

MED: 100-2,15,80; 100-4,3,10.4

86157	titer	Ⓐ ▣

MED: 100-2,15,80; 100-4,3,10.4

86160	Complement; antigen, each component	Ⓐ

MED: 100-2,15,80; 100-4,3,10.4

86161	functional activity, each component	Ⓐ

MED: 100-2,15,80; 100-4,3,10.4

86162	total hemolytic (CH50)	Ⓐ

MED: 100-2,15,80; 100-4,3,10.4

86171	Complement fixation tests, each antigen	Ⓐ

MED: 100-2,15,80; 100-4,3,10.4

If a Coombs test is performed, consult CPT codes 86880-86886.

86185	Counterimmunoelectrophoresis, each antigen	Ⓐ ▣

MED: 100-2,15,80; 100-4,3,10.4

To report antibodies to cryptococcus, consult CPT code 86641.

86200	Cyclic citrullinated peptide (CCP), antibody	Ⓐ

MED: 100-4,3,10.4

86215	Deoxyribonuclease, antibody	Ⓐ ▣

MED: 100-2,15,80; 100-4,3,10.4

86225	Deoxyribonucleic acid (DNA) antibody; native or double stranded	Ⓐ ▣

MED: 100-2,15,80; 100-4,3,10.4

To report antibodies to echinococcus, consult the appropriate code according to the specific method used. If an HIV antibody test is performed, consult CPT codes 86701-86703.

86226	single stranded	Ⓐ ▣

MED: 100-2,15,80; 100-4,3,10.4

To report fluorescent noninfectious agent antibody, consult CPT codes 86255 and 86256.

86235	Extractable nuclear antigen, antibody to, any method (eg, nRNP, SS-A, SS-B, Sm, RNP, Sc170, J01), each antibody	Ⓐ ▣

MED: 100-2,15,80; 100-3,220.8; 100-4,3,10.4

86243	Fc receptor	Ⓐ

MED: 100-2,15,80; 100-4,3,10.4

To report antibodies to filaria, consult the appropriate code according to the specific method used.

86255	Fluorescent noninfectious agent antibody; screen, each antibody	Ⓐ 80 ▣

MED: 100-2,15,80; 100-4,3,10.4; 100-4,12,60

AMA: 1998,Nov,27

86256	titer, each antibody	Ⓐ 80 ▣

MED: 100-2,15,80; 100-4,3,10.4; 100-4,12,60

To report fluorescent technique for antigen identification in tissue, consult CPT code 88346; for indirect fluorescence, consult CPT code 88347. If a confirmatory test is performed for treponema pallidum, (e.g., FTA), consult CPT code 86781. To report gel (agar) diffusion tests, consult CPT code 86331.

86277	Growth hormone, human (HGH), antibody	Ⓐ

MED: 100-2,15,80; 100-4,3,10.4

86280	Hemagglutination inhibition test (HAI)	Ⓐ

MED: 100-2,15,80; 100-4,3,10.4

To report rubella, consult CPT code 86762. To report antibodies to infectious agents, consult CPT codes 86602-86804. To report hepatitis delta agent, antibody, consult CPT code 86692.

86294	Immunoassay for tumor antigen, qualitative or semiquantitative (eg, bladder tumor antigen)	Ⓐ ✖

MED: 100-2,15,80; 100-4,3,10.4

86300	Immunoassay for tumor antigen, quantitative; CA 15-3 (27.29)	Ⓐ ▣

MED: 100-2,15,80; 100-3,190.29; 100-4,3,10.4

86301	CA 19-9	Ⓐ ▣

MED: 100-2,15,80; 100-3,190.30; 100-4,3,10.4

86304	CA 125	Ⓐ ▣

MED: 100-2,15,80; 100-3,190.28; 100-4,3,10.4

To report measurement of serum HER-2/neu oncoprotein, consult CPT code 83950. For hepatitis delta agent, antibody, consult CPT code 86692.

86308	Heterophile antibodies; screening	Ⓐ ✖

MED: 100-2,15,80; 100-4,3,10.4

To report antibodies to infectious agents, consult CPT codes 86602-86804.

86309	titer	Ⓐ

MED: 100-2,15,80; 100-4,3,10.4

86310	titers after absorption with beef cells and guinea pig kidney	Ⓐ

MED: 100-2,15,80; 100-4,3,10.4

AMA: 1993,Fall,26

To report antibodies to histoplasma, consult CPT code 86698. To report skin testing, consult CPT code 86510. To report antibodies to infectious agents, consult CPT codes 86602-86804. To report human growth hormone antibody, consult CPT code 86277.

86316	Immunoassay for tumor antigen, other antigen, quantitative (eg, CA 50, 72-4, 549), each	Ⓐ ▣

MED: 100-2,15,80; 100-4,3,10.4

AMA: 1999,Dec,10; 1999,Aug,5; 1998,Apr,15; 1996,May,11; 1996,Aug,11

86317	Immunoassay for infectious agent antibody, quantitative, not otherwise specified	Ⓐ ▣

MED: 100-2,15,80; 100-4,3,10.4

AMA: 1997,Nov,30-31

To report immunoassay techniques To report antigens, consult CPT codes 83516, 83518, 83519, 83520, 87301-87450, and 87810-87899. To report particle agglutination procedures, consult CPT code 86403.

86318	Immunoassay for infectious agent antibody, qualitative or semiquantitative, single step method (eg, reagent strip)	Ⓐ ✖

MED: 100-2,15,80; 100-4,3,10.4

86320	Immunoelectrophoresis; serum	Ⓐ 80 ▣

MED: 100-2,15,80; 100-4,3,10.4; 100-4,12,60

86325	other fluids (eg, urine, cerebrospinal fluid) with concentration	Ⓐ 80 ▣

MED: 100-2,15,80; 100-4,3,10.4; 100-4,12,60

86327	crossed (2-dimensional assay)	Ⓐ 80 ▣

MED: 100-2,15,80; 100-4,3,10.4; 100-4,12,60

86329	Immunodiffusion; not elsewhere specified	Ⓐ ▣

MED: 100-2,15,80; 100-4,3,10.4

AMA: 2000,Aug,11

86331	gel diffusion, qualitative (Ouchterlony), each antigen or antibody	Ⓐ ▣

MED: 100-2,15,80; 100-4,3,10.4

86332	Immune complex assay	Ⓐ

MED: 100-2,15,80; 100-4,3,10.4

Ⓖ Modifier 63 Exempt Code   ⊙ Conscious Sedation   + CPT Add-on Code   ⦰ Modifier 51 Exempt Code   ● New Code   ▲ Revised Code

Ⓜ Maternity Edit   Ⓐ Age Edit   ✖ CLIA Waived Test   Ⓐ-Ⓨ APC Status Indicators   ▣ CCI Comprehensive Code   80 Bilateral Procedure

© 2006 Ingenix *(Blue Ink)*   **CPT only © 2006 American Medical Association. All Rights Reserved.** *(Black Ink)*   **Path/Lab — 311**

86334 Immunofixation electrophoresis; serum Ⓐ 80 ▣
MED: 100-2,15,80; 100-4,3,10.4; 100-4,12,60

86335 other fluids with concentration (eg, urine, CSF) Ⓐ 80 ▣
MED: 100-4,3,10.4

86336 Inhibin A Ⓐ
MED: 100-2,15,80; 100-4,3,10.4

86337 Insulin antibodies Ⓐ
MED: 100-2,15,80; 100-4,3,10.4

86340 Intrinsic factor antibodies Ⓐ
MED: 100-2,15,80; 100-4,3,10.4
To report antibodies to leptospira, consult CPT code 86720. To report leukoagglutinins, consult CPT code 86021.

86341 Islet cell antibody Ⓐ
MED: 100-2,15,80; 100-4,3,10.4
AMA: 1994,Summer,6

86343 Leukocyte histamine release test (LHR) Ⓐ
MED: 100-2,15,80; 100-4,3,10.4

86344 Leukocyte phagocytosis Ⓐ ▣
MED: 100-2,15,80; 100-4,3,10.4

86353 Lymphocyte transformation, mitogen (phytomitogen) or antigen induced blastogenesis Ⓐ ▣
MED: 100-2,15,80; 100-3,190.8; 100-4,3,10.4
To report lymphocytes immunophenotyping, consult CPT codes 88182 and 88189 for cytometry and consult CPT codes 88342 and 88346 for microscopic techniques. To report malaria antibodies, consult CPT code 86750.

86355 B cells, total count Ⓐ
MED: 100-4,3,10.4

86357 Natural killer (NK) cells, total count Ⓐ
MED: 100-4,3,10.4

86359 T cells; total count Ⓐ ▣
MED: 100-2,15,80; 100-4,3,10.4
AMA: 1997,Nov,30

86360 absolute CD4 and CD8 count, including ratio Ⓐ ▣
MED: 100-2,15,80; 100-4,3,10.4
AMA: 1997,Nov,30

86361 absolute CD4 count Ⓐ ▣
MED: 100-2,15,80; 100-4,3,10.4
AMA: 1997,Nov,30

86367 Stem cells (ie, CD34), total count Ⓐ
MED: 100-4,3,10.4
To report flow cytometric immunophenotyping for the assessment of potential hematolymphoid neoplasia, consult CPT codes 88184-88189.

86376 Microsomal antibodies (eg, thyroid or liver-kidney), each Ⓐ ▣
MED: 100-2,15,80; 100-4,3,10.4

86378 Migration inhibitory factor test (MIF) Ⓐ ▣
MED: 100-2,15,80; 100-4,3,10.4
To report mitochondrial antibody, liver, consult CPT codes 86255 and 86256. To report mononucleosis, consult CPT codes 86308-86310.

86382 Neutralization test, viral Ⓐ ▣
MED: 100-2,15,80; 100-4,3,10.4

86384 Nitroblue tetrazolium dye test (NTD) Ⓐ ▣
MED: 100-2,15,80; 100-4,3,10.4
To report Ouchterlony diffusion, consult CPT code 86331. To report platelet antibodies, consult CPT codes 86022 and 86023.

86403 Particle agglutination; screen, each antibody Ⓐ
MED: 100-2,15,80; 100-4,3,10.4

86406 titer, each antibody Ⓐ
MED: 100-2,15,80; 100-4,3,10.4
If a pregnancy test is conducted, consult CPT codes 84702 and 84703. If a rapid plasma reagin test (RPR) is conducted, consult CPT codes 86592 and 86593.

86430 Rheumatoid factor; qualitative Ⓐ
MED: 100-2,15,80; 100-4,3,10.4

86431 quantitative Ⓐ
MED: 100-2,15,80; 100-4,3,10.4
If a serologic test is performed to test for syphilis, consult CPT codes 86592 and 86593.

86480 Tuberculosis test, cell mediated immunity measurement of gamma interferon antigen response Ⓐ
MED: 100-4,3,10.4

86485 Skin test; candida Ⓧ ▣TC 80
MED: 100-2,15,80; 100-4,3,10.4; 100-4,4,20.5
To report antibody, candida, consult CPT code 86628.

86490 coccidioidomycosis Ⓧ ▣TC 80
MED: 100-2,15,80; 100-4,3,10.4; 100-4,4,20.5

86510 histoplasmosis Ⓧ ▣TC 80
MED: 100-2,15,80; 100-4,3,10.4; 100-4,4,20.5
To report histoplasma, antibody, consult CPT code 86698.

86580 tuberculosis, intradermal Ⓧ ▣TC 80 ▣
MED: 100-2,15,80; 100-4,3,10.4; 100-4,4,20.5
Heaf test

86586 Unlisted antigen, each Ⓐ ▣
MED: 100-2,15,80; 100-4,3,10.4; 100-4,4,20.5
AMA: 1998,Jul,11

86590 Streptokinase, antibody Ⓐ
MED: 100-2,15,80; 100-4,3,10.4
To report antibodies to infectious agents, consult CPT codes 86602-86804. To report streptolysin O antibody, see antistreptolysin O codes 86060 and 86063.

86592 Syphilis test; qualitative (eg, VDRL, RPR, ART) Ⓐ
MED: 100-2,15,80; 100-4,3,10.4
To report antibodies to infectious agents, consult CPT codes 86602-86804.

Wasserman test

86593 quantitative Ⓐ
MED: 100-2,15,80; 100-4,3,10.4
To report antibodies to infectious agents, consult CPT codes 86602-86804.

To report tetanus antibody, consult 86774. To report Thyroglobulin antibody, consult 86800. To report Thyroglobulin, consult 84432. To report Thyroid microsomal antibody, consult 86376. To report toxoplasma antibody, consult 86777-86778.

Codes 86602-86804 represent qualitative or semiquantitative immunoassays performed by multiple step methods and are used for the detection of antibodies

㉖ Professional Component Only   80/ 80 Assist-at-Surgery Allowed/With Documentation   Unlisted   Not Covered

▣TC Technical Component Only   **MED:** Pub 100/NCD References   **AMA:** CPT Assistant References   ❶-❾ ASC Group   ♂ Male Only   ♀ Female Only

312 — CPT Expert   CPT only © 2006 American Medical Association. All Rights Reserved. *(Black Ink)*   © 2006 Ingenix *(Blue Ink)*

to infectious agents. To report immunoassays by single step method, consult code 86318. Codes for identification of antibodies should be as specific as possible. For example, an antibody to a virus could be coded with increasing specificity for virus, family, genus, species, or type. Sometimes it may be possible to add codes that specifiy the class of immunoglobulin being detected. When multiple tests are done to detect antibodies to organisms classified more precisely than the specificity allowed by the available codes, it is appropriate to separately code each service. For example, a test for antibody to an enterovirus is coded as 86658. Coxsackie viruses are enteroviruses, but there are no codes available for the individual species of enterovirus. If assays are performed for antibodies to coxasackie A and B species, each assay should be reported separately. Similarly, if multiple assays are performed for antibodies of different immunoglobulin classes, each assay should be reported separately. For reporting IgM specific antibodies, such as 86632, when the option is available, report the corrsponding nonspecific code such as 86631 when either an antibody analysis that is not specific for a particular immunoglobulin class or an IgG analysis is performed.

86602   **Antibody; actinomyces**   Ⓐ
> MED: 100-2,15,80; 100-4,3,10.4
> AMA: 1993,Fall,26

86603   **adenovirus**   Ⓐ
> MED: 100-2,15,80; 100-4,3,10.4
> AMA: 1993,Fall,26

86606   **Aspergillus**   Ⓐ
> MED: 100-2,15,80; 100-4,3,10.4
> AMA: 1993,Fall,26

86609   **bacterium, not elsewhere specified**   Ⓐ
> MED: 100-2,15,80; 100-4,3,10.4
> AMA: 1993,Fall,26

86611   **Bartonella**   Ⓐ
> MED: 100-2,15,80; 100-4,3,10.4
> AMA: 1993,Fall,26

86612   **Blastomyces**   Ⓐ
> MED: 100-2,15,80; 100-4,3,10.4
> AMA: 1993,Fall,26
> To report infectious agent/antigen detection, consult CPT codes 87620-87899.

86615   **Bordetella**   Ⓐ
> MED: 100-2,15,80; 100-4,3,10.4
> AMA: 1993,Fall,26

86617   **Borrelia burgdorferi (Lyme disease) confirmatory test (eg, Western Blot or immunoblot)**   Ⓐ
> MED: 100-2,15,80; 100-4,3,10.4
> AMA: 1993,Fall,26

86618   **Borrelia burgdorferi (Lyme disease)**   Ⓐ Ⓧ
> MED: 100-2,15,80; 100-4,3,10.4
> AMA: 1993,Fall,26

86619   **Borrelia (relapsing fever)**   Ⓐ
> MED: 100-2,15,80; 100-4,3,10.4
> AMA: 1993,Fall,26

86622   **Brucella**   Ⓐ
> MED: 100-2,15,80; 100-4,3,10.4
> AMA: 1993,Fall,26

86625   **Campylobacter**   Ⓐ
> MED: 100-2,15,80; 100-4,3,10.4
> AMA: 1993,Fall,26

86628   **Candida**   Ⓐ
> MED: 100-2,15,80; 100-4,3,10.4
> AMA: 1993,Fall,26
> To report a skin test for candida, consult CPT code 86485.

86631   **Chlamydia**   Ⓐ
> MED: 100-2,15,80; 100-4,3,10.4
> AMA: 1993,Fall,26
> To report infectious agent/antigen detection, consult CPT codes 87620-87899.

86632   **Chlamydia, IgM**   Ⓐ
> MED: 100-2,15,80; 100-4,3,10.4
> AMA: 1997,Nov,31; 1993,Fall,26
> To report chlamydia antigen, consult CPT codes 87270 and 87320. To report fluorescent antibody technique, consult CPT codes 86255 and 86256.

86635   **Coccidioides**   Ⓐ
> MED: 100-2,15,80; 100-4,3,10.4
> AMA: 1993,Fall,26
> To report infectious agent/antigen detection, consult CPT codes 87620-87899.

86638   **Coxiella burnetii (Q fever)**   Ⓐ
> MED: 100-2,15,80; 100-4,3,10.4
> AMA: 1993,Fall,26

86641   **Cryptococcus**   Ⓐ
> MED: 100-2,15,80; 100-4,3,10.4
> AMA: 1993,Fall,26

86644   **cytomegalovirus (CMV)**   Ⓐ
> MED: 100-2,15,80; 100-4,3,10.4
> AMA: 1993,Fall,26

86645   **cytomegalovirus (CMV), IgM**   Ⓐ
> MED: 100-2,15,80; 100-4,3,10.4
> AMA: 1993,Fall,26
> To report infectious agent/antigen detection, consult CPT codes 87620-87899.

86648   **Diphtheria**   Ⓐ
> MED: 100-2,15,80; 100-4,3,10.4
> AMA: 1993,Fall,26

86651   **encephalitis, California (La Crosse)**   Ⓐ
> MED: 100-2,15,80; 100-4,3,10.4
> AMA: 1993,Fall,26

86652   **encephalitis, Eastern equine**   Ⓐ
> MED: 100-2,15,80; 100-4,3,10.4
> AMA: 1993,Fall,26

86653   **encephalitis, St. Louis**   Ⓐ
> MED: 100-2,15,80; 100-4,3,10.4
> AMA: 1993,Fall,26

86654   **encephalitis, Western equine**   Ⓐ
> MED: 100-2,15,80; 100-4,3,10.4
> AMA: 1993,Fall,26

86658   **enterovirus (eg, coxsackie, echo, polio)**   Ⓐ
> MED: 100-2,15,80; 100-4,3,10.4
> AMA: 1993,Fall,26
> To report antibodies to trichinella, consult CPT code 86784. To report antibodies to trypanosoma, consult the code appropriate for the specific method used. If skin testing is performed for tuberculosis, consult CPT code 86580. To report viral antibodies, consult the code appropriate for the specific method used.

86663   **Epstein-Barr (EB) virus, early antigen (EA)**   Ⓐ
> MED: 100-2,15,80; 100-4,3,10.4
> AMA: 1993,Fall,26

86664   **Epstein-Barr (EB) virus, nuclear antigen (EBNA)**   Ⓐ
> MED: 100-2,15,80; 100-3,220.8; 100-4,3,10.4
> AMA: 1993,Fall,26

◎ Modifier 63 Exempt Code   ⊙ Conscious Sedation   + CPT Add-on Code   ⊘ Modifier 51 Exempt Code   ● New Code   ▲ Revised Code

Ⓜ Maternity Edit   Ⓐ Age Edit   Ⓧ CLIA Waived Test   Ⓐ-Ⓨ APC Status Indicators   ⒸⒸⒾ CCI Comprehensive Code   50 Bilateral Procedure

© 2006 Ingenix *(Blue Ink)*   **CPT only © 2006 American Medical Association. All Rights Reserved.** *(Black Ink)*   Path/Lab — 313

86665	Epstein-Barr (EB) virus, viral capsid (VCA)	A

MED: 100-2,15,80; 100-4,3,10.4
AMA: 1993,Fall,26

86666	Ehrlichia	A

MED: 100-2,15,80; 100-4,3,10.4
AMA: 1993,Fall,26

86668	Francisella tularensis	A

MED: 100-2,15,80; 100-4,3,10.4
AMA: 1993,Fall,26

86671	fungus, not elsewhere specified	A

MED: 100-2,15,80; 100-4,3,10.4
AMA: 1993,Fall,26

86674	Giardia lamblia	A

MED: 100-2,15,80; 100-4,3,10.4
AMA: 1993,Fall,26

86677	Helicobacter pylori	A

MED: 100-2,15,80; 100-4,3,10.4
AMA: 1993,Fall,26

86682	helminth, not elsewhere specified	A

MED: 100-2,15,80; 100-4,3,10.4
AMA: 1993,Fall,26

86684	Haemophilus influenza	A

MED: 100-2,15,80; 100-4,3,10.4
AMA: 1993,Fall,26

86687	HTLV-I	A

MED: 100-2,15,80; 100-4,3,10.4
AMA: 1993,Fall,26
To report infectious agent/antigen detection, consult CPT codes 87620-87899.

86688	HTLV-II	A

MED: 100-2,15,80; 100-4,3,10.4
AMA: 1993,Fall,26

86689	HTLV or HIV antibody, confirmatory test (eg, Western Blot)	A

MED: 100-2,15,80; 100-3,190.9; 100-3,190.14; 100-4,3,10.4
AMA: 1993,Fall,26

86692	hepatitis, delta agent	A

MED: 100-2,15,80; 100-4,3,10.4
AMA: 1997,Nov,31; 1993,Fall,26
To report hepatitis delta agent, antigen, consult CPT code 87380.

86694	herpes simplex, non-specific type test	A

MED: 100-2,15,80; 100-4,3,10.4
AMA: 1993,Fall,26

86695	herpes simplex, type 1	A

MED: 100-2,15,80; 100-4,3,10.4
AMA: 1993,Fall,26

86696	herpes simplex, type 2	A

MED: 100-2,15,80; 100-4,3,10.4
AMA: 1997,Nov,31; 1993,Fall,26

86698	histoplasma	A

MED: 100-2,15,80; 100-4,3,10.4
AMA: 1993,Fall,26

86701	HIV-1	A ✕

MED: 100-2,15,80; 100-3,190.9; 100-3,190.14; 100-4,3,10.4
AMA: 1993,Fall,26

86702	HIV-2	A

MED: 100-2,15,80; 100-3,190.9; 100-3,190.14; 100-4,3,10.4
AMA: 1993,Fall,26

86703	HIV-1 and HIV-2, single assay	A

MED: 100-2,15,80; 100-3,190.9; 100-3,190.14; 100-4,3,10.4
AMA: 1997,Nov,31; 1993,Fall,26
To report HIV-1 antigen, consult CPT code 87390. To report HIV-2 antigen, consult CPT code 87391. If a confirmatory test is conducted for the HIV antibody, (e.g., Western Blot), consult CPT code 86689.

86704	Hepatitis B core antibody (HBcAb); total	A

MED: 100-2,15,80; 100-4,3,10.4
AMA: 1997,Nov,31-32; 1993,Fall,26

86705	IgM antibody	A

MED: 100-2,15,80; 100-4,3,10.4
AMA: 1997,Nov,31-32; 1993,Fall,26

86706	Hepatitis B surface antibody (HBsAb)	A

MED: 100-2,15,80; 100-3,190.10; 100-4,3,10.4
AMA: 1997,Nov,31-32; 1993,Fall,26

86707	Hepatitis Be antibody (HBeAb)	A

MED: 100-2,15,80; 100-4,3,10.4
AMA: 1997,Nov,31-32; 1993,Fall,26

86708	Hepatitis A antibody (HAAb); total	A

MED: 100-2,15,80; 100-4,3,10.4
AMA: 2000,Jun,11; 1997,Nov,31-32; 1993,Fall,26

86709	IgM antibody	A

MED: 100-2,15,80; 100-4,3,10.4
AMA: 2000,Jun,11; 1997,Nov,31-32; 1993,Fall,26

86710	Antibody; influenza virus	A

MED: 100-2,15,80; 100-4,3,10.4
AMA: 1993,Fall,26

86713	Legionella	A

MED: 100-2,15,80; 100-4,3,10.4
AMA: 1993,Fall,26

86717	Leishmania	A

MED: 100-2,15,80; 100-4,3,10.4
AMA: 1993,Fall,26

86720	Leptospira	A

MED: 100-2,15,80; 100-4,3,10.4
AMA: 1993,Fall,26

86723	Listeria monocytogenes	A

MED: 100-2,15,80; 100-4,3,10.4
AMA: 1993,Fall,26

86727	lymphocytic choriomeningitis	A

MED: 100-2,15,80; 100-4,3,10.4
AMA: 1993,Fall,26

86729	lymphogranuloma venereum	A

MED: 100-2,15,80; 100-4,3,10.4
AMA: 1993,Fall,26

86732	mucormycosis	A

MED: 100-2,15,80; 100-4,3,10.4
AMA: 1993,Fall,26

86735	mumps	A

MED: 100-2,15,80; 100-4,3,10.4
AMA: 1993,Fall,26

86738	mycoplasma	A

MED: 100-2,15,80; 100-4,3,10.4
AMA: 1993,Fall,26

86741	Neisseria meningitidis	A

MED: 100-2,15,80; 100-4,3,10.4
AMA: 1993,Fall,26

86744	Nocardia	A

MED: 100-2,15,80; 100-4,3,10.4
AMA: 1993,Fall,26

---

26 Professional Component Only   80/ 80 Assist-at-Surgery Allowed/With Documentation   Unlisted   Not Covered

TC Technical Component Only   MED: Pub 100/NCD References   AMA: CPT Assistant References   1-9 ASC Group   ♂ Male Only   ♀ Female Only

314 — CPT Expert   CPT only © 2006 American Medical Association. All Rights Reserved. *(Black Ink)*   © *2006 Ingenix (Blue Ink)*

86747	**parvovirus**	Ⓐ

MED: 100-2,15,80; 100-4,3,10.4
AMA: 1993,Fall,26

| 86750 | **Plasmodium (malaria)** | Ⓐ |

MED: 100-2,15,80; 100-4,3,10.4
AMA: 1993,Fall,26

| 86753 | **protozoa, not elsewhere specified** | Ⓐ |

MED: 100-2,15,80; 100-4,3,10.4
AMA: 1993,Fall,26

| 86756 | **respiratory syncytial virus** | Ⓐ |

MED: 100-2,15,80; 100-4,3,10.4
AMA: 1993,Fall,26

| 86757 | **Rickettsia** | Ⓐ |

MED: 100-2,15,80; 100-4,3,10.4
AMA: 1993,Fall,26

| 86759 | **rotavirus** | Ⓐ |

MED: 100-2,15,80; 100-4,3,10.4
AMA: 1993,Fall,26

| 86762 | **rubella** | Ⓐ |

MED: 100-2,15,80; 100-4,3,10.4
AMA: 1993,Fall,26

| 86765 | **rubeola** | Ⓐ |

MED: 100-2,15,80; 100-4,3,10.4
AMA: 1993,Fall,26

| 86768 | **Salmonella** | Ⓐ |

MED: 100-2,15,80; 100-4,3,10.4
AMA: 1993,Fall,26

| 86771 | **Shigella** | Ⓐ |

MED: 100-2,15,80; 100-4,3,10.4
AMA: 1993,Fall,26

| 86774 | **tetanus** | Ⓐ |

MED: 100-2,15,80; 100-4,3,10.4
AMA: 1993,Fall,26

| 86777 | **Toxoplasma** | Ⓐ |

MED: 100-2,15,80; 100-4,3,10.4
AMA: 1993,Fall,26

| 86778 | **Toxoplasma, IgM** | Ⓐ |

MED: 100-2,15,80; 100-4,3,10.4
AMA: 1993,Fall,26

| 86781 | **Treponema pallidum, confirmatory test (eg, FTA-abs)** | Ⓐ |

MED: 100-2,15,80; 100-4,3,10.4
AMA: 1993,Fall,26

| 86784 | **Trichinella** | Ⓐ |

MED: 100-2,15,80; 100-4,3,10.4
AMA: 1993,Fall,26

| 86787 | **varicella-zoster** | Ⓐ |

MED: 100-2,15,80; 100-4,3,10.4
AMA: 1993,Fall,26

● 86788	**West Nile virus, IgM**	Ⓐ
● 86789	**West Nile virus**	Ⓐ
86790	**virus, not elsewhere specified**	Ⓐ

MED: 100-2,15,80; 100-4,3,10.4
AMA: 1993,Fall,26

| 86793 | **Yersinia** | Ⓐ |

MED: 100-2,15,80; 100-4,3,10.4
AMA: 1993,Fall,26

| 86800 | **Thyroglobulin antibody** | Ⓐ |

MED: 100-2,15,80; 100-4,3,10.4
AMA: 1993,Fall,26

To report thyroglobulin, consult CPT code 84432.

| 86803 | **Hepatitis C antibody;** | Ⓐ |

MED: 100-2,15,80; 100-4,3,10.4
AMA: 1997,Nov,31-32; 1993,Fall,26

| 86804 | **confirmatory test (eg, immunoblot)** | Ⓐ |

MED: 100-2,15,80; 100-4,3,10.4
AMA: 1997,Nov,31-32; 1993,Fall,26

TISSUE TYPING

| 86805 | **Lymphocytotoxicity assay, visual crossmatch; with titration** | Ⓐ 🄲 |

MED: 100-2,15,80; 100-4,3,10.4

| 86806 | **without titration** | Ⓐ |

MED: 100-2,15,80; 100-4,3,10.4

| 86807 | **Serum screening for cytotoxic percent reactive antibody (PRA); standard method** | Ⓐ |

MED: 100-2,15,80; 100-4,3,10.4
AMA: 2001,Jun,11

| 86808 | **quick method** | Ⓐ |

MED: 100-2,15,80; 100-4,3,10.4
AMA: 2001,Jun,11

| 86812 | **HLA typing; A, B, or C (eg, A10, B7, B27), single antigen** | Ⓐ |

MED: 100-2,15,80; 100-3,190.1; 100-4,3,10.4

| 86813 | **A, B, or C, multiple antigens** | Ⓐ 🄲 |

MED: 100-2,15,80; 100-3,190.1; 100-4,3,10.4

| 86816 | **DR/DQ, single antigen** | Ⓐ |

MED: 100-2,15,80; 100-3,190.1; 100-4,3,10.4

| 86817 | **DR/DQ, multiple antigens** | Ⓐ 🄲 |

MED: 100-2,15,80; 100-3,190.1; 100-4,3,10.4

| 86821 | **lymphocyte culture, mixed (MLC)** | Ⓐ |

MED: 100-2,15,80; 100-3,190.1; 100-3,190.8; 100-4,3,10.4

| 86822 | **lymphocyte culture, primed (PLC)** | Ⓐ |

MED: 100-2,15,80; 100-3,190.1; 100-3,190.8; 100-4,3,10.4

| 86849 | **Unlisted immunology procedure** | Ⓧ |

MED: 100-2,15,80; 100-4,3,10.4
AMA: 1998,Mar,10

TRANSFUSION MEDICINE

For apheresis, consult CPT code 36511 or 36512. For therapeutic phlebotomy, consult CPT code 99195.

| 86850 | **Antibody screen, RBC, each serum technique** | Ⓧ |

MED: 100-2,15,80; 100-4,3,10.4
AMA: 1993,Fall,25

| 86860 | **Antibody elution (RBC), each elution** | Ⓧ |

MED: 100-2,15,80; 100-4,3,10.4

| 86870 | **Antibody identification, RBC antibodies, each panel for each serum technique** | Ⓧ |

MED: 100-2,15,80; 100-4,3,10.4
AMA: 2001,Mar,10; 1993,Fall,25

| 86880 | **Antihuman globulin test (Coombs test); direct, each antiserum** | Ⓧ |

MED: 100-2,15,80; 100-4,3,10.4

| 86885 | **indirect, qualitative, each antiserum** | Ⓧ |

MED: 100-2,15,80; 100-4,3,10.4

| 86886 | **indirect, titer, each antiserum** | Ⓧ |

MED: 100-2,15,80; 100-4,3,10.4

Pathology and Laboratory

86890 — 87046

86890	**Autologous blood or component, collection processing and storage; predeposited** ☒ ▯
	MED: 100-1,3,20.5.2; 100-2,15,80; 100-3,110.7; 100-3,110.8; 100-4,3,10.4
	AMA: 1996,Apr,2
86891	**intra- or postoperative salvage** ☒ ▯
	MED: 100-1,3,20.5.2; 100-2,15,80; 100-3,110.7; 100-3,110.8; 100-4,3,10.4
	To report physician services to autologous donors, consult CPT codes 99201-99204.
86900	**Blood typing; ABO** ☒
	MED: 100-2,15,80; 100-4,3,10.4
86901	**Rh (D)** ☒
	MED: 100-2,15,80; 100-4,3,10.4
	AMA: 1993,Fall,25
86903	**antigen screening for compatible blood unit using reagent serum, per unit screened** ☒ ▯
	MED: 100-2,15,80; 100-4,3,10.4
86904	**antigen screening for compatible unit using patient serum, per unit screened** ☒
	MED: 100-2,15,80; 100-4,3,10.4
86905	**RBC antigens, other than ABO or Rh (D), each** ☒
	MED: 100-2,15,80; 100-4,3,10.4
86906	**Rh phenotyping, complete** ☒
	MED: 100-2,15,80; 100-4,3,10.4
86910	**Blood typing, for paternity testing, per individual; ABO, Rh and MN** Ⓔ
	MED: 100-2,15,80; 100-4,3,10.4
86911	**each additional antigen system** Ⓔ
	MED: 100-2,15,80; 100-4,3,10.4
86920	**Compatibility test each unit; immediate spin technique** ☒
	MED: 100-2,15,80; 100-4,3,10.4
86921	**incubation technique** ☒
	MED: 100-2,15,80; 100-4,3,10.4
86922	**antiglobulin technique** ☒
	MED: 100-2,15,80; 100-4,3,10.4
86923	**electronic** ☒
	MED: 100-4,3,10.4
	Code 86923 cannot be reported with 86920-86922 for same unit crossmatch.
86927	**Fresh frozen plasma, thawing, each unit** ☒
	MED: 100-2,15,80; 100-4,3,10.4
86930	**Frozen blood, each unit; freezing (includes preparation)** ☒
	MED: 100-2,15,80; 100-4,3,10.4
	AMA: 1996,Apr,2
86931	**thawing** ☒ ▯
	MED: 100-2,15,80; 100-4,3,10.4
86932	**freezing (includes preparation) and thawing** ☒ ▯
	MED: 100-2,15,80; 100-4,3,10.4
86940	**Hemolysins and agglutinins; auto, screen, each** Ⓐ
	MED: 100-2,15,80; 100-4,3,10.4
86941	**incubated** Ⓐ
	MED: 100-2,15,80; 100-4,3,10.4
86945	**Irradiation of blood product, each unit** ☒
	MED: 100-2,15,80; 100-4,3,10.4

86950	**Leukocyte transfusion** ☒ ▯
	MED: 100-1,3,20.5.2; 100-1,3,20.5.3; 100-2,15,80; 100-3,110.5; 100-3,110.7; 100-4,3,10.4
	To report leukapheresis, consult CPT code 36511.
86960	**Volume reduction of blood or blood product (eg, red blood cells or platelets), each unit** ☒
	MED: 100-4,3,10.4
86965	**Pooling of platelets or other blood products** ☒
	MED: 100-2,15,80; 100-3,110.8; 100-4,3,10.4
86970	**Pretreatment of RBCs for use in RBC antibody detection, identification, and/or compatibility testing; incubation with chemical agents or drugs, each** ☒
	MED: 100-2,15,80; 100-4,3,10.4
86971	**incubation with enzymes, each** ☒
	MED: 100-2,15,80; 100-4,3,10.4
86972	**by density gradient separation** ☒
	MED: 100-2,15,80; 100-4,3,10.4
86975	**Pretreatment of serum for use in RBC antibody identification; incubation with drugs, each** ☒
	MED: 100-2,15,80; 100-4,3,10.4
86976	**by dilution** ☒
	MED: 100-2,15,80; 100-4,3,10.4
86977	**incubation with inhibitors, each** ☒
	MED: 100-2,15,80; 100-4,3,10.4
86978	**by differential red cell absorption using patient RBCs or RBCs of known phenotype, each absorption** ☒
	MED: 100-2,15,80; 100-4,3,10.4
86985	**Splitting of blood or blood products, each unit** ☒
	MED: 100-2,15,80; 100-4,3,10.4
	AMA: 1996,Apr,2
86999	**Unlisted transfusion medicine procedure** ☒
	MED: 100-1,3,20.5; 100-1,3,20.5.2; 100-2,15,80; 100-4,3,10.4

MICROBIOLOGY

87001	**Animal inoculation, small animal; with observation** Ⓐ
	MED: 100-2,15,80; 100-4,3,10.4
87003	**with observation and dissection** Ⓐ ▯
	MED: 100-2,15,80; 100-4,3,10.4
87015	**Concentration (any type), for infectious agents** Ⓐ
	MED: 100-2,15,80; 100-4,3,10.4
	CPT code 87015 should not be reported in conjunction with CPT code 87177.
87040	**Culture, bacterial; blood, aerobic, with isolation and presumptive identification of isolates (includes anaerobic culture, if appropriate)** Ⓐ ▯
	MED: 100-2,15,80; 100-4,3,10.4
	AMA: 2002,Jun,1; 1997,Aug,18
87045	**stool, aerobic, with isolation and preliminary examination (eg, KIA, LIA), Salmonella and Shigella species** Ⓐ ▯
	MED: 100-2,15,80; 100-4,3,10.4
87046	**stool, aerobic, additional pathogens, isolation and presumptive identification of isolates, each plate** Ⓐ ▯
	MED: 100-2,15,80; 100-4,3,10.4

☎ Professional Component Only	⁸⁰/ ⁸⁰ Assist-at-Surgery Allowed/With Documentation	Unlisted	Not Covered
☎ Technical Component Only	**MED:** Pub 100/NCD References **AMA:** CPT Assistant References	**1**-**9** ASC Group ♂ Male Only	♀ Female Only

87070   any other source except urine, blood or stool, aerobic, with isolation and presumptive identification of isolates   [A]

MED: 100-2,15,80; 100-4,3,10.4
AMA: 2001,Nov,10; 1997,Aug,18
To report urine, consult CPT codes 87086-87088.

87071   quantitative, aerobic with isolation and presumptive identification of isolates, any source except urine, blood or stool   [A] [C]

MED: 100-2,15,80; 100-4,3,10.4
To report urine, consult CPT codes 87086-87088.

87073   quantitative, anaerobic with isolation and presumptive identification of isolates, any source except urine, blood or stool   [A] [C]

MED: 100-2,15,80; 100-4,3,10.4
To report definitive identification of isolates, consult CPT code 87076 or 87077. To report typing of isolates, consult CPT codes 87140-87158.

87075   any source, except blood, anaerobic with isolation and presumptive identification of isolates   [A]

MED: 100-2,15,80; 100-4,3,10.4

87076   anaerobic isolate, additional methods required for definitive identification, each isolate   [A]

MED: 100-2,15,80; 100-4,3,10.4
To report GLC (gas liquid chromatography) or HPLC (high pressure lipid chromatography) consult CPT code 87143.

87077   aerobic isolate, additional methods required for definitive identification, each isolate   [A] [X]

MED: 100-2,15,80; 100-4,3,10.4
AMA: 2001,Nov,10

87081   Culture, presumptive, pathogenic organisms, screening only;   [A] [C]

MED: 100-2,15,80; 100-4,3,10.4
AMA: 2001,Nov,10

87084   with colony estimation from density chart   [A] [C]

MED: 100-2,15,80; 100-4,3,10.4

87086   Culture, bacterial; quantitative colony count, urine   [A] [C]

MED: 100-2,15,80; 100-3,190.12; 100-4,3,10.4

▲ **87088**   with isolation and presumptive identification of each isolate, urine   [A] [C]

MED: 100-2,15,80; 100-3,190.12; 100-4,3,10.4

87101   Culture, fungi (mold or yeast) isolation, with presumptive identification of isolates; skin, hair, or nail   [A]

MED: 100-2,15,80; 100-4,3,10.4
AMA: 1999,Sep,10

87102   other source (except blood)   [A]

MED: 100-2,15,80; 100-4,3,10.4

87103   blood   [A]

MED: 100-2,15,80; 100-4,3,10.4

87106   Culture, fungi, definitive identification, each organism; yeast   [A] [C]

MED: 100-2,15,80; 100-4,3,10.4
Report CPT code 87106 in addition to CPT codes 87101, 87102 or 87103 when appropriate.

87107   mold   [A]

MED: 100-2,15,80; 100-4,3,10.4

87109   Culture, mycoplasma, any source   [A]

MED: 100-2,15,80; 100-4,3,10.4

87110   Culture, chlamydia, any source   [A]

MED: 100-2,15,80; 100-4,3,10.4
To report immunofluorescence staining of shell vials, consult CPT code 87140.

87116   Culture, tubercle or other acid-fast bacilli (eg, TB, AFB, mycobacteria) any source, with isolation and presumptive identification of isolates   [A]

MED: 100-2,15,80; 100-4,3,10.4

87118   Culture, mycobacterial, definitive identification, each isolate   [A]

MED: 100-2,15,80; 100-4,3,10.4
To report nucleic acid probe identification, consult CPT code 87149. To report GLC or HPLC identification consult CPT code 87143.

87140   Culture, typing; immunofluorescent method, each antiserum   [A] [C]

MED: 100-2,15,80; 100-4,3,10.4
AMA: 2001,Nov,10

87143   gas liquid chromatography (GLC) or high pressure liquid chromatography (HPLC) method   [A] [C]

MED: 100-2,15,80; 100-4,3,10.4

87147   immunologic method, other than immunofluoresence (eg, agglutination grouping), per antiserum   [A] [C]

MED: 100-2,15,80; 100-4,3,10.4
AMA: 2002,Apr,18

87149   identification by nucleic acid probe   [A] [C]

MED: 100-2,15,80; 100-4,3,10.4
AMA: 2001,Nov,10

87152   identification by pulse field gel typing   [A] [C]

MED: 100-2,15,80; 100-4,3,10.4

87158   other methods   [A] [C]

MED: 100-2,15,80; 100-4,3,10.4
AMA: 2001,Nov,10

87164   Dark field examination, any source (eg, penile, vaginal, oral, skin); includes specimen collection   [A] [80] [C]

MED: 100-2,15,80; 100-4,3,10.4; 100-4,12,60

87166   without collection   [A] [C]

MED: 100-2,15,80; 100-4,3,10.4

87168   Macroscopic examination; arthropod   [A] [C]

MED: 100-2,15,80; 100-4,3,10.4

87169   parasite   [A] [C]

MED: 100-2,15,80; 100-4,3,10.4

87172   Pinworm exam (eg, cellophane tape prep)   [A] [C]

MED: 100-2,15,80; 100-4,3,10.4

87176   Homogenization, tissue, for culture   [A]

MED: 100-2,15,80; 100-4,3,10.4

87177   Ova and parasites, direct smears, concentration and identification   [A] [C]

MED: 100-2,15,80; 100-4,3,10.4
Do not report CPT code 87177 in conjunction with CPT code 87015. For coccidia or microsporidia exam, consult CPT code 87207. To report complex special stains including trichrome, iron hematoxylin, consult CPT code 87209. For nucleic acid probes in cytologic material, consult CPT code 88365. For molecular diagnostics, consult CPT codes 83890-83898 and 87470-87799.

To report direct smears from a primary source, consult CPT code 87207.

---

⑥³ Modifier 63 Exempt Code   ⊙ Conscious Sedation   + CPT Add-on Code   ⊘ Modifier 51 Exempt Code   ● New Code   ▲ Revised Code

[M] Maternity Edit   [A] Age Edit   [X] CLIA Waived Test   [A]-[Y] APC Status Indicators   [C] CCI Comprehensive Code   [50] Bilateral Procedure

 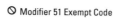

87181 Susceptibility studies, antimicrobial agent; agar dilution method, per agent (eg, antibiotic gradient strip) Ⓐ ▢

MED: 100-2,15,80; 100-4,3,10.4

AMA: 2001,Nov,10

87184 disk method, per plate (12 or fewer agents) Ⓐ ▢

MED: 100-2,15,80; 100-3,190.12; 100-4,3,10.4

AMA: 2001,Nov,10

87185 enzyme detection (eg, beta lactamase), per enzyme Ⓐ ▢

MED: 100-2,15,80; 100-4,3,10.4

AMA: 2001,Nov,10

87186 microdilution or agar dilution (minimum inhibitory concentration (MIC) or breakpoint), each multi-antimicrobial, per plate Ⓐ ▢

MED: 100-2,15,80; 100-3,190.12; 100-4,3,10.4

AMA: 2001,Nov,10

+ 87187 microdilution or agar dilution, minimum lethal concentration (MLC), each plate (List separately in addition to code for primary procedure) Ⓐ

MED: 100-2,15,80; 100-4,3,10.4

AMA: 2001,Nov,10

Note that 87187 is an add-on code and must be used in conjunction with CPT code 87186 or 87188.

87188 macrobroth dilution method, each agent Ⓐ ▢

MED: 100-2,15,80; 100-4,3,10.4

AMA: 2001,Nov,10

87190 mycobacteria, proportion method, each agent Ⓐ

MED: 100-2,15,80; 100-4,3,10.4

To report other mycobacterial susceptibility studies, consult CPT codes 87181, 87184, 87186 87188. For fungal susceptibility studies, consult CPT codes 87181, 87184, 87187 or 87188.

87197 Serum bactericidal titer (Schlicter test) Ⓐ

MED: 100-2,15,80; 100-4,3,10.4

87205 Smear, primary source with interpretation; Gram or Giemsa stain for bacteria, fungi, or cell types Ⓐ ▢

MED: 100-2,15,80; 100-4,3,10.4

87206 fluorescent and/or acid fast stain for bacteria, fungi, parasites, viruses or cell types Ⓐ ▢

MED: 100-2,15,80; 100-4,3,10.4

87207 special stain for inclusion bodies or parasites (eg, malaria, coccidia, microsporidia, trypanosomes, herpes viruses) Ⓐ 80 ▢

MED: 100-2,15,80; 100-4,3,10.4; 100-4,12,60

To report direct smears with concentration and identification, consult CPT code 87177.

For thick smear preparation, consult CPT code 87015. For complex special stains, consult CPT codes 88312 and 88313. For fat, meat, fibers, nasal eosinophils and starch, see Other Procedures section.

Tzank smear

87209 complex special stain (eg, trichrome, iron hemotoxylin) for ova and parasites Ⓐ

MED: 100-4,3,10.4

87210 wet mount for infectious agents (eg, saline, India ink, KOH preps) Ⓐ ▢ ✕

MED: 100-2,15,80; 100-4,3,10.4

To report KOH exam of skin, hair or nails, consult CPT code 87220.

87220 Tissue examination by KOH slide of samples from skin, hair, or nails for fungi or ectoparasite ova or mites (eg, scabies) Ⓐ ▢

MED: 100-2,15,80; 100-4,3,10.4

87230 Toxin or antitoxin assay, tissue culture (eg, Clostridium difficile toxin) Ⓐ

MED: 100-2,15,80; 100-4,3,10.4

87250 Virus isolation; inoculation of embryonated eggs, or small animal, includes observation and dissection Ⓐ

MED: 100-2,15,80; 100-4,3,10.4

87252 tissue culture inoculation, observation, and presumptive identification by cytopathic effect Herpes Ⓐ

MED: 100-2,15,80; 100-4,3,10.4

87253 tissue culture, additional studies or definitive identification (eg, hemabsorption, neutralization, immunofluoresence stain), each isolate Ⓐ ▢

MED: 100-2,15,80; 100-4,3,10.4

To report electron microscopy, consult CPT code 88348. To report inclusion bodies in tissue sections, consult CPT codes 88304-88309; in smears, consult CPT codes 87207-87210; in fluids, consult CPT code 88106.

87254 centrifuge enhanced (shell vial) technique, includes identification with immunofluorescence stain, each virus Ⓐ ▢

MED: 100-2,15,80; 100-4,3,10.4

Report CPT code 87254 in addition to CPT code 87252 as appropriate.

87255 including identification by non-immunologic method, other than by cytopathic effect (eg, virus specific enzymatic activity) Ⓐ ▢

MED: 100-4,3,10.4

87260 Infectious agent antigen detection by immunofluorescent technique; adenovirus Ⓐ ▢

MED: 100-2,15,80; 100-4,3,10.4

87265 Bordetella pertussis/parapertussis Ⓐ ▢

MED: 100-2,15,80; 100-4,3,10.4

AMA: 1997,Nov,32

87267 Enterovirus, direct fluorescent antibody (DFA) Ⓐ ▢

MED: 100-4,3,10.4

87269 Giardia Ⓐ ▢

MED: 100-4,3,10.4

87270 Chlamydia trachomatis Ⓐ ▢

MED: 100-2,15,80; 100-4,3,10.4

AMA: 1997,Nov,32

87271 Cytomegalovirus, direct fluorescent antibody (DFA) Ⓐ ▢

MED: 100-4,3,10.4

87272 cryptosporidium Ⓐ ▢

MED: 100-2,15,80; 100-4,3,10.4

AMA: 1997,Nov,32

87273 Herpes simplex virus type 2 Ⓐ ▢

MED: 100-2,15,80; 100-4,3,10.4

87274 Herpes simplex virus type 1 Ⓐ ▢

MED: 100-2,15,80; 100-4,3,10.4

AMA: 1997,Nov,32

87275 influenza B virus Ⓐ ▢

MED: 100-2,15,80; 100-4,3,10.4

26 Professional Component Only　　　　80/ 80 Assist-at-Surgery Allowed/With Documentation　　　Unlisted　　　Not Covered

TC Technical Component Only　　MED: Pub 100/NCD References　AMA: CPT Assistant References　1-9 ASC Group　♂ Male Only　♀ Female Only

318 — CPT Expert　　　　　CPT only © 2006 American Medical Association. All Rights Reserved. (Black Ink)　　　© 2006 Ingenix (Blue Ink)

87276   influenza A virus   Ⓐ ▣
>MED: 100-2,15,80; 100-4,3,10.4
>AMA: 1997,Nov,32

87277   Legionella micdadei   Ⓐ ▣
>MED: 100-2,15,80; 100-4,3,10.4

87278   Legionella pneumophila   Ⓐ ▣
>MED: 100-2,15,80; 100-4,3,10.4
>AMA: 1997,Nov,32

87279   Parainfluenza virus, each type   Ⓐ ▣
>MED: 100-2,15,80; 100-4,3,10.4

87280   respiratory syncytial virus   Ⓐ ▣
>MED: 100-2,15,80; 100-4,3,10.4
>AMA: 1997,Nov,32

87281   Pneumocystis carinii   Ⓐ ▣
>MED: 100-2,15,80; 100-4,3,10.4

87283   Rubeola   Ⓐ ▣
>MED: 100-2,15,80; 100-4,3,10.4

87285   Treponema pallidum   Ⓐ ▣
>MED: 100-2,15,80; 100-4,3,10.4
>AMA: 1997,Nov,32

87290   Varicella zoster virus   Ⓐ ▣
>MED: 100-2,15,80; 100-4,3,10.4
>AMA: 1997,Nov,32

87299   not otherwise specified, each organism   Ⓐ ▣
>MED: 100-2,15,80; 100-4,3,10.4
>AMA: 2001,Nov,10; 1997,Nov,32

87300   Infectious agent antigen detection by immunofluorescent technique, polyvalent for multiple organisms, each polyvalent antiserum   Ⓐ ▣
>MED: 100-2,15,80; 100-4,3,10.4
>To report physician evaluation of infectious disease agents by immunofluoroescence, consult CPT code 88346.

87301   Infectious agent antigen detection by enzyme immunoassay technique, qualitative or semiquantitative, multiple-step method; adenovirus enteric types 40/41   Ⓐ
>MED: 100-2,15,80; 100-4,3,10.4
>AMA: 1999,Nov,46; 1997,Nov,32

● 87305   Aspergillus   Ⓐ

87320   Chlamydia trachomatis   Ⓐ ▣
>MED: 100-2,15,80; 100-4,3,10.4
>AMA: 1997,Nov,32

87324   Clostridium difficile toxin(s)   Ⓐ ▣
>MED: 100-2,15,80; 100-4,3,10.4
>AMA: 1997,Nov,32

87327   Cryptococcus neoformans   Ⓐ
>MED: 100-2,15,80; 100-4,3,10.4
>To report Cryptococcus latex agglutination, consult CPT code 86403.

87328   cryptosporidium   Ⓐ ▣
>MED: 100-2,15,80; 100-4,3,10.4
>AMA: 1997,Nov,32

87329   giardia   Ⓐ ▣
>MED: 100-4,3,10.4

87332   cytomegalovirus   Ⓐ ▣
>MED: 100-2,15,80; 100-4,3,10.4
>AMA: 1997,Nov,32

87335   Escherichia coli 0157   Ⓐ
>MED: 100-2,15,80; 100-4,3,10.4
>AMA: 1997,Nov,32
>To report Giardia antigen, consult CPT code 87329.

87336   Entamoeba histolytica dispar group   Ⓐ
>MED: 100-2,15,80; 100-4,3,10.4

87337   Entamoeba histolytica group   Ⓐ
>MED: 100-2,15,80; 100-4,3,10.4

87338   Helicobacter pylori, stool   Ⓐ ▣
>MED: 100-2,15,80; 100-4,3,10.4
>AMA: 1999,Nov,46
>To report H. pylori, breath and blood by mass spectrometry, consult CPT codes 83013, 83014. To report H. pylori, liquid scintillation counter, consult CPT code 78267, 78268.

87339   Helicobacter pylori   Ⓐ ▣
>MED: 100-2,15,80; 100-4,3,10.4
>To report H. pylori, breath and blood by mass spectrometry, consult CPT codes 83013, 83014. To report H. pylori, liquid scintillation counter, consult CPT code 78267, 78268.
>
>To report H. pylori, stool, use CPT code 87338.

87340   hepatitis B surface antigen (HBsAg)   Ⓐ ▣
>MED: 100-2,15,80; 100-3,190.10; 100-4,3,10.4
>AMA: 2000,Jan,11; 1997,Nov,32

87341   hepatitis B surface antigen (HBsAg) neutralization   Ⓐ
>MED: 100-2,15,80; 100-4,3,10.4

87350   hepatitis Be antigen (HBeAg)   Ⓐ ▣
>MED: 100-2,15,80; 100-4,3,10.4
>AMA: 1997,Nov,32

87380   hepatitis, delta agent   Ⓐ
>MED: 100-2,15,80; 100-4,3,10.4
>AMA: 1997,Nov,32

87385   Histoplasma capsulatum   Ⓐ
>MED: 100-2,15,80; 100-4,3,10.4
>AMA: 1997,Nov,32

87390   HIV-1   Ⓐ ▣
>MED: 100-2,15,80; 100-3,190.14; 100-4,3,10.4
>AMA: 1997,Nov,32

87391   HIV-2   Ⓐ
>MED: 100-2,15,80; 100-3,190.14; 100-4,3,10.4
>AMA: 1997,Nov,32

87400   Influenza, A or B, each   Ⓐ ▣
>MED: 100-2,15,80; 100-4,3,10.4
>AMA: 2001,Jun,11; 2001,Dec,6

87420   respiratory syncytial virus   Ⓐ
>MED: 100-2,15,80; 100-4,3,10.4
>AMA: 1997,Nov,32

87425   rotavirus   Ⓐ ▣
>MED: 100-2,15,80; 100-4,3,10.4
>AMA: 1997,Nov,32

87427   Shiga-like toxin   Ⓐ
>MED: 100-2,15,80; 100-4,3,10.4

87430   Streptococcus, group A   Ⓐ ▣
>MED: 100-2,15,80; 100-4,3,10.4
>AMA: 1997,Nov,32

87449 Infectious agent antigen detection by enzyme immunoassay technique qualitative or semiquantitative; multiple step method, not otherwise specified, each organism ▲ ↻ ☒

MED: 100-2,15,80; 100-4,3,10.4

AMA: 2001,Nov,10; 2000,Jan,11; 1997,Nov,32

87450 single step method, not otherwise specified, each organism ▲

MED: 100-2,15,80; 100-4,3,10.4

AMA: 1997,Nov,33

87451 multiple step method, polyvalent for multiple organisms, each polyvalent antiserum ▲

MED: 100-2,15,80; 100-4,3,10.4

87470 Infectious agent detection by nucleic acid (DNA or RNA); Bartonella henselae and Bartonella quintana, direct probe technique ▲ ↻

MED: 100-2,15,80; 100-4,3,10.4

AMA: 1997,Nov,33-34

87471 Bartonella henselae and Bartonella quintana, amplified probe technique ▲ ↻

MED: 100-2,15,80; 100-4,3,10.4

AMA: 1997,Nov,33-34

87472 Bartonella henselae and Bartonella quintana, quantification ▲ ↻

MED: 100-2,15,80; 100-4,3,10.4

AMA: 1997,Nov,33-34

87475 Borrelia burgdorferi, direct probe technique ▲ ↻

MED: 100-2,15,80; 100-4,3,10.4

AMA: 1997,Nov,33-34

87476 Borrelia burgdorferi, amplified probe technique ▲ ↻

MED: 100-2,15,80; 100-4,3,10.4

AMA: 1997,Nov,33-34

87477 Borrelia burgdorferi, quantification ▲ ↻

MED: 100-2,15,80; 100-4,3,10.4

AMA: 1997,Nov,33-34

87480 Candida species, direct probe technique ▲ ↻

MED: 100-2,15,80; 100-4,3,10.4

AMA: 1997,Nov,33-34

87481 Candida species, amplified probe technique ▲ ↻

MED: 100-2,15,80; 100-4,3,10.4

AMA: 1997,Nov,33-34

87482 Candida species, quantification ▲ ↻

MED: 100-2,15,80; 100-4,3,10.4

AMA: 1997,Nov,33-34

87485 Chlamydia pneumoniae, direct probe technique ▲ ↻

MED: 100-2,15,80; 100-4,3,10.4

AMA: 1997,Nov,33-34

87486 Chlamydia pneumoniae, amplified probe technique ▲ ↻

MED: 100-2,15,80; 100-4,3,10.4

AMA: 1997,Nov,33-34

87487 Chlamydia pneumoniae, quantification ▲ ↻

MED: 100-2,15,80; 100-4,3,10.4

AMA: 1997,Nov,33-34

87490 Chlamydia trachomatis, direct probe technique ▲ ↻

MED: 100-2,15,80; 100-4,3,10.4

AMA: 1997,Nov,33-34

87491 Chlamydia trachomatis, amplified probe technique ▲ ↻

MED: 100-2,15,80; 100-4,3,10.4

AMA: 1997,Nov,33-34

87492 Chlamydia trachomatis, quantification ▲ ↻

MED: 100-2,15,80; 100-4,3,10.4

AMA: 1997,Nov,33-34

87495 cytomegalovirus, direct probe technique ▲ ↻

MED: 100-2,15,80; 100-4,3,10.4

AMA: 1997,Nov,33-34

87496 cytomegalovirus, amplified probe technique ▲ ↻

MED: 100-2,15,80; 100-4,3,10.4

AMA: 1997,Nov,33-34

87497 cytomegalovirus, quantification ▲ ↻

MED: 100-2,15,80; 100-4,3,10.4

AMA: 1997,Nov,33-34

● **87498** enterovirus, amplified probe technique ▲

87510 Gardnerella vaginalis, direct probe technique ▲ ↻

MED: 100-2,15,80; 100-4,3,10.4

AMA: 1997,Nov,33-34

87511 Gardnerella vaginalis, amplified probe technique ▲ ↻

MED: 100-2,15,80; 100-4,3,10.4

AMA: 1997,Nov,33-34

87512 Gardnerella vaginalis, quantification ▲ ↻

MED: 100-2,15,80; 100-4,3,10.4

AMA: 1997,Nov,33-34

87515 hepatitis B virus, direct probe technique ▲ ↻

MED: 100-2,15,80; 100-4,3,10.4

AMA: 1997,Nov,33-34

87516 hepatitis B virus, amplified probe technique ▲ ↻

MED: 100-2,15,80; 100-4,3,10.4

AMA: 1997,Nov,33-34

87517 hepatitis B virus, quantification ▲ ↻

MED: 100-2,15,80; 100-4,3,10.4

AMA: 1997,Nov,33-34

87520 hepatitis C, direct probe technique ▲ ↻

MED: 100-2,15,80; 100-4,3,10.4

AMA: 1997,Nov,33-34

87521 hepatitis C, amplified probe technique ▲ ↻

MED: 100-2,15,80; 100-4,3,10.4

AMA: 1997,Nov,33-34

87522 hepatitis C, quantification ▲ ↻

MED: 100-2,15,80; 100-4,3,10.4

AMA: 1997,Nov,33-34

87525 hepatitis G, direct probe technique ▲ ↻

MED: 100-2,15,80; 100-4,3,10.4

AMA: 1997,Nov,33-34

87526 hepatitis G, amplified probe technique ▲ ↻

MED: 100-2,15,80; 100-4,3,10.4

AMA: 1997,Nov,33-34

87527 hepatitis G, quantification ▲ ↻

MED: 100-2,15,80; 100-4,3,10.4

AMA: 1997,Nov,33-34

87528 Herpes simplex virus, direct probe technique ▲ ↻

MED: 100-2,15,80; 100-4,3,10.4

AMA: 1997,Nov,33-34

---

26 Professional Component Only   80/ 80 Assist-at-Surgery Allowed/With Documentation   Unlisted   Not Covered

TC Technical Component Only   **MED:** Pub 100/NCD References   **AMA:** CPT Assistant References   1-9 ASC Group   ♂ Male Only   ♀ Female Only

320 — CPT Expert   CPT only © 2006 American Medical Association. All Rights Reserved. (Black Ink)   © 2006 Ingenix (Blue Ink)

87529   Herpes simplex virus, amplified probe
         technique   A C

MED: 100-2,15,80; 100-4,3,10.4

AMA: 1997,Nov,33-34

87530   Herpes simplex virus, quantification   A C

MED: 100-2,15,80; 100-4,3,10.4

AMA: 1997,Nov,33-34

87531   Herpes virus-6, direct probe technique A C

MED: 100-2,15,80; 100-4,3,10.4

AMA: 1997,Nov,33-34

87532   Herpes virus-6, amplified probe technique A C

MED: 100-2,15,80; 100-4,3,10.4

AMA: 1997,Nov,33-34

87533   Herpes virus-6, quantification   A C

MED: 100-2,15,80; 100-4,3,10.4

AMA: 1997,Nov,33-34

87534   HIV-1, direct probe technique   A C

MED: 100-2,15,80; 100-3,190.14; 100-4,3,10.4

AMA: 1997,Nov,33-34

87535   HIV-1, amplified probe technique   A C

MED: 100-2,15,80; 100-3,190.14; 100-4,3,10.4

AMA: 1997,Nov,33-34

87536   HIV-1, quantification   A C

MED: 100-2,15,80; 100-3,190.13; 100-4,3,10.4

AMA: 1997,Nov,33-34

87537   HIV-2, direct probe technique   A C

MED: 100-2,15,80; 100-3,190.14; 100-4,3,10.4

AMA: 1997,Nov,33-34

87538   HIV-2, amplified probe technique   A C

MED: 100-2,15,80; 100-3,190.14; 100-4,3,10.4

AMA: 1997,Nov,33-34

87539   HIV-2, quantification   A C

MED: 100-2,15,80; 100-3,190.13; 100-4,3,10.4

AMA: 1997,Nov,33-34

87540   Legionella pneumophila, direct probe
         technique   A C

MED: 100-2,15,80; 100-4,3,10.4

AMA: 1997,Nov,33-34

87541   Legionella pneumophila, amplified probe
         technique   A C

MED: 100-2,15,80; 100-4,3,10.4

AMA: 1997,Nov,33-34

87542   Legionella pneumophila, quantification A C

MED: 100-2,15,80; 100-4,3,10.4

AMA: 1997,Nov,33-34

87550   Mycobacteria species, direct probe
         technique   A C

MED: 100-2,15,80; 100-4,3,10.4

AMA: 1997,Nov,33-34

87551   Mycobacteria species, amplified probe
         technique   A C

MED: 100-2,15,80; 100-4,3,10.4

AMA: 1997,Nov,33-34

87552   Mycobacteria species, quantification   A C

MED: 100-2,15,80; 100-4,3,10.4

AMA: 1997,Nov,33-34

87555   Mycobacteria tuberculosis, direct probe
         technique   A C

MED: 100-2,15,80; 100-4,3,10.4

AMA: 1997,Nov,33-34

87556   Mycobacteria tuberculosis, amplified probe
         technique   A C

MED: 100-2,15,80; 100-4,3,10.4

AMA: 1997,Nov,33-34

87557   Mycobacteria tuberculosis, quantification A C

MED: 100-2,15,80; 100-4,3,10.4

AMA: 1997,Nov,33-34

87560   Mycobacteria avium-intracellulare, direct probe
         technique   A C

MED: 100-2,15,80; 100-4,3,10.4

AMA: 1997,Nov,33-34

87561   Mycobacteria avium-intracellulare, amplified probe
         technique   A C

MED: 100-2,15,80; 100-4,3,10.4

AMA: 1997,Nov,33-34

87562   Mycobacteria avium-intracellulare,
         quantification   A C

MED: 100-2,15,80; 100-4,3,10.4

AMA: 1997,Nov,33-34

87580   Mycoplasma pneumoniae, direct probe
         technique   A C

MED: 100-2,15,80; 100-4,3,10.4

AMA: 1997,Nov,33-34

87581   Mycoplasma pneumoniae, amplified probe
         technique   A C

MED: 100-2,15,80; 100-4,3,10.4

AMA: 1997,Nov,33-34

87582   Mycoplasma pneumoniae, quantification A C

MED: 100-2,15,80; 100-4,3,10.4

AMA: 1997,Nov,33-34

87590   Neisseria gonorrhoeae, direct probe
         technique   A C

MED: 100-2,15,80; 100-4,3,10.4

AMA: 1997,Nov,33-34

87591   Neisseria gonorrhoeae, amplified probe
         technique   A C

MED: 100-2,15,80; 100-4,3,10.4

AMA: 1997,Nov,33-34

87592   Neisseria gonorrhoeae, quantification A C

MED: 100-2,15,80; 100-4,3,10.4

AMA: 1997,Nov,33-34

87620   papillomavirus, human, direct probe
         technique   A C

MED: 100-2,15,80; 100-4,3,10.4

AMA: 2002,Feb,10; 1997,Nov,33-34

87621   papillomavirus, human, amplified probe
         technique   A C

MED: 100-2,15,80; 100-4,3,10.4

AMA: 1997,Nov,33-34

87622   papillomavirus, human, quantification A C

MED: 100-2,15,80; 100-4,3,10.4

AMA: 1997,Nov,33-34

● 87640   Staphylococcus aureus, amplified probe
            technique   A

● 87641   Staphylococcus aureus, methicillin resistant,
            amplified probe technique   A

Use code 87341 for assays that detect methicillin
resistance and identify Staphylococcus aureus using a
single nuclic acid sequence.

87650   Streptococcus, group A, direct probe
         technique   A C

MED: 100-2,15,80; 100-4,3,10.4

AMA: 1997,Nov,33-34

Pathology and Laboratory

87651 — 88029

87651	Streptococcus, group A, amplified probe technique	Ⓐ ◫

MED: 100-2,15,80; 100-4,3,10.4
AMA: 1997,Nov,33-34

87652	Streptococcus, group A, quantification	Ⓐ ◫

MED: 100-2,15,80; 100-4,3,10.4
AMA: 1997,Nov,33-34

● 87653   Streptococcus, group B, amplified probe technique   Ⓐ

87660   Trichomonas vaginalis, direct probe technique   Ⓐ ◫

MED: 100-4,3,10.4

87797   Infectious agent detection by nucleic acid (DNA or RNA), not otherwise specified; direct probe technique, each organism   Ⓐ ◫

MED: 100-2,15,80; 100-4,3,10.4
AMA: 2001,Nov,10; 1997,Nov,34

87798   amplified probe technique, each organism   Ⓐ ◫

MED: 100-2,15,80; 100-4,3,10.4
AMA: 2001,Nov,10; 1997,Nov,34

87799   quantification, each organism   Ⓐ ◫

MED: 100-2,15,80; 100-4,3,10.4
AMA: 1997,Nov,34

87800   Infectious agent detection by nucleic acid (DNA or RNA), multiple organisms; direct probe(s) technique   Ⓐ ◫

MED: 100-2,15,80; 100-4,3,10.4

87801   amplified probe(s) technique   Ⓐ ◫

MED: 100-2,15,80; 100-4,3,10.4

See codes 87470-87660 for each specific organism nucleic acid detection from a primary source. For detection of specific infectious agents not otherwise specified, report codes 87797, 87798, or 87799 one time for each agent.

87802   Infectious agent antigen detection by immunoassay with direct optical observation; Streptococcus, group B   Ⓐ ◫

MED: 100-2,15,80; 100-4,3,10.4

87803   Clostridium difficile toxin A   Ⓐ ◫

MED: 100-2,15,80; 100-4,3,10.4

87804   Influenza   Ⓐ ◫ ☒

MED: 100-2,15,80; 100-4,3,10.4

87807   respiratory syncytial virus   Ⓐ ◫

MED: 100-4,3,10.4

● 87808   Trichomonas vaginalis   Ⓐ

87810   Infectious agent detection by immunoassay with direct optical observation; Chlamydia trachomatis   Ⓐ ◫

MED: 100-2,15,80; 100-4,3,10.4
AMA: 1998,Jan,6; 1997,Nov,34

87850   Neisseria gonorrhoeae   Ⓐ ◫

MED: 100-2,15,80; 100-4,3,10.4
AMA: 1998,Jan,6; 1997,Nov,34

87880   Streptococcus, group A   Ⓐ ◫ ☒

MED: 100-2,15,80; 100-4,3,10.4
AMA: 1998,Jan,6; 1998,Dec,8; 1997,Nov,34

87899   not otherwise specified   Ⓐ ◫ ☒

MED: 100-2,15,80; 100-4,3,10.4
AMA: 2001,Jun,11

87900   Infectious agent drug susceptibility phenotype prediction using regularly updated genotypic bioinformatics   Ⓐ

MED: 100-4,3,10.4

87901   Infectious agent genotype analysis by nucleic acid (DNA or RNA); HIV 1, reverse transcriptase and protease   Ⓐ ◫

MED: 100-2,15,80; 100-4,3,10.4

To report infectious agent drug susceptiblity phenotype prediction for HIV-1, consult CPT code 87900.

87902   Hepatitis C virus   Ⓐ ◫

MED: 100-2,15,80; 100-4,3,10.4

87903   Infectious agent phenotype analysis by nucleic acid (DNA or RNA) with drug resistance tissue culture analysis, HIV 1; first through 10 drugs tested   Ⓐ ◫

MED: 100-2,15,80; 100-4,3,10.4

+   87904   each additional drug tested (List separately in addition to code for primary procedure)   Ⓐ ◫

MED: 100-2,15,80; 100-4,3,10.4

Note that 87904 is an add-on code and must be used in conjunction with CPT code 87903.

87999   Unlisted microbiology procedure   ☒

MED: 100-2,15,80; 100-4,3,10.4

ANATOMIC PATHOLOGY

POSTMORTEM EXAMINATION

Codes 88000-88099 are used to report physician services only. For services performed by an outside laboratory, append modifier 90.

88000   Necropsy (autopsy), gross examination only; without CNS   Ⓔ

MED: 100-1,5,90.2; 100-2,15,80; 100-2,15,80.1; 100-4,16,10; 100-4,16,10.1; 100-4,16,110.4
AMA: 1993,Fall,26

88005   with brain   Ⓔ

MED: 100-2,15,80
AMA: 1993,Fall,26

88007   with brain and spinal cord   Ⓔ

MED: 100-2,15,80
AMA: 1993,Fall,26

88012   infant with brain   Ⓐ Ⓔ

MED: 100-2,15,80
AMA: 1993,Fall,26

88014   stillborn or newborn with brain   Ⓐ Ⓔ

MED: 100-2,15,80
AMA: 1993,Fall,26

88016   macerated stillborn   Ⓐ Ⓔ

MED: 100-2,15,80
AMA: 1993,Fall,26

88020   Necropsy (autopsy), gross and microscopic; without CNS   Ⓔ

MED: 100-1,5,90.2; 100-2,15,80; 100-2,15,80.1; 100-4,16,10; 100-4,16,10.1; 100-4,16,110.4
AMA: 1993,Fall,26

88025   with brain   Ⓔ

MED: 100-2,15,80
AMA: 1993,Fall,26

88027   with brain and spinal cord   Ⓔ

MED: 100-2,15,80
AMA: 1993,Fall,26

88028   infant with brain   Ⓐ Ⓔ

MED: 100-2,15,80
AMA: 1993,Fall,26

88029   stillborn or newborn with brain   Ⓐ Ⓔ

MED: 100-2,15,80
AMA: 1993,Fall,26

㉖ Professional Component Only	⑧⓪/ ⑧⑥ Assist-at-Surgery Allowed/With Documentation	Unlisted	Not Covered
㊀ Technical Component Only	MED: Pub 100/NCD References AMA: CPT Assistant References	❶-❾ ASC Group ♂ Male Only	♀ Female Only

322 — CPT Expert   CPT only © 2006 American Medical Association. All Rights Reserved. (Black Ink)   © 2006 Ingenix (Blue Ink)

88036 Necropsy (autopsy), limited, gross and/or microscopic; regional [E]

MED: 100-1,5,90.2; 100-2,15,80; 100-2,15,80.1; 100-4,16,10; 100-4,16,10.1; 100-4,16,110.4

AMA: 1993,Fall,26

88037 single organ [E]

MED: 100-2,15,80

AMA: 1993,Fall,26

88040 Necropsy (autopsy); forensic examination [E]

MED: 100-1,5,90.2; 100-2,15,80; 100-2,15,80.1; 100-4,16,10; 100-4,16,10.1; 100-4,16,110.4

AMA: 1993,Fall,26

88045 coroner's call [E]

MED: 100-2,15,80

AMA: 1993,Fall,26

88099 Unlisted necropsy (autopsy) procedure [E]

MED: 100-1,5,90.2; 100-2,15,80; 100-2,15,80.1; 100-4,16,10; 100-4,16,10.1; 100-4,16,110.4

AMA: 1993,Fall,26

CYTOPATHOLOGY

To report cytology specimen collection via mammary duct catheter lavage, consult CPT Category III codes 0046T and 0047T.

88104 Cytopathology, fluids, washings or brushings, except cervical or vaginal; smears with interpretation [X][80][⬛]

MED: 100-2,15,80; 100-4,4,20.5; 100-4,12,60

AMA: 1994,Fall,3; 1991,Spring,6

▲ **88106** simple filter method with interpretation [X][80]

MED: 100-2,15,80; 100-4,4,20.5; 100-4,12,60

AMA: 1994,Fall,3

▲ **88107** smears and simple filter preparation with interpretation [X][80][⬛]

MED: 100-2,15,80; 100-4,4,20.5; 100-4,12,60

AMA: 1994,Fall,3

88108 Cytopathology, concentration technique, smears and interpretation (eg, Saccomanno technique) [X][80][⬛]

MED: 100-2,15,80; 100-4,4,20.5; 100-4,12,60

AMA: 1998,Jan,6; 1997,Nov,34; 1994,Fall,3

To report gastric intubation with lavage, consult CPT codes 89130-89141 and 91055. To report cervical or vaginal smears, consult CPT code 88150-88155. To report x-ray localization, consult CPT code 74340.

88112 Cytopathology, selective cellular enhancement technique with interpretation (eg, liquid based slide preparation method), except cervical or vaginal [X][80][⬛]

MED: 100-4,4,20.5

Code 88112 cannot be reported in conjunction with 88108.

88125 Cytopathology, forensic (eg, sperm) [X][80]

MED: 100-2,15,80; 100-4,4,20.5; 100-4,12,60

88130 Sex chromatin identification; Barr bodies [A]

MED: 100-2,15,80; 100-4,3,10.4

88140 peripheral blood smear, polymorphonuclear drumsticks [A]

MED: 100-2,15,80; 100-4,3,10.4

AMA: 1998,Nov,27-28

To report Guard stain, consult CPT code 88313.

Report 88150-88154 for conventional Pap smears that are examined using the non-Bethesda method.

Report codes 88164-88167 for conventional Pap smears that are examined using the Bethesda method of reporting. Report 88142-88143 for liquid-based specimens processed as thin-layer preparations that are examined using any system of reporting. Report codes 88174-88175 for automated screening of liquid-based specimens. Report 88141 and 88155 in addition to the screening code selected when the additional services are provided. Manual rescreening requires a complete visual reassessment of the entire slide initially screened by either an automated or manual process. A manual review represents an assessment of selected cells or regions of a slide identified by an initial automated review.

88141 Cytopathology, cervical or vaginal (any reporting system), requiring interpretation by physician ♀ [N][26][80][⬛]

MED: 100-2,15,80; 100-3,190.2; 100-3,210.2

AMA: 1999,Nov,46; 1999,May,6; 1999,Jan,11; 1998,Jan,6; 1997,Nov,35

Note that 88141 is an add-on code and must be used in conjunction with 88142-88154, 88164-88167, and 88174-88175.

88142 Cytopathology, cervical or vaginal (any reporting system), collected in preservative fluid, automated thin layer preparation; manual screening under physician supervision ♀ [A][⬛]

MED: 100-2,15,80; 100-3,190.2; 100-3,210.2; 100-4,3,10.4

AMA: 1999,May,6; 1998,Nov,28; 1998,Jan,6; 1997,Nov,34-35

88143 with manual screening and rescreening under physician supervision ♀ [A][⬛]

MED: 100-2,15,80; 100-3,190.2; 100-3,210.2; 100-4,3,10.4

AMA: 1999,May,6; 1998,Nov,28; 1997,Nov,34-35

To report automated screening of automated thin layer prep, consult CPT codes 88174, 88175.

88147 Cytopathology smears, cervical or vaginal; screening by automated system under physician supervision ♀ [A][⬛]

MED: 100-2,15,80; 100-3,190.2; 100-3,210.2; 100-4,3,10.4

AMA: 1999,Nov,46; 1999,May,6; 1999,Jan,1; 1998,Nov,28; 1997,Nov,35

88148 screening by automated system with manual rescreening under physician supervision ♀ [A][⬛]

MED: 100-2,15,80; 100-3,190.2; 100-3,210.2; 100-4,3,10.4

AMA: 1999,Nov,46; 1999,May,6; 1999,Jan,1

88150 Cytopathology, slides, cervical or vaginal; manual screening under physician supervision ♀ [A][⬛]

MED: 100-2,15,80; 100-3,190.2; 100-3,210.2; 100-4,3,10.4

AMA: 1999,May,6; 1998,Nov,28; 1997,Nov,34-35; 1991,Winter,19

88152 with manual screening and computer-assisted rescreening under physician supervision ♀ [A][⬛]

MED: 100-2,15,80; 100-3,190.2; 100-3,210.2; 100-4,3,10.4

AMA: 1999,May,6; 1998,Jan,6; 1997,Nov,35

88153 with manual screening and rescreening under physician supervision ♀ [A][⬛]

MED: 100-2,15,80; 100-3,190.2; 100-3,210.2; 100-4,3,10.4

AMA: 1999,May,6; 1998,Nov,28; 1997,Nov,34-35

---

⑥³ Modifier 63 Exempt Code ⊙ Conscious Sedation + CPT Add-on Code ⊘ Modifier 51 Exempt Code ● New Code ▲ Revised Code

[M] Maternity Edit [A] Age Edit [X] CLIA Waived Test [A]-[Y] APC Status Indicators [⬛] CCI Comprehensive Code [50] Bilateral Procedure

© *2006 Ingenix (Blue Ink)* CPT only © 2006 American Medical Association. All Rights Reserved. *(Black Ink)* Path/Lab — 323

88154 with manual screening and computer-assisted rescreening using cell selection and review under physician supervision ♀ Ⓐ ▣

MED: 100-2,15,80; 100-3,190.2; 100-3,210.2; 100-4,3,10.4

AMA: 1999,May,6; 1998,Nov,28; 1997,Nov,34-35

+ **88155** Cytopathology, slides, cervical or vaginal, definitive hormonal evaluation (eg, maturation index, karyopyknotic index, estrogenic index) (List separately in addition to code(s) for other technical and interpretation services) ♀ Ⓐ ▣

MED: 100-2,15,80; 100-3,190.2; 100-3,210.2; 100-4,3,10.4

AMA: 1999,Nov,46; 1999,May,6; 1998,Nov,28; 1997,Nov,35

Note that 88155 is an add-on code and must be used in conjunction with 88142-88154, 88164-88167, and 88174-88175.

88160 Cytopathology, smears, any other source; screening and interpretation Ⓧ 80 ▣

MED: 100-2,15,80; 100-4,4,20.5; 100-4,12,60

88161 preparation, screening and interpretation Ⓧ 80 ▣

MED: 100-2,15,80; 100-4,4,20.5; 100-4,12,60

AMA: 1997,Aug,18

88162 extended study involving over 5 slides and/or multiple stains Ⓧ 80 ▣

MED: 100-2,15,80; 100-4,4,20.5

If specimen needs to be obtained, consult percutaneous needle biopsy under the individual organ in the Surgery section of the CPT book. For aerosol collection of sputum, consult CPT code 89220. For special stains, consult CPT codes 88312-88314.

88164 Cytopathology, slides, cervical or vaginal (the Bethesda System); manual screening under physician supervision ♀ Ⓐ ▣

MED: 100-2,15,80; 100-3,190.2; 100-3,210.2; 100-4,3,10.4; 100-4,4,20.5

AMA: 1999,May,6; 1998,Nov,28

88165 with manual screening and rescreening under physician supervision ♀ Ⓐ ▣

MED: 100-2,15,80; 100-3,190.2; 100-3,210.2; 100-4,3,10.4; 100-4,4,20.5

AMA: 1999,May,6; 1998,Nov,28

88166 with manual screening and computer-assisted rescreening under physician supervision ♀ Ⓐ ▣

MED: 100-2,15,80; 100-3,190.2; 100-3,210.2; 100-4,3,10.4; 100-4,4,20.5

AMA: 1999,May,6; 1998,Nov,28

88167 with manual screening and computer-assisted rescreening using cell selection and review under physician supervision ♀ Ⓐ ▣

MED: 100-2,15,80; 100-3,190.2; 100-3,210.2; 100-4,3,10.4; 100-4,4,20.5

AMA: 1999,May,6; 1998,Nov,28

88172 Cytopathology, evaluation of fine needle aspirate; immediate cytohistologic study to determine adequacy of specimen(s) Ⓧ 80 ▣

MED: 100-2,15,80; 100-4,4,20.5; 100-4,12,60

AMA: 1998,Dec,8; 1994,Fall,2; 1993,Fall,26

88173 interpretation and report Ⓧ 80 ▣

MED: 100-2,15,80; 100-4,4,20.5; 100-4,12,60

AMA: 1998,Dec,8; 1994,Fall,2; 1993,Fall,26

To report fine needle aspirate, consult CPT codes 10021, 10022.

Codes 88172 and 88173 should not be reported with codes 88333 and 88334 for the same specimen.

88174 Cytopathology, cervical or vaginal (any reporting system), collected in preservative fluid, automated thin layer preparation; screening by automated system, under physician supervision ♀ Ⓐ ▣

MED: 100-4,3,10.4; 100-4,4,20.5

88175 with screening by automated system and manual rescreening or review, under physician supervision ♀ Ⓐ ▣

MED: 100-4,3,10.4; 100-4,4,20.5

To report manual screening, consult CPT codes 88142, 88143.

88182 Flow cytometry, cell cycle or DNA analysis Ⓧ 80 ▣

MED: 100-2,15,80; 100-4,4,20.5; 100-4,12,60

To report tumor morphometry and DNA and ploidy analysis for imaging techniques, consult CPT code 88358.

88184 Flow cytometry, cell surface, cytoplasmic, or nuclear marker, technical component only; first marker Ⓧ TC 80 ▣

MED: 100-4,3,10.4; 100-4,4,20.5

+ **88185** each additional marker (List separately in addition to code for first marker) Ⓧ TC 80

MED: 100-4,3,10.4; 100-4,4,20.5

Note that 88185 is an add-on code and must be used in conjunction with code 88184.

88187 Flow cytometry, interpretation; 2 to 8 markers Ⓧ 26 80 ▣

MED: 100-4,3,10.4; 100-4,4,20.5

88188 9 to 15 markers Ⓧ 26 80 ▣

MED: 100-4,3,10.4; 100-4,4,20.5

88189 16 or more markers Ⓧ 26 80 ▣

MED: 100-4,3,10.4; 100-4,4,20.5

88199 Unlisted cytopathology procedure Ⓧ 80

MED: 100-2,15,80; 100-4,3,10.4; 100-4,4,20.5

To report electron microscopy, consult CPT codes 88348 and 88349.

CYTOGENETIC STUDIES

Report the appropriate modifier when molecular diagnostic procedures are performed to test for oncologic or inherited disorder to specify probe type or condition tested.

For acetylcholinesterase, consult CPT code 82013. For alpha-fetoprotein, serum or amniotic fluid, consult CPT codes 82105 and 82106.

For laser microdissection of cells from tissue sample, consult CPT code 88380.

88230 Tissue culture for non-neoplastic disorders; lymphocyte Ⓐ

MED: 100-2,15,80; 100-3,190.3; 100-3,190.8; 100-4,3,10.4

AMA: 1999,Oct,1; 1998,Nov,29

88233 skin or other solid tissue biopsy Ⓐ

MED: 100-2,15,80; 100-3,190.3; 100-4,3,10.4

AMA: 1999,Oct,1; 1998,Nov,29

88235 amniotic fluid or chorionic villus cells Ⓜ ♀ Ⓐ

MED: 100-2,15,80; 100-3,190.3; 100-4,3,10.4

AMA: 1999,Oct,1; 1998,Nov,29

88237 Tissue culture for neoplastic disorders; bone marrow, blood cells Ⓐ

MED: 100-1,5,90.2; 100-2,15,80; 100-2,15,80.1; 100-3,190.3; 100-4,3,10.4; 100-4,16,10; 100-4,16,10.1; 100-4,16,110.4

AMA: 1999,Oct,1; 1998,Nov,29

26 Professional Component Only   80/ 80 Assist-at-Surgery Allowed/With Documentation   Unlisted   Not Covered

TC Technical Component Only   MED: Pub 100/NCD References   AMA: CPT Assistant References   ❶-❾ ASC Group   ♂ Male Only   ♀ Female Only

324 — CPT Expert   CPT only © 2006 American Medical Association. All Rights Reserved. *(Black Ink)*   © 2006 Ingenix *(Blue Ink)*

Pathology and Laboratory

88154 — 88237

88239   solid tumor   A

MED: 100-2,15,80; 100-3,190.3; 100-4,3,10.4

AMA: 1999,Oct,1; 1998,Nov,29

88240   Cryopreservation, freezing and storage of cells, each cell line   A C

MED: 100-2,15,80; 100-3,190.3; 100-4,3,10.4

AMA: 1999,Oct,1; 1998,Nov,29

To report therapeutic cryopreservation and storage, consult CPT code 38207.

88241   Thawing and expansion of frozen cells, each aliquot   A C

MED: 100-2,15,80; 100-3,190.3; 100-4,3,10.4

AMA: 1999,Oct,1; 1998,Nov,29

To report therapeutic thawing of previous harvest, consult CPT code 38208.

88245   Chromosome analysis for breakage syndromes; baseline Sister Chromatid Exchange (SCE), 20-25 cells   A C

MED: 100-2,15,80; 100-3,190.3; 100-4,3,10.4

AMA: 1999,Oct,1; 1998,Nov,29

88248   baseline breakage, score 50-100 cells, count 20 cells, 2 karyotypes (eg, for ataxia telangiectasia, Fanconi anemia, fragile X)   A C

MED: 100-2,15,80; 100-3,190.3; 100-4,3,10.4

AMA: 1999,Oct,1; 1998,Nov,29

88249   score 100 cells, clastogen stress (eg, diepoxybutane, mitomycin C, ionizing radiation, UV radiation)   A C

MED: 100-2,15,80; 100-3,190.3; 100-4,3,10.4

AMA: 1999,Oct,1; 1998,Nov,29

88261   Chromosome analysis; count 5 cells, 1 karyotype, with banding   A C

MED: 100-2,15,80; 100-3,190.3; 100-4,3,10.4

AMA: 1999,Oct,1; 1998,Nov,29

88262   count 15-20 cells, 2 karyotypes, with banding   A C

MED: 100-2,15,80; 100-3,190.3; 100-4,3,10.4

AMA: 1999,Oct,1; 1998,Nov,29

88263   count 45 cells for mosaicism, 2 karyotypes, with banding   A C

MED: 100-2,15,80; 100-3,190.3; 100-4,3,10.4

AMA: 1999,Oct,1; 1998,Nov,29

88264   analyze 20-25 cells   A C

MED: 100-2,15,80; 100-3,190.3; 100-4,3,10.4

AMA: 1999,Oct,1; 1998,Nov,29

88267   Chromosome analysis, amniotic fluid or chorionic villus, count 15 cells, 1 karyotype, with banding   M ♀ A C

MED: 100-2,15,80; 100-3,190.3; 100-4,3,10.4

88269   Chromosome analysis, in situ for amniotic fluid cells, count cells from 6-12 colonies, 1 karyotype, with banding   M ♀ A C

MED: 100-2,15,80; 100-3,190.3; 100-4,3,10.4

88271   Molecular cytogenetics; DNA probe, each (eg, FISH)   A C

MED: 100-2,15,80; 100-3,190.3; 100-4,3,10.4

AMA: 1999,Oct,1; 1999,Mar,10; 1998,Nov,29

88272   chromosomal in situ hybridization, analyze 3-5 cells (eg, for derivatives and markers)   A C

MED: 100-2,15,80; 100-3,190.3; 100-4,3,10.4

AMA: 1999,Oct,1; 1999,Mar,10; 1998,Nov,29

88273   chromosomal in situ hybridization, analyze 10-30 cells (eg, for microdeletions)   A C

MED: 100-2,15,80; 100-3,190.3; 100-4,3,10.4

AMA: 1999,Oct,1; 1999,Mar,10; 1998,Nov,29

88274   interphase in situ hybridization, analyze 25-99 cells   A C

MED: 100-2,15,80; 100-3,190.3; 100-4,3,10.4

AMA: 1999,Oct,1; 1999,Mar,10; 1998,Nov,29

88275   interphase in situ hybridization, analyze 100-300 cells   A C

MED: 100-2,15,80; 100-3,190.3; 100-4,3,10.4

AMA: 1999,Oct,1; 1999,Mar,10; 1998,Nov,29

88280   Chromosome analysis; additional karyotypes, each study   A C

MED: 100-2,15,80; 100-3,190.3; 100-4,3,10.4

88283   additional specialized banding technique (eg, NOR, C-banding)   A C

MED: 100-2,15,80; 100-3,190.3; 100-4,3,10.4

88285   additional cells counted, each study   A C

MED: 100-2,15,80; 100-3,190.3; 100-4,3,10.4

88289   additional high resolution study   A C

MED: 100-2,15,80; 100-3,190.3; 100-4,3,10.4

AMA: 1999,Oct,1

88291   Cytogenetics and molecular cytogenetics, interpretation and report   M 26 80 C

MED: 100-2,15,80; 100-3,190.3; 100-4,3,10.4

AMA: 1999,Oct,1; 1998,Nov,29

88299   Unlisted cytogenetic study   X 80

MED: 100-2,15,80; 100-3,190.3; 100-4,3,10.4

SURGICAL PATHOLOGY

Codes 88300-88309 include accession, examination, and reporting. Codes 88311-88365 and 88399 are not included and should be reported separately when they are performed.

A specimen is defined as tissue(s) that is submitted for individual and separate attention, requiring individual examination and pathologic diagnosis. Report two or more specimens from the same patient, such as separate biopsies, are reported separately with the appropriate code.

Code 88300 should be reported for any specimen that in the opinion of the examining physician can be correctly diagnosed without microscopic examination. Report 88302 when gross and microscopic examination is performed on a specimen to confirm identification and the absence of disease. CPT code 88304-88309 describe all other specimens requiring gross and microscopic exam, and represent additional ascending levels of physician work. Levels 88302-88309 are specifically defined by the assigned specimen.

If a particular specimen is not defined in the description, report the code that closest reflects the physician work involved as compared to other specimens in that category.

Codes 88302-88309 should not be reported in addition to a specimen that is part of Mohs surgery.

88300   Level I - Surgical pathology, gross examination only   X 80

MED: 100-1,5,90.2; 100-2,15,80; 100-2,15,80.1; 100-4,4,20.5; 100-4,12,60; 100-4,16,10; 100-4,16,10.1; 100-4,16,110.4

AMA: 2000,Sep,10; 1991,Winter,18

⊛ Modifier 63 Exempt Code   ⊙ Conscious Sedation   + CPT Add-on Code   ⊘ Modifier 51 Exempt Code   ● New Code   ▲ Revised Code

M Maternity Edit   A Age Edit   ⊠ CLIA Waived Test   A-Y APC Status Indicators   C CCI Comprehensive Code   50 Bilateral Procedure

Pathology and Laboratory

88302 — 88307

88302 Level II - Surgical pathology, gross and microscopic examination ☒ 🔟

MED: 100-1,5,90.2; 100-2,15,80; 100-2,15,80.1; 100-4,4,20.5; 100-4,12,60; 100-4,16,10; 100-4,16,10.1; 100-4,16,110.4

AMA: 2000,Sep,10; 1991,Winter,18

Appendix, Incidental; Fallopian Tube, Sterilization; Fingers/Toes, Amputation,Traumatic; Foreskin, Newborn, Hernia Sac, Any Location; Hydrocele Sac; Nerve; Skin, Plastic Repair; Sympathetic Ganglion; Testis, Castration; Vaginal Mucosa, Incidental; Vas Deferens, Sterilization

88304 Level III - Surgical pathology, gross and microscopic examination ☒ 🔟 🔁

MED: 100-1,5,90.2; 100-2,15,80.1; 100-4,4,20.5; 100-4,12,60; 100-4,16,10; 100-4,16,10.1; 100-4,16,110.4

AMA: 2000,Sep,10; 1997,Aug,18; 1991,Winter,18; 1991,Spring,2

Abortion, Induced Abscess Aneurysm - Arterial/Ventricular Anus, Tag Appendix, Other than Incidental Artery, Atheromatous Plaque Bartholin's Gland Cyst Bone Fragment(s), Other than Pathologic Fracture Bursa/Synovial Cyst Carpal Tunnel Tissue Cartilage, Shavings Cholesteatoma Colon, Colostomy Stoma Conjunctiva - Biopsy/Pterygium Cornea Diverticulum - Esophagus/Small Intestine Dupuytren's Contracture Tissue Femoral Head, Other than Fracture Fissure/Fistula Foreskin, Other than Newborn Gallbladder Ganglion Cyst Hematoma Hemorrhoids Hydatid of Morgagni Intervertebral Disc Joint, Loose Body Meniscus Mucocele, Salivary Neuroma - Morton's/Traumatic Pilonidal Cyst/Sinus Polyps, Inflammatory - Nasal/Sinusoidal Skin - Cyst/Tag/Debridement Soft Tissue, Debridement Soft Tissue, Lipoma Spermatocele Tendon/Tendon Sheath Testicular Appendage Thrombus or Embolus Tonsil and/or Adenoids Varicocele Vas Deferens, Other than Sterilization Vein, Varicosity

88305 Level IV - Surgical pathology, gross and microscopic examination ☒ 🔟 🔁

MED: 100-1,5,90.2; 100-2,15,80; 100-2,15,80.1; 100-4,4,20.5; 100-4,12,60; 100-4,16,10; 100-4,16,10.1; 100-4,16,110.4

AMA: 2000,Sep,10; 2000,Jul,4; 2000,Dec,15; 1998,Nov,29-30; 1998,Jul,4; 1997,Aug,18; 1992,Winter,17; 1991,Winter,18; 1991,Spring,6

Abortion - Spontaneous/Missed Artery, Biopsy Bone Marrow, Biopsy Bone Exostosis Brain/Meninges, Other than for Tumor Resection Breast, Biopsy, Not Requiring Microscopic Evaluation of Surgical Margins Breast, Reduction Mammoplasty Bronchus, Biopsy Cell Block, Any Source Cervix, Biopsy Colon, Biopsy Duodenum, Biopsy Endocervix, Curettings/Biopsy Endometrium, Curettings/Biopsy Esophagus, Biopsy Extremity, Amputation, Traumatic Fallopian Tube, Biopsy Fallopian Tube, Ectopic Pregnancy Femoral Head, Fracture Fingers/Toes, Amputation, Non-traumatic Gingiva/Oral Mucosa, Biopsy Heart Valve Joint, Resection Kidney, Biopsy Larynx, Biopsy Leiomyoma(s), Uterine Myomectomy - without Uterus Lip, Biopsy/Wedge Resection Lung, Transbronchial Biopsy Lymph Node, Biopsy Muscle, Biopsy Nasal Mucosa, Biopsy Nasopharynx/Oropharynx, Biopsy Nerve, Biopsy Odontogenic/Dental Cyst Omentum, Biopsy Ovary with or without Tube, Non-neoplastic Ovary, Biopsy/Wedge Resection Parathyroid Gland Peritoneum, Biopsy Pituitary Tumor Placenta, Other than Third Trimester Pleura/Pericardium - Biopsy/Tissue Polyp, Cervical/Endometrial Polyp, Colorectal Polyp, Stomach/Small Intestine Prostate, Needle Biopsy Prostate, TUR Salivary Gland, Biopsy Sinus, Paranasal Biopsy Skin, Other than Cyst/Tag/Debridement/Plastic Repair Small Intestine, Biopsy Soft Tissue, Other than Tumor/Mass/Lipoma/Debridement Spleen Stomach, Biopsy Synovium Testis, Other than Tumor/Biopsy/Castration Thyroglossal Duct/Brachial Cleft Cyst Tongue, Biopsy Tonsil, Biopsy Trachea, Biopsy Ureter, Biopsy Urethra, Biopsy Urinary Bladder, Biopsy Uterus, with or without Tubes and Ovaries, for Prolapse Vagina, Biopsy Vulva/Labia, Biopsy

88307 Level V - Surgical pathology, gross and microscopic examination ☒ 🔟 🔁

MED: 100-1,5,90.2; 100-2,15,80; 100-2,15,80.1; 100-4,4,20.5; 100-4,12,60; 100-4,16,10; 100-4,16,10.1; 100-4,16,110.4

AMA: 2000,Sep,10; 2000,Jul,4; 2000,Dec,15; 1999,Jul,10; 1998,Nov,29-30; 1998,Jul,4; 1992,Winter,18; 1991,Winter,18

Adrenal, Resection; Bone - Biopsy/Curettings; Bone Fragment(s), Pathologic Fracture; Brain, Biopsy; Brain/Meninges, Tumor Resection; Breast, Excision of Lesion, Requiring Microscopic Evaluation of Surgical Margins; Breast, Mastectomy - Partial/Simple; Cervix, Conization; Colon, Segmental Resection, Other than for Tumor; Extremity, Amputation, Non-Traumatic; Eye, Enucleation; Kidney, Partial/Total Nephrectomy; Larynx, Partial/Total Resection; Liver, Biopsy - Needle/Wedge; Liver, Partial Resection; Lung, Wedge Biopsy; Lymph Nodes, Regional Resection; Mediastinum, Mass; Myocardium, Biopsy; Odontogenic Tumor; Ovary with or without Tube, Neoplastic; Pancreas, Biopsy; Placenta, Third Trimester; Prostate, Except Radical Resection; Salivary Gland; Sentinel Lymph Node; Small Intestine; Resection, Other than for Tumor; Soft Tissue Mass (except Lipoma) - Biopsy/Simple Excision; Stomach - Subtotal/Total Resection, Other than for Tumor; Testis, Biopsy; Thymus, Tumor; Thyroid, Total/Lobe; Ureter, Resection; Urinary Bladder, TUR; Uterus, with or without Tubes and Ovaries, Other than Neoplastic/Prolapse

---

26 Professional Component Only   **80**/ **80** Assist-at-Surgery Allowed/With Documentation   Unlisted   Not Covered

TC Technical Component Only   MED: Pub 100/NCD References   AMA: CPT Assistant References   **1-9** ASC Group   ♂ Male Only   ♀ Female Only

326 — CPT Expert   CPT only © 2006 American Medical Association. All Rights Reserved. *(Black Ink)*   © 2006 Ingenix *(Blue Ink)*

88309 Level VI - Surgical pathology, gross and microscopic examination ☒ 80 🗗

MED: 100-1,5,90.2; 100-2,15,80; 100-2,15,80.1; 100-4,4,20.5; 100-4,12,60; 100-4,16,10; 100-4,16,10.1; 100-4,16,110.4
AMA: 2000,Sep,10; 2000,Jul,4; 1993,Fall,"2, 26"; 1991,Winter,18; 1991,Spring,2

Bone Resection; Breast, Mastectomy - with Regional Lymph Nodes; Colon, Segmental Resection for Tumor; Colon, Total Resection; Esophagus, Partial/Total Resection; Extremity, Disarticulation; Fetus, with Dissection; Larynx, Partial/Total Resection - with Regional Lymph Nodes; Lung - Total/Lobe/Segment Resection; Pancreas, Total/Subtotal Resection; Prostate, Radical Resection; Small Intestine, Resection for Tumor; Soft Tissue Tumor, Extensive Resection; Stomach - Subtotal/Total Resection for Tumor; Testis, Tumor; Tongue/Tonsil - Resection for Tumor; Urinary Bladder, Partial/Total Resection; Uterus, with or without Tubes&Ovaries, Neoplastic; Vulva, Total/Subtotal Resection

To report fine needle aspiration, consult CPT codes 10021, 10022.

To report evaluation of fine needle aspirate, consult CPT codes 88172, 88173.

+ 88311 Decalcification procedure (List separately in addition to code for surgical pathology examination) ☒ 80

MED: 100-1,5,90.2; 100-2,15,80; 100-2,15,80.1; 100-4,4,20.5; 100-4,12,60; 100-4,16,10; 100-4,16,10.1; 100-4,16,110.4
AMA: 2002,Jun,11; 1998,Jul,4; 1992,Winter,18

+ 88312 Special stains (List separately in addition to code for primary service); Group I for microorganisms (eg, Gridley, acid fast, methenamine silver), each ☒ 80

MED: 100-4,4,20.5; 100-4,12,60
AMA: 2002,Jun,11

+ 88313 Group II, all other, (eg, iron, trichrome), except immunocytochemistry and immunoperoxidase stains, each ☒ 80 🗗

MED: 100-4,4,20.5; 100-4,12,60
AMA: 2002,Jun,11

If immunocytochemistry and immunoperoxidase tissue studies are performed, consult CPT code 88342.

+ 88314 histochemical staining with frozen section(s) ☒ 80

MED: 100-1,5,90.2; 100-2,15,80; 100-2,15,80.1; 100-4,4,20.5; 100-4,12,60; 100-4,16,10; 100-4,16,10.1; 100-4,16,110.4

88318 Determinative histochemistry to identify chemical components (eg, copper, zinc) ☒ 80

MED: 100-4,4,20.5; 100-4,12,60

88319 Determinative histochemistry or cytochemistry to identify enzyme constituents, each ☒ 80

MED: 100-4,4,20.5; 100-4,12,60

88321 Consultation and report on referred slides prepared elsewhere ☒ 80 🗗

MED: 100-4,4,20.5; 100-4,12,60
AMA: 2002,Dec,10; 2000,Oct,7; 1997,Apr,9; 1991,Winter,19

88323 Consultation and report on referred material requiring preparation of slides ☒ 80 🗗

MED: 100-4,4,20.5; 100-4,12,60
AMA: 2000,Oct,7; 1997,Apr,9; 1991,Winter,19

88325 Consultation, comprehensive, with review of records and specimens, with report on referred material ☒ 80 🗗

MED: 100-4,4,20.5; 100-4,12,60
AMA: 1997,Apr,9; 1991,Winter,19

88329 Pathology consultation during surgery; ☒ 80 🗗

MED: 100-4,4,20.5; 100-4,12,60
AMA: 1997,Aug,18; 1997,Apr,12; 1991,Winter,19

88331 first tissue block, with frozen section(s), single specimen ☒ 80 🗗

MED: 100-1,5,90.2; 100-2,15,80; 100-2,15,80.1; 100-4,4,20.5; 100-4,12,60; 100-4,16,10; 100-4,16,10.1; 100-4,16,110.4
AMA: 2002,Nov,5; 2000,Jul,4; 1997,Aug,18; 1997,Apr,12; 1991,Winter,19; 1991,Spring,2

88332 each additional tissue block with frozen section(s) ☒ 80 🗗

MED: 100-1,5,90.2; 100-2,15,80; 100-2,15,80.1; 100-4,4,20.5; 100-4,12,60; 100-4,16,10; 100-4,16,10.1; 100-4,16,110.4
AMA: 2000,Jul,4; 1997,Aug,18; 1997,Apr,12; 1991,Winter,19

88333 cytologic examination (eg, touch prep, squash prep), initial site ☒ 80

MED: 100-4,4,20.5

88334 cytologic examination (eg, touch prep, squash prep), each additional site ☒ 80

MED: 100-4,4,20.5

To report an intraoperative consultation on a specimen that requires both a frozen section and a cytologic evaluation, consult CPT codes 88331 and 88334.

To report a percutaneous needle biopsy that requires an intraprocedural cytologic examination, consult CPT code 88333.

Codes 88333 and 88334 cannot be reported for non-intraoperative cytologic examination; consult CPT codes 88160-88162.

Codes 88333 and 88334 cannot be reported for intraprocedural cytologic evaluation of fine needle aspirate; consult code 88172.

88342 Immunohistochemistry (including tissue immunoperoxidase), each antibody ☒ 80 🗗

MED: 100-4,4,20.5; 100-4,12,60
AMA: 2002,Nov,5; 2000,Jul,10

Code 88342 cannot be reported with CPT code 88360 or 88361 for the same antibody.

To report quantitative or semiquantitative immunohistochemistry, consult CPT codes 88360 and 88361.

88346 Immunofluorescent study, each antibody; direct method ☒ 80

MED: 100-4,4,20.5; 100-4,12,60

88347 indirect method ☒ 80

MED: 100-4,4,20.5; 100-4,12,60

88348 Electron microscopy; diagnostic ☒ 80 🗗

MED: 100-3,190.4; 100-4,4,20.5; 100-4,12,60

88349 scanning ☒ 80

MED: 100-3,190.4; 100-4,4,20.5; 100-4,12,60

88355 Morphometric analysis; skeletal muscle ☒ 80 🗗

MED: 100-4,4,20.5; 100-4,12,60

88356 nerve ☒ 80 🗗

MED: 100-4,4,20.5; 100-4,12,60

88358 tumor (eg, DNA ploidy) ☒ 80 🗗

MED: 100-4,4,20.5; 100-4,12,60
AMA: 2002,Jun,11; 1999,Jul,11; 1998,Jul,4

Code 88358 should not be reported with 88313 unless each procedure is for a different special stain.

88360   Morphometric analysis, tumor immunohistochemistry (eg, Her-2/neu, estrogen receptor/progesterone receptor), quantitative or semiquantitative, each antibody; manual   Ⓧ 80 ▱

88361   using computer-assisted technology   Ⓧ 80 ▱

Codes 88360 and 88361 should not be reported with 88342 unless each procedure is for a different antibody.

To report morphometric analysis in situ hybridization, consult CPT codes 88367and 88368.

If semi-thin plastic-embedded sections are performed with morphometric analysis, only the analysis should be reported; if performed as an independent procedure, consult CPT codes 88300-88309.

88362   Nerve teasing preparations   Ⓧ 80 ▱
     MED: 100-4,4,20.5; 100-4,12,60

88365   In situ hybridization (eg, FISH), each probe   Ⓧ 80 ▱
     MED: 100-4,4,20.5
     AMA: 2002,Jun,11
Code 88365 cannot be reported with CPT codes 88367, 88368, for the same probe.

88367   Morphometric analysis, in situ hybridization, (quantitative or semi-quantitative) each probe; using computer-assisted technology   Ⓧ 80 ▱

88368   manual   Ⓧ 80 ▱

88371   Protein analysis of tissue by Western Blot, with interpretation and report;   Ⓐ 80 ▱
     MED: 100-3,190.8

88372   immunological probe for band identification, each   Ⓐ 80 ▱
     MED: 100-3,190.8; 100-4,12,60

88380   Microdissection (eg, mechanical, laser capture)   Ⓝ 80
     AMA: 2002,Apr,17

88384   Array-based evaluation of multiple molecular probes; 11 through 50 probes   Ⓧ 80

88385   51 through 250 probes   Ⓧ 80

88386   251 through 500 probes   Ⓧ 80

To report preparation of array-based evaluation, consult CPT codes 83890-83892, 83898-83901.

To report preparation and analyses of less than 11 probes, consult codes 83890-83914.

88399   Unlisted surgical pathology procedure   Ⓧ 80
     MED: 100-1,5,90.2; 100-2,15,80; 100-2,15,80.1; 100-4,4,20.5; 100-4,16,10; 100-4,16,10.1; 100-4,16,110.4

TRANSCUTANEOUS PROCEDURES

88400   Bilirubin, total, transcutaneous   Ⓐ ▱
     MED: 100-4,3,10.4

OTHER PROCEDURES

89049   Caffeine halothane contracture test (CHCT) for malignant hyperthermia susceptibility, including interpretation and report   Ⓧ 80
     MED: 100-4,3,10.4

89050   Cell count, miscellaneous body fluids (eg, cerebrospinal fluid, joint fluid), except blood;   Ⓐ ▱
     MED: 100-2,15,80; 100-4,3,10.4

89051   with differential count   Ⓐ ▱
     MED: 100-2,15,80; 100-4,3,10.4

89055   Leukocyte assessment, fecal, qualitative or semiquantitative   Ⓐ
     MED: 100-4,3,10.4

▲ 89060   Crystal identification by light microscopy with or without polarizing lens analysis, tissue or any body fluid (except urine)   Ⓐ 80 ▱
     MED: 100-2,15,80; 100-4,3,10.4; 100-4,12,60
Do not report 89060 for crystal identification on paraffin-embedded tissue.

89100   Duodenal intubation and aspiration; single specimen (eg, simple bile study or afferent loop culture) plus appropriate test procedure   Ⓧ 80 ▱
     MED: 100-4,3,10.4

89105   collection of multiple fractional specimens with pancreatic or gallbladder stimulation, single or double lumen tube   Ⓧ 80 ▱
     MED: 100-4,3,10.4

To report radiological localization, consult CPT code 74340. If chemical analyses are necessary, consult the Chemistry section of the CPT book. If an electrocardiogram is performed, consult CPT codes 93000-93268. If an esophagus acid perfusion test (Bernstein) is performed, consult CPT code 91030.

89125   Fat stain, feces, urine, or respiratory secretions   Ⓐ ▱
     MED: 100-4,3,10.4

89130   Gastric intubation and aspiration, diagnostic, each specimen, for chemical analyses or cytopathology;   Ⓧ 80 ▱
     MED: 100-4,3,10.4

89132   after stimulation   Ⓧ 80 ▱
     MED: 100-4,3,10.4

89135   Gastric intubation, aspiration, and fractional collections (eg, gastric secretory study); one hour   Ⓧ 80 ▱
     MED: 100-4,3,10.4

89136   two hours   Ⓧ 80 ▱
     MED: 100-4,3,10.4

89140   two hours including gastric stimulation (eg, histalog, pentagastrin)   Ⓧ 80 ▱
     MED: 100-4,3,10.4

89141   three hours, including gastric stimulation   Ⓧ 80 ▱
     MED: 100-4,3,10.4

To report gastric lavage, therapeutic, consult CPT code 91105. To report radiologic localization of a gastric tube, consult CPT code 74340. If chemical analyses are necessary, consult CPT codes 82926 and 82928. To report joint fluid chemistry, consult the Chemistry section of the CPT book.

89160   Meat fibers, feces   Ⓐ ▱
     MED: 100-4,3,10.4

89190   Nasal smear for eosinophils   Ⓐ ▱
     MED: 100-4,3,10.4
To report occult blood, feces, consult CPT code 82270.

To report paternity tests, consult CPT code 86910.

89220   Sputum, obtaining specimen, aerosol induced technique (separate procedure)   Ⓧ ⓉⒸ 80
     MED: 100-4,3,10.4

89225   Starch granules, feces   Ⓐ ▱
     MED: 100-4,3,10.4

89230	**Sweat collection by iontophoresis**	☒ ☒ 80 ☒

MED: 100-4,3,10.4

89235	**Water load test**	☒ ☒

MED: 100-4,3,10.4

89240	**Unlisted miscellaneous pathology test**	☒ 80

MED: 100-4,3,10.4

If necessary to report basal metabolic rate, use CPT code 89240.

REPRODUCTIVE MEDICINE PROCEDURES

89250	**Culture of oocyte(s)/embryo(s), less than 4 days;**	♀ ☒

MED: 100-4,3,10.4

AMA: 1998,Oct,1; 1998,Jan,6; 1997,Nov,35-36

89251	**with co-culture of oocyte(s)/embryos**	♀ ☒ ☒

MED: 100-4,3,10.4

AMA: 1998,Oct,1; 1998,Jan,6; 1997,Nov,35-36
To report extended culture of oocyte(s)/embryo(s), consult CPT code 89272.

89253	**Assisted embryo hatching, microtechniques (any method)**	☒

MED: 100-4,3,10.4

AMA: 1998,Oct,1; 1998,Jan,6; 1997,Nov,35-36

89254	**Oocyte identification from follicular fluid**	♀ ☒

MED: 100-4,3,10.4

AMA: 1998,Oct,1; 1998,Jan,6; 1997,Nov,35-36

89255	**Preparation of embryo for transfer (any method)**	☒

MED: 100-4,3,10.4

AMA: 1998,Oct,1; 1998,Jan,6; 1997,Nov,35-36

89257	**Sperm identification from aspiration (other than seminal fluid)**	☒ ☒

MED: 100-4,3,10.4

AMA: 1998,Oct,1; 1998,Nov,30; 1998,Jan,6; 1997,Nov,35-36
If semen is analyzed, consult CPT codes 89300-89320. If sperm is identified from testis tissue, consult CPT code 89264.

89258	**Cryopreservation; embryo(s)**	☒

MED: 100-4,3,10.4

AMA: 1998,Oct,1; 1998,Jan,6; 1997,Nov,36

89259	**sperm**	☒

MED: 100-4,3,10.4

AMA: 1998,Oct,1; 1998,Jan,6; 1997,Nov,36
To report cryopreservation of reproductive tissue, testicular, consult CPT code 89335.

To report cryopreservation of reproductive tissue, ovarian, consult CPT Category III code 0058T.

To report cryopreservation of oocyte(s), consult CPT Category III code 0059T.

89260	**Sperm isolation; simple prep (eg, sperm wash and swim-up) for insemination or diagnosis with semen analysis**	☒ ☒

MED: 100-4,3,10.4

AMA: 1998,Jan,6; 1998,Oct,1; 1997,Nov,36

89261	**complex prep (eg, Percoll gradient, albumin gradient) for insemination or diagnosis with semen analysis**	☒ ☒

MED: 100-4,3,10.4

AMA: 1998,Oct,1; 1998,Jan,6; 1997,Nov,36
If semen is analyzed without sperm wash or swim-up, consult CPT code 89320.

89264	**Sperm identification from testis tissue, fresh or cryopreserved**	☒ ☒

MED: 100-4,3,10.4

AMA: 1998,Nov,30
If the testis is biopsied, consult CPT codes 54500 and 54505. If sperm is identified from aspiration, consult CPT code 89257. If semen is analyzed, consult CPT codes 89300-89320.

89268	**Insemination of oocytes**	♀ ☒

MED: 100-4,3,10.4

89272	**Extended culture of oocyte(s)/embryo(s), 4-7 days**	♀ ☒

MED: 100-4,3,10.4

89280	**Assisted oocyte fertilization, microtechnique; less than or equal to 10 oocytes**	♀ ☒

MED: 100-4,3,10.4

89281	**Assisted oocyte fertilization, microtechnique; greater than 10 oocytes**	♀ ☒

MED: 100-4,3,10.4

89290	**Biopsy, oocyte polar body or embryo blastomere, microtechnique (for pre-implantation genetic diagnosis); less than or equal to 5 embryos**	♀ ☒

MED: 100-4,3,10.4

89291	**Biopsy, oocyte polar body or embryo blastomere, microtechnique (for pre-implantation genetic diagnosis); greater than 5 embryos**	♀ ☒

MED: 100-4,3,10.4

89300	**Semen analysis; presence and/or motility of sperm including Huhner test (post coital)**	☒ ☒ ☒

MED: 100-2,15,20.1; 100-4,3,10.4

AMA: 1998,Oct,1; 1998,Jul,10; 1997,Nov,36

89310	**motility and count (not including Huhner test)**	☒ ☒

MED: 100-2,15,20.1; 100-4,3,10.4

89320	**complete (volume, count, motility and differential)**	☒ ☒

MED: 100-2,15,20.1; 100-4,3,10.4

To report skin tests, consult CPT codes 86485-86585 and 95010-95199.

89321	**Semen analysis, presence and/or motility of sperm**	☒ ☒

MED: 100-2,15,20.1; 100-4,3,10.4

To report Hyaluronan binding assay (HBA), consult Category III code 0087T.

89325	**Sperm antibodies**	☒ ☒

MED: 100-2,15,20.1; 100-4,3,10.4

To report medicolegal identification of sperm, consult CPT code 88125.

89329	**Sperm evaluation; hamster penetration test**	☒ ☒

MED: 100-4,3,10.4

89330	**cervical mucus penetration test, with or without spinnbarkeit test**	☒ ☒

MED: 100-4,3,10.4

㊿ Modifier 63 Exempt Code	⊙ Conscious Sedation	+ CPT Add-on Code

⊘ Modifier 51 Exempt Code   ● New Code   ▲ Revised Code

ⓜ Maternity Edit   Ⓐ Age Edit   ☒ CLIA Waived Test   Ⓐ-Ⓨ APC Status Indicators   ☒ CCI Comprehensive Code   50 Bilateral Procedure

89335   **Cryopreservation, reproductive tissue, testicular**   ☒

MED: 100-4,3,10.4

To report cryopreservation of embryo(s), consult CPT code 89258. To report cryopreservation of sperm, consult CPT code 89259.

To report cryopreservation of reproductive tissue, ovarian, consult CPT Category III code 0058T.

To report cryopreservation of oocyte(s), consult CPT Category III code 0059T.

89342   **Storage, (per year); embryo(s)**   ☒

MED: 100-4,3,10.4

89343   **sperm/semen**   ☒

MED: 100-4,3,10.4

89344   **reproductive tissue, testicular/ovarian**   ☒

MED: 100-4,3,10.4

89346   **oocyte(s)**   ♀ ☒

MED: 100-4,3,10.4

89352   **Thawing of cryopreserved; embryo(s)**   ☒

MED: 100-4,3,10.4

89353   **sperm/semen, each aliquot**   ☒

MED: 100-4,3,10.4

89354   **reproductive tissue, testicular/ovarian**   ☒

MED: 100-4,3,10.4

89356   **oocytes, each aliquot**   ☒

MED: 100-4,3,10.4

26 Professional Component Only   80/ 80 Assist-at-Surgery Allowed/With Documentation   Unlisted   Not Covered

TC Technical Component Only   MED: Pub 100/NCD References   AMA: CPT Assistant References   1-9 ASC Group   ♂ Male Only   ♀ Female Only

330 — CPT Expert   CPT only © 2006 American Medical Association. All Rights Reserved. *(Black Ink)*   © 2006 Ingenix *(Blue Ink)*

Medicine

CODING INFORMATION

ORGANIZATION

The medicine section (90281–99602) follows the pathology and laboratory section. The diagnostic and therapeutic services include immunizations, injections, specialty-specific codes, and special services.

Subsections within the medicine section are:

- Immune Globulins
- Immunization Administration for Vaccines/Toxoids
- Vaccines/Toxoids
- Hydration, Therapeutic, Prophylactic, and Diagnostic Injections and Infusions
- Psychiatry
- Dialysis
- Ophthalmology
- Special Otorhinolaryngologic Services
- Noninvasive Vascular Diagnostic Studies
- Echocardiography
- Cardiac Catheterization
- Intracardiac Electrophysiological Procedures/Studies
- Peripheral Arterial Disease Rehabilitation
- Cerebrovascular Arterial Studies
- Pulmonary
- Routine Electroencephalography (EEG)
- Electromyography and Nerve Conduction Tests
- Neurostimulators
- Functional Brain Mapping
- Medical Genetics and Genetic Counseling Services
- Central Nervous System Assessments and Tests
- Health and Behavior Assessment/Interventions
- Chemotherapy Administration
- Special Dermatological Procedures
- Physical Medicine and Rehabilitation
- Acupuncture
- Osteopathic Manipulative Treatment

- Chiropractic Manipulative Treatment
- Education and Training for Patient Self-Management
- Special Services, Procedures and Reports
- Moderate (Conscious) Sedation
- Home Health Procedures/Services
- Allergy and Clinical Immunology
- Neurology and Neuromuscular Procedures
- Health and Behavior Assessment/Intervention
- Chemotherapy Administration
- Photodynamic Therapy
- Special Dermatological Procedures
- Physical Medicine and Rehabilitation
- Medical Nutrition Therapy
- Osteopathic Manipulative Treatment
- Chiropractic Manipulative Treatment
- Special Services, Procedures and Reports
- Qualifying Circumstances for Anesthesia
- Sedation with or without Analgesia (Conscious Sedation)
- Other Services and Procedures
- Home Health Procedures/Services
- Home Infusion Procedures

RESULTS/TESTING/REPORTS

Results indicate the technical component of a procedure or service. Testing is the service that leads to the report and interpretation. Reports provide interpretation of the tests.

GUIDELINES

BUNDLED MEDICINE CODES

The process of coding integral services separately from a procedure or bundled service is called unbundling or fragmenting. If the component is considered part of the package or bundled service, do not code it individually. For example, 93015 includes all the components of a stress test and should be reported as such when the complete procedure is performed. If the components 93016, 93017 and 93018 are reported separately instead of the complete test (93015), the payer may rebundle the codes and reimburse for 93015. However, the payer may also simply deny the entire claim. It is important that you report only the services actually provided.

Medicine

90281 — 90471

IMMUNE GLOBULINS

Immune globulin codes (90281-90399) report only the supply of the immune globulin product that includes broad-spectrum and anti-infective immune globulins, antitoxins, and various other isoantibodies. Administration is reported separately with codes 90765-90768, 90772, 90774, 90775.

⊘ **90281** **Immune globulin (Ig), human, for intramuscular use** E
   MED: 100-2,15,50; 100-4,4,20.5
   AMA: 1999,Sep,10; 1999,Jan,1; 1998,Nov,30

⊘ **90283** **Immune globulin (IgIV), human, for intravenous use** E
   MED: 100-2,15,50; 100-4,4,20.5
   AMA: 1999,Jan,1; 1998,Nov,30

⊘ **90287** **Botulinum antitoxin, equine, any route** E
   MED: 100-2,15,50; 100-4,4,20.5
   AMA: 1999,Jan,1; 1998,Nov,30

⊘ **90288** **Botulism immune globulin, human, for intravenous use** E
   MED: 100-2,15,50; 100-4,4,20.5
   AMA: 1999,Jan,1; 1998,Nov,30

⊘ **90291** **Cytomegalovirus immune globulin (CMV-IgIV), human, for intravenous use** E
   MED: 100-2,15,50; 100-4,4,20.5
   AMA: 1999,Jan,1; 1998,Nov,30

⊘ **90296** **Diphtheria antitoxin, equine, any route** N
   MED: 100-2,15,50; 100-4,4,20.5
   AMA: 1999,Jan,1; 1998,Nov,30

⊘ **90371** **Hepatitis B immune globulin (HBIg), human, for intramuscular use** K
   MED: 100-2,15,50; 100-4,4,20.5; 100-4,4,230.1
   AMA: 1999,Jan,1; 1998,Nov,30

⊘ **90375** **Rabies immune globulin (RIg), human, for intramuscular and/or subcutaneous use** K ↵
   MED: 100-2,15,50; 100-4,4,20.5
   AMA: 1999,Jan,1; 1998,Nov,30

⊘ **90376** **Rabies immune globulin, heat-treated (RIg-HT), human, for intramuscular and/or subcutaneous use** K
   MED: 100-2,15,50; 100-4,4,20.5
   AMA: 1999,Jan,1; 1998,Nov,30

⊘ **90378** **Respiratory syncytial virus immune globulin (RSV-IgIM), for intramuscular use, 50 mg, each** E ↵
   MED: 100-2,15,50; 100-2,16,90; 100-4,4,20.5
   AMA: 1999,Jan,1; 1998,Nov,30

⊘ **90379** **Respiratory syncytial virus immune globulin (RSV-IgIV), human, for intravenous use** E
   MED: 100-2,15,50; 100-2,16,90; 100-4,4,20.5
   AMA: 1999,Jan,1; 1998,Nov,30

⊘ **90384** **Rho(D) immune globulin (RhIg), human, full-dose, for intramuscular use** E
   MED: 100-2,15,50; 100-4,4,20.5
   AMA: 1999,Jan,1; 1998,Nov,30

⊘ **90385** **Rho(D) immune globulin (RhIg), human, mini-dose, for intramuscular use** N
   MED: 100-2,15,50; 100-4,4,20.5
   AMA: 1999,Jan,1; 1998,Nov,30

⊘ **90386** **Rho(D) immune globulin (RhIgIV), human, for intravenous use** E
   MED: 100-2,15,50; 100-4,4,20.5
   AMA: 1999,Jan,1; 1998,Nov,30

⊘ **90389** **Tetanus immune globulin (TIg), human, for intramuscular use** E
   MED: 100-2,15,50; 100-4,4,20.5
   AMA: 1999,Jan,1; 1998,Nov,30

⊘ **90393** **Vaccinia immune globulin, human, for intramuscular use** N
   MED: 100-2,15,50; 100-4,4,20.5
   AMA: 1999,Jan,1; 1998,Nov,30

⊘ **90396** **Varicella-zoster immune globulin, human, for intramuscular use** K
   MED: 100-2,15,50; 100-4,4,20.5
   AMA: 1999,Jan,1; 1998,Nov,30

⊘ **90399** **Unlisted immune globulin** E
   MED: 100-2,15,50; 100-4,4,20.5
   AMA: 1999,Sep,10; 1999,Jan,1; 1999,Feb,11; 1998,Nov,30

IMMUNIZATION ADMINISTRATION FOR VACCINES/TOXOIDS

IMMUNIZATION ADMINISTRATION FOR VACCINES/TOXOIDS

Immunization administration codes (90465-90474) are reported separately in addition to the code for the vaccine or toxoid supply (90476-90749). Significant, separately identifiable E/M services should also be reported.

Codes 90465-90468 should be reported only when the physician provides face-to-face counseling of the patient and the family during the administration of the vaccine. Report 90471-90474 when immunization administration is not accompanied by face-to-face physician contact.

If allergy tests are conducted, consult CPT codes 95004 and subsequent codes. For skin testing of bacterial, viral, fungal, extracts, consult CPT codes 86485-86586. If therapeutic or diagnostic injections are administered, consult CPT codes 90772-90779.

▲ **90465** **Immunization administration younger than 8 years of age (includes percutaneous, intradermal, subcutaneous, or intramuscular injections) when the physician counsels the patient/family; first injection (single or combination vaccine/toxoid), per day** A B 80
   Code 90465 cannot be reported with CPT code 90467.

+ ▲ **90466** **each additional injection (single or combination vaccine/toxoid), per day (List separately in addition to code for primary procedure)** A B 80
   Note that 90466 is an add-on code and must be used in conjunction with code 90465 or 90467.

90467 **Immunization administration younger than age 8 years (includes intranasal or oral routes of administration) when the physician counsels the patient/family; first administration (single or combination vaccine/toxoid), per day** A B 80 ↵
   Code 90467 cannot be reported with CPT code 90465.

+ **90468** **each additional administration (single or combination vaccine/toxoid), per day (List separately in addition to code for primary procedure)** A B 80
   Note that 90468 is an add-on code and must be used in conjunction with code 90465 or 90467.

90471 **Immunization administration (includes percutaneous, intradermal, subcutaneous, or intramuscular injections); one vaccine (single or combination vaccine/toxoid)** S 80 ↵
   MED: 100-2,15,50; 100-4,4,240
   AMA: 2002,Nov,11; 2001,Jul,1; 2001,Feb,4; 2000,Nov,10; 1999,Nov,47-48; 1999,Jan,1; 1999,Apr,10; 1998,Nov,31
   Code 90471 cannot be reported with CPT code 90473.

---

26 Professional Component Only   80/80 Assist-at-Surgery Allowed/With Documentation   Unlisted   Not Covered
TC Technical Component Only   MED: Pub 100/NCD References   AMA: CPT Assistant References   1-9 ASC Group   ♂ Male Only   ♀ Female Only

+ **90472** each additional vaccine (single or combination vaccine/toxoid) (List separately in addition to code for primary procedure) ⑤ ⑧⓪

MED: 100-2,15,50

AMA: 2002,Nov,11; 2001,Jul,1; 2001,Feb,4; 2000,Nov,10; 1999,Nov,47-48; 1999,Jan,1; 1999,Apr,10; 1998,Nov,31
Note that 90472 is an add-on code and must be used in conjunction with 90471 or 90473.

If immune globulins are administered, use CPT codes 90281-90399 and consult CPT codes 90760, 90761, 90765-90768 and 90774. For intravesical administration of BCG vaccine, see CPT codes 51720, 90586.

90473 Immunization administration by intranasal or oral route; one vaccine (single or combination vaccine/toxoid) ⑤ ⑧⓪ ▣

MED: 100-2,15,50

AMA: 2002,Nov,11
Code 90473 cannot be reported with CPT code 90471.

+ **90474** each additional vaccine (single or combination vaccine/toxoid) (List separately in addition to code for primary procedure) ⑤ ⑧⓪

MED: 100-2,15,50

AMA: 2002,Nov,11
Note that 90474 is an add-on code and must be used in conjunction with code 90471 or 90473.

VACCINES, TOXOIDS
The AMA will be publishing new vaccine products before they have received FDA approval. The codes are identified with the symbol. Once they are approved, the symbol will be removed. Monitor the website at www.ama-assn.org/ama/pub/category/10902.html for the most up-to-date information on these codes. The AMA will use this site to give CPT users updates of the CPT Editorial Panel actions regarding these products. Codes will also be made available twice a year, July 1 and January 1, on the website. Report codes 90476-90748 recognize the vaccine product only. To report the administration of a vaccine/toxoid, the vaccine/toxoid product codes 90476-90749 must be used in addition to an immunization administration code(s) 90465-90474. Do not report modifier 51 to the vaccine/toxoid product code (90476-90749).

⊘ **90476** Adenovirus vaccine, type 4, live, for oral use Ⓝ

MED: 100-2,15,50; 100-4,4,20.5

AMA: 1999,Sep,10; 1999,Nov,48; 1999,Jan,1; 1998,Nov,31-33

⊘ **90477** Adenovirus vaccine, type 7, live, for oral use Ⓝ

MED: 100-2,15,50; 100-4,4,20.5

AMA: 1999,Nov,48; 1999,Jan,1; 1998,Nov,31-33

⊘ **90581** Anthrax vaccine, for subcutaneous use Ⓝ ▣

MED: 100-2,15,50; 100-4,4,20.5

AMA: 1999,Nov,48; 1999,Jan,1; 1998,Nov,31-33

⊘ **90585** Bacillus Calmette-Guerin vaccine (BCG) for tuberculosis, live, for percutaneous use Ⓚ ▣

MED: 100-4,4,20.5

AMA: 1999,Nov,48; 1999,Jan,1; 1998,Nov,31-33

⊘ **90586** Bacillus Calmette-Guerin vaccine (BCG) for bladder cancer, live, for intravesical use Ⓑ

MED: 100-2,15,50; 100-4,4,20.5

AMA: 1999,Nov,48; 1999,Jan,1; 1998,Nov,31-33

⊘ **90632** Hepatitis A vaccine, adult dosage, for intramuscular use Ⓝ ▣

MED: 100-2,15,50; 100-2,16,90; 100-4,4,20.5

AMA: 1999,Nov,48; 1999,Jan,1; 1998,Nov,31-33

⊘ **90633** Hepatitis A vaccine, pediatric/adolescent dosage-2 dose schedule, for intramuscular use Ⓝ ▣

MED: 100-2,15,50; 100-2,16,90; 100-4,4,20.5

AMA: 1999,Nov,48; 1999,Jan,1; 1998,Nov,31-33

⊘ **90634** Hepatitis A vaccine, pediatric/adolescent dosage-3 dose schedule, for intramuscular use Ⓝ ▣

MED: 100-2,15,50; 100-2,16,90; 100-4,4,20.5

AMA: 1999,Nov,48; 1999,Jan,1; 1998,Nov,31-33

⊘ **90636** Hepatitis A and hepatitis B vaccine (HepA-HepB), adult dosage, for intramuscular use Ⓝ ▣

MED: 100-2,15,50; 100-4,4,20.5

AMA: 1999,Nov,48; 1999,Jan,1; 1998,Nov,31-33

⊘ **90645** Hemophilus influenza b vaccine (Hib), HbOC conjugate (4 dose schedule), for intramuscular use Ⓝ ▣

MED: 100-2,15,50; 100-4,4,20.5

AMA: 1999,Nov,48; 1999,Jan,1; 1998,Nov,31-33

⊘ **90646** Hemophilus influenza b vaccine (Hib), PRP-D conjugate, for booster use only, intramuscular use Ⓝ ▣

MED: 100-2,15,50; 100-4,4,20.5

AMA: 1999,Nov,48; 1999,Jan,1; 1998,Nov,31-33

⊘ **90647** Hemophilus influenza b vaccine (Hib), PRP-OMP conjugate (3 dose schedule), for intramuscular use Ⓝ ▣

MED: 100-2,15,50; 100-4,4,20.5

AMA: 1999,Nov,48; 1999,Jan,1; 1998,Nov,31-33

⊘ **90648** Hemophilus influenza b vaccine (Hib), PRP-T conjugate (4 dose schedule), for intramuscular use Ⓝ ▣

MED: 100-2,15,50; 100-4,4,20.5

AMA: 1999,Nov,48; 1999,Jan,1; 1998,Nov,31-33

⊘ **90649** Human Papilloma virus (HPV) vaccine, types 6, 11, 16, 18 (quadrivalent), 3 dose schedule, for intramuscular use Ⓑ

MED: 100-4,4,20.5

⊘ ▲ **90655** Influenza virus vaccine, split virus, preservative free, when administered to children 6-35 months of age, for intramuscular use Ⓐ Ⓛ ▣

MED: 100-2,6,10; 100-4,4,20.5

⊘ ▲ **90656** Influenza virus vaccine, split virus, preservative free, when administered to 3 years and older, for intramuscular use Ⓛ ▣

MED: 100-2,6,10; 100-4,4,20.5

⊘ ▲ **90657** Influenza virus vaccine, split virus, when administered to children 6-35 months of age, for intramuscular use Ⓐ Ⓛ ▣

MED: 100-2,6,10; 100-2,15,50; 100-4,4,20.5; 100-4,4,240

AMA: 2002,Feb,10; 1999,Nov,48; 1999,Jan,1; 1998,Nov,31-33

⊘ ▲ **90658** Influenza virus vaccine, split virus, when administered to 3 years of age and older, for intramuscular use Ⓛ ▣

MED: 100-2,6,10; 100-2,15,50; 100-4,4,20.5; 100-4,4,240

AMA: 1999,Nov,48; 1999,Jan,1; 1998,Nov,31-33

⊘ **90660** Influenza virus vaccine, live, for intranasal use Ⓛ ▣

MED: 100-2,15,50; 100-4,4,20.5

AMA: 1999,Nov,48; 1999,Jan,1; 1998,Nov,31-33

⊘ **90665** Lyme disease vaccine, adult dosage, for intramuscular use Ⓝ ▣

MED: 100-2,15,50; 100-4,4,20.5

AMA: 1999,Nov,48; 1999,Jan,1; 1998,Nov,31-33

⊘ ▲ **90669** Pneumococcal conjugate vaccine, polyvalent, when administered to children younger than 5 years, for intramuscular use Ⓔ

MED: 100-2,15,50

AMA: 2000,Jun,10; 1999,Nov,48; 1999,Jan,1; 1998,Nov,31-33

⊘ **90675** Rabies vaccine, for intramuscular use Ⓚ ▣

MED: 100-2,15,50; 100-4,4,20.5

AMA: 1999,Nov,48; 1999,Jan,1; 1998,Nov,31-33

⊙③ Modifier 63 Exempt Code   ⊙ Conscious Sedation   + CPT Add-on Code   ⊘ Modifier 51 Exempt Code   ● New Code   ▲ Revised Code

Ⓜ Maternity Edit   Ⓐ Age Edit   Ⓐ-Ⓨ APC Status Indicators   ▣ CCI Comprehensive Code   ✏ Drug Not Approved by FDA   ⑤⓪ Bilateral Procedure

⊘ 90676 **Rabies vaccine, for intradermal use** Ⓚ ⬛
MED: 100-2,15,50; 100-4,4,20.5
AMA: 1999,Nov,48; 1999,Jan,1; 1998,Nov,31-33

⊘ 90680 **Rotavirus vaccine, pentavalent, 3 dose schedule, live, for oral use** Ⓝ
MED: 100-2,15,50; 100-4,4,20.5
AMA: 1999,Nov,48; 1999,Jan,1; 1998,Nov,31-33

⊘ 90690 **Typhoid vaccine, live, oral** Ⓝ
MED: 100-2,15,50; 100-4,4,20.5
AMA: 1999,Nov,48; 1999,Jan,1; 1998,Nov,31-33

⊘ 90691 **Typhoid vaccine, Vi capsular polysaccharide (ViCPs), for intramuscular use** Ⓝ ⬛
MED: 100-2,15,50; 100-4,4,20.5
AMA: 1999,Nov,48; 1999,Jan,1; 1998,Nov,31-33

⊘ 90692 **Typhoid vaccine, heat- and phenol-inactivated (H-P), for subcutaneous or intradermal use** Ⓝ ⬛
MED: 100-2,15,50; 100-4,4,20.5
AMA: 1999,Nov,48; 1999,Jan,1; 1998,Nov,31-33

⊘ 90693 **Typhoid vaccine, acetone-killed, dried (AKD), for subcutaneous use (U.S. military)** Ⓑ ⬛
MED: 100-2,15,50; 100-4,4,20.5
AMA: 1999,Nov,48; 1999,Jan,1; 1998,Nov,31-33

⊘ ✎ 90698 **Diphtheria, tetanus toxoids, acellular pertussis vaccine, haemophilus influenza Type B, and poliovirus vaccine, inactivated (DTaP - Hib - IPV), for intramuscular use** Ⓝ
MED: 100-4,4,20.5

⊘ ▲ 90700 **Diphtheria, tetanus toxoids, and acellular pertussis vaccine (DTaP), when administered to younger than 7 years, for intramuscular use** Ⓐ Ⓝ ⬛
MED: 100-2,15,50; 100-4,4,20.5
AMA: 1999,Nov,48; 1999,Jan,1; 1998,Nov,31-33; 1997,Feb,9; 1996,Jan,5

⊘ 90701 **Diphtheria, tetanus toxoids, and whole cell pertussis vaccine (DTP), for intramuscular use** Ⓝ ⬛
MED: 100-2,15,50; 100-4,4,20.5
AMA: 1999,Nov,48; 1999,Jan,1; 1998,Nov,31-33; 1996,Jan,6

⊘ ▲ 90702 **Diphtheria and tetanus toxoids (DT) adsorbed when administered to younger than 7 years, for intramuscular use** Ⓐ Ⓝ ⬛
MED: 100-2,15,50; 100-4,4,20.5
AMA: 2000,Jun,10; 1999,Sep,10; 1999,Nov,48; 1999,Jan,1; 1998,Nov,31-33; 1996,Jan,6

⊘ 90703 **Tetanus toxoid adsorbed, for intramuscular use** Ⓝ ⬛
MED: 100-2,15,50; 100-4,4,20.5
AMA: 1999,Sep,10; 1999,Nov,48; 1999,Jan,1; 1998,Nov,31-33; 1996,Jan,6

⊘ 90704 **Mumps virus vaccine, live, for subcutaneous use** Ⓝ ⬛
MED: 100-2,15,50; 100-2,16,90; 100-4,4,20.5
AMA: 1999,Nov,48; 1999,Jan,1; 1998,Nov,31-33

⊘ 90705 **Measles virus vaccine, live, for subcutaneous use** Ⓝ ⬛
MED: 100-2,15,50; 100-2,16,90; 100-4,4,20.5
AMA: 1999,Nov,48; 1999,Jan,1; 1998,Nov,31-33

⊘ 90706 **Rubella virus vaccine, live, for subcutaneous use** Ⓝ ⬛
MED: 100-2,15,50; 100-2,16,90; 100-4,4,20.5
AMA: 1999,Nov,48; 1999,Jan,1; 1998,Nov,31-33

⊘ 90707 **Measles, mumps and rubella virus vaccine (MMR), live, for subcutaneous use** Ⓝ ⬛
MED: 100-2,15,50; 100-2,16,90; 100-4,4,20.5
AMA: 1999,Nov,48; 1999,Jan,1; 1998,Nov,31-33; 1997,Apr,10; 1996,May,10; 1996,Jan,6

⊘ 90708 **Measles and rubella virus vaccine, live, for subcutaneous use** Ⓚ ⬛
MED: 100-2,15,50; 100-2,16,90; 100-4,4,20.5
AMA: 1999,Nov,48; 1999,Jan,1; 1998,Nov,31-33

⊘ 90710 **Measles, mumps, rubella, and varicella vaccine (MMRV), live, for subcutaneous use** Ⓝ ⬛
MED: 100-2,15,50; 100-2,16,90; 100-4,4,20.5
AMA: 1999,Nov,48; 1999,Jan,1; 1998,Nov,31-33; 1997,Apr,10; 1996,May,10

⊘ 90712 **Poliovirus vaccine, (any type(s)) (OPV), live, for oral use** Ⓝ ⬛
MED: 100-2,15,50; 100-2,16,90; 100-4,4,20.5
AMA: 1999,Nov,48; 1999,Jan,1; 1998,Nov,31-33; 1996,Jan,6

⊘ 90713 **Poliovirus vaccine, inactivated, (IPV), for subcutaneous or intramuscular use** Ⓝ ⬛
MED: 100-2,15,50; 100-2,16,90; 100-4,4,20.5
AMA: 1999,Nov,48; 1999,Jan,1; 1998,Nov,31-33

⊘ ▲ 90714 **Tetanus and diphtheria toxoids (Td) adsorbed, preservative free, when administered to 7 years or older, for intramuscular use** Ⓝ
MED: 100-4,4,20.5

⊘ ▲ 90715 **Tetanus, diphtheria toxoids and acellular pertussis vaccine (Tdap), when administered to 7 years or older, for intramuscular use** Ⓝ
MED: 100-4,4,20.5

⊘ 90716 **Varicella virus vaccine, live, for subcutaneous use** Ⓑ ⬛
MED: 100-2,15,50; 100-2,16,90; 100-4,4,20.5
AMA: 1999,Nov,48; 1999,Jan,1; 1998,Nov,31-33; 1997,Apr,10; 1996,May,10; 1996,Jan,6

⊘ 90717 **Yellow fever vaccine, live, for subcutaneous use** Ⓝ ⬛
MED: 100-4,4,20.5
AMA: 1999,Nov,48; 1999,Jan,1; 1998,Nov,31-33

⊘ ▲ 90718 **Tetanus and diphtheria toxoids (Td) adsorbed when administered to 7 years or older, for intramuscular use** Ⓝ ⬛
MED: 100-2,15,50; 100-2,16,90; 100-4,4,20.5
AMA: 2000,Jun,10; 1999,Nov,48; 1999,Jan,1; 1998,Nov,31-33; 1996,Aug,10

⊘ 90719 **Diphtheria toxoid, for intramuscular use** Ⓝ ⬛
MED: 100-2,15,50; 100-2,16,90; 100-4,4,20.5
AMA: 1999,Sep,10; 1999,Nov,48; 1999,Jan,1; 1998,Nov,31-33

⊘ 90720 **Diphtheria, tetanus toxoids, and whole cell pertussis vaccine and Hemophilus influenza B vaccine (DTP-Hib), for intramuscular use** Ⓚ ⬛
MED: 100-2,15,50; 100-2,16,90; 100-4,4,20.5
AMA: 1999,Nov,48; 1999,Jan,1; 1998,Nov,31-33; 1996,Jan,5

⊘ 90721 **Diphtheria, tetanus toxoids, and acellular pertussis vaccine and Hemophilus influenza B vaccine (DtaP-Hib), for intramuscular use** Ⓝ ⬛
MED: 100-2,15,50; 100-2,16,90; 100-4,4,20.5
AMA: 1999,Nov,48; 1999,Jan,1; 1998,Nov,31-33; 1996,Jan,5

⊘ 90723 **Diphtheria, tetanus toxoids, acellular pertussis vaccine, Hepatitis B, and poliovirus vaccine, inactivated (DtaP-HepB-IPV), for intramuscular use** Ⓔ
MED: 100-2,15,50; 100-2,16,90; 100-4,4,20.5
AMA: 1999,Nov,48

⊘ 90725 **Cholera vaccine for injectable use** Ⓝ ⬛
MED: 100-2,15,50; 100-4,4,20.5
AMA: 1999,Nov,48; 1999,Jan,1; 1998,Nov,31-33

⊘ 90727 **Plague vaccine, for intramuscular use** Ⓚ ⬛
MED: 100-2,15,50; 100-4,4,20.5
AMA: 1999,Nov,48; 1999,Jan,1; 1998,Nov,31-33

🖳 Professional Component Only   🖳 Technical Component Only   **MED:** Pub 100/NCD References   **AMA:** CPT Assistant References

⑧⓪/ ⑧⓪ Assist-at-Surgery Allowed/With Documentation   **❶-❾** ASC Group   Unlisted   Not Covered   ♂ Male Only   ♀ Female Only

334 — CPT Expert   CPT only © 2006 American Medical Association. All Rights Reserved. *(Black Ink)*   © 2006 Ingenix *(Blue Ink)*

⊘	▲ 90732	**Pneumococcal polysaccharide vaccine, 23-valent, adult or immunosuppressed patient dosage, when administered to 2 years or older, for subcutaneous or intramuscular use** L ⊡

> MED: 100-2,6,10; 100-2,15,50; 100-4,4,20.5; 100-4,4,240
> AMA: 1999,Nov,48; 1999,Jan,1; 1998,Nov,31-33

⊘	90733	**Meningococcal polysaccharide vaccine (any group(s)), for subcutaneous use** K ⊡

> MED: 100-2,15,50; 100-4,4,20.5
> AMA: 1999,Nov,48; 1999,Jan,1; 1999,Dec,7; 1998,Nov,31-33

⊘	90734	**Meningococcal conjugate vaccine, serogroups A, C, Y and W-135 (tetravalent), for intramuscular use** K ⊡

> MED: 100-4,4,20.5

⊘	90735	**Japanese encephalitis virus vaccine, for subcutaneous use** K ⊡

> MED: 100-2,15,50; 100-4,4,20.5
> AMA: 1999,Nov,48; 1999,Jan,1; 1998,Nov,31-33

⊘	90736	**Zoster (shingles) vaccine, live, for subcutaneous injection** B

> MED: 100-4,4,20.5

⊘	90740	**Hepatitis B vaccine, dialysis or immunosuppressed patient dosage (3 dose schedule), for intramuscular use** F

> MED: 100-2,6,10; 100-2,15,50; 100-3,190.10; 100-4,4,20.5; 100-4,4,240
> AMA: 2001,Apr,10; 1999,Nov,48

⊘	90743	**Hepatitis B vaccine, adolescent (2 dose schedule), for intramuscular use** F

> MED: 100-2,6,10; 100-2,15,50; 100-4,4,20.5; 100-4,4,240
> AMA: 1999,Nov,48

⊘	90744	**Hepatitis B vaccine, pediatric/adolescent dosage (3 dose schedule), for intramuscular use** F

> MED: 100-2,6,10; 100-2,15,50; 100-4,4,20.5; 100-4,4,240
> AMA: 2000,Jun,10; 1999,Nov,48-49; 1999,Nov,48; 1999,Jan,1; 1998,Nov,31-33; 1997,Jun,10; 1996,Jan,5

⊘	90746	**Hepatitis B vaccine, adult dosage, for intramuscular use** F

> MED: 100-2,6,10; 100-2,15,50; 100-4,4,20.5; 100-4,4,240
> AMA: 1999,Nov,48; 1999,Jan,1; 1998,Nov,31-33; 1996,Jan,5

⊘	90747	**Hepatitis B vaccine, dialysis or immunosuppressed patient dosage (4 dose schedule), for intramuscular use** F

> MED: 100-2,6,10; 100-2,15,50; 100-3,190.10; 100-4,4,20.5; 100-4,4,240
> AMA: 2001,Apr,10; 2000,Jun,10; 1999,Nov,48; 1999,Jan,1; 1998,Nov,31-33; 1997,Jun,10; 1996,Jan,5

⊘	90748	**Hepatitis B and Hemophilus influenza b vaccine (HepB-Hib), for intramuscular use** E

> MED: 100-2,15,50; 100-4,4,20.5
> AMA: 1999,Sep,10; 1999,Nov,48; 1999,Jan,1; 1998,Nov,31-33; 1997,Nov,37

⊘	90749	**Unlisted vaccine/toxoid** N

> MED: 100-2,15,50; 100-4,4,20.5
> AMA: 2002,Nov,11; 1999,Nov,48; 1999,Jan,1; 1998,Nov,31-33; 1997,Feb,9; 1996,Jan,6

HYDRATION, THERAPEUTIC, PROPHYLACTIC, AND DIAGNOSTIC INJECTIONS AND INFUSIONS (EXCLUDES CHEMOTHERAPY)

Physician work involved in hydration, therapeutic, prophylactic, and diagnostic injections and infusion services includes verification of a plan of treatment and direction of personnel.

To report an evaluation and management service in addition to hydration, therapeutic, prophylactic, and diagnostic injections and infusion services, consult the appropriate evaluation and management code. Append modifier 25 to evaluation and management code.

The following codes are included in the infusion or injection:

- Local anesthesia
- Starting the IV
- Access to catheter, IV, or port
- Routine tubing, syringe, and supplies
- Flushing at the completion of the infusion

For declotting of a catheter or port, consult CPT code 36550.

Report the materials or drugs in addition to the injection or infusion codes.

If multiple infusions, injections, or combination services are performed, only the initial code should be reported unless the procedure requires the use of two separate IV sites. Report subsequent or concurrent services using the code that most closely describes the main reason for the procedure even if that is not the order in which the services are performed.

When reporting codes for which time is an issue, use the actual time for the administration of the infusion.

HYDRATION

The following codes are used to report infusion of prepacked fluids and electrolytes, and not drugs or other substances. These services usually require the supervision of a physician to include consent, safety oversight, and supervision of personnel. There is typically little special handling required to prepare, deliver, or dispose of the IV, and the administration does not require any special training for the staff. There is usually little patient risk after the initial set-up, and special patient monitoring is usually not required.

	90760	**Intravenous infusion, hydration; initial, up to 1 hour** S 80

> Code 90760 cannot be reported when performed as a concurrent infusion service.

+ ▲	90761	**each additional hour (List separately in addition to code for primary procedure)** S 80

> Note that 90761 is an add-on code and should be reported in conjunction with 90760.
>
> Code 90761 should be reported for hydration infusion intervals of greater than 30 minutes beyond 1-hour increments.
>
> Code 90761 should be reported to identify hydration if provided as a secondary or subsequent service after a different initial service [90760, 90765, 90774, 96409, 96413] is provided.

THERAPEUTIC, PROPHYLACTIC, AND DIAGNOSTIC INJECTIONS AND INFUSIONS

The following codes are used to describe a therapeutic, prophylactic, or diagnostic IV infusion or injection administered for other than hydration. These codes are used for the administration of drugs, and the fluid in which the drug is mixed is incidental and not separately reportable. These services usually require the supervision of a physician to include all aspects of patient assessment , consent, safety oversight, and the supervision of personnel. The staff usually requires training to include how to assess the patient, dose, and dispose of drugs and supplies, and monitor the patient during the treatment.

An intravenous or intra-arterial push requires:

- The constant presence of the health care professional administering the substance or drug
- An infusion of 15 minutes or less

Codes 90765-90779 should not be reported with codes for which IV push or infusion is an intregral part of the procedure.

| ⊛ Modifier 63 Exempt Code | ⊙ Conscious Sedation | + CPT Add-on Code | ⊘ Modifier 51 Exempt Code | ● New Code | ▲ Revised Code |
| M Maternity Edit | A Age Edit | A-Y APC Status Indicators | ⊡ CCI Comprehensive Code | ⁄ Drug Not Approved by FDA | 50 Bilateral Procedure |

© 2006 Ingenix *(Blue Ink)*   CPT only © 2006 American Medical Association. All Rights Reserved. *(Black Ink)*   Medicine — 335

Medicine

90765 — 90802

90765   Intravenous infusion, for therapy, prophylaxis, or diagnosis (specify substance or drug); initial, up to 1 hour   ⑤ ⑧⓪

MED: 100-4,20,160.1

+ ▲ 90766   each additional hour (List separately in addition to code for primary procedure)   ⑤ ⑧⓪

Note that 90766 is an add-on code and should be reported in conjunction with 90765.

Code 90766 should be reported for additional hour(s) of sequential infusion.

Code 90766 should be reported for infusion intervals of greater than 30 minutes beyond 1-hour increments.

+ 90767   additional sequential infusion, up to 1 hour (List separately in addition to code for primary procedure)   ⑤ ⑧⓪

Code 90767 should be reported in conjunction with 90765, 90774, 96409, 96413 when provided as a secondary or subsequent service after a different initial service. Report 90767 only once per sequential infusion of same infusate mix.

+ 90768   concurrent infusion (List separately in addition to code for primary procedure)   Ⓝ ⑧⓪

Code 90768 should be reported only once per encounter.

Note that 90768 is an add-on code and should be reported in conjunction with 90765, 90766, 96413, 96415, 96416, 96422, and 96423.

90772   Therapeutic, prophylactic or diagnostic injection (specify substance or drug); subcutaneous or intramuscular   ⑤ ⑧⓪

MED: 100-4,4,20.5; 100-4,4,230.2.3

To report administration of vaccines/toxoids consult 90465-90466, 90471-90472.

Code 90772 should be reported for non-antineoplastic hormonal therapy injections.

Code 96401 should be reported for antineoplastic nonhormonal injection therapy.

Code 96402 should be reported for antineoplastic hormonal injection therapy.

Code 90772 cannot be reported for injections given without direct physician supervision; consult CPT code 99211.

90773   intra-arterial   ⑤ ⑧⓪

MED: 100-4,4,20.5; 100-4,4,230.2.3

90774   intravenous push, single or initial substance/drug   ⑤ ⑧⓪

MED: 100-4,4,20.5

Codes 90772-90774 do not include injections for allergen immunotherapy; consult CPT codes 95115-95117.

+ 90775   each additional sequential intravenous push of a new substance/drug (List separately in addition to code for primary procedure)   ⑤ ⑧⓪

Note that 90775 is an add-on code and must be used in conjunction with 90765, 90774, 96409, 96413.

Use code 90775 to report intravenous push of a new substance/drug when provided as a secondary or subsequent service after a different initial service has been provided.

90779   Unlisted therapeutic, prophylactic or diagnostic intravenous or intra-arterial injection or infusion   ⑤ ⑧⓪

MED: 100-4,4,20.5; 100-4,4,230.2.3

To report allergy immunizations, consult 95004 et seq.

PSYCHIATRY

Psychiatry codes include psychiatric diagnostic or evaluation interview procedures (90801-90802), and psychiatric therapeutic procedures (90804-90899).

Psychiatric diagnostic interview exam (90801) includes a history, mental status, and disposition, and may include communication with family or other sources and ordering/interpretation of diagnostic studies. An interactive psychiatric diagnostic interview (90802) is furnished to children and older individuals lacking expressive and receptive communication skills. These procedure codes are normally reported only on the initial visit.

The most frequently reported services are therapeutic psychiatric service codes (90804-90829) for individual psychotherapy. Individual psychotherapy services are organized first by place of service (office/outpatient, inpatient/partial hospital/residential care). Codes within these two subcategories are organized by type of psychotherapy service (insight oriented, behavior modifying, supportive, interactive), face-to-face time, and the provision of additional medical evaluation or management services.

Other psychotherapy services (90845-90857) are used to report family and group psychotherapy services. Psychiatric services and procedures (90862-90899) are used to report medication management, electroconvulsive therapy, and hypnotherapy.

Hospital inpatient service codes (99221-99233) in the E/M section of the CPT book should be reported when the physician is involved in the medical management of an inpatient (e.g., when the attending physician reviews laboratory tests or initiates the patient's treatment plan). However, do not use hospital inpatient service codes when both psychotherapy and E/M services are provided on the same day. Combined E/M and psychotherapy services should be reported with codes designated as such in the psychiatry section (90804-90829).

To report repetitive transcranial magnetic stimulation for treatment of clinical depression, consult CPT Category III code 0018T.

PSYCHIATRIC DIAGNOSTIC OR EVALUATIVE INTERVIEW PROCEDURES

90801   Psychiatric diagnostic interview examination   ⑤ ⑧⓪ ▣

MED: 100-3,10.3; 100-3,10.4; 100-3,20.10; 100-3,40.5; 100-3,130.1; 100-3,130.2; 100-3,130.3; 100-3,130.4; 100-3,130.5; 100-3,130.6; 100-4,4,20.5; 100-4,12,100; 100-4,12,100.1.7; 100-4,12,100.1.8; 100-4,12,110.2; 100-4,12,160; 100-4,12,160.1; 100-4,12,170; 100-4,12,190.7

AMA: 2001,Mar,5; 1997,Nov,37-38; 1992,Summer,12

90802   Interactive psychiatric diagnostic interview examination using play equipment, physical devices, language interpreter, or other mechanisms of communication   ⑤ ⑧⓪ ▣

MED: 100-3,10.3; 100-3,10.4; 100-3,20.10; 100-3,40.5; 100-3,130.1; 100-3,130.2; 100-3,130.3; 100-3,130.4; 100-3,130.5; 100-3,130.6; 100-4,4,20.5; 100-4,12,100; 100-4,12,100.1.7; 100-4,12,100.1.8; 100-4,12,110.2; 100-4,12,150; 100-4,12,160; 100-4,12,160.1; 100-4,12,170

AMA: 2001,Mar,5; 1997,Nov,37-38

㉖ Professional Component Only   ⑳/⑧⓪ Assist-at-Surgery Allowed/With Documentation   Unlisted   Not Covered

ⓉⒸ Technical Component Only   MED: Pub 100/NCD References   AMA: CPT Assistant References   ❶-❾ ASC Group   ♂ Male Only   ♀ Female Only

336 — CPT Expert   CPT only © 2006 American Medical Association. All Rights Reserved. (Black Ink)   © 2006 Ingenix (Blue Ink)

PSYCHIATRIC THERAPEUTIC PROCEDURES

OFFICE OR OTHER OUTPATIENT FACILITY

INSIGHT ORIENTED, BEHAVIOR MODIFYING AND/OR SUPPORTIVE PSYCHOTHERAPY

90804 Individual psychotherapy, insight oriented, behavior modifying and/or supportive, in an office or outpatient facility, approximately 20 to 30 minutes face-to-face with the patient; [S] [80] [□]

MED: 100-3,10.4; 100-3,20.10; 100-3,40.5; 100-3,130.2; 100-3,130.3; 100-3,130.4; 100-3,130.5; 100-3,130.6; 100-3,130.7; 100-4,4,20.5; 100-4,12,100; 100-4,12,100.1.7; 100-4,12,100.1.8; 100-4,12,110.2; 100-4,12,150; 100-4,12,160; 100-4,12,160.1; 100-4,12,170

AMA: 2002,Oct,11; 2001,Mar,5; 1999,Jul,10; 1997,Nov,39

90805   with medical evaluation and management services [S] [80] [□]

MED: 100-3,10.4; 100-3,20.10; 100-3,40.5; 100-3,130.2; 100-3,130.3; 100-3,130.4; 100-3,130.5; 100-3,130.6; 100-3,130.7; 100-4,4,20.5; 100-4,12,100; 100-4,12,100.1.7; 100-4,12,100.1.8; 100-4,12,110.2; 100-4,12,150; 100-4,12,160; 100-4,12,160.1; 100-4,12,170

AMA: 2001,Mar,5; 1999,Jul,10; 1997,Nov,39

90806 Individual psychotherapy, insight oriented, behavior modifying and/or supportive, in an office or outpatient facility, approximately 45 to 50 minutes face-to-face with the patient; [S] [80] [□]

MED: 100-3,10.4; 100-3,20.10; 100-3,40.5; 100-3,130.2; 100-3,130.3; 100-3,130.4; 100-3,130.5; 100-3,130.6; 100-3,130.7; 100-4,4,20.5; 100-4,12,100; 100-4,12,100.1.7; 100-4,12,100.1.8; 100-4,12,110.2; 100-4,12,150; 100-4,12,160; 100-4,12,160.1; 100-4,12,170

AMA: 2001,Mar,5; 1999,Jul,10; 1997,Nov,39

90807   with medical evaluation and management services [S] [80] [□]

MED: 100-3,10.4; 100-3,20.10; 100-3,40.5; 100-3,130.2; 100-3,130.3; 100-3,130.4; 100-3,130.5; 100-3,130.6; 100-3,130.7; 100-4,4,20.5; 100-4,12,100; 100-4,12,100.1.7; 100-4,12,100.1.8; 100-4,12,110.2; 100-4,12,150; 100-4,12,160; 100-4,12,160.1; 100-4,12,170

AMA: 1999,Jul,10; 1997,Nov,39

90808 Individual psychotherapy, insight oriented, behavior modifying and/or supportive, in an office or outpatient facility, approximately 75 to 80 minutes face-to-face with the patient; [S] [80] [□]

MED: 100-3,10.4; 100-3,20.10; 100-3,40.5; 100-3,130.2; 100-3,130.3; 100-3,130.4; 100-3,130.5; 100-3,130.6; 100-3,130.7; 100-4,4,20.5; 100-4,12,100; 100-4,12,100.1.7; 100-4,12,100.1.8; 100-4,12,110.2; 100-4,12,150; 100-4,12,160; 100-4,12,160.1; 100-4,12,170

AMA: 2001,Mar,5; 1999,Jul,10; 1997,Nov,39

90809   with medical evaluation and management services [S] [80] [□]

MED: 100-3,10.4; 100-3,20.10; 100-3,40.5; 100-3,130.2; 100-3,130.3; 100-3,130.4; 100-3,130.5; 100-3,130.6; 100-3,130.7; 100-4,4,20.5; 100-4,12,100; 100-4,12,100.1.7; 100-4,12,100.1.8; 100-4,12,110.2; 100-4,12,150; 100-4,12,160; 100-4,12,160.1; 100-4,12,170

AMA: 2001,Mar,5; 1999,Jul,10; 1997,Nov,39

INTERACTIVE PSYCHOTHERAPY

90810 Individual psychotherapy, interactive, using play equipment, physical devices, language interpreter, or other mechanisms of non-verbal communication, in an office or outpatient facility, approximately 20 to 30 minutes face-to-face with the patient; [S] [80] [□]

MED: 100-3,10.4; 100-3,20.10; 100-3,40.5; 100-3,130.2; 100-3,130.3; 100-3,130.4; 100-3,130.5; 100-3,130.6; 100-3,130.7; 100-4,12,100; 100-4,12,100.1.7; 100-4,12,100.1.8; 100-4,12,110.2; 100-4,12,150; 100-4,12,160; 100-4,12,160.1; 100-4,12,170

AMA: 2001,Mar,5; 1997,Nov,39

90811   with medical evaluation and management services [S] [80] [□]

MED: 100-3,10.4; 100-3,20.10; 100-3,40.5; 100-3,130.2; 100-3,130.3; 100-3,130.4; 100-3,130.5; 100-3,130.6; 100-3,130.7; 100-4,12,100; 100-4,12,100.1.7; 100-4,12,100.1.8; 100-4,12,110.2; 100-4,12,150; 100-4,12,160.1; 100-4,12,170

AMA: 2001,Mar,5

90812 Individual psychotherapy, interactive, using play equipment, physical devices, language interpreter, or other mechanisms of non-verbal communication, in an office or outpatient facility, approximately 45 to 50 minutes face-to-face with the patient; [S] [80] [□]

MED: 100-3,10.4; 100-3,20.10; 100-3,40.5; 100-3,130.2; 100-3,130.3; 100-3,130.4; 100-3,130.5; 100-3,130.6; 100-3,130.7; 100-4,4,20.5; 100-4,12,100; 100-4,12,100.1.7; 100-4,12,100.1.8; 100-4,12,110.2; 100-4,12,150; 100-4,12,160; 100-4,12,160.1; 100-4,12,170

AMA: 2001,Mar,5; 1997,Nov,39

90813   with medical evaluation and management services [S] [80] [□]

MED: 100-3,10.4; 100-3,20.10; 100-3,40.5; 100-3,130.2; 100-3,130.3; 100-3,130.4; 100-3,130.5; 100-3,130.6; 100-3,130.7; 100-4,4,20.5; 100-4,12,100; 100-4,12,100.1.7; 100-4,12,100.1.8; 100-4,12,110.2; 100-4,12,150; 100-4,12,160; 100-4,12,160.1; 100-4,12,170

AMA: 2001,Mar,5; 1997,Nov,39

90814 Individual psychotherapy, interactive, using play equipment, physical devices, language interpreter, or other mechanisms of non-verbal communication, in an office or outpatient facility, approximately 75 to 80 minutes face-to-face with the patient; [S] [80] [□]

MED: 100-3,10.4; 100-3,20.10; 100-3,40.5; 100-3,130.2; 100-3,130.3; 100-3,130.4; 100-3,130.5; 100-3,130.6; 100-3,130.7; 100-4,4,20.5; 100-4,12,100; 100-4,12,100.1.7; 100-4,12,100.1.8; 100-4,12,110.2; 100-4,12,150; 100-4,12,160; 100-4,12,170

AMA: 2001,Mar,5; 1997,Nov,39

90815   with medical evaluation and management services [S] [80] [□]

MED: 100-3,10.4; 100-3,20.10; 100-3,40.5; 100-3,130.2; 100-3,130.3; 100-3,130.4; 100-3,130.5; 100-3,130.6; 100-3,130.7; 100-4,4,20.5; 100-4,12,100; 100-4,12,100.1.7; 100-4,12,100.1.8; 100-4,12,110.2; 100-4,12,150; 100-4,12,160; 100-4,12,160.1; 100-4,12,170

AMA: 2001,Mar,5; 1997,Nov,39

INPATIENT HOSPITAL, PARTIAL HOSPITAL OR RESIDENTIAL CARE FACILITY

INSIGHT ORIENTED, BEHAVIOR MODIFYING AND/OR SUPPORTIVE PSYCHOTHERAPY

90816 Individual psychotherapy, insight oriented, behavior modifying and/or supportive, in an inpatient hospital, partial hospital or residential care setting, approximately 20 to 30 minutes face-to-face with the patient; [S] [80] [□]

MED: 100-2,15,60.3; 100-3,10.3; 100-3,20.10; 100-3,130.1; 100-3,130.3; 100-3,130.4; 100-3,130.6; 100-3,130.7; 100-4,4,20.5; 100-4,12,100; 100-4,12,100.1.7; 100-4,12,100.1.8; 100-4,12,110.2; 100-4,12,150; 100-4,12,160; 100-4,12,160.1; 100-4,12,170

AMA: 2001,Mar,5; 1997,Nov,39-40

90817   with medical evaluation and management services [S] [80] [□]

MED: 100-2,15,60.3; 100-3,10.3; 100-3,20.10; 100-3,130.1; 100-3,130.3; 100-3,130.4; 100-3,130.6; 100-3,130.7; 100-4,4,20.5; 100-4,12,100; 100-4,12,100.1.7; 100-4,12,100.1.8; 100-4,12,110.2

AMA: 2001,Mar,5; 1997,Nov,39-40

90818 Individual psychotherapy, insight oriented, behavior modifying and/or supportive, in an inpatient hospital, partial hospital or residential care setting, approximately 45 to 50 minutes face-to-face with the patient; [S] [80] [□]

MED: 100-2,15,60.3; 100-3,10.3; 100-3,20.10; 100-3,130.1; 100-3,130.3; 100-3,130.4; 100-3,130.6; 100-3,130.7; 100-4,4,20.5; 100-4,12,100; 100-4,12,100.1.7; 100-4,12,100.1.8; 100-4,12,110.2; 100-4,12,150; 100-4,12,160; 100-4,12,160.1; 100-4,12,170

AMA: 2001,Mar,5; 1997,Nov,39-40

⊛ Modifier 63 Exempt Code   ⊙ Conscious Sedation   + CPT Add-on Code   ⦸ Modifier 51 Exempt Code   ● New Code   ▲ Revised Code

[M] Maternity Edit   [A] Age Edit   [A]-[Y] APC Status Indicators   [□] CCI Comprehensive Code   ✗ Drug Not Approved by FDA   [50] Bilateral Procedure

© 2006 Ingenix *(Blue Ink)*   CPT only © 2006 American Medical Association. All Rights Reserved. *(Black Ink)*   Medicine — 337

Medicine

90819 — 90862

90819　with medical evaluation and management services　[S] [80] [↗]

MED: 100-2,15,60.3; 100-3,10.3; 100-3,20.10; 100-3,130.1; 100-3,130.3; 100-3,130.4; 100-3,130.6; 100-3,130.7; 100-4,4,20.5; 100-4,12,100; 100-4,12,100.1.7; 100-4,12,100.1.8; 100-4,12,110.2; 100-4,12,150; 100-4,12,160; 100-4,12,160.1; 100-4,12,170

AMA: 2001,Mar,5

90821　Individual psychotherapy, insight oriented, behavior modifying and/or supportive, in an inpatient hospital, partial hospital or residential care setting, approximately 75 to 80 minutes face-to-face with the patient;　[S] [80] [↗]

MED: 100-2,15,60.3; 100-3,10.3; 100-3,20.10; 100-3,130.1; 100-3,130.3; 100-3,130.4; 100-3,130.6; 100-3,130.7; 100-4,4,20.5; 100-4,12,100; 100-4,12,100.1.7; 100-4,12,100.1.8; 100-4,12,110.2; 100-4,12,150; 100-4,12,160; 100-4,12,160.1; 100-4,12,170

AMA: 2001,Mar,5; 1997,Nov,39-40

90822　with medical evaluation and management services　[S] [80] [↗]

MED: 100-2,15,60.3; 100-3,10.3; 100-3,20.10; 100-3,130.1; 100-3,130.3; 100-3,130.4; 100-3,130.6; 100-3,130.7; 100-4,4,20.5; 100-4,12,100; 100-4,12,100.1.7; 100-4,12,100.1.8; 100-4,12,110.2; 100-4,12,150; 100-4,12,160; 100-4,12,160.1; 100-4,12,170

AMA: 2001,Mar,5; 1997,Nov,39-40

INTERACTIVE PSYCHOTHERAPY

90823　Individual psychotherapy, interactive, using play equipment, physical devices, language interpreter, or other mechanisms of non-verbal communication, in an inpatient hospital, partial hospital or residential care setting, approximately 20 to 30 minutes face-to-face with the patient;　[S] [80] [↗]

MED: 100-2,15,60.3; 100-3,10.3; 100-3,20.10; 100-3,130.1; 100-3,130.3; 100-3,130.4; 100-3,130.6; 100-3,130.7; 100-4,4,20.5; 100-4,12,100; 100-4,12,100.1.7; 100-4,12,100.1.8; 100-4,12,110.2; 100-4,12,150; 100-4,12,160; 100-4,12,160.1; 100-4,12,170

AMA: 2001,Mar,5; 1997,Nov,40

90824　with medical evaluation and management services　[S] [80] [↗]

MED: 100-2,15,60.3; 100-3,10.3; 100-3,20.10; 100-3,130.1; 100-3,130.3; 100-3,130.4; 100-3,130.6; 100-3,130.7; 100-4,4,20.5; 100-4,12,100; 100-4,12,100.1.7; 100-4,12,100.1.8; 100-4,12,110.2; 100-4,12,150; 100-4,12,160; 100-4,12,160.1; 100-4,12,170

AMA: 2001,Mar,5

90826　Individual psychotherapy, interactive, using play equipment, physical devices, language interpreter, or other mechanisms of non-verbal communication, in an inpatient hospital, partial hospital or residential care setting, approximately 45 to 50 minutes face-to-face with the patient;　[S] [80] [↗]

MED: 100-2,15,60.3; 100-3,10.3; 100-3,20.10; 100-3,130.1; 100-3,130.3; 100-3,130.4; 100-3,130.6; 100-3,130.7; 100-4,4,20.5; 100-4,12,100; 100-4,12,100.1.7; 100-4,12,100.1.8; 100-4,12,110.2; 100-4,12,150; 100-4,12,160; 100-4,12,160.1; 100-4,12,170

AMA: 2001,Mar,5; 1997,Nov,40

90827　with medical evaluation and management services　[S] [80] [↗]

MED: 100-2,15,60.3; 100-3,10.3; 100-3,20.10; 100-3,130.1; 100-3,130.3; 100-3,130.4; 100-3,130.6; 100-3,130.7; 100-4,4,20.5; 100-4,12,100; 100-4,12,100.1.7; 100-4,12,100.1.8; 100-4,12,110.2; 100-4,12,150; 100-4,12,160; 100-4,12,160.1; 100-4,12,170

AMA: 2001,Mar,5; 1997,Nov,40

90828　Individual psychotherapy, interactive, using play equipment, physical devices, language interpreter, or other mechanisms of non-verbal communication, in an inpatient hospital, partial hospital or residential care setting, approximately 75 to 80 minutes face-to-face with the patient;　[S] [80] [↗]

MED: 100-2,15,60.3; 100-3,10.3; 100-3,20.10; 100-3,130.1; 100-3,130.3; 100-3,130.4; 100-3,130.6; 100-3,130.7; 100-4,4,20.5; 100-4,12,100; 100-4,12,100.1.7; 100-4,12,100.1.8; 100-4,12,110.2; 100-4,12,150; 100-4,12,160; 100-4,12,160.1; 100-4,12,170

AMA: 2001,Mar,5; 1997,Nov,40

90829　with medical evaluation and management services　[S] [80] [↗]

MED: 100-2,15,60.3; 100-3,10.3; 100-3,20.10; 100-3,130.1; 100-3,130.3; 100-3,130.4; 100-3,130.6; 100-3,130.7; 100-4,4,20.5; 100-4,12,110.2; 100-4,12,150; 100-4,12,160; 100-4,12,160.1; 100-4,12,170

AMA: 2001,Mar,5; 1997,Nov,40

OTHER PSYCHOTHERAPY

90845　Psychoanalysis　[S] [80] [↗]

MED: 100-2,15,160; 100-3,10.3; 100-3,10.4; 100-3,40.5; 100-3,130.1; 100-3,130.2; 100-3,130.3; 100-3,130.4; 100-3,130.5; 100-3,130.6; 100-3,130.7; 100-4,4,20.5; 100-4,12,110.2; 100-4,12,150; 100-4,12,160; 100-4,12,160.1; 100-4,12,170; 100-4,12,170.1

AMA: 2001,Mar,5; 1997,Nov,40-41; 1992,Summer,15

90846　Family psychotherapy (without the patient present)　[S] [80] [↗]

MED: 100-2,15,160; 100-3,10.3; 100-3,10.4; 100-3,40.5; 100-3,130.1; 100-3,130.2; 100-3,130.3; 100-3,130.4; 100-3,130.5; 100-3,130.6; 100-3,130.7; 100-4,4,20.5; 100-4,12,110.2; 100-4,12,150; 100-4,12,160; 100-4,12,160.1; 100-4,12,170; 100-4,12,170.1

AMA: 2001,Mar,5; 1997,Nov,40-41; 1992,Summer,15

90847　Family psychotherapy (conjoint psychotherapy) (with patient present)　[S] [80] [↗]

MED: 100-3,10.3; 100-3,10.4; 100-3,40.5; 100-3,130.1; 100-3,130.2; 100-3,130.3; 100-3,130.4; 100-3,130.5; 100-3,130.6; 100-3,130.7; 100-4,4,20.5; 100-4,12,70; 100-4,12,110.2; 100-4,12,150; 100-4,12,160; 100-4,12,160.1; 100-4,12,170; 100-4,13,20; 100-4,13,90

AMA: 2001,Mar,5; 1997,Nov,40-41; 1992,Summer,15

90849　Multiple-family group psychotherapy　[S] [80] [↗]

MED: 100-2,15,160; 100-3,10.3; 100-3,10.4; 100-3,40.5; 100-3,130.1; 100-3,130.2; 100-3,130.3; 100-3,130.4; 100-3,130.5; 100-3,130.6; 100-3,130.7; 100-4,4,20.5; 100-4,12,110.2; 100-4,12,150; 100-4,12,160; 100-4,12,160.1; 100-4,12,170; 100-4,12,170.1

AMA: 2001,Mar,5; 1997,Nov,40-41; 1992,Summer,15

90853　Group psychotherapy (other than of a multiple-family group)　[S] [80] [↗]

MED: 100-2,15,160; 100-3,10.3; 100-3,10.4; 100-3,40.5; 100-3,130.1; 100-3,130.2; 100-3,130.3; 100-3,130.4; 100-3,130.5; 100-3,130.6; 100-3,130.7; 100-4,4,20.5; 100-4,12,110.2; 100-4,12,150; 100-4,12,160; 100-4,12,160.1; 100-4,12,170; 100-4,12,170.1

AMA: 2001,Mar,5; 1997,Nov,40-41; 1992,Summer,15

90857　Interactive group psychotherapy　[S] [80] [↗]

MED: 100-2,15,160; 100-3,10.3; 100-3,10.4; 100-3,40.5; 100-3,130.1; 100-3,130.2; 100-3,130.3; 100-3,130.4; 100-3,130.5; 100-3,130.6; 100-3,130.7; 100-4,4,20.5; 100-4,12,110.2; 100-4,12,150; 100-4,12,160; 100-4,12,160.1; 100-4,12,170; 100-4,12,170.1

AMA: 2001,Mar,5; 1997,Nov,40-41; 1992,Summer,15

OTHER PSYCHIATRIC SERVICES OR PROCEDURES

To report repetitive transcranial magnetic stimulation for treatment of clinical depression, consult Category III codes 0160T, 0161T.

90862　Pharmacologic management, including prescription, use, and review of medication with no more than minimal medical psychotherapy　[X] [80] [↗]

MED: 100-2,15,160; 100-3,10.3; 100-3,10.4; 100-3,40.5; 100-3,130.1; 100-3,130.2; 100-3,130.3; 100-3,130.4; 100-3,130.5; 100-3,130.6; 100-3,130.7; 100-4,4,20.5; 100-4,12,160; 100-4,12,170; 100-4,12,170.1

AMA: 2001,Mar,5; 1997,Nov,40-41; 1992,Summer,16

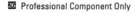
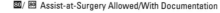

90865 Narcosynthesis for psychiatric diagnostic and therapeutic purposes (eg, sodium amobarbital (Amytal) interview) [S] [80] [CCI]

MED: 100-1,3,30; 100-1,3,30.1; 100-1,3,30.2; 100-1,3,30.3; 100-2,15,160; 100-2,15,170; 100-4,4,20.5; 100-4,12,150; 100-4,12,160; 100-4,12,160.1; 100-4,12,170; 100-4,12,170.1; 100-4,12,210

AMA: 2001,Mar,5; 1997,Nov,41

90870 Electroconvulsive therapy (includes necessary monitoring) [S] [80] [CCI]

MED: 100-1,3,30; 100-1,3,30.1; 100-1,3,30.2; 100-1,3,30.3; 100-2,15,160; 100-2,15,170; 100-4,4,20.5; 100-4,12,150; 100-4,12,160; 100-4,12,160.1; 100-4,12,170; 100-4,12,170.1; 100-4,12,210

AMA: 2001,Mar,5; 1992,Summer,16

90875 Individual psychophysiological therapy incorporating biofeedback training by any modality (face-to-face with the patient), with psychotherapy (eg, insight oriented, behavior modifying or supportive psychotherapy); approximately 20-30 minutes [E]

MED: 100-3,30.1; 100-3,30.1.1

AMA: 2001,Mar,5; 1999,Jun,5; 1998,Apr,14; 1997,Sep,11; 1997,Nov,41

90876 approximately 45-50 minutes [E]

MED: 100-1,3,30; 100-1,3,30.1; 100-1,3,30.2; 100-1,3,30.3; 100-2,15,160; 100-2,15,170; 100-3,30.1; 100-3,30.1.1; 100-4,12,150; 100-4,12,160; 100-4,12,160.1; 100-4,12,170; 100-4,12,170.1; 100-4,12,210

AMA: 2001,Mar,5; 1999,Jun,5; 1997,Sep,11; 1997,Nov,41

90880 Hypnotherapy [S] [80] [CCI]

MED: 100-1,3,30; 100-1,3,30.1; 100-1,3,30.2; 100-1,3,30.3; 100-2,15,160; 100-2,15,170; 100-4,4,20.5; 100-4,12,150; 100-4,12,160; 100-4,12,160.1; 100-4,12,170; 100-4,12,170.1; 100-4,12,210

AMA: 2001,Mar,5; 1997,Nov,41; 1992,Summer,16

90882 Environmental intervention for medical management purposes on a psychiatric patient's behalf with agencies, employers, or institutions [E]

AMA: 2001,Mar,5; 1992,Summer,16

90885 Psychiatric evaluation of hospital records, other psychiatric reports, psychometric and/or projective tests, and other accumulated data for medical diagnostic purposes [N]

MED: 100-1,3,30; 100-1,3,30.1; 100-1,3,30.2; 100-1,3,30.3; 100-2,15,160; 100-2,15,170; 100-4,12,150; 100-4,12,160; 100-4,12,160.1; 100-4,12,170; 100-4,12,170.1; 100-4,12,210

AMA: 2001,Mar,5; 1997,Nov,41

90887 Interpretation or explanation of results of psychiatric, other medical examinations and procedures, or other accumulated data to family or other responsible persons, or advising them how to assist patient [N]

MED: 100-1,3,30; 100-1,3,30.1; 100-1,3,30.2; 100-1,3,30.3; 100-2,15,160; 100-2,15,170; 100-3,70.1; 100-4,12,150; 100-4,12,160; 100-4,12,160.1; 100-4,12,170; 100-4,12,170.1; 100-4,12,210

AMA: 2002,Oct,11; 2001,Mar,5; 1992,Summer,17

90889 Preparation of report of patient's psychiatric status, history, treatment, or progress (other than for legal or consultative purposes) for other physicians, agencies, or insurance carriers [N]

MED: 100-1,3,30; 100-1,3,30.1; 100-1,3,30.2; 100-1,3,30.3; 100-2,15,160; 100-2,15,170; 100-4,12,150; 100-4,12,160; 100-4,12,170; 100-4,12,170.1; 100-4,12,210

AMA: 2001,Mar,5; 1992,Summer,17

90899 Unlisted psychiatric service or procedure [S] [80]

MED: 100-3,30.5; 100-4,4,20.5

AMA: 2001,Mar,5

BIOFEEDBACK

Biofeedback codes (90901-90911) may require prior authorization. If the payer does not cover biofeedback, enlist the help of the medical director or prior authorization (or utilization) review nurses for service coverage. Documentation may be required, such as articles or printed research material about the benefits of biofeedback.

If psychophysiological therapy is performed incorporating biofeedback training, consult CPT codes 90875 and 90876.

90901 Biofeedback training by any modality [A] [80] [CCI]

MED: 100-3,30.1; 100-3,30.1.1; 100-3,40.5; 100-3,130.5; 100-3,130.6; 100-3,160.2; 100-4,4,20.5

AMA: 2002,May,18; 1999,Jun,5; 1998,Jun,10; 1998,Apr,14; 1997,Sep,11

90911 Biofeedback training, perineal muscles, anorectal or urethral sphincter, including EMG and/or manometry [S] [80] [CCI]

MED: 100-3,30.1; 100-3,30.1.1; 100-3,40.5; 100-3,130.5; 100-3,130.6; 100-3,160.2; 100-4,4,20.5

AMA: 1999,Jun,5; 1998,Jun,10; 1997,Sep,11; 1997,Nov,41

To report pulsed magnetic neuromodulation to treat incontinence, consult CPT Category III code 0029T.

To report rectal sensation tone and compliance, consult 91120.

DIALYSIS

END STAGE RENAL DISEASE SERVICES

Dialysis services (90918-90999) are divided into end-stage renal disease (ESRD) services, hemodialysis, peritoneal dialysis, and miscellaneous dialysis procedures. Codes for the latter three services are selected according to whether the service includes single physician evaluations or repeated evaluations. Repeated evaluations are reported despite the lack of changes in the dialysis prescription.

Codes that report ESRD related services (90918-90921) are selected according to the age of the patient and reflect services for a full month. These services (90918-90921) should not be used if the physician is also submitting hospitalization codes during the month. For less than a full month, 90922-90925 are reported for each day ESRD service is provided. And the appropriate code from 90935-90947 should be reported for the inpatient dialysis services. Procedures for other medical problems and complications unrelated to ESRD are not included in the monthly ESRD service.

The dialysis procedure (90935-90947) includes all evaluation and management services related to the patient's ESRD rendered on a day dialysis is performed, as well as all other patient care services rendered during the dialysis procedure. Office and hospital visits are reported in addition to dialysis procedures only when they are unrelated to dialysis and cannot be rendered during a dialysis session.

For dialysis procedures other than hemodialysis provided during an inpatient hospital stay, consult CPT codes 90945-90947. For ESRD related services during an inpatient hospital stay, consult the appropriate Evaluation and Management codes.

Report CPT codes 90918-90921 one time per month for services performed in an outpatient setting. Do not use these codes if a hospitalization occurred during the month.

These procedures do not include dialysis treatment or services provided to the patient that are non-ESRD related. Report separately any non-ESRD related Evaluation and Management services that cannot be performed during the dialysis session.

90918 End-stage renal disease (ESRD) related services per full month; for patients younger than two years of age to include monitoring for the adequacy of nutrition, assessment of growth and development, and counseling of parents [A] [E]

MED: 100-3,110.15; 100-3,190.10; 100-3,230.14

AMA: 2003,Jan,22; 2002,May,17; 1996,May,4; 1993,Fall,5

⊛ Modifier 63 Exempt Code   ⊙ Conscious Sedation   + CPT Add-on Code   ⊘ Modifier 51 Exempt Code   ● New Code   ▲ Revised Code

[M] Maternity Edit   [A] Age Edit   [A]-[Y] APC Status Indicators   [CCI] CCI Comprehensive Code   ⚹ Drug Not Approved by FDA   [50] Bilateral Procedure

Medicine

90919 — 91000

90919   End-stage renal disease (ESRD) related services per full month; for patients between two and eleven years of age to include monitoring for the adequacy of nutrition, assessment of growth and development, and counseling of parents   ▲E

  MED: 100-3,110.15; 100-3,190.10; 100-3,230.14
  AMA: 2003,Jan,22; 2002,May,17; 1996,May,5; 1993,Fall,5

90920   End-stage renal disease (ESRD) related services per full month; for patients between twelve and nineteen years of age to include monitoring for the adequacy of nutrition, assessment of growth and development, and counseling of parents   ▲E

  MED: 100-3,110.15; 100-3,190.10; 100-3,230.14
  AMA: 2003,Jan,22; 2002,May,17; 1996,May,5; 1993,Fall,5

▲ **90921**   for patients twenty years of age and older   E

  MED: 100-3,110.15; 100-3,190.10; 100-3,230.14
  AMA: 2003,Jan,22; 2002,May,17; 1996,May,5; 1993,Fall,5

▲ **90922**   End-stage renal disease (ESRD) related services (less than full month), per day; for patients younger than two years of age   ▲E

  MED: 100-3,110.15; 100-3,190.10; 100-3,230.14
  AMA: 2003,Jan,22; 1996,May,5; 1993,Fall,5

90923   for patients between two and eleven years of age   ▲E

  MED: 100-3,110.15; 100-3,190.10; 100-3,230.14
  AMA: 2003,Jan,22; 2002,May,17; 1996,May,5

90924   for patients between twelve and nineteen years of age   ▲E

  MED: 100-3,110.15; 100-3,190.10; 100-3,230.14
  AMA: 2003,Jan,22; 2002,May,17; 1996,May,5

▲ **90925**   for patients twenty years of age and older   E

  MED: 100-3,110.15; 100-3,190.10; 100-3,230.14
  AMA: 2003,Jan,22; 2002,May,17; 1996,May,5

HEMODIALYSIS

Use CPT codes 90935-90937 for inpatient ESRD. Use CPT codes 90935-90937 to report the hemodialysis procedure and any Evaluation and Management service that is related to the patient's renal disorder provided on the day of the hemodialysis procedure.

For an unrelated Evaluation and Management service performed on the same day as hemodialysis, consult the appropriate Evaluation and Management code and append modifier 25 or code 09925.

For home visit hemodialysis services performed by a non-physician health care professional, use 99512.

If cannula declotting is performed, consult CPT codes 36831, 36833, 36860, and 36861. If a thrombolytic agent declots an implanted vascular access device or catheter, consult CPT code 36550. If the physician is in attendance for a prolonged period of time, consult CPT codes 99354-99360.

When collecting a blood specimen from a partially or completely implantable venous access device, consult CPT code 36540.

90935   Hemodialysis procedure with single physician evaluation   S 80

  MED: 100-2,1,10; 100-3,110.15; 100-3,130.8; 100-3,190.10; 100-3,230.14; 100-4,3,100.6; 100-4,4,20.5
  AMA: 2003,Jan,22; 2002,May,17; 1999,Nov,49; 1993,Fall,2

90937   Hemodialysis procedure requiring repeated evaluation(s) with or without substantial revision of dialysis prescription   B 80

  MED: 100-2,1,10; 100-3,110.15; 100-3,130.8; 100-3,190.10; 100-3,230.14; 100-4,3,100.6; 100-4,4,20.5
  AMA: 2003,Jan,22; 2002,May,17; 1999,Nov,49; 1993,Fall,2

90940   Hemodialysis access flow study to determine blood flow in grafts and arteriovenous fistulae by an indicator method   N

  MED: 100-4,3,100.6; 100-4,4,20.5
  AMA: 2003,Jan,22; 1999,Nov,49
  Consult CPT code 93990 to report duplex scan of hemodialysis access.

MISCELLANEOUS DIALYSIS PROCEDURES

If the physician is in attendance for a prolonged period of time, consult CPT codes 99354-99360. If an intraperitoneal cannula or catheter is inserted, consult CPT codes 49420 and 49421.

90945   Dialysis procedure other than hemodialysis (eg, peritoneal dialysis, hemofiltration, or other continuous renal replacement therapies), with single physician evaluation   S 80

  MED: 100-2,1,10; 100-3,110.15; 100-3,190.10; 100-3,230.14; 100-4,3,100.6; 100-4,4,20.5
  AMA: 2003,Jan,22; 2001,Oct,11; 1998,Jul,10; 1997,Nov,41; 1993,Fall,2
  To report home infusion of peritoneal dialysis, consult CPT codes 99601 and 99602.

90947   Dialysis procedure other than hemodialysis (eg, peritoneal dialysis, hemofiltration, or other continuous renal replacement therapies) requiring repeated physician evaluations, with or without substantial revision of dialysis prescription   B 80

  MED: 100-2,1,10; 100-3,110.15; 100-3,190.10; 100-3,230.14; 100-4,3,100.6; 100-4,4,20.5
  AMA: 2003,Jan,22; 2001,Oct,11; 1998,Jul,10; 1997,Nov,41; 1993,Fall,2

90989   Dialysis training, patient, including helper where applicable, any mode, completed course   B

  MED: 100-3,190.10; 100-4,3,100.6; 100-4,4,20.5
  AMA: 2001,Jun,10; 1993,Fall,5

90993   Dialysis training, patient, including helper where applicable, any mode, course not completed, per training session   B

  MED: 100-3,190.10; 100-4,3,100.6; 100-4,4,20.5
  AMA: 2001,Jun,10; 1993,Fall,5

90997   Hemoperfusion (eg, with activated charcoal or resin)   B 80

  MED: 100-3,110.15; 100-3,230.14; 100-4,3,100.6; 100-4,4,20.5

90999   Unlisted dialysis procedure, inpatient or outpatient   B 80

  MED: 100-3,190.10; 100-4,3,100.6; 100-4,4,20.5

GASTROENTEROLOGY

The diagnostic procedures (91000-91299) are frequently performed with consultations or other E/M services that are reported separately. Even though gastroenterology is a medicine subspecialty, the majority of procedures performed by gastroenterologists are endoscopic and listed in the surgery section.

If duodenal intubation and aspiration are performed, consult CPT codes 89100-89105. If gastrointestinal radiologic procedures are performed, consult CPT codes 74210-74363. If esophagoscopy procedures are performed, consult CPT codes 43200-43228; upper GI endoscopy 43234-43259; endoscopy, small bowel and stomal 44360-44393; proctosigmoidoscopy 45300-45321; sigmoidoscopy 45330-45339; colonoscopy 45355-45385; and anoscopy 46600-46615.

91000   Esophageal intubation and collection of washings for cytology, including preparation of specimens (separate procedure)   X 80

91010   **Esophageal motility (manometric study of the esophagus and/or gastroesophageal junction) study;**   X 80 ▣

     MED: 100-3,100.4
     AMA: 1997,Nov,42

91011   **with mecholyl or similar stimulant**   X 80 ▣

91012   **with acid perfusion studies**   X 80 ▣

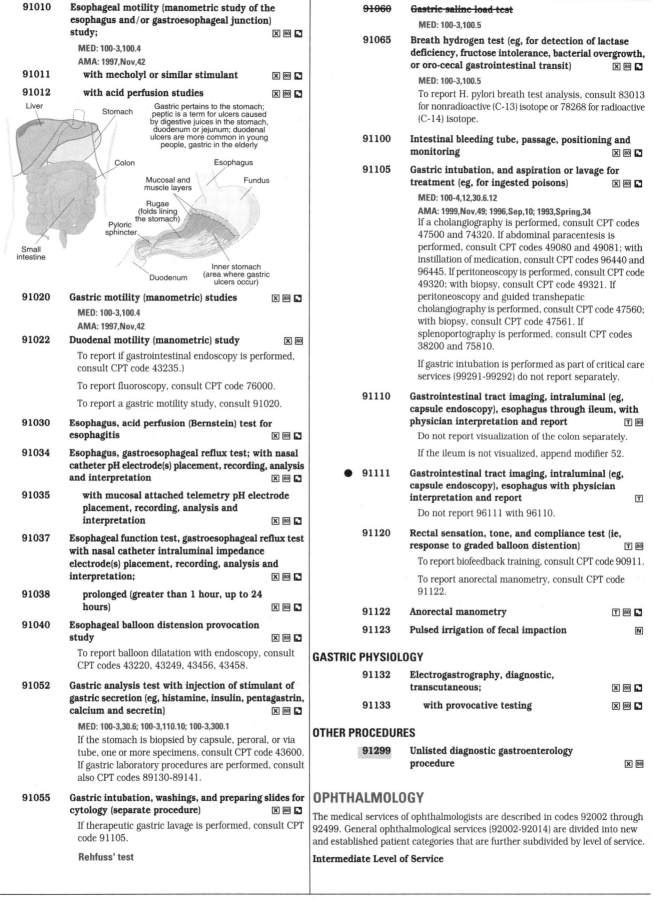

Gastric pertains to the stomach; peptic is a term for ulcers caused by digestive juices in the stomach, duodenum or jejunum; duodenal ulcers are more common in young people, gastric in the elderly

91020   **Gastric motility (manometric) studies**   X 80 ▣

     MED: 100-3,100.4
     AMA: 1997,Nov,42

91022   **Duodenal motility (manometric) study**   X 80

     To report if gastrointestinal endoscopy is performed, consult CPT code 43235.)

     To report fluoroscopy, consult CPT code 76000.

     To report a gastric motility study, consult 91020.

91030   **Esophagus, acid perfusion (Bernstein) test for esophagitis**   X 80 ▣

91034   **Esophagus, gastroesophageal reflux test; with nasal catheter pH electrode(s) placement, recording, analysis and interpretation**   X 80 ▣

91035   **with mucosal attached telemetry pH electrode placement, recording, analysis and interpretation**   X 80 ▣

91037   **Esophageal function test, gastroesophageal reflux test with nasal catheter intraluminal impedance electrode(s) placement, recording, analysis and interpretation;**   X 80 ▣

91038   **prolonged (greater than 1 hour, up to 24 hours)**   X 80 ▣

91040   **Esophageal balloon distension provocation study**   X 80 ▣

     To report balloon dilatation with endoscopy, consult CPT codes 43220, 43249, 43456, 43458.

91052   **Gastric analysis test with injection of stimulant of gastric secretion (eg, histamine, insulin, pentagastrin, calcium and secretin)**   X 80 ▣

     MED: 100-3,30.6; 100-3,110.10; 100-3,300.1
     If the stomach is biopsied by capsule, peroral, or via tube, one or more specimens, consult CPT code 43600. If gastric laboratory procedures are performed, consult also CPT codes 89130-89141.

91055   **Gastric intubation, washings, and preparing slides for cytology (separate procedure)**   X 80 ▣

     If therapeutic gastric lavage is performed, consult CPT code 91105.

     Rehfuss' test

~~91060~~   ~~Gastric saline load test~~

     MED: 100-3,100.5

91065   **Breath hydrogen test (eg, for detection of lactase deficiency, fructose intolerance, bacterial overgrowth, or oro-cecal gastrointestinal transit)**   X 80 ▣

     MED: 100-3,100.5

     To report H. pylori breath test analysis, consult 83013 for nonradioactive (C-13) isotope or 78268 for radioactive (C-14) isotope.

91100   **Intestinal bleeding tube, passage, positioning and monitoring**   X 80 ▣

91105   **Gastric intubation, and aspiration or lavage for treatment (eg, for ingested poisons)**   X 80 ▣

     MED: 100-4,12,30.6.12
     AMA: 1999,Nov,49; 1996,Sep,10; 1993,Spring,34
     If a cholangiography is performed, consult CPT codes 47500 and 74320. If abdominal paracentesis is performed, consult CPT codes 49080 and 49081; with instillation of medication, consult CPT codes 96440 and 96445. If peritoneoscopy is performed, consult CPT code 49320; with biopsy, consult CPT code 49321. If peritoneoscopy and guided transhepatic cholangiography is performed, consult CPT code 47560; with biopsy, consult CPT code 47561. If splenoportography is performed, consult CPT codes 38200 and 75810.

     If gastric intubation is performed as part of critical care services (99291-99292) do not report separately.

91110   **Gastrointestinal tract imaging, intraluminal (eg, capsule endoscopy), esophagus through ileum, with physician interpretation and report**   T 80

     Do not report visualization of the colon separately.

     If the ileum is not visualized, append modifier 52.

● 91111   **Gastrointestinal tract imaging, intraluminal (eg, capsule endoscopy), esophagus with physician interpretation and report**   T

     Do not report 96111 with 96110.

91120   **Rectal sensation, tone, and compliance test (ie, response to graded balloon distention)**   T 80

     To report biofeedback training, consult CPT code 90911.

     To report anorectal manometry, consult CPT code 91122.

91122   **Anorectal manometry**   T 80 ▣

91123   **Pulsed irrigation of fecal impaction**   N

GASTRIC PHYSIOLOGY

91132   **Electrogastrography, diagnostic, transcutaneous;**   X 80 ▣

91133   **with provocative testing**   X 80 ▣

OTHER PROCEDURES

91299   **Unlisted diagnostic gastroenterology procedure**   X 80

OPHTHALMOLOGY

The medical services of ophthalmologists are described in codes 92002 through 92499. General ophthalmological services (92002-92014) are divided into new and established patient categories that are further subdivided by level of service.

Intermediate Level of Service

⊛ Modifier 63 Exempt Code   ⊙ Conscious Sedation   + CPT Add-on Code   ⊘ Modifier 51 Exempt Code   ● New Code   ▲ Revised Code

M Maternity Edit   A Age Edit   A-Y APC Status Indicators   ▣ CCI Comprehensive Code   ✗ Drug Not Approved by FDA   50 Bilateral Procedure

Intermediate service codes (92002 and 92012) report the evaluation of new or existing conditions that have been complicated by a new diagnostic or management problem. This new complaint may relate to the primary diagnosis. Included in the evaluation are:

- History
- General medical observation
- External examination
- Ophthalmoscopy
- Other diagnostic procedures as indicated:
  ○ biomicroscopy
  ○ mydriasis
  ○ tonometry
- Initiation of diagnostic and treatment program

Comprehensive Level of Service

Comprehensive service codes (92004 and 92014) report the evaluation of the complete visual system. This is a single service that need not be performed at one session. Included in this evaluation are:

- History
- General medical observation
- General evaluation of the complete visual system to include:
  ○ external examination
  ○ ophthalmoscopy
  ○ gross visual field
  ○ basic sensorimotor examination
- Other diagnostic procedures as indicated:
  ○ biomicroscopy
  ○ dilation (cycloplegia)
  ○ mydriasis
  ○ tonometry
- Initiation of a diagnostic treatment program

GENERAL OPHTHALMOLOGICAL SERVICES

NEW PATIENT

Consult the glossary for terms and definitions and the front matter of this chapter for additional information.

If surgical procedures are performed, consult Eye and Ocular Adnexa in the Surgery section (65091 and subsequent codes).

92002 Ophthalmological services: medical examination and evaluation with initiation of diagnostic and treatment program; intermediate, new patient [V] [80] [⌐]
MED: 100-4,4,20.5; 100-4,4,160
AMA: 1998,Aug,1; 1997,Feb,6

92004 comprehensive, new patient, one or more visits [V] [80] [⌐]
MED: 100-4,4,20.5; 100-4,4,160
AMA: 1998,Aug,1; 1997,Feb,6

ESTABLISHED PATIENT

92012 Ophthalmological services: medical examination and evaluation, with initiation or continuation of diagnostic and treatment program; intermediate, established patient [V] [80] [⌐]
MED: 100-4,4,20.5; 100-4,4,160
AMA: 1998,Aug,1; 1997,Feb,6

92014 comprehensive, established patient, one or more visits [V] [80] [⌐]
MED: 100-4,4,20.5; 100-4,4,160
AMA: 1999,Dec,10; 1998,Aug,1; 1997,Feb,6

SPECIAL OPHTHALMOLOGICAL SERVICES

Refractions (92015) should be reported additionally when performed at the time of a general ophthalmological service (92002-92014). Medicare allows the reporting of refractions, a noncovered service, to minimize patient confusion.

Gross visual field testing is integral to the general ophthalmic service and should not be reported separately. However, more extensive visual field examinations should be reported separately with codes 92081-92083. The CPT book recognizes three coding levels for visual field exams. The three specific visual field tests (limited, intermediate, and extended) are described as unilateral or bilateral.

Fitting and provision of contact lenses, glasses, and ocular prostheses are reported with the CPT codes 92310-92396. Use modifier 26 with 92391 or 92396 to report the service of fitting without supply. All the codes in this section are bilateral. For prescription or fitting of one eye, append modifier 52.

92015 Determination of refractive state [E]
MED: 100-2,16,90; 100-4,4,20.5
AMA: 1998,Aug,1; 1997,Feb,6; 1996,Mar,11

92018 Ophthalmological examination and evaluation, under general anesthesia, with or without manipulation of globe for passive range of motion or other manipulation to facilitate diagnostic examination; complete [T] [80] [⌐]
MED: 100-4,4,20.5
AMA: 1997,Feb,6

92019 limited [T] [80] [⌐]
MED: 100-4,4,20.5
AMA: 1997,Feb,6

92020 Gonioscopy (separate procedure) [S] [80] [⌐]
MED: 100-4,4,20.5
AMA: 1997,Feb,6
If gonioscopy is performed under general anesthesia, consult CPT cde 92018.

● **92025** Computerized corneal topography, unilateral or bilateral, with interpretation and report [S]
Do not report code 92025 with codes 65710-65755.

Code 92025 is not used for manual keratoscopy, which is a part of a single system Evaluation and Management or ophthalmological service.

92060 Sensorimotor examination with multiple measurements of ocular deviation (eg, restrictive or paretic muscle with diplopia) with interpretation and report (separate procedure) [S] [80] [⌐]
MED: 100-4,4,20.5
AMA: 1997,Feb,6

92065 Orthoptic and/or pleoptic training, with continuing medical direction and evaluation [S] [80] [⌐]
MED: 100-4,4,20.5
AMA: 1998,Jun,10; 1997,Feb,6

92070 Fitting of contact lens for treatment of disease, including supply of lens [N] [80] [⌐]
MED: 100-3,80.1; 100-3,80.4; 100-3,80.9; 100-4,4,20.5
AMA: 1997,Feb,6

92081 Visual field examination, unilateral or bilateral, with interpretation and report; limited examination (eg, tangent screen, Autoplot, arc perimeter, or single stimulus level automated test, such as Octopus 3 or 7 equivalent) [S] [80] [⌐]
MED: 100-3,80.9; 100-4,4,20.5
AMA: 1997,Feb,6

92082	intermediate examination (eg, at least 2 isopters on Goldmann perimeter, or semiquantitative, automated suprathreshold screening program, Humphrey suprathreshold automatic diagnostic test, Octopus program 33) [S] [80] [C]

MED: 100-3,80.9; 100-4,4,20.5

AMA: 1997,Feb,6

92083	extended examination (eg, Goldmann visual fields with at least 3 isopters plotted and static determination within the central 30°, or quantitative, automated threshold perimetry, Octopus program G-1, 32 or 42, Humphrey visual field analyzer full threshold programs 30-2, 24-2, or 30/60-2) [S] [80] [C]

MED: 100-3,80.9; 100-4,4,20.5

AMA: 1997,Feb,6

Note that gross visual field testing (e.g., confrontation testing) is a part of general ophthalmological services and is not reported separately.

92100	Serial tonometry (separate procedure) with multiple measurements of intraocular pressure over an extended time period with interpretation and report, same day (eg, diurnal curve or medical treatment of acute elevation of intraocular pressure) [N] [80] [C]

MED: 100-4,4,20.5

AMA: 1998,Jun,10; 1997,Feb,6

92120	Tonography with interpretation and report, recording indentation tonometer method or perilimbal suction method [S] [80] [C]

MED: 100-4,4,20.5

AMA: 1997,Feb,6

92130	Tonography with water provocation [S] [80] [C]

MED: 100-4,4,20.5

AMA: 1997,Feb,6

92135	Scanning computerized ophthalmic diagnostic imaging (eg, scanning laser) with interpretation and report, unilateral [S] [C]

MED: 100-4,4,20.5

AMA: 1999,Mar,10; 1999,Apr,10; 1998,Nov,33

92136	Ophthalmic biometry by partial coherence interferometry with intraocular lens power calculation [S] [80] [C]

MED: 100-3,10.1; 100-4,4,20.5

AMA: 2002,Apr,18

Open-angle is the most common type of glaucoma; the disease occurs most frequently in people over age 60

Cornea

Trabecular meshwork

Anterior chamber angle

Schlemm's canal

Iris

Schematic of anterior chamber

Lens

Normal flow of aqueous humor from behind lens to Schlemm's canal

Glaucoma is caused by excessive intraocular pressure and abnormal accumulation of aqueous humor in the anterior chamber of the eye; pressure reduces blood supply to the optic nerve and causes nerve damage

92140	Provocative tests for glaucoma, with interpretation and report, without tonography [S] [80] [C]

MED: 100-4,4,20.5

AMA: 1998,Aug,1; 1997,Feb,6

OPHTHALMOSCOPY

Routine ophthalmoscopy is considered part of special or general ophthalmologic services when indicated and not separately reported.

92225	Ophthalmoscopy, extended, with retinal drawing (eg, for retinal detachment, melanoma), with interpretation and report; initial [S] [80] [C]

MED: 100-4,4,20.5

AMA: 1999,Dec,10; 1998,Aug,1; 1997,Feb,6

92226	subsequent [S] [80] [C]

MED: 100-4,4,20.5

AMA: 1998,Aug,1; 1997,Feb,6

92230	Fluorescein angioscopy with interpretation and report [S] [80] [C]

MED: 100-4,4,20.5

AMA: 1997,Feb,6

92235	Fluorescein angiography (includes multiframe imaging) with interpretation and report [S] [80] [C]

MED: 100-4,4,20.5

AMA: 1997,Feb,6

92240	Indocyanine-green angiography (includes multiframe imaging) with interpretation and report [S] [80] [C]

MED: 100-3,80.6; 100-4,4,20.5

92250	Fundus photography with interpretation and report [S] [80] [C]

MED: 100-3,80.6; 100-4,4,20.5

AMA: 1999,Apr,10; 1997,Feb,6

92260	Ophthalmodynamometry [S] [80] [C]

MED: 100-4,4,20.5

AMA: 1997,Feb,6

If ophthalmoscopy is performed under general anesthesia, consult CPT code 92018.

OTHER SPECIALIZED SERVICES

92265	Needle oculoelectromyography, one or more extraocular muscles, one or both eyes, with interpretation and report [S] [80] [C]

MED: 100-4,4,20.5

AMA: 1997,Feb,6

92270	Electro-oculography with interpretation and report [S] [80] [C]

MED: 100-4,4,20.5

AMA: 1997,Feb,6

92275	Electroretinography with interpretation and report [S] [80] [C]

MED: 100-4,4,20.5

AMA: 1997,Feb,6

If electronystagmography is performed for vestibular function studies, consult CPT codes 92541 and subsequent codes. If ophthalmic echography is performed (diagnostic ultrasound), consult CPT codes 76511-76529.

92283	Color vision examination, extended, eg, anomaloscope or equivalent [S] [80] [C]

MED: 100-4,4,20.5

AMA: 1997,Feb,6

Note that color vision testing with pseudoisochromatic plates (such as HRR or Ishihara) is not reported separately. It is included in the appropriate general or ophthalmological service.

Farnsworth-Munsell color test

92284	Dark adaptation examination with interpretation and report [S] [80] [C]

MED: 100-4,4,20.5

AMA: 1997,Feb,6

---

⑥³ Modifier 63 Exempt Code ⊙ Conscious Sedation ✛ CPT Add-on Code ⊘ Modifier 51 Exempt Code ● New Code ▲ Revised Code

[M] Maternity Edit [A] Age Edit [A]-[Y] APC Status Indicators [C] CCI Comprehensive Code ✗ Drug Not Approved by FDA [50] Bilateral Procedure

CPT only © 2006 American Medical Association. All Rights Reserved. (Black Ink)

92285   External ocular photography with interpretation and report for documentation of medical progress (eg, close-up photography, slit lamp photography, goniophotography, stereo-photography)   S 80 ▣

     MED: 100-3,80.8; 100-4,4,20.5
     AMA: 1997,Sep,10; 1997,Feb,6

92286   Special anterior segment photography with interpretation and report; with specular endothelial microscopy and cell count   S 80 ▣

     MED: 100-4,4,20.5
     AMA: 1997,Feb,6

92287   with fluorescein angiography   S 80 ▣

     MED: 100-4,4,20.5
     AMA: 1997,Feb,6

CONTACT LENS SERVICES

Report the following contact lens codes separately from other ophthalmological services.

Fitting of contact lenses includes patient training and instruction as well as incidental revision of the contacts during the training period.

For therapeutic or surgical use of contact lens, consult CPT codes 68340 and 92970.

92310   Prescription of optical and physical characteristics of and fitting of contact lens, with medical supervision of adaptation; corneal lens, both eyes, except for aphakia   E

     MED: 100-3,80.1; 100-3,80.4; 100-4,4,20.5
     AMA: 1997,Feb,6
     To report prescription and fitting of one eye, append modifier 52.

92311   corneal lens for aphakia, one eye   X 80 ▣

     MED: 100-3,80.1; 100-3,80.4; 100-4,4,20.5
     AMA: 1997,Feb,6

92312   corneal lens for aphakia, both eyes   X 80 ▣

     MED: 100-3,80.1; 100-3,80.4; 100-4,4,20.5
     AMA: 1997,Feb,6

92313   corneoscleral lens   X 80 ▣

     MED: 100-3,80.1; 100-3,80.4; 100-4,4,20.5
     AMA: 1997,Feb,7

92314   Prescription of optical and physical characteristics of contact lens, with medical supervision of adaptation and direction of fitting by independent technician; corneal lens, both eyes except for aphakia   E

     MED: 100-3,80.1; 100-3,80.4; 100-4,4,20.5
     AMA: 1997,Feb,7
     To report prescription and fitting of one eye, append modifier 52.

92315   corneal lens for aphakia, one eye   X 80 ▣

     MED: 100-3,80.1; 100-3,80.4; 100-4,4,20.5
     AMA: 1997,Feb,7

92316   corneal lens for aphakia, both eyes   X 80 ▣

     MED: 100-3,80.1; 100-3,80.4; 100-4,4,20.5
     AMA: 1997,Feb,7

92317   corneoscleral lens   X 80 ▣

     MED: 100-3,80.1; 100-3,80.4; 100-4,4,20.5
     AMA: 1997,Feb,7

92325   Modification of contact lens (separate procedure), with medical supervision of adaptation   X 80 ▣

     MED: 100-3,80.1; 100-3,80.4; 100-4,4,20.5
     AMA: 1997,Feb,7
     To report therapeutic or surgical use of contact lens, consult CPT codes 68340 and 92970.

92326   Replacement of contact lens   X 80 ▣

     MED: 100-3,80.1; 100-3,80.4; 100-4,4,20.5
     AMA: 1997,Feb,7
     To report the prescription, fitting, and/or medical supervision of ocular prosthetic adaptation by the physician, consult the E/M codes or 92002-92004.

SPECTACLE SERVICES (INCLUDING PROSTHESIS FOR APHAKIA)

92340   Fitting of spectacles, except for aphakia; monofocal   E

     MED: 100-4,4,20.5
     AMA: 1998,Aug,1; 1997,Feb,7

92341   bifocal   E

     MED: 100-4,4,20.5
     AMA: 1997,Feb,7

92342   multifocal, other than bifocal   E

     MED: 100-4,4,20.5
     AMA: 1997,Feb,7

92352   Fitting of spectacle prosthesis for aphakia; monofocal   X

     MED: 100-2,15,120; 100-4,1,30.3.5; 100-4,4,20.5
     AMA: 1997,Feb,7

92353   multifocal   X

     MED: 100-2,15,120; 100-4,1,30.3.5; 100-4,4,20.5
     AMA: 1997,Feb,7

92354   Fitting of spectacle mounted low vision aid; single element system   X

     MED: 100-4,4,20.5
     AMA: 1997,Feb,7

92355   telescopic or other compound lens system   X

     MED: 100-4,4,20.5
     AMA: 1997,Feb,7

92358   Prosthesis service for aphakia, temporary (disposable or loan, including materials)   X

     MED: 100-2,15,120; 100-4,1,30.3.5; 100-4,4,20.5
     AMA: 1997,Feb,7

92370   Repair and refitting spectacles; except for aphakia   E

     MED: 100-4,4,20.5
     AMA: 1997,Feb,7

92371   spectacle prosthesis for aphakia   X

     MED: 100-2,15,120; 100-4,1,30.3.5; 100-4,4,20.5
     AMA: 1998,Aug,1; 1997,Feb,7
     Report the appropriate supply codes for spectacles or contact lenses.

OTHER PROCEDURES

92499   Unlisted ophthalmological service or procedure   S 80

     MED: 100-4,4,20.5
     AMA: 1997,Feb,7

SPECIAL OTORHINOLARYNGOLOGIC SERVICES

Otorhinolaryngologic codes (92502-92700) identify the special diagnostic and treatment services not usually included in a comprehensive otorhinolaryngologic evaluation. Comprehensive ear, nose, and throat (ENT) evaluations include basic diagnostic procedures such as otoscopy and rhinoscopy. These services are an integral part of the evaluation and management service and are not itemized separately. Special services not generally included in this total evaluation are reported separately with 92502-92700, such as audiologic function tests (92551-92597). Hearing tests using calibrated electronic equipment are reportable; use of a tuning fork is not.

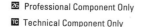
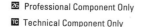
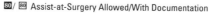

Hearing test codes are inherently bilateral (binaural, both ears). If only one ear is tested, the reduced service is reported with modifier 52. Codes 92590, 92592, and 92594 are the exceptions, identified in CPT as monaural (one ear). If binaural, report with 92591, 92593, or 92595.

If laryngoscopy is performed with stroboscopy, consult CPT code 31579.

92502   Otolaryngologic examination under general anesthesia   T 80 ▣
MED: 100-4,4,20.5

92504   Binocular microscopy (separate diagnostic procedure)   N 80 ▣
MED: 100-4,4,20.5

92506   Evaluation of speech, language, voice, communication, and/or auditory processing   A 80 ▣
MED: 100-3,170.3; 100-4,4,20.5; 100-4,32,100

92507   Treatment of speech, language, voice, communication, and/or auditory processing disorder; individual   A 80 ▣
MED: 100-2,15,230.3; 100-3,50.3; 100-4,4,20.5; 100-4,32,100

92508   group, 2 or more individuals   A 80 ▣
MED: 100-2,15,230.3; 100-3,50.3; 100-4,4,20.5

92511   Nasopharyngoscopy with endoscope (separate procedure)   T 80 ▣
MED: 100-4,4,20.5

92512   Nasal function studies (eg, rhinomanometry)   X 80
MED: 100-4,4,20.5

92516   Facial nerve function studies (eg, electroneuronography)   X 80
MED: 100-4,4,20.5

92520   Laryngeal function studies (ie, aerodynamic testing and acoustic testing)   X 80 ▣
MED: 100-4,4,20.5

To report a single test, use modifier 52.

To report a flexible fiber optic laryngeal evaluation of swallowing and laryngeal sensory testing, consult CPT codes 92611-92617.

To report other testing of laryngeal function (eg. electroglottography), consult CPT code 92700.

92526   Treatment of swallowing dysfunction and/or oral function for feeding   A 80 ▣
MED: 100-3,170.3; 100-4,4,20.5

VESTIBULAR FUNCTION TESTS

WITH OBSERVATION AND EVALUATION BY PHYSICIAN, WITHOUT ELECTRICAL RECORDING

92531   Spontaneous nystagmus, including gaze   N
MED: 100-4,4,20.5

92532   Positional nystagmus test   N
MED: 100-4,4,20.5

92533   Caloric vestibular test, each irrigation (binaural, bithermal stimulation constitutes four tests)   N
MED: 100-4,4,20.5
AMA: 1996,May,5
Barany caloric test

92534   Optokinetic nystagmus test   N
MED: 100-4,4,20.5

WITH RECORDING (EG, ENG, PENG), AND MEDICAL DIAGNOSTIC EVALUATION

92541   Spontaneous nystagmus test, including gaze and fixation nystagmus, with recording   X 80 ▣
MED: 100-4,4,20.5

92542   Positional nystagmus test, minimum of 4 positions, with recording   X 80
MED: 100-4,4,20.5

92543   Caloric vestibular test, each irrigation (binaural, bithermal stimulation constitutes four tests), with recording   X 80 ▣
MED: 100-4,4,20.5
AMA: 1996,May,5

92544   Optokinetic nystagmus test, bidirectional, foveal or peripheral stimulation, with recording   X 80
MED: 100-4,4,20.5

92545   Oscillating tracking test, with recording   X 80
MED: 100-4,4,20.5

92546   Sinusoidal vertical axis rotational testing   X 80
MED: 100-4,4,20.5

+ **92547**   Use of vertical electrodes (List separately in addition to code for primary procedure)   X TC 80
MED: 100-4,4,20.5

Note that 92547 is an add-on code and must be used in conjunction with 92541-92546. If vestibular tests are unlisted, consult CPT code 92700.

92548   Computerized dynamic posturography   X 80
MED: 100-4,4,20.5

AUDIOLOGIC FUNCTION TESTS WITH MEDICAL DIAGNOSTIC EVALUATION

The following codes describe the use of electronic equipment and differ from other otorhinolaryngologic services that include the use of tuning forks, clapping, whispering, and other stimuli. All CPT codes in this section are considered bilateral. Use modifier 52 if the test is performed on one ear only.

If speech, language, and/or hearing problems are evaluated through observation and assessment of performance, consult CPT code 92506.

92551   Screening test, pure tone, air only   E
MED: 100-2,15,80.3; 100-4,4,20.5

92552   Pure tone audiometry (threshold); air only   X TC 80 ▣
MED: 100-2,15,80.3; 100-4,4,20.5

92553   air and bone   X TC 80 ▣
MED: 100-2,15,80.3; 100-4,4,20.5

92555   Speech audiometry threshold;   X TC 80 ▣
MED: 100-2,15,80.3; 100-4,4,20.5

92556   with speech recognition   X TC 80 ▣
MED: 100-2,15,80.3; 100-4,4,20.5

92557   Comprehensive audiometry threshold evaluation and speech recognition (92553 and 92556 combined)   X TC 80 ▣
MED: 100-4,4,20.5

To report hearing aid evaluation and selection, consult CPT codes 92590-92595.

92559   Audiometric testing of groups   E
MED: 100-4,4,20.5

92560   Bekesy audiometry; screening   E
MED: 100-2,15,80.3; 100-4,4,20.5

92561   diagnostic   X TC 80 ▣
MED: 100-2,15,80.3; 100-4,4,20.5

⊕ Modifier 63 Exempt Code   ☉ Conscious Sedation   + CPT Add-on Code   ⊘ Modifier 51 Exempt Code   ● New Code   ▲ Revised Code

M Maternity Edit   A Age Edit   A-Y APC Status Indicators   ▣ CCI Comprehensive Code   ⚕ Drug Not Approved by FDA   50 Bilateral Procedure

92562	Loudness balance test, alternate binaural or monaural	⊠ TC 80 ↻
	MED: 100-4,4,20.5	
92563	Tone decay test	⊠ TC 80 ↻
	MED: 100-4,4,20.5	
92564	Short increment sensitivity index (SISI)	⊠ TC 80 ↻
	MED: 100-4,4,20.5	
	AMA: 1996,Oct,9	
92565	Stenger test, pure tone	⊠ TC 80 ↻
	MED: 100-4,4,20.5	
92567	Tympanometry (impedance testing)	⊠ TC 80 ↻
	MED: 100-4,4,20.5	
92568	Acoustic reflex testing; threshold	⊠ TC 80 ↻
	MED: 100-4,4,20.5	
92569	decay	⊠ TC 80 ↻
	MED: 100-4,4,20.5	
92571	Filtered speech test	⊠ TC 80 ↻
	MED: 100-4,4,20.5	
92572	Staggered spondaic word test	⊠ TC 80 ↻
	MED: 100-4,4,20.5	
~~92573~~	~~Lombard test~~	
	Use 92700.	
92575	Sensorineural acuity level test	⊠ TC 80 ↻
	MED: 100-4,4,20.5	
92576	Synthetic sentence identification test	⊠ TC 80 ↻
	MED: 100-4,4,20.5	
92577	Stenger test, speech	⊠ TC 80 ↻
	MED: 100-4,4,20.5	
92579	Visual reinforcement audiometry (VRA)	⊠ TC 80 ↻
	MED: 100-4,4,20.5	
92582	Conditioning play audiometry	⊠ TC 80 ↻
	MED: 100-4,4,20.5	
92583	Select picture audiometry	⊠ TC 80 ↻
	MED: 100-4,4,20.5	
92584	Electrocochleography	⊠ TC 80 ↻
	MED: 100-3,160.10; 100-4,4,20.5	
92585	Auditory evoked potentials for evoked response audiometry and/or testing of the central nervous system; comprehensive	S 80 ↻
	MED: 100-3,160.10; 100-4,4,20.5	
92586	limited	S TC 80 ↻
	MED: 100-3,160.10; 100-4,4,20.5	
92587	Evoked otoacoustic emissions; limited (single stimulus level, either transient or distortion products)	⊠ 80 ↻
	MED: 100-4,4,20.5	
92588	comprehensive or diagnostic evaluation (comparison of transient and/or distortion product otoacoustic emissions at multiple levels and frequencies)	⊠ 80 ↻
	MED: 100-4,4,20.5	
92590	Hearing aid examination and selection; monaural	E
	MED: 100-2,15,80.3; 100-4,4,20.5	
92591	binaural	E
	MED: 100-2,15,80.3; 100-4,4,20.5	
92592	Hearing aid check; monaural	E
	MED: 100-2,15,80.3; 100-4,4,20.5	

92593	binaural	E
	MED: 100-2,15,80.3; 100-4,4,20.5	
92594	Electroacoustic evaluation for hearing aid; monaural	E
	MED: 100-2,15,80.3; 100-4,4,20.5	
92595	binaural	E
	MED: 100-2,15,80.3; 100-4,4,20.5	
92596	Ear protector attenuation measurements	⊠ TC 80 ↻
	MED: 100-2,15,80.3; 100-4,4,20.5	
92597	Evaluation for use and/or fitting of voice prosthetic device to supplement oral speech	A 80 ↻

To report augmentative and alternative communication device services, consult CPT codes 92605, 92607, and 92608.

EVALUATIVE AND THERAPEUTIC SERVICES

CPT codes 92601 and 92603 are used to report post-operative analysis and fitting of previously placed external devices, connection to the cochlear implant, and stimulator programming. CPT codes 92602 and 92604 are used to report subsequent sessions for measurements and adjustments of the external transmitter and internal stimulator.

To report placement of cochlear implant, consult CPT code 69930.

▲ 92601	Diagnostic analysis of cochlear implant, patient younger than 7 years of age; with programming	A ⊠ 80 ↻
	MED: 100-2,15,80.3; 100-3,50.3; 100-4,32,100	
▲ 92602	subsequent reprogramming	A ⊠ 80 ↻
	MED: 100-2,15,80.3; 100-3,50.3; 100-4,32,100	

Do not report 92602 with CPT code 92601.

To report aural rehabilitation services after a cochlear implant consult CPT codes 92626-92627, 92630-92633.

92603	Diagnostic analysis of cochlear implant, age 7 years or older; with programming	⊠ 80 ↻
	MED: 100-2,15,80.3; 100-3,50.3; 100-4,32,100	
92604	subsequent reprogramming	⊠ 80 ↻
	MED: 100-2,15,80.3; 100-3,50.3; 100-4,32,100	

Do not report 92604 with CPT code 92603.

92605	Evaluation for prescription of non-speech-generating augmentative and alternative communication device	A
	MED: 100-2,15,230.3; 100-3,50.2; 100-3,50.3	
92606	Therapeutic service(s) for the use of non-speech-generating device, including programming and modification	A
	MED: 100-2,15,230.3; 100-3,50.3	
92607	Evaluation for prescription for speech-generating augmentative and alternative communication device, face-to-face with the patient; first hour	A 80 ↻
	MED: 100-2,15,230.3; 100-3,50.1; 100-3,50.2; 100-3,50.3	

To report evaluation for prescription of a non-speech generating device, consult CPT code 92605.

| + 92608 | each additional 30 minutes (List separately in addition to code for primary procedure) | A 80 ↻ |
| | MED: 100-2,15,230.3; 100-3,50.2; 100-3,50.3 | |

Note that 92608 is an add-on code and must be used in conjunction with CPT code 92607.

---

26 Professional Component Only   80/ 80 Assist-at-Surgery Allowed/With Documentation   Unlisted   Not Covered

TC Technical Component Only   MED: Pub 100/NCD References   AMA: CPT Assistant References   1-9 ASC Group   ♂ Male Only   ♀ Female Only

346 — CPT Expert   CPT only © 2006 American Medical Association. All Rights Reserved. (Black Ink)   © 2006 Ingenix (Blue Ink)

92609 Therapeutic services for the use of speech-generating device, including programming and modification ☐A☐ 80 ☐

MED: 100-2,15,230.3; 100-3,50.1; 100-3,50.2; 100-3,50.3

To report therapeutic service(s) for the use of a non-speech generating device, consult CPT code 92606.

92610 Evaluation of oral and pharyngeal swallowing function ☐A☐ 80 ☐

MED: 100-2,15,230.3; 100-3,50.3; 100-3,170.3

To report motion fluoroscopic evaluation of swallowing function, consult CPT code 92611.

To report flexible endoscopic examination, consult CPT codes 92612-92617.

92611 Motion fluoroscopic evaluation of swallowing function by cine or video recording ☐A☐ 80 ☐

MED: 100-2,15,230.3; 100-3,50.3; 100-3,170.3

To report radiological supervision and interpretation, consult CPT code 74230.

To report evaluation of oral and pharyngeal swallowing functions, consult CPT code 92610.

92612 Flexible fiberoptic endoscopic evaluation of swallowing by cine or video recording; ☐A☐ 80 ☐

MED: 100-2,15,230.3; 100-3,50.3; 100-3,170.3

To report flexible fiberoptic or endoscopic swallowing evaluation performed without cine or video recording, consult CPT code 92700.

To report flexible fiberoptic diagnostic laryngoscopy, consult CPT code 31575. Code 31575 cannot be reported with 92612-92617.

92613 physician interpretation and report only ☐B☐ 80 ☐

MED: 100-2,15,230.3; 100-3,50.3; 100-3,170.3

To report evaluation of oral and pharyngeal swallowing function, consult CPT code 92610.

To report motion fluoroscopic evaluation of swallowing function, consult CPT code 92611.

92614 Flexible fiberoptic endoscopic evaluation, laryngeal sensory testing by cine or video recording; ☐A☐ 80 ☐

MED: 100-2,15,230.3; 100-3,50.3; 100-3,170.3

If flexible fiberoptic or endoscopic evaluation of swallowing is performed without cine or video recording, use 92700

92615 physician interpretation and report only ☐E☐ 80 ☐

MED: 100-2,15,230.3; 100-3,50.3; 100-3,170.3

92616 Flexible fiberoptic endoscopic evaluation of swallowing and laryngeal sensory testing by cine or video recording; ☐A☐ 80 ☐

MED: 100-2,15,230.3; 100-3,50.3; 100-3,170.3

To report flexible fiberoptic endoscopic swallowing evaluation performed without cine or video recording, consult CPT code 92700.

92617 physician interpretation and report only ☐E☐ 80 ☐

MED: 100-2,15,230.3; 100-3,50.3; 100-3,170.3

92620 Evaluation of central auditory function, with report; initial 60 minutes ☐X☐ TC 80 ☐

92621 each additional 15 minutes ☐N☐ TC 80 ☐

Codes 92620, 92621 cannot be reported with CPT code 92506.

92625 Assessment of tinnitus (includes pitch, loudness matching, and masking) ☐X☐ TC 80 ☐

Code 92625 cannot be reported with CPT code 92562.

If the procedure is performed unilaterally, append with modifier 52.

92626 Evaluation of auditory rehabilitation status; first hour ☐X☐ TC 80 ☐

+ **92627** each additional 15 minutes (List separately in addition to code for primary procedure) ☐N☐ TC 80 ☐

Note that 92627 is an add-on code and must be used in conjunction with 92626.

Codes 92626, 92627 are used to report the face-to-face time with the patient or family.

92630 Auditory rehabilitation; prelingual hearing loss ☐E☐

92633 postlingual hearing loss ☐E☐

SPECIAL DIAGNOSTIC PROCEDURES

● **92640** Diagnostic analysis with programming of auditory brainstem implant, per hour ☐X☐

Report nonprogramming services separately, e.g. cardiac monitoring.

OTHER PROCEDURES

92700 Unlisted otorhinolaryngological service or procedure ☐X☐ 80

MED: 100-2,15,230.3; 100-3,50.3; 100-3,170.3

CARDIOVASCULAR

Cardiovascular services (92950-93799) include diagnostic and therapeutic services.

THERAPEUTIC SERVICES AND PROCEDURES

Therapeutic services are performed for treatment of a specific condition, disorder, or disease. Some of the more frequently performed services include percutaneous placement of intracoronary stents, percutaneous transluminal coronary angioplasty (PTCA), and percutaneous transluminal coronary arthrectomy.

Percutaneous placement of coronary stents (92980-92981) includes therapeutic procedures such as PTCA and arthrectomy. Do not report stent placements for procedures 92982, 92984, 92995, and 92996.

PTCA (92982-92984) is used to treat coronary artery obstruction. A balloon catheter is placed in the affected artery and the balloon is inflated to flatten the plaque against the wall of the artery and open the obstruction.

Percutaneous transluminal coronary arthrectomy (92995-92996) may be used instead of the PTCA to treat coronary artery obstruction. Arthrectomy involves placing a catheter into the affected artery and using a rotary cutter to remove the plaque. When arthrectomy is performed with a PTCA, the PTCA is not reported separately as it is included in procedures 92995 and 92996.

For non-surgical septal reduction therapy (e.g., alcohol ablation), consult CPT Category III code 0024T.

92950 Cardiopulmonary resuscitation (eg, in cardiac arrest) ☐S☐ 80 ☐

MED: 100-4,4,20.5
AMA: 1996,Jan,7
Consult also critical care services 99291 and 99292.

⊙ **92953** Temporary transcutaneous pacing ☐S☐ 80 ☐

MED: 100-4,4,20.5; 100-4,12,30.6.12

To report physician direction of ambulance or rescue personnel outside the hospital, consult CPT code 99288.

If temporary transcutaneous pacing is performed as part of critical care services (99291-99292) do not report separately.

Medicine

92960 — 92995

⊙ **92960** Cardioversion, elective, electrical conversion of arrhythmia; external ⑤ 80 ⬚

MED: 100-4,4,20.5

AMA: 2001,Jul,11; 2000,Nov,9; 2000,Jun,5; 1999,Nov,49; 1993,Summer,13

⊙ **92961** internal (separate procedure) ⑤ ⬚

MED: 100-4,4,20.5

AMA: 2000,Nov,9; 2000,Jun,5; 2000,Jul,5; 1999,Nov,49; 1993,Summer,13

Note that 92961 cannot be reported in addition to CPT codes 93618-93624, 93631, 93640-93642, 93650-93652, 93662, and 93741-93744.

92970 Cardioassist-method of circulatory assist; internal ⓒ 80 ⬚

92971 external ⓒ 80 ⬚

If a balloon atrial-septostomy is performed, consult CPT code 92992. If catheters are placed for use in circulatory assist devices such as an intra-aortic balloon pump, consult CPT code 33970.

+ ⊙ **92973** Percutaneous transluminal coronary thrombectomy (List separately in addition to code for primary procedure) ⓣ 80 ⬚

AMA: 2002,Mar,10; 2002,Mar,1

Note that 92973 is an add-on code and must be used in conjunction with codes 92980, 92982.

+ ⊙ **92974** Transcatheter placement of radiation delivery device for subsequent coronary intravascular brachytherapy (List separately in addition to code for primary procedure) ⓣ 80 ⬚

AMA: 2002,Mar,1

Note that 92974 is an add-on code and must be used in conjunction with codes 92980, 92982, 92995, 93508.

For intravascular radioelement application, see 77781-77784.

⊙ **92975** Thrombolysis, coronary; by intracoronary infusion, including selective coronary angiography ⓒ 80 ⬚

92977 by intravenous infusion ⓣ 80 ⬚

If thrombolysis is performed of vessels other than coronary, consult CPT codes 37201 and 75896. If cerebral thrombolysis is performed, consult CPT code 37195.

+ ⊙ **92978** Intravascular ultrasound (coronary vessel or graft) during diagnostic evaluation and/or therapeutic intervention including imaging supervision, interpretation and report; initial vessel (List separately in addition to code for primary procedure) ⑤ 80 ⬚

MED: 100-3,220.5

AMA: 1999,Nov,49; 1997,Nov,43-44

Note that intravascular ultrasound services include all transducer manipulations and repositioning within the specific vessel being examined, both before and after therapeutic intervention (e.g., stent placement).

Note that 92978 is an add-on code that must be used in conjunction with the appropriate code for the primary procedure. This code cannot be reported alone.

+ ⊙ **92979** each additional vessel (List separately in addition to code for primary procedure) ⑤ 80

MED: 100-3,220.5

AMA: 1999,Nov,49; 1997,Nov,43-44

Note that 92979 is an add-on code and must be used in conjunction with 92978.

⊙ **92980** Transcatheter placement of an intracoronary stent(s), percutaneous, with or without other therapeutic intervention, any method; single vessel ⓣ 80 ⬚

AMA: 2001,Mar,11; 2001,Apr,10; 1998,Aug,3; 1998,Apr,9; 1996,Dec,11; 1996,Aug,2

+ ⊙ **92981** each additional vessel (List separately in addition to code for primary procedure) ⓣ 80 ⬚

MED: 100-3,20.7

AMA: 2001,Mar,11; 2001,Apr,10

Note that 92981 is an add-on code and must be used in conjunction with 92980.

Use 92980, 92981 to report coronary artery stenting. If coronary angioplasty (92982, 92984) or atherectomy (92995, 92996) is performed in the same artery, it is considered part of the stenting procedure and should not be reported separately. Codes 92973 (percutaneous transluminal coronary thrombectomy), 92974 (coronary brachytherapy) and 92978, 92979 (intravascular ultrasound) should be used in addition to reporting the procedure for coronary stenting, atherectomy, and angioplasty and are not included in the therapeutic interventions in 92980.

If additional vessels are treated by angioplasty or atherectomy during the same session, consult CPT codes 92984 and 92996.

To report transcatheter placement of radiation delivery device for coronary intravascular brachytherapy, use 92974.

For intravascular radioelement application, consult CPT codes 77781-77784.

⊙ **92982** Percutaneous transluminal coronary balloon angioplasty; single vessel ⓣ 80 ⬚

MED: 100-3,20.7; 100-4,4,61.2

AMA: 1997,Apr,10; 1996,Aug,2; 1992,Winter,15

+ ⊙ **92984** each additional vessel (List separately in addition to code for primary procedure) ⓣ 80 ⬚

MED: 100-3,20.7; 100-4,4,61.2

AMA: 1997,Apr,10; 1996,Dec,11; 1996,Aug,2; 1992,Winter,15

Note that 92984 is an add-on code and must be used in conjunction with 92980, 92982, or 92995. If a stent is placed following the completion of angioplasty or atherectomy, consult CPT codes 92980 and 92981.

To report transcatheter placement of radiation delivery device for coronary intravascular brachytherapy, use 92974.

For intravascular radioelement application, see 77781-77784.

⊙ **92986** Percutaneous balloon valvuloplasty; aortic valve ⓣ 80 ⬚

⊙ **92987** mitral valve ⓣ 80 ⬚

92990 pulmonary valve ⓣ 80 ⬚

92992 Atrial septectomy or septostomy; transvenous method, balloon (eg, Rashkind type) (includes cardiac catheterization) ⓒ 80 ⬚

AMA: 1998,Apr,3, 10; 1997,Nov,44

92993 blade method (Park septostomy) (includes cardiac catheterization) ⓒ 80 ⬚

AMA: 1998,Apr,3, 10

⊙ **92995** Percutaneous transluminal coronary atherectomy, by mechanical or other method, with or without balloon angioplasty; single vessel ⓣ 80 ⬚

MED: 100-3,20.7; 100-4,4,61.2

AMA: 1992,Winter,15

26 Professional Component Only   80/ 80 Assist-at-Surgery Allowed/With Documentation   Unlisted   Not Covered

TC Technical Component Only   MED: Pub 100/NCD References   AMA: CPT Assistant References   1-9 ASC Group   ♂ Male Only   ♀ Female Only

348 — CPT Expert   CPT only © 2006 American Medical Association. All Rights Reserved. *(Black Ink)*   © 2006 Ingenix *(Blue Ink)*

+ ⊙ 92996   each additional vessel (List separately in addition to code for primary procedure)   T 80 ⬛

MED: 100-4,4,61.2

AMA: 1998,Apr,3; 1992,Winter,15

Note that 92996 is an add-on code and must be used in conjunction with 92982, 92982, or 92995. If a stent is placed following the completion of angioplasty or atherectomy, consult CPT codes 92980 and 92981. If additional vessels are treated by angioplasty or atherectomy during the same session, consult CPT code 92984.

92997   Percutaneous transluminal pulmonary artery balloon angioplasty; single vessel   T 80 ⬛

MED: 100-3,20.7; 100-4,4,61.2

AMA: 1997,Nov,44

+ 92998   each additional vessel (List separately in addition to code for primary procedure)   T 80 ⬛

MED: 100-3,20.7; 100-4,4,61.2

AMA: 1997,Nov,44

Note that 92998 is an add-on code and must be used in conjunction with 92997.

CARDIOGRAPHY

Cardiography services include electrocardiogram (ECG), cardiovascular stress tests, and electrocardiographic (Holter) monitoring. The Holter monitor is a diagnostic tool that creates a continuous record of the heart's electrical activity during the patient"s normal activities for a 24-hour period. Cardiography codes include both a professional and a technical component. These codes have separate listings for the total component, the recording (technical component), and the review and interpretation (professional component). For example, code 93015 identifies the total service (global) for a cardiovascular stress test and includes the following components:

- Tracing (the technical component only (93017)
- Supervision of the procedure (a portion of the professional component) (93016)
- Interpretation and report (a portion of the professional component) (93018)

If echocardiography is performed, consult CPT codes 93303-93350.

93000   Electrocardiogram, routine ECG with at least 12 leads; with interpretation and report   B 80 ⬛

MED: 100-3,20.15; 100-3,160.17; 100-4,12,30.6.12; 100-4,13,100

AMA: 1997,Aug,9

93005   tracing only, without interpretation and report   S TC 80 ⬛

MED: 100-3,20.15; 100-4,4,20.5; 100-4,13,100

AMA: 1997,Aug,9

If echocardiography is performed, consult CPT codes 93303-93350.

93010   interpretation and report only   B 26 80 ⬛

MED: 100-3,20.15; 100-4,12,30.6.12; 100-4,13,100

AMA: 1997,Aug,9

If ECG monitoring is needed, consult CPT codes 99354-99360.

93012   Telephonic transmission of post-symptom electrocardiogram rhythm strip(s), 24-hour attended monitoring, per 30 day period of time; tracing only   N TC 80 ⬛

MED: 100-3,20.15

AMA: 1996,Jun,2

93014   Telephonic transmission of post-symptom electrocardiogram rhythm strip(s), 24-hour attended monitoring, per 30 day period of time; physician review with interpretation and report only   B 26 80 ⬛

MED: 100-3,20.15

AMA: 1996,Jun,2

If echocardiography is performed, consult CPT codes 93303-93350.

93015   Cardiovascular stress test using maximal or submaximal treadmill or bicycle exercise, continuous electrocardiographic monitoring, and/or pharmacological stress; with physician supervision, with interpretation and report   B 80 ⬛

MED: 100-2,15,60.3; 100-3,20.10; 100-3,20.15; 100-4,3,40.3; 100-4,4,20.5

AMA: 2002,Aug,10; 1996,Jun,10; 1996,Apr,11

93016   physician supervision only, without interpretation and report   B 26 80 ⬛

MED: 100-2,15,60.3; 100-3,20.10; 100-3,20.15; 100-4,4,20.5

AMA: 2002,Aug,10; 1996,Apr,11

93017   tracing only, without interpretation and report   X TC 80 ⬛

MED: 100-2,15,60.3; 100-3,20.10; 100-3,20.15; 100-4,4,20.5

AMA: 2002,Aug,10

93018   interpretation and report only   B 26 80 ⬛

MED: 100-2,15,60.3; 100-3,20.10; 100-3,20.15; 100-4,4,20.5

AMA: 1996,Jun,10; 1996,Apr,11

To report the inert gas rebreathing measurement, consult Category III codes 0104T, 0105T.

93024   Ergonovine provocation test   X 80 ⬛

MED: 100-3,20.15; 100-4,4,20.5

93025   Microvolt T-wave alternans for assessment of ventricular arrhythmias   X 80 ⬛

AMA: 2002,Mar,1

93040   Rhythm ECG, one to three leads; with interpretation and report   B 80 ⬛

MED: 100-2,15,60.3; 100-3,20.10; 100-3,20.15; 100-4,4,20.5; 100-4,12,30.6.12; 100-4,13,100

93041   tracing only without interpretation and report   S TC 80

MED: 100-2,15,60.3; 100-3,20.10; 100-3,20.15; 100-4,4,20.5; 100-4,13,100

93042   interpretation and report only   B 26 80 ⬛

MED: 100-2,15,60.3; 100-3,20.10; 100-3,20.15; 100-4,4,20.5; 100-4,12,30.6.12; 100-4,13,100

93224   Electrocardiographic monitoring for 24 hours by continuous original ECG waveform recording and storage, with visual superimposition scanning; includes recording, scanning analysis with report, physician review and interpretation   B 80 ⬛

MED: 100-3,20.15; 100-4,4,20.5

93225   recording (includes hook-up, recording, and disconnection)   X TC 80 ⬛

MED: 100-3,20.15; 100-4,4,20.5

93226   scanning analysis with report   X TC 80 ⬛

MED: 100-3,20.15

93227   physician review and interpretation   B 26 80 ⬛

MED: 100-3,20.15

⊛ Modifier 63 Exempt Code   ⊙ Conscious Sedation   + CPT Add-on Code   ⊘ Modifier 51 Exempt Code   ● New Code   ▲ Revised Code

M Maternity Edit   A Age Edit   A-Y APC Status Indicators   ⬛ CCI Comprehensive Code   ⁄ Drug Not Approved by FDA   50 Bilateral Procedure

93230 Electrocardiographic monitoring for 24 hours by continuous original ECG waveform recording and storage without superimposition scanning utilizing a device capable of producing a full miniaturized printout; includes recording, microprocessor-based analysis with report, physician review and interpretation B 80 ◻
MED: 100-3,20.15; 100-4,4,20.5

93231 recording (includes hook-up, recording, and disconnection) X TC 80 ◻
MED: 100-3,20.15

93232 microprocessor-based analysis with report X TC 80 ◻
MED: 100-3,20.15

93233 physician review and interpretation B 26 80 ◻
MED: 100-3,20.15

93235 Electrocardiographic monitoring for 24 hours by continuous computerized monitoring and non-continuous recording, and real-time data analysis utilizing a device capable of producing intermittent full-sized waveform tracings, possibly patient activated; includes monitoring and real-time data analysis with report, physician review and interpretation B 80 ◻
MED: 100-3,20.15; 100-4,4,20.5
Holter monitor procedure

93236 monitoring and real-time data analysis with report X TC 80 ◻
MED: 100-3,20.15

93237 physician review and interpretation B 26 80 ◻
MED: 100-3,20.15

93268 Patient demand single or multiple event recording with presymptom memory loop, 24-hour attended monitoring, per 30 day period of time; includes transmission, physician review and interpretation B 80 ◻
MED: 100-3,20.15
AMA: 1999,Nov,49-50; 1996,Jun,2
If postsymptom recording is needed, consult CPT codes 93012 and 93014. If implanted patient activated cardiac event recording is needed, consult CPT codes 33282 and 93727.

93270 recording (includes hook-up, recording, and disconnection) X TC 80 ◻
MED: 100-3,20.15
AMA: 1996,Jun,2

93271 monitoring, receipt of transmissions, and analysis X TC 80 ◻
MED: 100-3,20.15
AMA: 1996,Jun,2

93272 physician review and interpretation only B 26 80 ◻
MED: 100-3,20.15
AMA: 1999,Nov,49-50; 1998,Apr,14; 1996,Jun,2

93278 Signal-averaged electrocardiography (SAECG), with or without ECG S 80 ◻
MED: 100-3,20.15; 100-4,4,20.5
To report only the interpretation and report, append modifier 26.

ECHOCARDIOGRAPHY

This ultrasound technique of visualizing the heart and great arteries provides the physician with two-dimensional images and/or Doppler signals.

If fetal echocardiography is performed, consult CPT codes 76825-76828.

To report only the interpretation and report, append modifier 26. Report an echocardiography code for an ultrasound evaluation of the cardiac chambers and valves, the adjacent great vessels, and the pericardium. A complete transthoracic echocardiogram (93307) is a service that includes 2-dimensional and selected M-mode examination of the left and right atria, left and right ventricles, the aortic, mitral, and tricuspid valves, the pericardium, and adjacent portions of the aorta. These structures are evaluated using multiple views as required to obtain a complete functional and anatomic evaluation, and appropriate measurements are obtained and recorded. Identification and measurement of some structures may not always be possible in spite of significant effort. In these cases, the reason the a structure could not be visualized such as pulmonary veins, pulmonary artery, pulmonic valve, or inferior vena cava should be documented. Visualization of additional structures is included in this service.

Report a limited or follow-up study with code 93308. This is an examination that does not evaluate or document the attempt to evaluate all the structures that make up the complete echocardiography. When a repeat complete exam is not necessary, a follow up exam may be performed to do a more focused review. This is typically done in the follow up of a complete exam.

An echocardiography, either complete or limited must include an interpretation of all information obtained, documentation of all clinically relevant findings including quantitative measurements obtained, plus a description of any recognized abnormalities. The pertinent images, videotape, and/or digital data must be permanently stored and available for review. Do not separately report echocardiography that does not meet this criteria.

Do not report an ultrasound without a thorough examination of the organ(s) or anatomic region, documentation of the image, and a final written report.

93303 Transthoracic echocardiography for congenital cardiac anomalies; complete S 80 ◻
MED: 100-4,4,20.5; 100-4,12,30.4
AMA: 1997,Nov,44; 1997,Dec,5

93304 follow-up or limited study S 80 ◻
MED: 100-4,4,20.5; 100-4,12,30.4
AMA: 1997,Nov,44; 1997,Dec,5

93307 Echocardiography, transthoracic, real-time with image documentation (2D) with or without M-mode recording; complete S 80 ◻
MED: 100-4,3,40.3; 100-4,4,20.5; 100-4,12,30.4
AMA: 2000,Apr,1; 1997,Dec,5

93308 follow-up or limited study S 80 ◻
MED: 100-4,3,40.3; 100-4,4,20.5; 100-4,12,30.4
AMA: 1997,Dec,5

⊙ **93312** Echocardiography, transesophageal, real time with image documentation (2D) (with or without M-mode recording); including probe placement, image acquisition, interpretation and report S 80 ◻
MED: 100-4,4,20.5; 100-4,12,30.4
AMA: 2000,Jan,10; 1997,Dec,5

⊙ **93313** placement of transesophageal probe only S 80 ◻
MED: 100-4,4,20.5; 100-4,12,30.4
AMA: 1997,Dec,5

⊙ **93314** image acquisition, interpretation and report only N 80 ◻
MED: 100-4,4,20.5; 100-4,12,30.4
AMA: 2000,Jan,10; 1997,Dec,5

⊙ **93315** Transesophageal echocardiography for congenital cardiac anomalies; including probe placement, image acquisition, interpretation and report S 80 ◻
MED: 100-4,4,20.5; 100-4,12,30.4
AMA: 1997,Nov,44; 1997,Dec,5

⊙ **93316** placement of transesophageal probe only S 80 ◻
MED: 100-4,4,20.5; 100-4,12,30.4
AMA: 1997,Nov,44; 1997,Dec,5

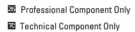 Professional Component Only
TC Technical Component Only

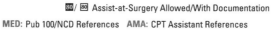 80/ 80 Assist-at-Surgery Allowed/With Documentation
MED: Pub 100/NCD References AMA: CPT Assistant References 1 - 9 ASC Group

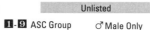 Unlisted   Not Covered
♂ Male Only   ♀ Female Only

350 — CPT Expert   CPT only © 2006 American Medical Association. All Rights Reserved. *(Black Ink)*   © 2006 Ingenix *(Blue Ink)*

⊙ 93317   image acquisition, interpretation and report only   N 80 ▣

     MED: 100-4,4,20.5; 100-4,12,30.4

     AMA: 1997,Nov,44; 1997,Dec,5

⊙ 93318   Echocardiography, transesophageal (TEE) for monitoring purposes, including probe placement, real time 2-dimensional image acquisition and interpretation leading to ongoing (continuous) assessment of (dynamically changing) cardiac pumping function and to therapeutic measures on an immediate time basis   S 80 ▣

     MED: 100-4,4,20.5

+ 93320   Doppler echocardiography, pulsed wave and/or continuous wave with spectral display (List separately in addition to codes for echocardiographic imaging); complete   S 80 ▣

     MED: 100-3,220.5; 100-4,3,40.3; 100-4,4,20.5; 100-4,12,30.4

     AMA: 1997,Nov,44; 1997,Dec,5

     Note that 93320 is an add-on code and must be used in conjunction with 93303, 93304, 93307, 93308, 93312, 93314, 93315, 93317, and 93350.

+ 93321   follow-up or limited study (List separately in addition to codes for echocardiographic imaging)   S 80 ▣

     MED: 100-4,4,20.5; 100-4,12,30.4

     AMA: 1997,Nov,44; 1997,Dec,5

     Note that 93321 is an add-on code and must be used in conjunction with 93303, 93304, 93307, 93308, 93312, 93314, 93315, 93317, and 93350.

+ 93325   Doppler echocardiography color flow velocity mapping (List separately in addition to codes for echocardiography)   S 80 ▣

     MED: 100-3,220.5; 100-4,4,20.5; 100-4,12,30.4

     AMA: 1997,Nov,44; 1997,Dec,5

     Note that 93325 is an add-on code and must be used in conjunction with 76825, 76826, 76827, 76828, 93303, 93304, 93307, 93308, 93312, 93314, 93315, 93317, 93320, 93321, and 93350.

93350   Echocardiography, transthoracic, real-time with image documentation (2D), with or without M-mode recording, during rest and cardiovascular stress test using treadmill, bicycle exercise and/or pharmacologically induced stress, with interpretation and report   S 80 ▣

     MED: 100-4,4,20.5; 100-4,12,30.4

     AMA: 2002,Aug,11

     Consult CPT codes 93015-93018 for the appropriate stress testing code that needs to be reported in addition to 93350 to capture the exercise stress portion of the study.

CARDIAC CATHETERIZATION

Cardiac catheterizations are invasive procedures used to visualize the heart chambers, valves, great vessels, and coronary arteries. Catheter procedures produce pressure measurements and blood volumes used to evaluate cardiac function and valve patency.

The three major components of cardiac catheterization include: introduction and positioning of the catheter (93501-93533) including repositioning, injection procedures (93539-93545) and imaging supervision, interpretation, and report (93555-93556).

Supervision and interpretation codes related to cardiac catheterization (93555 and 93556) are used with imaging performed as part of cardiac catheterization procedures. The plural presentation of the word "procedure(s)" as well as the "and/or" terminology in the descriptions of imaging services suggest the codes include imaging of one or more areas.

Aortic root aortography (93544) is the injection of a large bolus of dye into the proximal ascending aorta, just above the aortic valve. When thoracic aortography is performed without a cardiac catheterization, it should be reported using procedure 36200 and the appropriate radiologic supervision/interpretation(75600 or 75605).

A number of services rely on the following cardiac catheterization codes. The procedure itself includes introduction, positioning, gauging pressure, and procuring samples.

⊘ ⊙ 93501   Right heart catheterization   T 80 ▣

     MED: 100-4,3,40.3; 100-4,4,20.5

     AMA: 2000,Apr,10; 1998,Apr,1; 1994,Spring,24

     To report bundle of His recording, consult CPT code 93600.

⊘ 93503   Insertion and placement of flow directed catheter (eg, Swan-Ganz) for monitoring purposes   T 80 ▣

     MED: 100-4,3,40.3; 100-4,4,20.5

     AMA: 1998,Apr,1; 1995,Fall,8

     If subsequent monitoring is needed, consult CPT codes 99356-99357.

ENDOMYOCARDIAL BIOPSY

Biopsy of the inside and middle layers of the heart is a separately reportable service. It may be performed in surgery or in the cardiac cath lab with the patient under local anesthesia. The sample is usually taken from the right or left ventricle. The patient is monitored constantly with both intracardiac and external ECG leads to record cardiac response.

⊘ ⊙ 93505   Endomyocardial biopsy   T 80 ▣

     MED: 100-4,3,40.3; 100-4,4,20.5

     AMA: 2000,Apr,10; 1998,Apr,1

⊘ ⊙ 93508   Catheter placement in coronary artery(s), arterial coronary conduit(s), and/or venous coronary bypass graft(s) for coronary angiography without concomitant left heart catheterization   T 80 ▣

     MED: 100-4,4,20.5

     AMA: 2000,Aug,11; 2000,Apr,10; 1998,Apr,1; 1997,Nov,44-45

     Note that 93508 is to be used only when left heart catheterization is not performed (CPT codes 93510, 93511, 93524, and 93526). Also note that 93508 is to be used only once per procedure.

     To report transcatheter placement of radiation delivery device for coronary intravascular brachytherapy, consult CPT code 92974.

     For intravascular radioelement application, consult CPT code 77781-77784.

⊘ ⊙ 93510   Left heart catheterization, retrograde, from the brachial artery, axillary artery or femoral artery; percutaneous   T 80 ▣

     MED: 100-4,3,40.3; 100-4,4,20.5

     AMA: 1998,Apr,1; 1997,Nov,44-45; 1994,Spring,26

⊘ ⊙ 93511   by cutdown   T 80 ▣

     MED: 100-4,4,20.5

     AMA: 1998,Apr,1; 1997,Nov,44-45; 1994,Spring,24

⊘ ⊙ 93514   Left heart catheterization by left ventricular puncture   T 80 ▣

     MED: 100-4,4,20.5

     AMA: 1998,Apr,1; 1994,Spring,24

⊘ ⊙ 93524   Combined transseptal and retrograde left heart catheterization   T 80 ▣

     MED: 100-4,4,20.5

     AMA: 1998,Apr,1; 1997,Nov,44-45; 1994,Spring,24

⊛ Modifier 63 Exempt Code   ⊙ Conscious Sedation   + CPT Add-on Code   ⊘ Modifier 51 Exempt Code   ● New Code   ▲ Revised Code

M Maternity Edit   A Age Edit   A-Y APC Status Indicators   ▣ CCI Comprehensive Code   ✗ Drug Not Approved by FDA   50 Bilateral Procedure

© 2006 Ingenix (Blue Ink)   CPT only © 2006 American Medical Association. All Rights Reserved. (Black Ink)   Medicine — 351

Medicine

93526 — 93571

⊘ ⊙ **93526** **Combined right heart catheterization and retrograde left heart catheterization** ⊤ 80 ▣

MED: 100-4,3,40.3; 100-4,4,20.5

AMA: 1998,Apr,1; 1997,Nov,44-45; 1994,Spring,28

⊘ ⊙ **93527** **Combined right heart catheterization and transseptal left heart catheterization through intact septum (with or without retrograde left heart catheterization)** ⊤ 80 ▣

MED: 100-4,4,20.5

AMA: 1998,Apr,1

⊘ ⊙ **93528** **Combined right heart catheterization with left ventricular puncture (with or without retrograde left heart catheterization)** ⊤ 80 ▣

MED: 100-4,4,20.5

AMA: 1998,Apr,1

⊘ ⊙ **93529** **Combined right heart catheterization and left heart catheterization through existing septal opening (with or without retrograde left heart catheterization)** ⊤ 80 ▣

MED: 100-4,4,20.5

AMA: 1998,Apr,1

⊘ ⊙ **93530** **Right heart catheterization, for congenital cardiac anomalies** ⊤ 80 ▣

MED: 100-4,4,20.5

AMA: 1998,Mar,11; 1998,Apr,3, 6-7; 1997,Nov,45

⊘ **93531** **Combined right heart catheterization and retrograde left heart catheterization, for congenital cardiac anomalies** ⊤ 80 ▣

MED: 100-4,4,20.5

AMA: 1998,Mar,11; 1998,Apr,8, 10-11; 1997,Nov,45

⊘ **93532** **Combined right heart catheterization and transseptal left heart catheterization through intact septum with or without retrograde left heart catheterization, for congenital cardiac anomalies** ⊤ 80 ▣

MED: 100-4,4,20.5

AMA: 1998,Mar,11; 1998,Apr,10-11; 1997,Nov,45

⊘ **93533** **Combined right heart catheterization and transseptal left heart catheterization through existing septal opening, with or without retrograde left heart catheterization, for congenital cardiac anomalies** ⊤ 80 ▣

MED: 100-4,4,20.5

AMA: 1998,Mar,11; 1998,Apr,12, 13; 1997,Nov,45

⊘ ⊙ **93539** **Injection procedure during cardiac catheterization; for selective opacification of arterial conduits (eg, internal mammary), whether native or used for bypass** N 80 ▣

MED: 100-4,4,20.5

AMA: 2001,Oct,11; 1998,Apr,3; 1997,Nov,44-45; 1994,Spring,27
When injection procedures are performed in conjunction with cardiac catheterization, these services do not include introduction of catheters but do include repositioning of catheters when necessary and use of automatic power injectors. Injection procedures represent separate identifiable services and may be coded in conjunction with one another when appropriate. The technical details of angiography, which include supervision of filming and processing and interpretation and report are not included. To report the technical details, consult CPT code 93555 and/or 93556. Note that modifier 51 should not be appended to these procedures.

⊘ ⊙ **93540** **for selective opacification of aortocoronary venous bypass grafts, one or more coronary arteries** N 80 ▣

MED: 100-4,4,20.5

AMA: 1998,Apr,3; 1997,Nov,44-45; 1994,Spring,27

⊘ ⊙ **93541** **for pulmonary angiography** N 80 ▣

MED: 100-4,3,40.3; 100-4,4,20.5

AMA: 1998,Apr,3; 1997,Nov,44-45; 1994,Spring,28

⊘ ⊙ **93542** **for selective right ventricular or right atrial angiography** N 80 ▣

MED: 100-4,3,40.3; 100-4,4,20.5

AMA: 1998,Apr,3; 1997,Nov,44-45; 1994,Spring,24

⊘ ⊙ **93543** **for selective left ventricular or left atrial angiography** N 80 ▣

MED: 100-4,3,40.3; 100-4,4,20.5

AMA: 1998,Apr,3; 1997,Nov,44-45; 1994,Spring,28

⊘ ⊙ **93544** **for aortography** N 80 ▣

MED: 100-4,3,40.3; 100-4,4,20.5

AMA: 1998,Apr,3; 1997,Nov,44-45; 1994,Spring,28

⊘ ⊙ **93545** **for selective coronary angiography (injection of radiopaque material may be by hand)** N 80 ▣

MED: 100-4,3,40.3; 100-4,4,20.5

AMA: 2002,Nov,10; 1998,Apr,3; 1997,Nov,44-45; 1994,Spring,28

⊘ ⊙ **93555** **Imaging supervision, interpretation and report for injection procedure(s) during cardiac catheterization; ventricular and/or atrial angiography** N 80 ▣

MED: 100-4,4,20.5

AMA: 1998,Apr,3, 11, 12; 1997,Oct,10; 1997,Nov,44-45; 1994,Spring,28

⊘ ⊙ **93556** **pulmonary angiography, aortography, and/or selective coronary angiography including venous bypass grafts and arterial conduits (whether native or used in bypass)** N 80 ▣

MED: 100-4,4,20.5

AMA: 1998,Apr,3, 11, 12; 1997,Oct,10; 1997,Nov,44-45; 1994,Spring,28

⊙ **93561** **Indicator dilution studies such as dye or thermal dilution, including arterial and/or venous catheterization; with cardiac output measurement (separate procedure)** N 80 ▣

MED: 100-4,3,40.3; 100-4,4,20.5; 100-4,12,30.6.12

AMA: 1991,Winter,25
If cardiac output measurements are done as part of critical care services (99291-99292), do not report separately.

Note that 93561 and 93562 are not to be used with cardiac catheterization codes. If radioisotope method is used for cardiac output, consult CPT code 78472, 78473, or 78481.

⊙ **93562** **subsequent measurement of cardiac output** N 80 ▣

MED: 100-4,3,40.3; 100-4,4,20.5; 100-4,12,30.6.12

AMA: 1991,Winter,25

+ ⊙ **93571** **Intravascular Doppler velocity and/or pressure derived coronary flow reserve measurement (coronary vessel or graft) during coronary angiography including pharmacologically induced stress; initial vessel (List separately in addition to code for primary procedure)** S 80 ▣

MED: 100-3,220.5; 100-4,4,20.5

AMA: 2000,Apr,1; 1998,Nov,33
Note that 93571 is an add-on code that must be used in conjunction with the appropriate code for the primary procedure. This code cannot be reported alone.

+ ⊙   **93572**   **each additional vessel (List separately in addition to code for primary procedure)** S 80

MED: 100-3,220.5; 100-4,4,20.5

AMA: 2000,Apr,1; 1998,Nov,34

Note that measurements of intravascular distal coronary blood flow velocity include all Doppler transducer manipulations and repositioning within the specific vessel being examined, during coronary angiography or therapeutic intervention (e.g., angioplasty). If an unlisted cardiac catheterization procedure is performed, consult CPT code 93799.

Note that 93572 is an add-on code that must be used in conjunction with code 93571.

REPAIR OF SEPTAL DEFECT

To report echocardiographic services performed in conjunction with 93580-93581, consult CPT codes 93303-93317 and 93662 as appropriate.

   93580   **Percutaneous transcatheter closure of congenital interatrial communication (ie, Fontan fenestration, atrial septal defect) with implant** T 80

CPT code 93580 includes right heart catheterization and contrast injections for atrial and ventricular angiograms. Do not report 93501, 93529-93533, 93539, 93543 or 93555 in conjunction with CPT code 93580.

   93581   **Percutaneous transcatheter closure of a congenital ventricular septal defect with implant** T 80

CPT code 93581 includes right heart catheterization and contrast injections for atrial and ventricular angiograms. Do not report 93501, 93529-93533, 93539, 93543 or 93555 in conjunction with CPT code 93581.

See codes 0166T and 0167T for vetricular septal defect closure via transmyocardial implant delivery.

INTRACARDIAC ELECTROPHYSIOLOGICAL PROCEDURES/STUDIES

ELECTROPHYSIOLOGIC STUDIES (EPS)

EPS evaluates the electrical conduction system of the heart. An electrode is placed and the patient is monitored constantly with both intracardiac external ECG leads to record the cardiac response. Programmed electrical stimulation is delivered through an electrode catheter to evaluate electrical conduction pathways, formation of dysrhythmia, and automaticity and refractoriness of myocardial cells. These procedures may include induction of arrhythmia to isolate the origin of the conduction problem.

⊘   **93600**   **Bundle of His recording** T 80

MED: 100-3,20.12; 100-3,20.13; 100-4,4,20.5; 100-4,4,61.2

AMA: 1997,Aug,9; 1994,Summer,12

⊘   **93602**   **Intra-atrial recording** T 80

MED: 100-4,4,20.5; 100-4,4,61.2

AMA: 1997,Aug,9; 1994,Summer,12

⊘   **93603**   **Right ventricular recording** T 80

MED: 100-4,4,20.5; 100-4,4,61.2

AMA: 1997,Aug,9; 1994,Summer,12

+ ⊙   **93609**   **Intraventricular and/or intra-atrial mapping of tachycardia site(s) with catheter manipulation to record from multiple sites to identify origin of tachycardia (List separately in addition to code for primary procedure)** T 80

MED: 100-3,20.12; 100-4,4,20.5; 100-4,4,61.2

AMA: 1997,Aug,9; 1994,Summer,12

Note that 93609 is an add-on code and must be used in conjunction with codes 93620, 93651, 93652.

Do not report 93609 in conjunction wit CPT code 93613.

⊘   **93610**   **Intra-atrial pacing** T 80

MED: 100-3,20.12; 100-4,4,20.5; 100-4,4,61.2

AMA: 1997,Aug,9; 1994,Summer,12

⊘   **93612**   **Intraventricular pacing** T 80

MED: 100-3,20.12; 100-4,4,20.5; 100-4,4,61.2

AMA: 1997,Aug,9; 1994,Summer,12

Do not report 93612 in conjunction with codes 93620, 93651, 93652.

+ ⊙   **93613**   **Intracardiac electrophysiologic 3-dimensional mapping (List separately in addition to code for primary procedure)** T 80

MED: 100-3,20.12; 100-4,4,20.5; 100-4,4,61.2

Note that 93613 is an add-on code and must be used in conjunction with codes 93620, 93651, 93652.

Do not report 93613 in conjunction with CPT code 93609.

⊘ ⊙   **93615**   **Esophageal recording of atrial electrogram with or without ventricular electrogram(s);** T 80

MED: 100-4,4,20.5; 100-4,4,61.2

AMA: 1997,Aug,9; 1994,Summer,12

⊘ ⊙   **93616**   **with pacing** T 80

MED: 100-4,4,20.5; 100-4,4,61.2

AMA: 1997,Aug,9; 1994,Summer,12

⊘ ⊙   **93618**   **Induction of arrhythmia by electrical pacing** T 80

MED: 100-4,4,20.5; 100-4,4,61.2

AMA: 2000,Jun,5; 1999,Apr,10; 1997,Aug,9; 1994,Summer,12

If an intracardiac phonocardiogram is performed, consult CPT code 93799.

⊘ ⊙   **93619**   **Comprehensive electrophysiologic evaluation with right atrial pacing and recording, right ventricular pacing and recording, His bundle recording, including insertion and repositioning of multiple electrode catheters, without induction or attempted induction of arrhythmia** T 80

MED: 100-3,20.12; 100-4,4,20.5

AMA: 1997,Aug,9

Code 93619 should not be used in conjunction with codes 93600, 93602, 93610, 93612, 93618, or 93620-93622.

⊘ ⊙   **93620**   **Comprehensive electrophysiologic evaluation including insertion and repositioning of multiple electrode catheters with induction or attempted induction of arrhythmia; with right atrial pacing and recording, right ventricular pacing and recording, His bundle recording** T 80

MED: 100-3,20.12; 100-4,4,20.5

AMA: 1998,Jul,10; 1997,Oct,10; 1997,Aug,9; 1994,Summer,12

Code 93620 should not be used in conjunction with codes 93600, 93602, 93610, 93612, 93618, or 93619.

+ ⊙   **93621**   **with left atrial pacing and recording from coronary sinus or left atrium (List separately in addition to code for primary procedure)** T 80

MED: 100-3,20.12; 100-4,4,20.5

AMA: 1998,Nov,34; 1998,Jul,10; 1997,Oct,10; 1997,Aug,9; 1994,Summer,12

Note that 93621 is an add-on code and must be used in conjunction with 93620.

+ ⊙ **93622** with left ventricular pacing and recording (List separately in addition to code for primary procedure) T 80 ◨

MED: 100-3,20.12; 100-4,4,20.5

AMA: 1998,Nov,34; 1998,Jul,10; 1997,Oct,10; 1997,Aug,9; 1994,Summer,14

Note that 93622 is an add-on code and must be used in conjunction with 93620.

+ **93623** Programmed stimulation and pacing after intravenous drug infusion (List separately in addition to code for primary procedure) T 80 ◨

MED: 100-3,20.12; 100-4,4,20.5; 100-4,4,61.2

AMA: 1997,Aug,9; 1994,Summer,14

Note that 93623 is an add-on code and must be used in conjunction with 93619, 93620.

⊘ ⊙ **93624** Electrophysiologic follow-up study with pacing and recording to test effectiveness of therapy, including induction or attempted induction of arrhythmia T 80 ◨

MED: 100-3,20.11; 100-3,20.12; 100-4,4,20.5; 100-4,4,61.2

AMA: 1997,Aug,9; 1994,Summer,14

⊘ **93631** Intra-operative epicardial and endocardial pacing and mapping to localize the site of tachycardia or zone of slow conduction for surgical correction T 80 ◨

MED: 100-3,20.11; 100-3,20.12; 100-4,4,20.5; 100-4,4,61.2

AMA: 1997,Aug,9; 1994,Summer,14

⊘ ⊙ **93640** Electrophysiologic evaluation of single or dual chamber pacing cardioverter-defibrillator leads including defibrillation threshold evaluation (induction of arrhythmia, evaluation of sensing and pacing for arrhythmia termination) at time of initial implantation or replacement; N 80 ◨

MED: 100-3,20.12; 100-4,4,20.5

AMA: 1999,Nov,50; 1999,Apr,10; 1997,Aug,9; 1994,Summer,14

If subsequent or periodic electronic analysis and/or reprogramming of single or dual-chamber pacing cardioverter-defibrillators is needed, consult CPT codes 93642 and 92741-93744.

⊘ ⊙ **93641** with testing of single or dual chamber pacing cardioverter-defibrillator pulse generator N 80 ◨

MED: 100-3,20.8.2; 100-3,20.12; 100-4,4,20.5

AMA: 2000,Jun,5; 2000,Jul,5; 1999,Nov,50; 1999,Apr,10; 1997,Aug,9; 1994,Summer,14

⊘ ⊙ **93642** Electrophysiologic evaluation of single or dual chamber pacing cardioverter-defibrillator (includes defibrillation threshold evaluation, induction of arrhythmia, evaluation of sensing and pacing for arrhythmia termination, and programming or reprogramming of sensing or therapeutic parameters) S 80 ◨

MED: 100-3,20.8.2; 100-3,20.12; 100-4,4,20.5

AMA: 2000,Jun,5; 1999,Nov,50; 1997,Aug,9; 1994,Summer,14

⊘ ⊙ **93650** Intracardiac catheter ablation of atrioventricular node function, atrioventricular conduction for creation of complete heart block, with or without temporary pacemaker placement T 80 ◨

MED: 100-4,4,20.5

AMA: 1997,Aug,9; 1994,Summer,15

⊘ ⊙ **93651** Intracardiac catheter ablation of arrhythmogenic focus; for treatment of supraventricular tachycardia by ablation of fast or slow atrioventricular pathways, accessory atrioventricular connections or other atrial foci, singly or in combination T 80 ◨

MED: 100-4,4,20.5

AMA: 1997,Aug,9; 1994,Summer,15

⊘ ⊙ **93652** for treatment of ventricular tachycardia T 80 ◨

MED: 100-4,4,20.5

AMA: 1997,Aug,9; 1994,Summer,15

⊘ **93660** Evaluation of cardiovascular function with tilt table evaluation, with continuous ECG monitoring and intermittent blood pressure monitoring, with or without pharmacological intervention S 80 ◨

MED: 100-4,4,20.5

If testing is performed of the autonomic nervous system function, consult CPT codes 95921-95923.

+ **93662** Intracardiac echocardiography during therapeutic/diagnostic intervention, including imaging supervision and interpretation (List separately in addition to code for primary procedure) S 80 ◨

MED: 100-4,4,20.5

Note that 93662 is an add-on code and must be used in conjunction with 93580, 93581, 93621, 93622, 93651 or 93652 as appropriate.

Do not report CPT code 92961 in addition to CPT code 93662.

PERIPHERAL ARTERIAL DISEASE REHABILITATION

Code 93668 identifies a service where the patient exercises under medical supervision for several sessions until symptoms of the disease abate. Each session is 45 to 60 minutes long.

93668 Peripheral arterial disease (PAD) rehabilitation, per session E

MED: 100-3,20.14; 100-4,4,20.5

NONINVASIVE PHYSIOLOGIC STUDIES AND PROCEDURES

If arterial cannulization and recording is performed of direct arterial pressure, consult CPT code 36620. If radiographic injection procedures are performed, consult CPT codes 36000-36299. If hemodialysis is performed for vascular cannulization, consult CPT codes 36800-36821. If chemotherapy is needed for a malignant disease, consult CPT codes 96408-96549. If penile plethysmography is performed, consult CPT code 54240.

93701 Bioimpedance, thoracic, electrical S 80

MED: 100-3,20.16; 100-4,4,20.5

AMA: 2002,Mar,1

93720 Plethysmography, total body; with interpretation and report B 80 ◨

MED: 100-3,20.14; 100-4,4,20.5

AMA: 1999,Mar,10

93721 tracing only, without interpretation and report X TC 80

MED: 100-3,20.14; 100-4,4,20.5

AMA: 1999,Mar,10

93722 interpretation and report only B 26 80

MED: 100-3,20.8; 100-3,20.8.1; 100-3,20.14; 100-4,4,20.5

AMA: 1999,Mar,10

If regional plethysmography is performed, consult CPT codes 93875-93931.

93724 Electronic analysis of antitachycardia pacemaker system (includes electrocardiographic recording, programming of device, induction and termination of tachycardia via implanted pacemaker, and interpretation of recordings) S 80 ◨

MED: 100-3,20.8; 100-3,20.8.1; 100-3,20.8.2; 100-3,20.15; 100-4,4,20.5

AMA: 1994,Summer,23

---

26 Professional Component Only   80/ 80 Assist-at-Surgery Allowed/With Documentation   Unlisted   Not Covered

TC Technical Component Only   MED: Pub 100/NCD References   AMA: CPT Assistant References   1 - 9 ASC Group   ♂ Male Only   ♀ Female Only

354 — CPT Expert   CPT only © 2006 American Medical Association. All Rights Reserved. (Black Ink)   © 2006 Ingenix (Blue Ink)

93727	Electronic analysis of implantable loop recorder (ILR) system (includes retrieval of recorded and stored ECG data, physician review and interpretation of retrieved ECG data and reprogramming)	S 26 ⬚

MED: 100-3,20.8; 100-3,20.8.1; 100-3,20.15; 100-4,4,20.5
AMA: 2000,Jul,5; 1999,Nov,50

93731	Electronic analysis of dual-chamber pacemaker system (includes evaluation of programmable parameters at rest and during activity where applicable, using electrocardiographic recording and interpretation of recordings at rest and during exercise, analysis of event markers and device response); without reprogramming	S 80 ⬚

MED: 100-3,20.8; 100-3,20.8.1; 100-3,20.8.2; 100-3,20.15; 100-4,4,20.5
AMA: 1998,Feb,11; 1994,Summer,23

93732	with reprogramming	S 80 ⬚

MED: 100-3,20.8; 100-3,20.8.1; 100-3,20.8.2; 100-3,20.15; 100-4,4,20.5
AMA: 2000,Mar,10; 1998,Feb,11; 1994,Summer,23

93733	Electronic analysis of dual chamber internal pacemaker system (may include rate, pulse amplitude and duration, configuration of wave form, and/or testing of sensory function of pacemaker), telephonic analysis	S 80 ⬚

MED: 100-3,20.8; 100-3,20.8.1; 100-3,20.8.2; 100-3,20.15; 100-4,4,20.5
AMA: 1994,Summer,23

93734	Electronic analysis of single chamber pacemaker system (includes evaluation of programmable parameters at rest and during activity where applicable, using electrocardiographic recording and interpretation of recordings at rest and during exercise, analysis of event markers and device response); without reprogramming	S 80 ⬚

MED: 100-3,20.8; 100-3,20.8.1; 100-3,20.8.2; 100-3,20.15; 100-4,4,20.5
AMA: 1998,Feb,11; 1994,Summer,23

93735	with reprogramming	S 80 ⬚

MED: 100-3,20.8; 100-3,20.8.1; 100-3,20.8.2; 100-3,20.15; 100-4,4,20.5
AMA: 1998,Feb,11; 1994,Summer,23

93736	Electronic analysis of single chamber internal pacemaker system (may include rate, pulse amplitude and duration, configuration of wave form, and/or testing of sensory function of pacemaker), telephonic analysis	S 80 ⬚

MED: 100-3,20.8; 100-3,20.8.1; 100-3,20.8.2; 100-3,20.15; 100-4,4,20.5
AMA: 1994,Summer,23

93740	Temperature gradient studies	X

MED: 100-4,4,20.5

93741	Electronic analysis of pacing cardioverter-defibrillator (includes interrogation, evaluation of pulse generator status, evaluation of programmable parameters at rest and during activity where applicable, using electrocardiographic recording and interpretation of recordings at rest and during exercise, analysis of event markers and device response); single chamber or wearable cardioverter-defibrillator system, without reprogramming	S ⬚

MED: 100-3,20.15; 100-4,4,20.5
AMA: 2000,Jul,5; 1999,Nov,50-51
Code 93741 cannot be reported with CPT code 93745.

93742	single chamber or wearable cardioverter-defibrillator system, with reprogramming	S ⬚

MED: 100-3,20.15; 100-4,4,20.5
AMA: 2000,Jul,5; 1999,Nov,50-51
Code 93742 cannot be reported with CPT code 93745.

93743	dual chamber, without reprogramming	S ⬚

MED: 100-3,20.15; 100-4,4,20.5
AMA: 2000,Jul,5; 1999,Nov,50-51

93744	dual chamber, with reprogramming	S ⬚

MED: 100-3,20.15; 100-3,220.11; 100-4,4,20.5
AMA: 2000,Jul,5; 1999,Nov,50-51

93745	Initial set-up and programming by a physician of wearable cardioverter-defibrillator includes initial programming of system, establishing baseline electronic ECG, transmission of data to data repository, patient instruction in wearing system and patient reporting of problems or events	S 80 ⬚

MED: 100-4,4,20.5
Code 93745 cannot be reported with 93741, 93742.

93760	Thermogram; cephalic	E

MED: 100-3,220.11; 100-4,4,20.5

93762	peripheral	E

MED: 100-3,220.11; 100-4,4,20.5

93770	Determination of venous pressure	N

MED: 100-3,20.19; 100-4,4,20.5
If central venous cannulization and pressure measurements are taken, consult CPT codes 36500 and 36555-36556.

93784	Ambulatory blood pressure monitoring, utilizing a system such as magnetic tape and/or computer disk, for 24 hours or longer; including recording, scanning analysis, interpretation and report	E 80 ⬚

MED: 100-3,20.19; 100-4,4,20.5; 100-4,32,10.1

93786	recording only	X TC 80

MED: 100-3,20.19; 100-4,4,20.5; 100-4,32,10.1

93788	scanning analysis with report	X TC 80

MED: 100-3,20.19; 100-4,4,20.5; 100-4,32,10.1

93790	physician review with interpretation and report	B 26 80

MED: 100-3,20.19; 100-4,4,20.5; 100-4,32,10.1

OTHER PROCEDURES

93797	Physician services for outpatient cardiac rehabilitation; without continuous ECG monitoring (per session)	S 80 ⬚

MED: 100-2,15,60.3; 100-3,20.10; 100-4,4,20.5

93798	with continuous ECG monitoring (per session)	S 80 ⬚

MED: 100-2,15,60.3; 100-3,20.10; 100-4,4,20.5

93799	Unlisted cardiovascular service or procedure	X 80

MED: 100-4,4,20.5
AMA: 1998,Mar,11

NON-INVASIVE VASCULAR DIAGNOSTIC STUDIES

Noninvasive vascular study codes (93875-93990) include the patient care required to supervise the studies and interpret the results.

A Duplex scan combines both two-dimensional structure of motion with time and Doppler ultrasonic signal documentation with spectral analysis and color flow velocity mapping or imaging to produce a real-time video display of organ structure and motion.

◎ Modifier 63 Exempt Code ☉ Conscious Sedation + CPT Add-on Code ⊘ Modifier 51 Exempt Code ● New Code ▲ Revised Code

M Maternity Edit A Age Edit A-Y APC Status Indicators ⬚ CCI Comprehensive Code ⚡ Drug Not Approved by FDA 80 Bilateral Procedure

A vascular study must produce a hard copy with data analysis for the patient's record, including bidirectional vascular flow or imaging when provided. Simple hand-held (screening) devices do not meet these requirements and are not reported separately.

Report 93886 for a complete transcranial Doppler (TCD) study. A complete study includes an ultrasound evaluation of the right and left anterior circulation territories and the posterior circulation territories and the posterior circulation (which includes the vertebral arteries and the basilar artery). A limited TCD study (93888) is comprised of an ultrasound evaluation of two or fewer of these territories. For a TCD, ultrasound study is a reasonable and concerted attempt to identify arterial signals through an acoustic window.

CEREBROVASCULAR ARTERIAL STUDIES

93875 Noninvasive physiologic studies of extracranial arteries, complete bilateral study (eg, periorbital flow direction with arterial compression, ocular pneumoplethysmography, Doppler ultrasound spectral analysis) S 80
> MED: 100-3,20.14; 100-3,20.17; 100-4,4,20.5
> AMA: 2000,Apr,1; 1997,Dec,10; 1996,Jun,9

93880 Duplex scan of extracranial arteries; complete bilateral study S 80
> MED: 100-3,20.17; 100-4,4,20.5
> AMA: 1996,Jun,9

93882 unilateral or limited study S 80
> MED: 100-3,20.17; 100-4,4,20.5
> AMA: 1996,Jun,9

93886 Transcranial Doppler study of the intracranial arteries; complete study S 80
> MED: 100-3,20.17; 100-4,4,20.5
> AMA: 1996,Jun,9

93888 limited study S 80
> MED: 100-3,20.17; 100-4,4,20.5
> AMA: 1996,Jun,9

93890 vasoreactivity study S 80
> MED: 100-4,4,20.5

93892 emboli detection without intravenous microbubble injection S 80
> MED: 100-4,4,20.5

93893 emboli detection with intravenous microbubble injection S 80
> MED: 100-4,4,20.5
> Codes 93890-93893 cannot be reported with CPT code 93888.

EXTREMITY ARTERIAL STUDIES (INCLUDING DIGITS)

93922 Noninvasive physiologic studies of upper or lower extremity arteries, single level, bilateral (eg, ankle/brachial indices, Doppler waveform analysis, volume plethysmography, transcutaneous oxygen tension measurement) S 80
> MED: 100-3,20.14; 100-4,4,20.5
> AMA: 1996,Jun,9

93923 Noninvasive physiologic studies of upper or lower extremity arteries, multiple levels or with provocative functional maneuvers, complete bilateral study (eg, segmental blood pressure measurements, segmental Doppler waveform analysis, segmental volume plethysmography, segmental transcutaneous oxygen tension measurements, measurements with postural provocative tests, measurements with reactive hyperemia) S 80
> MED: 100-3,20.14; 100-4,4,20.5
> AMA: 2001,Jun,10; 1996,Jun,9

93924 Noninvasive physiologic studies of lower extremity arteries, at rest and following treadmill stress testing, complete bilateral study S 80
> MED: 100-3,20.14; 100-4,4,20.5
> AMA: 1996,Jun,9

93925 Duplex scan of lower extremity arteries or arterial bypass grafts; complete bilateral study S 80
> MED: 100-3,20.14; 100-4,4,20.5
> AMA: 1996,Jun,9

93926 unilateral or limited study S 80
> MED: 100-3,20.14; 100-4,4,20.5
> AMA: 2001,Oct,1; 1996,Jun,9

93930 Duplex scan of upper extremity arteries or arterial bypass grafts; complete bilateral study S 80
> MED: 100-3,20.14; 100-4,4,20.5
> AMA: 1996,Jun,9

93931 unilateral or limited study S 80
> MED: 100-3,20.14; 100-4,4,20.5
> AMA: 2001,Oct,1; 1996,Jun,9

EXTREMITY VENOUS STUDIES (INCLUDING DIGITS)

93965 Noninvasive physiologic studies of extremity veins, complete bilateral study (eg, Doppler waveform analysis with responses to compression and other maneuvers, phleborheography, impedance plethysmography) S 80
> MED: 100-3,20.14; 100-4,4,20.5
> AMA: 1996,Jun,9

93970 Duplex scan of extremity veins including responses to compression and other maneuvers; complete bilateral study S 80
> MED: 100-4,4,20.5
> AMA: 1996,Jun,9

93971 unilateral or limited study S 80
> MED: 100-4,4,20.5
> AMA: 2001,Oct,1; 1996,Jun,9

VISCERAL AND PENILE VASCULAR STUDIES

93975 Duplex scan of arterial inflow and venous outflow of abdominal, pelvic, scrotal contents and/or retroperitoneal organs; complete study S 80
> MED: 100-4,4,20.5
> AMA: 1996,Jun,9; 1996,Apr,11

93976 limited study S 80
> MED: 100-4,4,20.5
> AMA: 1996,Jun,9; 1996,Apr,11

93978 Duplex scan of aorta, inferior vena cava, iliac vasculature, or bypass grafts; complete study S 80
> MED: 100-4,4,20.5
> AMA: 1996,Jun,9

93979 unilateral or limited study S 80
> MED: 100-4,4,20.5
> AMA: 1996,Jun,9

93980 Duplex scan of arterial inflow and venous outflow of penile vessels; complete study ♂ S 80
> MED: 100-4,4,20.5
> AMA: 1996,Jun,9

93981 follow-up or limited study ♂ S 80
> MED: 100-4,4,20.5
> AMA: 1996,Jun,9

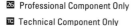

EXTREMITY ARTERIAL-VENOUS STUDIES

93990 **Duplex scan of hemodialysis access (including arterial inflow, body of access and venous outflow)** Ⓢ 80 🔲

MED: 100-4,4,20.5

AMA: 1996,Jun,9

When using indicator dilution methods for measurement of hemodialysis access flow, consult CPT code 90940.

PULMONARY

Pulmonary codes (94010-94799) include both diagnostic and therapeutic services. All procedures include laboratory services, interpretation, and physician services. List hospital inpatient visits, consultations, emergency department services, or office visits separately when performed on the same date as a diagnostic pulmonary service. Specify the procedures that may be performed in requesting prior authorization for pulmonary testing. If ordering tests for a patient and unsure about which test should be performed, contact the pulmonary laboratory for clarification and CPT code numbers. Include that information in documentation for prior authorization and claim review.

CPT codes 94010-94799 include laboratory procedures and interpretation of results. Consult the appropriate Evaluation and Management CPT code and report it in addition to 94010-94799 when separate identifiable Evaluation and Management services are provided.

VENTILATOR MANAGEMENT

● **94002** **Ventilation assist and management, initiation of pressure or volume preset ventilators for assisted or controlled breathing; hospital inpatient/observation, initial day** Ⓢ

● **94003** **hospital inpatient/observation, each subsequent day** Ⓢ

● **94004** **nursing facility, per day** Ⓑ

Do not report codes 94002-94004 with Evaluation and Management services 99201-99499.

● **94005** **Home ventilator management care plan oversight of a patient (patient not present) in home, domiciliary or rest home (eg, assisted living) requiring review of status, review of laboratories and other studies and revision of orders and respiratory care plan (as appropriate), within a calendar month, 30 minutes or more** Ⓔ

Do not report code 94005 with codes 99339, 99340, or 99374-99378.

Ventilator management care plan oversight is reported separately from home, domiciliary, or rest home (e.g. assisted living) services. A physician may report 94005, when performed, including when a different physician reports 99339, 99340, or 99374-99378 for the same 30 days.

OTHER PROCEDURES

Spirometry (94010-94070) measures lung capacity. Code 94010 refers to the measurement of the lung's capacity and flow measurements using a spirometer. Expiratory flow rate is calculated generally in terms of liters per second. Maximal voluntary ventilation is included in this service. The graphic record produced by the spirometer goes into the patient's record.

Codes 94014-94016 report patient initiated spirometric recording per 30 day time period.

Bronchospasm evaluation (94060) includes spirometry before and after the use of a bronchodilator. The final codes in this series report prolonged evaluation with multiple spirometric determinations.

94010 **Spirometry, including graphic record, total and timed vital capacity, expiratory flow rate measurement(s), with or without maximal voluntary ventilation** ⊠ 80 🔲

MED: 100-4,4,20.5

AMA: 1999,Jan,8; 1999,Feb,9; 1998,Nov,35; 1997,Nov,45; 1996,Mar,10; 1996,Feb,9; 1995,Summer,4

94014 **Patient-initiated spirometric recording per 30-day period of time; includes reinforced education, transmission of spirometric tracing, data capture, analysis of transmitted data, periodic recalibration and physician review and interpretation** ⊠ 80 🔲

MED: 100-4,4,20.5

AMA: 1999,Jan,8; 1999,Feb,9; 1998,Nov,34; 1996,Mar,10; 1996,Feb,9; 1995,Summer,4

94015 **recording (includes hook-up, reinforced education, data transmission, data capture, trend analysis, and periodic recalibration)** ⊠ TC 80 🔲

MED: 100-4,4,20.5

AMA: 1999,Jan,8; 1999,Feb,9; 1998,Nov,34; 1996,Mar,10; 1996,Feb,9; 1995,Summer,4

94016 **physician review and interpretation only** Ⓐ 26 80 🔲

MED: 100-4,4,20.5

AMA: 1999,Jan,8; 1999,Feb,9; 1998,Nov,34; 1996,Mar,10; 1996,Feb,9; 1995,Summer,4

94060 **Bronchodilation responsiveness, spirometry as in 94010, pre- and post-bronchodilator administration** ⊠ 80 🔲

MED: 100-4,4,20.5

AMA: 1999,Jan,8; 1999,Feb,9; 1998,Nov,34; 1997,Feb,10; 1996,Mar,10; 1996,Feb,9; 1995,Summer,4

If a bronchodilator supply is used, report with CPT code 99070 or applicable supply code.

If a prolonged exercise test is conducted for bronchospasm with pre- and post-spirometry, consult CPT code 94620.

94070 **Bronchospasm provocation evaluation, multiple spirometric determinations as in 94010, with administered agents (eg, antigen(s), cold air, methacholine)** ⊠ 80 🔲

MED: 100-4,4,20.5

AMA: 1999,Jan,8; 1999,Feb,9; 1997,Nov,45; 1996,Mar,10; 1996,Feb,9

Antigen administration should be reported separately with CPT code 99070 or applicable supply code.

94150 **Vital capacity, total (separate procedure)** ⊠

MED: 100-4,4,20.5

AMA: 1999,Jan,8; 1999,Feb,9; 1996,Mar,10; 1996,Feb,9; 1995,Summer,4

94200 **Maximum breathing capacity, maximal voluntary ventilation** ⊠ 80

MED: 100-4,4,20.5

AMA: 1999,Jan,8; 1999,Feb,9; 1996,Mar,10; 1996,Feb,9; 1995,Summer,4

94240 **Functional residual capacity or residual volume: helium method, nitrogen open circuit method, or other method** ⊠ 80 🔲

MED: 100-4,4,20.5

AMA: 1999,Jan,8; 1999,Feb,9; 1996,Mar,10; 1996,Feb,9; 1995,Summer,4

94250 **Expired gas collection, quantitative, single procedure (separate procedure)** ⊠ 80

MED: 100-4,4,20.5

AMA: 1999,Jan,8; 1999,Feb,9; 1996,Mar,10; 1996,Feb,9; 1995,Summer,4

⊛ Modifier 63 Exempt Code   ⊙ Conscious Sedation   ✛ CPT Add-on Code   ⊘ Modifier 51 Exempt Code   ● New Code   ▲ Revised Code

Ⓜ Maternity Edit   Ⓐ Age Edit   Ⓐ-Ⓨ APC Status Indicators   🔲 CCI Comprehensive Code   ✗ Drug Not Approved by FDA   50 Bilateral Procedure

94260 Thoracic gas volume $\boxed{X}$ $\boxed{80}$ $\boxed{\square}$

MED: 100-4,4,20.5

AMA: 1999,Jan,8; 1999,Feb,9; 1996,Mar,10; 1996,Feb,9; 1995,Summer,4

If plethysmography is performed, consult CPT codes 93720-93722.

94350 Determination of maldistribution of inspired gas: multiple breath nitrogen washout curve including alveolar nitrogen or helium equilibration time $\boxed{X}$ $\boxed{80}$ $\boxed{\square}$

MED: 100-4,4,20.5

AMA: 1999,Jan,8; 1999,Feb,9; 1996,Mar,10; 1996,Feb,9; 1995,Summer,4

94360 Determination of resistance to airflow, oscillatory or plethysmographic methods $\boxed{X}$ $\boxed{80}$ $\boxed{\square}$

MED: 100-4,4,20.5

AMA: 1999,Jan,8; 1999,Feb,9; 1996,Mar,10; 1996,Feb,9; 1995,Summer,4

94370 Determination of airway closing volume, single breath tests $\boxed{X}$ $\boxed{80}$ $\boxed{\square}$

MED: 100-4,4,20.5

AMA: 1999,Jan,8; 1999,Feb,9; 1996,Mar,10; 1996,Feb,9; 1995,Summer,4

94375 Respiratory flow volume loop $\boxed{X}$ $\boxed{80}$ $\boxed{\square}$

MED: 100-4,4,20.5

AMA: 1999,Jan,8; 1999,Feb,9; 1996,Mar,10; 1996,Feb,9; 1995,Summer,4

94400 Breathing response to CO2 (CO2 response curve) $\boxed{X}$ $\boxed{80}$ $\boxed{\square}$

MED: 100-4,4,20.5

AMA: 1999,Jan,8; 1999,Feb,9; 1996,Mar,10; 1996,Feb,9; 1995,Summer,4

94450 Breathing response to hypoxia (hypoxia response curve) $\boxed{X}$ $\boxed{80}$ $\boxed{\square}$

MED: 100-4,4,20.5

AMA: 1999,Jan,8; 1999,Feb,9; 1996,Mar,10; 1996,Feb,9; 1995,Summer,4

To report high altitude simulation test (HAST), consult CPT codes 94452, 94453.

94452 High altitude simulation test (HAST), with physician interpretation and report; $\boxed{X}$ $\boxed{80}$ $\boxed{\square}$

MED: 100-4,4,20.5

To report obtaining arterial blood gases, consult CPT code 36600.

Code 94452 cannot be reported with CPT codes 94453, 94760, 94761.

94453 with supplemental oxygen titration $\boxed{X}$ $\boxed{80}$ $\boxed{\square}$

MED: 100-4,4,20.5

To report obtaining arterial blood gases, consult CPT code 36600.

Code 94453 cannot be reported with CPT codes 94452, 94760, 94761.

$\oslash$ ● **94610** Intrapulmonary surfactant administration by a physician through endotracheal tube $\boxed{S}$

Do not report code 94610 with codes 99293-99296.

Use code 31500 for endotracheal intubation.

Report 94610 once per dosing episode.

▲ **94620** Pulmonary stress testing; simple (eg, 6-minute walk test, prolonged exercise test for bronchospasm with pre- and post-spirometry and oximetry) $\boxed{X}$ $\boxed{80}$ $\boxed{\square}$

MED: 100-3,240.7; 100-4,4,20.5

AMA: 1999,Jan,8; 1999,Feb,9; 1998,Nov,35; 1996,Mar,10; 1996,Feb,9; 1995,Summer,4

94621 complex (including measurements of CO2 production, O2 uptake, and electrocardiographic recordings) $\boxed{X}$ $\boxed{80}$ $\boxed{\square}$

MED: 100-3,20.15; 100-4,4,20.5

AMA: 2002,Aug,10; 1999,Jan,8; 1999,Feb,9; 1998,Nov,35; 1996,Mar,10; 1996,Feb,9; 1995,Summer,4

94640 Pressurized or nonpressurized inhalation treatment for acute airway obstruction or for sputum induction for diagnostic purposes (eg, with an aerosol generator, nebulizer, metered dose inhaler or intermittent positive pressure breathing [IPPB] device) $\boxed{S}$ $\boxed{80}$ $\boxed{\square}$

MED: 100-4,4,20.5

AMA: 2000,Apr,11; 1999,Jan,8; 1999,Feb,9; 1998,May,10; 1996,Mar,10; 1996,Feb,9; 1995,Summer,4

To report more than one inhalation treatment on the same day, append modifier 76 to code 94640.

See codes 94644 and 94645 for continuous inhalation treatment of one hour or more.

94642 Aerosol inhalation of pentamidine for pneumocystis carinii pneumonia treatment or prophylaxis $\boxed{S}$ $\boxed{80}$ $\boxed{\square}$

MED: 100-4,4,20.5

AMA: 1999,Jan,8; 1999,Feb,9; 1996,Mar,10; 1996,Feb,9; 1995,Summer,4

● **94644** Continuous inhalation treatment with aerosol medication for acute airway obstruction; first hour $\boxed{S}$

Use 94640 for services less than one hour.

+ ● **94645** each additional hour (List separately in addition to code for primary procedure) $\boxed{S}$

Note that 94645 is an add-on code and must be reported with code 94644.

~~**94656** Ventilation assist and management, initiation of pressure or volume preset ventilators for assisted or controlled breathing; first day~~

Use 94002-94005.

~~**94657** subsequent days~~

Use 94002-94005.

94660 Continuous positive airway pressure ventilation (CPAP), initiation and management $\boxed{S}$ $\boxed{80}$

MED: 100-4,4,20.5; 100-4,12,30.6.12

AMA: 1999,Jan,10; 1999,Feb,9; 1996,Mar,10; 1996,Feb,9; 1995,Summer,4; 1992,Fall,30

If CPAP is performed as part of critical care services (99291-99292) do not report separately.

94662 Continuous negative pressure ventilation (CNP), initiation and management $\boxed{S}$ $\boxed{80}$ $\boxed{\square}$

MED: 100-4,4,20.5; 100-4,12,30.6.12

AMA: 1999,Jan,8; 1999,Feb,9; 1996,Mar,10; 1996,Feb,9; 1995,Summer,4; 1992,Fall,30

If CNP is performed as part of critical care services (99291-99292) do not report separately.

94664 Demonstration and/or evaluation of patient utilization of an aerosol generator, nebulizer, metered dose inhaler or IPPB device $\boxed{S}$ $\boxed{80}$ $\boxed{\square}$

MED: 100-4,4,20.5

AMA: 2000,Apr,11; 1999,Jan,8; 1999,Feb,9; 1998,May,10; 1996,Mar,10; 1996,Feb,9; 1995,Summer,4

Report 94664 only once per date of service.

94667 Manipulation chest wall, such as cupping, percussing, and vibration to facilitate lung function; initial demonstration and/or evaluation $\boxed{S}$ $\boxed{80}$ $\boxed{\square}$

MED: 100-3,150.1; 100-3,240.7; 100-4,4,20.5

AMA: 1999,Jan,8; 1999,Feb,9; 1996,Mar,10; 1996,Feb,9; 1995,Summer,4

94668   subsequent   S 80 ▣

MED: 100-3,150.1; 100-3,240.7; 100-4,4,20.5

AMA: 1999,Jan,8; 1999,Feb,9; 1996,Mar,10; 1996,Feb,9; 1995,Summer,4

94680   Oxygen uptake, expired gas analysis; rest and exercise, direct, simple   X 80 ▣

MED: 100-4,4,20.5

AMA: 1999,Jan,8; 1999,Feb,9; 1996,Mar,10; 1996,Feb,9; 1995,Summer,4

94681   including CO2 output, percentage oxygen extracted   X 80 ▣

MED: 100-4,4,20.5

AMA: 1999,Jan,8; 1999,Feb,9; 1996,Mar,10; 1996,Feb,9; 1995,Summer,4

To report blood gases consult CPT codes 82800-82810.

94690   rest, indirect (separate procedure)   X 80 ▣

MED: 100-4,4,20.5

AMA: 1999,Jan,8; 1999,Feb,9; 1996,Mar,10; 1996,Feb,9; 1995,Summer,4

If a single arterial procedure is performed, consult CPT code 36600.

94720   Carbon monoxide diffusing capacity (eg, single breath, steady state)   X 80 ▣

MED: 100-4,4,20.5

AMA: 1999,Jan,8; 1999,Feb,9; 1996,Mar,10; 1996,Feb,9; 1995,Summer,4

94725   Membrane diffusion capacity   X 80 ▣

MED: 100-4,4,20.5

AMA: 1999,Jan,8; 1999,Feb,9; 1996,Mar,10; 1996,Feb,9; 1995,Summer,4

94750   Pulmonary compliance study (eg, plethysmography, volume and pressure measurements)   X 80 ▣

MED: 100-4,4,20.5

AMA: 1999,Jan,8; 1999,Feb,9; 1996,Mar,10; 1996,Feb,9; 1995,Summer,4

94760   Noninvasive ear or pulse oximetry for oxygen saturation; single determination   N TC 80 ▣

MED: 100-4,4,20.5; 100-4,12,30.6.12

AMA: 1999,Jan,8; 1999,Feb,9; 1998,Jul,1; 1997,Feb,10; 1996,Mar,10; 1996,Feb,9; 1995,Summer,4

To report blood gases, consult CPT codes 82800-82810.

94761   multiple determinations (eg, during exercise)   N TC 80 ▣

MED: 100-4,4,20.5

AMA: 1999,Jun,10; 1999,Jan,8; 1999,Feb,9; 1998,Jul,1; 1996,Mar,10; 1996,Feb,9; 1995,Summer,4

94762   by continuous overnight monitoring (separate procedure)   Q TC 80 ▣

MED: 100-4,4,20.5; 100-4,12,30.6.12

AMA: 1999,Jan,8; 1999,Feb,9; 1998,Jul,1; 1996,Mar,10; 1996,Feb,9; 1995,Summer,4

94770   Carbon dioxide, expired gas determination by infrared analyzer   X 80 ▣

MED: 100-4,4,20.5

AMA: 1999,Jan,8; 1999,Feb,9; 1996,Mar,10; 1996,Feb,9; 1995,Summer,4

If bronchoscopy is performed, consult CPT codes 31622-31659. If a flow directed catheter is placed, consult CPT code 93503. If venipuncture is performed, consult CPT code 36410. If a central venous catheter is placed, consult CPT codes 36488-36491. If an arterial puncture is performed, consult CPT code 36600. If arterial catheterization is performed, consult CPT code 36620. If thoracentesis is performed, consult CPT code 32000. If a therapeutic phlebotomy is performed, consult CPT code 99195. If a needle biopsy is performed on the lung, consult CPT code 32405. If orotracheal or nasotracheal intubation is necessary, consult CPT code 31500.

94772   Circadian respiratory pattern recording (pediatric pneumogram), 12-24 hour continuous recording, infant   A X 80 ▣

MED: 100-4,4,20.5

AMA: 1999,Jan,8; 1999,Feb,9; 1996,Mar,10; 1996,Feb,9; 1995,Summer,4

Separate procedure codes for electromyograms, EEG, ECG, and recordings of respiration cannot be reported with this procedural code.

● 94774   Pediatric home apnea monitoring event recording including respiratory rate, pattern and heart rate per 30-day period of time; includes monitor attachment, download of data, physician review, interpretation, and preparation of a report   B

Do not report code 94774 with codes 94775-94777 during the same reporting period.

● 94775   monitor attachment only (includes hook-up, initiation of recording and disconnection)   X

● 94776   monitoring, download of information, receipt of transmission(s) and analyses by computer only   X

● 94777   physician review, interpretation and preparation of report only   B

Do not report oxygen saturation monitoring separately when used in addition to heart rate and respiratory monitoring.

Do not report codes 94774-94777 with codes 93224-3272.

Do not report apnea recording device separately.

Use codes 95805-95811 for sleep study.

94799   Unlisted pulmonary service or procedure   X 80

MED: 100-4,4,20.5

AMA: 1999,Jan,8; 1999,Feb,9; 1996,Mar,10; 1996,Feb,9; 1995,Summer,4

ALLERGY AND CLINICAL IMMUNOLOGY

Allergy testing and immunology treatment (95004-95199) is performed according to the patient's history, physical findings, and clinical judgment of the provider. Specify the number of tests performed in the unit area of the claim or electronic billing form. Significant, separately identifiable E/M services should be reported in addition to allergen testing and immunotherapy.

Allergy sensitivity tests (95004-95075) reports the performance and evaluation of cutaneous and mucous membrane tests, the number of tests performed is based on clinical judgment, patient history and physical findings.

Immunotherapy (95115-95199) is the administration of allergenic extracts as antigens at periodic intervals in increasing dosages to a maintenance therapy

---

◎ Modifier 63 Exempt Code   ⊙ Conscious Sedation   + CPT Add-on Code   ⊘ Modifier 51 Exempt Code   ● New Code   ▲ Revised Code

M Maternity Edit   A Age Edit   A-Y APC Status Indicators   ▣ CCI Comprehensive Code   ⁄ Drug Not Approved by FDA   80 Bilateral Procedure

© 2006 Ingenix (Blue Ink)   CPT only © 2006 American Medical Association. All Rights Reserved. (Black Ink)   Medicine — 359

level. If significant, separately identifiable evaluation and management services are provided in addition to immunotherapy, report the appropriate E/M code and append modifier 25.

ALLERGY TESTING

95004   Percutaneous tests (scratch, puncture, prick) with allergenic extracts, immediate type reaction, specify number of tests   ☒ 80 ☐

MED: 100-2,15,20.2; 100-2,15,20.3; 100-4,4,20.5; 100-4,12,200

AMA: 1991,Summer,15

95010   Percutaneous tests (scratch, puncture, prick) sequential and incremental, with drugs, biologicals or venoms, immediate type reaction, specify number of tests   ☒ 80 ☐

MED: 100-2,15,20.2; 100-2,15,20.3; 100-4,4,20.5; 100-4,12,200

AMA: 1991,Summer,15

● 95012   Nitric oxide expired gas determination   ☒

Use code 0064T for nitric oxide determination by spectroscopy.

95015   Intracutaneous (intradermal) tests, sequential and incremental, with drugs, biologicals, or venoms, immediate type reaction, specify number of tests   ☒ 80 ☐

MED: 100-2,15,20.2; 100-2,15,20.3; 100-4,4,20.5; 100-4,12,200

AMA: 1991,Summer,15

95024   Intracutaneous (intradermal) tests with allergenic extracts, immediate type reaction, specify number of tests   ☒ 80 ☐

MED: 100-2,15,20.2; 100-2,15,20.3; 100-4,4,20.5; 100-4,12,200

AMA: 1991,Summer,15

95027   Intracutaneous (intradermal) tests, sequential and incremental, with allergenic extracts for airborne allergens, immediate type reaction, specify number of tests   ☒ TC 80 ☐

MED: 100-2,15,20.2; 100-2,15,20.3; 100-4,4,20.5; 100-4,12,200

AMA: 1997,Jun,10; 1991,Summer,15

95028   Intracutaneous (intradermal) tests with allergenic extracts, delayed type reaction, including reading, specify number of tests   ☒ TC 80 ☐

MED: 100-2,15,20.2; 100-2,15,20.3; 100-4,4,20.5; 100-4,12,200

AMA: 1991,Summer,14

95044   Patch or application test(s) (specify number of tests)   ☒ 80 ☐

MED: 100-2,15,20.2; 100-2,15,20.3; 100-4,4,20.5; 100-4,12,200

AMA: 1994,Spring,31; 1991,Summer,15

95052   Photo patch test(s) (specify number of tests)   ☒ 80 ☐

MED: 100-2,15,20.2; 100-2,15,20.3; 100-4,4,20.5; 100-4,12,200

AMA: 1994,Spring,31

95056   Photo tests   ☒ 80 ☐

MED: 100-2,15,20.2; 100-2,15,20.3; 100-4,4,20.5; 100-4,12,200

AMA: 1991,Summer,16

95060   Ophthalmic mucous membrane tests   ☒ TC 80

MED: 100-2,15,20.2; 100-2,15,20.3; 100-4,4,20.5; 100-4,12,200

AMA: 1991,Summer,16

95065   Direct nasal mucous membrane test   ☒ TC 80 ☐

MED: 100-2,15,20.2; 100-2,15,20.3; 100-4,4,20.5; 100-4,12,200

AMA: 1991,Summer,16

95070   Inhalation bronchial challenge testing (not including necessary pulmonary function tests); with histamine, methacholine, or similar compounds   ☒ TC 80 ☐

MED: 100-2,15,20.2; 100-2,15,20.3; 100-4,4,20.5; 100-4,12,200

AMA: 1991,Summer,16

95071   with antigens or gases, specify   ☒ TC 80 ☐

MED: 100-2,15,20.2; 100-2,15,20.3; 100-3,110.12; 100-4,4,20.5; 100-4,12,200

AMA: 1991,Summer,16

If pulmonary function tests are performed, consult CPT codes 94060 and 94070.

95075   Ingestion challenge test (sequential and incremental ingestion of test items, eg, food, drug or other substance such as metabisulfite)   ☒ 80

MED: 100-2,15,20.2; 100-2,15,20.3; 100-3,110.12; 100-4,4,20.5; 100-4,12,200

AMA: 2002,Oct,11; 2001,Sep,10; 1991,Summer,16

~~95078   Provocative testing (eg, Rinkel test)~~

MED: 100-3,110.11

ALLERGEN IMMUNOTHERAPY

95115   Professional services for allergen immunotherapy not including provision of allergenic extracts; single injection   ☒ 80 ☐

MED: 100-2,15,20.2; 100-2,15,20.3; 100-4,12,200

AMA: 2000,Apr,4; 1998,Nov,35; 1996,May,1; 1995,Summer,4; 1994,Spring,30; 1991,Fall,19

CPT codes 95115-95199 include all professional services needed for allergen immunotherapy. Office visits may be reported in addition to immunotherapy if other separately identifiable E/M services are rendered at the same time.

95117   two or more injections   ☒ 80 ☐

MED: 100-2,15,20.2; 100-2,15,20.3; 100-4,12,200

AMA: 2000,Apr,4; 1998,Nov,35; 1996,May,1; 1996,Aug,10; 1994,Spring,30; 1991,Fall,19

95120   Professional services for allergen immunotherapy in prescribing physicians office or institution, including provision of allergenic extract; single injection   ☒

MED: 100-2,15,20.2; 100-2,15,20.3; 100-4,12,200

AMA: 1998,Nov,35; 1996,May,2; 1994,Spring,30; 1991,Fall,19

95125   two or more injections   ☒

MED: 100-2,15,20.2; 100-2,15,20.3; 100-4,12,200

AMA: 1998,Nov,35; 1996,May,2; 1996,Aug,10; 1994,Spring,30; 1991,Fall,19

95130   single stinging insect venom   ☒

MED: 100-2,15,20.2; 100-2,15,20.3; 100-4,12,200

AMA: 1999,Sep,10; 1998,Nov,35; 1996,May,2; 1996,Jun,10; 1991,Fall,19

95131   two stinging insect venoms   ☒

MED: 100-2,15,20.2; 100-2,15,20.3; 100-4,12,200

AMA: 1999,Sep,10; 1998,Nov,35; 1996,May,2; 1996,Jun,10; 1991,Fall,19

95132   three stinging insect venoms   ☒

MED: 100-2,15,20.2; 100-2,15,20.3; 100-4,12,200

AMA: 1999,Sep,11; 1998,Nov,35; 1996,May,2; 1991,Fall,19

95133   four stinging insect venoms   ☒

MED: 100-2,15,20.2; 100-2,15,20.3; 100-4,12,200

AMA: 1999,Sep,11; 1998,Nov,35; 1996,May,2; 1991,Fall,19

95134   five stinging insect venoms   ☒

MED: 100-2,15,20.2; 100-2,15,20.3; 100-4,12,200

AMA: 1999,Sep,11; 1998,Nov,35; 1996,May,2; 1991,Fall,19

95144   Professional services for the supervision of preparation and provision of antigens for allergen immunotherapy, single dose vial(s) (specify number of vials)   ☒ 80 ☐

MED: 100-2,15,20.2; 100-2,15,20.3; 100-3,110.9; 100-4,4,20.5; 100-4,12,200

AMA: 1998,Nov,35; 1996,May,10; 1994,Spring,30; 1991,Fall,19

A single dose vial is defined as a single dose of antigen administered in one injection.

26 Professional Component Only   80/ 80 Assist-at-Surgery Allowed/With Documentation   Unlisted   Not Covered

TC Technical Component Only   MED: Pub 100/NCD References   AMA: CPT Assistant References   1 - 9 ASC Group   ♂ Male Only   ♀ Female Only

360 — CPT Expert   CPT only © 2006 American Medical Association. All Rights Reserved. (Black Ink)   © 2006 Ingenix (Blue Ink)

95145 Professional services for the supervision of preparation and provision of antigens for allergen immunotherapy (specify number of doses); single stinging insect venom ⓢ ⑧⓪ ▣

MED: 100-2,15,20.2; 100-2,15,20.3; 100-3,110.9; 100-4,4,20.5; 100-4,12,200

AMA: 1998,Nov,35; 1996,May,1; 1991,Fall,19

95146 two single stinging insect venoms ⓢ ⑧⓪ ▣

MED: 100-2,15,20.2; 100-2,15,20.3; 100-4,4,20.5; 100-4,12,200

AMA: 1998,Nov,35; 1996,May,11; 1991,Fall,19

95147 three single stinging insect venoms ⓢ ⑧⓪ ▣

MED: 100-2,15,20.2; 100-2,15,20.3; 100-3,110.9; 100-4,4,20.5; 100-4,12,200

AMA: 1998,Nov,35; 1996,May,11; 1991,Fall,19

95148 four single stinging insect venoms ⓢ ⑧⓪ ▣

MED: 100-2,15,20.2; 100-2,15,20.3; 100-3,110.9; 100-4,4,20.5; 100-4,12,200

AMA: 1998,Nov,35; 1996,May,11; 1991,Fall,19

95149 five single stinging insect venoms ⓢ ⑧⓪ ▣

MED: 100-2,15,20.2; 100-2,15,20.3; 100-3,110.9; 100-4,4,20.5; 100-4,12,200

AMA: 1998,Nov,35; 1996,May,11; 1991,Fall,19

95165 Professional services for the supervision of preparation and provision of antigens for allergen immunotherapy; single or multiple antigens (specify number of doses) ⓢ ⑧⓪ ▣

MED: 100-2,15,20.2; 100-2,15,20.3; 100-3,110.9; 100-4,4,20.5; 100-4,12,200

AMA: 2001,Apr,11; 2000,Apr,4; 1998,Nov,35; 1996,May,11; 1994,Spring,30; 1991,Fall,19

95170 whole body extract of biting insect or other arthropod (specify number of doses) ⓢ ⑧⓪ ▣

MED: 100-2,15,20.2; 100-2,15,20.3; 100-3,110.9; 100-4,4,20.5; 100-4,12,200

AMA: 2001,Apr,11; 1996,May,12; 1994,Spring,30; 1991,Fall,19

When reporting allergy immunotherapy, a dose is the amount of antigen(s) administered in a single injection from a multiple dose vial.

95180 Rapid desensitization procedure, each hour (eg, insulin, penicillin, equine serum) ⓧ ⑧⓪ ▣

MED: 100-2,15,20.2; 100-2,15,20.3; 100-4,4,20.5

95199 Unlisted allergy/clinical immunologic service or procedure ⓧ ⑧⓪

MED: 100-2,15,20.2; 100-2,15,20.3; 100-3,110.12; 100-4,4,20.5

AMA: 1998,Nov,35; 1995,Summer,4

If skin testing for bacterial, viral, and fungal extracts is performed, consult CPT codes 86485-86586 and 95028. If special reports are filed for an allergy patient, consult CPT code 99080. If testing procedures such as allergosorbent testing (RAST), rat mast cell technique (RMCT), mast cell degranulation test (MCDT), lymphocytic transformation test (LTT), leukocyte histamine release (LHR), migration inhibitory factor test (MIF), transfer factor test (TFT), or nitroblue tetrazolium dye test (NTD) are performed, consult the Immunology section in Pathology or use 95199.

ENDOCRINOLOGY

95250 Ambulatory continuous glucose monitoring of interstitial tissue fluid via a subcutaneous sensor for up to 72 hours; sensor placement, hook-up, calibration of monitor, patient training, removal of sensor, and printout of recording ⓧ ⓣⓒ ⑧⓪ ▣

Code 95250 should not be used in conjunction with 99091.

To report physician review, interpretation and written report associated with code 95250, see Evaluation and Management services section.

95251 physician interpretation and report Ⓑ ②⑥ ⑧⓪

Codes 95250, 95251 cannot be used in conjunction with 99091.

NEUROLOGY AND NEUROMUSCULAR PROCEDURES

Appropriate levels of consultation codes 99241-99255 may be used as neurologic services are typically consultative in nature.

In addition, services outlined in the evaluation and management guidelines applicable to a neurologic illness may be reported.

Included in the EEG is autonomic function, evoked potentials, reflex tests, EMG, NCV, and MEG services (codes 95812-95829 and 95860-95967). These include the recording, interpretation by a physician and report. For interpretation only, append modifier 26.

SLEEP TESTING

Sleep services (95805-95811) include sleep studies and polysomnography. Both types of services include continuous and simultaneous monitoring and recording of selected physiological and pathophysiological sleep parameters for a minimum of six hours. For studies of less than six hours append modifier 52. These services are global and include tracing, interpretation, and report. For interpretation only, append modifier 26. These studies are performed to diagnose a variety of sleep disorders and to evaluate a patient's response to therapies such as nasal continuous positive airway pressure (NCPAP).

Polysomnography is distinguished from sleep studies by the inclusion of sleep staging, which is defined to include:

- 1-4 lead electroencephalogram (EEG)
- Electro-oculogram (EOG)
- Submental electromyogram (EMG)

Additional parameters of sleep include:

- Electrocardiogram (ECG)
- Airflow
- Ventilation and respiratory effort
- Gas exchange by oximetry, transcutaneous monitoring, or end tidal gas analysis
- Extremity muscle activity, motor activity-movement
- Extended electroencephalogram (EEG) monitoring
- Penile tumescence
- Gastroesophageal reflux
- Continuous blood pressure monitoring
- Snoring
- Body positions

95805 Multiple sleep latency or maintenance of wakefulness testing, recording, analysis and interpretation of physiological measurements of sleep during multiple trials to assess sleepiness ⓢ ⑧⓪ ▣

MED: 100-4,4,20.5

AMA: 2002,Sep,1; 2001,Dec,3; 1998,Nov,35; 1997,Nov,45-46

---

⑥③ Modifier 63 Exempt Code ⊙ Conscious Sedation ✛ CPT Add-on Code ⊘ Modifier 51 Exempt Code ● New Code ▲ Revised Code

Ⓜ Maternity Edit Ⓐ Age Edit Ⓐ-Ⓨ APC Status Indicators ▣ CCI Comprehensive Code ⚕ Drug Not Approved by FDA ⑤⓪ Bilateral Procedure

© 2006 Ingenix (Blue Ink)   CPT only © 2006 American Medical Association. All Rights Reserved. (Black Ink)   Medicine — 361

Medicine

95806 — 95865

95806   Sleep study, simultaneous recording of ventilation, respiratory effort, ECG or heart rate, and oxygen saturation, unattended by a technologist   [S] [80] [↻]

     MED: 100-4,4,20.5

     AMA: 1998,Nov,35; 1998,Aug,10; 1997,Nov,45-46

95807   Sleep study, simultaneous recording of ventilation, respiratory effort, ECG or heart rate, and oxygen saturation, attended by a technologist   [S] [80] [↻]

     MED: 100-4,4,20.5

     AMA: 1998,Nov,35; 1997,Nov,46

95808   Polysomnography; sleep staging with 1-3 additional parameters of sleep, attended by a technologist   [S] [80] [↻]

     MED: 100-4,4,20.5

     AMA: 2002,Sep,1; 1998,Nov,35; 1998,Feb,6; 1997,Nov,46; 1996,Sep,11

95810   sleep staging with 4 or more additional parameters of sleep, attended by a technologist   [S] [80] [↻]

     MED: 100-4,4,20.5

     AMA: 2002,Sep,1; 1998,Nov,35; 1998,Feb,6

95811   sleep staging with 4 or more additional parameters of sleep, with initiation of continuous positive airway pressure therapy or bilevel ventilation, attended by a technologist   [S] [80] [↻]

     MED: 100-4,4,20.5

     AMA: 2002,Sep,1; 1998,Nov,35; 1998,Feb,6; 1997,Nov,46

ROUTINE ELECTROENCEPHALOGRAPHY (EEG)

CPT codes 95812-95822 include hyperventilation and/or photic stimulation procedures, do not report separately. Standard EEG services 95816-95822 include recording of 20-40 minutes. To report recordings of longer than 40 minutes, consult CPT codes 95812-95813.

95812   Electroencephalogram (EEG) extended monitoring; 41-60 minutes   [S] [80] [↻]

     MED: 100-3,160.21; 100-4,4,20.5

     AMA: 1998,Nov,35; 1994,Winter,18

95813   greater than one hour   [S] [80] [↻]

     MED: 100-4,4,20.5

     AMA: 1998,Nov,35; 1994,Winter,18

95816   Electroencephalogram (EEG); including recording awake and drowsy   [S] [80] [↻]

     MED: 100-3,160.21; 100-4,4,20.5

     AMA: 2000,Jul,1; 1999,Nov,51; 1998,Nov,35; 1996,Sep,11

95819   including recording awake and asleep   [S] [80] [↻]

     MED: 100-3,160.21; 100-4,4,20.5

     AMA: 2000,Jul,1; 1999,Nov,51; 1998,Nov,35

95822   recording in coma or sleep only   [S] [80]

     MED: 100-3,160.21; 100-4,4,20.5

     AMA: 1998,Nov,35

95824   cerebral death evaluation only   [S] [80] [↻]

     MED: 100-4,4,20.5

     AMA: 1998,Nov,35

95827   all night recording   [S] [80] [↻]

     MED: 100-4,4,20.5

     AMA: 1998,Nov,35

If ambulatory 24 hour EEG monitoring is needed, consult CPT code 95950-95953 or 95956. If an EEG is performed during nonintracranial surgery, consult CPT code 95955. If a Wada test is performed, consult CPT code 95958. If circadian respiratory patterns of infants are recorded, consult CPT code 94772.

To report digital analysis of EEG, consult CPT code 95957.

95829   Electrocorticogram at surgery (separate procedure)   [S] [80] [↻]

     MED: 100-4,4,20.5

     AMA: 1998,Nov,35

95830   Insertion by physician of sphenoidal electrodes for electroencephalographic (EEG) recording   [B] [80] [↻]

     MED: 100-3,160.21; 100-4,4,20.5

MUSCLE AND RANGE OF MOTION TESTING

95831   Muscle testing, manual (separate procedure) with report; extremity (excluding hand) or trunk   [A] [80] [↻]

     MED: 100-2,15,230.4; 100-4,4,20.5; 100-4,5,20

     AMA: 2001,Nov,4; 2000,Mar,11; 2000,Jul,1; 1999,Nov,51; 1999,Dec,10

95832   hand, with or without comparison with normal side   [A] [80] [↻]

     MED: 100-2,15,230.4; 100-4,4,20.5; 100-4,5,20

     AMA: 2001,Nov,4; 2000,Mar,11; 2000,Jul,1; 1999,Nov,51; 1999,Dec,10

95833   total evaluation of body, excluding hands   [A] [80] [↻]

     MED: 100-2,15,230.4; 100-4,4,20.5; 100-4,5,20

     AMA: 2001,Nov,4; 1999,Nov,51; 1999,Dec,10

95834   total evaluation of body, including hands   [A] [80] [↻]

     MED: 100-2,15,230.4; 100-4,4,20.5; 100-4,5,20

     AMA: 2001,Nov,4; 2000,Jul,1; 1999,Nov,51; 1999,Dec,10

95851   Range of motion measurements and report (separate procedure); each extremity (excluding hand) or each trunk section (spine)   [A] [80]

     MED: 100-2,15,230.4; 100-4,4,20.5; 100-4,5,20

     AMA: 2001,Nov,4; 1999,Sep,10

95852   hand, with or without comparison with normal side   [A] [80]

     MED: 100-2,15,230.4; 100-4,4,20.5; 100-4,5,20

     AMA: 2001,Nov,4

95857   Tensilon test for myasthenia gravis   [S] [80] [↻]

     MED: 100-4,4,20.5

ELECTROMYOGRAPHY AND NERVE CONDUCTION TESTS

95860   Needle electromyography; one extremity with or without related paraspinal areas   [S] [80] [↻]

     MED: 100-2,15,80; 100-2,15,230.4; 100-4,4,20.5

     AMA: 2002,Apr,1; 2000,Jul,1; 1997,Nov,46

95861   two extremities with or without related paraspinal areas   [S] [80] [↻]

     MED: 100-2,15,80; 100-2,15,230.4; 100-4,4,20.5

     AMA: 2002,Apr,1; 2000,Jul,1; 1997,Nov,46

To report dynamic electromyography performed during motion analysis studies, consult CPT code 96002-96003.

95863   three extremities with or without related paraspinal areas   [S] [80] [↻]

     MED: 100-2,15,80; 100-2,15,230.4; 100-4,4,20.5

     AMA: 2002,Apr,1; 2000,Jul,1; 1997,Nov,46

95864   four extremities with or without related paraspinal areas   [S] [80] [↻]

     MED: 100-2,15,80; 100-2,15,230.4; 100-4,4,20.5

     AMA: 2002,Jan,11; 2002,Apr,1; 2000,Jul,1; 1997,Nov,46

95865   larynx   [S] [80]

     MED: 100-4,4,20.5

Modifier 50 cannot be used with 95865.

Report modifier 52 with 95865 to report a unilateral procedure.

	95866	hemidiaphragm	S 80 50

MED: 100-4,4,20.5

	95867	cranial nerve supplied muscle(s), unilateral	S 80 ⌧

MED: 100-2,15,80; 100-2,15,230.4; 100-4,4,20.5
AMA: 2002,Apr,1

	95868	cranial nerve supplied muscles, bilateral	S 80 ⌧

MED: 100-2,15,80; 100-2,15,230.4; 100-4,4,20.5
AMA: 2002,Apr,1

	95869	thoracic paraspinal muscles (excluding T1 or T12)	S 80 ⌧

MED: 100-2,15,80; 100-2,15,230.4; 100-4,4,20.5
AMA: 2002,Apr,1; 1997,Nov,46

	95870	limited study of muscles in one extremity or non-limb (axial) muscles (unilateral or bilateral), other than thoracic paraspinal, cranial nerve supplied muscles, or sphincters	S 80

MED: 100-2,15,80; 100-2,15,230.4; 100-4,4,20.5
AMA: 2002,Apr,1; 2000,Jul,1; 1999,Nov,51; 1997,Nov,46
Adson test

	95872	Needle electromyography using single fiber electrode, with quantitative measurement of jitter, blocking and/or fiber density, any/all sites of each muscle studied	S 80

MED: 100-2,15,80; 100-2,15,230.4; 100-4,4,20.5
AMA: 2002,Apr,1

+	95873	Electrical stimulation for guidance in conjunction with chemodenervation (List separately in addition to code for primary procedure)	S 80

MED: 100-4,4,20.5

+	95874	Needle electromyography for guidance in conjunction with chemodenervation (List separately in addition to code for primary procedure)	S 80

MED: 100-4,4,20.5

Note that 95873, 95874 are add-on codes and must be used in conjunction with 64612-64614.

Code 95874 cannot be used with 95873.

Codes 95873, 95874 cannot be used with 95860-95870.

	95875	Ischemic limb exercise test with serial specimen(s) acquisition for muscle(s) metabolite(s)	S 80 ⌧

MED: 100-2,15,80; 100-2,15,230.4; 100-4,4,20.5

⊘	95900	Nerve conduction, amplitude and latency/velocity study, each nerve; motor, without F-wave study	S 80

MED: 100-2,15,230.4; 100-4,4,20.5
AMA: 2002,Apr,1; 2000,Jul,1; 2000,Jan,10; 1999,Nov,51-52; 1996,Jan,2

⊘	95903	motor, with F-wave study	S 80 ⌧

MED: 100-2,15,80; 100-2,15,230.4; 100-4,4,20.5
AMA: 2002,Apr,1; 2000,Jan,10; 1999,Nov,51-52; 1996,Jan,2

⊘	95904	sensory	S 80

MED: 100-2,15,80; 100-2,15,230.4; 100-4,4,20.5
AMA: 2002,Apr,1; 1999,Sep,11; 1999,Nov,51-52; 1996,Jan,2
Note that 95900, 95903, and 95904 are to be reported only once when multiple sites on the same nerve are stimulated or recorded.

INTRAOPERATIVE NEUROPHYSIOLOGY

+	95920	Intraoperative neurophysiology testing, per hour (List separately in addition to code for primary procedure)	S 80 ⌧

MED: 100-2,15,80; 100-2,15,230.4; 100-4,4,20.5
AMA: 1999,Nov,52; 1998,Nov,35-36

Note that 95920 is an add-on code and must be used in conjunction with the study performed 92585, 95822, 95860, 95861, 95867, 95868, 95870, 95900, 95904, 95904, 95925-95937.

Code 95920 describes ongoing electrophysiologic testing and monitoring performed during surgical procedures. Code 95920 is reported per hour of service, and includes only the ongoing electrophysiologic monitoring time distinct from performance of specific type(s) of baseline electrophysiologic study(ies) (95860, 95861, 95867, 95868, 95870, 95900, 95904, 95928, 95929, 95933-95937) or interpretation of specific type(s) of baseline electrophysiologic study(ies) (92585, 95822, 95870, 95925-95928, 95929, 95930). The time spent performing or interpreting the baseline electrophysiologic study(ies) should not be counted as intraoperative monitoring, but represents separately reportable procedures. Code 95920 should be used once per hour even if multiple electrophysiologic studies are performed. The baseline electrophysiologic study(ies) should be used once per operative session.

To report electrocorticography, consult CPT code 95829. To report intraoperative EEG during nonintracranial surgery, consult CPT code 95955.

To report intraoperative functional cortical or subcortical mapping, consult CPT codes 95961-95962. To report intraoperative neurostimulator programming and analysis, consult CPT codes 95970-95975.

AUTONOMIC FUNCTION TESTS

	95921	Testing of autonomic nervous system function; cardiovagal innervation (parasympathetic function), including two or more of the following: heart rate response to deep breathing with recorded R-R interval, Valsalva ratio, and 30:15 ratio	S 80 ⌧

MED: 100-4,4,20.5
AMA: 2002,Apr,1; 1998,Nov,35-36

	95922	vasomotor adrenergic innervation (sympathetic adrenergic function), including beat-to-beat blood pressure and R-R interval changes during Valsalva maneuver and at least five minutes of passive tilt	S 80 ⌧

AMA: 2002,Apr,1; 1998,Nov,35-36

	95923	sudomotor, including one or more of the following: quantitative sudomotor axon reflex test (QSART), silastic sweat imprint, thermoregulatory sweat test, and changes in sympathetic skin potential	S 80 ⌧

MED: 100-3,190.5; 100-4,4,20.5
AMA: 2002,Apr,1; 1998,Nov,35-36

EVOKED POTENTIALS AND REFLEX TESTS

	95925	Short-latency somatosensory evoked potential study, stimulation of any/all peripheral nerves or skin sites, recording from the central nervous system; in upper limbs	S 80

MED: 100-2,15,80; 100-2,15,230.4; 100-3,160.10; 100-4,4,20.5
AMA: 2002,Apr,1; 1998,Nov,35-36

Medicine

95926 — 95966

95926   in lower limbs   [S] [80]

MED: 100-2,15,80; 100-2,15,230.4; 100-3,160.10; 100-4,4,20.5

AMA: 2002,Apr,1; 2001,May,11

95927   in the trunk or head   [S] [80]

MED: 100-2,15,80; 100-2,15,230.4; 100-3,160.10; 100-4,4,20.5

AMA: 2002,Apr,1

If this procedure is performed unilaterally, append modifier 52 to the procedural code. If visual evoked potential testing is performed on the central nervous system, consult CPT code 95930. If brainstem evoked response recording takes place, consult CPT code 92585. If auditory evoked potentials testing is conducted on the central nervous system, consult CPT code 92585.

95928   Central motor evoked potential study (transcranial motor stimulation); upper limbs   [S] [80]

MED: 100-4,4,20.5

95929   lower limbs   [S] [80]

MED: 100-4,4,20.5

95930   Visual evoked potential (VEP) testing central nervous system, checkerboard or flash   [S] [80]

MED: 100-2,15,80; 100-2,15,230.4; 100-3,160.10; 100-4,4,20.5

95933   Orbicularis oculi (blink) reflex, by electrodiagnostic testing   [S] [80]

MED: 100-2,15,80; 100-2,15,230.4; 100-4,4,20.5

AMA: 1998,Nov,35-36

95934   H-reflex, amplitude and latency study; record gastrocnemius/soleus muscle   [S] [80] [50]

MED: 100-2,15,80; 100-2,15,230.4; 100-4,4,20.5

AMA: 2002,Apr,1; 2001,Jul,11; 1998,Nov,35-36; 1996,Jan,3

95936   record muscle other than gastrocnemius/soleus muscle   [S] [80] [50]

MED: 100-2,15,80; 100-2,15,230.4; 100-4,4,20.5

AMA: 2002,Apr,1; 1996,Jan,3

If this procedure is performed bilaterally, append modifier 50 to the procedural code.

95937   Neuromuscular junction testing (repetitive stimulation, paired stimuli), each nerve, any one method   [S] [80] [▣]

MED: 100-2,15,80; 100-2,15,230.4; 100-4,4,20.5

AMA: 2002,Apr,1; 1998,Nov,35-36

SPECIAL EEG TESTS

95950   Monitoring for identification and lateralization of cerebral seizure focus, electroencephalographic (eg, 8 channel EEG) recording and interpretation, each 24 hours   [S] [80] [▣]

MED: 100-3,160.21; 100-3,160.22; 100-4,4,20.5

AMA: 1998,Nov,35

95951   Monitoring for localization of cerebral seizure focus by cable or radio, 16 or more channel telemetry, combined electroencephalographic (EEG) and video recording and interpretation (eg, for presurgical localization), each 24 hours   [S] [80] [▣]

MED: 100-3,160.21; 100-3,160.22; 100-4,4,20.5

AMA: 1998,Nov,35

95953   Monitoring for localization of cerebral seizure focus by computerized portable 16 or more channel EEG, electroencephalographic (EEG) recording and interpretation, each 24 hours   [S] [80] [▣]

MED: 100-3,160.21; 100-3,160.22; 100-4,4,20.5

AMA: 1998,Nov,35

95954   Pharmacological or physical activation requiring physician attendance during EEG recording of activation phase (eg, thiopental activation test)   [S] [80] [▣]

MED: 100-4,4,20.5

AMA: 1998,Nov,35; 1994,Winter,18

If an EEG is analyzed digitally, consult CPT code 95957.

95955   Electroencephalogram (EEG) during nonintracranial surgery (eg, carotid surgery)   [S] [80] [▣]

MED: 100-3,160.8; 100-3,160.9; 100-3,160.21; 100-3,160.22; 100-4,4,20.5

AMA: 1998,Nov,35

95956   Monitoring for localization of cerebral seizure focus by cable or radio, 16 or more channel telemetry, electroencephalographic (EEG) recording and interpretation, each 24 hours   [S] [80] [▣]

MED: 100-3,160.21; 100-3,160.22; 100-4,4,20.5

AMA: 1998,Nov,35

95957   Digital analysis of electroencephalogram (EEG) (eg, for epileptic spike analysis)   [S] [80] [▣]

MED: 100-3,160.21; 100-3,160.22; 100-4,4,20.5

AMA: 1998,Nov,35; 1994,Winter,18

95958   Wada activation test for hemispheric function, including electroencephalographic (EEG) monitoring   [S] [80] [▣]

MED: 100-3,130.5; 100-3,130.6; 100-3,160.2; 100-3,160.21; 100-3,160.22; 100-4,4,20.5

AMA: 1998,Nov,35

95961   Functional cortical and subcortical mapping by stimulation and/or recording of electrodes on brain surface, or of depth electrodes, to provoke seizures or identify vital brain structures; initial hour of physician attendance   [S] [80] [▣]

MED: 100-3,160.2; 100-3,160.7; 100-4,4,20.5; 100-4,32,50

AMA: 1999,Nov,52-53; 1998,Nov,35; 1994,Winter,18

+ **95962**   each additional hour of physician attendance (List separately in addition to code for primary procedure)   [S] [80] [▣]

MED: 100-4,4,20.5; 100-4,32,50

AMA: 1999,Nov,52-53; 1998,Nov,35; 1994,Winter,18

Note that 95962 is an add-on code and must be used in conjunction with 95961.

95965   Magnetoencephalography (MEG), recording and analysis; for spontaneous brain magnetic activity (eg, epileptic cerebral cortex localization)   [S] [80] [▣]

95966   for evoked magnetic fields, single modality (eg, sensory, motor, language, or visual cortex localization)   [S] [80] [▣]

[26] Professional Component Only   [80]/ [80] Assist-at-Surgery Allowed/With Documentation   Unlisted   Not Covered

[TC] Technical Component Only   **MED:** Pub 100/NCD References   **AMA:** CPT Assistant References   [1]-[9] ASC Group   ♂ Male Only   ♀ Female Only

364 — CPT Expert   CPT only © 2006 American Medical Association. All Rights Reserved. *(Black Ink)*   © 2006 Ingenix *(Blue Ink)*

+ **95967** for evoked magnetic fields, each additional modality (eg, sensory, motor, language, or visual cortex localization) (List separately in addition to code for primary procedure) [S] [80]

Note that 95967 is an add-on code and must be used in conjunction with code 95966.

For electroencephalography performed in addition to magnetoencephalography, consult CPT codes 95812-95827.

For somatosensory evoked potentials, auditory evoked potentials, and visual evoked potentials performed in addition to magnetic evoked field responses, consult CPT codes 92585, 95925, 95926, and/or 95930.

For computed tomography performed in addition to magnetoencephalography, consult CPT codes 70450-70470, 70496.

To report MRI performed in addition to magnetoencephalography, consult CPT codes 70551-70553.

NEUROSTIMULATORS, ANALYSIS-PROGRAMMING

The following codes discuss the analysis and programming of neurostimulators. Neurostimulator pulse generators and transmitters affect pulse amplitude, duration, and frequency; more than eight electrode contacts; cycling; stimulation duration and spacing; number of programs and channels; phase angle; alternating polarities; configuration of wave form; and more than one clinical symptom.

CPT defines a simple neurostimulator as affecting up to three of these and a complex neurostimulator as affecting three or more.

Codes 95978 and 95979 describe initial or subsequent electronic analysis of an implanted brain neurostimulator pulse generator system, with programming.

If a neurostimulator pulse generator is inserted, consult CPT codes 61885, 63685, 63688, and 64590. If a neurostimulator pulse generator or receiver is revised or removed, consult CPT codes 61888, 63688, and 64595. If neurostimulator electrodes are implanted, consult CPT codes 43647, 43881, 61850-61875, 63650-63655, 64553-64580, 0155T, 0157T. If neurostimulator electrodes are revised or removed, consult CPT codes 43648, 43882, 61880, 63660, 64585, 0156T, and 0158T

95970 Electronic analysis of implanted neurostimulator pulse generator system (eg, rate, pulse amplitude and duration, configuration of wave form, battery status, electrode selectability, output modulation, cycling, impedance and patient compliance measurements); simple or complex brain, spinal cord, or peripheral (ie, cranial nerve, peripheral nerve, autonomic nerve, neuromuscular) neurostimulator pulse generator/transmitter, without reprogramming [S] [80] [✪]

MED: 100-3,160.13; 100-4,4,20.5; 100-4,32,50
AMA: 1999,Sep,1; 1999,Nov,53-54; 1998,Nov,36-37

95971 simple spinal cord, or peripheral (ie, peripheral nerve, autonomic nerve, neuromuscular) neurostimulator pulse generator/transmitter, with intraoperative or subsequent programming [S] [80] [✪]

MED: 100-3,160.13; 100-4,4,20.5; 100-4,32,50
AMA: 1999,Sep,1; 1999,Nov,53-54; 1998,Nov,36-37

95972 complex spinal cord, or peripheral (except cranial nerve) neurostimulator pulse generator/transmitter, with intraoperative or subsequent programming, first hour [S] [80] [✪]

MED: 100-4,4,20.5; 100-4,32,50
AMA: 1999,Sep,1; 1999,Nov,53-54; 1998,Nov,36-37

+ **95973** complex spinal cord, or peripheral (except cranial nerve) neurostimulator pulse generator/transmitter, with intraoperative or subsequent programming, each additional 30 minutes after first hour (List separately in addition to code for primary procedure) [S] [80]

MED: 100-4,4,20.5; 100-4,32,50
AMA: 1999,Sep,1; 1999,Nov,53-54; 1998,Nov,36-37
Note that 95973 is an add-on code and must be used in conjunction with 95972.

95974 complex cranial nerve neurostimulator pulse generator/transmitter, with intraoperative or subsequent programming, with or without nerve interface testing, first hour [S] [80]

MED: 100-4,4,20.5
AMA: 1999,Sep,1; 1999,Nov,53-54; 1998,Nov,36-37

+ **95975** complex cranial nerve neurostimulator pulse generator/transmitter, with intraoperative or subsequent programming, each additional 30 minutes after first hour (List separately in addition to code for primary procedure) [S] [80]

MED: 100-4,4,20.5
AMA: 1999,Sep,1; 1999,Nov,53-54; 1998,Nov,36-37
Note that 95975 is an add-on code and must be used in conjunction with 95974.

Use code 0162T for electronic analysis, programming, and reprogramming of gastric neurostimulator pulse generator, lesser curvaluture (morbid obesity).

95978 Electronic analysis of implanted neurostimulator pulse generator system (eg, rate, pulse amplitude and duration, battery status, electrode selectability and polarity, impedance and patient compliance measurements), complex deep brain neurostimulator pulse generator/transmitter, with initial or subsequent programming; first hour [S] [80] [✪]

MED: 100-4,4,20.5

+ **95979** each additional 30 minutes after first hour (List separately in addition to code for primary procedure) [S] [80]

MED: 100-4,4,20.5
Note that 95979 os am add-on code and must be used in conjunction with 95978.

OTHER PROCEDURES

95990 Refilling and maintenance of implantable pump or reservoir for drug delivery, spinal (intrathecal, epidural) or brain (intraventricular); [T] [80] [✪]

MED: 100-3,280.14; 100-4,4,20.5
To report analysis and/or reprogramming of implantable infusion pump, consult CPT codes 62367-62368.

To report refill/maintenance of implanted infusion pump or reservoir for systemic drug therapy (e.g. shemotherapy or insulin), use code 96522.

95991 administered by physician [T] [80] [✪]

MED: 100-3,280.14; 100-4,4,20.5

95999 Unlisted neurological or neuromuscular diagnostic procedure [S] [80]

MED: 100-4,4,20.5
AMA: 1999,Feb,11

MOTION ANALYSIS

Report codes 96000-96004 for services performed as part of major therapeutic or diagnostic decision making. Motion analysis is performed in a dedicated motion analysis department. This includes a facility capable of performing videotaping

⦾ Modifier 63 Exempt Code   ⊙ Conscious Sedation   + CPT Add-on Code   ⊘ Modifier 51 Exempt Code   ● New Code   ▲ Revised Code

[M] Maternity Edit   [A] Age Edit   [A-Y] APC Status Indicators   [✪] CCI Comprehensive Code   ✗ Drug Not Approved by FDA   [50] Bilateral Procedure

© 2006 Ingenix (Blue Ink)   CPT only © 2006 American Medical Association. All Rights Reserved. (Black Ink)   Medicine — 365

from the front, back and both sides, computerized 3-D kinematics, 3-D kinetics and dynamic electromyography. 3-D kinetics and stride characteristics may be included in code 96000.

96000 Comprehensive computer-based motion analysis by video-taping and 3-D kinematics; S 80 ▯

MED: 100-2,15,80; 100-2,15,230.4

AMA: 2002,Aug,5

96001 with dynamic plantar pressure measurements during walking S 80 ▯

MED: 100-2,15,80; 100-2,15,230.4

AMA: 2002,Aug,5

96002 Dynamic surface electromyography, during walking or other functional activities, 1-12 muscles S 80 ▯

MED: 100-2,15,80; 100-2,15,230.4

AMA: 2002,Aug,5

96003 Dynamic fine wire electromyography, during walking or other functional activities, 1 muscle S 80 ▯

MED: 100-2,15,80; 100-2,15,230.4

AMA: 2002,Aug,5

Codes 96002 and 96003 cannot be used with codes 95860-95864, 95869-95872.

96004 Physician review and interpretation of comprehensive computer-based motion analysis, dynamic plantar pressure measurements, dynamic surface electromyography during walking or other functional activities, and dynamic fine wire electromyography, with written report B 26 80 ▯

AMA: 2002,Aug,5

FUNCTIONAL BRAIN MAPPING

Functional brain mapping codes include the selection and administration of testing of language, memory, cognition, movement, sensation, and other neurological functions when conducted in connection to functional neuroimaging, performance monitoring of this testing, and determining the validity of neurofunctional testing relative to separately interpreted functional magnetic resonance images.

● 96020 Neurofunctional testing selection and administration during noninvasive imaging functional brain mapping, with test administered entirely by a physician or psychologist, with review of test results and report X

Use code 70555 for functional magnetic resonance imaging (MRI), brain.

Do not report code 96020 with code 70544.

Do not report code 96020 in conjunction with codes 96101-96103 or 96166-96120.

Evaluation and Management service codes should not be reported on the same day as 96020.

MEDICAL GENETICS AND GENETIC COUNSELING SERVICES

These codes describe services that are provided by a trained genetic counselor and may include obtaining a structural family genetic history, pedigree construction, analysis for genetic risk assessment, and counseling of the patient and family. These activities may be provided during one or more sessions and may include the review of medical data and family information, face-to-face interviews, and counseling services.

● 96040 Medical genetics and genetic counseling services, each 30 minutes face-to-face with patient/family E

When genetic counseling and education is provided by a physician to an individual, consult the appropriate Evaluation and Management codes.

When genetic counseling and education is provided by a physician to a group, use code 99078.

See codes 98961 and 98962 for education regarding genetic risks provided by a nonphysician to a group.

Consult codes 99401-99412 for genetic counseling and/or risk factor reduction intervention provided by a physician to patient(s) without symptoms or established disease.

CENTRAL NERVOUS SYSTEM ASSESSMENTS/TESTS (EG, NEURO-COGNITIVE, MENTAL STATUS, SPEECH TESTING)

The reports resulting from the following tests address the cognitive function of the patient.

To report development of cognitive skills, consult CPT codes 97532 and 97533.

96101 Psychological testing (includes psychodiagnostic assessment of emotionality, intellectual abilities, personality and psychopathology, eg, MMPI, Rorschach, WAIS), per hour of the psychologist's or physician's time, both face-to-face time with the patient and time interpreting test results and preparing the report X 80

MED: 100-4,4,20.5

96102 Psychological testing (includes psychodiagnostic assessment of emotionality, intellectual abilities, personality and psychopathology, eg, MMPI and WAIS), with qualified health care professional interpretation and report, administered by technician, per hour of technician time, face-to-face X 80

MED: 100-4,4,20.5

96103 Psychological testing (includes psychodiagnostic assessment of emotionality, intellectual abilities, personality and psychopathology, eg, MMPI), administered by a computer, with qualified health care professional interpretation and report X 80

MED: 100-4,4,20.5

96105 Assessment of aphasia (includes assessment of expressive and receptive speech and language function, language comprehension, speech production ability, reading, spelling, writing, eg, by Boston Diagnostic Aphasia Examination) with interpretation and report, per hour A 80 ▯

MED: 100-1,3,30; 100-1,3,30.1; 100-1,3,30.2; 100-1,3,30.3; 100-2,15,80.2; 100-2,15,160; 100-2,15,170; 100-4,4,20.5; 100-4,5,20; 100-4,12,150; 100-4,12,160; 100-4,12,170; 100-4,12,170.1; 100-4,12,210

AMA: 1996,Jul,8

96110 Developmental testing; limited (eg, Developmental Screening Test II, Early Language Milestone Screen), with interpretation and report X 80 ▯

MED: 100-1,3,30; 100-1,3,30.1; 100-1,3,30.2; 100-1,3,30.3; 100-2,15,80.2; 100-2,15,160; 100-2,15,170; 100-4,4,20.5; 100-4,5,20; 100-4,12,150; 100-4,12,160; 100-4,12,170; 100-4,12,170.1; 100-4,12,210

AMA: 1996,Jul,9

26 Professional Component Only

80/ 80 Assist-at-Surgery Allowed/With Documentation

Unlisted

Not Covered

TC Technical Component Only MED: Pub 100/NCD References AMA: CPT Assistant References 1 - 9 ASC Group ♂ Male Only ♀ Female Only

366 — CPT Expert CPT only © 2006 American Medical Association. All Rights Reserved. (Black Ink) © 2006 Ingenix (Blue Ink)

96111   **extended (includes assessment of motor, language, social, adaptive and/or cognitive functioning by standardized developmental instruments) with interpretation and report** [X] [80] [↻]

MED: 100-1,3,30; 100-1,3,30.1; 100-1,3,30.2; 100-1,3,30.3; 100-2,15,80.2; 100-2,15,160; 100-2,15,170; 100-4,4,20.5; 100-4,5,20; 100-4,12,150; 100-4,12,160; 100-4,12,170; 100-4,12,170.1; 100-4,12,210

AMA: 1996,Jul,9

96116   **Neurobehavioral status exam (clinical assessment of thinking, reasoning and judgment, eg, acquired knowledge, attention, language, memory, planning and problem solving, and visual spatial abilities), per hour of the psychologist's or physician's time, both face-to-face time with the patient and time interpreting test results and preparing the report** [X] [80]

MED: 100-4,4,20.5

96118   **Neuropsychological testing (eg, Halstead-Reitan Neuropsychological Battery, Wechsler Memory Scales and Wisconsin Card Sorting Test), per hour of the psychologist's or physician's time, both face-to-face time with the patient and time interpreting test results and preparing the report** [X] [80]

MED: 100-4,4,20.5

96119   **Neuropsychological testing (eg, Halstead-Reitan Neuropsychological Battery, Wechsler Memory Scales and Wisconsin Card Sorting Test), with qualified health care professional interpretation and report, administered by technician, per hour of technician time, face-to-face** [X] [80]

MED: 100-4,4,20.5

96120   **Neuropsychological testing (eg, Wisconsin Card Sorting Test), administered by a computer, with qualified health care professional interpretation and report** [X] [80]

MED: 100-4,4,20.5

HEALTH AND BEHAVIOR ASSESSMENT/INTERVENTION

Health and behavior assessment/intervention (96150-96155), are procedures used to identify the psychological, behavioral, emotional, cognitive, and social factors important to the prevention, treatment, or management of physical health problems. The codes include health and behavior assessment as well as health and behavior intervention, of which the latter is reported in 15-minute increments of direct face-to-face contact with the individual, a group, or the family of the individual.

For health and behavior assessment and/or intervention performed by a physician, consult Evaluation and Management or Preventive Medicine services codes.

96150   **Health and behavior assessment (eg, health-focused clinical interview, behavioral observations, psychophysiological monitoring, health-oriented questionnaires), each 15 minutes face-to-face with the patient; initial assessment** [S] [80] [↻]

AMA: 2002,Mar,4

96151   **re-assessment** [S] [80] [↻]

AMA: 2002,Mar,4

96152   **Health and behavior intervention, each 15 minutes, face-to-face; individual** [S] [80] [↻]

AMA: 2002,Mar,4

96153   **group (2 or more patients)** [S] [80] [↻]

AMA: 2002,Mar,4

96154   **family (with the patient present)** [S] [80] [↻]

AMA: 2002,Mar,4

96155   **family (without the patient present)** [E]

AMA: 2002,Mar,4

CHEMOTHERAPY ADMINISTRATION

The following codes describe intravenous, subcutaneous, intramuscular, intra-arterial, and other than oral types of chemotherapy administration. This also includes administration of chemotherapy for noncancer diagnoses or monoclonal antibody agents, and other biologic response modifiers. These are complex services and usually require highly trained personnel to administer, mix, and dispose of the drug or substance. They require the direct supervision of the physician, including patient assessment, consent, supervision, and oversight during the procedure. The patient will usually require frequent monitoring during the infusion.

The following services are included in the administration codes:

- Use of a local anesthesia
- Starting the IV
- Access to IV, catheter, or port
- Routine tubing, syringe, and supplies
- Preparation of drug(s)
- Flushing at the completion of the infusion
- Hydration fluid

(For declotting of a catheter or port consult 36550.)

Report separate codes for each method of administration given by different techniques. For administration of other non-chemotherapy agents (e.g., antibiotics, analgesics, and steroids), consult CPT codes 90760, 90761, 90765, and 90779. These should be reported separately if administered as supportive management of the chemotherapy administration.

Report the drug separately. Fluid used for hydration is considered incidental.

If multiple infusions, injections, or combinations services are performed, only the initial code should be reported unless the procedure requires the use of two separate IV sites. Report the code that most closely describes the main reason for the procedure even if that is not the order in which the services are performed.

When reporting codes for which time is an issue, use the actual time for the administration of the infusion.

To report an evaluation and management service in addition to hydration, therapeutic, prophylactic, and diagnostic injections and infusion services, consult the appropriate evaluation and management codes. For an E/M service on the same day, append modifier 25 to 96401-96549. A different diagnosis is not required.

Report regional or isolation chemotherapy with codes for arterial infusion (96420-96425). Consult surgery codes from the Cardiovascular Surgery section to report placement of the catheter. To report placement of arterial and venous cannula(s) for extracorporeal circulation via a membrane oxygenator perfusion pump, consult 36823. This code includes dose calculation and the administration of chemotherapy by injection into the perfusate. Do not report codes 96409-96425 with 36823.

(For home infusion services, consult CPT codes 99601-99602.)

INJECTION AND INTRAVENOUS INFUSION CHEMOTHERAPY

An intravenous or intra-arterial push requires:

- The constant presence of the health care professional administering the substance or drug
- An infusion of 15 minutes or less

96401   **Chemotherapy administration, subcutaneous or intramuscular; non-hormonal anti-neoplastic** [S] [80]

MED: 100-4,4,230.2.2

96402   **hormonal anti-neoplastic** [S] [80]

MED: 100-4,4,230.2.2

96405   **Chemotherapy administration; intralesional, up to and including 7 lesions** [S] [↻]

MED: 100-3,110.6; 100-4,4,230.2.2; 100-4,12,30.5

AMA: 2001,Jul,1; 2001,Feb,10; 1997,Aug,19; 1996,Sep,5

---

⑥ Modifier 63 Exempt Code   ⊙ Conscious Sedation   + CPT Add-on Code   ⊘ Modifier 51 Exempt Code   ● New Code   ▲ Revised Code

[M] Maternity Edit   [A] Age Edit   [A]-[Y] APC Status Indicators   [↻] CCI Comprehensive Code   ✗ Drug Not Approved by FDA   [50] Bilateral Procedure

© 2006 Ingenix (Blue Ink)   CPT only © 2006 American Medical Association. All Rights Reserved. (Black Ink)   Medicine — 367

Medicine

| | 96406 | intralesional, more than 7 lesions ⑤ 🔲 |

MED: 100-4,4,230.2.2; 100-4,12,30.5

AMA: 2001,Jul,1; 2001,Feb,10; 1997,Aug,19; 1996,Sep,5

| | 96409 | intravenous, push technique, single or initial substance/drug ⑤ ⑧⓪ |

| + | 96411 | intravenous, push technique, each additional substance/drug (List separately in addition to code for primary procedure) ⑤ ⑧⓪ |

Note that 96411 is an add-on code and must be used in conjunction with 96409, 96413.

| | 96413 | **Chemotherapy administration, intravenous infusion technique; up to 1 hour, single or initial substance/drug** ⑤ ⑧⓪ |

| + ▲ | 96415 | **each additional hour (List separately in addition to code for primary procedure)** ⑤ ⑧⓪ |

Note that 96415 is an add-on code and must be used in conjunction with 96413.

Code 96415 should be used for infusion intervals of greater than 30 minutes beyond 1-hour increments.

Code 90761 should be used to identify hydration, or 90766, 90767, 90775 to identify therapeutic, prophylactic, or diagnostic drug infusion or injection, if provided as a secondary or subsequent service in addition to 96413.

| | 96416 | **initiation of prolonged chemotherapy infusion (more than 8 hours), requiring use of a portable or implantable pump** ⑤ ⑧⓪ |

MED: 100-4,4,230.2.1; 100-4,4,230.2.2

To report refilling and maintenance of a portable pump or an implantable infusion pump or reservoir for drug delivery, consult 96521-96523.

| + | 96417 | **each additional sequential infusion (different substance/drug), up to 1 hour (List separately in addition to code for primary procedure)** ⑤ ⑧⓪ |

Note that 96417 is an add-on code and must be used in conjunction with 96413.

This code should be used only once per sequential infusion. Report code 96415 for additional hour(s) of sequential infusion.

INTRA-ARTERIAL CHEMOTHERAPY

| | 96420 | **Chemotherapy administration, intra-arterial; push technique** ⑤ ⑧⓪ 🔲 |

MED: 100-3,110.2; 100-3,110.6; 100-4,4,230.2.2; 100-4,12,30.5

AMA: 2001,Jul,1; 2001,Feb,10; 1999,Nov,54; 1998,Nov,37; 1997,Aug,19

| | 96422 | infusion technique, up to one hour ⑤ ⑧⓪ 🔲 |

MED: 100-3,110.6; 100-4,4,230.2.2; 100-4,12,30.5

AMA: 2001,Jul,1; 2001,Feb,10; 1998,Nov,37; 1997,Aug,19; 1996,Dec,10

| + ▲ | 96423 | **infusion technique, each additional hour (List separately in addition to code for primary procedure)** ⑤ ⑧⓪ 🔲 |

MED: 100-3,110.6; 100-4,4,230.2.2; 100-4,12,30.5

AMA: 2001,Jul,1; 2001,Feb,10; 1998,Nov,37; 1996,Dec,10

Note that 96423 is an add-on code and must be used in conjunction with 96422.

Code 96423 should be reported for infusion intervals of greater than 30 minutes beyond 1-hour increments

| | 96425 | **infusion technique, initiation of prolonged infusion (more than 8 hours), requiring the use of a portable or implantable pump** ⑤ ⑧⓪ |

MED: 100-3,110.6; 100-4,4,230.2.1; 100-4,12,30.5

AMA: 2001,Jul,1; 2001,Feb,10; 1999,Nov,54

If an implanted pump or reservoir is refilled, consult CPT codes 96521-96523.

OTHER CHEMOTHERAPY

| | 96440 | **Chemotherapy administration into pleural cavity, requiring and including thoracentesis** ⑤ ⑧⓪ 🔲 |

MED: 100-3,110.2; 100-3,110.6; 100-4,4,230.2.2; 100-4,12,30.5

AMA: 2001,Jul,1; 2001,Feb,10

| | 96445 | **Chemotherapy administration into peritoneal cavity, requiring and including peritoneocentesis** ⑤ ⑧⓪ 🔲 |

MED: 100-3,110.2; 100-3,110.6; 100-4,4,230.2.2; 100-4,12,30.5

AMA: 2001,Jul,1; 2001,Feb,10

| | 96450 | **Chemotherapy administration, into CNS (eg, intrathecal), requiring and including spinal puncture** ⑤ ⑧⓪ 🔲 |

MED: 100-3,110.2; 100-3,110.6; 100-4,4,230.2.2; 100-4,12,30.5

AMA: 2001,Jul,1; 2001,Feb,10

If intravesical (bladder) chemotherapy is administered, consult CPT code 51720. If a subarachnoid catheter and reservoir is inserted for drug infusion, consult CPT codes 62350, 62351, and 62360-62362. If an intraventricular catheter and reservoir is inserted, consult CPT codes 61210 and 61215.

| | 96521 | **Refilling and maintenance of portable pump** ⑤ ⑧⓪ |

MED: 100-4,4,230.2.1

| | 96522 | **Refilling and maintenance of implantable pump or reservoir for drug delivery, systemic (eg, intravenous, intra-arterial)** ⑤ ⑧⓪ |

MED: 100-4,4,230.2.1

For refilling and maintenance of an implantable infusion pump for a spinal or brain drug infusion, use 95990-95991.

| | 96523 | **Irrigation of implanted venous access device for drug delivery systems** ⓠ ⑧⓪ |

MED: 100-4,4,230.2.1

Code 96523 cannot be reported if an injection or infusion is provided on the same date of service.

| | 96542 | **Chemotherapy injection, subarachnoid or intraventricular via subcutaneous reservoir, single or multiple agents** ⑤ ⑧⓪ 🔲 |

MED: 100-3,110.2; 100-3,110.6; 100-4,4,230.2.2; 100-4,12,30.5

AMA: 2001,Jul,1; 1997,Aug,19

| | 96549 | **Unlisted chemotherapy procedure** ⑤ ⑧⓪ |

MED: 100-3,110.6; 100-4,4,230.2.2; 100-4,12,30.5

AMA: 2001,Jul,1; 1997,Aug,19

PHOTODYNAMIC THERAPY

These three codes (96567-96571) report photodynamic therapy either by external application of light to destroy malignancies or by endoscopic application of light that activates photosensitive drugs to destroy abnormal tissue.

For reporting ocular photodynamic therapy consult CPT code 67221.

| | 96567 | **Photodynamic therapy by external application of light to destroy premalignant and/or malignant lesions of the skin and adjacent mucosa (eg, lip) by activation of photosensitive drug(s), each phototherapy exposure session** ⓣ ⑧⓪ 🔲 |

MED: 100-3,80.2; 100-3,80.3

+ **96570**   Photodynamic therapy by endoscopic application of light to ablate abnormal tissue via activation of photosensitive drug(s); first 30 minutes (List separately in addition to code for endoscopy or bronchoscopy procedures of lung and esophagus)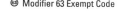

> MED: 100-3,80.2; 100-3,80.3; 100-3,100.2; 100-4,4,20.5
> AMA: 2000,Sep,5; 1999,Nov,54
> Note that 96570 and 96571 are to be used in addition to bronchoscopy, endoscopy codes. Note that 96570-96571 are add-on codes and must be used in conjunction with 31641 or 43228 as appropriate.

+ **96571**   each additional 15 minutes (List separately in addition to code for endoscopy or bronchoscopy procedures of lung and esophagus) ⊤

> MED: 100-3,80.2; 100-3,80.3; 100-3,100.2; 100-4,4,20.5
> AMA: 2000,Sep,5; 1999,Nov,54
> Note that 96570 and 96571 are to be used in addition to bronchoscopy, endoscopy codes. Note that 96570-96571 are add-on codes and must be used in conjunction with 31641 or 43228 as appropriate.

SPECIAL DERMATOLOGICAL PROCEDURES

If intralesional injections are administered, consult CPT codes 11900 and 11901. If a Tzanck smear is performed, consult CPT code 87207.

96900   Actinotherapy (ultraviolet light) ⓢ 80

> MED: 100-4,4,20.5

96902   Microscopic examination of hairs plucked or clipped by the examiner (excluding hair collected by the patient) to determine telogen and anagen counts, or structural hair shaft abnormality ⓝ

> MED: 100-3,190.6; 100-4,4,20.5
> AMA: 1997,Nov,46-47

● **96904**   Whole body integumentary photography, for monitoring of high risk patients with dysplastic nevus syndrome or a history of dysplastic nevi, or patients with a personal or familial history of melanoma ⓝ

96910   Photochemotherapy; tar and ultraviolet B (Goeckerman treatment) or petrolatum and ultraviolet B ⓢ 80

> MED: 100-3,250.1; 100-3,250.4; 100-4,4,20.5

96912   psoralens and ultraviolet A (PUVA) ⓢ 80

> MED: 100-3,250.1; 100-3,250.4; 100-4,4,20.5

96913   Photochemotherapy (Goeckerman and/or PUVA) for severe photoresponsive dermatoses requiring at least four to eight hours of care under direct supervision of the physician (includes application of medication and dressings) ⓢ 80

> MED: 100-3,250.1; 100-3,250.4; 100-4,4,20.5

96920   Laser treatment for inflammatory skin disease (psoriasis); total area less than 250 sq cm ⊤

> MED: 100-4,4,20.5

96921   250 sq. cm to 500 sq. cm ⊤

> MED: 100-4,4,20.5

96922   over 500 sq cm ⊤

> MED: 100-4,4,20.5

96999   Unlisted special dermatological service or procedure ⊤ 80

> MED: 100-4,4,20.5

PHYSICAL MEDICINE AND REHABILITATION

EVALUATION SERVICES

Codes 97001-97006 report evaluation and re-evaluation services for physical, occupational, and athletic therapy. Codes 97001, 97003, and 97005 indicate the initial evaluation service. Re-evaluation services should be reported with codes 97002, 97004, and 97006.

97001   Physical therapy evaluation Ⓐ 80

> MED: 100-2,15,60.3; 100-2,15,230.4; 100-3,20.10; 100-4,4,240; 100-4,5,10; 100-4,5,20
> AMA: 2002,Oct,11; 2001,Sep,10; 2000,Feb,11; 1997,Nov,47

97002   Physical therapy re-evaluation Ⓐ 80

> MED: 100-2,15,60.3; 100-2,15,230.4; 100-3,20.10; 100-4,4,240; 100-4,5,10; 100-4,5,20
> AMA: 2002,Oct,11; 2001,Sep,10; 2000,Feb,11; 1997,Nov,47

97003   Occupational therapy evaluation Ⓐ 80

> MED: 100-2,15,60.3; 100-2,15,230.4; 100-3,20.10; 100-4,4,240; 100-4,5,10; 100-4,5,20
> AMA: 2002,Oct,11; 1997,Nov,47

97004   Occupational therapy re-evaluation Ⓐ 80

> MED: 100-2,15,60.3; 100-2,15,230.4; 100-3,20.10; 100-4,4,240; 100-4,5,10; 100-4,5,20
> AMA: 2002,Oct,11; 1997,Nov,47

97005   Athletic training evaluation Ⓔ

> MED: 100-2,15,230.4; 100-4,5,10
> AMA: 2002,Jun,9

97006   Athletic training re-evaluation Ⓔ

> MED: 100-2,15,230.4; 100-4,5,10
> AMA: 2002,Jun,9

MODALITIES

The modality range is organized into two groups. The first group (97010-97028) describes supervised procedures that do not require direct (one-on-one) patient contact. The second group (97032-97039) requires constant attendance and direct (one-on-one) patient contact.

The description for all treatment modalities specifies application of a modality to one or more areas. In other words, when hot or cold packs are applied to the arm, leg, and neck, code 97010 should be reported once. However, when different modalities are used, such as 97010 that reports the application of hot or cold pack, 97014 that reports the application of electrical stimulation, and 97022 for whirlpool therapy, each is reported separately.

Time should be reported in 15-minute increments for treatment modalities requiring constant attendance. If more than 15 minutes are required (i.e., 30 minutes) report two units on the CMS-1500 claim form. For less than 15 minutes, append the reduced service modifier 52 and adjust the usual cost of the code based on the time actually spent.

SUPERVISED

97010   Application of a modality to one or more areas; hot or cold packs Ⓐ

> MED: 100-2,15,60.3; 100-2,15,230; 100-2,15,230.1; 100-2,15,230.2; 100-2,15,230.4; 100-3,20.10; 100-4,5,10; 100-4,5,20
> AMA: 2002,Aug,11; 2001,Nov,4; 1998,Dec,1; 1997,Nov,47; 1996,Apr,10; 1995,Summer,5

97012   traction, mechanical Ⓐ 80

> MED: 100-2,15,60.3; 100-2,15,230; 100-2,15,230.1; 100-2,15,230.2; 100-2,15,230.4; 100-3,20.10; 100-4,5,10; 100-4,5,20
> AMA: 2002,Aug,11; 2001,Nov,4; 1998,Dec,1; 1997,Nov,47; 1995,Summer,5

⊚ Modifier 63 Exempt Code   ⊙ Conscious Sedation   + CPT Add-on Code   ⊘ Modifier 51 Exempt Code   ● New Code   ▲ Revised Code

Ⓜ Maternity Edit   Ⓐ Age Edit   Ⓐ-ⓨ APC Status Indicators   ⓒ CCI Comprehensive Code   ↗ Drug Not Approved by FDA   50 Bilateral Procedure

© 2006 Ingenix (Blue Ink)   CPT only © 2006 American Medical Association. All Rights Reserved. (Black Ink)   Medicine — 369

Medicine

97014 — 97140

97014   **electrical stimulation (unattended)**   [E]

MED: 100-2,15,60.3; 100-2,15,230; 100-3,20.10; 100-3,160.12; 100-3,160.15; 100-3,270.1

AMA: 2002,Aug,11; 2002,Apr,18; 2001,Nov,4; 1998,May,10; 1997,Nov,47; 1995,Summer,5

To report acupuncture is performed with electrical stimulation, consult CPT code 97813, 97814.

97016   **vasopneumatic devices**   [A] [80] [↻]

MED: 100-2,15,60.3; 100-2,15,230; 100-2,15,230.1; 100-2,15,230.2; 100-2,15,230.4; 100-3,20.10; 100-4,5,10; 100-4,5,20

AMA: 2002,Aug,11; 2001,Nov,4; 1998,Dec,1; 1995,Summer,6

97018   **paraffin bath**   [A] [80] [↻]

MED: 100-2,15,60.3; 100-2,15,230; 100-2,15,230.1; 100-2,15,230.2; 100-2,15,230.4; 100-3,20.10; 100-4,5,10; 100-4,5,20

AMA: 2002,Aug,11; 2001,Nov,4; 1998,Dec,1; 1995,Summer,6

97022   **whirlpool**   [A] [80] [↻]

MED: 100-2,15,60.3; 100-2,15,230; 100-2,15,230.1; 100-3,20.10; 100-3,150.5; 100-3,160.2; 100-3,270.4; 100-4,5,20

AMA: 2002,Aug,11; 2001,Nov,4; 1998,May,10; 1998,Dec,1; 1995,Summer,6

97024   **diathermy (eg, microwave)**   [A] [80] [↻]

MED: 100-2,15,60.3; 100-2,15,230; 100-2,15,230.1; 100-3,20.10; 100-3,150.5; 100-3,240.4; 100-4,5,20

AMA: 2002,Aug,11; 2001,Nov,4; 1998,Dec,1; 1995,Summer,6

97026   **infrared**   [A] [80] [↻]

MED: 100-2,15,60.3; 100-2,15,230; 100-2,15,230.1; 100-2,15,230.2; 100-2,15,230.4; 100-3,20.10; 100-4,5,10; 100-4,5,20

AMA: 2002,Aug,11; 2001,Nov,4; 1998,Dec,1; 1995,Summer,6

97028   **ultraviolet**   [A] [80] [↻]

MED: 100-2,15,60.3; 100-2,15,230; 100-2,15,230.1; 100-2,15,230.2; 100-2,15,230.4; 100-3,20.10; 100-4,5,10; 100-4,5,20

AMA: 2002,Aug,11; 2001,Nov,4; 1998,Dec,1; 1996,Apr,11; 1995,Summer,6

CONSTANT ATTENDANCE

97032   **Application of a modality to one or more areas; electrical stimulation (manual), each 15 minutes**   [A] [80] [↻]

MED: 100-2,15,60.3; 100-2,15,230; 100-3,20.10; 100-3,160.12; 100-3,160.15; 100-3,270.1; 100-4,5,20

AMA: 2002,Apr,18; 2001,Nov,4; 1998,Dec,1; 1995,Summer,6

97033   **iontophoresis, each 15 minutes**   [A] [80] [↻]

MED: 100-2,15,60.3; 100-2,15,230; 100-2,15,230.1; 100-2,15,230.2; 100-2,15,230.4; 100-3,20.10; 100-4,5,10; 100-4,5,20

AMA: 2001,Nov,4; 1998,Dec,1; 1995,Summer,7

97034   **contrast baths, each 15 minutes**   [A] [80] [↻]

MED: 100-2,15,60.3; 100-2,15,230; 100-2,15,230.1; 100-2,15,230.2; 100-2,15,230.4; 100-3,20.10; 100-4,5,10; 100-4,5,20

AMA: 2001,Nov,4; 1998,Dec,1; 1995,Summer,7

97035   **ultrasound, each 15 minutes**   [A] [80] [↻]

MED: 100-2,15,60.3; 100-2,15,230; 100-2,15,230.1; 100-2,15,230.2; 100-3,20.10; 100-3,240.3

AMA: 2001,Nov,4; 1998,Dec,1; 1996,Sep,10; 1995,Summer,7

97036   **Hubbard tank, each 15 minutes**   [A] [80] [↻]

MED: 100-2,15,60.3; 100-2,15,230; 100-2,15,230.1; 100-2,15,230.2; 100-3,20.10; 100-3,160.2; 100-3,250.1; 100-3,250.4; 100-3,270.4

AMA: 2001,Nov,4; 1998,Dec,1; 1995,Summer,7

97039   **Unlisted modality (specify type and time if constant attendance)**   [A] [80] [↻]

MED: 100-2,15,60.3; 100-2,15,230; 100-2,15,230.1; 100-2,15,230.2; 100-2,15,230.4; 100-3,20.10; 100-4,5,10; 100-4,5,20

AMA: 2001,Nov,4; 2000,Jan,10; 1998,May,10; 1998,Dec,1; 1995,Summer,7

THERAPEUTIC PROCEDURES

Therapeutic procedures describe the application of clinical skills or services to improve function. These procedures require direct (one-on-one) patient contact.

Some therapeutic procedures have a time component and should be reported once for each 15 minutes of treatment. Others do not have a time component and should be reported only once per visit. For work hardening/conditioning (97545-97546), report 97545 for the initial two hours and 97546 for each additional hour. Procedure 97546 is considered an "add on" procedure. "Add on" procedures are never reduced in value and modifier 51 multiple procedures should not be appended.

Report codes 97001-97555 for each distinct procedure performed. Modifier 51 should not be used with codes 97001-97555.

If muscles are tested for range of joint motion, electromyography, consult CPT codes 95831 and subsequent codes. For biofeedback training by EMG, consult CPT code 90901. For transcutaneous nerve stimulation (TNS), consult CPT code 64550.

97110   **Therapeutic procedure, one or more areas, each 15 minutes; therapeutic exercises to develop strength and endurance, range of motion and flexibility**   [A] [80] [↻]

MED: 100-2,15,60.3; 100-2,15,230; 100-2,15,230.1; 100-2,15,230.2; 100-2,15,230.4; 100-3,20.10; 100-4,5,10; 100-4,5,20

AMA: 1999,Dec,11; 1998,Nov,37; 1995,Summer,7

97112   **neuromuscular reeducation of movement, balance, coordination, kinesthetic sense, posture, and/or proprioception for sitting and/or standing activities**   [A] [80] [↻]

MED: 100-2,15,60.3; 100-2,15,230; 100-2,15,230.1; 100-2,15,230.2; 100-2,15,230.4; 100-3,20.10; 100-4,5,10; 100-4,5,20

AMA: 1995,Summer,7

97113   **aquatic therapy with therapeutic exercises**   [A] [80] [↻]

MED: 100-2,15,60.3; 100-2,15,230; 100-2,15,230.1; 100-2,15,230.2; 100-2,15,230.4; 100-3,20.10; 100-4,5,10; 100-4,5,20

AMA: 1995,Summer,7

97116   **gait training (includes stair climbing)**   [A] [80] [↻]

MED: 100-2,15,60.3; 100-2,15,230; 100-2,15,230.1; 100-2,15,230.2; 100-2,15,230.4; 100-3,20.10; 100-4,5,10; 100-4,5,20

AMA: 1996,Sep,7; 1995,Summer,8

To report comprehensive gait and motion analysis procedures, consult CPT codes 96000-96003.

97124   **massage, including effleurage, petrissage and/or tapotement (stroking, compression, percussion)**   [A] [80] [↻]

MED: 100-2,15,60.3; 100-2,15,230; 100-2,15,230.1; 100-2,15,230.2; 100-2,15,230.4; 100-3,20.10; 100-4,5,10; 100-4,5,20

AMA: 1999,Dec,7; 1996,May,10; 1995,Summer,8

To report myofascial release, consult CPT code 97140.

97139   Unlisted therapeutic procedure (specify)   [A] [80] [↻]

MED: 100-2,15,60.3; 100-2,15,230; 100-2,15,230.1; 100-2,15,230.2; 100-2,15,230.4; 100-3,20.10; 100-4,5,10; 100-4,5,20

AMA: 1995,Summer,8

97140   Manual therapy techniques (eg, mobilization/ manipulation, manual lymphatic drainage, manual traction), one or more regions, each 15 minutes   [A] [80] [↻]

MED: 100-2,15,60.3; 100-2,15,230; 100-2,15,230.1; 100-2,15,230.2; 100-2,15,230.4; 100-3,20.10; 100-4,5,10; 100-4,5,20

AMA: 2001,Aug,10; 1999,Mar,1; 1999,Jul,11; 1999,Feb,10; 1998,Nov,37

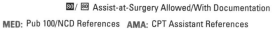

CPT only © 2006 American Medical Association. All Rights Reserved. *(Black Ink)*   © 2006 Ingenix *(Blue Ink)*

97150 Therapeutic procedure(s), group (2 or more individuals) Ⓐ 80 🗗

MED: 100-2,15,60.3; 100-2,15,230; 100-2,15,230.1; 100-2,15,230.2; 100-3,20.10; 100-4,5,20; 100-4,5,100.10

AMA: 1999,Oct,10; 1999,Nov,54-55; 1999,Dec,11; 1997,Feb,10; 1996,Dec,10; 1995,Summer,8

Note that 97150 is reported for each member of the group. Group therapy procedures involve constant attendance of the physician or therapist, but by definition do not require one-on-one patient contact by the physician or therapist. If manipulation under general anesthesia is performed, consult the appropriate anatomic section in Musculoskeletal System. If osteopathic manipulative treatment (OMT) is given, consult CPT codes 98925-98929.

97530 Therapeutic activities, direct (one-on-one) patient contact by the provider (use of dynamic activities to improve functional performance), each 15 minutes Ⓐ 80 🗗

MED: 100-2,15,60.3; 100-2,15,230; 100-2,15,230.1; 100-2,15,230.2; 100-2,15,230.4; 100-3,20.10; 100-4,5,10; 100-4,5,20

AMA: 2001,Dec,6; 1995,Summer,9

97532 Development of cognitive skills to improve attention, memory, problem solving, (includes compensatory training), direct (one-on-one) patient contact by the provider, each 15 minutes Ⓐ 80 🗗

MED: 100-2,15,230; 100-2,15,230.1; 100-2,15,230.2; 100-2,15,230.4; 100-3,20.10; 100-4,5,10

AMA: 2001,Dec,1

97533 Sensory integrative techniques to enhance sensory processing and promote adaptive responses to environmental demands, direct (one-on-one) patient contact by the provider, each 15 minutes Ⓐ 80 🗗

MED: 100-2,15,230; 100-2,15,230.1; 100-2,15,230.2; 100-2,15,230.4; 100-3,20.10; 100-4,5,10; 100-4,5,20

AMA: 2001,Dec,1

97535 Self-care/home management training (eg, activities of daily living (ADL) and compensatory training, meal preparation, safety procedures, and instructions in use of assistive technology devices/adaptive equipment) direct one-on-one contact by provider, each 15 minutes Ⓐ 80 🗗

MED: 100-2,15,60.3; 100-2,15,230; 100-2,15,230.1; 100-2,15,230.2; 100-2,15,230.4; 100-3,20.10; 100-4,5,10; 100-4,5,20

AMA: 2000,Apr,11; 1996,Sep,7

97537 Community/work reintegration training (eg, shopping, transportation, money management, avocational activities and/or work environment/modification analysis, work task analysis, use of assistive technology device/adaptive equipment), direct one-on-one contact by provider, each 15 minutes Ⓐ 80 🗗

MED: 100-2,15,60.3; 100-2,15,230; 100-2,15,230.1; 100-2,15,230.2; 100-2,15,230.4; 100-3,20.10; 100-4,5,10; 100-4,5,20

AMA: 1996,Sep,7

If wheelchair management/propulsion training is conducted, consult CPT code 97542.

97542 Wheelchair management (eg, assessment, fitting, training), each 15 minutes Ⓐ 80 🗗

MED: 100-2,15,60.3; 100-2,15,230; 100-2,15,230.1; 100-2,15,230.2; 100-2,15,230.4; 100-3,20.10; 100-4,5,10; 100-4,5,20

AMA: 1996,Sep,8

97545 Work hardening/conditioning; initial 2 hours Ⓐ 80 🗗

MED: 100-2,15,60.3; 100-2,15,230; 100-2,15,230.1; 100-2,15,230.2; 100-2,15,230.4; 100-3,20.10; 100-4,5,10

+ 97546 each additional hour (List separately in addition to code for primary procedure) Ⓐ 80

MED: 100-2,15,60.3; 100-2,15,230; 100-2,15,230.1; 100-2,15,230.2; 100-2,15,230.4; 100-3,20.10; 100-4,5,10

Note that 97546 is an add-on code and must be used in conjunction with 97545.

ACTIVE WOUND CARE MANAGEMENT

Codes 97597-97606 report procedures that promote healing. Since the codes involve selective and nonselective debridement techniques, do not report codes 11040-11044 from the surgery section in addition to these codes.

97597 Removal of devitalized tissue from wound(s), selective debridement, without anesthesia (eg, high pressure waterjet with/without suction, sharp selective debridement with scissors, scalpel and forceps), with or without topical application(s), wound assessment, and instruction(s) for ongoing care, may include use of a whirlpool, per session; total wound(s) surface area less than or equal to 20 square centimeters Ⓣ 80 🗗

MED: 100-4,5,20

Codes 97597-97602 cannot be reported with CPT codes 11040-11044.

97598 total wound(s) surface area greater than 20 square centimeters Ⓣ 80 🗗

MED: 100-4,5,20

97602 Removal of devitalized tissue from wound(s), non-selective debridement, without anesthesia (eg, wet-to-moist dressings, enzymatic, abrasion), including topical application(s), wound assessment, and instruction(s) for ongoing care, per session Ⓧ

MED: 100-2,15,230.4; 100-3,250.1; 100-3,250.4; 100-3,270.1; 100-3,270.2; 100-3,270.4; 100-4,5,10; 100-4,5,20

AMA: 2002,May,5

Do not report CPT codes 97601, 97602 when reporting CPT codes 11040-11044.

97605 Negative pressure wound therapy (eg, vacuum assisted drainage collection), including topical application(s), wound assessment, and instruction(s) for ongoing care, per session; total wound(s) surface area less than or equal to 50 square centimeters Ⓣ 80

MED: 100-4,5,20

97606 total wound(s) surface area greater than 50 square centimeters Ⓣ 80

MED: 100-4,5,20

TESTS AND MEASUREMENTS

These services require direct on-on-one patient contact.

To report muscle testing, range of motion, electromyography or nerve velocity determinations, consult CPT codes 95831-95904.

97750 Physical performance test or measurement (eg, musculoskeletal, functional capacity), with written report, each 15 minutes Ⓐ 80 🗗

MED: 100-2,15,230; 100-2,15,230.1; 100-2,15,230.2; 100-2,15,230.4; 100-3,20.10; 100-4,5,10; 100-4,5,20

AMA: 2002,May,18; 2001,Nov,4; 2000,Mar,11; 1998,Aug,11; 1997,Feb,10; 1995,Summer,5

97755 Assistive technology assessment (eg, to restore, augment or compensate for existing function, optimize functional tasks and/or maximize environmental accessibility), direct one-on-one contact by provider, with written report, each 15 minutes Ⓐ 80 🗗

When reporting augmentative and alternative communication devices, consult CPT codes 92605 or 92607.

ORTHOTIC MANAGEMENT AND PROSTHETIC MANAGEMENT

97760 Orthotic(s) management and training (including assessment and fitting when not otherwise reported), upper extremity(s), lower extremity(s) and/or trunk, each 15 minutes Ⓐ 80

> Code 97760 cannot be reported with 97116 for the same extremity.

97761 Prosthetic training, upper and/or lower extremity(s), each 15 minutes Ⓐ 80

97762 Checkout for orthotic/prosthetic use, established patient, each 15 minutes Ⓐ 80

OTHER PROCEDURES

For extracorporeal shock wave musculoskeletal therapy, consult CPT Category III code 0019T, 0101T, 0102T.

97799 Unlisted physical medicine/rehabilitation service or procedure Ⓐ 80

> MED: 100-2,15,230.4; 100-4,5,10; 100-4,5,20
> AMA: 1999,Oct,10; 1995,Summer,5

MEDICAL NUTRITION THERAPY

Three codes, 97802-97804, report medical nutrition therapy face-to-face with the patient, each 15 minutes (97802) or a face-to-face reassessment and intervention, each 15 minutes (97803). Report 97804 for therapy involving two or more patients, each 30-minute period.

Consult Evaluation and Management or Preventive Medicine service codes for medical nutrition therapy assessment and/or intervention performed by physician.

97802 Medical nutrition therapy; initial assessment and intervention, individual, face-to-face with the patient, each 15 minutes Ⓐ 80 🔲

> MED: 100-3,40.1; 100-3,40.5; 100-3,180.1; 100-4,4,300

97803 re-assessment and intervention, individual, face-to-face with the patient, each 15 minutes Ⓐ 80 🔲

> MED: 100-3,40.1; 100-3,40.5; 100-3,180.1; 100-4,4,300

97804 group (2 or more individual(s)), each 30 minutes Ⓐ 80

> MED: 100-3,40.1; 100-3,40.5; 100-3,180.1; 100-4,4,300

ACUPUNCTURE

Report acupuncture services based on 15-minute increments. This must be face-to-face contact with the patient and not the duration of the needle placement.

Report only one code per 15-minute increment. Report either 97810 or 97813 for the initial 15-minute increment. Use only one initial code per day.

Evaluation and management codes may be reported separately with modifier 25 if the patient's condition justifies the service.

97810 Acupuncture, 1 or more needles; without electrical stimulation, initial 15 minutes of personal one-on-one contact with the patient Ⓔ

+ **97811** without electrical stimulation, each additional 15 minutes of personal one-on-one contact with the patient, with re-insertion of needle(s) (List separately in addition to code for primary procedure) Ⓔ

Note that 97811 is an add-on code and must be used in conjunction with 97810, 97813.

If evaluation and management services are performed separately, they can be coded with modifier 25 appended. The patient's condition must warrant such services. The time of the E/M service is not included in the time of the acupuncture.

97813 with electrical stimulation, initial 15 minutes of personal one-on-one contact with the patient Ⓔ

Code 97813 cannot be used in conjunction with 97810.

+ **97814** with electrical stimulation, each additional 15 minutes of personal one-on-one contact with the patient, with re-insertion of needle(s) (List separately in addition to code for primary procedure) Ⓔ

Note that 97814 is an add-on code and must be used in conjunction with 97810, 97813.

If evaluation and management services are performed separately, they can be coded with modifier 25 appended. The patient's condition must warrant such services. The time of the E/M service is not included in the time of the acupuncture.

OSTEOPATHIC MANIPULATIVE TREATMENT

Codes 98925-98929 report inpatient or outpatient osteopathic manipulative treatment (OMT), which is a form of manual treatment applied by a physician to eliminate or alleviate somatic dysfunction and related disorders.

The number of body regions involved in the treatment differentiate the codes (i.e., head, cervical, thoracic, lumbar, sacral, pelvic, lower extremities, upper extremities, rib cage, and abdomen and viscera). OMT includes a component of E/M service to ascertain the effectiveness of the therapy and may be identified separately when:

- A physician diagnoses the condition requiring manipulative therapy and provides the therapy during the same visit.
- The condition requiring manipulative therapy fails to respond to the therapy or the condition significantly changes or intensifies and requires E/M services beyond the usual pre- and post-service work associated with the procedure.
- The physician treats a condition unrelated to the one requiring manipulative therapy during the same visit.

Consult the appropriate Evaluation and Management CPT code and append modifier 25 (or 09925) in addition to the code for OMT when separately identifiable Evaluation and Management services, above and beyond any pre or post service work associated with OMT, are provided.

Consult the glossary for terms and definitions and the front matter of this chapter for additional information.

98925 Osteopathic manipulative treatment (OMT); one to two body regions involved Ⓢ 80 🔲

> MED: 100-3,150.1; 100-4,4,20.5
> AMA: 2000,Dec,15; 2000,Aug,11; 1998,Nov,37-38; 1998,Jul,10; 1997,Jan,8, 10; 1996,May,10

98926 three to four body regions involved Ⓢ 80 🔲

> MED: 100-3,150.1; 100-4,4,20.5
> AMA: 2000,Dec,15; 2000,Aug,11; 1998,Nov,37-38; 1997,Jan,8; 1996,May,10

98927	five to six body regions involved	S 80 CCI

MED: 100-3,150.1; 100-4,4,20.5

AMA: 2000,Dec,15; 2000,Aug,11; 1998,Nov,37-38; 1997,Jan,8; 1996,May,10

98928	seven to eight body regions involved	S 80 CCI

MED: 100-3,150.1; 100-4,4,20.5

AMA: 2000,Dec,15; 2000,Aug,11; 1998,Nov,37-38; 1997,Jan,8; 1996,May,10

98929	nine to ten body regions involved	S 80 CCI

MED: 100-3,150.1; 100-4,4,20.5

AMA: 2000,Aug,11; 1998,Nov,37-38; 1997,Jan,8,10; 1996,May,10

CHIROPRACTIC MANIPULATIVE TREATMENT

Chiropractic manipulative treatment (CMT), reported with codes 98940-98943, is a form of manual treatment performed to influence joint and neurophysical function. CMT codes include a premanipulation patient assessment. Evaluation and management services should not be reported separately unless the patient's condition requires a separately identifiable E/M service beyond the usual pre- and post-service work normally associated with the procedure.

CMT codes are reported by region. The five spinal regions are cervical (includes atlanto-occipital joint); thoracic (includes costovertebral and costotransverse joints); lumbar, sacral; and pelvic (includes sacroiliac joint). The five extraspinal regions are defined as follows: head (including temporomandibular joint); lower extremities; upper extremities; rib cage, and abdomen.

Consult the appropriate Evaluation and Management CPT code and append modifier 25 (or 09925) in addition to the code for CMT when separately identifiable Evaluation and Management services, above and beyond any pre or post service work associated with CMT, are provided.

Consult the glossary for terms and definitions and the front matter of this chapter for additional information.

98940	Chiropractic manipulative treatment (CMT); spinal, one to two regions	S 80 CCI

MED: 100-1,5,70.6; 100-3,150.1; 100-4,4,20.5

AMA: 2000,Dec,15; 1999,Feb,10; 1998,Nov,38; 1997,Jan,7, 11

98941	spinal, three to four regions	S 80 CCI

MED: 100-1,5,70.6; 100-3,150.1; 100-4,4,20.5

AMA: 2000,Dec,15; 1999,Feb,10; 1998,Nov,38; 1997,Mar,10; 1997,Jan,7, 11

98942	spinal, five regions	S 80 CCI

MED: 100-1,5,70.6; 100-3,150.1; 100-4,4,20.5

AMA: 2000,Dec,15; 1999,Feb,10; 1998,Nov,38; 1997,Jan,7, 11

98943	extraspinal, one or more regions	E

MED: 100-1,5,70.6; 100-3,150.1

AMA: 2000,Dec,15; 1999,Feb,10; 1997,Mar,10; 1997,Jan,7, 11

EDUCATION AND TRAINING FOR PATIENT SELF-MANAGEMENT

The education and training for patient self-management codes are used to report education and training services prescribed by a physician and provided by a qualified nonphysician health care provider. These codes may be used only when using a standardized curriculum that may be modified as necessary for the clinical needs, cultural norms, and health literacy of the patient(s).

The purpose of the educational and training services is to teach the patient how to manage the illness or delay the comorbidity(s).

98960	Education and training for patient self-management by a qualified, nonphysician health care professional using a standardized curriculum, face-to-face with the patient (could include caregiver/family) each 30 minutes; individual patient	E
98961	2-4 patients	E
98962	5-8 patients	E

SPECIAL SERVICES, PROCEDURES AND REPORTS

Special services and reports (99000-99091) allow supplemental reporting for services adjunct to the basic services provided. These services can be reported by both physicians and other qualified health care professionals. To justify use of these codes, identify the medical necessity of special circumstances. Document the information clearly and completely in the patient's medical record.

Code 99024 reports a postoperative follow-up visit included in the global service period. Codes 99050-99058 identify emergency office calls and services provided after hours, on Sundays, or on holidays. Other codes in this category identify medical testimony, unusual travel requirements (e.g., escorting a patient on a trip of more than 10 miles), and educational services. Codes for transportation of specimens (99000-99001) should be reported only once per visit, regardless of the number of specimens. Code (99091) reports the collection and interpretation of physiologic data, with instructions to report the code only once in a 30-day period.

MISCELLANEOUS SERVICES

The following codes are for use for reporting services that are adjunct to the basic service performed.

99000	Handling and/or conveyance of specimen for transfer from the physician's office to a laboratory	E

AMA: 2002,May,19; 1999,Oct,11; 1999,Feb,10; 1994,Winter,26

99001	Handling and/or conveyance of specimen for transfer from the patient in other than a physician's office to a laboratory (distance may be indicated)	E

AMA: 2002,May,19; 1994,Winter,26

99002	Handling, conveyance, and/or any other service in connection with the implementation of an order involving devices (eg, designing, fitting, packaging, handling, delivery or mailing) when devices such as orthotics, protectives, prosthetics are fabricated by an outside laboratory or shop but which items have been designed, and are to be fitted and adjusted by the attending physician	B

AMA: 1994,Winter,26

To report a routine collection of venous blood, consult CPT code 36415.

99024	Postoperative follow-up visit, normally included in the surgical package, to indicate that an evaluation and management service was performed during a postoperative period for a reason(s) related to the original procedure	B

AMA: 2002,May,19; 1997,Sep,10; 1994,Winter,26

Note that 99024 is a component of a surgical package. Consult surgery guidelines.

99026	Hospital mandated on call service; in-hospital, each hour	E
99027	out-of-hospital, each hour	E

To report physician standby services requiring prolonged attendance, consult CPT code 99360, as appropriate.

99050	Services provided in the office at times other than regularly scheduled office hours, or days when the office is normally closed (eg, holidays, Saturday or Sunday), in addition to basic service	B

MED: 100-4,12,70; 100-4,13,20; 100-4,13,90

AMA: 2002,May,19; 1994,Winter,27

99051	Service(s) provided in the office during regularly scheduled evening, weekend, or holiday office hours, in addition to basic service	B
99053	Service(s) provided between 10:00 PM and 8:00 AM at 24-hour facility, in addition to basic service	B

⊛ Modifier 63 Exempt Code   ⊙ Conscious Sedation   + CPT Add-on Code   ⊘ Modifier 51 Exempt Code   ● New Code   ▲ Revised Code

M Maternity Edit   A Age Edit   A-Y APC Status Indicators   CCI CCI Comprehensive Code   ∕ Drug Not Approved by FDA   50 Bilateral Procedure

99056   Service(s) typically provided in the office, provided out of the office at request of patient, in addition to basic service   B

AMA: 2002,May,19; 1994,Winter,27

99058   Service(s) provided on an emergency basis in the office, which disrupts other scheduled office services, in addition to basic service   B

MED: 100-4,12,70; 100-4,13,20; 100-4,13,90
AMA: 2002,May,19; 1994,Winter,27

99060   Service(s) provided on an emergency basis, out of the office, which disrupts other scheduled office services, in addition to basic service   B

99070   Supplies and materials (except spectacles), provided by the physician over and above those usually included with the office visit or other services rendered (list drugs, trays, supplies, or materials provided)   B

AMA: 2002,May,19; 2002,Aug,11; 2001,Jul,1, 3; 2000,Jun,11; 1999,Jun,10; 1998,May,10; 1994,Winter,28
To report a supply of spectacles, consult CPT codes 92390-92395.

99071   Educational supplies, such as books, tapes, and pamphlets, provided by the physician for the patient's education at cost to physician   B

MED: 100-2,15,60.3; 100-3,20.10; 100-4,12,70; 100-4,13,20; 100-4,13,90
AMA: 2002,May,19; 1994,Winter,28

99075   Medical testimony   E

MED: 100-3,40.1
AMA: 2002,May,19; 1994,Winter,28

99078   Physician educational services rendered to patients in a group setting (eg, prenatal, obesity, or diabetic instructions)   N

MED: 100-2,15,60.3; 100-3,20.10; 100-3,40.1
AMA: 2002,May,19; 1998,Jan,12; 1994,Winter,28

99080   Special reports such as insurance forms, more than the information conveyed in the usual medical communications or standard reporting form   B

AMA: 2002,May,19; 1994,Winter,28
Code 99080 cannot be reported in conjunction with 99455, 99456 for the completion of Workers' Compensation forms.

99082   Unusual travel (eg, transportation and escort of patient)   B 80

MED: 100-4,12,80.3
AMA: 2003,Jan,24; 2002,May,19

99090   Analysis of clinical data stored in computers (eg, ECGs, blood pressures, hematologic data)   B

MED: 100-4,12,30.6.12; 100-4,12,70; 100-4,13,20; 100-4,13,90
AMA: 2002,May,19; 1994,Winter,28
To report physician/health care professional collection and interpretation of physiologic data stored/transmitted by patient/caregiver, see 99091.

Do not report 99090 if other more specific CPT codes exist, e.g., 93014, 93227, 93233, 93272 for cardiographic services; 95250 for continuous glucose monitoring, 97750 for musculoskeletal function testing.

99091   Collection and interpretation of physiologic data (eg, ECG, blood pressure, glucose monitoring) digitally stored and/or transmitted by the patient and/or caregiver to the physician or other qualified health care professional, requiring a minimum of 30 minutes of time   N

AMA: 2002,May,19

QUALIFYING CIRCUMSTANCES FOR ANESTHESIA

If an explanation is needed for these services, consult the Anesthesia guidelines.

+   99100   Anesthesia for patient of extreme age, younger than 1 year and older than 70 (List separately in addition to code for primary anesthesia procedure)   B

MED: 100-4,12,50; 100-4,12,140; 100-4,12,140.2; 100-4,12,140.3.2
To procedure performed on infant one year of age or younger, consult CPT codes 00326, 00561, 00834, 00836.

+   99116   Anesthesia complicated by utilization of total body hypothermia (List separately in addition to code for primary anesthesia procedure)   B

MED: 100-4,12,50; 100-4,12,140; 100-4,12,140.2; 100-4,12,140.3.2

+   99135   Anesthesia complicated by utilization of controlled hypotension (List separately in addition to code for primary anesthesia procedure)   B

MED: 100-4,12,50; 100-4,12,140; 100-4,12,140.2; 100-4,12,140.3.2

+   99140   Anesthesia complicated by emergency conditions (specify) (List separately in addition to code for primary anesthesia procedure)   B

MED: 100-4,12,50; 100-4,12,140; 100-4,12,140.2; 100-4,12,140.3.2
AMA: 2001,Mar,10; 2001,Mar,10
An emergency exists when a delay in treatment would lead to a significant increase in the threat to life or body part.

MODERATE (CONSCIOUS) SEDATION

Moderate (conscious) sedation includes the following services:

- Patient assessment
- IV access
- Administration of medication
- Maintenance of sedation
- Monitoring of oxygen saturation, heart rate, and blood pressure
- Recovery (not included in intraservice time)

Intraservice time begins when medication is given to start the sedation and requires continuous face-to-face attendance and ends when the physician is no longer in attendance.

Do not report 99143-99150 with 94760-94762.

When a physician other than a physician performing the procedure administers the moderate sedation in the facility setting, the second physician reports his/her services with codes 99148-99150. In the non-facility setting, codes 99148-99150 would not be used.

⊘   99143   Moderate sedation services (other than those services described by codes 00100-01999) provided by the same physician performing the diagnostic or therapeutic service that the sedation supports, requiring the presence of an independent trained observer to assist in the monitoring of the patient's level of consciousness and physiological status; younger than 5 years of age, first 30 minutes intra-service time   N 80

⊘   99144   age 5 years or older, first 30 minutes intra-service time   N 80

+   99145   each additional 15 minutes intra-service time (List separately in addition to code for primary service)   N 80

Note that 99145 is an add-on code and must be used in conjunction with 99143, 99144.

| | 99148 | Moderate sedation services (other than those services described by codes 00100-01999), provided by a physician other than the health care professional performing the diagnostic or therapeutic service that the sedation supports; younger than 5 years of age, first 30 minutes intra-service time |
|⊘| | N 80 |

| | 99149 | age 5 years or older, first 30 minutes intra-service time |
|⊘| | N 80 |

| | 99150 | each additional 15 minutes intra-service time (List separately in addition to code for primary service) |
| | | N 80 |

Note that 99150 is an add-on code and must be used in conjunction with 99148, 99149.

OTHER SERVICES AND PROCEDURES

Codes 99170-99199 report services such as anogenital examinations in cases of suspected child sexual abuse, medical intervention, and observation of patient following suspected cases of poisoning, and therapeutic phlebotomy.

| 99170 | Anogenital examination with colposcopic magnification in childhood for suspected trauma   A T ⬛ |

MED: 100-4,4,20.5
AMA: 1999,Nov,55

| 99172 | Visual function screening, automated or semi-automated bilateral quantitative determination of visual acuity, ocular alignment, color vision by pseudoisochromatic plates, and field of vision (may include all or some screening of the determination(s) for contrast sensitivity, vision under glare)   E |

MED: 100-2,16,90
AMA: 2001,Feb,7

This service MUST consist of graduated visual acuity stimuli that allow a quantitative determination of visual acuity (e.g., Snellen chart).

This service may not be used in addition to a general opthalmological service or an E/M service.

CPT code 99172 must not be used in conjunction with CPT code 99173.

| 99173 | Screening test of visual acuity, quantitative, bilateral   E |

MED: 100-2,16,90
AMA: 1999,Nov,55

CPT code 99173 must not be used in conjunction with CPT code 99172.

| 99175 | Ipecac or similar administration for individual emesis and continued observation until stomach adequately emptied of poison   N 80 |

If diagnostic intubation is needed, consult CPT codes 82926-82928 and 89130-89141. If gastric lavage is used for diagnostic purposes, consult CPT code 91055.

| 99183 | Physician attendance and supervision of hyperbaric oxygen therapy, per session   B 80 |

MED: 100-3,20.29; 100-4,32,30
AMA: 2003,Jan,23

Note that Evaluation and Management services and/or procedures (e.g., wound debridement) provided in a hyperbaric oxygen treatment facility in conjunction with a hyperbaric oxygen therapy session should be reported separately.

| 99185 | Hypothermia; regional   N 80 |

MED: 100-3,110.6; 100-4,4,20.5; 100-4,12,70; 100-4,13,20; 100-4,13,90

| | 99186 | total body   N 80 ⬛ |

MED: 100-4,4,20.5

| | 99190 | Assembly and operation of pump with oxygenator or heat exchanger (with or without ECG and/or pressure monitoring); each hour   C ⬛ |

| ▲ | 99191 | 45 minutes   C ⬛ |

| ▲ | 99192 | 30 minutes   C ⬛ |

| | 99195 | Phlebotomy, therapeutic (separate procedure)   X 80 ⬛ |

MED: 100-4,4,20.5
AMA: 1996,Jun,10; 1996,Apr,3

| | 99199 | Unlisted special service, procedure or report   B 80 |

AMA: 1999,Nov,55

HOME HEALTH PROCEDURES/SERVICES

Codes 99500-99600 report various home health procedures and services that are to be used by nonphysician health care providers. The codes report services delivered in the patient's home, which includes a private home, an assisted living apartment, a group home, a custodial care facility, or a school.

| 99500 | Home visit for prenatal monitoring and assessment to include fetal heart rate, non-stress test, uterine monitoring, and gestational diabetes monitoring   M ♀ E |

| 99501 | Home visit for postnatal assessment and follow-up care   ♀ E |

| 99502 | Home visit for newborn care and assessment   A E |

| 99503 | Home visit for respiratory therapy care (eg, bronchodilator, oxygen therapy, respiratory assessment, apnea evaluation)   E |

| 99504 | Home visit for mechanical ventilation care   E |

| 99505 | Home visit for stoma care and maintenance including colostomy and cystostomy   E |

| 99506 | Home visit for intramuscular injections   E |

| 99507 | Home visit for care and maintenance of catheter(s) (eg, urinary, drainage, and enteral)   E |

| 99509 | Home visit for assistance with activities of daily living and personal care   E |

To report self-care/home management training, see 97535.

To report home medical nutrition assessment and intervention services, see 97802-97804.

To report home speech therapy services, see 92507-92508.

| 99510 | Home visit for individual, family, or marriage counseling   E |

| 99511 | Home visit for fecal impaction management and enema administration   E |

| 99512 | Home visit for hemodialysis   E |

To report home infusion of peritoneal dialysis, consult CPT codes 99601 and 99602.

| 99600 | Unlisted home visit service or procedure   E |

HOME INFUSION PROCEDURES/SERVICES

The home infusion procedures (99601-99602) should be used to report the home administration of a variety of drugs and medications. These codes do not include the patient's self-administration of the medication.

| ⊛ Modifier 63 Exempt Code | ⊙ Conscious Sedation | + CPT Add-on Code | ⊘ Modifier 51 Exempt Code | ● New Code | ▲ Revised Code |

| M Maternity Edit | A Age Edit | A-Y APC Status Indicators | ⬛ CCI Comprehensive Code | ⟋ Drug Not Approved by FDA | 50 Bilateral Procedure |

These services are used to report home infusion, per visit. Any solutions, supplies, drugs or equipment provided the patient are not included in these codes and should be reported separately. To report more than two hours of home infusion, report 99601 for the first two hours and 99602 for each additional hour.

99601   **Home infusion/specialty drug administration, per visit (up to 2 hours);**   E

+   **99602**   **each additional hour (List separately in addition to primary procedure)**   E

Note that 99602 is an add-on code that must be used in conjunction with code 99601.

CATEGORY II CODES

The following section contains codes that describe services that may be considered parts of an evaluation and management service or clinical service and, as such, do not have a relative value associated with them. They may include results of a laboratory or radiology tests and other procedures, or safety practices or services reflecting compliance with state or federal law.

The codes include components that are usually part of another service and, do not have a relative value attached. The codes may also describe results from laboratory tests and other procedures, services intended to address patient safety practices, or services that demonstrate compliance with state or federal laws.

Codes are comprised of alpha numeric characters (i.e., 4 digits followed by the letter F).

Composite Measures 0001F

Patient Management 0500F

Patient History 1000F

Physical Examination 2000F

Diagnostic/Screening Processes or Results 3000F

Therapeutic, Preventive or Other Interventions 4000F

Follow-up or Other Outcomes 5000F

Patient Safety 6000F

Cross references to the measures associated with each Category II code and their source are included in the Apendix of this book. Acronyms for the related diseases or clinical conditions are found at the end of each code descriptor to identify the topic or clinical condition category in which that code is included. A complete listing of these acronyms can be found in the Appendix of this book.

Category II codes are reviewed by the Performance Measurements Advisory Group (PMAG), which is an advisory body to the CPT Editorial Panel and the CPT/HCPAC Advisory Committee. The PMAG is comprised of performance measurement experts representing the Agency for Healthcare Research and Quality (AHRQ), the American Medical Association (AMA), the Centers for Medicare and Medicaid Services (CMS), the Joint Commission on Accreditation of Healthcare Organizations (JCAHO), the National Committee for Quality Assurance (NCQA), and the Physician Consortium for Performance Improvement. The PMAG may also seek advice and input from other national health care organizations, as needed, with regard to the development of Category II codes. Other sources may include national medical specialty societies, other national health care professional associations, accrediting bodies, and federal regulatory agencies.

The Category II codes are published during the year. Go to "www.ama-assn.org/go/cpt" for the most current listing.

Modifiers

The following performance measurement modifiers may be used for Category II codes to indicate that a service specified in the associate measure(s) was considered but not provided due to either medical, patient, or system situation(s)documented in the medical record. These modifiers function to exclude denominators from the performance measure. Category II modifiers can be reported only with Category II codes and cannot be reported with Category I or Category III codes. Unless otherwise noted in the special guidelines, reporting instructions, code specific notes or code descriptions.

1P Performance Measure Exclusion Modifier due to Medical Reasons:

Includes:

- Not indicated (absence of the organ/limb, already received/performed, other)
- Contraindicated (patient allergic history, potential adverse drug interaction, other)

2P Performance Measure Exclusion Modifier due to Patient Reasons:
Includes:

- Patient declined
- Economic, social, or religious reasons
- Other patient reasons

3P Performance Measure Exclusion Modifier due to System Reasons:

Includes:

- Resources to perform the services not available
- Insurance coverage/payor-related limitations
- Other reasons attributable to health care delivery system

COMPOSITE CODES

Composite measures codes combine several measures grouped within a single code descriptor to make possible reporting for clinical conditions when all of the components have been met. Report separately services that are provided in addition to those that are included in the composite code.

▲ **0001F** **Heart failure assessed (includes assessment of all the following components): Blood pressure measured (2000F) Level of activity assessed (1003F) Clinical symptoms of volume overload (excess) assessed (1004F) Weight, recorded (2001F) Clinical signs of volume overload (excess) assessed (2002F)** Ⓜ

▲ **0005F** **Osteoarthritis assessed Includes assessment of all the following components: Osteoarthritis symptoms and functional status assessed (1006F) Use of anti-inflammatory or over-the-counter (OTC) analgesic medications assessed (1007F) Initial examination of the involved joint(s) (includes visual inspection, palpation, range of motion) (2004F)** Ⓜ

● **0012F** **Community-acquired bacterial pneumonia assessment (includes all of the following components) Co-morbid conditions assessed (1026F) Vital signs recorded (2010F) Mental status assessed (2014F) Hydration status assessed (2018F)** Ⓜ

PATIENT MANAGEMENT

The codes in this section describe encounters with healthcare professionals for the purpose of specific clinical indications, such as obstetrical care. The codes are used to track utilization of these services.

▲ **0500F** **Initial prenatal care visit (report at first prenatal encounter with health care professional providing obstetrical care. Report also date of visit and, in a separate field, the date of the last menstrual period-LMP) (Prenatal)[2]** Ⓜ ♀ Ⓜ

▲ **0501F** **Prenatal flow sheet documented in medical record by first prenatal visit (documentation includes at minimum blood pressure, weight, urine protein, uterine size, fetal heart tones, and estimated date of delivery). Report also: date of visit and, in a separate field, the date of the last menstrual period - LMP (Note: If reporting 0501F Prenatal flow sheet, it is not necessary to report 0500F Initial prenatal care visit) (Prenatal)[1]** Ⓜ ♀ Ⓜ

▲ **0502F** **Subsequent prenatal care visit (Prenatal)[2]** Ⓜ ♀ Ⓜ

Excludes: patients who are seen for a condition unrelated to pregnancy or prenatal care (eg, an upper respiratory infection; patients seen for consultation only, not for continuing care)

▲ **0503F** **Postpartum care visit (Prenatal)[2]** Ⓜ ♀ Ⓜ

FOOTNOTES:

[1] Physician Consortium for Performance Improvement, www. physicianconsortium.org

[2] National Committee on Quality Assurance (NCOA), Health Employer Data Information Set (HEDIS®), www.ncqa.org

---

Category II Codes

1000F — 3021F

PATIENT HISTORY

This section of codes is used to describe measures for specific aspects of a patient history or for a review of systems.

▲ 1000F   Tobacco use assessed (CAD, CAP, COPD, PV)[1] (DM)[4]   Ⓜ

    1001F   Tobacco use, non-smoking, assessed

▲ 1002F   Anginal symptoms and level of activity assessed (CAD)[1]   Ⓜ

▲ 1003F   Level of activity assessed (HF)[1]   Ⓜ

▲ 1004F   Clinical symptoms of volume overload (excess) assessed (HF)[1]   Ⓜ

▲ 1005F   Asthma symptoms evaluated (includes physician documentation of numeric frequency of symptoms or patient completion of an asthma assessment tool/survey/questionnaire) (Asthma)[1]   Ⓜ

▲ 1006F   Osteoarthritis symptoms and functional status assessed (may include the use of a standardized scale or the completion of an assessment questionnaire, such as the SF-36, AAOS Hip & Knee Questionnaire) (OA)[1]   Ⓜ

    Instructions: Report when osteoarthritis is addressed during the patient encounter

▲ 1007F   Use of anti-inflammatory or analgesic over-the-counter (OTC) medications for symptom relief assessed (OA)[1]   Ⓜ

▲ 1008F   Gastrointestinal and renal risk factors assessed for patients on prescribed or OTC non-steroidal anti-inflammatory drug (NSAID) (OA)[1]   Ⓜ

● 1015F   Chronic obstructive pulmonary disease (COPD) symptoms assessed (Includes assessment of at least one of the following: dyspnea, cough/sputum, wheezing), or respiratory symptom assessment tool completed (COPD)[1]   Ⓜ

● 1018F   Dyspnea assessed, not present (COPD)[1]   Ⓜ

● 1019F   Dyspnea assessed, present (COPD)[1]   Ⓜ

● 1022F   Pneumococcus immunization status assessed (CAP, COPD)[1]   Ⓜ

● 1026F   Co-morbid conditions assessed (eg, includes assessment for presence or absence of: malignancy, liver disease, congestive heart failure, cerebrovascular disease, renal disease, chronic obstructive pulmonary disease, asthma, diabetes, other co-morbid conditions) (CAP)[1]   Ⓜ

● 1030F   Influenza immunization status assessed (CAP)[1]   Ⓜ

● 1034F   Current tobacco smoker (CAD, CAP, COPD, PV)[1] (DM)[4]   Ⓜ

● 1035F   Current smokeless tobacco user (eg, chew, snuff) (PV)[1]   Ⓜ

● 1036F   Current tobacco non-user (CAD, CAP, COPD, PV)[1] (DM)[4]   Ⓜ

● 1038F   Persistent asthma (mild, moderate or severe) (Asthma)[1]   Ⓜ

● 1039F   Intermittent asthma (Asthma)[1]   Ⓜ

PHYSICAL EXAMINATION

This section of codes is used to describe measures for specific aspects of a physical examination.

▲ 2000F   Blood pressure, measured (HF, CAD, HTN)[1]   Ⓜ

▲ 2001F   Weight recorded (HF, PAG)[1]   Ⓜ

▲ 2002F   Clinical signs of volume overload (excess) assessed (HF)[1]   Ⓜ

  ~~2003F   Auscultation of the heart performed~~

▲ 2004F   Initial examination of the involved joint(s) (includes visual inspection, palpation, range of motion) (OA)[1]   Ⓜ

    Instructions: Report only for initial osteoarthritis visit or for visits for new joint involvement

● 2010F   Vital signs recorded (includes at minimum: temperature, pulse, respiration, and blood pressure)(CAP)[1]   Ⓜ

● 2014F   Mental status assessed (normal/mildly impaired/severely impaired) (CAP)[1]   Ⓜ

● 2018F   Hydration status assessed (normal/mildly dehydrated/severely dehydrated) (CAP)[1]   Ⓜ

● 2022F   Dilated retinal eye exam with interpretation by an ophthalmologist or optometrist documented and reviewed (DM)[4]   Ⓜ

● 2024F   Seven standard field stereoscopic photos with interpretation by an ophthalmologist or optometrist documented and reviewed (DM)[4]   Ⓜ

● 2026F   Eye imaging validated to match diagnosis from seven standard field stereoscopic photos results documented and reviewed (DM)[4]   Ⓜ

● 2028F   Foot examination performed (includes examination through visual inspection, sensory exam with monofilament, and pulse exam – report when any of the three components are completed) (DM)[4]   Ⓜ

DIAGNOSTIC/SCREENING PROCESSES OR RESULTS

Diagnostic/screening processes or results codes describe the results of tests that are ordered such as clinical laboratory tests as well as radiological and other procedural examinations.

● 3006F   Chest X-ray results documented and reviewed (CAP)[1]   Ⓜ

● 3011F   Lipid panel results documented and reviewed (must include total cholesterol, HDL-C, triglycerides and calculated LDL-C) (CAD)[1]   Ⓜ

● 3014F   Screening mammography results documented and reviewed (PV)[1]   Ⓜ

● 3017F   Colorectal cancer screening results documented and reviewed (PV)[1]   Ⓜ

● 3020F   Left ventricular function (LVF) assessment (eg, echocardiography, nuclear test, or ventriculography) documented in the medical record (includes: quantitative or qualitative assessment results) (HF)[1]   Ⓜ

● 3021F   Left ventricular ejection fraction (LVEF) < 40% or documentation of moderately or severely depressed left ventricular systolic function (CAD, HF)[1]   Ⓜ

FOOTNOTES:

[1] Physician Consortium for Performance Improvement, www. physicianconsortium.org

[4] National Diabetes Quality Improvement Alliance (NDQIA), www.nationaldiabetesalliance.org

---

26 Professional Component Only   80/80 Assist-at-Surgery Allowed/With Documentation | Unlisted | Not Covered

TC Technical Component Only   **MED:** Pub 100/NCD References   **AMA:** CPT Assistant References   1-9 ASC Group   ♂ Male Only   ♀ Female Only

● **3022F** Left ventricular ejection fraction (LVEF) ≥ 40% or documentation as normal or mildly depressed left ventricular systolic function (CAD, HF)[1]) Ⓜ

● **3023F** Spirometry results documented and reviewed (COPD)[1] Ⓜ

● **3025F** Spirometry test results demonstrate $FEV_1/FVC < 70\%$ with COPD symptoms (eg, dyspnea, cough/sputum, wheezing) (CAP, COPD)[1]) Ⓜ

● **3027F** Spirometry test results demonstrate $FEV_1/FVC \geq 70\%$ or patient does not have COPD symptoms (COPD)[1] Ⓜ

● **3028F** Oxygen saturation results documented and reviewed (Includes assessment through pulse oximetry or arterial blood gas measurement) (CAP, COPD)[1] Ⓜ

● **3035F** Oxygen saturation ≤ 88% or a $PaO_2 \leq 55$ mm Hg (COPD)[1] Ⓜ

● **3037F** Oxygen saturation > 88% or $PaO_2 > 55$ mmHg (COPD)[1] Ⓜ

● **3040F** Functional expiratory volume (FEV_1) < 40% of predicted value (COPD)[1] Ⓜ

● **3042F** Functional expiratory volume (FEV_1) ≥ 40% of predicted value (COPD)[1] Ⓜ

● **3046F** Most recent hemoglobin A1c level > 9.0% (DM)[4] Ⓜ

● **3047F** Most recent hemoglobin A1c level ≤ 9.0% (DM)[4] Ⓜ

● **3048F** Most recent LDL-C < 100 mg/dL (DM)[4] Ⓜ

● **3049F** Most recent LDL-C 100-129 mg/dL (DM)[4] Ⓜ

● **3050F** Most recent LDL-C ≥ 130 mg/dL (DM)[4] Ⓜ

● **3060F** Positive microalbuminuria test result documented and reviewed (DM)[4] Ⓜ

● **3061F** Negative microalbuminuria test result documented and reviewed (DM)[4] Ⓜ

● **3062F** Positive macroalbuminuria test result documented and reviewed (DM)[4] Ⓜ

● **3066F** Documentation of treatment for nephropathy (eg, patient receiving dialysis, patient being treated for ESRD, CRF, ARF, or renal insufficiency, any visit to a nephrologist) (DM)[4] Ⓜ

● **3072F** Low risk for retinopathy (no evidence of retinopathy in the prior year) (DM)[4] Ⓜ

● **3076F** Most recent systolic blood pressure < 140 mm Hg (DM[4] HTN[1]) Ⓜ

● **3077F** Most recent systolic blood pressure ≥ 140 mm Hg (HTN)[1] (DM)[4] Ⓜ

● **3078F** Most recent diastolic blood pressure < 80 mm Hg (DM[4], HTN[1]) Ⓜ

● **3079F** Most recent diastolic blood pressure 80-89 mm Hg (HTN)[1] (DM)[4] Ⓜ

● **3080F** Most recent diastolic blood pressure ≥ 90 mm Hg (HTN)[1] (DM)[4] Ⓜ

THERAPEUTIC, PREVENTIVE OR OTHER INTERVENTIONS

This section of codes is used to describe therapeutic, preventive or other interventions such as patient education and counseling for tobacco use and medication therapy.

FOOTNOTES:

[1] Physician Consortium for Performance Improvement, www.physicianconsortium.org

[3] Joint Commission on Accreditation of Healthcare Organizations (JCAHO), ORYX Initiative Performance Measures, www.JointCommission.org

[4] National Diabetes Quality Improvement Alliance (NDQIA), www.nationaldiabetesalliance.org

▲ **4000F** Tobacco use cessation intervention, counseling (COPD, CAP, CAD)[1] Ⓜ

▲ **4001F** Tobacco use cessation intervention, pharmacologic therapy (COPD, CAD, CAP, PV)[1] (DM)[4] Ⓜ

▲ **4002F** Statin therapy, prescribed (CAD)[1] Ⓜ

▲ **4003F** Patient education, written/oral, appropriate for patients with heart failure, performed (HF)[1] Ⓜ

▲ **4006F** Beta-blocker therapy, prescribed (CAD, HF)[1] Ⓜ

▲ **4009F** Angiotensin converting enzyme (ACE) inhibitor or angiotensin receptor blocker (ARB) therapy, prescribed (HF, CAD)[1] Ⓜ

▲ **4011F** Oral antiplatelet therapy prescribed (eg, aspirin, clopidogrel/Plavix, or combination of aspirin and dipyridamole/Aggrenox) (CAD)[1] Ⓜ

▲ **4012F** Warfarin therapy prescribed (CHF)[1] Ⓜ

4014F Written discharge instructions provided to heart failure patients discharged home. (Instructions include all of the following components: activity level, diet, discharge medications, follow-up appointment, weight monitoring, what to do if symptoms worsen)[3] Ⓜ

Excludes patients 18 years of age

▲ **4015F** Persistent asthma, preferred long term control medication or an acceptable alternative treatment, prescribed (Asthma)[1] Ⓜ

Note: There are no medical exclusion criteria

Modifier 1P cannot be used with 4015F.

Modifier 2P should be used to report patient reasons for not prescribing.

▲ **4016F** Anti-inflammatory/analgesic agent prescribed (OA)[1] Ⓜ

Use for prescribed or continued medication[s], including over-the-counter medication[s]

▲ **4017F** Gastrointestinal prophylaxis for NSAID use prescribed (OA)[1] Ⓜ

▲ **4018F** Therapeutic exercise for the involved joint(s) instructed or physical or occupational therapy prescribed (OA)[1] Ⓜ

● **4025F** Inhaled bronchodilator prescribed (COPD)[1] Ⓜ

● **4030F** Long-term oxygen therapy prescribed (more than 15 hours per day) (COPD)[1] Ⓜ

● **4033F** Pulmonary rehabilitation exercise training recommended (COPD)[1] Ⓜ

● **4035F** Influenza immunization recommended (COPD)[1] Ⓜ

● **4037F** Influenza immunization ordered or administered (COPD, PV)[1] Ⓜ

● **4040F** Pneumococcal immunization ordered or administered (COPD)[1] Ⓜ

● **4045F** Appropriate empiric antibiotic prescribed (See measure developer's Web site for definition of appropriate antibiotic) (CAP)[1] Ⓜ

● **4050F** Hypertension plan of care documented as appropriate (HTN)[1] Ⓜ

---

⑥③ Modifier 63 Exempt Code   ⊙ Conscious Sedation   + CPT Add-on Code   ⊘ Modifier 51 Exempt Code   ● New Code   ▲ Revised Code

Ⓜ Maternity Edit   Ⓐ Age Edit   Ⓐ-Ⓨ APC Status Indicators   Ⓒ CCI Comprehensive Code   ⑤⓪ Bilateral Procedure

FOLLOW-UP OR OTHER OUTCOMES

Follow-up or other outcomes Category II codes designate the review and communication of test results to patients, patient satisfaction or experience with care, patient functional status, and patient morbidity and mortality.

No codes at this time.

PATIENT SAFETY

Category II codes that describe patient safety practices.

● **6005F**   **Rationale (eg, severity of illness and safety) for level of care (eg, home, hospital) documented (CAP)**[1]   Ⓜ

FOOTNOTES:

[1] Physician Consortium for Performance Improvement, www. physicianconsortium.org

CATEGORY III CODES

The following is taken from information provided by the American Medical Association (AMA).

Category III codes are alphanumeric codes intended to allow data collection for the services and procedures below. This is an activity that is critically important in the evaluation of health care delivery and the formation of public and private policy. The use of the codes in this section will allow physicians and other qualified health care professionals, payers, health services researchers, and health policy experts to identify emerging technology, services, and procedures for clinical efficacy, utilization and outcomes. Category III codes are comprised of alpha-numeric characters (i.e. 4 digits followed by the letter T).

Category I codes are the long-used, five-digit codes that make up the rest of the book. **If a Category III code is available for a given service or procedure, use the Category III code instead of a Category I unlisted code.**

The inclusion of a service or procedure in this section neither implies nor endorses clinical efficacy, safety or the applicability to clinical practice. The codes in this section do not conform to the usual requirements for CPT Category I codes. For Category I codes, the AMA requires that the service or procedure be performed by many health care professionals in clinical practice in multiple locations and that necessary FDA approval has already been received. The nature of emerging technology, services, and procedures is that these requirements may not be met. New temporary codes for emerging technology, services, and procedures have been placed in a separate section of the CPT book and the codes are differentiated from Category I CPT codes by the use of alphanumeric characters.

Since these are temporary codes, they may or may not receive placement in the CPT book; and, those not adopted as permanent codes will be archived by the AMA after five years unless it is believed the temporary code is still needed. If made a permanent code in the CPT book, the existing numbers do not imply where they will be placed.

Category III codes are released twice a year. The codes can be reviewed at the AMA website 222.ama-assn.org/go/cpt.

CATEGORY III CODES

0003T ~~Cervicography~~

0008T ~~Upper gastrointestinal endoscopy including esophagus, stomach, and either the duodenum and/or jejunum as appropriate, with suturing of the esophagogastric junction~~

0016T Destruction of localized lesion of choroid (eg, choroidal neovascularization), transpupillary thermotherapy T 80 50 ◫

0017T Destruction of macular drusen, photocoagulation T 80 50 ◫
MED: 100-3,80.3

0018T Delivery of high power, focal magnetic pulses for direct stimulation to cortical neurons

0019T Extracorporeal shock wave involving musculoskeletal system, not otherwise specified, low energy A 80
To report the application of high energy extracorporeal shock wave involving the musculoskeletal system not otherwise specified, consult Category III code 0101T.
To report the application of high energy extracorporeal shock wave that involves the lateral humeral epicondyle, consult Category III code 0102T.

0021T ~~Insertion of transcervical or transvaginal fetal oximetry sensor~~

0024T Non-surgical septal reduction therapy (eg, alcohol ablation), for hypertrophic obstructive cardiomyopathy, with coronary arteriograms, with or without temporary pacemaker C 80 ◫

0026T Lipoprotein, direct measurement, intermediate density lipoproteins (IDL) (remnant lipoproteins) A 80

0027T Endoscopic lysis of epidural adhesions with direct visualization using mechanical means (eg, spinal endoscopic catheter system) or solution injection (eg, normal saline) including radiologic localization and epidurography T 80
To report diagnostic epidurography, consult CPT code 64999.

0028T Dual energy x-ray absorptiometry (DEXA) body composition study, one or more sites N 80

0029T Treatment(s) for incontinence, pulsed magnetic neuromodulation, per day A 80

0030T Antiprothrombin (phospholipid cofactor) antibody, each Ig class A 80

0031T Speculoscopy; ♀ N 80

0032T with directed sampling ♀ N 80 ◫

0041T Urinalysis infectious agent detection, semi-quantitative analysis of volatile compounds A 80

0042T Cerebral perfusion analysis using computed tomography with contrast administration, including post-processing of parametric maps with determination of cerebral blood flow, cerebral blood volume, and mean transit time N 80 ◫

0043T Carbon monoxide, expired gas analysis (eg, ETCOc/hemolysis breath test) A 80

0044T ~~Whole body integumentary photography, at request of a physician, for monitoring of high-risk patients; with dysplastic nevus syndrome or familial melanoma~~
Use 96904.

0045T ~~with history of dysplastic nevi or personal history of melanoma~~
Use 96904.

0046T Catheter lavage of a mammary duct(s) for collection of cytology specimen(s), in high risk individuals (GAIL risk scoring or prior personal history of breast cancer), each breast; single duct ♀ T 80 ◫

0047T each additional duct ♀ T 80 ◫

0048T Implantation of a ventricular assist device, extracorporeal, percutaneous transseptal access, single or dual cannulation C 80 ◫
MED: 100-4,3,90.2.1

+ 0049T Prolonged extracorporeal percutaneous transseptal ventricular assist device, greater than 24 hours, each subsequent 24 hour period (List separately in addition to code for primary procedure) C 80
Note that 0049T is an add-on code that must be used in conjunction with code 0048T.

0050T Removal of a ventricular assist device, extracorporeal, percutaneous transseptal access, single or dual cannulation C 80 ◫

0051T Implantation of a total replacement heart system (artificial heart) with recipient cardiectomy C 80 ◫
MED: 100-4,3,90.2.1
To report implantation of heart assist or ventricular assist device, consult CPT codes 33975, 33976.

⊛ Modifier 63 Exempt Code   ⊙ Conscious Sedation   + CPT Add-on Code   ⊘ Modifier 51 Exempt Code   ● New Code   ▲ Revised Code
Ⓜ Maternity Edit   Ⓐ Age Edit   A-Y APC Status Indicators   ◫ CCI Comprehensive Code   50 Bilateral Procedure

CPT only © 2006 American Medical Association. All Rights Reserved. (Black Ink)

0052T Replacement or repair of thoracic unit of a total replacement heart system (artificial heart) [C] [80] [symbol]

MED: 100-4,3,90.2.1

To report replacement or repair of other implantable components in a total replacement heart system (artificial heart), consult CPT Category III code 0053T.

0053T Replacement or repair of implantable component or components of total replacement heart system (artificial heart), excluding thoracic unit [C] [80] [symbol]

MED: 100-4,3,90.2.1

To report replacement or repair of a thoracic unit of a total replacement heart system (artificial heart), consult CPT Category III code 0052T.

+ **0054T** Computer-assisted musculoskeletal surgical navigational orthopedic procedure, with image-guidance based on fluoroscopic images (List separately in addition to code for primary procedure) [S] [80] [symbol]

Note that 0054T is an add-on code that must be used in conjunction with the appropriate code for the primary procedure. This code cannot be reported alone.

+ **0055T** Computer-assisted musculoskeletal surgical navigational orthopedic procedure, with image-guidance based on CT/MRI images (List separately in addition to code for primary procedure) [S] [80] [symbol]

Note that 0055T is an add-on code that must be used in conjunction with the appropriate code for the primary procedure. This code cannot be reported alone.

When CT and MRI are both eprformed, report 0055T only once.

+ **0056T** Computer-assisted musculoskeletal surgical navigational orthopedic procedure, image-less (List separately in addition to code for primary procedure) [S] [80]

Note that 0056T is an add-on code that must be used in conjunction with the appropriate code for the primary procedure. This code cannot be reported alone.

0058T Cryopreservation; reproductive tissue, ovarian [X] [80]

0059T oocyte(s) [X] [80]

To report cryopreservation of embryo(s), sperm and testicular reproductive tissue, consult CPT codes 89258, 89259, 89335.

0060T Electrical impedance scan of the breast, bilateral (risk assessment device for breast cancer) [B] [80]

0061T Destruction/reduction of malignant breast tumor including breast carcinoma cells in the margins, microwave phased array thermotherapy, disposable catheter with combined temperature monitoring probe and microwave sensor, externally applied microwave energy, including interstitial placement of sensor [B] [80] [symbol]

To report imaging guidance, consult CPT codes 76942, 76986.

▲ **0062T** Percutaneous intradiscal annuloplasty, any method except electrothermal, unilateral or bilateral including fluoroscopic guidance; single level [T] [80] [symbol]

+ ▲ **0063T** 1 or more additional levels (List separately in addition to 0062T for primary procedure) [T] [80]

To report CT or MRI guidance and localization for needle placement and annuloplasty in conjunction with 0062T, 0063T, consult CPT codes 76360, 76393.

0064T Spectroscopy, expired gas analysis (eg, nitric oxide/carbon dioxide test) [X] [80]

0065T Ocular photoscreening, with interpretation and report, bilateral [E] [80]

Code 0065T cannot be reported with CPT code 99172 or 99173.

0066T Computed tomographic (CT) colonography (ie, virtual colonoscopy); screening [E]

0067T diagnostic [S] [80]

Codes 0066T and 0067T cannot be reported with CPT codes 72192-72194, 74150-74170.

+ ▲ **0068T** Acoustic heart sound recording and computer analysis; with interpretation and report [B] [80]

+ ▲ **0069T** acoustic heart sound recording and computer analysis only [N] [80]

+ **0070T** interpretation and report only (List separately in addition to codes for electrocardiography) [B] [80]

Note that 0070T is an add-on code and must be reported with 93010.

0071T Focused ultrasound ablation of uterine leiomyomata, including MR guidance; total leiomyomata volume less than 200 cc of tissue [♀] [T] [80] [symbol]

0072T total leiomyomata volume greater or equal to 200 cc of tissue [♀] [T] [80] [symbol]

Code 0071T, 0072T cannot be reported with CPT codes 51702 or 76394.

0073T Compensator-based beam modulation treatment delivery of inverse planned treatment using three or more high resolution (milled or cast) compensator convergent beam modulated fields, per treatment session [S] [TC] [80] [symbol]

MED: 100-4,4,220.1

To report treatment planning, consult code 77301.

Code 0073T cannot be reported with CPT codes 77401-77416, 77418.

ONLINE MEDICAL EVALUATION

A medical evaluation provided online is a service provided to a patient using internet resources. This service is provided as a response to a patient's inquiry online to a physician or a qualified healthcare professional. The physician or qualified healthcare professional must keep a permanent record of the encounter. These codes should not be to report routine services that would be included in other evaluation and management services. The codes include all communication including telephone calls, prescriptions, and laboratory orders related to the online evaluation.

0074T Online evaluation and management service, per encounter, provided by a physician, using the Internet or similar electronic communications network, in response to a patient's request, established patient [E]

0075T Transcatheter placement of extracranial vertebral or intrathoracic carotid artery stent(s), including radiologic supervision and interpretation, percutaneous; initial vessel [C] [80] [symbol]

[2G] Professional Component Only   [80]/[80] Assist-at-Surgery Allowed/With Documentation   Unlisted   Not Covered

[TC] Technical Component Only   MED: Pub 100/NCD References   AMA: CPT Assistant References   [1]-[9] ASC Group   ♂ Male Only   ♀ Female Only

382 — CPT Expert   CPT only © 2006 American Medical Association. All Rights Reserved. *(Black Ink)*   © 2006 Ingenix *(Blue Ink)*

+ 0076T **each additional vessel (List separately in addition to code for primary procedure)** [C] [80]

Note 0076T must be used with code 0075T.

When the ipsilateral extracranial vertebral or intrathoracic carotid arteriogram (including imaging and selective catheterization) confirms the need for stenting, then 0075T and 0076T include all the ipsilateral extracranial vertebral or intrathoracic selective carotid catheterization, all diagnostic imaging for ipsilateral extracranial vertebral or intrathoracic carotid artery stenting, and all related radiologic supervision and interpretation. Use the appropriate codes for selective catheterization and imaging instead of 0075T or 0076T if stenting is not indicated.

0077T **Implanting and securing cerebral thermal perfusion probe, including twist drill or burr hole, to measure absolute cerebral tissue perfusion** [C] [80] [CCI]

Report 0078T-0081T according to the Endovascular Abdominal Aneurysm Repair guidelines set up for 34800-34826.

0078T **Endovascular repair using prosthesis of abdominal aortic aneurysm, pseudoaneurysm or dissection, abdominal aorta involving visceral branches (superior mesenteric, celiac and/or renal artery(s))** [C] [80] [CCI]

Code 0078T cannot be reported with CPT codes 34800-34805, 35081, 35102, 35452, 35454, 35472, 37205-37208.

Note 0078T must be used with 35454, 37205-37208, when these procedures are performed outside the target zone of the endoprosthesis.

+ 0079T **Placement of visceral extension prosthesis for endovascular repair of abdominal aortic aneurysm involving visceral vessels, each visceral branch (List separately in addition to code for primary procedure)** [C] [80] [CCI]

Note 0079T must be used with 0078T.

Code 0079T cannot be reported with 34800-34805, 35081, 35102, 35452, 35454, 35472, 37205-37208.

Note 0079T must be used with 35454, 37205-37208 when these procedures are performed outside the target zone of the endoprosthesis.

0080T **Endovascular repair of abdominal aortic aneurysm, pseudoaneurysm or dissection, abdominal aorta involving visceral vessels (superior mesenteric, celiac or renal), using fenestrated modular bifurcated prosthesis (two docking limbs), radiological supervision and interpretation** [C] [80] [CCI]

Code 0080T cannot be reported with CPT codes 34800-34805, 35801, 35102, 35452, 35472, 37205-37208.

Note 0080T must be used with 35454, 37205-37208, when these procedures are performed outside the target zone of the endoprosthesis.

+ 0081T **Placement of visceral extension prosthesis for endovascular repair of abdominal aortic aneurysm involving visceral vessels, each visceral branch, radiological supervision and interpretation (List separately in addition to code for primary procedure)** [C] [80] [CCI]

Not 0081T must be used with 0080T.

Code 00081T cannot be used with CPT codes 34800-34805, 35081, 35102, 35452, 35454, 35472, 37205-37208.

Note 0081T must be used with 35454, 37205-37208, when these procedures are performed outside the target zone of the endoprosthesis

~~0082T~~ ~~Stereotactic body radiation therapy, treatment delivery, one or more treatment areas, per day~~

Use 77371-77373.

~~0083T~~ ~~Stereotactic body radiation therapy, treatment management, per day~~

Use 77371-77373.

0084T **Insertion of a temporary prostatic urethral stent** ♂ [T] [80] [CCI]

0085T **Breath test for heart transplant rejection** [X] [80]

0086T **Left ventricular filling pressure indirect measurement by computerized calibration of the arterial waveform response to Valsalva maneuver** [N] [80]

▲ **0087T** **Sperm evaluation, Hyaluronan binding assay** [X] [80]

0088T **Submucosal radiofrequency tissue volume reduction of tongue base, one or more sites, per session (ie, for treatment of obstructive sleep apnea syndrome)** [T] [80] [CCI]

0089T **Actigraphy testing, recording, analysis and interpretation (minimum of three-day recording)** [S] [80]

▲ **0090T** **Total disc arthroplasty (artificial disc), anterior approach, including discectomy to prepare interspace (other than for decompression) cervical; single interspace** [E] [80]

~~0091T~~ ~~single interspace, lumbar~~

+ ▲ **0092T** **each additional interspace (List separately in addition to code for primary procedure)** [C] [80]

Note that 0092T is an add-on code and must be used in conjunction with 0090T, 0091T.

▲ **0093T** **Removal of total disc arthroplasty, anterior approach cervical; single interspace** [C] [80]

To report removal of total disc lumbar arthroplasty, consult code 22865.

~~0094T~~ ~~single interspace, lumbar~~

+ **0095T** **each additional interspace (List separately in addition to code for primary procedure)** [C] [80]

Note that 0095T is an add-on code and must be used in conjunction with 0093T, 0094T.

▲ **0096T** **Revision of total disc arthroplasty, anterior approach cervical; single interspace** [C] [80]

~~0097T~~ ~~single interspace, lumbar~~

\+ **0098T** **each additional interspace (List separately in addition to code for primary procedure)** C 80

Note that 0098T is an add-on code and must be used in conjunction with 0096T, 0097. Code 0098T cannot be used with 0095T. Code 0090T-0097T cannot be used with 22851, 49010 when performed at the same level.

Codes 0090T-0097T include fluoroscopy.

To report decompression, consult CPT codes 63001-63048.

0099T **Implantation of intrastromal corneal ring segments** T 80

0100T **Placement of a subconjunctival retinal prosthesis receiver and pulse generator, and implantation of intra-ocular retinal electrode array, with vitrectomy** T 80

0101T **Extracorporeal shock wave involving musculoskeletal system, not otherwise specified, high energy** T 80

To report the application of low energy musculoskeletal system extracorporeal shock wave, consult Category III code 0019T.

0102T **Extracorporeal shock wave, high energy, performed by a physician, requiring anesthesia other than local, involving lateral humeral epicondyle** T 80

To report the application of low energy musculoskeletal system extracorporeal shock wave, consult Category III code 0019T.

0103T **Holotranscobalamin, quantitative** A 80

0104T **Inert gas rebreathing for cardiac output measurement; during rest** A 80

0105T **during exercise** A 80

0106T **Quantitative sensory testing (QST), testing and interpretation per extremity; using touch pressure stimuli to assess large diameter sensation** X 80

0107T **using vibration stimuli to assess large diameter fiber sensation** X 80

0108T **using cooling stimuli to assess small nerve fiber sensation and hyperalgesia** X 80

0109T **using heat-pain stimuli to assess small nerve fiber sensation and hyperalgesia** X 80

0110T **using other stimuli to assess sensation** X 80

0111T **Long-chain (C20-22) omega-3 fatty acids in red blood cell (RBC) membranes** A 80

To report very long chain fatty acids, consult CPT code 82726.

0115T **Medication therapy management service(s) provided by a pharmacist, individual, face-to-face with patient, initial 15 minutes, with assessment, and intervention if provided; initial encounter** B 80

0116T **subsequent encounter** B 80

\+ **0117T** **each additional 15 minutes (List separately in addition to code for primary service)** B 80

Note that 0117T is an add-on code and must be used in conjunction with 0115T, 0116T.

~~0120T~~ ~~Ablation, cryosurgical, of fibroadenoma, including ultrasound guidance, each fibroadenoma~~

0123T **Fistulization of sclera for glaucoma, through ciliary body** T 80

0124T **Conjunctival incision with posterior juxtascleral placement of pharmacological agent (does not include supply of medication)** T 80

0126T **Common carotid intima-media thickness (IMT) study for evaluation of atherosclerotic burden or coronary heart disease risk factor assessment** N 80

0130T **Validated, statistically reliable, randomized, controlled, single-patient clinical investigation of FDA approved chronic care drugs, provided by a pharmacist, interpretation and report to the prescribing health care professional** B 80

0133T **Upper gastrointestinal endoscopy, including esophagus, stomach, and either the duodenum and/or jejunum as appropriate, with injection of implant material into and along the muscle of the lower esophageal sphincter (eg, for treatment of gastroesophageal reflux disease)** T 80

0135T **Ablation, renal tumor(s), unilateral, percutaneous, cryotherapy** T 80

0137T **Biopsy, prostate, needle, saturation sampling for prostate mapping** T 80

Code 0137T cannot be used with 76942.

0140T **Exhaled breath condensate pH** A 80

0141T **Pancreatic islet cell transplantation through portal vein, percutaneous** E 80

To report open approach, consult, 0142T. Use 0143T for laparoscopic approach.

Use 75887 for radiological supervision and interpretation.

Report 36481 for percuatenous portal vein catheterization.

0142T **Pancreatic islet cell transplantation through portal vein, open** E 80

0143T **Laparoscopy, surgical, pancreatic islet cell transplantation through portal vein** E 80

0144T **Computed tomography, heart, without contrast material, including image postprocessing and quantitative evaluation of coronary calcium** S 80

Do not report 0144T with 0145T-0151T.

0145T **Computed tomography, heart, without contrast material followed by contrast material(s) and further sections, including cardiac gating and 3D image postprocessing; cardiac structure and morphology** S 80

0146T **computed tomographic angiography of coronary arteries (including native and anomalous coronary arteries, coronary bypass grafts), without quantitative evaluation of coronary calcium** S 80

0147T **computed tomographic angiography of coronary arteries (including native and anomalous coronary arteries, coronary bypass grafts), with quantitative evaluation of coronary calcium** S 80

▲ **0148T** **cardiac structure and morphology and computed tomographic angiography of coronary arteries (including native and anomalous coronary arteries, coronary bypass grafts), without quantitative evaluation of coronary calcium** S 80

▲ 0149T   cardiac structure and morphology and computed
            tomographic angiography of coronary arteries
            (including native and anomalous coronary arteries,
            coronary bypass grafts), with quantitative
            evaluation of coronary calcium   Ⓢ 80

    Do not report 0149T with 0144T.

▲ 0150T   cardiac structure and morphology in congenital
            heart disease   Ⓢ 80

▲ 0151T   Computed tomography, heart, without contrast
            material followed by contrast material(s) and further
            sections, including cardiac gating and 3D image
            postprocessing, function evaluation (left and right
            ventricular function, ejection-fraction and segmental
            wall motion) (List separately in addition to code for
            primary procedure)   Ⓢ 80

~~0152T~~   ~~Computer aided detection (computer algorithm
            analysis of digital image data for lesion detection)
            with further physician review for interpretation, with
            or without digitization of film radiographic images;
            chest radiograph(s) (List separately in addition to code
            for primary procedure)~~

+ ▲ 0153T   Transcatheter placement of wireless physiologic sensor
            in aneurysmal sac during endovascular repair,
            including radiological supervision and interpretation
            and instrument calibration (List separately in addition
            to code for primary procedure)   Ⓒ 80

    0154T   Noninvasive physiologic study of implanted wireless
            pressure sensor in aneurysmal sac following
            endovascular repair, complete study including
            recording, analysis of pressure and waveform tracings,
            interpretation and report   Ⓧ 80

    Do not report 0154T with 0153T.

● 0155T   Laparoscopy, surgical; implantation or replacement
            of gastric stimulation electrodes, lesser curvature (ie,
            morbid obesity)   Ⓣ 80

● 0156T   revision or removal of gastric stimulation
            electrodes, lesser curvature (ie, morbid
            obesity)   Ⓣ 80

    Use 0157T, 0158T for open approach.

    Use 64590 for insertion of gastric neurostimulator pulse
    generator. Use 64595 for revision or removal of gastric
    neurostimulator pulse generator.

    Consult 95999 for electronic analysis and programming
    of gastric neurostimulator pulse generator.

● 0157T   Laparotomy, implantation or replacement of gastric
            stimulation electrodes, lesser curvature (ie, morbid
            obesity)   Ⓒ 80

● 0158T   Laparotomy, revision or removal of gastric stimulation
            electrodes, lesser curvature (ie, morbid
            obesity)   Ⓒ 80

    Consult 0155T, 0156T for laparoscopic approach.

    Consult 64590 for insertion of gastric neurostimulator
    pulse generator. Use 64595 for revision or removal of
    gastric neurostimulator pulse generator.

    To report electronic analysis and programming of gastric
    neurostimulator pulse generator, consult 95999. Use
    0162T for electronic analysis, programming, and
    reprogramming of gastric neurostimulator.

+ ● 0159T   Computer-aided detection, including computer
            algorithm analysis of MRI image data for lesion
            detection/characterization, pharmacokinetic analysis,
            with further physician review for interpretation, breast
            MRI (List separately in addition to code for primary
            procedure)   Ⓝ 80

● 0160T   Therapeutic repetitive transcranial magnetic
            stimulation treatment planning   Ⓢ 80

● 0161T   Therapeutic repetitive transcranial magnetic
            stimulation treatment delivery and management, per
            session   Ⓢ 80

● 0162T   Electronic analysis and programming, reprogramming
            of gastric neurostimulator (ie, morbid obesity)   Ⓢ

+ ● 0163T   Total disc arthroplasty (artificial disc), anterior
            approach, including discectomy to prepare interspace
            (other than for decompression), lumbar, each
            additional interspace   Ⓒ

    Note that 0163T is an add-on code and must be reported
    with 22857.

+ ● 0164T   Removal of total disc arthroplasty, anterior approach,
            lumbar, each additional interspace   Ⓒ

    Note that 0164T is an add-on code and must be reported
    with 22865.

+ ● 0165T   Revision of total disc arthroplasty, anterior approach,
            lumbar, each additional interspace   Ⓒ

● 0166T   Transmyocardial transcatheter closure of ventricular
            septal defect, with implant; without cardiopulmonary
            bypass   Ⓒ

● 0167T   with cardiopulmonary bypass   Ⓒ

    Do not report 0166T, 0167T with 32020, 33210, or
    33211.

    Use 93581 for ventricular septal defect closure via
    percutaneous transcatheter implant delivery.

● 0168T   Rhinophototherapy, intranasal application of
            ultraviolet and visible light, bilateral   Ⓣ

● 0169T   Stereotactic placement of infusion catheter(s) in the
            brain for delivery of therapeutic agent(s), including
            computerized stereotactic planning and burr
            hole(s)   Ⓒ

    Do not report 0169T with 20660, 61107, or 61795.

● 0170T   Repair of anorectal fistula with plug (eg, porcine small
            intestine submucosa [SIS])   Ⓣ

    For repair of anal fistula using fibrin glue, consult 46706

    Do not report 0170T in conjunction with 15430 or
    15431.

UNPUBLISHED CODES EFFECTIVE JANUARY 1, 2007

The following codes were announced by the AMA July 1, 2006 for implementation
January 1, 2007, but were adopted too late for publication in the AMA's CPT
manual. For more information, consult the AMA Web site, www.ama-assn.org.
These codes are valid, but unpublished in the AMA's CPT Manual.

● 0171T   Insertion of posterior spinous process distraction
            device (including necessary removal of bone or
            ligament for insertion and imaging guidance), lumbar;
            single level   Ⓣ

● 0172T   each additional level (List separately in addition
            to code for primary procedure)   Ⓣ

● 0173T   Monitoring of intraocular pressure during vitrectomy
            surgery (List separately in addition to code for primary
            procedure)   Ⓝ

● 0174T   Computer aided detection (CAD) (computer algorithm analysis of digital image data for lesion detection) with further physician review for interpretation and report, with or without digitization of film radiographic images, chest radiograph(s), performed concurrent with primary interpretation (List separately in addition to code for primary procedure)   N

● 0175T   Computer aided detection (CAD) (computer algorithm analysis of digital image data for lesion detection) with further physician review for interpretation and report, with or without digitization of film radiographic images, chest radiograph(s), performed remote from primary interpretation   N

● 0176T   Transluminal dilation of aqueous outflow canal; without retention of device or stent   9 T

● 0177T   with retention of device or stent   9 T

APPENDIX A — MODIFIERS

CPT Modifiers

This list includes all of the modifiers applicable to CPT codes.

21   **Prolonged Evaluation and Management Services:** When the face-to-face or floor/unit service(s) provided is prolonged or otherwise greater than that usually required for the highest level of evaluation and management service within a given category, it may be identified by adding modifier 21 to the evaluation and management code number. A report may also be appropriate.

22   **Unusual Procedural Services:** When the service(s) provided is greater than that usually required for the listed procedure, it may be identified by adding modifier 22 to the usual procedure number. A report may also be appropriate.

23   **Unusual Anesthesia:** Occasionally, a procedure, which usually requires either no anesthesia or local anesthesia, because of unusual circumstances must be done under general anesthesia. This circumstance may be reported by adding modifier 23 to the procedure code of the basic service.

24   **Unrelated Evaluation and Management Service by the Same Physician During a Postoperative Period:** The physician may need to indicate that an evaluation and management service was performed during a postoperative period for a reason(s) unrelated to the original procedure. This circumstance may be reported by adding modifier 24 to the appropriate level of E/M service.

25   **Significant, Separately Identifiable Evaluation and Management Service by the Same Physician on the Same Day of the Procedure or Other Service:** The physician may need to indicate that on the day a procedure or service identified by a CPT code was performed, the patient's condition required a significant, separately identifiable E/M service above and beyond the other service provided or beyond the usual preoperative and postoperative care associated with the procedure that was performed. A significant, separately identifiable E/M service is defined or substantiated by documentationthat satisfies the relevant criteria for the respective E/M wervices to be reported (see Evaluation and Management Services Guidelines for instructions on determining level of E/M service.) The E/M service may be prompted by the symptom or condition for which the procedure and/or service was provided. As such, different diagnoses are not required for reporting of the E/M services on the same date. This circumstance may be reported by adding modifier 25 to the appropriate level of E/M service. Note: This modifier is not used to report an E/M service that resulted in a decision to perform surgery. See modifier 57.

26   **Professional Component:** Certain procedures are a combination of a physician component and a technical component. When the physician component is reported separately, the service may be identified by adding modifier 26 to the usual procedure number.

32   **Mandated Services:** Services related to mandated consultation and/or related services (eg, PRO, third party payer, governmental, legislative, or regulatory requirement) may be identified by adding modifier 32 to the basic procedure.

47   **Anesthesia by Surgeon:** Regional or general anesthesia provided by the surgeon may be reported by adding modifier 47 to the basic service. (This does not include local anesthesia.) Note: Modifier 47 would not be used as a modifier for the anesthesia procedures 00100-01999.

50   **Bilateral Procedure:** Unless otherwise identified in the listings, bilateral procedures that are performed at the same operative session should be identified by adding modifier 50 to the appropriate five digit code.

51   **Multiple Procedures:** When multiple procedures, other than Evaluation and Management Services, are performed at the same session by the same provider, the primary procedure or service may be reported as listed. The additional procedure(s) or service(s) may be identified by appending modifier 51 to the additional procedure or service code(s). Note: This modifier should not be appended to designated "add-on" codes.

52   **Reduced Services:** Under certain circumstances a service or procedure is partially reduced or eliminated at the physician's discretion. Under these circumstances the service provided can be identified by its usual procedure number and the addition of modifier 52, signifying that the service is reduced. This provides a means of reporting reduced services without disturbing the identification of the basic service. Note: For hospital outpatient reporting of a previously scheduled procedure/service that is partially reduced or cancelled as a result of extenuating circumstances or those that threaten the well-being of the patient prior to or after administration of anesthesia, see modifiers 73 and 74 (see modifiers approved for ASC hospital outpatient use).

53   **Discontinued Procedure:** Under certain circumstances, the physician may elect to terminate a surgical or diagnostic procedure. Due to extenuating circumstances or those that threaten the well being of the patient, it may be necessary to indicate that a surgical or diagnostic procedure was started but discontinued. This circumstance may be reported by adding modifier 53 to the code reported by the physician for the discontinued procedure. Note: This modifier is not used to report the elective cancellation of a procedure prior to the patient's anesthesia induction and/or surgical preparation in the operating suite. For outpatient hospital/ambulatory surgery center (ASC) reporting of a previously scheduled procedure/service that is partially reduced or cancelled as a result of extenuating circumstances or those that threaten the well being of the patient prior to or after administration of anesthesia, see modifiers 73 and 74 (see modifiers approved for ASC hospital outpatient use).

54   **Surgical Care Only:** When one physician performs a surgical procedure and another provides preoperative and/or postoperative management, surgical services may be identified by adding modifier 54 to the usual procedure number.

55   **Postoperative Management Only:** When one physician performs the postoperative management and another physician has performed the surgical procedure, the postoperative component may be identified by adding modifier 55 to the usual procedure number.

56   **Preoperative Management Only:** When one physician performs the preoperative care and evaluation and another physician performs the surgical procedure, the preoperative component may be identified by adding modifier 56 to the usual procedure number.

57   **Decision for Surgery:** An evaluation and management service that resulted in the initial decision to perform the surgery may be identified by adding modifier 57 to the appropriate level of E/M service.

58   **Staged or Related Procedure or Service by the Same Physician During the Postoperative Period:** The physician may need to indicate that the performance of a procedure or service during the postoperative period was: a) planned prospectively at the time of the original procedure (staged); b) more extensive than the original procedure; or c) for therapy following a diagnostic surgical procedure. This circumstance may be reported by adding modifier 58 to the staged or related procedure. Note: This modifier is not used to report the treatment of a problem that requires a return to the operating room. See modifier 78.

59   **Distinct Procedural Service:** Under certain circumstances, the physician may need to indicate that a procedure or service was distinct or independent from other services performed on the same day. Modifier 59 is used to identify procedures/services that are not normally reported together, but are appropriate under the circumstances. This may represent a different session or patient encounter, different procedure or surgery, different site or organ system, separate incision/excision, separate lesion, or separate injury (or area of injury in extensive injuries) not ordinarily encountered or performed on the same day by the same physician. However, when another already established modifier is appropriate it should be used rather than modifier 59. Only if no more descriptive modifier is available, and the use of modifier 59 best explains the circumstances, should modifier 59 be used.

62   **Two Surgeons:** When two surgeons work together as primary surgeons performing distinct part(s) of a procedure, each surgeon should report his/her distinct operative work by adding modifier 62 to the procedure code and any associated add-on code(s) for that procedure as long as both surgeons continue to work together as primary surgeons. Each surgeon should report the co-surgery once using the same procedure code. If an additional procedure(s) (including an add-on procedure(s)) is performed during the same surgical session, a separate code(s) may be reported with the modifier 62 added. Note: If a co-surgeon acts as an assistant in the performance of an additional procedure(s) during the same surgical session, the service(s) may be reported using a separate procedure code(s) with modifier 80 or modifier 82 added, as appropriate.

63   **Procedure Performed on Infants less than 4 kg:** Procedures performed on neonates and infants up to a present body weight of 4 kg may involve significantly increased complexity and physician work commonly associated with these patients. This circumstance may be reported by adding the modifier 63 to the procedure number. Note: Unless otherwise designated, this modifier may only be appended to procedures/services listed in the 20000-69999 code series. Modifier 63 should not be appended to any CPT codes in the E/M, Anesthesia, Radiology, Pathology/Laboratory or Medicine sections.

66   **Surgical Team:** Under some circumstances, highly complex procedures (requiring the concomitant services of several physicians, often of different specialties, plus other highly skilled, specially trained personnel, various types of complex equipment) are carried out under the "surgical team" concept. Such circumstances may be identified by each participating physician with the addition of modifier 66 to the basic procedure number used for reporting services.

76 Repeat Procedure by Same Physician: The physician may need to indicate that a procedure or service was repeated subsequent to the original procedure or service. This circumstance may be reported by adding modifier 76 to the repeated procedure/service.

77 Repeat Procedure by Another Physician: The physician may need to indicate that a basic procedure or service performed by another physician had to be repeated. This situation may be reported by adding modifier 77 to the repeated procedure/service.

78 Return to the Operating Room for a Related Procedure During the Postoperative Period: The physician may need to indicate that another procedure was performed during the postoperative period of the initial procedure. When this subsequent procedure is related to the first, and requires the use of the operating room, it may be reported by adding modifier 78 to the related procedure. (For repeat procedures on the same day, see modifier 76.)

79 Unrelated Procedure or Service by the Same Physician During the Postoperative Period: The physician may need to indicate that the performance of a procedure or service during the postoperative period was unrelated to the original procedure. This circumstance may be reported by using modifier 79. (For repeat procedures on the same day, see modifier 76.)

80 Assistant Surgeon: Surgical assistant services may be identified by adding modifier 80 to the usual procedure number(s).

81 Minimum Assistant Surgeon: Minimum surgical assistant services are identified by adding modifier 81 to the usual procedure number.

82 Assistant Surgeon (when qualified resident surgeon not available): The unavailability of a qualified resident surgeon is a prerequisite for use of modifier 82 appended to the usual procedure code number(s).

90 Reference (Outside) Laboratory: When laboratory procedures are performed by a party other than the treating or reporting physician, the procedure may be identified by adding modifier 90 to the usual procedure number.

91 Repeat Clinical Diagnostic Laboratory Test: In the course of treatment of the patient, it may be necessary to repeat the same laboratory test on the same day to obtain subsequent (multiple) test results. Under these circumstances, the laboratory test performed can be identified by its usual procedure number and the addition of modifier 91. Note: This modifier may not be used when tests are rerun to confirm initial results; due to testing problems with specimens or equipment; or for any other reason when a normal, one-time, reportable result is all that is required. This modifier may not be used when another code(s) describes a series of test results (eg, glucose tolerance tests, evocative/suppression testing). This modifier may only be used for a laboratory test(s) performed more than once on the same day on the same patient.

99 Multiple Modifiers: Under certain circumstances two or more modifiers may be necessary to completely delineate a service. In such situations, modifier 99 should be added to the basic procedure and other applicable modifiers may be listed as part of the description of the service.

Anesthesia Physical Status Modifiers

All anesthesia services are reported by use of the five-digit anesthesia procedure code with the appropriate physical status modifier appended.

Under certain circumstances, when other modifier(s) are appropriate, they should be reported in addition to the physical status modifier.

P1 A normal healthy patient

P2 A patient with mild systemic disease

P3 A patient with severe systemic disease

P4 A patient with severe systemic disease that is a constant threat to life

P5 A moribund patient who is not expected to survive without the operation

P6 A declared brain-dead patient whose organs are being removed for donor purposes

MODIFIERS APPROVED FOR AMBULATORY SURGERY CENTER (ASC) HOSPITAL OUTPATIENT USE

CPT Level I Modifiers

25 Significant, Separately Identifiable Evaluation and Management Service by the Same Physician on the Same Day of the Procedure or Other Service: The physician may need to indicate that on the day a procedure or service identified by a CPT code was performed, the patient's condition required a significant, separately identifiable E/M service above and beyond the other service provided or beyond the usual preoperative and postoperative care associated with the procedure that was performed. A significant, separately identifiable E/M service is defined or substantiated by documentationthat satisfies the relevant criteria for the respective E/M wervices to be reported (see Evaluation and Management Services Guidelines for instructions on determining level of E/M service.) The E/M service may be prompted by the symptom or condition for which the procedure and/or service was provided. As such, different diagnoses are not required for reporting of the E/M services on the same date. This circumstance may be reported by adding modifier 25 to the appropriate level of E/M service. Note: This modifier is not used to report an E/M service that resulted in a decision to perform surgery. See modifier 57.

27 Multiple Outpatient Hospital E/M Encounters on the Same Date: For hospital outpatient reporting purposes, utilization of hospital resources related to separate and distinct E/M encounters performed in multiple outpatient hospital settings on the same date may be reported by adding modifier 27 to each appropriate level outpatient and/or emergency department E/M code(s). This modifier provides a means of reporting circumstances involving evaluation and management services provided by a physician(s) in more than one (multiple) outpatient hospital setting(s) (eg, hospital emergency department, clinic). Note: This modifier is not to be used for physician reporting of multiple E/M services performed by the same physician on the same date. For physician reporting of all outpatient evaluation and management services provided by the same physician on the same date and performed in multiple outpatient settings (eg, hospital emergency department, clinic), see Evaluation and Management, Emergency Department, or Preventive Medicine Services codes.

50 Bilateral Procedure: Unless otherwise identified in the listings, bilateral procedures that are performed at the same operative session should be identified by adding modifier 50 to the appropriate five digit code.

52 Reduced Services: Under certain circumstances a service or procedure is partially reduced or eliminated at the physician's discretion. Under these circumstances the service provided can be identified by its usual procedure number and the addition of modifier 52, signifying that the service is reduced. This provides a means of reporting reduced services without disturbing the identification of the basic service. Note: For hospital outpatient reporting of a previously scheduled procedure/service that is partially reduced or cancelled as a result of extenuating circumstances or those that threaten the well-being of the patient prior to or after administration of anesthesia, see modifiers 73 and 74 (see modifiers approved for ASC hospital outpatient use).

58 Staged or Related Procedure or Service by the Same Physician During the Postoperative Period: The physician may need to indicate that the performance of a procedure or service during the postoperative period was: a) planned prospectively at the time of the original procedure (staged); b) more extensive than the original procedure; or c) for therapy following a diagnostic surgical procedure. This circumstance may be reported by adding modifier 58 to the staged or related procedure. Note: This modifier is not used to report the treatment of a problem that requires a return to the operating room. See modifier 78.

59 Distinct Procedural Service: Under certain circumstances, the physician may need to indicate that a procedure or service was distinct or independent from other services performed on the same day. Modifier 59 is used to identify procedures/services that are not normally reported together, but are appropriate under the circumstances. This may represent a different session or patient encounter, different procedure or surgery, different site or organ system, separate incision/excision, separate lesion, or separate injury (or area of injury in extensive injuries) not ordinarily encountered or performed on the same day by the same physician. However, when another already established modifier is appropriate it should be used rather than modifier 59. Only if no more descriptive modifier is available, and the use of modifier 59 best explains the circumstances, should modifier 59 be used.

73 Discontinued Out-Patient Hospital/Ambulatory Surgery Center (ASC) Procedure Prior to the Administration of Anesthesia: Due to extenuating circumstances or those that threaten the well being of the patient, the physician may cancel a surgical or diagnostic procedure subsequent to the patient's surgical preparation (including sedation when provided, and being taken to the room where the procedure is to be performed), but prior to the administration of anesthesia (local, regional block(s), or general). Under these circumstances, the intended service that is prepared for but cancelled can be reported by its usual procedure number and the addition of modifier 73. Note: The elective cancellation of a service prior to the administration of anesthesia and/or surgical preparation of the patient should not be reported. For physician reporting of a discontinued procedure, see modifier 53.

74 **Discontinued Out-Patient Hospital/Ambulatory Surgery Center (ASC) Procedure After Administration of Anesthesia:** Due to extenuating circumstances or those that threaten the well being of the patient, the physician may terminate a surgical or diagnostic procedure after the administration of anesthesia (local, regional block(s), general) or after the procedure was started (incision made, intubation started, scope inserted, etc.). Under these circumstances, the procedure started but terminated can be reported by its usual procedure number and the addition of modifier 74. Note: The elective cancellation of a service prior to the administration of anesthesia and/or surgical preparation of the patient should not be reported. For physician reporting of a discontinued procedure, see modifier 53.

76 **Repeat Procedure by Same Physician:** The physician may need to indicate that a procedure or service was repeated subsequent to the original procedure or service. This circumstance may be reported by adding modifier 76 to the repeated procedure/service.

77 **Repeat Procedure by Another Physician:** The physician may need to indicate that a basic procedure or service performed by another physician had to be repeated. This situation may be reported by adding modifier 77 to the repeated procedure/service.

78 **Return to the Operating Room for a Related Procedure During the Postoperative Period:** The physician may need to indicate that another procedure was performed during the postoperative period of the initial procedure. When this subsequent procedure is related to the first, and requires the use of the operating room, it may be reported by adding modifier 78 to the related procedure. (For repeat procedures on the same day, see modifier 76.)

79 **Unrelated Procedure or Service by the Same Physician During the Postoperative Period:** The physician may need to indicate that the performance of a procedure or service during the postoperative period was unrelated to the original procedure. This circumstance may be reported by using modifier 79. (For repeat procedures on the same day, see modifier 76.)

91 **Repeat Clinical Diagnostic Laboratory Test:** In the course of treatment of the patient, it may be necessary to repeat the same laboratory test on the same day to obtain subsequent (multiple) test results. Under these circumstances, the laboratory test performed can be identified by its usual procedure number and the addition of modifier 91. Note: This modifier may not be used when tests are rerun to confirm initial results; due to testing problems with specimens or equipment; or for any other reason when a normal, one-time, reportable result is all that is required. This modifier may not be used when another code(s) describe a series of test results (eg, glucose tolerance tests, evocative/suppression testing). This modifier may only be used for a laboratory test(s) performed more than once on the same day on the same patient.

Level II (HCPCS/National) Modifiers

Anatomical Modifiers

E1 Upper left, eyelid

E2 Lower left, eyelid

E3 Upper right, eyelid

E4 Lower right, eyelid

F1 Left hand, second digit

F2 Left hand, third digit

F3 Left hand, fourth digit

F4 Left hand, fifth digit

F5 Right hand, thumb

F6 Right hand, second digit

F7 Right hand, third digit

F8 Right hand, fourth digit

F9 Right hand, fifth digit

FA Left hand, thumb

LT Left side (used to identify procedures performed on the left side of the body)

RT Right side (used to identify procedures performed on the right side of the body)

T1 Left foot, second digit

T2 Left foot, third digit

T3 Left foot, fourth digit

T4 Left foot, fifth digit

T5 Right foot, great toe

T6 Right foot, second digit

T7 Right foot, third digit

T8 Right foot, fourth digit

T9 Right foot, fifth digit

TA Left foot, great toe

Ambulance Modifiers

GM Multiple patients on one ambulance trip

QM Ambulance service provided under arrangement by a provider of services

QN Ambulance service furnished directly by a provider of services

QL Patient pronounced dead after ambulance called

HCPCS Level II codes for ambulance services must be reported with modifiers that indicate pick-up origins and destinations. The modifier describing the arrangement (QM, QN) is listed second. The modifiers describing the origin and destination are listed second. Origin and destination modifiers are created by combining two alpha characters from the following list. Each alpha character, with the exception of X, represents either an origin or a destination. Each pair of alpha characters creates one modifier. The first position represents the origin and the second the destination.

D Diagnostic or therapeutic site other than "P" or "H" when these are used as origin codes

E Residential, domiciliary, custodial facility (other than an 1819 facility)

G Hospital-based dialysis facility (hospital or hospital-related)

H Hospital

I Site of transfer (e.g., airport or helicopter pad) between modes of ambulance transport

J Nonhospital-based dialysis facility

N SNF (1819 facility)

P Physician's office (includes HMO nonhospital facility, clinic, etc.)

R Residence

S Scene of accident or acute event

X Destination code only. Intermediate stop at physician's office enroute to the hospital (includes HMO nonhospital facility, clinic, etc.)

Anesthesia Modifiers

AA Anesthesia services performed personally by anesthesiologist

AD Medical supervision by a physician: more than four concurrent anesthesia procedures

G8 Monitored anesthesia care (MAC) for deep complex, complicated, or markedly invasive surgical procedure

G9 Monitored anesthesia care for patient who has history of severe cardio-pulmonary condition

QK Medical direction of two, three, or four concurrent anesthesia procedures involving qualified individuals

QS Monitored anesthesia care service

QY Medical direction of one certified registered nurse anesthetist (CRNA) by an anesthesiologist

QZ CRNA service: without medical direction by a physician

P1 A normal healthy patient

P2 A patient with mild systemic disease

P3 A patient with severe systemic disease

P4 A patient with severe systemic disease that is a constant threat to life

P5 A moribund patient who is not expected to survive without the operation

P6 A declared brain-dead patient whose organs are being removed for donor purposes

Coronary Artery Modifiers

LC Left circumflex coronary artery (Hospitals use with codes 92980-92984, 92995, 92996)

LD Left anterior descending coronary artery (Hospitals use with codes 92980-92984, 92995, 92996)

RC Right coronary artery (Hospitals use with codes 92980-92984, 92995, 92996)

Ophthalmology Modifiers

AP Determination of refractive state was not performed in the course of diagnostic ophthalmological examination

LS FDA-monitored intraocular lens implant

PL Progressive addition lenses

VP Aphakic patient

Professional Services

AE Registered dietician

AF Specialty physician

AG Primary physician

AH Clinical psychologist

AJ Clinical social worker

AK Non participating physician

AM Physician, team member service

AQ Physician providing a service in an unlisted health professional shortage area (HPSA)

AR Physician provider services in a physician scarcity area

AS Physician assistant, nurse practitioner, or clinical nurse specialist services for assistant at surgery

AT Acute treatment (this modifier should be used when reporting service 98940, 98941, 98942)

BL Special acquisition of blood and blood products

CA Procedure payable only in the inpatient setting when performed emergently on an outpatient who expires prior to admission

CB Service ordered by a renal dialysis facility (RDF) physician as part of the esrd beneficiary's dialysis benefit, is not part of the composite rate, and is separately reimbursable

CC Procedure code change (use 'CC' when the procedure code submitted was changed either for administrative reasons or because an incorrect code was filed)

CG Innovator drug dispensed

CR Catastrophe/disaster related

EP Service provided as part of medicaid early periodic screening diagnosis and treatment (EPSDT) program

ET Emergency services

FB Item provided without cost to provider, supplier or practitioner (examples, but not limited to: covered under warranty, replaced due to defect, free samples)

G7 Pregnancy resulted from rape or incest or pregnancy certified by physician as life threatening

GA Waiver of liability statement on file

GB Claim being resubmitted for payment because it is no longer covered under a global payment demonstration

GC This service has been performed in part by a resident under the direction of a teaching physician

GE This service has been performed by a resident without the presence of a teaching physician under the primary care exception

GF Non-physician (e.g. nurse practitioner (NP), certified registered nurse anaesthetist (CRNA), certified registered nurse (CRN), clinical nurse specialist (CNS), physician assistant (PA)) services in a critical access hospital

GG Performance and payment of a screening mammogram and diagnostic mammogram on the same patient, same day

GH Diagnostic mammogram converted from screening mammogram on same day

GJ "OPT OUT" physician or practitioner emergency or urgent service

GK Actual item/service ordered byphysician, item associated with GA or GZ modifier

GL Medically unnecessary upgrade provided instead of standard item, no charge, no advance beneficiary notice (ABN)

GN Service delivered under an outpatient speech-language pathology plan of care

GO Service delivered an outpatient occupational therapy plan of care

GP Service delivered under an outpatient physical therapy plan of care

GQ Via asynchronous telecommunications system

GR This service was performed in whole or in part by a resident in a department of veterans affairs medical center or clinic, supervised in accordance with VA policy

GT Via interactive audio and video telecommunication systems

GV Attending physician not employed or paid under arrangement by the patient's hospice provider

GW Service not related to the hospice patient's terminal condition

GY Item or service statutorily excluded or does not meet the definition of any medicare benefit

GZ Item or service expected to be denied as not reasonable and necessary

H9 Court-ordered

HA Child/adolescent program

HB Adult program, non geriatric

HC Adult program, geriatric

HD Pregnant/parenting women's program

HE Mental health program

HF Substance abuse program

HG Opioid addiction treatment program

HH Integrated mental health/substance abuse program

HI Integrated mental health and mental retardation/developmental disabilities program

HJ Employee assistance program

HK Specialized mental health programs for high-risk populations

HL Intern

HM Less than bachelor degree level

HN Bachelors degree level

HO Masters degree level

HP Doctoral level

HQ Group setting

HR Family/couple with client present

HS Family/couple without client present

HT Multi-disciplinary team

HU Funded by child welfare agency

HV Funded state addictions agency

HW Funded by state mental health agency

HX Funded by county/local agency

HY Funded by juvenile justice agency

HZ Funded by criminal justice agency

JA Administered intravenously

JB Administered subcutaneously

KB Beneficiary requested upgrade for ABN, more than four modifiers identified on claim

KC Replacement of special power wheelchair interface

KF Item designated by FDA as class III device

KX Specific required documentation on file

KZ New coverage not implemented by managed care

Q4 Service for ordering/referring physician qualifies as a service exemption

Q5 Service furnished by a substitute physician under a reciprocal billing arrangement

Q6 Service furnished by a locum tenens physician

QJ Services/items provided to a prisoner or patient in state or local custody, however the state or local government, as applicable, meets the requirements in 42 cfr 411.4 (b)

QP Documentation is on file showing that the laboratory test(s) was ordered individually or ordered as a CPT-recognized panel other than automated profile codes 80002-80019, G0058, G0059, and G0060

QR Repeat laboratory test performed on the same day

QS Monitored anesthesia care service

QV Item or service provided as routine care in a Medicare qualifying clinical trial

QW CLIA waived test

QX CRNA service: with medical direction by a physician

QY Medical direction of one certified registered nurse anesthetist (CRNA) by an anesthesiologist

QZ CRNA service: without medical direction by a physician

SA Nurse practitioner rendering service in collaboration with a physician

SB Nurse Midwife

SC Medically necessary service or supply

SD Services provided by registered nurse with specialized, highly technical home infusion training

SE State and/or federally funded programs/services

SG Ambulatory surgical center (ASC) facility service

SH Second concurrently administered infusion therapy

SJ Third or more concurrently administered infusion therapy

SK Member of high risk population (use only with codes for immunization)

SL State supplied vaccine

SM Second surgical opinion

SN Third surgical opinion

SQ Item ordered by home health

ST Related to trauma or injury

SU Procedure performed in physician's office (to denote use of facility and equipment)

SW Services provided by a certified diabetic educator

SY Persons who are in close contact with member of high-risk population (use only with codes for immunization)

TC Technical component. Under certain circumstances, a charge may be made for the technical component alone. Under those circumstances the technical component charge is identified by adding modifier 'TC' to the usual procedure number. Technical component charges are institutional charges and not billed separately by physicians. However, portable x-ray suppliers only bill for technical component and should utilize modifier TC. The charge data from portable x-ray suppliers will then be used to build customary and prevailing profiles.

TD RN

TE LPN/LVN

TF Intermediate level of care

TG Complex/high level of care

TH Obstetrical treatment/services, prenatal or postpartum

TJ Program group, child and/or adolescent

TL Early intervention/individualized family service plan (IFSP)

TM Individualized education program (IEP)

TN Rural/outside providers' customary service area

TP Medical transport, unloaded vehicle

TQ Basic life support transport by a volunteer ambulance provider

TS Follow-up service

TT Individualized service provided to more than one patient in same setting

TU Special payment rate, overtime

TV Special payment rates, holidays/weekends

U1 Medicaid level of care 1, as defined by each state

U2 Medicaid level of care 2, as defined by each state

U3 Medicaid level of care 3, as defined by each state

U4 Medicaid level of care 4, as defined by each state

U5 Medicaid level of care 5, as defined by each state

U6 Medicaid level of care 6, as defined by each state

U7 Medicaid level of care 7, as defined by each state

U8 Medicaid level of care 8, as defined by each state

U9 Medicaid level of care 9, as defined by each state

UA Medicaid level of care 10, as defined by each state

UB Medicaid level of care 11, as defined by each state

UC Medicaid level of care 12, as defined by each state

UD Medicaid level of care 13, as defined by each state

UF Services provided in the morning

UG Services provided in the afternoon

UH Services provided in the evening

UJ Services provided at night

UK Services provided on behalf of the client to someone other than the client (collateral relationship)

UN Two patients served

UP Three patients served

UQ Four patients served

UR Five patients served

US Six or more patients served

1P Performance Measure Exclusion Modifier Due to Medical Reasons; Includes: Not indicated (absence of the organ/limb, already received/performed, other); Contraindicated (patient allergic history, potential adverse drug interaction, other

2P Performance Measure Exclusion Modifier Due to Patient Reasons; Includes: Patient declined; Economic, social, or religious reasons; Other patient reasons

3P Performance Measure Exclusion Modifier Due to System Reasons; Resources to perform the services not available; Insurance coverage/payor-related limitations; Other reasons attributable to health care delivery system

ESRD Modifiers

EJ Subsequent claims for a defined course of therapy, e.g., EPO, sodium hyaluronate, infliximab

EM Emergency reserve supply (for ESRD benefit only)

G1 Most recent urea reduction ratio (URR) reading of less than 60

G2 Most recent urea reduction ration (URR) reading of 60 to 64.9

G3 Most recent urea reduction ratio (URR) reading of 65 to 69.9

G4 Most recent urea reduction ratio (URR) reading of 70 to 74.9

G5 Most recent urea reduction ratio (URR) reading of 75 or greater

G6 ESRD patient for whom less than six dialysis sessions have been provided in a month

GS Dosage of EPO or darbepoietin alfa has been reduced and maintained in response to hematocrit or hemoglobin level

Q3 Live kidney donor: services associated with postoperative medical complications directly related to the donation

Dental Modifiers
ET Emergency services (dental procedures performed in emergency situations should show the modifier 'ET')

Dressings Modifiers
A1 Dressing for one wound

A2 Dressing for two wounds

A3 Dressing for three wounds

A4 Dressing for four wounds

A5 Dressing for five wounds

A6 Dressing for six wounds

A7 Dressing for seven wounds

A8 Dressing for eight wounds

A9 Dressing for nine or more wounds

Drug Modifiers
J1 Competitive acquisition program no-pay submission for a prescription number

J2 Competitive acquisition program, restocking of emergency drugs after emergency administration

J3 Competitive acquisition program (CAP), drug not available through CAP as written, reimbursed under average sales price methodology

JW Drug amount discarded/not administered to any patient

KD Drug or biological infused through DME

RD Drug provided to beneficiary, but not administered "incident-to"

Genetic Testing Modifiers
The ten disease categories are:

0 Neoplasia (solid tumor, excluding sarcoma and lymphoma)

1 Neoplasia (sarcoma)

2 Neoplasia (lymphoid/hematopoietic)

3 Non-neoplastic hematology/coagulation

4 Histocompatibility/blood typing/identity/micorsatellite

5 Neurologic, non-neoplastic

6 Muscular, non-neoplastic

7 Metabolic, other

8 Metabolic, transport

9 Metabolic-pharmacogenetics (9A-9L)

9 Dysmorphology (9M-9Z)

The modifiers are:

0A BRCA1 (Hereditary breast/ovarian cancer)

0B BRCA1 (Hereditary breast cancer)

0C Neurofibromin (Neurofibromatosis, type 1)

0D Merlin (Neurofibromatosis, type 2)

0E c-RET (Multiple endocrine neoplasia, types 2A/B, familial medullary thyroid carcinoma)

0F VHL (Von Hippel Lindau disease)

0G SDHD (Hereditary paraganglioma)

0H SDHB (Hereditary paraganglioma)

0I ERRB2, commonly called Her-2/neu

0J MLH1 (HNPCC mismatch repair genes)

0K MSH2, MSH6, or PMS2 (HNPCC, mismatch repair genes)

0L APC (Hereditary polyposis coli)

0M Rb (Retinoblastoma)

0N TP53, commonly called p53

0O PTEN (Cowden's syndrome0

0P KIT, also called CD 117 (gastrointestinal stromal tumor)

0Z Solid tumor gene, not otherwise specified

1A WT1 or WT2 (Wilm's tumor)

1B PAX3, PAX7, or FOX01A (Alveolar rhabdomyosarcoma)

1C FLI1, ERG, ETV1, or EWSR1 (Ewing's sarcoma, desmoplastic round cell)

1D DDIT3 or FUS (Myxoid liposarcoma)

1E NR4A3, RBF56, or TCF12 (Myxoid chondrosarcoma)

1F SSX1, SSX2, or SYT (Synovial sarcoma)

1G MYCN (Neuroblastoma)

1H COL1A1 or PDGFB (Dermatofibrosarcoma protuberans)

1I TFE3 or ASPSCR1 (Alveolar soft parts sarcoma)

1J JAZF1 or JJAZ1 (Endometrial stromal sarcoma)

1Z Solid tumor, not otherwise specified

2A RUNX1 or CBFA2T1, commonly called AML1 or ETO, (genes associated with t(8;21) AML1–also ETO (Acute myeloid leukemia)

2B BCR–also ABL, genes associated with t(9;22) (Chronic myelogenous or acute leukemia)_ BCR—also ABL (Chronic myeloid, acute lymphoid leukemia)

2C PBX1 or TCF3, genes associated with t(1;19) (Acaute lymphoblastic leukemia)CGF-1

2D CBFB or MYH11, genes associated with inv 16 (AQcute myelogenous leukemia)CBF beta (Leukemia)

2E MML (Leukemia)

2F PML or RARAgenes associated with t(15;17) (Acute promyelocytic leukemia)PML/RAR alpha (Promyelocytic leukemia)

2G ETV6, commonly called TEL, gene associated with t(12;210 (acute leukemia)TEL (Leukemia)

2H BCL2 (B cell lymphoma, follicle center cell origin) bcl-2 (Lymphoma)

2I CCND1, commonly called BCL1, cyclin D1 (Mantle cell lymphoma, myeloma) bcl-1 (Lymphoma)

2J MYC (Burkitt lymphoma) c-myc (Lymphoma)

2K IgH (Lymphoma/leukemia)

2L IGK (Lymphoma/leukemia)

2M TRB, T cell receptor beta (Lymphoma/leukemia)

2N TRG, T cell receptor gamma (Lymphoma/leukemia)

2O SIL or TAL1 (T cell leukemia)

2T BCL6 (B cell lymphoma)

2Q API1 or MALT1 (MALT lymphoma)

2R NPM or ALK, genes associated with t(2;5)

2S FLT3 (Acute myelogenous leukemia)

2Z Lymphoid/hematopoetic neoplasia, not otherwise specified

3A F5, commonly called Factor V (Leiden, others) (Hypercoagulable state)

3B FACC (Fanconi anemia)

3C FACD (Fanconi anemia)

3D HBB, Beta globin (Thalassemia, Sickle cell anemia, other hemoglobinopathies)

3E HBA, commonly called alpha globin (thalassemia)

3F MTHFR (Elevated homocysteine)

3G F2, commonly called prothrombin (20210, others) (Hypercoagulable state)Prothrombin (Factor II, 20210A) (Hypercoagulable state)

3H F8, commonly called Factor VII (Hemophilia A/VWF)

3I F9, commonly called Factor IX (Hemophilia B)

3K F13, commonly called Factor XII (bleeding or hypercoagulable state) Beta globin

3Z Non-neoplastic hematology/coagulation, not otherwise specified

4A HLA-A

4B HLA-B

4C HLA-C

4D HLA-D

4E HLA-DR

4F HLA-DQ

4G HLA-DP

4H Kell

4I Fingerprint for engraftment (post-allogenic progenitor cell transplant)

4J Fingerprint for donor allelotype (allogeneic transplant)

4K Fingerprint for recipient allelotype (allogeneic transplant)

4L fingerprint for leukocyte chimerism (allogeneic solid organ transplant)

4M fingerprint for maternal versus fetal origin

4N Microsatellite instability

4O Microsatelite loss (loss of heterozygosity)

4Z Histocompatibility/blood typing, not otherwise specified

5A ASPA, commonly calledAspartoacylase A (Canavan disease)

5B FMR-1 (Fragile X, FRAXA, syndrome)

5C FRDA, commonly calledFrataxin (Freidreich's ataxia)

5D HD, commonly called Huntington (Huntington's disease)

5E GABRA, NIPA1, UBE3A, or ANCR GABRA (Prader Willi-Angelman syndrome)

5F GJB2, commonly called Connexin-26 (Hereditary hearing loss) Connexin-26 (GJB2) (Hereditary deafness)

5G GJB1, commonly calledConnexin-32 (X-linked Charcot-Marie-Tooth disease)

5H SNRPN (Prader Willi-Angelman syndrome)

5I SCA1, commonly called Ataxin-1 (Spinocerebellar ataxia, type 1)

5J SCA2, commonly calledAtaxin-2 (Spinocerebellar ataxia, type 2)

5K MJD, commonly called Ataxin-3 (Spinocerebellar ataxia, type 3, Machado-Joseph disease)

5L CACNA1A (Spinocerebellar ataxia, type 6)

5M ATXN7 Ataxin-7 (Spinocerebellar ataxia, type 7)

5N PMP-22 (Charcot-Marie-Tooth disease, type 1A)

5O MECP1 (Rett syndrome)

5Z Neurologic, non-neoplastic, not otherwise specified

6A DMD, commonly called Dystrophin (Duchenne/Becker muscular dystrophy)

6B DMPK (Myotonic dystrophy, type 1)

6C ZNF-9 (Myotonic dystrophy, type 2)

6D SMN1/SMN2 (Autosomal recessive spinal muscular atrophy)

6E MTTK, commonly called tRNAlys (mytonic epilepsy, MERRF)

6F MTTL1, commonly called tRNAleu (mitochondrial encephalomyopathy, MELAS)

6Z Muscular, not otherwise specified

7A APOE, commonly calledApolipoprotein E (Cardiovascular disease, Alzheimer's disease)

7B NPC1 or NPC2, commonly called sphingomyelin phosphodiesterase (Nieman-Pick disease)

7C GBA, commonly called Acid Beta Glucosidase (Gaucher disease)

7D HFE (Hemochromatosis)

7E HEXA, commonly called Hexosaminidase A (Tay-Sachs disease)

7F ACADM (medium chain acyl CoA dhydrogenase deficiency)

7Z Metabolic, other, not otherwise specified

8A CFTR (Cystic fibrosis)

8B PRSS1 (Hereditary pancreatitis)

8Z Metabolic, transport, not otherwise specified)

9A TPMT (thiopurine methyltransferase) (patients on antimetabolite therapy)

9B CYP2 genes, commonly called cytochrome p450 (drug metabolism)

9C ABCB1, commonly called MDR1 or p-glycoprotein (drug transport)

9D NAT2 (drug metabolism)

9L Metabolic-pharmacogenetics, not otherwise specified

9M FGFR-1 (Pfeiffer and Kallmann syndromes)

9N FGFR2 (Crouzon, Jackson-Weiss, Apert, Saethre-Chotzen syndromes)

9O FGFR3 (Achondroplasia, Hypochondroplasia, Thanatophoric dysplasia, types I and II, Crouzon syndrome with acanthosis nigricans, Muencke syndromes)

9P TWIST (Saethre-Chotzen syndrome)

9Q DCGR, commonly called CATCH-22 (22q11 deletion syndromes)

9Z Dysmorphology, not otherwise specified

APPENDIX B — NEW, CHANGED, DELETED, AND MODIFIED CODES

The following lists include codes ear-marked as new, changed, and deleted. Codes specified as add-on, exempt from Modifier 51 and 63, and include conscious sedation are listed. The lists are designed to be read left to right rather than vertically.

New Codes

0012F 00625 00626 0155T 0156T 0157T 0158T
0159T 0160T 0161T 0162T 0163T 0164T 0165T
0166T 0167T 0168T 0169T 0170T 0171T 0172T
0173T 0174T 0175T 0176T 0177T 0505F 0507F
1015F 1018F 1019F 1022F 1026F 1030F 1034F
1035F 1036F 1038F 1039F 1040F 15002 15003
15004 15005 15731 15830 15847 17311 17312
17313 17314 17315 19105 19300 19301 19302
19303 19304 19305 19306 19307 2010F 2014F
2018F 2022F 2024F 2026F 2028F 2030F 2031F
22526 22527 22857 22862 22865 25109 25606
25607 25608 25609 27325 27326 28055 3006F
3011F 3014F 3017F 3020F 3021F 3022F 3023F
3025F 3027F 3028F 3035F 3037F 3040F 3042F
3046F 3047F 3048F 3049F 3050F 3060F 3061F
3062F 3066F 3072F 3076F 3077F 3078F 3079F
3080F 3082F 3083F 3084F 3085F 3088F 3089F
3090F 3091F 3092F 3093F 32998 33202 33203
33254 33255 33256 33265 33266 33675 33676
33677 33724 33726 35302 35303 35304 35305
35306 35537 35538 35539 35540 35637 35638
35883 35884 37210 4025F 4030F 4033F 4035F
4037F 4040F 4045F 4050F 4051F 4052F 4053F
4054F 4055F 4056F 4058F 4060F 4062F 4064F
4065F 4066F 4067F 43647 43648 43881 43882
44157 44158 47719 48105 48548 49324 49325
49326 49402 49435 49436 54865 55875 55876
56442 57296 57558 58541 58542 58543 58544
58548 58957 58958 6005F 64910 64911 67346
70554 70555 72291 72292 76776 76813 76814
76998 77001 77002 77003 77011 77012 77013
77014 77021 77022 77031 77032 77051 77052
77053 77054 77055 77056 77057 77058 77059
77071 77072 77073 77074 77075 77076 77077
77078 77079 77080 77081 77082 77083 77084
77371 77372 77373 77435 82107 83688 83913
86788 86789 87305 87498 87640 87641 87653
87808 91111 92025 92640 94002 94003 94004
94005 94610 94644 94645 94774 94775 94776
94777 95012 96020 96040 96904 99363 99364

Changed Codes

0001F 0005F 00326 00561 0062T 0063T 0068T
0069T 0070T 0093T 0096T 01230 01232 01234 01340
01360 0148T 0149T 0150T 0151T 0153T 01905
0500F 0501F 0502F 0503F 1000F 1002F 1003F
1004F 1005F 1006F 1007F 1008F 15110 15111
15115 15116 15120 15121 15130 15131 15135
15136 15152 15157 15170 15171 15175 15176
15300 15301 15320 15321 15330 15331 15335
15336 15360 15361 15365 15366 15400 15401
15420 15421 15430 15431 15832 15833 15834
15835 15836 15837 15838 15839 17000 17003
17004 17110 17111 17380 19120 19361 2000F
2001F 2002F 2004F 22220 22222 22224 22226
22532 22533 22534 25600 26170 26180 31601
33681 35301 35501 35506 35509 35601 36400
36405 36406 36420 36440 36555 36557 36560
36568 36570 4000F 4001F 4002F 4003F 4006F
4009F 4011F 4012F 4015F 4016F 4017F 4018F
42820 42825 42830 42835 44211 49491 49492
49495 49496 49500 49501 49505 49507 49580
49582 49585 49587 51720 52204 54150 54160
54161 58140 58145 58146 58260 58262 58263
58267 58270 58950 58951 58952 61105 61107
61210 64590 64595 69633 69637 70540 70542
70543 71275 72285 72295 76506 76536 76604
76645 76700 76705 76770 76775 76856 76857
76880 76940 77327 77328 78700 78701 78707
78708 78709 78710 78730 78761 82105 82106
82652 87088 88106 88107 89060 90465 90466
90655 90656 90657 90658 90669 90700 90702
90714 90715 90718 90732 90761 90766 90921
90922 90925 92601 92602 94620 96415 96423
99191 99192 99218 99251 99252 99253 99254
99255

Deleted Codes

0003T 0008T 0018T 0021T 0044T 0045T 0082T
0083T 0091T 0094T 0097T 0120T 0152T 01995
1001F 15000 15001 15831 17304 17305 17306
17307 17310 19140 19160 19162 19180 19182
19200 19220 19240 2003F 21300 25611 25620
26504 27315 27320 28030 3000F 3002F 31700
31708 31710 33200 33201 33245 33246 33253
35381 35507 35541 35546 35641 44152 44153
47716 48005 48180 49085 54152 54820 55859
56720 57820 67350 75998 76003 76005 76006
76012 76013 76020 76040 76061 76062 76065
76066 76070 76071 76075 76076 76077 76078
76082 76083 76086 76088 76090 76091 76092
76093 76094 76095 76096 76355 76360 76362
76370 76393 76394 76400 76778 76986 78704
78715 78760 91060 92573 94656 94657 95078

Add-On Codes

0049T 0054T 0055T 0056T 0063T 0068T 0069T
0070T 0076T 0079T 0081T 0092T 0095T 0098T
0117T 0153T 0159T 0163T 0164T 0165T 01953
01968 01969 11001 11008 11101 11201 11732
11922 13102 13122 13133 13153 15003 15005
15101 15111 15116 15121 15131 15136 15151
15152 15156 15157 15171 15176 15201 15221
15241 15261 15301 15321 15331 15336 15341
15361 15366 15401 15421 15431 15787 15831
15847 16036 17003 17312 17314 17315 19001
19126 19291 19295 19297 22103 22116 22216
22226 22328 22522 22525 22527 22534 22585
22614 22632 26125 26861 26863 27358 27692
31620 31632 31633 31637 32501 33141 33225
33508 33530 33572 33768 33884 33924 33961
34808 34813 34826 35306 35390 35400 35500
35572 35681 35682 35683 35685 35686 35697
35700 36218 36248 36476 36479 37185 37186
37206 37208 37250 37251 38102 38746 38747
43635 44015 44121 44128 44139 44203 44213
44701 44955 47001 47550 48400 49435 49568
49905 56606 57267 58110 58611 59525 60512
61316 61517 61609 61610 61611 61612 61641
61642 61795 61864 61868 62148 62160 63035
63043 63044 63048 63057 63066 63076 63078
63082 63086 63088 63091 63103 63295 63308
64472 64476 64480 64484 64623 64627 64727
64778 64783 64787 64832 64837 64859 64872
64874 64876 64901 64902 66990 67225 67320
67331 67332 67334 67335 67340 69990 74301
75774 75946 75964 75968 75993 75996 76802
76125 76802 76810 76812 76814 76937 77001
77051 77052 78020 78478 78480 78496 78730
83901 87187 87904 88155 88185 88311 88312
88313 88314 90466 90468 90472 90474 90761
90766 90767 90768 90775 92547 92608 92627
92973 92974 92978 92979 92981 92984 92996
92998 93320 93321 93325 93571 93572 93609
93613 93621 93622 93623 93662 94645 95873
95874 95920 95962 95967 95973 95975 95979
96411 96415 96417 96423 96570 96571 97546
97811 97814 99100 99116 99135 99140 99145
99290 99292 99354 99355 99356 99357 99358
99359 99602

Modifier 51 Exempt Codes

17004 20660 20690 20692 20900 20902 20910
20912 20920 20922 20924 20926 20930 20931
20936 20937 20938 20974 20975 22840 22841
22842 22843 22844 22845 22846 22847 22848
22851 31500 32000 32002 32020 33517 33518
33519 33521 33522 33523 35600 36620 36660
38792 44500 61107 61210 62284 90281 90283
90287 90288 90291 90296 90371 90375 90376
90378 90379 90384 90385 90386 90389 90393
90396 90399 90476 90477 90581 90585 90586
90632 90633 90634 90636 90645 90646 90647
90648 90649 90655 90656 90657 90658 90660
90665 90669 90675 90676 90680 90690 90691
90692 90693 90698 90700 90701 90702 90703
90704 90705 90706 90707 90708 90710 90712
90713 90714 90715 90716 90717 90718 90719
90720 90721 90723 90725 90727 90732 90733
90734 90735 90736 90740 90743 90744 90746
90747 90748 90749 93501 93503 93505 93508
93510 93511 93514 93524 93526 93527 93528
93529 93530 93531 93532 93533 93539 93540
93541 93542 93543 93544 93545 93555 93556

93600	93602	93603	93610	93612	93615	93616
93618	93619	93620	93624	93631	93640	93641
93642	93650	93651	93652	93660	94610	95900
95903	95904	99143	99144	99148	99149	

Modifier 63 Exempt Codes

30540	30545	31520	33401	33403	33470	33472
33502	33503	33505	33506	33610	33611	33619
33647	33670	33690	33694	33730	33732	33735
33736	33750	33755	33762	33778	33786	33922
33960	33961	36415	36420	36450	36460	36510
36660	39503	43313	43314	43520	43831	44055
44126	44127	44128	46070	46705	46715	46716
46730	46735	46740	46742	46744	47700	47701
49215	49491	49492	49495	49496	49600	49605
49606	49610	49611	53025	54000	54150	54160
63700	63702	63704	63706	65820		

Conscious Sedation Codes

19298	20982	22526	22527	31615	31620	31622
31623	31624	31625	31628	31629	31635	31645
31646	31656	31725	32019	32020	32201	33010
33011	33206	33207	33208	33210	33211	33212
33213	33214	33216	33217	33218	33220	33222
33223	33233	33234	33235	33240	33241	33244
33249	35470	35471	35472	35473	35474	35475
35476	36555	36557	36558	36560	36561	36563
36565	36566	36568	36570	36571	36576	36578
36581	36582	36583	36585	36590	36870	37184
37185	37186	37187	37188	37203	37215	37216

43200	43201	43202	43204	43205	43215	43216
43217	43219	43220	43226	43227	43228	43231
43232	43234	43235	43236	43237	43238	43239
43240	43241	43242	43243	43244	43245	43246
43247	43248	43249	43250	43251	43255	43256
43257	43258	43259	43260	43261	43262	43263
43264	43265	43267	43268	43269	43271	43272
43453	43456	43458	43750	44360	44361	44363
44364	44365	44366	44369	44370	44372	44373
44376	44377	44378	44379	44380	44382	44383
44385	44386	44388	44389	44390	44391	44392
44393	44394	44397	44500	44901	45303	45305
45307	45308	45309	45315	45317	45320	45321
45327	45332	45333	45334	45335	45337	45338
45339	45340	45341	45342	45345	45355	45378
45379	45380	45381	45382	45383	45384	45385
45386	45387	45391	45392	47011	48511	49021
49041	49061	50021	50382	50384	50387	50592
58823	66720	69300	77600	77605	77610	77615
92953	92960	92961	92973	92974	92975	92978
92979	92980	92981	92982	92984	92986	92987
92995	92996	93312	93313	93314	93315	93316
93317	93318	93501	93505	93508	93510	93511
93514	93524	93526	93527	93528	93529	93530
93539	93540	93541	93542	93543	93544	93545
93555	93556	93561	93562	93571	93572	93609
93613	93615	93616	93618	93619	93620	93621
93622	93624	93640	93641	93642	93650	93651
93652						

APPENDIX C — PLACE OF SERVICE AND TYPE OF SERVICE

Place of Service Codes for Professional Claims

Database (last updated September 1, 2006)

Listed below are place of service codes and descriptions. These codes should be used on professional claims to specify the entity where service(s) were rendered. Check with individual payers (e.g., Medicare, Medicaid, other private insurance) for reimbursement policies regarding these codes. If you would like to comment on a code(s) or description(s), please send your request to posinfo@cms.hhs.gov.

01	Pharmacy	A facility or location where drus and other medically related items and services are sold, dispensed, or otherwise provided directly to patients.
02	Unassigned	N/A
03	School	A facility whose primary purpose is education.
04	Homeless Shelter	A facility or location whose primary purpose is to provide temporary housing to homeless individuals (e.g., emergency shelters, individual or family shelters).
05	Indian Health Service Free-standing Facility	A facility or location, owned and operated by the Indian Health Service, which provides diagnostic, therapeutic (surgical and non-surgical), and rehabilitation services to American Indians and Alaska Natives who do not require hospitalization.
06	Indian Health Service Provider-based Facility	A facility or location, owned and operated by the Indian Health Service, which provides diagnostic, therapeutic (surgical and non-surgical), and rehabilitation services rendered by, or under the supervision of, physicians to American Indians and Alaska Natives admitted as inpatients or outpatients.
07	Tribal 638 Free-standing Facility	A facility or location owned and operated by a federally recognized American Indian or Alaska Native tribe or tribal organization under a 638 agreement, which provides diagnostic, therapeutic (surgical and non-surgical), and rehabilitation services to tribal members who do not require hospitalization.
08	Tribal 638 Provider-based Facility	A facility or location owned and operated by a federally recognized American Indian or Alaska Native tribe or tribal organization under a 638 agreement, which provides diagnostic, therapeutic (surgical and non-surgical), and rehabilitation services to tribal members admitted as inpatients or outpatients.
09	Prison/Correctional Facility	A prison, jail, reformatory, work farm, detention center, or any other similar facility maintained by either Federal, State or local authorities for the purpose of confinement or rehabilitation of adult or juvenile criminal offenders. (effective July 1, 2006)
10	Unassigned	N/A
11	Office	Location, other than a hospital, skilled nursing facility (SNF), military treatment facility, community health center, State or local public health clinic, or intermediate care facility (ICF), where the health professional routinely provides health examinations, diagnosis, and treatment of illness or injury on an ambulatory basis.
12	Home	Location, other than a hospital or other facility, where the patient receives care in a private residence.
13	Assisted Living Facility	Congregate residential facility with self-contained living units providing assessment of each resident's needs and on-site support 24 hours a day, 7 days a week, with the capacity to deliver or arrange for services including some health care and other services.
14	Group Home	A residence, with shared living areas, where clients receive supervision and other services such as social and/or behavioral services, custodial service, and minimal services (e.g., medication administration).
15	Mobile Unit	A facility/unit that moves from place-to-place equipped to provide preventive, screening, diagnostic, and/or treatment services.
16-19	Unassigned	N/A
20	Urgent Care Facility	Location, distinct from a hospital emergency room, an office, or a clinic, whose purpose is to diagnose and treat illness or injury for unscheduled, ambulatory patients seeking immediate medical attention.
21	Inpatient Hospital	A facility, other than psychiatric, which primarily provides diagnostic, therapeutic (both surgical and nonsurgical), and rehabilitation services by, or under, the supervision of physicians to patients admitted for a variety of medical conditions.

22	Outpatient Hospital	A portion of a hospital which provides diagnostic, therapeutic (both surgical and nonsurgical), and rehabilitation services to sick or injured persons who do not require hospitalization or institutionalization.
23	Emergency Room - Hospital	A portion of a hospital where emergency diagnosis and treatment of illness or injury is provided.
24	Ambulatory Surgical Center	A freestanding facility, other than a physician's office, where surgical and diagnostic services are provided on an ambulatory basis.
25	Birthing Center	A facility, other than a hospital's maternity facilities or a physician's office, which provides a setting for labor, delivery, and immediate post-partum care as well as immediate care of new born infants.
26	Military Treatment Facility	A medical facility operated by one or more of the Uniformed Services. Military Treatment Facility (MTF) also refers to certain former U.S. Public Health Service (USPHS) facilities now designated as Uniformed Service Treatment Facilities (USTF).
27-30	Unassigned	N/A
31	Skilled Nursing Facility	A facility which primarily provides inpatient skilled nursing care and related services to patients who require medical, nursing, or rehabilitative services but does not provide the level of care or treatment available in a hospital.
32	Nursing Facility	A facility which primarily provides to residents skilled nursing care and related services for the rehabilitation of injured, disabled, or sick persons, or, on a regular basis, health-related care services above the level of custodial care to other than mentally retarded individuals.
33	Custodial Care Facility	A facility which provides room, board and other personal assistance services, generally on a long-term basis, and which does not include a medical component.
34	Hospice	A facility, other than a patient's home, in which palliative and supportive care for terminally ill patients and their families are provided.
35-40	Unassigned	N/A
41	Ambulance - Land	A land vehicle specifically designed, equipped and staffed for lifesaving and transporting the sick or injured.
42	Ambulance - Air or Water	An air or water vehicle specifically designed, equipped and staffed for lifesaving and transporting the sick or injured.
43-48	Unassigned	N/A
49	Independent Clinic	A location, not part of a hospital and not described by any other Place of Service code, that is organized and operated to provide preventive, diagnostic, therapeutic, rehabilitative, or palliative services to outpatients only.
50	Federally Qualified Health Center	A facility located in a medically underserved area that provides Medicare beneficiaries preventive primary medical care under the general direction of a physician.
51	Inpatient Psychiatric Facility	A facility that provides inpatient psychiatric services for the diagnosis and treatment of mental illness on a 24-hour basis, by or under the supervision of a physician.
52	Psychiatric Facility-Partial Hospitalization	A facility for the diagnosis and treatment of mental illness that provides a planned therapeutic program for patients who do not require full time hospitalization, but who need broader programs than are possible from outpatient visits to a hospital-based or hospital-affiliated facility.
53	Community Mental Health Center	A facility that provides the following services: outpatient services, including specialized outpatient services for children, the elderly, individuals who are chronically ill, and residents of the CMHC's mental health services area who have been discharged from inpatient treatment at a mental health facility; 24 hour a day emergency care services; day treatment, other partial hospitalization services, or psychosocial rehabilitation services; screening for patients being considered for admission to State mental health facilities to determine the appropriateness of such admission; and consultation and education services.
54	Intermediate Care Facility/Mentally Retarded	A facility which primarily provides health-related care and services above the level of custodial care to mentally retarded individuals but does not provide the level of care or treatment available in a hospital or SNF.

55	Residential Substance Abuse Treatment Facility	A facility which provides treatment for substance (alcohol and drug) abuse to live-in residents who do not require acute medical care. Services include individual and group therapy and counseling, family counseling, laboratory tests, drugs and supplies, psychological testing, and room and board.
56	Psychiatric Residential Treatment Center	A facility or distinct part of a facility for psychiatric care which provides a total 24-hour therapeutically planned and professionally staffed group living and learning environment.
57	Non-residential Substance Abuse Treatment Facility	A location which provides treatment for substance (alcohol and drug) abuse on an ambulatory basis. Services include individual and group therapy and counseling, family counseling, laboratory tests, drugs and supplies, and psychological testing.
58-59	Unassigned	N/A
60	Mass Immunization Center	A location where providers administer pneumococcal pneumonia and influenza virus vaccinations and submit these services as electronic media claims, paper claims, or using the roster billing method. This generally takes place in a mass immunization setting, such as, a public health center, pharmacy, or mall but may include a physician office setting.
61	Comprehensive Inpatient Rehabilitation Facility	A facility that provides comprehensive rehabilitation services under the supervision of a physician to inpatients with physical disabilities. Services include physical therapy, occupational therapy, speech pathology, social or psychological services, and orthotics and prosthetics services.
62	Comprehensive Outpatient Rehabilitation Facility	A facility that provides comprehensive rehabilitation services under the supervision of a physician to outpatients with physical disabilities. Services include physical therapy, occupational therapy, and speech pathology services.
63-64	Unassigned	N/A
65	End-Stage Renal Disease Treatment Facility	A facility other than a hospital, which provides dialysis treatment, maintenance, and/or training to patients or caregivers on an ambulatory or home-care basis.
66-70	Unassigned	N/A

71	Public Health Clinic	A facility maintained by either State or local health departments that provides ambulatory primary medical care under the general direction of a physician. (effective 10/1/03)
72	Rural Health Clinic	A certified facility which is located in a rural medically underserved area that provides ambulatory primary medical care under the general direction of a physician.
73-80	Unassigned	N/A
81	Independent Laboratory	A laboratory certified to perform diagnostic and/or clinical tests independent of an institution or a physician's office.
82-98	Unassigned	N/A
99	Other Place of Service	Other place of service not identified above.

Type of Service

Common Working File Type of Service (TOS) Indicators

For submitting a claim to the Common Working File (CWF), use the following table to assign the proper TOS. Some procedures may have more than one applicable TOS. CWF will reject alerts on codes with incorrect TOS designations. CWF is rejecting claims with incorrect TOS designations.

The only exceptions to this table are:

- Surgical services billed with the ASC facility service modifier SG must be reported as TOS F. The indicator F does not appear on the TOS table because its use is dependent upon the use of the SG modifier.

- Surgical services billed with an assistant-at-surgery modifier (80-82, AS,) must be reported with TOS 8. The 8 indicator does not appear on the TOS table because its use is dependent upon the use of the appropriate modifier. (See Medicare Claims Processing Manual, Chapter 12, "Physician/Practitioner Billing," for instructions on when assistant-at-surgery is allowable.)

- Psychiatric treatment services that are subject to the outpatient mental health treatment limitation should be reported with TOS T.

- TOS H appears in the list of descriptors. However, it does not appear in the table. In CWF, "H" is used only as an indicator for hospice. The carrier should not submit TOS H to CWF at this time.

- When these specific transfusion medicine codes appear on the claim (86880, 86885, 86886, 86900, 86903, 86904, 86905, and 86906 that also contains a blood product (P9010-P9022)), the transfusion medicine codes are paid under reasonable charge. When these services are to be paid under reasonable charge, use TOS 1. When paid under reasonable charge, tests are paid at 80 percent. Coinsurance and deductible also apply.

NOTE: For injection codes with more than one possible TOS designation, use the following guidelines when assigning the TOS:

When the choice is L or 1,

- Use TOS L when the drug is used related to ESRD; or

- Use TOS 1 when the drug is not related to ESRD and is administered in the office.

When the choice is G or 1:

- Use TOS G when the drug is an immunosuppressive drug; or

- Use TOS 1 when the drug is used for other than immunosuppression.

When the choice is P or 1,

- Use TOS P if the drug is administered through durable medical equipment (DME); or

- Use TOS 1 if the drug is administered in the office.

The place of service or diagnosis may be considered when determining the appropriate TOS. The descriptors for each of the TOS codes listed in the following table are:

0   Whole Blood

1   Medical Care

2   Surgery

3   Consultation

4   Diagnostic Radiology

5   Diagnostic Laboratory

6   Therapeutic Radiology

7   Anesthesia

8   Assistant at Surgery

9   Other Medical Items or Services

A   Used DME

B   High Risk Screening Mammography

C   Low Risk Screening Mammography

D   Ambulance

E   Enteral/Parenteral Nutrients/Supplies

F   Ambulatory Surgical Center (Facility Usage for Surgical Services)

G   Immunosuppressive Drugs

H   Hospice

J   Diabetic Shoes

K   Hearing Items and Services

L   ESRD Supplies

M   Monthly Capitation Payment for Dialysis

N   Kidney Donor

P   Lump Sum Purchase of DME, Prosthetics, Orthotics

Q   Vision Items or Services

R   Rental of DME

S   Surgical Dressings or Other Medical Supplies

T   Outpatient Mental Health Treatment Limitation

U   Occupational Therapy

V   Pneumococcal/Flu Vaccine

W   Physical Therapy

Berenson-Eggers Type of Service (BETOS) Codes

The BETOS coding system was developed primarily for analyzing the growth in Medicare expenditures. The coding system covers all HCPCS codes; assigns a HCPCS code to only one BETOS code; consists of readily understood clinical categories (as opposed to statistical or financial categories); consists of categories that permit objective assignment; is stable over time; and is relatively immune to minor changes in technology or practice patterns.

BETOS CODES AND DESCRIPTIONS:

1. Evaluation And Management

    1.   M1A Office Visits—New

    2.   M1B Office Visits—Established

    3.   M2A Hospital Visit—Initial

    4.   M2B Hospital Visit—Subsequent

    5.   M2C Hospital Visit—Critical Care

    6.   M3 Emergency Room Visit

    7.   M4A Home Visit

    8.   M4B Nursing Home Visit

    9.   M5A Specialist—Pathology

    10. M5B Specialist—Psychiatry

    11. M5C Specialist—Ophthalmology

    12. M5D Specialist—Other

    13. M6 Consultations

2. Procedures

    1.   P0 Anesthesia

    2.   P1A Major Procedure—Breast

    3.   P1B Major Procedure—Colectomy

    4.   P1C Major Procedure—Cholecystectomy

    5.   P1D Major Procedure—Turp

    6.   P1E Major Procedure—Hysterectomy

    7.   P1F Major Procedure—Explor/Decompr/Excisdisc

    8.   P1G Major Procedure—Other

    9.   P2A Major Procedure, Cardiovascular—CABG

    10. P2B Major Procedure, Cardiovascular—Aneurysm Repair

    11. P2C Major Procedure, Cardiovascular—Thromboendarterectomy

    12. P2D Major Procedure, Cardiovascular—Coronary Angioplasty (PTCA)

    13. P2E Major Procedure, Cardiovascular—Pacemaker Insertion

    14. P2F Major Procedure, Cardiovascular—Other

    15. P3Aa Major Procedure, Orthopedic—Hip Fracture Repair

    16. P3B Major Procedure, Orthopedic—Hip Replacement

    17. P3C Major Procedure, Orthopedic—Knee Replacement

    18. P3D Major Procedure, Orthopedic—Other

    19. P4A Eye Procedure—Corneal Transplant

    20. P4B Eye Procedure—Cataract Removal/Lens Insertion

    21. P4C Eye Procedure—Retinal Detachment

    22. P4D Eye Procedure—Treatment Of Retinal Lesions

    23. P4E Eye Procedure—Other

    24. P5A Ambulatory Procedures—Skin

    25. P5B Ambulatory Procedures—Musculoskeletal

    26. P5C Ambulatory Procedures—Inguinal Hernia Repair

    27. P5D Ambulatory Procedures—Lithotripsy

    28. P5E Ambulatory Procedures—Other

    29. P6A Minor Procedures—Skin

    30. P6B Minor Procedures—Musculoskeletal

    31. P6C Minor Procedures—Other (Medicare Fee Schedule)

    32. P6D Minor Procedures—Other (Non-Medicare Fee Schedule)

    33. P7A Oncology—Radiation Therapy

    34. P7B Oncology—Other

    35. P8A Endoscopy—Arthroscopy

    36. P8B Endoscopy—Upper Gastrointestinal

    37. P8C Endoscopy—Sigmoidoscopy

    38. P8D Endoscopy—Colonoscopy

    39. P8E Endoscopy—Cystoscopy

    40. P8F Endoscopy—Bronchoscopy

41. P8G Endoscopy—Laparoscopic Cholecystectomy

42. P8H Endoscopy—Laryngoscopy

43. P8I Endoscopy—Other

44. P9A Dialysis Services (Medicare Fee Schedule)

45. P9B Dialysis Services (Non-Medicare Fee Schedule)

3. Imaging

1. I1A Standard Imaging—Chest

2. I1B Standard Imaging—Musculoskeletal

3. I1C Standard Imaging—Breast

4. I1D Standard Imaging—Contrast Gastrointestinal

5. I1E Standard Imaging—Nuclear Medicine

6. I1F Standard Imaging—Other

7. I2A Advanced Imaging—CAT/CT/CTA; Brain/Head/Neck

8. I2B Advanced Imaging—CAT/CT/CTA; Other

9. I2C Advanced Imaging—MRI/MRA; Brain/Head/Neck

10. I2D Advanced Imaging—MRI/MRA; Other

11. I3A Echography—Eye

12. I3B Echography—Abdomen/Pelvis

13. I3C Echography—Heart

14. I3D Echography—Carotid Arteries

15. I3E Echography—Prostate, Transrectal

16. I3F Echography—Other

17. I4A Imaging/Procedure—Heart,Including Cardiac Catheterization

18. I4B Imaging/Procedure—Other

4. Tests

1. T1A Lab Tests—Routine Venipuncture (Non-Medicare Fee Schedule)

2. T1B Lab Tests—Automated General Profiles

3. T1C Lab Tests—Urinalysis

4. T1D Lab Tests—Blood Counts

5. T1E Lab Tests—Glucose

6. T1F Lab Tests—Bacterial Cultures

7. T1G Lab Tests—Other (Medicare Fee Schedule)

8. T1H Lab Tests—Other (Non-Medicare Fee Schedule)

9. T2A Other Tests—Electrocardiograms

10. T2B Other Tests—Cardiovascular Stress Tests

11. T2C Other Tests—Ekg Monitoring

12. T2D Other Tests—Other

5. Durable Medical Equipment

1. D1A Medical/Surgical Supplies

2. D1B Hospital Beds

3. D1C Oxygen And Supplies

4. D1D Wheelchairs

5. D1E Other DME

6. D1F Orthotic Devices

7. D1G Drugs Administered through DME

6. Other

1. O1A Ambulance

2. O1B Chiropractic

3. O1C Enteral And Parenteral

4. O1D Chemotherapy

5. O1E Other Drugs

6. O1F Vision, Hearing And Speech Services

7. O1G Influenza Immunization

7. Exceptions/Unclassified

1. Y1 Other—Medicare Fee Schedule

2. Y2 Other—Non-Medicare Fee Schedule

3. Z1 Local Codes

4. Z2 Undefined Codes

APPENDIX D — PUB 100 REFERENCES
REVISIONS TO THE CMS MANUAL SYSTEM

The Centers for Medicare and Medicaid Services (CMS) initiated its long awaited transition from a paper-based manual system to a Web-based system on October 1, 2003, which updates and restructures all manual instructions. The new system, called the online CMS Manual system, combines all of the various program instructions into an electronic manual, which can be found at http://www.cms.hhs.gov/manuals.

Effective September 30, 2003, the former method of publishing program memoranda (PMs) to communicate program instructions was replaced by the following four templates:

- One-time notification:

- Manual revisions:

- Business requirement:

- Confidential requirements:

The Office of Strategic Operations and Regulatory Affairs (OSORA), Division of Issuances, will continue to communicate advanced program instructions to the regions and contractor community every Friday as it currently does. These instructions will also contain a transmittal sheet to identify changes pertaining to a specific manual, requirement, or notification.

The Web-based system has been organized by functional area (e.g., eligibility, entitlement, claims processing, benefit policy, program integrity) in an effort to eliminate redundancy within the manuals, simplify the updating process, and make CMS program instructions available in a more timely manner. The initial release will include Pub. 100, Pub. 100-02, Pub. 100-03, Pub. 100-04, Pub. 100-05, Pub. 100-09, Pub. 100-15, and Pub. 100-20.

The Web-based system contains the functional areas included in the table below:

Publication #	Title
Pub. 100	Introduction
Pub. 100-1	Medicare General Information, Eligibility, and Entitlement
Pub. 100-2	Medicare Benefit Policy (basic coverage rules)
Pub. 100-3	Medicare National Coverage Determinations (national coverage decisions)
Pub. 100-4	Medicare Claims Processing (includes appeals, contractor interface with CWF, and MSN)
Pub. 100-5	Medicare Secondary Payer
Pub. 100-6	Medicare Financial Management (includes Intermediary Desk Review and Audit)
Pub. 100-7	Medicare State Operations
Pub. 100-8	Medicare Program Integrity
Pub. 100-9	Medicare Contractor Beneficiary and Provider Communications
Pub. 100-10	Medicare Quality Improvement Organization
Pub. 100-11	Reserved
Pub. 100-12	State Medicaid
Pub. 100-13	Medicaid State Children's Health Insurance Program
Pub. 100-14	Medicare End Stage Renal Disease Network
Pub. 100-15	Medicare State Buy-In
Pub. 100-16	Medicare Managed Care
Pub. 100-17	Medicare Business Partners Systems Security
Pub. 100-18	Medicare Business Partners Security Oversight
Pub. 100-19	Demonstrations
Pub. 100-20	One-Time Notification

Table of Contents

The table below shows the paper-based manuals used to construct the Web-based system. Although this is just an overview, CMS is in the process of developing detailed crosswalks to guide you from a specific section of the old manuals to the appropriate area of the new manual, as well as to show how the information in each section was derived.

Paper-Based Manuals	Internet-Only Manuals
Pub. 06 — Medicare Coverage Issues	Pub. 100-01 — Medicare General Information, Eligibility, and Entitlement
Pub. 09 — Medicare Outpatient Physical Therapy	Pub. 100-02 — Medicare Benefit Policy
Pub. 10 — Medicare Hospital	Pub. 100-03 — Medicare National Coverage Determinations
Pub. 11 — Medicare Home Health Agency	Pub. 100-04 — Medicare Claims Processing
Pub. 12 — Medicare Skilled Nursing Facility	Pub. 100-05 — Medicare Secondary Payer
Pub. 13 — Medicare Intermediary Manual, Parts 1, 2, 3, and 4	Pub. 100-06 — Medicare Financial Management
Pub. 14 — Medicare Carriers Manual, Parts 1, 2, 3, and 4	Pub. 100-08 — Medicare Program Integrity
Pub. 21 — Medicare Hospice	Pub. 100-09 — Medicare Contractor Beneficiary and Provider Communications
Pub. 27 — Medicare Rural Health Clinic and Federally Qualified Health Center	
Pub. 29 — Medicare Renal Dialysis Facility	

Program Memoranda

Pub. 60A — Intermediaries
Pub. 60B — Carriers
Pub. 60AB — Intermediaries/Carriers
NOTE: Information derived from Pub. 06 to Pub. 60AB was used to develop Pub. 100-01 to Pub. 100-09 for the Internet-only manual.

Paper-Based Manuals	Internet-Only Manuals
Pub. 19 — Medicare Peer Review	Pub. 100-10 — Medicare Quality Organization Improvement Organization
Pub. 07 — Medicare State Operations	Pub. 100-07 — Medicare State Operations
Pub. 45 — State Medicaid	Pub. 100-12 — State Medicaid
Pub. 81 — Medicare End Stage Renal Disease	Pub. 100-13 — Medicaid State Children's Health Insurance Program
Pub. 24 — Medicare State Buy-In	Pub. 100-14 — Medicare End Stage Renal Disease Network Organizations Network Organizations
Pub. 75 — Health Maintenance Organization/Competitive Medical Plan Care	Pub. 100-15 — Medicare State Buy-In
Pub. 76 — Health Maintenance Organization/Competitive Medical Plan (PM)	Pub. 100-16 — Medicare Managed

Paper-Based Manuals	Internet-Only Manuals
Pub. 77 — Manual for Federally Qualified Health Maintenance Organizations	Pub. 100-17 — Business Partners Systems Security
Pub. 13 — Medicare Intermediaries Manual, Part 2	Pub. 100-18 — Business Partners Security Oversight
Pub. 14 — Medicare Carriers Manual, Part 2	Pub 100-19 — Demonstrations
Pub. 13 — Medicare Intermediaries Manual, Part 2	Pub 100-20 — One-Time
Pub. 14 — Medicare Carriers Manual, Part 2	
Demonstrations (PMs)	

Program instructions that impact multiple manuals or have no manual impact.

NATIONAL COVERAGE DETERMINATIONS MANUAL

The National Coverage Determinations Manual (NCD), which is the electronic replacement for the Coverage Issues Manual (CIM), is organized according to categories such as diagnostic services, supplies, and medical procedures. The table of contents lists each category and subject within that category. A revision transmittal sheet will identify any new material and recap the changes as well as provide an effective date for the change and any background information. At any time, one can refer to a transmittal indicated on the page of the manual to view this information.

By the time it is complete, the book will contain two chapters. Chapter 1 includes a description of national coverage determinations that have been made by CMS. When available, chapter 2 will contain a list of HCPCS codes related to each coverage determination. To make the manual easier to use, it is organized in accordance with CPT category sequences. Where there is no national coverage determination that affects a particular CPT category, the category is listed as reserved in the table of contents.

The following table is the crosswalk of the NCD to the CIM. However, at this time, many of the NCD policies are not yet available. The CMS Web site also contains a crosswalk of the CIM to the NCD.

MEDICARE BENEFIT POLICY MANUAL

The Medicare Benefit Policy Manual replaces current Medicare general coverage instructions that are not national coverage determinations. As a general rule, in the past these instructions have been found in chapter II of the Medicare Carriers Manual, the Medicare Intermediary Manual, other provider manuals, and program memoranda. New instructions will be published in this manual. As new transmittals are included they will be identified.

On the CMS Web site, a crosswalk from the new manual to the source manual is provided with each chapter and may be accessed from the chapter table of contents. In addition, the crosswalk for each section is shown immediately under the section heading.

The list below is the table of contents for the Medicare Benefit Policy Manual:

Chapter	Title
One	Inpatient Hospital Services
Two	Inpatient Psychiatric Hospital Services
Three	Duration of Covered Inpatient Services
Four	Inpatient Psychiatric Benefit Days Reduction and Lifetime Limitation
Five	Lifetime Reserve Days
Six	Hospital Services Covered Under Part B
Seven	Home Health Services
Eight	Coverage of Extended Care (SNF) Services Under Hospital Insurance
Chapter	Title
Nine	Coverage of Hospice Services Under Hospital Insurance
Ten	Ambulance Services
Eleven	End Stage Renal Disease (ESRD)
Twelve	Comprehensive Outpatient Rehabilitation Facility (CORF) Coverage
Thirteen	Rural Health Clinic (RHC) and Federally Qualified Health Center (FQHC) Services
Fourteen	Medical Devices
Fifteen	Covered Medical and Other Health Services
Sixteen	General Exclusions from Coverage

PUB100 REFERENCES

Pub. 100-1, Chapter 3, Section 20.5

Blood Deductibles (Part A and Part B)

Program payment may not be made for the first 3 pints of whole blood or equivalent units of packed red cells received under Part A and Part B combined in a calendar year. However, blood processing (e.g., administration, storage) is not subject to the deductible.

The blood deductibles are in addition to any other applicable deductible and coinsurance amounts for which the patient is responsible.

The deductible applies only to the first 3 pints of blood furnished in a calendar year, even if more than one provider furnished blood.

Pub. 100-1, Chapter 3, Section 20.5.2

Part B Blood Deductible

Blood is furnished on an outpatient basis or is subject to the Part B blood deductible and is counted toward the combined limit. It should be noted that payment for blood may be made to the hospital under Part B only for blood furnished in an outpatient setting. Blood is not covered for inpatient Part B services.

Pub. 100-1, Chapter 3, Section 20.5.3

Items Subject to Blood Deductibles

The blood deductibles apply only to whole blood and packed red cells. The term whole blood means human blood from which none of the liquid or cellular components have been removed. Where packed red cells are furnished, a unit of packed red cells is considered equivalent to a pint of whole blood. Other components of blood such as platelets, fibrinogen, plasma, gamma globulin, and serum albumin are not subject to the blood deductible. However, these components of blood are covered as biologicals.

Refer to Pub. 100-04, Medicare Claims Processing Manual, chapter 4, §231 regarding billing for blood and blood products under the Hospital Outpatient Prospective Payment System (OPPS).

Pub. 100-1, Chapter 3, Section 30

Outpatient Mental Health Treatment Limitation

Regardless of the actual expenses a beneficiary incurs for treatment of mental, psychoneurotic, and personality disorders while the beneficiary is not an inpatient of a hospital at the time such expenses are incurred, the amount of those expenses that may be recognized for Part B deductible and payment purposes is limited to 62.5 percent of the Medicare allowed amount for these services. The limitation is called the outpatient mental health treatment limitation. Since Part B deductible also applies the program pays for about half of the allowed amount recognized for mental health therapy services.

Expenses for diagnostic services (e.g., psychiatric testing and evaluation to diagnose the patient's illness) are not subject to this limitation. This limitation applies only to therapeutic services and to services performed to evaluate the progress of a course of treatment for a diagnosed condition.

Pub. 100-1, Chapter 3, Section 30.1

Status of Patient

The limitation is applicable to expenses incurred in connection with the treatment of an individual who is not an inpatient of a hospital. Thus, the limitation applies to mental health services furnished to a person in a physician's office, in the patient's home, in a skilled nursing facility, as an outpatient, and so forth. The term "hospital" in this context means an institution which is primarily engaged in providing to inpatients, by or under the supervision of a physician(s):

- Diagnostic and therapeutic services for medical diagnosis, and treatment, and care of injured, disabled, or sick persons;

- Rehabilitation services for injured, disabled, or sick persons; or

- Psychiatric services for the diagnosis and treatment of mentally ill patients.

Pub. 100-1, Chapter 3, Section 30.2

Disorders Subject to Mental Health Limitation

The term "mental, psychoneurotic, and personality disorders" is defined as the specific psychiatric conditions described in the American Psychiatric Association's Diagnostic and Statistical Manual of Mental Disorders, Third Edition - Revised (DSM-III-R).

If the treatment services rendered are for both a psychiatric condition and one or more nonpsychiatric conditions, the charges are separated to apply the limitation only to the mental health charge. Normally HCPCS code and diagnoses are used. Where HCPCS code is not available on the claim, revenue code is used.

If the service is primarily on the basis of a diagnosis of Alzheimer's Disease (coded 331.0 in the International Classification of Diseases, 9th Revision) or Alzheimer's or other disorders (coded 290.XX in DSM-III-R), treatment typically represents medical management of the patient's condition (rather than psychiatric treatment) and is not subject to the limitation.

Pub. 100-1, Chapter 3, Section 30.3

Diagnostic Services

The mental health limitation does not apply to tests and evaluations performed to establish or confirm the patient's diagnosis. Diagnostic services include psychiatric or psychological tests and interpretations, diagnostic consultations, and initial evaluations. However, testing services performed to evaluate a patient's progress during treatment are considered part of treatment and are subject to the limitation.

Pub. 100-1, Chapter 5, Section 70

Physician means doctor of medicine, doctor of osteopathy (including osteopathic practitioner), doctor of dental surgery or dental medicine (within the limitations in subsection §70.2), doctor of podiatric medicine (within the limitations in subsection §70.3), or doctor of optometry (within the limitations of subsection §70.5), and, with respect to certain specified treatment, a doctor of chiropractic legally authorized to practice by a State in which he/she performs this function. The services performed by a physician within these definitions are subject to any limitations imposed by the State on the scope of practice.

The issuance by a State of a license to practice medicine constitutes legal authorization. Temporary State licenses also constitute legal authorization to practice medicine. If State law authorizes local political subdivisions to establish higher standards for medical practitioners than those set by the State licensing board, the local standards determine whether a particular physician has legal authorization. If State licensing law limits the scope of practice of a particular type of medical practitioner, only the services within the limitations are covered.

The issuance by a State of a license to practice medicine constitutes legal authorization. Temporary State licenses also constitute legal authorization to practice medicine. If State law authorizes local political subdivisions to establish higher standards for medical practitioners than those set by the State licensing board, the local standards determine whether a particular physician has legal authorization. If State licensing law limits the scope of practice of a particular type of medical practitioner, only the services within the limitations are covered.

NOTE: The term physician does not include such practitioners as a Christian Science practitioner or naturopath.

Pub. 100-1, Chapter 5, Section 70.6

A. General

A licensed chiropractor who meets uniform minimum standards (see subsection C) is a physician for specified services. Coverage extends only to treatment by means of manual manipulation of the spine to correct a subluxation demonstrated by X-ray, provided such treatment is legal in the State where performed. All other services furnished or ordered by chiropractors are not covered. An X-ray obtained by a chiropractor for his or her own diagnostic purposes before commencing treatment may suffice for claims documentation purposes. This means that if a chiropractor orders, takes, or interprets an X-ray to demonstrate a subluxation of the spine, the X-ray can be used for claims processing purposes. However, there is no coverage or payment for these services or for any other diagnostic or therapeutic service ordered or furnished by the chiropractor.

In addition, in performing manual manipulation of the spine, some chiropractors use manual devices that are hand-held with the thrust of the force of the device being controlled manually. While such manual manipulation may be covered, there is no separate payment permitted for use of this device.

B. Licensure and Authorization to Practice

A chiropractor must be licensed or legally authorized to furnish chiropractic services by the State or jurisdiction in which the services are furnished.

C. Uniform Minimum Standards

I. Prior to July 1, 1974, Chiropractors licensed or authorized to practice prior to July 1, 1974, and those individuals who commenced their studies in a chiropractic college before that date must meet all of the following minimum standards to render payable services under the program:

a. Preliminary education equal to the requirements for graduation from an accredited high school or other secondary school;

b. Graduation from a college of chiropractic approved by the State's chiropractic examiners that included the completion of a course of study covering a period of not less than 3 school years of 6 months each year in actual continuous attendance covering adequate course of study in the subjects of anatomy, physiology, symptomatology and diagnosis, hygiene and sanitation, chemistry, histology, pathology, and principles and practice of chiropractic, including clinical instruction in vertebral palpation, nerve tracing and adjusting; and

c. Passage of an examination prescribed by the State's chiropractic examiners covering the subjects listed in subsection b.

2. After June 30, 1974 - Individuals commencing their studies in a chiropractic college after June 30, 1974, must meet all of the following additional requirements:

a. Satisfactory completion of 2 years of pre-chiropractic study at the college level;

b. Satisfactory completion of a 4-year course of 8 months each year (instead of a 3-year course of 6 months each year) at a college or school of chiropractic that includes not less than 4,000 hours in the scientific and chiropractic courses specified in subsection 1.b, plus courses in the use and effect of X-ray and chiropractic analysis; and

c. The practitioner must be over 21 years of age.

Pub. 100-1, Chapter 5, Section 90.2

Laboratory means a facility for the biological, microbiological, serological, chemical, immuno-hematological, hematological, biophysical, cytological, pathological, or other examination of materials derived from the human body for the purpose of providing information for the diagnosis, prevention, or treatment of any disease or impairment of, or the assessment of the health of, human beings. These examinations also include procedures to determine, measure, or otherwise describe the presence or absence of various substances or organisms in the body. Facilities only collecting or preparing specimens (or both) or only serving as a mailing service and not performing testing are not considered laboratories.

Pub. 100-2, Chapter 1, Section 10

Covered Inpatient Hospital Services Covered Under Part A

A3-3101, HO-210

Patients covered under hospital insurance are entitled to have payment made on their behalf for inpatient hospital services. (Inpatient hospital services do not include extended care services provided by hospitals pursuant to swing bed approvals. See Pub. 100-1, Chapter 8, §10.1, "Hospital Providers of Extended Care Services.") However, both inpatient hospital and inpatient SNF benefits are provided under Part A - Hospital Insurance Benefits for the Aged and Disabled, of Title XVIII).

Additional information concerning the following topics can be found in the following manual chapters:

- Benefit periods is found in Chapter 3, "Duration of Covered Inpatient Services";

- Copayment days is found in Chapter 2, "Duration of Covered Inpatient Services";

- Lifetime reserve days is found in Chapter 5, "Lifetime Reserve Days";

- Related payment information is housed in the Provider Reimbursement Manual.

Blood must be furnished on a day which counts as a day of inpatient hospital services to be covered as a Part A service and to count toward the blood deductible. Thus, blood is not covered under Part A and does not count toward the Part A blood deductible when furnished to an inpatient after the inpatient has exhausted all benefit days in a benefit period, or where the individual has elected not to use lifetime reserve days. However, where the patient is discharged on their first day of entitlement or on the hospital's first day of participation, the hospital is permitted to submit a billing form with no accommodation charge, but with ancillary charges including blood.

The records for all Medicare hospital inpatient discharges are maintained in CMS for statistical analysis and use in determining future PPS DRG classifications and rates.

Non-PPS hospitals do not pay for noncovered services generally excluded from coverage in the Medicare Program. This may result in denial of a part of the billed charges or in denial of the entire admission, depending upon circumstance. In PPS hospitals, the following are also possible:

1. In appropriately admitted cases where a noncovered procedure was performed, denied services may result in payment of a different DRG (i.e., one which excludes payment for the noncovered procedure); or

2. In appropriately admitted cases that become cost outlier cases, denied services may lead to denial of some or all of an outlier payment.

The following examples illustrate this principle. If care is noncovered because a patient does not need to be hospitalized, the intermediary denies the admission and makes no Part A (i.e., PPS) payment unless paid under limitation on liability. Under limitation on liability, Medicare payment may be made when the provider and the beneficiary were not aware the services were not necessary and could not reasonably be expected to know that he services were not necessary. For detailed instructions, see the Medicare Claims Processing Manual, Chapter 30,"Limitation on Liability." If a patient is appropriately hospitalized but receives (beyond routine services) only noncovered care, the admission is denied.

NOTE: The intermediary does not deny an admission that includes covered care, even if noncovered care was also rendered. Under PPS, Medicare assumes that it is paying for only the covered care rendered whenever covered services needed to treat and/or diagnose the illness were in fact provided.

If a noncovered procedure is provided along with covered nonroutine care, a DRG change rather than an admission denial might occur. If noncovered procedures are elevating costs into the cost outlier category, outlier payment is denied in whole or in part.

When the hospital is included in PPS, most of the subsequent discussion regarding coverage of inpatient hospital services is relevant only in the context of determining the appropriateness of admissions, which DRG, if any, to pay, and the appropriateness of payment for any outlier cases.

If a patient receives items or services in excess of, or more expensive than, those for which payment can be made, payment is made only for the covered items or services or for only the appropriate prospective payment amount. This provision applies not only to inpatient services, but also to all hospital services under Parts A and B of the program. If the items or services were requested by the patient, the hospital may charge him the difference between the amount customarily charged for the services requested and the amount customarily charged for covered services.

An inpatient is a person who has been admitted to a hospital for bed occupancy for purposes of receiving inpatient hospital services. Generally, a patient is considered an inpatient if formally admitted as inpatient with the expectation that he or she will remain at least overnight and occupy a bed even though it later develops that the patient can be discharged or transferred to another hospital and not actually use a hospital bed overnight.

The physician or other practitioner responsible for a patient's care at the hospital is also responsible for deciding whether the patient should be admitted as an inpatient. Physicians should use a 24-hour period as a benchmark, i.e., they should order admission for patients who are expected to need hospital care for 24 hours or more, and treat other patients on an outpatient basis. However, the decision to admit a patient is a complex medical judgment which can be made only after the physician has considered a number of factors, including the patient's medical history and current medical needs, the types of facilities available to inpatients and to outpatients, the hospital's by-laws and admissions policies, and the relative appropriateness of treatment in each setting. Factors to be considered when making the decision to admit include such things as:

- The severity of the signs and symptoms exhibited by the patient;

- The medical predictability of something adverse happening to the patient;

- The need for diagnostic studies that appropriately are outpatient services (i.e., their performance does not ordinarily require the patient to remain at the hospital for 24 hours or more) to assist in assessing whether the patient should be admitted; and

- The availability of diagnostic procedures at the time when and at the location where the patient presents.

Admissions of particular patients are not covered or noncovered solely on the basis of the length of time the patient actually spends in the hospital. In certain specific situations coverage of services on an inpatient or outpatient basis is determined by the following rules:

Minor Surgery or Other Treatment - When patients with known diagnoses enter a hospital for a specific minor surgical procedure or other treatment that is expected to keep them in the hospital for only a few hours (less than 24), they are considered outpatients for coverage purposes regardless of: the hour they came to the hospital, whether they used a bed, and whether they remained in the hospital past midnight.

Renal Dialysis - Renal dialysis treatments are usually covered only as outpatient services but may under certain circumstances be covered as inpatient services depending on the patient's condition. Patients staying at home, who are ambulatory, whose conditions are stable and who come to the hospital for routine chronic dialysis treatments, and not for a diagnostic workup or a change in therapy, are considered outpatients. On the other hand, patients undergoing short-term dialysis until their kidneys recover from an acute illness (acute dialysis), or persons with borderline renal failure who develop acute renal failure every time they have an illness and require dialysis (episodic dialysis) are usually inpatients. A patient may begin dialysis as an inpatient and then progress to an outpatient status.

Under original Medicare, the Quality Improvement Organization (QIO), for each hospital is responsible for deciding, during review of inpatient admissions on a case-by-case basis, whether the admission was medically necessary. Medicare law authorizes the QIO to make these judgments, and the judgments are binding for purposes of Medicare coverage. In making these judgments, however, QIOs consider only the medical evidence which was available to the physician at the time an admission decision had to be made. They do not take into account other information (e.g., test results) which became available only after admission, except in cases where considering the post-admission information would support a finding that an admission was medically necessary.

Refer to Parts 4 and 7 of the QIO Manual with regard to initial determinations for these services. The QIO will review the swing bed services in these PPS hospitals as well.

NOTE: When patients requiring extended care services are admitted to beds in a hospital, they are considered inpatients of the hospital. In such cases, the services furnished in the hospital will not be considered extended care services, and payment may not be made under the program for such services unless the services are extended care services furnished pursuant to a swing bed agreement granted to the hospital by the Secretary of Health and Human Services.

Pub. 100-2, Chapter 1, Section 90

Termination of Pregnancy

B3-4276.1,.2

Effective for services furnished on or after October 1, 1998, Medicare will cover abortions procedures in the following situations:

1. If the pregnancy is the result of an act or rape or incest; or

2. In the case where a woman suffers from a physical disorder, physical injury, or physical illness, including a life-endangering physical condition caused by the pregnancy itself that would, as certified by a physician, place the woman in danger of death unless an abortion is performed.

NOTE: The "G7" modifier must be used with the following CPT codes in order for these services to be covered when the pregnancy resulted from rape or incest, or the pregnancy is certified by a physician as life threatening to the mother:

59840

59841

59850

59851

59852

59855

59856

59857

59866

Pub. 100-2, Chapter 6, Section 10

Medical and Other Health Services Furnished to Inpatients of Participating Hospitals

Payment may be made under Part B for physician services and for the nonphysician medical and other health services listed below when furnished by a participating hospital (either directly or under arrangements) to an inpatient of the hospital, but only if payment for these services cannot be made under Part A.

In PPS hospitals, this means that Part B payment could be made for these services if:

- No Part A prospective payment is made at all for the hospital stay because of patient exhaustion of benefit days before admission;

- The admission was disapproved as not reasonable and necessary (and waiver of liability payment was not made);

- The day or days of the otherwise covered stay during which the services were provided were not reasonable and necessary (and no payment was made under waiver of liability);

- The patient was not otherwise eligible for or entitled to coverage under Part A (See the Medicare Benefit Policy Manual, Chapter 1, §150, for services received as a result of noncovered services); or

- No Part A day outlier payment is made (for discharges before October 1997) for one or more outlier days due to patient exhaustion of benefit days after admission but before the case's arrival at outlier status, or because outlier days are otherwise not covered and waiver of liability payment is not made.

However, if only day outlier payment is denied under Part A (discharges before October 1997), Part B payment may be made for only the services covered under Part B and furnished on the denied outlier days.

In non-PPS hospitals, Part B payment may be made for services on any day for which Part A payment is denied (i.e., benefit days are exhausted; services are not at the hospital level of care; or patient is not otherwise eligible or entitled to payment under Part A).

Services payable are:

- Diagnostic x-ray tests, diagnostic laboratory tests, and other diagnostic tests;

- X-ray, radium, and radioactive isotope therapy, including materials and services of technicians;

- Surgical dressings, and splints, casts, and other devices used for reduction of fractures and dislocations;

- Prosthetic devices (other than dental) which replace all or part of an internal body organ (including contiguous tissue), or all or part of the function of a permanently inoperative or malfunctioning internal body organ, including replacement or repairs of such devices;

- Leg, arm, back, and neck braces, trusses, and artificial legs, arms, and eyes including adjustments, repairs, and replacements required because of breakage, wear, loss, or a change in the patient's physical condition;

- Outpatient physical therapy, outpatient speech-language pathology services, and outpatient occupational therapy (see the Medicare Benefit Policy Manual, Chapter 15, "Covered Medical and Other Health Services," §§220 and 230);

- Screening mammography services;

- Screening pap smears;

- Influenza, pneumococcal pneumonia, and hepatitis B vaccines;

- Colorectal screening;

- Bone mass measurements;

- Diabetes self-management;

- Prostate screening;

- Ambulance services;

- Hemophilia clotting factors for hemophilia patients competent to use these factors without supervision);

- Immunosuppressive drugs;

- Oral anti-cancer drugs;

- Oral drug prescribed for use as an acute anti-emetic used as part of an anti-cancer chemotherapeutic regimen; and

- Epoetin Alfa (EPO).

Coverage rules for these services are described in the Medicare Benefit Policy Manual, Chapters 11, "End Stage Renal Disease (ESRD);" 14, "Medical Devices;" or 15, "Medical and Other Health Services."

For services to be covered under Part A or Part B, a hospital must furnish nonphysician services to its inpatients directly or under arrangements. A nonphysician service is one which does not meet the criteria defining physicians' services specifically provided for in regulation at 42 CFR 415.102. Services "incident to" physicians' services (except for the services of nurse anesthetists employed by anesthesiologists) are nonphysician services for purposes of this provision. This provision is applicable to all hospitals participating in Medicare, including those paid under alternative arrangements such as State cost control systems, and to emergency hospital services furnished by nonparticipating hospitals.

In all hospitals, every service provided to a hospital inpatient other than those listed in the next paragraph must be treated as an inpatient hospital service to be paid for under Part A, if Part A coverage is available and the beneficiary is entitled to Part A. This is because every hospital must provide directly or arrange for any nonphysician service rendered to its inpatients, and a hospital can be paid under Part B for a service provided in this manner only if Part A coverage does not exist.

These services, when provided to a hospital inpatient, may be covered under Part B, even though the patient has Part A coverage for the hospital stay. This is because these services are covered under Part B and not covered under Part A. They are:

Physicians' services (including the services of residents and interns in unapproved teaching programs);

Influenza vaccine;

Pneumoccocal vaccine and its administration;

Hepatitis B vaccine and its administration;

Screening mammography services;

Screening pap smears and pelvic exams;

Colorectal screening;

Bone mass measurements;

Diabetes self management training services; and

Prostate screening.

However, note that in order to have any Medicare coverage at all (Part A or Part B), any nonphysician service rendered to a hospital inpatient must be provided directly or arranged for by the hospital.

Pub. 100-2, Chapter 13, Section 30

Rural Health Clinic and Federally Qualified Health Center Service Defined

Payments for covered RHC/FQHC services furnished to Medicare beneficiaries are made on the basis of an all-inclusive rate per covered visit (except for pneumococcal and influenza vaccines and their administration, which is paid at 100 percent of reasonable cost). The term "visit" is defined as a face-to-face encounter between the patient and a physician, physician assistant, nurse practitioner, certified nurse midwife, visiting nurse, clinical psychologist, or clinical social worker during which an RHC/FQHC service is rendered. As a result of section 5114 of the Deficit Reduction Act of 2005 (DRA), the FQHC definition of a face-to-face encounter is expanded to include encounters with qualified practitioners of Outpatient Diabetes Self-Management Training Services (DSMT) and medical nutrition therapy (MNT) services when the FQHC meets all relevant program requirements for the provision of such services.

Encounters with (1) more than one health professional; and (2) multiple encounters with the same health professional which take place on the same day and at a single location, constitute a single visit. An exception occurs in cases in which the patient, subsequent to the first encounter, suffers an illness or injury requiring additional diagnosis or treatment.

Pub. 100-2, Chapter 15, Section 20.1

Physician Expense for Surgery, Childbirth, and Treatment for Infertility

B3-2005.l

A. Surgery and Childbirth

Skilled medical management is covered throughout the events of pregnancy, beginning with diagnosis, continuing through delivery and ending after the necessary postnatal care. Similarly, in the event of termination of pregnancy, regardless of whether terminated spontaneously or for therapeutic reasons (i.e., where the life of the mother would be endangered if the fetus were brought to term), the need for skilled medical management and/or medical services is equally important as in those cases carried to full term. After the infant is delivered and is a separate individual, items and services furnished to the infant are not covered on the basis of the mother's eligibility.

Most surgeons and obstetricians bill patients an all-inclusive package charge intended to cover all services associated with the surgical procedure or delivery of the child. All expenses for surgical and obstetrical care, including preoperative/prenatal examinations and tests and post-operative/postnatal services, are considered incurred on the date of surgery or delivery, as appropriate. This policy applies whether the physician bills on a package charge basis, or itemizes the bill separately for these items.

Occasionally, a physician's bill may include charges for additional services not directly related to the surgical procedure or the delivery. Such charges are considered incurred on the date the additional services are furnished.

The above policy applies only where the charges are imposed by one physician or by a clinic on behalf of a group of physicians. Where more than one physician imposes charges for surgical or obstetrical services, all preoperative/prenatal and post-operative/postnatal services performed by the physician who performed the surgery or delivery are considered incurred on the date of the surgery or delivery. Expenses for services rendered by other physicians are considered incurred on the date they were performed.

B. Treatment for Infertility

Reasonable and necessary services associated with treatment for infertility are covered under Medicare. Infertility is a condition sufficiently at variance with the usual state of health to make it appropriate for a person who normally is expected to be fertile to seek medical consultation and treatment.

Pub. 100-2, Chapter 15, Section 20.2

Physician Expense for Allergy Treatment

B3-2005.2, B3-4145

Allergists commonly bill separately for the initial diagnostic workup and for the treatment (See §60.2). Where it is necessary to provide treatment over an extended period, the allergist may submit a single bill for all of the treatments, or may bill periodically. In either case the Form CMS-1500 claim shows the Healthcare Common Procedure Coding System (HCPCS) codes and from and through dates of service, or the Form CMS-1450 outpatient claim shows the HCPCS code and date of service (except for critical access hospital (CAH) claims).

Pub. 100-2, Chapter 15, Section 20.3

Artificial Limbs, Braces, and Other Custom Made Items Ordered But Not Furnished

B3-2005.3

A. Date of Incurred Expense

If a custom-made item was ordered but not furnished to a beneficiary because the individual died or because the order was canceled by the beneficiary or because the beneficiary's condition changed and the item was no longer reasonable and necessary or appropriate, payment can be made based on the supplier's expenses. (See subsection B for determination of the allowed amount.) In such cases, the expense is considered incurred on the date the beneficiary died or the date the supplier learned of the cancellation or that the item was no longer reasonable and necessary or appropriate for the beneficiary's condition. If the beneficiary died or the beneficiary's condition changed and the item was no longer reasonable and necessary or appropriate, payment can be made on either an assigned or unassigned claim. If the beneficiary, for any other reason, canceled the order, payment can be made to the supplier only.

B. Determination of Allowed Amount

The allowed amount is based on the services furnished and materials used, up to the date the supplier learned of the beneficiary's death or of the cancellation or that the item was no longer reasonable and necessary or appropriate. The Durable Medical Equipment Regional Carrier (DMERC), carrier or intermediary, as appropriate, determines the services performed and the allowable amount appropriate in the particular situation. It takes into account any salvage value of the device to the supplier.

Where a supplier breaches an agreement to make a prosthesis, brace, or other custom-made device for a Medicare beneficiary, e.g., an unexcused failure to provide the article within the time specified in the contract, payment may not be made for any work or material expended on the item. Whether a particular supplier has lived up to its agreement, of course, depends on the facts in the individual case.

Pub. 100-2, Chapter 15, Section 30

Physician Services

B3-2020, B3-4142

A. General

Physician services are the professional services performed by a physician or physicians for a patient including diagnosis, therapy, surgery, consultation, and care plan oversight. The physician must render the service for the service to be covered. (See Publication 100-1, the Medicare General Information, Eligibility, and Entitlement Manual, Chapter 5, §70, for definition of physician.) A service may be considered to be a physician's service where the physician either examines the patient in person or is able to visualize some aspect of the patient's condition without the interposition of a third person's judgment. Direct visualization would be possible by means of x-rays, electrocardiogram and electroencephalogram tapes, tissue samples, etc.

For example, the interpretation by a physician of an actual electrocardiogram or electroencephalogram reading that has been transmitted via telephone (i.e., electronically rather than by means of a verbal description) is a covered service.

Professional services of the physician are covered if provided within the United States, and may be performed in a home, office, institution, or at the scene of an accident. A patient's home, for this purpose, is anywhere the patient makes his or her residence, e.g., home for the aged, a nursing home, a relative's home.

B. Telephone Services

Services by means of a telephone call between a physician and a beneficiary, or between a physician and a member of a beneficiary's family, are covered under Medicare, but carriers may not make separate payment for these services under the program. The physician work resulting from telephone calls is considered to be an integral part of the prework and postwork of other physician services, and the fee schedule amount for the latter services already includes payment for the telephone calls. See the Medicare Benefit Policy Manual, Chapter 15, "Covered Medical and Other Health Services," §270, for coverage of telehealth services.

C. Consultations

A consultation may be paid when the consulting physician initiates treatment on the same day as the consultation. It is only after a transfer of care has occurred that evaluation and management (E&M) services may not be billed as consultations; they must be billed as subsequent office/outpatient visits.

Therefore, if covered, a consultation is reimbursable when it is a professional service furnished a patient by a second physician at the request of the attending physician. Such a consultation includes the history and examination of the patient as well as the written report, which is furnished to the attending physician for inclusion in the patient's permanent medical record. These reports must be prepared and submitted to the provider for retention when they involve patients of institutions responsible for maintaining such records, and submitted to the attending physician's office for other patients.

To reimburse laboratory consultations, the services must:

- Be requested by the patient's attending physician;

- Relate to a test result that lies outside of the clinically significant normal or expected/established range relative to the condition of the patient;

- Result in a written narrative report included in the patient's medical record; and

- Require medical judgment by the consultant physician.

A consultation must involve a medical judgment that ordinarily requires a physician. Where a nonphysician laboratory specialist could furnish the information, the service of the physician is not a consultation payable under Part B.

The following indicators can ordinarily distinguish attending physician's claims:

- Therapeutic services are included on the bill in addition to an examination;

- The patient's history is before the examiner while the claim is reviewed and the billing physician has previously rendered other services to the patient; or

- Information in the file indicates that the patient was not referred.

The attending physician may remove himself from the care of the patient and turn the patient over to the person who performed a consultation service. In this situation, the initial examination would be a consultation if the above requirements were met at that time.

D. Patient-Initiated Second Opinions

Patient-initiated second opinions that relate to the medical need for surgery or for major nonsurgical diagnostic and therapeutic procedures (e.g., invasive diagnostic techniques such as cardiac catheterization and gastroscopy) are covered under Medicare. In the event that the recommendation of the first and second physician differs regarding the need for surgery (or other major procedure), a third opinion is also covered. Second and third opinions are covered even though the surgery or other procedure, if performed, is determined not covered. Payment may be made for the history and examination of the patient, and for other covered diagnostic services required to properly evaluate the patient's need for a procedure and to render a professional opinion. In some cases, the results of tests done by the first physician may be available to the second physician.

E. Concurrent Care

Concurrent care exists where more than one physician renders services more extensive than consultative services during a period of time. The reasonable and necessary services of each physician rendering concurrent care could be covered where each is required to play an active role in the patient's treatment, for example, because of the existence of more than one medical condition requiring diverse specialized medical services.

In order to determine whether concurrent physicians' services are reasonable and necessary, the carrier must decide the following:

1. Whether the patient's condition warrants the services of more than one physician on an attending (rather than consultative) basis, and

2. Whether the individual services provided by each physician are reasonable and necessary.

In resolving the first question, the carrier should consider the specialties of the physicians as well as the patient's diagnosis, as concurrent care is usually (although not always) initiated because of the existence of more than one medical condition requiring diverse specialized medical or surgical services. The specialties of the physicians are an indication of the necessity for concurrent services, but the patient's condition and the inherent reasonableness and necessity of the services, as determined by the carrier's medical staff in accordance with locality norms, must also be considered. For example, although cardiology is a sub-specialty of internal medicine, the treatment of both diabetes and of a serious heart condition might require the concurrent services of two physicians, each practicing in internal medicine but specializing in different sub-specialties.

While it would not be highly unusual for concurrent care performed by physicians in different specialties (e.g., a surgeon and an internist) or by physicians in different sub-specialties of the same specialty (e.g., an allergist and a cardiologist) to be found medically necessary, the need for such care by physicians in the same specialty or sub-specialty (e.g., two internists or two cardiologists) would occur infrequently since in most cases both physicians would possess the skills and knowledge necessary to treat the patient. However, circumstances could arise which would necessitate such care. For example, a patient may require the services of two physicians in the same specialty or sub-specialty when one physician has further limited his or her practice to some unusual aspect of that specialty, e.g., tropical medicine. Similarly, concurrent services provided by a family physician and an internist may or may not be found to be reasonable and necessary, depending on the circumstances of the specific case. If it is determined that the services of one of the physicians are not warranted by the patient's condition, payment may be made only for the other physician's (or physicians') services.

Once it is determined that the patient requires the active services of more than one physician, the individual services must be examined for medical necessity, just as where a single physician provides the care. For example, even if it is determined that the patient requires the concurrent services of both a cardiologist and a surgeon, payment may not be made for any services rendered by either physician which, for that condition, exceed normal frequency or duration unless there are special circumstances requiring the additional care.

The carrier must also assure that the services of one physician do not duplicate those provided by another, e.g., where the family physician visits during the post-operative period primarily as a courtesy to the patient.

Hospital admission services performed by two physicians for the same beneficiary on the same day could represent reasonable and necessary services, provided, as stated above, that the patient's condition necessitates treatment by both physicians. The level of difficulty of the service provided may vary between the physicians, depending on the severity of the complaint each one is treating and that physician's prior contact with the patient. For example, the admission services performed by a physician who has been treating a patient over a period of time for a chronic condition would not be as involved as the services performed by a physician who has had no prior contact with the patient and who has been called in to diagnose and treat a major acute condition.

Carriers should have sufficient means for identifying concurrent care situations. A correct coverage determination can be made on a concurrent care case only where the claim is sufficiently documented for the carrier to determine the role each physician played in the patient's care (i.e., the condition or conditions for which the physician treated the patient). If, in any case, the role of each physician involved is not clear, the carrier should request clarification.

F. Completion of Claims Forms

Separate charges for the services of a physician in completing a Form CMS-1500, a statement in lieu of a Form CMS-1500, or an itemized bill are not covered. Payment for completion of the Form CMS-1500 claim form is considered included in the fee schedule amount.

G. Care Plan Oversight Services

Care plan oversight is supervision of patients under care of home health agencies or hospices that require complex and multidisciplinary care modalities involving regular physician development and/or revision of care plans, review of subsequent reports of patient status, review of laboratory and other studies, communication with other health professionals not employed in the same practice who are involved in the patient's care, integration of new information into the care plan, and/or adjustment of medical therapy.

Such services are covered for home health and hospice patients, but are not covered for patients of skilled nursing facilities (SNFs), nursing home facilities, or hospitals.

These services are covered only if all the following requirements are met:

1. The beneficiary must require complex or multi-disciplinary care modalities requiring ongoing physician involvement in the patient's plan of care;

2. The care plan oversight (CPO) services should be furnished during the period in which the beneficiary was receiving Medicare covered HHA or hospice services;

3. The physician who bills CPO must be the same physician who signed the home health or hospice plan of care;

4. The physician furnished at least 30 minutes of care plan oversight within the calendar month for which payment is claimed. Time spent by a physician's nurse or the time spent consulting with one's nurse is not countable toward the 30-minute threshold. Low-intensity services included as part of other evaluation and management services are not included as part of the 30 minutes required for coverage;

5. The work included in hospital discharge day management (codes 99238-99239) and discharge from observation (code 99217) is not countable toward the 30 minutes per month required for work on the same day as discharge but only for those services separately documented as occurring after the patient is actually physically discharged from the hospital;

6. The physician provided a covered physician service that required a face-to-face encounter with the beneficiary within the six months immediately preceding the first care plan oversight service. Only evaluation and management services are acceptable prerequisite face-to-face encounters for CPO. EKG, lab, and surgical services are not sufficient face-to-face services for CPO;

7. The care plan oversight billed by the physician was not routine post-operative care provided in the global surgical period of a surgical procedure billed by the physician;

8. If the beneficiary is receiving home health agency services, the physician did not have a significant financial or contractual interest in the home health agency. A physician who is an employee of a hospice, including a volunteer medical director, should not bill CPO services. Payment for the services of a physician employed by the hospice is included in the payment to the hospice;

9. The physician who bills the care plan oversight services is the physician who furnished them;

10. Services provided incident to a physician's service do not qualify as CPO and do not count toward the 30-minute requirement;

11. The physician is not billing for the Medicare end stage renal disease (ESRD) capitation payment for the same beneficiary during the same month; and

12. The physician billing for CPO must document in the patient's record the services furnished and the date and length of time associated with those services.

Pub. 100-2, Chapter 15, Section 50

Drugs and Biologicals

B3-2049, A3-3112.4.B, HO-230.4.B

The Medicare program provides limited benefits for outpatient drugs. The program covers drugs that are furnished "incident to" a physician's service provided that the drugs are not usually self-administered by the patients who take them.

Generally, drugs and biologicals are covered only if all of the following requirements are met:

- They meet the definition of drugs or biologicals (see §50.1);

- They are of the type that are not usually self-administered. (see §50.2);

- They meet all the general requirements for coverage of items as incident to a physician's services (see §§50.1 and 50.3);

- They are reasonable and necessary for the diagnosis or treatment of the illness or injury for which they are administered according to accepted standards of medical practice (see §50.4);

- They are not excluded as noncovered immunizations (see §50.4.2); and

- They have not been determined by the FDA to be less than effective. (See §§50.4.4).

Medicare Part B does generally not cover drugs that can be self-administered, such as those in pill form, or are used for self-injection. However, the statute provides for the coverage of some self-administered drugs. Examples of self-administered drugs that are covered include blood-clotting factors, drugs used in immunosuppressive therapy, erythropoietin for dialysis patients, osteoporosis drugs for certain homebound patients, and certain oral cancer drugs. (See §110.3 for coverage of drugs, which are necessary to the effective use of Durable Medical Equipment (DME) or prosthetic devices.)

Pub. 100-2, Chapter 15, Section 50.5

Administered Drugs and Biologicals

B3-2049.5

Medicare Part B does not cover drugs that are usually self-administered by the patient unless the statute provides for such coverage. The statute explicitly provides coverage, for blood clotting factors, drugs used in immunosuppressive therapy, erythropoietin for dialysis patients, certain oral anti-cancer drugs and anti-emetics used in certain situations.

Pub. 100-2, Chapter 15, Section 60.3

Incident to Physician's Service in Clinic

B3-2050.3

Services and supplies incident to a physician's service in a physician directed clinic or group association are generally the same as those described above.

A physician directed clinic is one where:

1. A physician (or a number of physicians) is present to perform medical (rather than administrative) services at all times the clinic is open;

2. Each patient is under the care of a clinic physician; and

3. The nonphysician services are under medical supervision.

In highly organized clinics, particularly those that are departmentalized, direct physician supervision may be the responsibility of several physicians as opposed to an individual attending physician. In this situation, medical management of all services provided in the clinic is assured. The physician ordering a particular service need not be the physician who is supervising the service. Therefore, services performed by auxiliary personnel and other aides are covered even though they are performed in another department of the clinic.

Supplies provided by the clinic during the course of treatment are also covered. When the auxiliary personnel perform services outside the clinic premises, the services are covered only if performed under the direct supervision of a clinic physician. If the clinic refers a patient for auxiliary services performed by personnel who are not supervised by clinic physicians, such services are not incident to a physician's service.

Pub. 100-2, Chapter 15, Section 80

Ray, Diagnostic Laboratory, and Other Diagnostic Tests

B3-2070

This section describes the levels of physician supervision required for furnishing the technical component of diagnostic tests for a Medicare beneficiary who is not a hospital inpatient or outpatient. Section 410.32(b) of the Code of Federal Regulations (CFR) requires that diagnostic tests covered under §1861(s)(3) of the Act (the Act) and payable under the physician fee schedule, with certain exceptions listed in the regulation, have to be performed under the supervision of an individual meeting the definition of a physician (§1861(r) of the Act) to be considered reasonable and necessary and, therefore, covered under Medicare. The regulation defines these levels of physician supervision for diagnostic tests as follows:

General Supervision - means the procedure is furnished under the physician's overall direction and control, but the physician's presence is not required during the performance of the procedure. Under general supervision, the training of the nonphysician personnel who actually performs the diagnostic procedure and the maintenance of the necessary equipment and supplies are the continuing responsibility of the physician.

Direct Supervision - in the office setting means the physician must be present in the office suite and immediately available to furnish assistance and direction throughout the performance of the procedure. It does not mean that the physician must be present in the room when the procedure is performed.

Personal Supervision - means a physician must be in attendance in the room during the performance of the procedure.

One of the following numerical levels is assigned to each CPT or HCPCS code in the Medicare Physician Fee Schedule Database:

0	Procedure is not a diagnostic test or procedure is a diagnostic test which is not subject to the physician supervision policy.
1	Procedure must be performed under the general supervision of a physician.
2	Procedure must be performed under the direct supervision of a physician.
3	Procedure must be performed under the personal supervision of a physician.
4	Physician supervision policy does not apply when procedure is furnished by a qualified, independent psychologist or a clinical psychologist; otherwise must be performed under the general supervision of a physician.
5	Physician supervision policy does not apply when procedure is furnished by a qualified audiologist; otherwise must be performed under the general supervision of a physician.
6	Procedure must be performed by a physician or by a physical therapist (PT) who is certified by the American Board of Physical Therapy Specialties (ABPTS) as a qualified

electrophysiologic clinical specialist and is permitted to provide the procedure under State law.

6a	Supervision standards for level 66 apply; in addition, the PT with ABPTS certification may supervise another PT but only the PT with ABPTS certification may bill.
7a	Supervision standards for level 77 apply; in addition, the PT with ABPTS certification may supervise another PT but only the PT with ABPTS certification may bill.
9	Concept does not apply.
21	Procedure must be performed by a technician with certification under general supervision of a physician; otherwise must be performed under direct supervision of a physician.
22	Procedure may be performed by a technician with on-line real-time contact with physician.
66	Procedure must be performed by a physician or by a PT with ABPTS certification and certification in this specific procedure.
77	Procedure must be performed by a PT with ABPTS certification or by a PT without certification under direct supervision of a physician, or by a technician with certification under general supervision of a physician.

Nurse practitioners, clinical nurse specialists, and physician assistants are not defined as physicians under §1861(r) of the Act. Therefore, they may not function as supervisory physicians under the diagnostic tests benefit (§1861(s)(3) of the Act). However, when these practitioners personally perform diagnostic tests as provided under §1861(s)(2)(K) of the Act, §1861(s)(3) does not apply and they may perform diagnostic tests pursuant to State scope of practice laws and under the applicable State requirements for physician supervision or collaboration.

Because the diagnostic tests benefit set forth in §1861(s)(3) of the Act is separate and distinct from the incident to benefit set forth in §1861(s)(2) of the Act, diagnostic tests need not meet the incident to requirements. Diagnostic tests may be furnished under situations that meet the incident to requirements but this is not required. However, carriers must not scrutinize claims for diagnostic tests utilizing the incident to requirements.

Pub. 100-2, Chapter 15, Section 80.1

Clinical Laboratory Services

B3-2070.1

Section 1833 and 1861 of the Act provides for payment of clinical laboratory services under Medicare Part B. Clinical laboratory services involve the biological, microbiological, serological, chemical, immunohematological, hematological, biophysical, cytological, pathological, or other examination of materials derived from the human body for the diagnosis, prevention, or treatment of a disease or assessment of a medical condition. Laboratory services must meet all applicable requirements of the Clinical Laboratory Improvement Amendments of 1988 (CLIA), as set forth at 42 CFR part 493. Section 1862(a)(1)(A) of the Act provides that Medicare payment may not be made for services that are not reasonable and necessary. Clinical laboratory services must be ordered and used promptly by the physician who is treating the beneficiary as described in 42 CFR 410.32(a), or by a qualified nonphysician practitioner, as described in 42 CFR 410.32(a)(3).

See the Medicare Claims Processing Manual Chapter 16 for related claims processing instructions.

Pub. 100-2, Chapter 15, Section 80.2

Psychological Tests and Neuropsychological Tests

Medicare Part B coverage of psychological tests and neuropsychological tests is authorized under section 1861(s)(2)(C) of the Social Security Act. Payment for psychological and neuropsychological tests is authorized under section 1842(b)(2)(A) of the Social Security Act. The payment amounts for the new psychological and neuropsychological tests (CPT codes 96102, 96103, 96119 and 96120) that are effective January 1, 2006, and are billed for tests administered by a technician or a computer reflect a site of service payment differential for the facility and non-facility settings. Additionally, there is no authorization for payment for diagnostic tests when performed on an "incident to" basis.

Under the diagnostic tests provision, all diagnostic tests are assigned a certain level of supervision. Generally, regulations governing the diagnostic tests provision require that only physicians can provide the assigned level of supervision for diagnostic tests. However, there is a regulatory exception to the supervision requirement for diagnostic psychological and neuropsychological tests in terms of who can provide the supervision. That is, regulations allow a clinical psychologist (CP) or a physician to perform the general supervision assigned to diagnostic psychological and neuropsychological tests.

In addition, nonphysician practitioners such as nurse practitioners (NPs), clinical nurse specialists (CNSs) and physician assistants (PAs) who personally perform diagnostic psychological and neuropsychological tests are excluded from having to perform these tests under the general supervision of a physician or a CP. Rather, NPs and CNSs must perform such tests under the requirements of their respective benefit instead of the requirements for diagnostic psychological and neuropsychological tests. Accordingly, NPs and CNSs must perform tests in collaboration (as defined under Medicare law at section 1861(aa)(6) of the Act) with a physician. PAs perform tests under the general supervision of a physician as required for services furnished under the PA benefit.

Furthermore, physical therapists (PTs), occupational therapists (OTs) and speech language pathologists (SLPs) are authorized to bill three test codes as "sometimes therapy" codes. Specifically, CPT codes 96105, 96110 and 96111 may be performed by these therapists. However, when PTs, OTs and SLPs perform these three tests, they must be performed under the general supervision of a physician or a CP.

Who May Bill for Diagnostic Psychological and Neuropsychological Tests

- CPs — see qualifications under chapter 15, section 160 of the Benefits Policy Manual, Pub. 100-02.
- NPs — to the extent authorized under State scope of practice. See qualifications under chapter 15, section 200 of the Benefits Policy Manual, Pub. 100-02.
- CNSs — to the extent authorized under State scope of practice. See qualifications under chapter 15, section 210 of the Benefits Policy Manual, Pub. 100-02.
- PAs — to the extent authorized under State scope of practice. See qualifications under chapter 15, section 190 of the Benefits Policy Manual, Pub. 100-02.
- Independently Practicing Psychologists (IPPs)
- PTs, OTs and SLPs — see qualifications under chapter 15, sections 220-230.6 of the Benefits Policy Manual, Pub. 100-02.

Psychological and neuropsychological tests performed by a psychologist (who is not a CP) practicing independently of an institution, agency, or physician's office are covered when a physician orders such tests. An IPP is any psychologist who is licensed or certified to practice psychology in the State or jurisdiction where furnishing services or, if the jurisdiction does not issue licenses, if provided by any practicing psychologist. (It is CMS' understanding that all States, the District of Columbia, and Puerto Rico license psychologists, but that some trust territories do not. Examples of psychologists, other than CPs, whose psychological and neuropsychological tests are covered under the diagnostic tests provision include, but are not limited to, educational psychologists and counseling psychologists.)

The carrier must secure from the appropriate State agency a current listing of psychologists holding the required credentials to determine whether the tests of a particular IPP are covered under Part B in States that have statutory licensure or certification. In States or territories that lack statutory licensing or certification, the carrier checks individual qualifications before provider numbers are issued. Possible reference sources are the national directory of membership of the American Psychological Association, which provides data about the educational background of individuals and indicates which members are board-certified, the records and directories of the State or territorial psychological association, and the National Register of Health Service Providers. If qualification is dependent on a doctoral degree from a currently accredited program, the carrier verifies the date of accreditation of the school involved, since such accreditation is not retroactive. If the listed reference sources do not provide enough information (e.g., the psychologist is not a member of one of these sources), the carrier contacts the psychologist personally for the required information. Generally, carriers maintain a continuing list of psychologists whose qualifications have been verified.

NOTE: When diagnostic psychological tests are performed by a psychologist who is not practicing independently, but is on the staff of an institution, agency, or clinic, that entity bills for the psychological tests.

The carrier considers psychologists as practicing independently when:

- They render services on their own responsibility, free of the administrative and professional control of an employer such as a physician, institution or agency;
- The persons they treat are their own patients; and
- They have the right to bill directly, collect and retain the fee for their services.

A psychologist practicing in an office located in an institution may be considered an independently practicing psychologist when both of the following conditions exist:

- The office is confined to a separately-identified part of the facility which is used solely as the psychologist's office and cannot be construed as extending throughout the entire institution; and
- The psychologist conducts a private practice, i.e., services are rendered to patients from outside the institution as well as to institutional patients.

Payment for Diagnostic Psychological and Neuropsychological Tests

Expenses for diagnostic psychological and neuropsychological tests are not subject to the outpatient mental health treatment limitation, that is, the payment limitation on treatment services for mental, psychoneurotic and personality disorders as authorized under Section 1833(c) of the Act. The payment amount for the new psychological and neuropsychological tests (CPT codes 96102, 96103, 96119 and 96120) that are billed for tests performed by a technician or a computer reflect a site of service payment differential for the facility and non-facility settings. CPs, NPs, CNSs and PAs are required by law to accept assigned payment for psychological and neuropsychological tests. However, while IPPs are not required by law to accept assigned payment for these tests, they must report the name and address of the physician who ordered the test on the claim form when billing for tests.

CPT Codes for Diagnostic Psychological and Neuropsychological Tests

The range of CPT codes used to report psychological and neuropsychological tests is 96101-96120. CPT codes 96101, 96102, 96103, 96105, 96110, and 96111 are appropriate for use when billing for psychological tests. CPT codes 96116, 96118, 96119 and 96120 are appropriate for use when billing for neuropsychological tests.

All of the tests under this CPT code range 96101-96120 are indicated as active codes under the physician fee schedule database and are covered if medically necessary.

Payment and Billing Guidelines for Psychological and Neuropsychological Tests

The technician and computer CPT codes for psychological and neuropsychological tests include practice expense, malpractice expense and professional work relative value units. Accordingly, CPT psychological test code 96101 should not be paid when billed for the same tests or services performed under psychological test codes 96102 or 96103. CPT neuropsychological test code 96118 should not be paid when billed for the same tests or services performed under neuropsychological test codes 96119 or 96120. However, CPT codes 96101 and 96118 can be paid separately on the rare occasion when billed on the same date of service for different and separate tests from 96102, 96103, 96119 and 96120.

Under the physician fee schedule, there is no payment for services performed by students or trainees. Accordingly, Medicare does not pay for services represented by CPT codes 96102 and 96119 when performed by a student or a trainee. However, the presence of a student or a trainee while the test is being administered does not prevent a physician, CP, IPP, NP, CNS or PA from performing and being paid for the psychological test under 96102 or the neuropsychological test under 96119.

Pub. 100-2, Chapter 15, Section 80.3

Otologic Evaluations

B3-2070.3, PM-B-01-34, B-02-004, PM AB-02-080

Diagnostic testing, including hearing and balance assessment services, performed by a qualified audiologist is covered as "other diagnostic tests" under §1861(s)(3) of the Act when a physician orders such testing for the purpose of obtaining information necessary for the physician's diagnostic evaluation or to determine the appropriate medical or surgical treatment of a hearing deficit or related medical problem. Services are excluded by virtue of §1862(a)(7) of the Act when the diagnostic information required to determine the appropriate medial or surgical treatment is already known to the physician, or the diagnostic services are performed only to determine the need for or the appropriate type of hearing aid.

Diagnostic services performed by a qualified audiologist and meeting the above requirements are payable as "other diagnostic tests". The payment for these services is determined by the reason the tests were performed, rather than the diagnosis or the patient's condition. Payment for these services is based on the physician fee schedule amount except for audiology services furnished in a hospital outpatient department which are paid under the Outpatient Prospective Payment System. Nonhospital entities billing for the audiologist's services may accept assignment under the usual procedure or, if not accepting assignment, may charge the patient and submit a nonassigned claim on their behalf.

If a physician refers a beneficiary to an audiologist for evaluation of signs or symptoms associated with hearing loss or ear injury, the audiologist's diagnostic services should be covered even if the only outcome is the prescription of a hearing aid. If a beneficiary undergoes diagnostic testing performed by an audiologist without a physician referral, the tests are not covered even if the audiologist discovers a pathologic condition.

Pub. 100-2, Chapter 15, Section 100

Surgical Dressings, Splints, Casts, and Other Devices Used for Reductions of Fractures and Dislocations

B3-2079, A3-3110.3, HO-228.3,

Surgical dressings are limited to primary and secondary dressings required for the treatment of a wound caused by, or treated by, a surgical procedure that has been performed by a physician or other health care professional to the extent permissible under State law. In addition, surgical dressings required after debridement of a wound are also covered, irrespective of the type of debridement, as long as the debridement was reasonable and necessary and was performed by a health care professional acting within the scope of his/her legal authority when performing this function. Surgical dressings are covered for as long as they are medically necessary.

Primary dressings are therapeutic or protective coverings applied directly to wounds or lesions either on the skin or caused by an opening to the skin. Secondary dressing materials that serve a therapeutic or protective function and that are needed to secure a primary dressing are also covered. Items such as adhesive tape, roll gauze, bandages, and disposable compression material are examples of secondary dressings. Elastic stockings, support hose, foot coverings, leotards, knee supports, surgical leggings, gauntlets, and pressure garments for the arms and hands are examples of items that are not ordinarily covered as surgical dressings. Some items, such as transparent film, may be used as a primary or secondary dressing.

If a physician, certified nurse midwife, physician assistant, nurse practitioner, or clinical nurse specialist applies surgical dressings as part of a professional service that is billed to Medicare, the surgical dressings are considered incident to the professional services of the health care practitioner. (See §§60.1, 180, 190, 200, and 210.) When surgical dressings are not covered incident to the services of a health care practitioner and are obtained by the patient from a supplier (e.g., a drugstore, physician, or other health care practitioner that qualifies as a supplier) on an order from a physician or other health care professional authorized under State law or regulation to make such an order, the surgical dressings are covered separately under Part B.

Splints and casts, and other devices used for reductions of fractures and dislocations are covered under Part B of Medicare. This includes dental splints.

Pub. 100-2, Chapter 15, Section 120

Prosthetic Devices

B3-2130, A3-3110.4, HO-228.4, A3-3111, HO-229

A. General

Prosthetic devices (other than dental) which replace all or part of an internal body organ (including contiguous tissue), or replace all or part of the function of a permanently inoperative or malfunctioning internal body organ are covered when furnished on a physician's order. This does not require a determination that there is no possibility that the patient's condition may improve sometime in the future. If the medical record, including the judgment of the attending physician, indicates the condition is of long and indefinite duration, the test of permanence is considered met. (Such a device may also be covered under §60.l as a supply when furnished incident to a physician's service.)

Examples of prosthetic devices include artificial limbs, parenteral and enteral (PEN) nutrition, cardiac pacemakers, prosthetic lenses (see subsection B), breast prostheses (including a surgical brassiere) for postmastectomy patients, maxillofacial devices, and devices which replace all or part of the ear or nose. A urinary collection and retention system with or without a tube is a prosthetic device replacing bladder function in case of permanent urinary incontinence. The foley catheter is also considered a prosthetic device when ordered for a patient with permanent urinary incontinence. However, chucks, diapers, rubber sheets, etc., are supplies that are not covered under this provision. Although hemodialysis equipment is a prosthetic device, payment for the rental or purchase of such equipment in the home is made only for use under the provisions for payment applicable to durable medical equipment.

An exception is that if payment cannot be made on an inpatient's behalf under Part A, hemodialysis equipment, supplies, and services required by such patient could be covered under Part B as a prosthetic device, which replaces the function of a kidney. See the Medicare Benefit Policy Manual, Chapter 11, "End Stage Renal Disease," for payment for hemodialysis equipment used in the home. See the Medicare Benefit Policy Manual, Chapter 1, "Inpatient Hospital Services," §10, for additional instructions on hospitalization for renal dialysis.

NOTE: Medicare does not cover a prosthetic device dispensed to a patient prior to the time at which the patient undergoes the procedure that makes necessary the use of the device. For example, the carrier does not make a separate Part B payment for an intraocular lens (IOL) or pacemaker that a physician, during an office visit prior to the actual surgery, dispenses to the patient for his or her use. Dispensing a prosthetic device in this manner raises health and safety issues. Moreover, the need for the device cannot be clearly established until the procedure that makes its use possible is successfully performed. Therefore, dispensing a prosthetic device in this manner is not considered reasonable and necessary for the treatment of the patient's condition.

Colostomy (and other ostomy) bags and necessary accouterments required for attachment are covered as prosthetic devices. This coverage also includes irrigation and flushing equipment and other items and supplies directly related to ostomy care, whether the attachment of a bag is required.

Accessories and/or supplies which are used directly with an enteral or parenteral device to achieve the therapeutic benefit of the prosthesis or to assure the proper functioning of the device may also be covered under the prosthetic device benefit subject to the additional guidelines in the Medicare National Coverage Determinations Manual.

Covered items include catheters, filters, extension tubing, infusion bottles, pumps (either food or infusion), intravenous (I.V.) pole, needles, syringes, dressings, tape, Heparin Sodium (parenteral only), volumetric monitors (parenteral only), and parenteral and enteral nutrient solutions. Baby food and other regular grocery products that can be blenderized and used with the enteral system are not covered. Note that some of these items, e.g., a food pump and an I.V. pole, qualify as DME. Although coverage of the enteral and parenteral nutritional therapy systems is provided on the basis of the prosthetic device benefit, the payment rules relating to lump sum or monthly payment for DME apply to such items.

The coverage of prosthetic devices includes replacement of and repairs to such devices as explained in subsection D.

Finally, the Benefits Improvement and Protection Act of 2000 amended §1834(h)(1) of the Act by adding a provision (1834 (h)(1)(G)(i)) that requires Medicare payment to be made for the replacement of prosthetic devices which are artificial limbs, or for the replacement of any part of such devices, without regard to continuous use or useful lifetime restrictions if an ordering physician determines that the replacement device, or replacement part of such a device, is necessary.

Payment may be made for the replacement of a prosthetic device that is an artificial limb, or replacement part of a device if the ordering physician determines that the replacement device or part is necessary because of any of the following:

1. A change in the physiological condition of the patient;

2. An irreparable change in the condition of the device, or in a part of the device; or

3. The condition of the device, or the part of the device, requires repairs and the cost of such repairs would be more than 60 percent of the cost of a replacement device, or, as the case may be, of the part being replaced.

This provision is effective for items replaced on or after April 1, 2001. It supersedes any rule that that provided a 5-year or other replacement rule with regard to prosthetic devices.

B. Prosthetic Lenses

The term "internal body organ" includes the lens of an eye. Prostheses replacing the lens of an eye include post-surgical lenses customarily used during convalescence from eye surgery in which the lens of the eye was removed. In addition, permanent lenses are also covered when required by an individual lacking the organic lens of the eye because of surgical removal or congenital absence. Prosthetic lenses obtained on or after the beneficiary's date of entitlement to supplementary medical insurance benefits may be covered even though the surgical removal of the crystalline lens occurred before entitlement.

1. Prosthetic Cataract Lenses

One of the following prosthetic lenses or combinations of prosthetic lenses furnished by a physician (see §30.4 for coverage of prosthetic lenses prescribed by a doctor of optometry) may be covered when determined to be reasonable and necessary to restore essentially the vision provided by the crystalline lens of the eye:

- Prosthetic bifocal lenses in frames;

- Prosthetic lenses in frames for far vision, and prosthetic lenses in frames for near vision; or

- When a prosthetic contact lens(es) for far vision is prescribed (including cases of binocular and monocular aphakia), make payment for the contact lens(es) and prosthetic lenses in frames for near vision to be worn at the same time as the contact lens(es), and prosthetic lenses in frames to be worn when the contacts have been removed.

Lenses which have ultraviolet absorbing or reflecting properties may be covered, in lieu of payment for regular (untinted) lenses, if it has been determined that such lenses are medically reasonable and necessary for the individual patient.

Medicare does not cover cataract sunglasses obtained in addition to the regular (untinted) prosthetic lenses since the sunglasses duplicate the restoration of vision function performed by the regular prosthetic lenses.

2. Payment for Intraocular Lenses (IOLs) Furnished in Ambulatory Surgical Centers (ASCs)

Effective for services furnished on or after March 12, 1990, payment for intraocular lenses (IOLs) inserted during or subsequent to cataract surgery in a Medicare certified ASC is included with the payment for facility services that are furnished in connection with the covered surgery.

Refer to the Medicare Claims Processing Manual, Chapter 14, "Ambulatory Surgical Centers," for more information.

3. Limitation on Coverage of Conventional Lenses

One pair of conventional eyeglasses or conventional contact lenses furnished after each cataract surgery with insertion of an IOL is covered.

C. Dentures

Dentures are excluded from coverage. However, when a denture or a portion of the denture is an integral part (built-in) of a covered prosthesis (e.g., an obturator to fill an opening in the palate), it is covered as part of that prosthesis.

D. Supplies, Repairs, Adjustments, and Replacement

Supplies are covered that are necessary for the effective use of a prosthetic device (e.g., the batteries needed to operate an artificial larynx). Adjustment of prosthetic devices required by wear or by a change in the patient's condition is covered when ordered by a physician. General provisions relating to the repair and replacement of durable medical equipment in §110.2 for the repair and replacement of prosthetic devices are applicable. (See the Medicare Benefit Policy Manual, Chapter 16, "General Exclusions from Coverage," §40.4, for payment for devices replaced under a warranty.) Replacement of conventional eyeglasses or contact lenses furnished in accordance with §120.B.3 is not covered.

Necessary supplies, adjustments, repairs, and replacements are covered even when the device had been in use before the user enrolled in Part B of the program, so long as the device continues to be medically required.

Pub. 100-2, Chapter 15, Section 150
Dental Services
B3-2136

As indicated under the general exclusions from coverage, items and services in connection with the care, treatment, filling, removal, or replacement of teeth or structures directly supporting the teeth are not covered. "Structures directly supporting the teeth" means the periodontium, which includes the gingivae, dentogingival junction, periodontal membrane, cementum of the teeth, and alveolar process.

In addition to the following, see Pub 100-01, the Medicare General Information, Eligibility, and Entitlement Manual, Chapter 5, Definitions and Pub 3, the Medicare National Coverage Determinations Manual for specific services which may be covered when furnished by a dentist. If an otherwise noncovered procedure or service is performed by a dentist as incident to and as an integral part of a covered procedure or service performed by the dentist, the total service performed by the dentist on such an occasion is covered.

EXAMPLE 1:

The reconstruction of a ridge performed primarily to prepare the mouth for dentures is a noncovered procedure. However, when the reconstruction of a ridge is performed as a result of and at the same time as the surgical removal of a tumor (for other than dental purposes), the totality of surgical procedures is a covered service.

EXAMPLE 2:

Medicare makes payment for the wiring of teeth when this is done in connection with the reduction of a jaw fracture.

The extraction of teeth to prepare the jaw for radiation treatment of neoplastic disease is also covered. This is an exception to the requirement that to be covered, a noncovered procedure or service performed by a dentist must be an incident to and an integral part of a covered procedure or service performed by the dentist. Ordinarily, the dentist extracts the patient's teeth, but another physician, e.g., a radiologist, administers the radiation treatments.

When an excluded service is the primary procedure involved, it is not covered, regardless of its complexity or difficulty. For example, the extraction of an impacted tooth is not covered. Similarly, an alveoplasty (the surgical improvement of the shape and condition of the alveolar process) and a frenectomy are excluded from coverage when either of these procedures is performed in connection with an excluded service, e.g., the preparation of the mouth for dentures. In a like manner, the removal of a torus palatinus (a bony protuberance of the hard palate) may be a covered service. However, with rare exception, this surgery is performed in connection with an excluded service, i.e., the preparation of the mouth for dentures. Under such circumstances, Medicare does not pay for this procedure.

Dental splints used to treat a dental condition are excluded from coverage under 1862(a)(12) of the Act. On the other hand, if the treatment is determined to be a covered medical condition (i.e., dislocated upper/lower jaw joints), then the splint can be covered.

Whether such services as the administration of anesthesia, diagnostic x-rays, and other related procedures are covered depends upon whether the primary procedure being performed by the dentist is itself covered. Thus, an x-ray taken in connection with the reduction of a fracture of the jaw or facial bone is covered. However, a single x-ray or x-ray survey taken in connection with the care or treatment of teeth or the periodontium is not covered.

Medicare makes payment for a covered dental procedure no matter where the service is performed. The hospitalization or nonhospitalization of a patient has no direct bearing on the coverage or exclusion of a given dental procedure.

Payment may also be made for services and supplies furnished incident to covered dental services. For example, the services of a dental technician or nurse who is under the direct supervision of the dentist or physician are covered if the services are included in the dentist's or physician's bill.

Pub. 100-2, Chapter 15, Section 160

Clinical Psychologist Services

B3-2150

A. Clinical Psychologist (CP) Defined

To qualify as a clinical psychologist (CP), a practitioner must meet the following requirements:

- Hold a doctoral degree in psychology;

- Be licensed or certified, on the basis of the doctoral degree in psychology, by the State in which he or she practices, at the independent practice level of psychology to furnish diagnostic, assessment, preventive, and therapeutic services directly to individuals.

B. Qualified Clinical Psychologist Services Defined

Effective July 1, 1990, the diagnostic and therapeutic services of CPs and services and supplies furnished incident to such services are covered as the services furnished by a physician or as incident to physician's services are covered. However, the CP must be legally authorized to perform the services under applicable licensure laws of the State in which they are furnished.

C. Types of Clinical Psychologist Services That May Be Covered

The CPs may provide the following services:

- Diagnostic and therapeutic services that the CP is legally authorized to perform in accordance with State law and/or regulation. Carriers pay all qualified CPs based on the physician fee schedule for the diagnostic and therapeutic services. (Psychological tests by practitioners who do not meet the requirements for a CP may be covered under the provisions for diagnostic tests as described in §80.2.)

- Services and supplies furnished incident to a CP's services are covered if the requirements that apply to services incident to a physician's services, as described in §60 are met. These services must be:

- Mental health services that are commonly furnished in CPs' offices;

- An integral, although incidental, part of professional services performed by the CP;

- Performed under the direct personal supervision of the CP; i.e., the CP must be physically present and immediately available; and

- Furnished without charge or included in the CP's bill.

Any person involved in performing the service must be an employee of the CP (or an employee of the legal entity that employs the supervising CP) under the common law control test of the Act, as set forth in 20 CFR 404.1007 and §RS 2101.020 of the Retirement and Survivors Insurance part of the Social Security Program Operations Manual System.

Carriers are required to familiarize themselves with appropriate State laws and/or regulations governing a CP's scope of practice.

D. Noncovered Services

The services of CPs are not covered if the service is otherwise excluded from Medicare coverage even though a clinical psychologist is authorized by State law to perform them. For example, §1862(a)(1)(A) of the Act excludes from coverage services that are not "reasonable and necessary for the diagnosis or treatment of an illness or injury or to improve the functioning of a malformed body member." Therefore, even though the services are authorized by State law, the services of a CP that are determined to be not reasonable and necessary are not covered. Additionally, any therapeutic services that are billed by CPs under CPT psychotherapy codes that include medical evaluation and management services are not covered.

E. Requirement for Consultation

When applying for a Medicare provider number, a CP must submit to the carrier a signed Medicare provider/supplier enrollment form that indicates an agreement to the effect that, contingent upon the patient's consent, the CP will attempt to consult with the patient's attending or primary care physician in accordance with accepted professional ethical norms, taking into consideration patient confidentiality.

If the patient assents to the consultation, the CP must attempt to consult with the patient's physician within a reasonable time after receiving the consent. If the CP's attempts to consult directly with the physician are not successful, the CP must notify the physician within a reasonable time that he or she is furnishing services to the patient. Additionally, the CP must document, in the patient's medical record, the date the patient consented or declined consent to consultations, the date of consultation, or, if attempts to consult did not succeed, that date and manner of notification to the physician.

The only exception to the consultation requirement for CPs is in cases where the patient's primary care or attending physician refers the patient to the CP. Also, neither a CP nor a primary care nor attending physician may bill Medicare or the patient for this required consultation.

F. Outpatient Mental Health Services Limitation

All covered therapeutic services furnished by qualified CPs are subject to the outpatient mental health services limitation in Pub 100-1, Medicare General Information, Eligibility, and Entitlement Manual, Chapter 3, "Deductibles, Coinsurance Amounts, and Payment Limitations," §30, (i.e., only 62 1/2 percent of expenses for these services are considered incurred expenses for Medicare purposes). The limitation does not apply to diagnostic services.

G. Assignment Requirement

Assignment is required.

Pub. 100-2, Chapter 15, Section 170

Clinical Social Worker (CSW) Services

B3-2152

See the Medicare Claims Processing Manual Chapter 12, Physician/Nonphysician Practitioners, §150, "Clinical Social Worker Services," for payment requirements.

A. Clinical Social Worker Defined

Section 1861(hh) of the Act defines a "clinical social worker" as an individual who:

- Possesses a master's or doctor's degree in social work;

- Has performed at least two years of supervised clinical social work; and

- Is licensed or certified as a clinical social worker by the State in which the services are performed; or

- In the case of an individual in a State that does not provide for licensure or certification, has completed at least 2 years or 3,000 hours of post master's degree supervised clinical social work practice under the supervision of a master's level social worker in an appropriate setting such as a hospital, SNF, or clinic.

B. Clinical Social Worker Services Defined

Section 1861(hh)(2) of the Act defines "clinical social worker services" as those services that the CSW is legally authorized to perform under State law (or the State regulatory mechanism provided by State law) of the State in which such services are performed for the diagnosis and treatment of mental illnesses. Services furnished to an inpatient of a hospital or an inpatient of a SNF that the SNF is required to provide as a requirement for participation are not included. The services that are covered are those that are otherwise covered if furnished by a physician or as incident to a physician's professional service.

C. Covered Services

Coverage is limited to the services a CSW is legally authorized to perform in accordance with State law (or State regulatory mechanism established by State law). The services of a CSW may be covered under Part B if they are:

- The type of services that are otherwise covered if furnished by a physician, or as incident to a physician's service. (See §30 for a description of physicians' services and §70 of Pub 100-1, the Medicare General Information, Eligibility, and Entitlement Manual, Chapter 5, for the definition of a physician.);

- Performed by a person who meets the definition of a CSW (See subsection A.); and

- Not otherwise excluded from coverage.

Carriers should become familiar with the State law or regulatory mechanism governing a CSW's scope of practice in their service area.

D. Noncovered Services

Services of a CSW are not covered when furnished to inpatients of a hospital or to inpatients of a SNF if the services furnished in the SNF are those that the SNF is required to furnish as a condition of participation in Medicare. In addition, CSW services are not covered if they are otherwise excluded from Medicare coverage even though a CSW is authorized by State law to perform them. For example, the Medicare law excludes from coverage services that are not "reasonable and necessary for the diagnosis or treatment of an illness or injury or to improve the functioning of a malformed body member."

E. Outpatient Mental Health Services Limitation

All covered therapeutic services furnished by qualified CSWs are subject to the outpatient psychiatric services limitation in Pub 100-01, Medicare General Information, Eligibility, and Entitlement Manual, Chapter 3, "Deductibles, Coinsurance Amounts, and Payment Limitations," §30, (i.e., only 62 1/2 percent of expenses for these services are considered incurred expenses for Medicare purposes). The limitation does not apply to diagnostic services.

F. Assignment Requirement

Assignment is required.

Pub. 100-2, Chapter 15, Section 180

Midwife (CNM) Services

B3-2154

A. General

Effective on or after July 1, 1988, the services provided by a certified nurse-midwife or incident to the certified nurse-midwife's services are covered. Payment is made under assignment only.

See the Medicare Claims Processing Manual, Chapter 12, "Physician and Nonphysician Practitioners," §130, for payment methodology for nurse midwife services.

B. Certified Nurse-Midwife Defined

A certified nurse-midwife is a registered nurse who has successfully completed a program of study and clinical experience in nurse-midwifery, meeting guidelines prescribed by the Secretary, or who has been certified by an organization recognized by the Secretary. The Secretary has recognized certification by the American College of Nurse-Midwives and State qualifying requirements in those States that specify a program of education and clinical experience for nurse-midwives for these purposes. A nurse-midwife must:

- Be currently licensed to practice in the State as a registered professional nurse; and

- Meet one of the following requirements:

1. Be legally authorized under State law or regulations to practice as a nurse-midwife and have completed a program of study and clinical experience for nurse-midwives, as specified by the State; or

2. If the State does not specify a program of study and clinical experience that nurse-midwives must complete to practice in that State, the nurse-midwife must:

a. Be currently certified as a nurse-midwife by the American College of Nurse-Midwives;

b. Have satisfactorily completed a formal education program (of at least one academic year) that, upon completion, qualifies the nurse to take the certification examination offered by the American College of Nurse-Midwives; or

c. Have successfully completed a formal education program for preparing registered nurses to furnish gynecological and obstetrical care to women during pregnancy, delivery, and the postpartum period, and care to normal newborns, and have practiced as a nurse-midwife for a total of 12 months during any 18-month period from August 8, 1976, to July 16, 1982.

C. Covered Services

1. General - Effective January 1, 1988, through December 31, 1993, the coverage of nurse-midwife services was restricted to the maternity cycle. The maternity cycle is a period that includes pregnancy, labor, and the immediate postpartum period.

Beginning with services furnished on or after January 1, 1994, coverage is no longer limited to the maternity cycle. Coverage is available for services furnished by a nurse-midwife that he or she is legally authorized to perform in the State in which the services are furnished and that would otherwise be covered if furnished by a physician, including obstetrical and gynecological services.

2. Incident To - Services and supplies furnished incident to a nurse midwife's service are covered if they would have been covered when furnished incident to the services of a doctor of medicine or osteopathy, as described in §60.

D. Noncovered Services

The services of nurse-midwives are not covered if they are otherwise excluded from Medicare coverage even though a nurse-midwife is authorized by State law to perform them. For example, the Medicare program excludes from coverage routine physical checkups and services that are not reasonable and necessary for the diagnosis or treatment of an illness or injury or to improve the functioning of a malformed body member.

Coverage of service to the newborn continues only to the point that the newborn is or would normally be treated medically as a separate individual. Items and services furnished the newborn from that point are not covered on the basis of the mother's eligibility.

E. Relationship With Physician

Most States have licensure and other requirements applicable to nurse-midwives. For example, some require that the nurse-midwife have an arrangement with a physician for the referral of the patient in the event a problem develops that requires medical attention. Others may require that the nurse-midwife function under the general supervision of a physician. Although these and similar State requirements must be met in order for the nurse-midwife to provide Medicare covered care, they have no effect on the nurse-midwife's right to personally bill for and receive direct Medicare payment. That is, billing does not have to flow through a physician or facility.

See §60.2 for coverage of services performed by nurse-midwives incident to the service of physicians.

F. Place of Service

There is no restriction on place of service. Therefore, nurse-midwife services are covered if provided in the nurse-midwife's office, in the patient's home, or in a hospital or other facility, such as a clinic or birthing center owned or operated by a nurse-midwife.

G. Assignment Requirement

Assignment is required.

Pub. 100-2, Chapter 15, Section 230

Language Pathology

Pub. 100-2, Chapter 15, Section 230.1

Practice of Physical Therapy

A. General

Physical therapy services are those services provided within the scope of practice of physical therapists and necessary for the diagnosis and treatment of impairments, functional limitations, disabilities or changes in physical function and health status. (See Pub. 100-03, the Medicare National Coverage Determinations Manual, for specific conditions or services.)

B. Qualified Physical Therapist Defined

Reference: 42CFR484.4

A qualified physical therapist for program coverage purposes is a person who is licensed as a physical therapist by the state in which he or she is practicing and meets one of the following requirements:

- Has graduated from a physical therapy curriculum approved by (1) the American Physical Therapy Association, or by (2) the Committee on Allied Health Education and Accreditation of the American Medical Association, or (3) Council on Medical Education of the American Medical Association, and the American Physical Therapy Association; or

- Prior to January 1, 1966, (1) was admitted to membership by the American Physical Therapy Association, or (2) was admitted to registration by the American Registry of Physical Therapists, or (3) has graduated from a physical therapy curriculum in a 4-year college or university approved by a state department of education; or

- Has 2 years of appropriate experience as a physical therapist and has achieved a satisfactory grade on a proficiency examination conducted, approved or sponsored by the Public Health Service, except that such determinations of proficiency do not apply with respect to persons initially licensed by a state or seeking qualification as a physical therapist after December 31, 1977; or

- Was licensed or registered prior to January 1, 1966, and prior to January 1, 1970, had 15 years of full-time experience in the treatment of illness or injury through the practice of physical therapy in which services were rendered under the order and direction of attending and referring doctors of medicine or osteopathy; or

- If trained outside the United States, (1) was graduated since 1928 from a physical therapy curriculum approved in the country in which the curriculum was located and in which there is a member organization of the World Confederation for Physical Therapy, (2) meets the requirements for membership in a member organization of the World Confederation for Physical Therapy.

C. Services of Physical Therapy Support Personnel

Reference: 42CFR 484.4

A physical therapist assistant (PTA) is a person who is licensed as a physical therapist assistant, if applicable, by the State in which practicing, and

- Has graduated from a 2-year college-level program approved by the American Physical Therapy Association; or

- Has 2 years of appropriate experience as a physical therapist assistant, and has achieved a satisfactory grade on a proficiency examination conducted, approved, or sponsored by the U.S. Public Health Service, except that these determinations of proficiency do not apply with respect to persons initially licensed by a State or seeking initial qualification as a PTA after December 31, 1977.

The services of PTAs used when providing covered therapy benefits are included as part of the covered service. These services are billed by the supervising physical therapist. PTAs may not provide evaluation services, make clinical judgments or decisions or take responsibility for the service. They act at the direction and under the supervision of the treating physical therapist and in accordance with state laws.

A physical therapist must supervise PTAs. The level and frequency of supervision differs by setting (and by state or local law). General supervision is required for PTAs in all settings except private practice (which requires direct supervision) unless state practice requirements are more stringent, in which case state or local requirements must be followed. See specific settings for details. For example, in clinics, rehabilitation agencies, and public health agencies, 42CFR485.713 indicates that when a PTA provides services, either on or off the organization's premises, those services are supervised by a qualified physical therapist who makes an onsite supervisory visit at least once every 30 days or more frequently if required by state or local laws or regulation.

The services of a PTA shall not be billed as services incident to a physician/NPP's service, because they do not meet the qualifications of a therapist.

The cost of supplies (e.g., theraband, hand putty, electrodes) used in furnishing covered therapy care is included in the payment for the HCPCS codes billed by the physical therapist, and are, therefore, not separately billable. Separate coverage and billing provisions apply to items that meet the definition of brace in §130.

Services provided by aides, even if under the supervision of a therapist, are not therapy services in the outpatient setting and are not covered by Medicare. Although an aide may help the therapist by providing unskilled services, those services that are unskilled are not covered by Medicare and shall be denied as not reasonable and necessary if they are billed as therapy services.

D. Application of Medicare Guidelines to PT Services

This subsection will be used in the future to illustrate the application of the above guidelines to some of the physical therapy modalities and procedures utilized in the treatment of patients.

Pub. 100-2, Chapter 15, Section 230.2

Practice of Occupational Therapy

A. General

Occupational therapy services are those services provided within the scope of practice of occupational therapists and necessary for the diagnosis and treatment of impairments, functional disabilities or changes in physical function and health status. (See Pub. 100-03, the Medicare National Coverage Determinations Manual, for specific conditions or services.)

Occupational therapy is medically prescribed treatment concerned with improving or restoring functions which have been impaired by illness or injury or, where function has been permanently lost or reduced by illness or injury, to improve the individual's ability to perform those tasks required for independent functioning. Such therapy may involve:

- The evaluation, and reevaluation as required, of a patient's level of function by administering diagnostic and prognostic tests;

- The selection and teaching of task-oriented therapeutic activities designed to restore physical function; e.g., use of woodworking activities on an inclined table to restore shoulder, elbow, and wrist range of motion lost as a result of burns;

- The planning, implementing, and supervising of individualized therapeutic activity programs as part of an overall "active treatment" program for a patient with a diagnosed psychiatric illness; e.g., the use of sewing activities which require following a pattern to reduce confusion and restore reality orientation in a schizophrenic patient;

- The planning and implementing of therapeutic tasks and activities to restore sensory-integrative function; e.g., providing motor and tactile activities to increase sensory input and improve response for a stroke patient with functional loss resulting in a distorted body image;

- The teaching of compensatory technique to improve the level of independence in the activities of daily living, for example:

    — Teaching a patient who has lost the use of an arm how to pare potatoes and chop vegetables with one hand;

    — Teaching an upper extremity amputee how to functionally utilize a prosthesis;

    — Teaching a stroke patient new techniques to enable the patient to perform feeding, dressing, and other activities as independently as possible; or

    — Teaching a patient with a hip fracture/hip replacement techniques of standing tolerance and balance to enable the patient to perform such functional activities as dressing and homemaking tasks.

- The designing, fabricating, and fitting of orthotics and self-help devices; e.g., making a hand splint for a patient with rheumatoid arthritis to maintain the hand in a functional position or constructing a device which would enable an individual to hold a utensil and feed independently; or

- Vocational and prevocational assessment and training, subject to the limitations specified in item B below.

Only a qualified occupational therapist has the knowledge, training, and experience required to evaluate and, as necessary, reevaluate a patient's level of function, determine whether an occupational therapy program could reasonably be expected to improve, restore, or compensate for lost function and, where appropriate, recommend to the physician/NPP a plan of treatment.

B. Qualified Occupational Therapist Defined

Reference: 42CFR484.4

A qualified occupational therapist for program coverage purposes is an individual who meets one of the following requirements:

- Is a graduate of an occupational therapy curriculum accredited jointly by the Committee on Allied Health Education of the American Medical Association and the American Occupational Therapy Association;

- Is eligible for the National Registration Examination of the American Occupational Therapy Association; or

- Has 2 years of appropriate experience as an occupational therapist, and has achieved a satisfactory grade on a proficiency examination conducted, approved, or sponsored by the U.S. Public Health Service, except that such determinations of proficiency do not apply with respect to persons initially licensed by a State or seeking initial qualification as an occupational therapist after December 31, 1977.

C. Services of Occupational Therapy Support Personnel

Reference: 42CFR 484.4

An occupational therapy assistant (OTA) is a person who:

- Meets the requirements for certification as an occupational therapy assistant established by the American Occupational Therapy Association; or

- Has 2 years of appropriate experience as an occupational therapy assistant and has achieved a satisfactory grade on a proficiency examination conducted, approved, or sponsored by the U.S. Public Health Service, except that such determinations of proficiency do not apply with respect to persons initially licensed by a State or seeking initial qualification as an occupational therapy assistant after December 31, 1977.

The services of OTAs used when providing covered therapy benefits are included as part of the covered service. These services are billed by the supervising occupational therapist. OTAs may not provide evaluation services, make clinical judgments or decisions or take responsibility for the service. They act at the direction and under the supervision of the treating occupational therapist and in accordance with state laws.

An occupational therapist must supervise OTAs. The level and frequency of supervision differs by setting (and by state or local law). General supervision is required for OTAs in all settings except private practice (which requires direct supervision) unless state practice requirements are more stringent, in which case state or local requirements must be followed. See specific settings for details. For example, in clinics, rehabilitation agencies, and public health agencies, 42CFR485.713 indicates that when an OTA provides services, either on or off the organization's premises, those services are supervised by a qualified occupational therapist who makes an onsite supervisory visit at least once every 30 days or more frequently if required by state or local laws or regulation.

The services of an OTA shall not be billed as services incident to a physician/NPP's service, because they do not meet the qualifications of a therapist.

The cost of supplies (e.g., looms, ceramic tiles, or leather) used in furnishing covered therapy care is included in the payment for the HCPCS codes billed by the occupational therapist and are, therefore, not separately billable. Separate coverage and billing provisions apply to items that meet the definition of brace in §130 of this manual.

Services provided by aides, even if under the supervision of a therapist, are not therapy services in the outpatient setting and are not covered by Medicare. Although an aide may help the therapist by providing unskilled services, those services that are unskilled are not covered by Medicare and shall be denied as not reasonable and necessary if they are billed as therapy services.

D. Application of Medicare Guidelines to Occupational Therapy Services

Occupational therapy may be required for a patient with a specific diagnosed psychiatric illness. If such services are required, they are covered assuming the coverage criteria are met. However,

where an individual's motivational needs are not related to a specific diagnosed psychiatric illness, the meeting of such needs does not usually require an individualized therapeutic program. Such needs can be met through general activity programs or the efforts of other professional personnel involved in the care of the patient. Patient motivation is an appropriate and inherent function of all health disciplines, which is interwoven with other functions performed by such personnel for the patient. Accordingly, since the special skills of an occupational therapist are not required, an occupational therapy program for individuals who do not have a specific diagnosed psychiatric illness is not to be considered reasonable and necessary for the treatment of an illness or injury. Services furnished under such a program are not covered.

Occupational therapy may include vocational and prevocational assessment and training. When services provided by an occupational therapist are related solely to specific employment opportunities, work skills, or work settings, they are not reasonable or necessary for the diagnosis or treatment of an illness or injury and are not covered. However, carriers and intermediaries exercise care in applying this exclusion, because the assessment of level of function and the teaching of compensatory techniques to improve the level of function, especially in activities of daily living, are services which occupational therapists provide for both vocational and nonvocational purposes. For example, an assessment of sitting and standing tolerance might be nonvocational for a mother of young children or a retired individual living alone, but could also be a vocational test for a sales clerk. Training an amputee in the use of prosthesis for telephoning is necessary for everyday activities as well as for employment purposes. Major changes in life style may be mandatory for an individual with a substantial disability. The techniques of adjustment cannot be considered exclusively vocational or nonvocational.

Pub. 100-2, Chapter 15, Section 230.3

Language Pathology

A. General

Speech-language pathology services are those services provided within the scope of practice of speech-language pathologists and necessary for the diagnosis and treatment of speech and language disorders, which result in communication disabilities and for the diagnosis and treatment of swallowing disorders (dysphagia), regardless of the presence of a communication disability. (See Pub. 100-03, chapter 1, §170.3)

B. Qualified Speech-Language Pathologist Defined

A qualified speech-language pathologist for program coverage purposes meets one of the following requirements:

- The education and experience requirements for a Certificate of Clinical Competence in (speech-language pathology or audiology) granted by the American Speech-Language Hearing Association; or

- Meets the educational requirements for certification and is in the process of accumulating the supervised experience required for certification.

Speech-language pathologists may not enroll and submit claims directly to Medicare. The services of speech-language pathologists may be billed by providers such as rehabilitation agencies, HHAs, CORFs, hospices, outpatient departments of hospitals, and suppliers such as physicians, NPPs, physical and occupational therapists in private practice.

C. Services of Speech-Language Pathology Support Personnel

Services of speech-language pathology assistants are not recognized for Medicare coverage. Services provided by speech-language pathology assistants, even if they are licensed to provide services in their states, will be considered unskilled services and denied as not reasonable and necessary if they are billed as therapy services.

Services provided by aides, even if under the supervision of a therapist, are not therapy services and are not covered by Medicare. Although an aide may help the therapist by providing unskilled services, those services are not covered by Medicare and shall be denied as not reasonable and necessary if they are billed as therapy services.

D. Application of Medicare Guidelines to Speech-Language Pathology Services

1. Evaluation Services

Speech-language pathology evaluation services are covered if they are reasonable and necessary and not excluded as routine screening by §1862(a)(7) of the Act. The speech-language pathologist employs a variety of formal and informal speech, language, and dysphagia assessment tests to ascertain the type, causal factor(s), and severity of the speech and language or swallowing disorders. Reevaluation of patients for whom speech, language and swallowing were previously contraindicated is covered only if the patient exhibits a change in medical condition. However, monthly reevaluations; e.g., a Western Aphasia Battery, for a patient undergoing a rehabilitative speech-language pathology program, are considered a part of the treatment session and shall not be covered as a separate evaluation for billing purposes. Although hearing screening by the speech-language pathologist may be part of an evaluation, it is not billable as a separate service.

2. Therapeutic Services

The following are examples of common medical disorders and resulting communication deficits, which may necessitate active rehabilitative therapy. This list is not all-inclusive:

- Cerebrovascular disease such as cerebral vascular accidents presenting with dysphagia, aphasia/dysphasia, apraxia, and dysarthria;

- Neurological disease such as Parkinsonism or Multiple Sclerosis with dysarthria, dysphagia, inadequate respiratory volume/control, or voice disorder; or

- Laryngeal carcinoma requiring laryngectomy resulting in aphonia.

3. Aural Rehabilitation

Aural rehabilitation may be covered and medically necessary when it has been determined by a speech-language pathologist in collaboration with an audiologist that the beneficiary's current amplification options (hearing aid, other amplification device or cochlear implant) will not sufficiently meet the patient's functional communication needs.

Assessment for the need for aural rehabilitation may be done by a speech language pathologist and includes evaluation of comprehension and production of language in oral, signed or written modalities, speech and voice production, listening skills, speech reading, communications strategies, and the impact of the hearing loss on the patient/client and family.

Aural rehabilitation consists of treatment that focuses on comprehension, and production of language in oral, signed or written modalities; speech and voice production, auditory training, speech reading, multimodal (e.g., visual, auditory-visual, and tactile) training, communication strategies, education and counseling. In determining the necessity for treatment, the beneficiary's performance in both clinical and natural environment should be considered.

4. Dysphagia

Dysphagia, or difficulty in swallowing, can cause food to enter the airway, resulting in coughing, choking, pulmonary problems, aspiration or inadequate nutrition and hydration with resultant weight loss, failure to thrive, pneumonia and death. It is most often due to complex neurological and/or structural impairments including head and neck trauma, cerebrovascular accident, neuromuscular degenerative diseases, head and neck cancer, dementias, and encephalopathies. For these reasons, it is important that only qualified professionals with specific training and experience in this disorder provide evaluation and treatment.

The speech-language pathologist performs clinical and instrumental assessments and analyzes and integrates the diagnostic information to determine candidacy for intervention as well as appropriate compensations and rehabilitative therapy techniques. The equipment that is used in the examination may be fixed, mobile or portable. Professional guidelines recommend that the service be provided in a team setting with a physician/NPP who provides supervision of the radiological examination and interpretation of medical conditions revealed in it.

Swallowing assessment and rehabilitation are highly specialized services. The professional rendering care must have education, experience and demonstrated competencies. Competencies include but are not limited to: identifying abnormal upper aerodigestive tract structure and function; conducting an oral, pharyngeal, laryngeal and respiratory function examination as it relates to the functional assessment of swallowing; recommending methods of oral intake and risk precautions; and developing a treatment plan employing appropriate compensations and therapy techniques.

Pub. 100-2, Chapter 15, Section 230.4

Services Furnished by a Physical or Occupational Therapist in Private Practice

A. General

In order to qualify to bill Medicare directly as a therapist, each individual must be enrolled as a private practitioner and employed in one of the following practice types: an unincorporated solo practice, unincorporated partnership, unincorporated group practice, physician/NPP group or groups that are not professional corporations, if allowed by state and local law. Physician/NPP group practices may employ physical therapists in private practice (PTPP) and/or occupational therapists in private practice (OTPP) if state and local law permits this employee relationship.

For purposes of this provision, a physician/NPP group practice is defined as one or more physicians/NPPs enrolled with Medicare who may bill as one entity. For further details on issues concerning enrollment, see the provider enrollment Web site at www.cms.hhs.gov/providers/enrollment.

Private practice also includes therapists who are practicing therapy as employees of another supplier, of a professional corporation or other incorporated therapy practice. Private practice does not include individuals when they are working as employees of an institutional provider.

Services should be furnished in the therapist's or group's office or in the patient's home. The office is defined as the location(s) where the practice is operated, in the state(s) where the therapist (and practice, if applicable) is legally authorized to furnish services, during the hours that the therapist engages in the practice at that location. If services are furnished in a private practice office space, that space shall be owned, leased, or rented by the practice and used for the exclusive purpose of operating the practice. For example, a therapist in private practice may furnish aquatic therapy in a community center pool. As required in other settings (such as rehabilitation agencies and CORFs), the practice would have to rent or lease the pool for those hours, and the use of the pool during that time would have to be restricted to the therapist's patients, in order to recognize the pool as part of the therapist's own practice office during those hours. Therapists in private practice must be approved as meeting certain requirements, but do not execute a formal provider agreement with the Secretary.

If therapists who have their own Medicare Personal Identification number (PIN) or National Provider Identifier (NPI) are employed by therapist groups, physician/NPP groups, or groups that are not professional organizations, the requirement that therapy space be owned, leased, or rented may be satisfied by the group that employs the therapist. Each physical or occupational therapist employed by a group should enroll as a PT or OT in private practice.

When therapists with a Medicare PIN/NPI provide services in the physician's/NPP's office in which they are employed, and bill using their PIN/NPI for each therapy service, then the direct supervision requirement for PTAs and OTAs apply.

When the PT or OT who has a Medicare PIN/ NPI is employed in a physician's/NPP's office the services are ordinarily billed as services of the PT or OT, with the PT or OT identified on the claim as the supplier of services. However, services of the PT or OT who has a Medicare PIN/NPI may also be billed by the physician/NPP as services incident to the physician's/NPP's service. (See §230.5 for rules related to PTA and OTA services incident to a physician.) In that case, the physician/NPP is the supplier of service, the Unique Provider Identification Number (UPIN) or NPI of the physician/NPP (ordering or supervising, as indicated) is reported on the claim with the service and all the rules for incident to services (§230.5) must be followed.

B. Private Practice Defined

Reference: Federal Register November, 1998, pages 58863-58869; 42CFR 410.38(b)

The carrier considers a therapist to be in private practice if the therapist maintains office space at his or her own expense and furnishes services only in that space or the patient's home. Or, a therapist is employed by another supplier and furnishes services in facilities provided at the expense of that supplier.

The therapist need not be in full-time private practice but must be engaged in private practice on a regular basis; i.e., the therapist is recognized as a private practitioner and for that purpose has access to the necessary equipment to provide an adequate program of therapy.

The physical or occupational therapy services must be provided either by or under the direct supervision of the therapist in private practice. Each physical or occupational therapist in a practice should be enrolled as a Medicare provider. If a physical or occupational therapist is not enrolled, the services of that therapist must be directly supervised by an enrolled physical or occupational therapist. Direct supervision requires that the supervising private practice therapist be present in the office suite at the time the service is performed. These direct supervision requirements apply only in the private practice setting and only for physical therapists and occupational therapists and their assistants. In other outpatient settings, supervision rules differ. The services of support personnel must be included in the therapist's bill. The supporting personnel, including other therapists, must be W-2 or 1099 employees of the therapist in private practice or other qualified employer.

Coverage of outpatient physical therapy and occupational therapy under Part B includes the services of a qualified therapist in private practice when furnished in the therapist's office or the beneficiary's home. For this purpose, "home" includes an institution that is used as a home, but not a hospital, CAH or SNF, (Federal Register Nov. 2, 1998, pg 58869). Place of Service (POS) includes:

- 03/School, only if residential,
- 04/Homeless Shelter,
- 12/Home, other than a facility that is a private residence,
- 14/Group Home,
- 33/Custodial Care Facility.

C. Assignment

Reference: Nov. 2, 1998 Federal Register, pg. 58863

See also Pub. 100-04 chapter 1, §30.2.

When physicians, NPPs, PTPPs or OTPPs obtain provider numbers, they have the option of accepting assignment (participating) or not accepting assignment (nonparticipating). In contrast, providers, such as outpatient hospitals, SNFs, rehabilitation agencies, and CORFs, do not have the option. For these providers, assignment is mandatory.

If physicians/NPPs, PTPPs or OTPPs accept assignment (are participating), they must accept the Medicare Physician Fee Schedule amount as payment. Medicare pays 80% and the patient is responsible for 20%. In contrast, if they do not accept assignment, Medicare will only pay 95% of the fee schedule amount. However, when these services are not furnished on an assignment-related basis, the limiting charge applies. (See §1848(g)(2)(c) of the Act.)

NOTE: Services furnished by a therapist in the therapist's office under arrangements with hospitals in rural communities and public health agencies (or services provided in the beneficiary's home under arrangements with a provider of outpatient physical or occupational therapy services) are not covered under this provision. See section 230.6.

Pub. 100-2, Chapter 15, Section 260

Ambulatory Surgical Center Services

B3-2265

Facility services furnished by ambulatory surgical centers (ASCs) in connection with certain surgical procedures are covered under Part B. To receive coverage of and payment for its services under this provision, a facility must be certified as meeting the requirements for an ASC and enter into a written agreement with CMS. Medicare periodically updates the list of covered procedures and related payment amounts through release of regulations and Program Memoranda. The ASC must accept Medicare's payment for such procedures as payment in full with respect to those services defined as ASC facility services.

Where services are performed in an ASC, the physician and others who perform covered services may also be paid for his/her professional services; however, the "professional" rate is then adjusted since the ASC incurs the facility costs.

Pub. 100-2, Chapter 16, Section 10

General Exclusions From Coverage

A3-3150, HO-260, HHA-232, B3-2300

No payment can be made under either the hospital insurance or supplementary medical insurance program for certain items and services, when the following conditions exist:

- Not reasonable and necessary (§20);
- No legal obligation to pay for or provide (§40);
- Paid for by a governmental entity (§50);
- Not provided within United States (§60);
- Resulting from war (§70);
- Personal comfort (§80);
- Routine services and appliances (§90);

- Custodial care (§110);
- Cosmetic surgery (§120);
- Charges by immediate relatives or members of household (§130);
- Dental services (§140);
- Paid or expected to be paid under workers' compensation (§150);
- Nonphysician services provided to a hospital inpatient that were not provided directly or arranged for by the hospital (§170);
- Services Related to and Required as a Result of Services Which are not Covered

Under Medicare (§180);

- Excluded foot care services and supportive devices for feet (§30); or

Excluded investigational devices (See Chapter 14, §30).

Pub. 100-2, Chapter 16, Section 90

Routine Services and Appliances

A3-3157, HO-260.7, B3-2320, R-1797A3 - 5/00

Routine physical checkups; eyeglasses, contact lenses, and eye examinations for the purpose of prescribing, fitting, or changing eyeglasses; eye refractions by whatever practitioner and for whatever purpose performed; hearing aids and examinations for hearing aids; and immunizations are not covered.

The routine physical checkup exclusion applies to (a) examinations performed without relationship to treatment or diagnosis for a specific illness, symptom, complaint, or injury; and (b) examinations required by third parties such as insurance companies, business establishments, or Government agencies.

If the claim is for a diagnostic test or examination performed solely for the purpose of establishing a claim under title IV of Public Law 91-173, "Black Lung Benefits," the service is not covered under Medicare and the claimant should be advised to contact their Social Security office regarding the filing of a claim for reimbursement under the "Black Lung" program.

The exclusions apply to eyeglasses or contact lenses, and eye examinations for the purpose of prescribing, fitting, or changing eyeglasses or contact lenses for refractive errors. The exclusions do not apply to physicians' services (and services incident to a physicians' service) performed in conjunction with an eye disease, as for example, glaucoma or cataracts, or to post-surgical prosthetic lenses which are customarily used during convalescence from eye surgery in which the lens of the eye was removed, or to permanent prosthetic lenses required by an individual lacking the organic lens of the eye, whether by surgical removal or congenital disease. Such prosthetic lens is a replacement for an internal body organ - the lens of the eye. (See the Medicare Benefit Policy Manual, Chapter 15, "Covered Medical and Other Health Services," §120).

Expenses for all refractive procedures, whether performed by an ophthalmologist (or any other physician) or an optometrist and without regard to the reason for performance of the refraction, are excluded from coverage.

A. Immunizations

Vaccinations or inoculations are excluded as immunizations unless they are either

- Directly related to the treatment of an injury or direct exposure to a disease or condition, such as antirabies treatment, tetanus antitoxin or booster vaccine, botulin antitoxin, antivenin sera, or immune globulin.(In the absence of injury or direct exposure, preventive immunization (vaccination or inoculation) against such diseases as smallpox, polio, diphtheria, etc., is not covered.); or
- Specifically covered by statute, as described in the Medicare Benefit Policy Manual, Chapter 15, "Covered Medical and Other Health Services," §50.

B. Antigens

Prior to the Omnibus Reconciliation Act of 1980, a physician who prepared an antigen for a patient could not be reimbursed for that service unless the physician also administered the antigen to the patient. Effective January 1, 1981, payment may be made for a reasonable supply of antigens that have been prepared for a particular patient even though they have not been administered to the patient by the same physician who prepared them if:

- The antigens are prepared by a physician who is a doctor of medicine or osteopathy, and
- The physician who prepared the antigens has examined the patient and has determined a plan of treatment and a dosage regimen.

A reasonable supply of antigens is considered to be not more than a 12-week supply of antigens that has been prepared for a particular patient at any one time. The purpose of the reasonable supply limitation is to assure that the antigens retain their potency and effectiveness over the period in which they are to be administered to the patient. (See the Medicare Benefit Policy Manual, Chapter 15, "Covered Medical and Other Health Services," §50.4.4.2)

Pub. 100-2, Chapter 16, Section 100

Hearing Aids andAuditoryImplants

Section 1862(a)(7) of the Social Security Act states that no payment may be made under part A or part B for any expenses incurred for items or services "where such expenses are for hearing aids or examinations therefore." This policy is further reiterated at 42 CFR 411.15(d) which specifically states that "hearing aids or examination for the purpose of prescribing, fitting, or changing hearing aids" are excluded from coverage.

Hearing aids are amplifying devices that compensate for impaired hearing. Hearing aids include air conduction devices that provide acoustic energy to the cochlea via stimulation of the tympanic membrane with amplified sound. They also include bone conduction devices that provide mechanical energy to the cochlea via stimulation of the scalp with amplified mechanical vibration or by direct contact with the tympanic membrane or middle ear ossicles.

Certain devices that produce perception of sound by replacing the function of the middle ear, cochlea or auditory nerve are payable by Medicare as prosthetic devices. These devices are indicated only when hearing aids are medically inappropriate or cannot be utilized due to congenital malformations, chronic disease, severe sensorineural hearing loss or surgery.

The following are prosthetic devices:

- Cochlear implants and auditory brainstem implants, i.e., devices that replace the function of cochlear structures or auditory nerve and provide electrical energy to auditory nerve fibers and other neural tissue via implanted electrode arrays.
- Osseointegrated implants, i.e., devices implanted in the skull that replace the function of the middle ear and provide mechanical energy to the cochlea via a mechanical transducer.

Medicare contractors deny payment for an item or service that is associated with any hearing aid as defined above. See §180 for policy for the medically necessary treatment of complications of implantable hearing aids, such as medically necessary removals of implantable hearing aids due to infection.

Pub. 100-2, Chapter 16, Section 120

Cosmetic Surgery

A3-3160, HO-260.11, B3-2329

Cosmetic surgery or expenses incurred in connection with such surgery is not covered.

Cosmetic surgery includes any surgical procedure directed at improving appearance, except when required for the prompt (i.e., as soon as medically feasible) repair of accidental injury or for the improvement of the functioning of a malformed body member. For example, this exclusion does not apply to surgery in connection with treatment of severe burns or repair of the face following a serious automobile accident, or to surgery for therapeutic purposes which coincidentally also serves some cosmetic purpose.

Pub. 100-2, Chapter 16, Section 180

Services Related to and Required as a Result of Services Which Are Not Covered Under Medicare

B3-2300.1, A3-3101.14, HO-210.12

Medical and hospital services are sometimes required to treat a condition that arises as a result of services that are not covered because they are determined to be not reasonable and necessary or because they are excluded from coverage for other reasons. Services "related to" noncovered services (e.g., cosmetic surgery, noncovered organ transplants, noncovered artificial organ implants, etc.), including services related to follow-up care and complications of noncovered services which require treatment during a hospital stay in which the noncovered service was performed, are not covered services under Medicare. Services "not related to" noncovered services are covered under Medicare.

Following are examples of services "related to" and "not related to" noncovered services while the beneficiary is an inpatient:

- A beneficiary was hospitalized for a noncovered service and broke a leg while in the hospital. Services related to care of the broken leg during this stay is a clear example of "not related to" services and are covered under Medicare.
- A beneficiary was admitted to the hospital for covered services, but during the course of hospitalization became a candidate for a noncovered transplant or implant and actually received the transplant or implant during that hospital stay. When the original admission was entirely unrelated to the diagnosis that led to a recommendation for a noncovered transplant or implant, the services related to the admitting condition would be covered.
- A beneficiary was admitted to the hospital for covered services related to a condition which ultimately led to identification of a need for transplant and receipt of a transplant during the same hospital stay. If, on the basis of the nature of the services and a comparison of the date they are received with the date on which the beneficiary is identified as a transplant candidate, the services could reasonably be attributed to preparation for the noncovered transplant, the services would be "related to" noncovered services and would also be noncovered.

Following is an example of services received subsequent to a noncovered inpatient stay:

After a beneficiary has been discharged from the hospital stay in which the beneficiary received noncovered services, medical and hospital services required to treat a condition or complication that arises as a result of the prior noncovered services may be covered when they are reasonable and necessary in all other respects. Thus, coverage could be provided for subsequent inpatient stays or outpatient treatment ordinarily covered by Medicare, even if the need for treatment arose because of a previous noncovered procedure. Some examples of services that may be found to be covered under this policy are the reversal of intestinal bypass surgery for obesity, repair of complications from transsexual surgery or from cosmetic surgery, removal of a noncovered bladder stimulator, or treatment of any infection at the surgical site of a noncovered transplant that occurred following discharge from the hospital.

However, any subsequent services that could be expected to have been incorporated into a global fee are considered to have been paid in the global fee, and may not be paid again. Thus, where a patient undergoes cosmetic surgery and the treatment regimen calls for a series of postoperative visits to the surgeon for evaluating the patient's progress, these visits are not paid.

Pub. 100-3, Section 10.1

Use of Visual Tests Prior to and General Anesthesia During Cataract Surgery

A - Pre-Surgery Evaluations

Cataract surgery with an intraocular lens (IOL) implant is a high volume Medicare procedure. Along with the surgery, a substantial number of preoperative tests are available to the surgeon. In most cases, a comprehensive eye examination (ocular history and ocular examination) and a single scan to determine the appropriate pseudophakic power of the IOL are sufficient. In most cases involving a simple cataract, a diagnostic ultrasound A-scan is used. For patients with a dense cataract, an ultrasound B-scan is used.

Accordingly, where the only diagnosis is cataract(s), Medicare does not routinely cover testing other than one comprehensive eye examination (or a combination of a brief/intermediate examination not to exceed the charge of a comprehensive examination) and an A-scan or, if medically justified, a B-scan. Claims for additional tests are denied as not reasonable and necessary unless there is an additional diagnosis and the medical need for the additional tests is fully documented.

Because cataract surgery is an elective procedure, the patient may decide not to have the surgery until later, or to have the surgery performed by a physician other than the diagnosing physician. In these situations, it may be medically appropriate for the operating physician to conduct another examination. To the extent the additional tests are considered reasonable and necessary by the carrier's medical staff, they are covered.

B - General Anesthesia

The use of general anesthesia in cataract surgery may be considered reasonable and necessary if, for particular medical indications, it is the accepted procedure among ophthalmologists in the local community to use general anesthesia.

Pub. 100-3, Section 10.2

Transcutaneous Electrical Nerve Stimulation (TENS) for Acute Post-Operative Pain

The use of TENS for the relief of acute post-operative pain is covered under Medicare. TENS may be covered whether used as an adjunct to the use of drugs, or as an alternative to drugs, in the treatment of acute pain resulting from surgery.

TENS devices, whether durable or disposable, may be used in furnishing this service. When used for the purpose of treating acute post-operative pain, TENS devices are considered supplies. As such they may be hospital supplies furnished inpatients covered under Part A, or supplies incident to a physician's service when furnished in connection with surgery done on an outpatient basis, and covered under Part B.

It is expected that TENS, when used for acute post-operative pain, will be necessary for relatively short periods of time, usually 30 days or less. In cases when TENS is used for longer periods, contractors should attempt to ascertain whether TENS is no longer being used for acute pain but rather for chronic pain, in which case the TENS device may be covered as durable medical equipment as described in §280.13.

Pub. 100-3, Section 10.3

Inpatient Hospital Pain Rehabilitation Programs

Since pain rehabilitation programs of a lesser scope than that described above would raise a question as to whether the program could be provided in a less intensive setting than on an inpatient hospital basis, carefully evaluate such programs to determine whether the program does, in fact, necessitate a hospital level of care. Some pain rehabilitation programs may utilize services and devices which are excluded from coverage, e.g., acupuncture (see §35-8), biofeedback (see §35-27), dorsal column stimulator (see §65-8), and family counseling services (see §35-14). In determining whether the scope of a pain program does necessitate inpatient hospital care, evaluate only those services and devices which are covered. Although diagnostic tests may be an appropriate part of pain rehabilitation programs, such tests would be covered in an individual case only where they can be reasonably related to a patient's illness, complaint, symptom, or injury and where they do not represent an unnecessary duplication of tests previously performed.

An inpatient program of 4 weeks' duration is generally required to modify pain behavior. After this period it would be expected that any additional rehabilitation services which might be required could be effectively provided on an outpatient basis under an outpatient pain rehabilitation program (see §10.4 of the NCD Manual) or other outpatient program. The first 7-10 days of such an inpatient program constitute, in effect, an evaluation period. If a patient is unable to adjust to the program within this period, it is generally concluded that it is unlikely that the program will be effective and the patient is discharged from the program. On occasions a program longer than 4 weeks may be required in a particular case. In such a case there should be documentation to substantiate that inpatient care beyond a 4-week period was reasonable and necessary. Similarly, where it appears that a patient participating in a program is being granted frequent outside passes, a question would exist as to whether an inpatient program is reasonable and necessary for the treatment of the patient's condition.

An inpatient hospital stay for the purpose of participating in a pain rehabilitation program would be covered as reasonable and necessary to the treatment of a patient's condition where the pain is attributable to a physical cause, the usual methods of treatment have not been successful in alleviating it, and a significant loss of ability to function independently has resulted from the pain. Chronic pain patients often have psychological problems which accompany or stem from the physical pain and it is appropriate to include psychological treatment in the multidisciplinary approach. However, patients whose pain symptoms result from a mental condition, rather than from any physical cause, generally cannot be succesfully treated in a pain rehabilitation program.

Pub. 100-3, Section 10.4

Outpatient Hospital Pain Rehabilitation Programs

Coverage of services furnished under outpatient hospital pain rehabilitation programs, including services furnished in group settings under individualized plans of treatment, is available if the patient's pain is attributable to a physical cause, the usual methods of treatment have not been successful in alleviating it, and a significant loss of ability by the patient to function independently has resulted from the pain. If a patient meets these conditions and the program provides services of the types discussed in §10.3 of the NCD Manual, the services provided

under the program may be covered. Noncovered services (e.g., vocational counseling, meals for outpatients, or acupuncture) continue to be excluded from coverage, and intermediaries would not be precluded from finding, in the case of particular patients, that the pain rehabilitation program is not reasonable and necessary under §1862(a)(1) of the Act for the treatment of their conditions.

Pub. 100-3, Section 10.5

Autogenous Epidural Blood Graft

Autogenous epidural blood grafts are considered a safe and effective remedy for severe headaches that may occur after performance of spinal anesthesia, spinal taps or myelograms, and are covered.

Pub. 100-3, Section 20.1

Vertebral Artery Surgery

These procedures can be medically reasonable and necessary, but only if each of the following conditions is met:

* Symptoms of vertebral artery obstruction exist;

* Other causes have been considered and ruled out;

* There is radiographic evidence of a valid vertebral artery obstruction; and

* Contraindications to the procedure do not exist, such as coexistent obstructions of multiple cerebral vessels.

Angiograms documenting a valid obstruction should show not only the aortic arch with the vessels off the arch, but also show the vessels in the neck and head (providing biplane views of the carotid and vertebral vascular system). In addition, serial views are needed to diagnose "subclavian steal," the condition in which subclavian artery obstruction causes the symptoms of vertebral artery obstruction. Because the symptoms are not specific for vertebral artery obstruction, other causes must be considered. In addition to vertebral artery obstruction, the differential diagnosis should include various degenerative disorders of the brain, orthostatic hypotension, acoustic neuroma, labyrinthitis, diabetes mellitus and hypoglycemia related disorders.

Obstructions which can cause symptoms of blocked vertebral artery blood flow and which can be documented by an angiogram include:

* Intravascular obstructions - arteriosclerotic lesions within the vertebral artery or in other arteries.

* Extravascular obstructions.

* Bony tissue or osteophytes, located laterally in the C6(C7)-C2 cervical vertebral area course of the vertebral artery, most commonly at C5 -C6.

Anatomical variations - Anomalous location of the origin of the vertebral artery, a congenital aberration, and tortuosity and kinks of the vertebral artery.

Fibrous tissue - Tissue changed as a result of manipulation of the neck for neck pain or injury associated with hematoma; external bands, tendinous slings, and fibrous bands.

The most controversial obstructions include vertebral artery tortuosity and kinks and connective tissue along the course of the vertebral artery, and variously called external bands, tendinous slings and fibrous bands. In the absence of symptoms of vertebral artery obstruction, vascular surgeons feel such abnormalities are insignificant. Vascular surgery experts, however, agree that these abnormalities in very rare cases do cause symptoms of vertebral artery obstruction and do necessitate surgical correction.

Vertebral artery construction and vertebral artery surgery are phrases which most physicians interpret to include only surgical cleaning (endarterectomy) and bypass (resection) procedures. However, some physicians who use these terms mean all operative manipulations which remove vertebral artery blood flow obstructions. Also, some physicians use general terms of vascular surgery, such as endarterectomy when vertebral artery related surgery is performed. Use of the above terminology specifies neither the surgical procedure performed nor its relationship to the vertebral artery. Therefore, in developing claims for this type of procedure, require specific identification of the obstruction in question and the surgical procedure performed. Also, in view of the specific coverage criteria given, develop all claims for vertebral artery surgery on a case-by-case basis.

Make payment for a surgical procedure listed above if: (1) it is reasonable and necessary for the individual patient to have the surgery performed to remove or relieve an obstruction to vertebral artery flow, and (2) the four conditions noted are met.

In all other cases, these procedures cannot be considered reasonable and necessary within the meaning of §1862(a)(1) of the Act and are not reimbursable under the program.

Pub. 100-3, Section 20.3

Thoracic Duct Drainage (TDD) in Renal Transplants

TDD is performed on an inpatient basis, and the inpatient stay is covered for patients admitted for treatment in advance of a kidney transplant as well as for those receiving it post-transplant. TDD is a covered technique when furnished to a kidney transplant recipient or an individual approved to receive kidney transplantation in a hospital approved to perform kidney transplantation.

Pub. 100-3, Section 20.4

Implantable Automatic Defibrillators

A. Covered Indications

1. Documented episode of cardiac arrest due to ventricular fibrillation (VF), not due to a transient or reversible cause (effective July 1, 1991).

2. Documented sustained ventricular tachyarrhythmia (VT), either spontaneous or induced by an electrophysiology (EP) study, not associated with an acute myocardial infarction (MI) and not due to a transient or reversible cause (effective July 1, 1999).

3. Documented familial or inherited conditions with a high risk of life-threatening VT, such as long QT syndrome or hypertrophic cardiomyopathy (effective July 1, 1999).

Additional indications effective for services performed on or after October 1, 2003:

4. Coronary artery disease with a documented prior MI, a measured left ventricular ejection fraction (LVEF) <0.35, and inducible, sustained VT or VF at EP study. (The MI must have occurred more than 40 days prior to defibrillator insertion. The EP test must be performed more than 4 weeks after the qualifying MI.)

5. Documented prior MI and a measured LVEF <0.30 and a QRS duration of >120 milliseconds (the QRS restriction does not apply to services performed on or after January 27, 2005). Patients must not have:

a. New York Heart Association (NYHC) classification IV;

b. Cardiogenic shock or symptomatic hypotension while in a stable baseline rhythm;

c. Had a coronary artery bypass graft (CABG) or percutaneous transluminal coronary angioplasty (PTCA) within past 3 months;

d. Had an enzyme positive MI within past month (Effective for services on or after January 27, 2005, patients must not have an acute MI in the past 40 days);

e. Clinical symptoms or findings that would make them a candidate for coronary revascularization; or

f. Any disease, other than cardiac disease (e.g., cancer, uremia, liver failure), associated with a likelihood of survival less than 1 year.

Additional indications effective for services performed on or after January 27, 2005:

6. Patients with ischemic dilated cardiomyopathy (IDCM), documented prior MI, NYHA Class II and III heart failure, and measured LVEF <35%;

7. Patients with non-ischemic dilated cardiomyopathy (NIDCM) >9 months, NYHA Class II and III heart failure, and measured LVEF <35%;

8. Patients who meet all current Centers for Medicare & Medicaid Services (CMS) coverage requirements for a cardiac resynchronization therapy (CRT) device and have NYHA Class IV heart failure;

All indications must meet the following criteria:

a. Patients must not have irreversible brain damage from preexisting cerebral disease;

b. MIs must be documented and defined according to the consensus document of the Joint European Society of Cardiology/American College of Cardiology Committee for the Redefinition of Myocardial Infarction;

Indications 3 - 8 (primary prevention of sudden cardiac death) must also meet the following criteria:

a. Patients must be able to give informed consent;

b. Patients must not have:

— Cardiogenic shock or symptomatic hypotension while in a stable baseline rhythm;

— Had a CABG or PTCA within the past 3 months;

— Had an acute MI within the past 40 days;

— Clinical symptoms or findings that would make them a candidate for coronary revascularization;

— Any disease, other than cardiac disease (e.g., cancer, uremia, liver failure), associated with a likelihood of survival less than 1 year;

c. Ejection fractions must be measured by angiography, radionuclide scanning, or echocardiography;

d. The beneficiary receiving the defibrillator implantation for primary prevention is enrolled in either a Food and Drug Administration (FDA)-approved category B investigational device exemption (IDE) clinical trial (42 CFR §405.201), a trial under the CMS Clinical Trial Policy (National Coverage Determination (NCD) Manual §310.1) or a qualifying data collection system including approved clinical trials and registries. Initially, an implantable cardiac defibrillator (ICD) database will be maintained using a data submission mechanism that is already in use by Medicare participating hospitals to submit data to the Iowa Foundation for Medical Care (IFMC) – a Quality Improvement Organization (QIO) contractor – for determination of reasonable and necessary and quality improvement. Initial hypothesis and data elements are specified in this decision (Appendix VI) and are the minimum necessary to ensure that the device is reasonable and necessary. Data collection will be completed using the ICDA (ICD Abstraction Tool) and transmitted via QNet (Quality Network Exchange) to the IFMC who will collect and maintain the database. Additional stakeholder-developed data collection systems to augment or replace the initial QNet system, addressing at a minimum the hypotheses specified in this decision, must meet the following basic criteria:

- Written protocol on file;

- Institutional review board review and approval;

- Scientific review and approval by two or more qualified individuals who are not part of the research team;

- Certification that investigators have not been disqualified.

For purposes of this coverage decision, CMS will determine whether specific registries or clinical trials meet these criteria.

e. Providers must be able to justify the medical necessity of devices other than single lead devices. This justification should be available in the patient's medical record.

9. Patients with NIDCM >3 months, NYHA Class II or III heart failure, and measured LVEF <35%, only if the following additional criteria are also met:

a. Patients must be able to give informed consent;

b. Patients must not have:

- Cardiogenic shock or symptomatic hypotension while in a stable baseline rhythm;

- Had a CABG or PTCA within the past 3 months;

- Had an acute MI within the past 40 days;

- Clinical symptoms or findings that would make them a candidate for coronary revascularization;

- Irreversible brain damage from preexisting cerebral disease;

- Any disease, other than cardiac disease (e.g. cancer, uremia, liver failure), associated with a likelihood of survival less than 1 year;

c. Ejection fractions must be measured by angiography, radionuclide scanning, or echocardiography;

d. MIs must be documented and defined according to the consensus document of the Joint European Society of Cardiology/American College of Cardiology Committee for the Redefinition of Myocardial Infarction;

e. The beneficiary receiving the defibrillator implantation for this indication is enrolled in either an FDA-approved category B IDE clinical trial (42 CFR §405.201), a trial under the CMS Clinical Trial Policy (NCD Manual §310.1), or a prospective data collection system meeting the following basic criteria:

- Written protocol on file;

- Institutional Review Board review and approval;

- Scientific review and approval by two or more qualified individuals who are not part of the research team;

- Certification that investigators have not been disqualified.

- For purposes of this coverage decision, CMS will determine whether specific registries or clinical trials meet these criteria.

f. Providers must be able to justify the medical necessity of devices other than single lead devices. This justification should be available in the patient's medical record.

C. Other Indications

All other indications for implantable automatic defibrillators not currently covered in accordance with this decision will continue to be covered under Category B IDE trials (42 CFR §405.201) and the CMS routine clinical trials policy (NCD §310.1).

(This NCD last reviewed February 2005.)

Pub. 100-3, Section 20.5

Extracorporeal Immunoadsorption (ECI) Using Protein A Columns

For claims with dates of service on or after January 1, 2001, Medicare covers the use of Protein A columns for the treatment of ITP. In addition, Medicare will cover Protein A columns for the treatment of rheumatoid arthritis (RA) under the following conditions:

1. Patient has severe RA. Patient disease is active, having >5 swollen joints, >20 tender joints, and morning stiffness >60 minutes.

2. Patient has failed an adequate course of a minimum of 3 Disease Modifying Anti-Rheumatic Drugs (DMARDs). Failure does not include intolerance.

Other uses of these columns are currently considered to be investigational and, therefore, not reasonable and necessary under the Medicare law. (See §1862(a)(1)(A) of the Act.)

Pub. 100-3, Section 20.6

Transmyocardial Revascularization (TMR)

CMS therefore covers TMR as a late or last resort for patients with severe (Canadian Cardiovascular Society classification Classes III or IV) angina (stable or unstable), which has been found refractory to standard medical therapy, including drug therapy at the maximum tolerated or maximum safe dosages. In addition, the angina symptoms must be caused by areas of the heart not amenable to surgical therapies such as percutaneous transluminal coronary angioplasty, stenting, coronary atherectomy or coronary bypass. Coverage is further limited to those uses of the laser used in performing the procedure which have been approved by the Food and Drug Administration for the purpose for which they are being used.

Patients would have to meet the following additional selection guidelines:

1. An ejection fraction of 25% or greater;

2. Have areas of viable ischemic myocardium (as demonstrated by diagnostic study) which are not capable of being revascularized by direct coronary intervention; and

3. Have been stabilized, or have had maximal efforts to stabilize acute conditions such as severe ventricular arrhythmias, decompensated congestive heart failure or acute myocardial infarction.

Coverage is limited to physicians who have been properly trained in the procedure. Providers of this service is performed must also document that all ancillary personnel, including physicians, nurses, operating room personnel and technicians, are trained in the procedure and the proper use of the equipment involved. Coverage is further limited to providers which have dedicated cardiac care units, including the diagnostic and support services necessary for care of patients undergoing this therapy. In addition, these providers must conform to the standards for laser safety set by the American National Standards Institute, ANSIZ1363.

Pub. 100-3, Section 20.7

Percutaneous Transluminal Angioplasty (PTA)

B. Nationally Covered Indications

The PTA is covered to treat the following indications:

1. Atherosclerotic obstructive lesions:

- In the lower extremities, i.e., the iliac, femoral, and popliteal arteries, or in the upper extremities, i.e., the innominate, subclavian, axillary, and brachial arteries. The upper extremities do not include head or neck vessels.

- Of a single coronary artery for patients for whom the likely alternative treatment is coronary bypass surgery and who exhibit the following characteristics:
  - Angina refractory to optimal medical management;
  - Objective evidence of myocardial ischemia; and
  - Lesions amenable to angioplasty.

- Of the renal arteries for patients in whom there is an inadequate response to a thorough medical management of symptoms and for whom surgery is the likely alternative. The PTA for this group of patients is an alternative to surgery, not simply an addition to medical management.

- Of arteriovenous dialysis fistulas and grafts when performed through either a venous or arterial approach.

2. Effective July 1, 2001, Medicare covers PTA of the carotid artery concurrent with carotid stent placement when furnished in accordance with the Food and Drug Administration (FDA)-approved protocols governing Category B Investigational Device Exemption (IDE) clinical trials. The PTA of the carotid artery, when provided solely for the purpose of carotid artery dilation concurrent with carotid stent placement, is considered to be a reasonable and necessary service only when provided in the context of such a clinical trial.

3. Effective October 12, 2004, Medicare covers PTA of the carotid artery concurrent with the placement of an FDA-approved carotid stent for an FDA-approved indication when furnished in accordance with FDA-approved protocols governing post-approval studies. CMS determines that coverage of PTA of the carotid artery is reasonable and necessary under these circumstances.

4. Effective March 17, 2005, Medicare covers PTA of the carotid artery concurrent with the placement of an FDA-approved carotid stent with embolic protection for the following:

- Patients who are at high risk for carotid endarterectomy (CEA) and who also have symptomatic carotid artery stenosis >70%. Coverage is limited to procedures performed using FDA-approved carotid artery stenting systems and embolic protection devices;

- Patients who are at high risk for CEA and have symptomatic carotid artery stenosis between 50% and 70%, in accordance with the Category B IDE clinical trials regulation (42 CFR 405.201), as a routine cost under the clinical trials policy (Medicare National Coverage Determinations Manual (NCD), 310.1), or in accordance with the NCD on carotid artery stenting (CAS) post-approval studies (Medicare NCD Manual 20.7);

- Patients who are at high risk for CEA and have asymptomatic carotid artery stenosis >80%, in accordance with the Category B IDE clinical trials regulation (42 CFR 405.201), as a routine cost under the clinical trials policy (Medicare NCD Manual 310.1), or in accordance with the NCD on CAS post- approval studies (Medicare NCD Manual 20.7).

- Patients at high risk for CEA are defined as having significant comorbidities and/or anatomic risk factors (i.e., recurrent stenosis and/or previous radical neck dissection), and would be poor candidates for CEA in the opinion of a surgeon.

Significant comorbid conditions include but are not limited to:

- congestive heart failure (CHF) class III/IV;
- left ventricular ejection fraction (LVEF) <30%;
- unstable angina;
- contralateral carotid occlusion;
- recent myocardial infarction (MI);
- previous CEA with recurrent stenosis;
- prior radiation treatment to the neck; and
- other conditions that were used to determine patients at high risk for CEA in the prior CAS trials and studies, such as ARCHER, CABERNET, SAPPHIRE, BEACH, and MAVERIC II.

Symptoms of carotid artery stenosis include carotid transient ischemic attack (distinct focal neurologic dysfunction persisting less than 24 hours), focal cerebral ischemia producing a nondisabling stroke (modified Rankin scale <3 with symptoms for 24 hours or more),1 and transient monocular blindness (amaurosis fugax). Patients who have had a disabling stroke (modified Rankin scale >3) would be excluded from coverage.

The determination that a patient is at high risk for CEA and the patient's symptoms of carotid artery stenosis should be available in the patient medical records prior to performing any procedure.

The degree of carotid artery stenosis should be measured by duplex Doppler ultrasound or carotid artery angiography and recorded in the patient medical records. If the stenosis is measured by ultrasound prior to the procedure, then the degree of stenosis must be confirmed by angiography at the start of the procedure. If the stenosis is determined to be less than 70% by angiography, then CAS should not proceed.

In addition, CMS determines that CAS with embolic protection is reasonable and necessary only if performed in facilities that have been determined to be competent in performing the evaluation, procedure, and follow-up necessary to ensure optimal patient outcomes. Standards to determine competency will include specific physician training standards, facility support requirements, and data collection to evaluate outcomes during a required reevaluation.

The CMS created a list of minimum standards modeled in part on professional society statements on competency. All facilities must at least meet CMS's standards in order to receive coverage for CAS for high risk patients.

Facilities must have necessary imaging equipment, device inventory, staffing, and infrastructure to support a dedicated carotid stent program. Specifically, high-quality X-ray imaging equipment is a critical component of any carotid interventional suite, such as high resolution digital imaging systems with the capability of subtraction, magnification, road mapping, and orthogonal angulation.

Advanced physiologic monitoring must be available in the interventional suite. This includes real time and archived physiologic, hemodynamic, and cardiac rhythm monitoring equipment, as well as support staff who are capable of interpreting the findings and responding appropriately.

Emergency management equipment and systems must be readily available in the interventional suite such as resuscitation equipment, a defibrillator, vasoactive and antiarrhythmic drugs, endotracheal intubation capability, and anesthesia support.

Each institution should have a clearly delineated program for granting carotid stent privileges and for monitoring the quality of the individual interventionalists and the program as a whole. The oversight committee for this program should be empowered to identify the minimum case volume for an operator to maintain privileges, as well as the (risk-adjusted) threshold for complications that the institution will allow before suspending privileges or instituting measures for remediation. Committees are encouraged to apply published standards from national specialty societies recognized by the American Board of Medical Specialties to determine appropriate physician qualifications. Examples of standards and clinical competence guidelines include those published in the December 2004 edition of the American Journal of Neuroradiology, and those published in the August 18, 2004, Journal of the American College of Cardiology.

To continue to receive Medicare payment for CAS under this decision, the facility or a contractor to the facility must collect data on all CAS procedures done at that particular facility. This data must be analyzed routinely to ensure patient safety, and will also be used in the process of re-credentialing the facility. This data must be made available to CMS upon request. The interval for data analysis will be determined by the facility but should not be less frequent than every 6 months.

Since there currently is no recognized entity that evaluates CAS facilities, CMS established a mechanism for evaluating facilities. Facilities must provide written documentation to CMS that the facility meets one of the following:

1. The facility was an FDA-approved site that enrolled patients in prior CAS IDE trials, such as SAPPHIRE, and ARCHER;

2. The facility is an FDA-approved site that is participating and enrolling patients in ongoing CAS IDE trials, such as CREST;

3. The facility is an FDA-approved site for one or more FDA post-approval studies; or,

4. The facility has provided a written affidavit to CMS attesting that the facility has met the minimum facility standards. This should be sent to:Director, Coverage and Analysis Group7500 Security Boulevard, Mailstop C1-09-06Baltimore, MD 21244.

The letter must include the following information:Facility's name and complete address;Facility's Medicare provider number;Point-of-contact for questions with telephone number;Mechanism of data collection of CAS procedures; and,Signature of a senior facility administrative official.

A list of approved facilities will be made available and viewable at http://www.cms.hhs.gov/MedicareApprovedFacilitie/CASF/list.asp#TopOfPage. In addition, CMS will publish a list of approved facilities in the Federal Register. A new affidavit is required every two years to ensure that facilities maintain high standards.

C. Nationally Noncovered Indications

Performance of PTA to treat obstructive lesions of the vertebral and cerebral arteries remains noncovered. The safety and efficacy of these procedures are not established.

D. Other

All other indications for PTA for which CMS has not specifically indicated coverage remain noncovered.

(This NCD last reviewed April 2005.)

Pub. 100-3, Section 20.8

Cardiac Pacemakers

Cardiac pacemakers are covered as prosthetic devices under the Medicare program, subject to the following conditions and limitations. While cardiac pacemakers have been covered under Medicare for many years, there were no specific guidelines for their use other than the general Medicare requirement that covered services be reasonable and necessary for the treatment of the condition. Services rendered for cardiac pacing on or after the effective dates of this instruction are subject to these guidelines, which are based on certain assumptions regarding the clinical goals of cardiac pacing. While some uses of pacemakers are relatively certain or unambiguous, many other uses require considerable expertise and judgment.

Consequently, the medical necessity for permanent cardiac pacing must be viewed in the context of overall patient management. The appropriateness of such pacing may be conditional on other diagnostic or therapeutic modalities having been undertaken. Although significant complications and adverse side effects of pacemaker use are relatively rare, they cannot be ignored when considering the use of pacemakers for dubious medical conditions, or marginal clinical benefit.

These guidelines represent current concepts regarding medical circumstances in which permanent cardiac pacing may be appropriate or necessary. As with other areas of medicine, advances in knowledge and techniques in cardiology are expected. Consequently, judgments about the medical necessity and acceptability of new uses for cardiac pacing in new classes of patients may change as more more conclusive evidence becomes available. This instruction applies only to permanent cardiac pacemakers, and does not address the use of temporary, non-implanted pacemakers.

The two groups of conditions outlined below deal with the necessity for cardiac pacing for patients in general. These are intended as guidelines in assessing the medical necessity for pacing therapies, taking into account the particular circumstances in each case. However, as a general rule, the two groups of current medical concepts may be viewed as representing:

Group I: Single-Chamber Cardiac Pacemakers — a) conditions under which single chamber pacemaker claims may be considered covered without further claims development; and b) conditions under which single-chamber pacemaker claims would be denied unless further claims development shows that they fall into the covered category, or special medical circumstances exist of the sufficiency to convince the contractor that the claim should be paid.

Group II: Dual-Chamber Cardiac Pacemakers - a) conditions under which dual-chamber pacemaker claims may be considered covered without further claims development, and b) conditions under which dual-chamber pacemaker claims would be denied unless further claims development shows that they fall into the covered categories for single- and dual-chamber pacemakers, or special medical circumstances exist sufficient to convince the contractor that the claim should be paid.

CMS opened the NCD on Cardiac Pacemakers to afford the public an opportunity to comment on the proposal to revise the language contained in the instruction. The revisions transfer the focus of the NCD from the actual pacemaker implantation procedure itself to the reasonable and necessary medical indications that justify cardiac pacing. This is consistent with our findings that pacemaker implantation is no longer considered routinely harmful or an experimental procedure.

Group I: Single-Chamber Cardiac Pacemakers (Effective March 16, 1983)

A. Nationally Covered Indications

Conditions under which cardiac pacing is generally considered acceptable or necessary, provided that the conditions are chronic or recurrent and not due to transient causes such as acute myocardial infarction, drug toxicity, or electrolyte imbalance. (In cases where there is a rhythm disturbance, if the rhythm disturbance is chronic or recurrent, a single episode of a symptom such as syncope or seizure is adequate to establish medical necessity.)

1. Acquired complete (also referred to as third-degree) AV heart block.

2. Congenital complete heart block with severe bradycardia (in relation to age), or significant physiological deficits or significant symptoms due to the bradycardia.

3. Second-degree AV heart block of Type II (i.e., no progressive prolongation of P-R interval prior to each blocked beat. P-R interval indicates the time taken for an impulse to travel from the atria to the ventricles on an electrocardiogram).

4. Second-degree AV heart block of Type I (i.e., progressive prolongation of P-R interval prior to each blocked beat) with significant symptoms due to hemodynamic instability associated with the heart block.

5. Sinus bradycardia associated with major symptoms (e.g., syncope, seizures, congestive heart failure); or substantial sinus bradycardia (heart rate less than 50) associated with dizziness or confusion. The correlation between symptoms and bradycardia must be documented, or the symptoms must be clearly attributable to the bradycardia rather than to some other cause.

6. In selected and few patients, sinus bradycardia of lesser severity (heart rate 50-59) with dizziness or confusion. The correlation between symptoms and bradycardia must be documented, or the symptoms must be clearly attributable to the bradycardia rather than to some other cause.

7. Sinus bradycardia is the consequence of long-term necessary drug treatment for which there is no acceptable alternative when accompanied by significant symptoms (e.g., syncope, seizures, congestive heart failure, dizziness or confusion). The correlation between symptoms and bradycardia must be documented, or the symptoms must be clearly attributable to the bradycardia rather than to some other cause.

8. Sinus node dysfunction with or without tachyarrhythmias or AV conduction block (i.e., the bradycardia-tachycardia syndrome, sino-atrial block, sinus arrest) when accompanied by significant symptoms (e.g., syncope, seizures, congestive heart failure, dizziness or confusion).

9. Sinus node dysfunction with or without symptoms when there are potentially life-threatening ventricular arrhythmias or tachycardia secondary to the bradycardia (e.g., numerous premature ventricular contractions, couplets, runs of premature ventricular contractions, or ventricular tachycardia).

10. Bradycardia associated with supraventricular tachycardia (e.g., atrial fibrillation, atrial flutter, or paroxysmal atrial tachycardia) with high-degree AV block which is unresponsive to appropriate pharmacological management and when the bradycardia is associated with significant symptoms (e.g., syncope, seizures, congestive heart failure, dizziness or confusion).

11. The occasional patient with hypersensitive carotid sinus syndrome with syncope due to bradycardia and unresponsive to prophylactic medical measures.

12. Bifascicular or trifascicular block accompanied by syncope which is attributed to transient complete heart block after other plausible causes of syncope have been reasonably excluded.

13. Prophylactic pacemaker use following recovery from acute myocardial infarction during which there was temporary complete (third-degree) and/or Mobitz Type II second-degree AV block in association with bundle branch block.

14. In patients with recurrent and refractory ventricular tachycardia, "overdrive pacing" (pacing above the basal rate) to prevent ventricular tachycardia.

(Effective May 9, 1985)

15. Second-degree AV heart block of Type I with the QRS complexes prolonged.

B. Nationally Noncovered Indications

Conditions which, although used by some physicians as a basis for permanent cardiac pacing, are considered unsupported by adequate evidence of benefit and therefore should not generally be considered appropriate uses for single-chamber pacemakers in the absence of the above indications. Contractors should review claims for pacemakers with these indications to determine the need for further claims development prior to denying the claim, since additional claims development may be required. The object of such further development is to establish whether the particular claim actually meets the conditions in a) above. In claims where this is not the case or where such an event appears unlikely, the contractor may deny the claim

1. Syncope of undetermined cause.

2. Sinus bradycardia without significant symptoms.

3. Sino-atrial block or sinus arrest without significant symptoms.

4. Prolonged P-R intervals with atrial fibrillation (without third-degree AV block) or with other causes of transient ventricular pause.

5. Bradycardia during sleep.

6. Right bundle branch block with left axis deviation (and other forms of fascicular or bundle branch block) without syncope or other symptoms of intermittent AV block).

7. Asymptomatic second-degree AV block of Type I unless the QRS complexes are prolonged or electrophysiological studies have demonstrated that the block is at or beyond the level of the His bundle (a component of the electrical conduction system of the heart).

Effective October 1, 2001

8. Asymptomatic bradycardia in post-mycardial infarction patients about to initiate long-term beta-blocker drug therapy.

Group II: Dual-Chamber Cardiac Pacemakers — (Effective May 9, 1985)

A. Nationally Covered Indications

Conditions under dual-chamber cardiac pacing are considered acceptable or necessary in the general medical community unless conditions 1 and 2 under Group II. B., are present:

1. Patients in who single-chamber (ventricular pacing) at the time of pacemaker insertion elicits a definite drop in blood pressure, retrograde conduction, or discomfort.

2. Patients in whom the pacemaker syndrome (atrial ventricular asynchrony), with significant symptoms, has already been experienced with a pacemaker that is being replaced.

3. Patients in whom even a relatively small increase in cardiac efficiency will importantly improve the quality of life, e.g., patients with congestive heart failure despite adequate other medical measures.

4. Patients in whom the pacemaker syndrome can be anticipated, e.g., in young and active people, etc.

Dual-chamber pacemakers may also be covered for the conditions, as listed in Group I. A., if the medical necessity is sufficiently justified through adequate claims development. Expert physicians differ in their judgments about what constitutes appropriate criteria for dual-chamber pacemaker use. The judgment that such a pacemaker is warranted in the patient meeting accepted criteria must be based upon the individual needs and characteristics of that patient, weighing the magnitude and likelihood of anticipated benefits against the magnitude and likelihood of disadvantages to the patient.

B. Nationally Noncovered Indications

Whenever the following conditions (which represent overriding contraindications) are present, dual-chamber pacemakers are not covered:

1. Ineffective atrial contractions (e.g., chronic atrial fibrillation or flutter, or giant left atrium).

2. Frequent or persistent supraventricular tachycardias, except where the pacemaker is specifically for the control of the tachycardia.

3. A clinical condition in which pacing takes place only intermittently and briefly, and which is not associated with a reasonable likelihood that pacing needs will become prolonged, e.g., the occasional patient with hypersensitive carotid sinus syndrome with syncope due to bradycardia and unresponsive to prophylactic medical measures.

4. Prophylactic pacemaker use following recovery from acute myocardial infarction during which there was temporary complete (third-degree) and/or Type II second-degree AV block in association with bundle branch block.

C. Other

All other indications for dual-chamber cardiac pacing for which CMS has not specifically indicated coverage remain nationally noncovered, ecept for Category B IDE clinical trails, or as routine costs of dual-chamber cardiac pacing associated with clinical trials, in accordance with section 310.1 of the NCD Manual.

(This NCD last reviewed June 2004.)

Pub. 100-3, Section 20.8.1

Cardiac Pacemaker Evaluation Services

Medicare covers a variety of services for the post-implant follow-up and evaluation of implanted cardiac pacemakers. The following guidelines are designed to assist contractors in identifying and processing claims for such services.

NOTE: These new guidelines are limited to lithium battery-powered pacemakers, because mercury-zinc battery-powered pacemakers are no longer being manufactured and virtually all have been replaced by lithium units. Contractors still receiving claims for monitoring such units should continue to apply the guidelines published in 1980 to those units until they are replaced.

One fact of which contractors should be aware is that many dual-chamber units may be programmed to pace only the ventricles; this may be done either at the time the pacemaker is implanted or at some time afterward. In such cases, a dual-chamber unit, when programmed or reprogrammed for ventricular pacing, should be treated as a single-chamber pacemaker in applying screening guidelines.

The decision as to how often any patient's pacemaker should be monitored is the responsibility of the patient's physician who is best able to take into account the condition and circumstances of the individual patient. These may vary over time, requiring modifications of the frequency with which the patient should be monitored. In cases where monitoring is done by some entity other than the patient's physician, such as a commercial monitoring service or hospital outpatient department, the physician's prescription for monitoring is required and should be periodically renewed (at least annually) to assure that the frequency of monitoring is proper for the patient. When a patient is monitored both during clinica visits and transtelephonically, the contractor should be sure to include frequency data on both ypes of monitoring in evaluating the reasonableness of the frequency of monitoring services received by the patient.

Since there are over 200 pacemaker models in service at any given point, and a variety of patient conditions that give rise to the need for pacemakers, the question of the appropriate frequency of monitorings is a complex one. Nevertheless, it is possible to develop guidelines within which the vast majority of pacemaker monitorings will fall and contractors should do this, using their own data and experience, as well as the frequency guidelines which follow, in order to limit extensive claims development to those cases requiring special attention.

Pub. 100-3, Section 20.8.2

Self-Contained Pacemaker Monitors

Self-contained pacemaker monitors are accepted devices for monitoring cardiac pacemakers. Accordingly, program payment may be made for the rental or purchase of either of the following pacemaker monitors when it is prescribed by a physician for a patient with a cardiac pacemaker:

A. Digital Electronic Pacemaker Monitor. — This device provides the patient with an instantaneous digital readout of his pacemaker pulse rate. Use of this device does not involve professional services until there has been a change of five pulses (or more) per minute above or below the initial rate of the pacemaker; when such change occurs, the patient contacts his physician.

B. Audible/Visible Signal Pacemaker Monitor. — This device produces an audible and visible signal which indicates the pacemaker rate. Use of this device does not involve professional services until a change occurs in these signals; at such time, the patient contacts his physician.

NOTE: The design of the self-contained pacemaker monitor makes it possible for the patient to monitor his pacemaker periodically and minimizes the need for regular visits to the outpatient department of the provider.Therefore, documentation of the medical necessity for pacemaker evaluation in the outpatient department of the provider should be obtained where such evaluation is employed in addition to the self-contained pacemaker monitor used by the patient in his home.

Pub. 100-3, Section 20.8.3

Anesthesia in Cardiac Pacemaker Surgery

The use of general or monitored anesthesia during transvenous cardiac pacemaker surgery may be reasonable and necessary and therefore covered under Medicare only if adequate documentation of medical necessity is provided on a case-by-case basis. Obtain advice from your medical consultants or from appropriate specialty physicians or groups in your locality regarding the adequacy of documentation before deciding whether a particular claim should be covered.

A second type of pacemaker surgery that is sometimes performed involves the use of the thoracic method of implantation, which requires open surgery. Where the thoracic method is employed, general anesthesia is always used and should not require special medical documentation.

Pub. 100-3, Section 20.10

Cardiac Rehabilitation Programs

Indications and Limitations of Coverage

B. Nationally Covered Indications

Effective for services performed on or after March 22, 2006, Medicare coverage of cardiac rehabilitation programs is considered reasonable and necessary only for patients who: (1) have a documented diagnosis of acute myocardial infarction within the preceding 12 months; or (2) have had coronary bypass surgery; or (3) have stable angina pectoris; or (4) have had heart valve repair/replacement; or (5) have had percutaneous transluminal coronary angioplasty (PTCA) or coronary stenting; or (6) have had a heart or heart-lung transplant.

1. Program Requirements

a. Duration

Services provided in connection with a cardiac rehabilitation exercise program may be considered reasonable and necessary for up to 36 sessions. Patients generally receive 2 to 3 sessions per week for 12 to 18 weeks. Coverage of additional sessions is discussed in section D below.

b. Components

Cardiac rehabilitation programs must be comprehensive and to be comprehensive they must include a medical evaluation, a program to modify cardiac risk factors (e.g., nutritional counseling), prescribed exercise, education, and counseling.

c. Facility

The facility must have available for immediate use the necessary cardio-pulmonary, emergency, diagnostic, and therapeutic life-saving equipment accepted by the medical community as medically necessary, e.g., oxygen, cardiopulmonary resuscitation equipment, or defibrillator.

d. Staff

The program must be staffed by personnel necessary to conduct the program safely and effectively, who are trained in both basic and advanced life support techniques and in exercise therapy for coronary disease. The program must be under the direct supervision of a physician, as defined in 42 CFR §410.26(a)(2) (defined through cross reference to 42 CFR §410.32(b)(3)(ii), or 42 CFR §410.27(f)).

C. Nationally Non-Covered Indications

Except as provided in section D., all other indications are not covered.

D. Other

The contractor has the discretion to cover cardiac rehabilitation services beyond 18 weeks. Coverage must not exceed a total of 72 sessions for 36 weeks.

(This NCD last reviewed March 2006.)

Pub. 100-3, Section 20.11

Intraoperative Ventricular Mapping

The intraoperative ventricular mapping procedure is covered under Medicare only for the uses and medical conditions described below:

- Localize accessory pathways associated with the Wolff-Parkinson-White (WPW) and other preexcitation syndromes;

- Map the sequence of atrial and ventricular activation for drug-resistant supraventricular tachycardias;

- Delineate the anatomical course of His bundle and/or bundle branches during corrective cardiac surgery for congenital heart diseases; and:

- Direct the surgical treatment of patients with refractory ventricular tachyarrhythmias.

Pub. 100-3, Section 20.12

Diagnostic Endocardial Electrical Stimulation (Pacing)

Diagnostic endocardial electrical stimulation (EES), also called programmed electrical stimulation of the heart, is covered under Medicare when used for patients with severe cardiac arrhythmias.

Pub. 100-3, Section 20.13

HIS Bundle Study

Medicare coverage of the procedure would be limited to selected patients: those with complex ongoing acute arrhythmias, those with intermittent or permanent heart block in whom pacemaker implantation is being considered, and those patients who have recently developed heart block secondary to a myocardial infarction. When heart catheterization and the HIS Bundle Study are performed at the same time, the program will cover only one catheterization and a small additional charge for the study.

When a HIS bundle cardiogram is obtained as part of a diagnostic endocardial electrical stimulation, no separate charge will be recognized for the His bundle study.

Pub. 100-3, Section 20.14

Plethysmography

Medicare coverage is extended to those procedures listed in Category I below when used for the accepted medical indications mentioned above. The procedures in Category II are still considered experimental and are not covered at this time. Denial of claims because a noncovered procedure was used or because there was no medical indication for plethysmographic evaluation of any type should be based on §1862(a)(1) of the Act.

Category I - Covered

1. Segmental Plethysmography - Included under this procedure are services performed with a regional plethysmograph, differential plethysmograph, recording oscillometer, and a pulse volume recorder.

2. Electrical Impedance Plethysmography

3. Ultrasonic Measurement of Blood Flow (Doppler) - While not strictly a plethysmographic method, this is also a useful tool in the evaluation of suspected peripheral vascular disease or preoperative screening of podiatric patients with suspected peripheral vascular compromise. (See §50-7 for the applicable coverage policy on this procedure.)

4. Oculoplethysmography - See NCD on Noninvasive Tests of Carotid Function, §20.17.

5. Strain Gauge Plethysmography - This test is based on recording the non-pulsatile aspects of inflowing blood at various points on an extremity by a mercury-in-silastic strain gauge sensor. The instrument consists of a chart recorder, an automatic cuff inflation and deflation system, and a recording manometer.

Category II - Experimental

The following methods have not yet reached a level of development such as to allow their routine use in the evaluation of suspected peripheral vascular disease.

1. Inductance Plethysmography - This method is considered experimental and does not provide reproducible results.

2. Capacitance Plethysmography - This method is considered experimental and does not provide reproducible results.

3. Mechanical Oscillometry - This is a non-standardized method which offers poor sensitivity and is not considered superior to the simple measurement of peripheral blood pressure.

4. Photoelectric Plethysmography - This method is considered useful only in determining whether or not a pulse is present and does not provide reproducible measurements of blood flow.Differential plethysmography, on the other hand, is a system which uses an impedance technique to compare pulse pressures at various points along a limb, with a reference pressure at the mid-brachial or wrist level. It is not clear whether this technique, as usually performed in the physician's office, meets the definition of plethysmography because quantitative measurements of blood flow are usually not made. It has been concluded, in any event, that the differential plethysmography system is a blood pulse recorder of undetermined value, which has the potential for significant overutilization. Therefore, reimbursement for studies done by techniques other than venous occlusive pneumoplethysmography should be denied, at least until additional data on these devices, including controlled clinical studies, become available.

Pub. 100-3, Section 20.15

Electrocardiographic Services

B. Nationally Covered Indications

The following indications are covered nationally unless otherwise indicated:

a. Computer analysis of EKGs when furnished in a setting and under the circumstances required for coverage of other EKG services.

b. EKG services rendered by an independent diagnostic testing facility (IDTF), including physician review and interpretation. Separate physician services are not covered unless he/she is the patient's attending or consulting physician.

c. Emergency EKGs (i.e., when the patient is or may be experiencing a lifethreatening event) performed as a laboratory or diagnostic service by a portable x-ray supplier only when a physician is in attendance at the time the service is performed or immediately thereafter.

d. Home EKG services with documentation of medical necessity.

e. Trans-telephonic EKG transmissions (effective March 1, 1980) as a diagnostic service for the indications described below, when performed with equipment meeting the standards described below, subject to the limitations and conditions specified below. Coverage is further limited to the amounts payable with respect to the physician's service in interpreting the results of such transmissions, including charges for rental of the equipment. The device used by the beneficiary is part of a total diagnostic system and is not considered DME separately.

Covered uses are to:

a.Detect, characterize, and document symptomatic transient arrhythmias;

b.Initiate, revise, or discontinue arrhythmic drug therapy; or,

c.Carry out early post-hospital monitoring of patients discharged after myocardial infarction (MI); (only if 24-hour coverage is provided, see C.5. below).

Certain uses other than those specified above may be covered if, in the judgment of the local contractor, such use is medically necessary.Additionally, the transmitting devices must meet at least the following criteria:

a.They must be capable of transmitting EKG Leads, I, II, or III; and,

b.The tracing must be sufficiently comparable to a conventional EKG.24-hour attended coverage used as early post-hospital monitoring of patients discharged after MI is only covered if provision is made for such 24-hour attended coverage in the manner described below:24-hour attended coverage means there must be, at a monitoring site or central data center, an EKG technician or other non-physician, receiving calls and/or EKG data; tape recording devices do not meet this requirement. Further, such technicians should have immediate, 24-hour access to a physician to review transmitted data and make clinical decisions regarding the patient. The technician should also be instructed as to when and how to contact available facilities to assist the patient in case of emergencies.

C. Nationally Non-covered Indications

The following indications are non-covered nationally unless otherwise specified below:

a. The time-sampling mode of operation of ambulatory EKG cardiac event monitoring/recording.

b. Separate physician services other than those rendered by an IDTF unless rendered by the patient's attending or consulting physician.

c. Home EKG services without documentation of medical necessity.

d. Emergency EKG services by a portable x-ray supplier without a physician in attendance at the time of service or immediately thereafter.

e. 24-hour attended coverage used as early post-hospital monitoring of patients discharged after MI unless provision is made for such 24-hour attended coverage in the manner described in section B.5. above.

f. Any marketed Food and Drug Administration (FDA)-approved ambulatory cardiac monitoring device or service that cannot be categorized according to the framework below.

D. OtherAmbulatory cardiac monitoring performed with a marketed, FDA-approved device, is eligible for coverage if it can be categorized according to the framework below. Unless there is a specific NCD for that device or service, determination as to whether a device or service that fits into the framework is reasonable and necessary is according to local contractor discretion.

Electrocardiographic Services Framework

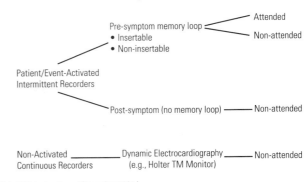

(This NCD last reviewed December 2004.)

Pub. 100-3, Section 20.16

Cardiac Output Monitoring by Thoracic Electrical Bioimpedance (TEB)

A. Covered Indications

1. TEB is covered for the following uses:

a. Differentiation of cardiogenic from pulmonary causes of acute dyspnea when medical history, physical examination, and standard assessment tools provide insufficient information, and the treating physician has determined that TEB hemodynamic data are necessary for appropriate management of the patient.

b. Optimization of atrioventricular (A/V) interval for patients with A/V sequential cardiac pacemakers when medicalhistory, physical examination, and standard assessment tools provide insufficient information, and the treating physician has determined that TEB hemodynamic data are necessary for appropriate management of the patient.

c. Monitoring of continuous inotropic therapy for patients with terminal congestive heart failure, when those patients have chosen to die with comfort at home, or for patients waiting at home for a heart transplant.

d. Evaluation for rejection in patients with a heart transplant as a predetermined alternative to a myocardial biopsy. Medical necessity must be documented should a biopsy be performed after TEB.

e. Optimization of fluid management in patients with congestive heart failure when medical history, physical examination, and standard assessment tools provide insufficient information, and the treating physician has determined that TEB hemodynamic data are necessary for appropriate management of the patient.

2. Contractors have discretion to determine whether the use of TEB for the management of drug-resistant hypertension is reasonable and necessary. Drug resistant hypertension is defined as failure to achieve goal BP in patients who are adhering to full doses of an appropriate three-drug regimen that includes a diuretic.

B. Noncovered Indications

1. TEB is noncovered when used for patients:

a. With proven or suspected disease involving severe regurgitation of the aorta;

b. With minute ventilation (MV) sensor function pacemakers, since the device may adversely affect the functioning of that type of pacemaker;

c. During cardiac bypass surgery; or

d. In the management of all forms of hypertension (with the exception of drug-resistant hypertension as outlined above).

2. All other uses of TEB not otherwise specified remain non-covered. (This NCD last reviewed January 2004.)

Pub. 100-3, Section 20.17

Noninvasive Tests of Carotid Function

It is important to note that the names of these tests are not standardized. Following are some of the acceptable tests, recognizing that this list is not inclusive and that determinations should be made by local medical consultants:

DIRECT TESTS

Carotid Phonoangiography

Direct Bruit Analysis

Spectral Bruit Analysis

Doppler Flow Velocity

Ultrasound Imaging including Real Time

B-Scan and Doppler Devices

INDIRECT TESTS

Periorbital Directional Doppler Ultrasonography

Oculoplethysmography

Ophthalmodynamometry

Pub. 100-3, Section 20.18

Carotid Body Resection/Carotid Body Denervation

Carotid body resection is occasionally used to relieve pulmonary symptoms, including asthma, but has been shown to lack general acceptance of the professional medical community. In addition, controlled clinical studies establishing the safety and effectiveness of this procedure are needed. Therefore, all carotid body resections to relieve pulmonary symptoms must be considered investigational and cannot be considered reasonable and necessary within the meaning of section 1862(a)(l) of the law. No program reimbursement may be made in such cases.

There is, however, one instance where carotid body resection has been accepted by the medical community as effective. That instance is when evidence of a mass in the carotid body,with or without symptoms, indicates the need for surgery to remove the carotid body tumor.

Denervation of a carotid sinus to treat hypersensitive carotid sinus reflex is another procedure performed in the area of the carotid body. In the case of hypersensitive carotid sinus, light pressure on the upper part of the neck (such as might be experienced when turning or raising one's head) results in symptoms such as dizziness or syncope due to hypotension and slowed heart rate. Failure of medical therapy and continued deterioration in the condition of the patient in such cases may indicate need for surgery. Denervation of the carotid sinus is rarely performed, but when elected as the therapy of choice with the above indications, this procedure may be considered reasonable and necessary.

Pub. 100-3, Section 20.19

Ambulatory Blood Pressure Monitoring

ABPM must be performed for at least 24 hours to meet coverage criteria.

ABPM is only covered for those patients with suspected white coat hypertension. Suspected white coat hypertension is defined as

1) office blood pressure >140/90 mm Hg on at least three separate clinic/office visits with two separate measurements made at each visit;

2) at least two documented blood pressure measurements taken outside the office which are <140/90 mm Hg; and

3) no evidence of end-organ damage.

The information obtained by ABPM is necessary in order to determine the appropriate management of the patient. ABPM is not covered for any other uses. In the rare circumstance that ABPM needs to be performed more than once in a patient, the qualifying criteria described above must be met for each subsequent ABPM test.

For those patients that undergo ABPM and have an ambulatory blood pressure of <135/85 with no evidence of end-organ damage, it is likely that their cardiovascular risk is similar to that of normotensives. They should be followed over time. Patients for which ABPM demonstrates a blood pressure of >135/85 may be at increased cardiovascular risk, and a physician may wish to consider antihypertensive therapy.

Pub. 100-3, Section 20.23

Fabric Wrapping of Abdominal Aneurysms

Fabric wrapping of abdominal aneurysms is not a covered Medicare procedure. This is a treatment for abdominal aneurysms which involves wrapping aneurysms with cellophane or fascia lata. This procedure has not been shown to prevent eventual rupture. In extremely rare instances, external wall reinforcement may be indicated when the current accepted treatment (excision of the aneurysm and reconstruction with synthetic materials) is not a viable alternative, but external wall reinforcement is not fabric wrapping. Accordingly, fabric wrapping of abdominal aneurysms is not considered reasonable and necessary within the meaning of §1862(a)(1) of the Act.

Pub. 100-3, Section 20.28

Therapeutic Embolization

Therapeutic embolization is covered when done for hemorrhage, and for other conditions amenable to treatment by the procedure, when reasonable and necessary for the individual patient. Renal embolization for the treatment of renal adenocarcinoma continues to be covered, effective December 15, 1978, as one type of therapeutic embolization, to:

- Reduce tumor vascularity preoperatively;

- Reduce tumor bulk in inoperable cases; or

- Palliate specific symptoms.

Pub. 100-3, Section 20.29

Hyperbaric Oxygen Therapy

A. Covered Conditions

Program reimbursement for HBO therapy will be limited to that which is administered in a chamber (including the one man unit) and is limited to the following conditions:

1. Acute carbon monoxide intoxication,

2. Decompression illness,

3. Gas embolism,

4. Gas gangrene,

5. Acute traumatic peripheral ischemia. HBO therapy is a valuable adjunctive treatment to be used in combination with accepted standard therapeutic measures when loss of function, limb, or life is threatened.

6. Crush injuries and suturing of severed limbs. As in the previous conditions, HBO therapy would be an adjunctive treatment when loss of function, limb, or life is threatened.

7. Progressive necrotizing infections (necrotizing fasciitis),

8. Acute peripheral arterial insufficiency,

9. Preparation and preservation of compromised skin grafts (not for primary management of wounds),

10. Chronic refractory osteomyelitis, unresponsive to conventional medical and surgical management,

11. Osteoradionecrosis as an adjunct to conventional treatment,

12. Soft tissue radionecrosis as an adjunct to conventional treatment,

13. Cyanide poisoning,

14. Actinomycosis, only as an adjunct to conventional therapy when the disease process is refractory to antibiotics and surgical treatment,

15. Diabetic wounds of the lower extremities in patients who meet the following three criteria:

a. Patient has type I or type II diabetes and has a lower extremity wound that is due to diabetes;

b. Patient has a wound classified as Wagner grade III or higher; and

c. Patient has failed an adequate course of standard wound therapy.

The use of HBO therapy is covered as adjunctive therapy only after there are no measurable signs of healing for at least 30 — days of treatment with standard wound therapy and must be used in addition to standard wound care. Standard wound care in patients with diabetic wounds includes: assessment of a patient's vascular status and correction of any vascular problems in the affected limb if possible, optimization of nutritional status, optimization of glucose control, debridement by any means to remove devitalized tissue, maintenance of a clean, moist bed of granulation tissue with appropriate moist dressings, appropriate off-loading, and necessary treatment to resolve any infection that might be present. Failure to respond to standard wound care occurs when there are no measurable signs of healing for at least 30 consecutive days. Wounds must be evaluated at least every 30 days during administration of HBO therapy. Continued treatment with HBO therapy is not covered if measurable signs of healing have not been demonstrated within any 30-day period of treatment.

B. Noncovered Conditions

All other indications not specified under §270.4(A) are not covered under the Medicare program. No program payment may be made for any conditions other than those listed in §270.4(A).

No program payment may be made for HBO in the treatment of the following conditions:

1. Cutaneous, decubitus, and stasis ulcers.

2. Chronic peripheral vascular insufficiency.

3. Anaerobic septicemia and infection other than clostridial.

4. Skin burns (thermal).

5. Senility.

6. Myocardial infarction.

7. Cardiogenic shock.

8. Sickle cell anemia.

9. Acute thermal and chemical pulmonary damage, i.e., smoke inhalation with pulmonary insufficiency.

10. Acute or chronic cerebral vascular insufficiency.

11. Hepatic necrosis.

12. Aerobic septicemia.

13. Nonvascular causes of chronic brain syndrome (Pick's disease, Alzheimer's disease, Korsakoff's disease).

14. Tetanus.

15. Systemic aerobic infection.

16. Organ transplantation.

17. Organ storage.

18. Pulmonary emphysema.

19. Exceptional blood loss anemia.

20. Multiple Sclerosis.

21. Arthritic Diseases.

22. Acute cerebral edema.

C. Topical Application of Oxygen

This method of administering oxygen does not meet the definition of HBO therapy as stated above. Also, its clinical efficacy has not been established. Therefore, no Medicare reimbursement may be made for the topical application of oxygen.

Pub. 100-3, Section 30.1

Biofeedback Therapy

Biofeedback therapy is covered under Medicare only when it is reasonable and necessary for the individual patient for muscle re-education of specific muscle groups or for treating pathological muscle abnormalities of spasticity, incapacitating muscle spasm, or weakness, and more conventional treatments (heat, cold, massage, exercise, support) have not been successful. This therapy is not covered for treatment of ordinary muscle tension states or for psychosomatic conditions. (See the Medicare Benefit Policy Manual, Chapter 15, for general coverage requirements about physical therapy requirements.)

Pub. 100-3, Section 30.1.1

Biofeedback Therapy for the Treatment of Urinary Incontinence

This policy applies to biofeedback therapy rendered by a practitioner in an office or other facility setting.

Biofeedback is covered for the treatment of stress and/or urge incontinence in cognitively intact patients who have failed a documented trial of pelvic muscle exercise (PME)training. Biofeedback is not a treatment, per se, but a tool to help patients learn how to perform PME. Biofeedback-assisted PME incorporates the use of an electronic or mechanical device to relay visual and/or auditory evidence of pelvic floor muscle tone, in order to improve awareness of pelvic floor musculature and to assist patients in the performance of PME.

A failed trial of PME training is defined as no clinically significant improvement in urinary incontinence after completing 4 weeks of an ordered plan of pelvic muscle exercises to increase periurethral muscle strength.

Contractors may decide whether or not to cover biofeedback as an initial treatment modality.

Home use of biofeedback therapy is not covered.

Pub. 100-3, Section 30.5

Transcendental Meditation

After review of this issue, HCFA has concluded that the evidence concerning the medical efficacy of TM is incomplete at best and does not demonstrate effectiveness and that a professional level of skill is not required for the training of patients to engage in TM.

Although many articles have been written about application of TM for patients with certain forms of hypertension and anxiety, there are no rigorous scientific studies that demonstrate the effectiveness of TM for use as an adjunct medical therapy for such conditions. Accordingly, neither TM nor the training of patients for its use are covered under the Medicare program.

Pub. 100-3, Section 30.6

Intravenous Histamine Therapy

However, there is no scientifically valid clinical evidence that histamine therapy is effective for any condition regardless of the method of administration, nor is it accepted or widely used by the medical profession. Therefore, histamine therapy cannot be considered reasonable and necessary, and program payment for such therapy is not made.

Pub. 100-3, Section 30.7

Laetrile and Related Substances

The FDA has determined that neither Laetrile nor any other drug called by the various terms mentioned above, nor any other product which might be characterized as a "nitriloside" is generally recognized (by experts qualified by scientific training and experience to evaluate the safety and effectiveness of drugs) to be safe and effective for any therapeutic use. Therefore, use of this drug cannot be considered to be reasonable and necessary within the meaning of §1862(a)(1) of the Act and program payment may not be made for its use or any services furnished in connection with its administration.

A hospital stay only for the purpose of having laetrile (or any other drug called by the terms mentioned above) administered is not covered. Also, program payment may not be made for laetrile (or other drug noted above) when it is used during the course of an otherwise covered hospital stay, since the FDA has found such drugs to not be safe and effective for any therapeutic purpose.

Pub. 100-3, Section 40.1

Diabetes Outpatient Self-Management Training

Please refer to 42 CFR 410.140 - 410.146 for conditions that must be met for Medicare coverage.

Pub. 100-3, Section 40.5

Treatment of Obesity

B. Nationally Covered Indications

Certain designated surgical services for the treatment of obesity are covered for Medicare beneficiaries who have a BMI >35, have at least one co-morbidity related to obesity and have been previously unsuccessful with the medical treatment of obesity. See §100.1.

C. Nationally Noncovered Indications

1. Treatments for obesity alone remain non-covered.

2. Supplemented fasting is not covered under the Medicare program as a general treatment for obesity (see section D. below for discretionary local coverage).

D. Other

Where weight loss is necessary before surgery in order to ameliorate the complications posed by obesity when it coexists with pathological conditions such as cardiac and respiratory diseases, diabetes, or hypertension (and other more conservative techniques to achieve this end are not regarded as appropriate), supplemented fasting with adequate monitoring of the patient is eligible for coverage on a case-by-case basis or pursuant to a local coverage determination. The risks associated with the achievement of rapid weight loss must be carefully balanced against the risk posed by the condition requiring surgical treatment.

(This NCD last reviewed February 2006.)

Pub. 100-3, Section 50.1

Speech Generating Devices

Effective January 1, 2001, augmentative and alternative communication devices or communicators, which are hereafter referred to as "speech generating devices" are now considered to fall within the DME benefit category established by §1861(n) of the Social Security Act. They may be covered if the contractor's medical staff determines that the patient suffers from a severe speech impairment and that the medical condition warrants the use of a device based on the following definitions.

Pub. 100-3, Section 50.2

Electronic Speech Aids

Electronic speech aids are covered under Part B as prosthetic devices when the patient has had a laryngectomy or his larynx is permanently inoperative.

Pub. 100-3, Section 50.3

Cochlear Implantation

B. Nationally Covered Indications

1. Effective for services performed on or after April 4, 2005, cochlear implantation may be covered for treatment of bilateral pre- or post-linguistic, sensorineural, moderate-to-profound hearing loss in individuals who demonstrate limited benefit from amplification. Limited benefit from amplification is defined by test scores of less than or equal to 40% correct in the best-aided listening condition on tape-recorded tests of open-set sentence cognition. Medicare coverage is provided only for those patients who meet all of the following selection guidelines.

- Diagnosis of bilateral moderate-to-profound sensorineural hearing impairment with limited benefit from appropriate hearing (or vibrotactile) aids;

- Cognitive ability to use auditory clues and a willingness to undergo an extended program of rehabilitation;

- Freedom from middle ear infection, an accessible cochlear lumen that is structurally suited to implantation, and freedom from lesions in the auditory nerve and acoustic areas of the central nervous system;

- No contraindications to surgery; and

- The device must be used in accordance with Food and Drug Administration (FDA)-approved labeling.

2. Effective for services performed on or after April 4, 2005, cochlear implantation may be covered for individuals meeting the selection guidelines above and with hearing test scores of greater than 40% and less than or equal to 60% only when the provider is participating in, and patients are enrolled in, either an FDA-approved category B investigational device exemption clinical trial as defined at 42 CFR 405.201, a trial under the Centers for Medicare & Medicaid (CMS) Clinical Trial Policy as defined at section 310.1 of the National Coverage Determinations Manual, or a prospective, controlled comparative trial approved by CMS as consistent with the evidentiary requirements for National Coverage Analyses and meeting specific quality standards.

C. Nationally Noncovered Indications

Medicare beneficiaries not meeting all of the coverage criteria for cochlear implantation listed are deemed not eligible for Medicare coverage under section 1862(a)(1)(A) of the Social Security Act.

D. Other

All other indications for cochlear implantation not otherwise indicated as nationally covered or non-covered above remain at local contractor discretion.

(This NCD last reviewed May 2005.)

Pub. 100-3, Section 70.1

Consultations with a Beneficiary's Family and Associates

In certain types of medical conditions, including when a patient is withdrawn and uncommunicative due to a mental disorder or comatose, the physician may contact relatives and close associates to secure background information to assist in diagnosis and treatment planning. When a physician contacts his patient's relatives or associates for this purpose, expenses of such interviews are properly chargeable as physician's services to the patient on whose behalf the information was secured. If the beneficiary is not an inpatient of a hospital, Part B reimbursement for such an interview is subject to the special limitation on payments for physicians' services in connection with mental, psychoneurotic, and personality disorders.

A physician may also have contacts with a patient's family and associates for purposes other than securing background information. In some cases, the physician will provide counseling to members of the household. Family counseling services are covered only where the primary purpose of such counseling is the treatment of the patient's condition. For example, two situations where family counseling services would be appropriate are as follows: (1) where there is a need to observe the patient's interaction with family members; and/or (2) where there is a need to assess the capability of and assist the family members in aiding in the management of the patient. Counseling principally concerned with the effects of the patient's condition on the individual being interviewed would not be reimbursable as part of the physician's personal services to the patient. While to a limited degree, the counseling described in the second situation may be used to modify the behavior of the family members, such services nevertheless are covered because they relate primarily to the management of the patient's problems and not to the treatment of the family member's problems.

Pub. 100-3, Section 70.2

Consultation Services Rendered by a Podiatrist in a Skilled Nursing Facility

Consultation services rendered by a podiatrist in a skilled nursing facility are covered if the services are reasonable and necessary and do not come within any of the specific statutory exclusions. Section I862(a)(13) of the Act excludes payment for the treatment of flat foot conditions, the treatment of subluxations of the foot, and routine foot care. To determine whether the consultation comes within the foot care exclusions, apply the same rule as for initial diagnostic examinations, i.e., where services are performed in connection with specific symptoms or complaints which suggest the need for covered services, the services are covered regardless of the resulting diagnosis. The exclusion of routine physician examinations is also pertinent and would generally exclude podiatric consultation performed on all patients in a skilled nursing facility on a routine basis for screening purposes, except in those cases where a specific foot ailment is involved. Section 1862(a)(7) of the Act excludes payment for routine physical checkups.

Pub. 100-3, Section 70.2.1

Services Provided for the Diagnosis and Treatment of Diabetic Sensory Neuropathy with Loss of Protective Sensation (AKA Diabetic Peripheral Neuropathy)

Diabetic sensory neuropathy with LOPS is a localized illness of the feet and falls within the regulation's exception to the general exclusionary rule [see 42 CFR §411.15(I)(1)(i)]. Foot exams for people with diabetic sensory neuropathy with LOPS are reasonable and necessary to allow for early intervention in serious complications that typically afflict diabetics with the disease.

Effective for services furnished on or after July 1, 2002, Medicare covers, as a physician service, an evaluation (examination and treatment) of the feet no more often than every six months for individuals with a documented diagnosis of diabetic sensory neuropathy and LOPS, as long as the beneficiary has not seen a foot care specialist for some other reason in the interim. LOPS shall be diagnosed through sensory testing with the 5.07 monofilament using established guidelines, such as those developed by the National Institute of Diabetes and Digestive and Kidney Diseases guidelines. Five sites should be tested on the plantar surface of each foot, according to the National Institute of Diabetes and Digestive and Kidney Diseases guidelines. The areas must be tested randomly since the loss of protective sensation may be patchy in distribution, and the patient may get clues if the test is done rhythmically. Heavily callused areas should be avoided. As suggested by the American Podiatric Medicine Association, an absence of sensation at two or more sites out of 5 tested on either foot when tested with the 5.07 Semmes-Weinstein monofilament must be present and documented to diagnose peripheral neuropathy with loss of protective sensation.

A. The examination includes:

1) a patient history, and

2) a physical examination that must consist of at least the following elements:

a. visual inspection of forefoot and hindfoot (including toe web spaces);

b. evaluation of protective sensation;

c. evaluation of foot structure and biomechanics;

d. evaluation of vascular status and skin integrity;

e. evaluation of the need for special footwear; and

3) patient education.

B. Treatment includes, but is not limited to:

1) local care of superficial wounds;

2) debridement of corns and calluses; and

3) trimming and debridement of nails.

The diagnosis of diabetic sensory neuropathy with LOPS should be established and documented prior to coverage of foot care. Other causes of peripheral neuropathy should be considered and investigated by the primary care physician prior to initiating or referring for foot care for persons with LOPS.

Pub. 100-3, Section 80.1

Hydrophilic Contact Lens For Corneal Bandage
Payment may be made under §1861(s)(2) of the Act for a hydrophilic contact les approved by the Food and Drug Administration (FDA) and used as a supply incident to a pphyscian's service. Payment for the lens is included in the payment for the physician's service to which the lens is incident. Contractors are authorized to accept an FDA letter of approval or other FDA published material as evidence of FDA approval. (See §80.4 of the NCD Manual for coverage of a hydrophilic contact lens as prosthetic device.)

Pub. 100-3, Section 80.2

Ocular Photodynamic Therapy
B - Covered Indications

Effective April 1, 2004, OPT with verteporfin continues to be approved for a diagnosis of neovascular AMD with predominately classic subfoveal CNV lesions (where the area of classic CNV occupies >= 50% of the area of the entire lesion) at the initial visit as determined by a fluorescein angiogram. (CNV lesions are comprised of classic and/or occult components.) Subsequent follow-up visits require a fluorescein angiogram prior to treatment. There are no requirements regarding visual acuity, lesion size, and number of re-treatments when treating predominately classic lesions.

In addition, after thorough review and reconsideration of the August 20, 2002, noncoverage policy, CMS determines that the evidence is adequate to conclude that OPT with verteporfin is reasonable and necessary for treating:

1. Subfoveal occult with no classic CNV associated with AMD; and,

2. Subfoveal minimally classic CNV (where the area of classic CNV occupies <50% of the area of the entire lesion) associated with AMD.

The above 2 indications are considered reasonable and necessary only when:

1. The lesions are small (4 disk areas or less in size) at the time of initial treatment or within the 3 months prior to initial treatment; and,

2. The lesions have shown evidence of progression within the 3 months prior to initial treatment. Evidence of progression must be documented by deterioration of visual acuity (at least 5 letters on a standard eye examination chart), lesion growth (an increase in at least 1 disk area), or the appearance of blood associated with the lesion.

C - Noncovered Indications

Other uses of OPT with verteporfin to treat AMD not already addressed by CMS will continue to be noncovered. These include, but are not limited to, the following AMD indications:

Juxtafoveal or extrafoveal CNV lesions (lesions outside the fovea),

Inability to obtain a fluorescein angiogram,

Atrophic or "dry" AMD.

D - Other

OPT with verteporfin for other ocular indications, such as pathologic myopia or presumed ocular histoplasmosis syndrome, continue to be eligible for local coverage determinations through individual contractor discretion.

Pub. 100-3, Section 80.3

Verteporfin
B - Covered Indications

Effective April 1, 2004, OPT with verteporfin is covered for patients with a diagnosis of neovascular age-related macular degeneration (AMD) with:

Predominately classic subfoveal choroidal neovascularization (CNV) lesions (where the area of classic CNV occupies >= 50% of the area of the entire lesion) at the initial visit as determined by a fluorescein angiogram. (CNV lesions are comprised of classic and/or occult components.) Subsequent follow-up visits require a fluorescein angiogram prior to treatment. There are no requirements regarding visual acuity, lesion size, and number of retreatments when treating predominately classic lesions.

Subfoveal occult with no classic associated with AMD.

Subfoveal minimally classic CNV CNV (where the area of classic CNV occupies <50% of the area of the entire lesion) associated with AMD.

The above 2 indications are considered reasonable and necessary only when:

1. The lesions are small (4 disk areas or less in size) at the time of initial treatment or within the 3 months prior to initial treatment; and,

2. The lesions have shown evidence of progression within the 3 months prior to initial treatment. Evidence of progression must be documented by deterioration of visual acuity (at least 5 letters on a standard eye examination chart), lesion growth (an increase in at least 1 disk area), or the appearance of blood associated with the lesion.

C - Noncovered Indications

Other uses of OPT with verteporfin to treat AMD not already addressed by CMS will continue to be noncovered. These include, but are not limited to, the following AMD indications: juxtafoveal or extrafoveal CNV lesions (lesions outside the fovea), inability to obtain a fluorescein angiogram, or atrophic or "dry" AMD.

D - Other

OPT with verteporfin for other ocular indications, such as pathologic myopia or presumed ocular histoplasmosis syndrome, continue to be eligible for local coverage determinations through individual contractor discretion.

Pub. 100-3, Section 80.4

Hydrophilic Contact Lenses
Hydrophilic contact lenses are eyeglasses within the meaning of the exclusion in §1862(a)(7) of the Act and are not covered when used in the treatment of nondiseased eyes with spherical ametrophia, refractive astigmatism, and/or corneal astigmatism. Payment may be made under the prosthetic device benefit, however, for hydrophilic contact lenses when prescribed for an aphakic patient.

Contractors are authorized to accept an FDA letter of approval or other FDA published material as evidence of FDA approval. (See §80.1 of the NCD Manual for coverage of a hydrophilic lens as a corneal bandage.)

Pub. 100-3, Section 80.6

Intraocular Photography
Intraocular photography is covered when used for the diagnosis of such conditions as macular degeneration, retinal neoplasms, choroid disturbances and diabetic retinopathy, or to identify glaucoma, multiple sclerosis and other central nervous system abnormalities. Make Medicare payment for the use of this procedure by an opthalmologist in these situations when it is reasonable and necessary for the individual patient to receive these services.

Pub. 100-3, Section 80.7

Refractive Keratoplasty
The correction of common refractive errors by eyeglasses, contact lenses or other prosthetic devices is specifically excluded from coverage. The use of radial keratotomy and/or keratoplasty for the purpose of refractive error compensation is considered a substitute or alternative to eye glasses or contact lenses, which are specifically excluded by §1862(a)(7) of the Act (except in certain cases in connection with cataract surgery). In addition, many in the medical community

consider such procedures cosmetic surgery, which is excluded by section §1862(a)(10) of the Act. Therefore, radial keratotomy and keratoplasty to treat refractive defects are not covered.

Keratoplasty that treats specific lesions of the cornea, such as phototherapeutic keratectomy that removes scar tissue from the visual field, deals with an abnormality of the eye and is not cosmetic surgery. Such cases may be covered under §1862(a)(1)(A) of the Act.

The use of lasers to treat ophthalmic disease constitutes opthalmalogic surgery. Coverage is restricted to practitioners who have completed an approved training program in ophthalmologic surgery.

Pub. 100-3, Section 80.8

Endothelial Cell Photography

Endothelial cell photography is a covered procedure under Medicare when reasonable and necessary for patients who meet one or more of the following criteria:

- Have slit lamp evidence of endothelial dystrophy (cornea guttata),

- Have slit lamp evidence of corneal edema (unilateral or bilateral),

- Are about to undergo a secondary intraocular lens implantation,

- Have had previous intraocular surgery and require cataract surgery,

- Are about to undergo a surgical procedure associated with a higher risk to corneal endothelium; i.e., phacoemulsification, or refractive surgery (see §35-54 for excluded refractive procedures),

- With evidence of posterior polymorphous dystrophy of the cornea or irido-corneal-endothelium syndrome, or

- Are about to be fitted with extended wear contact lenses after intraocular surgery.

When a pre-surgical examination for cataract surgery is performed and the conditions of this section are met, if the only visual problem is cataracts, endothelial cell photography is covered as part of the presurgical comprehensive eye examination or combination brief/intermediate examination provided prior to cataract surgery, and not in addition to it. (See §10.1)

Pub. 100-3, Section 80.9

Computer Enhanced Perimetry

It is a covered service when used in assessing visual fields in patients with glaucoma or other neuropathologic defects.

Pub. 100-3, Section 80.10

Phaco-Emulsification procedure - cataract extraction

In view of recommendations of authoritative sources in the field of ophthalmology, the subject technique is viewed as an accepted procedure for removal of cataracts. Accordingly, program reimbursement may be made for necessary services furnished in connection with cataract extraction utilizing the phaco-emulsification procedure.

Pub. 100-3, Section 80.11

Vitrectomy

Vitrectomy may be considered reasonable and necessary for the following conditions: vitreous loss incident to cataract surgery, vitreous opacities due to vitreous hemorrhage or other causes, retinal detachments secondary to vitreous strands, proliferative retinopathy, and vitreous retraction. See Chapter 23 of the Medicare Claims Manual for how to determine payment for physician vitrectomy services and Chapter 14 §40 for how to determine payment for ASC facility vitrectomy services. Also, see Chapter 23 §20.9 to identify when, for Medicare payment purposes, certain vitrectomy codes are included in other codes or when codes for other services include vitrectomy codes.

Pub. 100-3, Section 100.1

Gastric Bypass Surgery for Obesity

Gastric bypass surgery for extreme obesity is covered under the program if (1) it is medically appropriate for the individual to have such surgery; and (2) the surgery is to correct an illness which caused the obesity or was aggravated by the obesity.

Pub. 100-3, Section 100.2

Endoscopy

Endoscopic procedures are covered when reasonable and necessary for the individual patient.

Pub. 100-3, Section 100.4

Esophageal Manometry

Esophageal manometry is covered under Medicare where it is determined to be reasonable and necessary for the individual patient.

Pub. 100-3, Section 100.5

Diagnostic Breath Analyses

The Following Breath Test is Covered:

- Lactose breath hydrogen to detect lactose malabsorption.

The Following Breath Tests are Excluded from Coverage;

- Lactulose breath hydrogen for diagnosing small bowel bacterial overgrowth and measuring small bowel transit time.

- CO_2 for diagnosing bile acid malabsorption.

- CO_2 for diagnosing fat malabsorption.

Pub. 100-3, Section 100.8

Intestinal By-Pass Surgery

The safety of intestinal bypass surgery for treatment of obesity has not been demonstrated. Severe adverse reactions such as steatorrhea, electrolyte depletion, liver failure, arthralgia, hypoplasia of bone marrow, and avitaminosis have sometimes occurred as a result of this procedure. It does not meet the reasonable and necessary provisions of §1862(a)(1) of the Act and is not a covered Medicare procedure.

Pub. 100-3, Section 100.10

Injection Sclerotherapy for Esophageal Variceal Bleeding

This procedure is covered under Medicare.

Pub. 100-3, Section 100.12

Gastrophotography

Gastrophotography is an accepted procedure for diagnosis and treatment of gastrointestinal disorders. The photographic record provided by this procedure is often necessary for consultation and/or followup purposes and when required for such purposes, is more valuable than a conventional gastroscopic examination. Such a record facilitates the documentation and evaluation (healing or worsening) of lesions such as the gastric ulcer, facilitates consultation between physicians concerning difficult-to-interpret lesions, provides preoperative characterization for the surgeon, and permits better diagnosis of postoperative gastric bleeding to help determine whether there is a need for reoperation. Therefore, program reimbursement may be made for this procedure.

Pub. 100-3, Section 100.13

Laparoscopic Cholecystectomy

Laparoscopic cholecystectomy is a covered surgical procedure in which a diseased gall bladder is removed through the use of instruments introduced via cannulae, with vision of the operative field maintained by use of a high-resolution television camera-monitor system (video laparoscope). For inpatient claims, use ICD-9-CM code 51.23, Laparoscopic cholecystectomy. For all other claims, use CPT codes 49310 for laparoscopy, surgical; cholecystectomy (any method), and 49311 for laparoscopy, surgical: cholecystectomy with cholangiography.

Pub. 100-3, Section 110.1

Hyperthermia for Treatment of Cancer

Local hyperthermia is covered under Medicare when used in connection with radiation therapy for the treatment of primary or metastatic cutaneous or subcutaneous superficial malignancies. It is not covered when used alone or in connection with chemotherapy.

Pub. 100-3, Section 110.2

Certain Drugs Distributed by the National Cancer Institute

A physician is eligible to receive Group C drugs from the Divison of Cancer Treatment only if the following requirements are met:

- A physician must be registered with the NCI as an investigator by having completed an FD-Form 1573;

- A written request for the drug, indicating the disease to be treated, must be submitted to the NCI;

- The use of the drug must be limited to indications outlined in the NCI's guidelines; and

- All adverse reactions must be reported to the Investigational Drug Branch of the Division of Cancer Treatment.

In view of these NCI controls on distribution and use of Group C drugs, intermediaries may assume, in the absence of evidence to the contrary, that a Group C drug and the related hospital stay are covered if all other applicable coverage requirements are satisfied.

If there is reason to question coverage in a particular case, the matter should be resolved with the assistance of the Quality improvemetn organization (QIO), or if there is none, the assistance of your medical consultants.

Information regarding those drugs which are classified as Group C drugs may be obtained from:

Office of the Chief, Investigational Drug Branch

Division of Cancer Treatment, CTEP, Landow Building

Room 4C09, National Cancer Institute

Bethesda, Maryland 20205

Pub. 100-3, Section 110.3

Anti-Inhibitor Coagulant Complex (AICC)

Anti-inhibitor coagulant complex, AICC, is a drug used to treat hemophilia in patients with factor VIII inhibitor antibodies. AICC has been shown to be safe and effective and has Medicare coverage when furnished to patients with hemophilia A and inhibitor antibodies to factor VIII who have major bleeding episodes and who fail to respond to other, less expensive therapies.

Pub. 100-3, Section 110.4

Extracorporeal Photopheresis

Extracorporeal photopheresis is covered by Medicare only when used in the palliative treatment of the skin manifestations of CTCL that has not responded to other therapy.

Pub. 100-3, Section 110.5

Granulocyte Transfusions

Granulocyte transfusions to patients suffering from severe infection and granulocytopenia are a covered service under Medicare. Granulocytopenia is usually identified as fewer than 500 granulocytes/mm 3 whole blood. Accepted indications for granulocyte transfusions include:

Granulocytopenia with evidence of gram negative sepsis; and

Granulocytopenia in febrile patients with local progressive infections unresponsive to appropriate antibiotic therapy, thought to be due to gram negative organisms.

Pub. 100-3, Section 110.6

Scalp Hypothermia During Chemotherapy, to Prevent Hair Loss

While ice-filled bags or bandages or other devices used for scalp hypothermia during chemotherapy may be covered as supplies of the kind commonly furnished without a separate charge, no separate charge for them would be recognized.

Pub. 100-3, Section 110.7

Blood Transfusions

B. Policy Governing Transfusions

For Medicare coverage purposes, it is important to distinguish between a transfusion itself and preoperative blood services; e.g., collection, processing, storage. Medically necessary transfusion of blood, regardless of the type, may generally be a covered service under both Part A and Part B of Medicare. Coverage does not make a distinction between the transfusion of homologous, autologous, or donor-directed blood. With respect to the coverage of the services associated with the preoperative collection, processing, and storage of autologous and donor-directed blood, the following policies apply.

1. Hospital Part A and B Coverage and Payment

Under §1862(a)(14) of the Act, non-physician services furnished to hospital patients are covered and paid for as hospital services. As provided in §1886 of the Act, under the prospective [payment system (PPS) the diagnosis related group (DRG) payment to the hospital includes all covered blood and blood processing expenses, whether or not the blood is eventually used.

Under its provider agreement, a hospital is required to furnish or arrange for all covered services furnished to hospital patients. medicare payment is made to the hospital, under PPS or cost reimbursement, for covered inpatient services, and it is intended to reflect payment for all costs of furnishing those services.

2. Nonhospital Part B Coverage

Under Part B, to be eligible for separate coverage, a service must fit the definition of one of the services authorized by §1832 of the Act. These services are defined in 42 CFR 410.10 and do not include a separate category for a supplier's services associated with blood donation services, either autologous or donor-directed. That is, the collection, processing, and storage of blood for later transfusion into the beneficiary is not recognized as a separate service under Part B. Therefore, there is no avenue through which a blood supplier can receive direct payment under Part B for blood donation services.

C.Perioperative Blood Salvage

When the perioperative blood salvage process is used in surgery on a hospital patient, payment made to the hospital (under PPS or through cost reimbursement) for the procedure in which that process is used is intended to encompass payment for all costs relating to that process.

Pub. 100-3, Section 110.8

Blood Platelet Transfusions

Blood platelet transplants are safe and effective for the correction of thrombocytopenia and other blood defects. It is covered under Medicare when treatment is reasonable and necessary for the individual patient.

Pub. 100-3, Section 110.8.1

Stem Cell Transplantation

1. Allogeneic Stem Cell Transplantation

Allogeneic stem cell transplantation is a procedure in which a portion of a healthy donor's stem cell or bone marrow is obtained and prepared for intravenous infusion.

a. Covered Indications

The following uses of allogeneic bone marrow transplantation are covered under Medicare:

- Effective for services performed on or after August 1, 1978, for the treatment of leukemia, leukemia in remission, or aplastic anemia when it is reasonable and necessary; and

- Effective for services performed on or after June 3, 1985, for the treatment of severe combined immunodeficiency disease (SCID), and for the treatment of Wiskott-Aldrich syndrome.

b. Noncovered Indications

Effective for services performed on or after May 24, 1996, allogeneic stem cell transplantation is not covered as treatment for multiple myeloma.

2. Autologous Stem Cell Transplantation (AuSCT)

Autologous stem cell transplantation (AuSCT) is a technique for restoring stem cells using the patient's own previously stored cells.

a. Covered Indications

Effective for services performed on or after April 28, 1989, AuSCT is considered reasonable and necessary under §1862(a)(1)(A) of the Social Security Act (the Act) for the following conditions and is covered under Medicare for patients with:

- Acute leukemia in remission who have a high probability of relapse and who have no human leucocyte antigens (HLA)-matched;

- Resistant non-Hodgkin's lymphomas or those presenting with poor prognostic features following an initial response;

- Recurrent or refractory neuroblastoma; or

- Advanced Hodgkin's disease who have failed conventional therapy and have no HLA-matched donor.

Effective October 1, 2000, single AuSCT is only covered for Durie-Salmon Stage II or III patients that fit the following requirements:

- Newly diagnosed or responsive multiple myeloma. This includes those patients with previously untreated disease, those with at least a partial response to prior chemotherapy (defined as a 50% decrease either in measurable paraprotein [serum and/or urine] or in bone marrow infiltration, sustained for at least 1 month), and those in responsive relapse; and

- Adequate cardiac, renal, pulmonary, and hepatic function.

Effective for services performed on or after March 15, 2005, when recognized clinical risk factors are employed to select patients for transplantation, high dose melphalan (HDM) together with AuSCT is reasonable and necessary for Medicare beneficiaries of any age group with primary amyloid light chain (AL) amyloidosis who meet the following criteria:

- Amyloid deposition in 2 or fewer organs; and,

- Cardiac left ventricular ejection fraction (EF) greater than 45%.

b. Noncovered Indications

Insufficient data exist to establish definite conclusions regarding the efficacy of AuSCT for the following conditions:

- Acute leukemia not in remission;

- Chronic granulocytic leukemia;

- Solid tumors (other than neuroblastoma);

- Up to October 1, 2000, multiple myeloma;

- Tandem transplantation (multiple rounds of AuSCT) for patients with multiple myeloma;

- Effective October 1, 2000, non primary AL amyloidosis; and,

- Effective October 1, 2000, thru March 14, 2005, primary AL amyloidosis for Medicare beneficiaries age 64 or older.

In these cases, AuSCT is not considered reasonable and necessary within the meaning of §1862(a)(1)(A) of the Act and is not covered under Medicare.

B. Other

All other indications for stem cell transplantation not otherwise noted above as covered or noncovered nationally remain at local contractor discretion.

(This NCD last reviewed November 2005.)

Pub. 100-3, Section 110.9

Antigens Prepared for Sublingual Administration

For antigens provided to patients on or after November 17, 1996, Medicare does not cover such antigens if they are to be administered sublingually, i.e., by placing drops under the patient's tongue. This kind of allergy therapy has not been proven to be safe and effective. Antigens are covered only if they are administered by injection.

Pub. 100-3, Section 110.10

Intravenous Iron Therapy

A. Effective December 1, 2000, Medicare covers sodium ferric gluconate complex in sucrose injection as a first line treatment of iron deficiency anemia when furnished intravenously to patients undergoing chronic hemodialysis who are receiving supplemental erythropoeitin therapy.

B. Effective October 1, 2001, Medicare also covers iron sucrose injection as a first line treatment of iron deficiency anemia when furnished intravenously to patients undergoing chronic hemodialysis who are receiving supplemental erythropoeitin therapy.

Pub. 100-3, Section 110.11

Food Allergy Testing and Treatment

Effective October 31, 1988, sublingual intracutaneous and subcutaneous provocative and neutralization testing and neutralization therapy for food allergies are excluded from Medicare coverage because available evidence does not show that these tests and therapies are effective. This exclusion was published as a Final Notice in the "Federal Register" on September 29, 1988.

Pub. 100-3, Section 110.12

Challenge Ingestion Food Testing

This procedure is covered when it is used on an outpatient basis if it is reasonable and necessary for the individual patient.

Challenge ingestion food testing has not been proven to be effective in the diagnosis of rheumatoid arthritis, depression, or respiratory disorders. Accordingly, its use in the diagnosis of these conditions is not reasonable and necessary within the meaning of section 1862(a)(1) of the Medicare law, and no program payment is made for this procedure when it is so used.

Pub. 100-3, Section 110.13

Cytotoxic Food Tests

Prior to August 5, 1985, Medicare covered cytotoxic food tests as an adjunct to in vivo clinical allergy tests in complex food allergy problems. Effective August 5, l985, cytotoxic leukocyte tests for food allergies are excluded from Medicare coverage because available evidence does not show that these tests are safe and effective. This exclusion was published as a CMS Ruling in the "Federal Register" on July 5, 1985.

Pub. 100-3, Section 110.14

Apheresis (Therapeutic Pheresis)

B. Indications

Apheresis is covered for the following indications:

- Plasma exchange for acquired myasthenia gravis;
- Leukapheresis in the treatment of leukemekia
- Plasmapheresis in the treatment of primary macroglobulinemia (Waldenstrom);
- Treatment of hyperglobulinemias, including (but not limited to) multiple myelomas, cryoglobulinemia and hyperviscosity syndromes;
- Plasmapheresis or plasma exchange as a last resort treatment of thromobotic thrombocytopenic purpura (TTP);
- Plasmapheresis or plasma exchange in the last resort treatment of life threatening rheumatoid vasculitis;
- Plasma perfusion of charcoal filters for treatment of pruritis of cholestatic liver disease;
- Plasma exchange in the treatment of Goodpasture's Syndrome;
- Plasma exchange in the treatment of glomerulonephritis associated with antiglomerular basement membrane antibodies and advancing renal failure or pulmonary hemorrhage;
- Treatment of chronic relapsing polyneuropathy for patients with severe or life threatening symptoms who have failed to respond to conventional therapy;
- Treatment of life threatening scleroderma and polymyositis when the patient is unresponsive to conventional therapy;
- Treatment of Guillain-Barre Syndrome; and
- Treatment of last resort for life threatening systemic lupus erythematosus (SLE) when conventional therapy has failed to prevent clinical deterioration.

C. Settings

Apheresis is covered only when performed in a hospital setting (either inpatient or outpatient). or in a nonhospital setting. e.g. physician directed clinic when the following conditions are met:

- A physician (or a number of physicians) is present to perform medical services and to respond to medical emergencies at all times during patient care hours;
- Each patient is under the care of a physician; and
- All nonphysician services are furnished under the direct, personal supervision of a physician.

Pub. 100-3, Section 110.15

Ultrafiltration, Hemoperfusion and Hemofiltration

A. Ultrafiltration. — This is a process for removing excess fluid from the blood through the dialysis membrane by means of pressure. It is not a substitute for dialysis. Ultrafiltration is utilized in cases where excess fluid cannot be removed easily during the regular course of hemodialysis. When it is performed, it is commonly done during the first hour or two of each hemodialysis on patients who, e.g., have refractory edema. Ultrafiltration is a covered procedure under the Medicare program (effective for services performed on and after 9/1/79).

Predialysis Ultrafiltration. — While this procedure requires additional staff care, the facility dialysis rate is intended to cover the full range of complicated and uncomplicated nonacute dialysis treatments. Therefore, no additional facility charge is recognized for predialysis ultrafiltration. The physician's role in ultrafiltration varies with the stability of the patient's condition. In unstable patients, the physician may need to be present at the initiation of dialysis, and available either in- house or in close proximity to monitor the patient carefully. In patients who are relatively stable, but who seem to accumulate excessive weight gain, the procedure requires only a modest increase in physician involvement over routine outpatient hemodialysis.

Occasionally, medical complications may occur which require that ultrafiltration be performed separate from the dialysis treatment, and in these cases an additional charge can be recognized. However, the claim must be documented as to why the ultrafiltration could not have been performed at the same time as the dialysis.

B. Hemoperfusion. — This is a process which removes substances from the blood using a charcoal or resin artificial kidney. When used in the treatment of life threatening drug overdose, hemoperfusion is a covered service for patients with or without renal failure (effective for services performed on and after 9/1/79). Hemoperfusion generally requires a physician to be present to initiate treatment and to be present in the hospital or an adjacent medical office during the entire procedure, as changes may be sudden. Special staff training and equipment are required.

Develop charges for hemoperfusion in the same manner as for any new or unusual service. One or two treatments are usually all that is necessary to remove the toxic compound; document additional treatments. Hemoperfusion may be performed concurrently with dialysis, and in those cases payment for the hemoperfusion reflects only the additional care rendered over and above the care given with dialysis.

The effects of using hemoperfusion to improve the results of chronic hemodialysis are not known. Therefore, hemoperfusion is not a covered service when used to improve the results of hemodialysis. In addition, it has not been demonstrated that the use of hemoperfusion in conjunction with deferoxamine (DFO), in treating symptomatic patients with iron overload, is efficacious. There is also a paucity of data regarding its efficacy in treating asymptomatic patients with iron overload. Therefore, hemoperfusion used in conjunction with DFO in treating patients with iron overload is not a covered service; i.e., it is not considered reasonable and necessary within the meaning of §1862(a)(1) of the Act.

However, the use of hemoperfusion in conjunction with DFO for the treatment of patients with aluminum toxicity has been demonstrated to be clinically efficacious and is therefore regarded as a covered service.

C. Hemofiltration. — This is a process which removes fluid, electrolytes and other low molecular weight toxic substances from the blood by filtration through hollow artificial membranes and may be routinely performed in 3 weekly sessions. Hemofiltration (which is also known as diafiltration) is a covered procedure under Medicare and is a safe and effective technique for the treatment of ESRD patients and an alternative to peritoneal dialysis and hemodialysis (effective for services performed on and after August 20, 1987). In contrast to both hemodialysis and peritoneal dialysis treatments, which eliminate dissolved substances via diffusion across semipermeable membranes, hemofiltration mimics the filtration process of the normal kidney. The technique requires an arteriovenous access. Hemofiltration may be performed either in facility or at home.

The procedure is most advantageous when applied to high-risk unstable patients, such as older patients with cardiovascular diseases or diabetes, because there are fewer side effects such as hypotension, hypertension or volume overload.

Pub. 100-3, Section 110.16

Nonselective (Random) Transfusions and Living Related Donor Specific Transfusions (DST) in Kidney Transplantation

These pretransplant transfusions are covered under Medicare without a specific limitation on the number of transfusions, subject to the normal Medicare blood deductible provisions. Where blood is given directly to the transplant patient; e.g., in the case of donor specific transfusions, the blood is considered replaced for purposes of the blood deductible provisions.

Pub. 100-3, Section 130.1

Inpatient Hospital Stays for the Treatment of Alcoholism

A. Inpatient Hospital Stay for Alcohol Detoxification

Many hospitals provide detoxification services during the more acute stages of alcoholism or alcohol withdrawal. When the high probability or occurrence of medical complications (e.g., delirium, confusion, trauma, or unconsciousness) during detoxification for acute alcoholism or alcohol withdrawal necessitates the constant availability of physicians and/or complex medical equipment found only in the hospital setting, inpatient hospital care during this period is considered reasonable and necessary and is therefore covered under the program. Generally, detoxification can be accomplished within 2-3 days with an occasional need for up to 5 days where the patient's condition dictates. This limit (5 days) may be extended in an individual case where there is a need for a longer period for detoxification for a particular patient. In such cases, however, there should be documentation by a physician which substantiates that a longer period of detoxification was reasonable and necessary. When the detoxification needs of an individual no longer require an inpatient hospital setting, coverage should be denied on the basis that inpatient hospital care is not reasonable and necessary as required by section l862(a)(l) of the Act. Following detoxification a patient may be transferred to an inpatient rehabilitation unit or discharged to a residential treatment program or outpatient treatment setting.

B. Inpatient Hospital Stay for Alcohol Rehabilitation

Hospitals may also provide structured inpatient alcohol rehabilitation programs to the chronic alcoholic. These programs are composed primarily of coordinated educational and psychotherapeutic services provided on a group basis. Depending on the subject matter, a series of lectures, discussions, films, and group therapy sessions are led by either physicians, psychologists, or alcoholism counselors from the hospital or various outside organizations. In addition, individual psychotherapy and family counseling (see §70.1 of the NCD Manual) may be provided in selected cases. These programs are conducted under the supervision and direction of a physician. Patients may directly enter an inpatient hospital rehabilitation program after having undergone detoxification in the same hospital or in another hospital or may enter an inpatient hospital rehabilitation program without prior hospitalization for detoxification.Alcohol rehabilitation can be provided in a variety of settings other than the hospital setting. In order for an inpatient hospital stay for alcohol rehabilitation to be covered under Medicare it must be medically necessary for the care to be provided in the inpatient hospital setting rather than in a less costly facility or on an outpatient basis. Inpatient hospital care for receipt of an alcohol rehabilitation program would generally be medically necessary where either (l) there is documentation by the physician that recent alcohol rehabilitation services in a less intensive setting or on an outpatient basis have proven unsuccessful and, as a consequence, the patient requires the supervision and intensity of services which can only be found in the controlled environment of the hospital, or (2) only the hospital environment can assure the medical management or control of the patient's concomitant conditions during the course of alcohol rehabilitation. (However, a patient's concomitant condition may make the use of certain alcohol treatment modalities medically inappropriate.) In addition, the "active treatment" criteria (see the Medicare Benefit Policy Manual, Chapter 2, "Inpatient Psychiatric Hospital Services," §20) should be applied to psychiatric care in the general hospital as well as to psychiatric care in a psychiatric hospital. Since alcoholism is classifiable as a psychiatric condition the "active treatment" criteria must also be met in order for alcohol rehabilitation services to be covered under Medicare. (Thus, it is the combined need for "active treatment" and for covered care which can only be provided in the inpatient hospital setting, rather than the fact that rehabilitation immediately follows a period of detoxification, which provides the basis for coverage of inpatient hospital alcohol rehabilitation programs.)Generally 16-19 days of rehabilitation services are sufficient to bring a patient to a point where care could be continued in other than an inpatient hospital setting. An inpatient hospital stay for alcohol rehabilitation may be extended beyond this limit in an individual case where a longer period of alcohol rehabilitation is medically necessary. In such cases, however, there should be documentation by a physician which substantiates the need for such care. Where the rehabilitation needs of an individual no longer require an inpatient hospital setting, coverage should be denied on the basis that inpatient hospital care is not reasonable and necessary as required by section l862(a)(l) of the Act.Subsequent admissions to the inpatient hospital setting for alcohol rehabilitation followup, reinforcement, or "recap" treatments are considered to be readmissions (rather than an extension of the original stay) and must meet the requirements of this section for coverage under Medicare. Prior admissions to the inpatient hospital setting — either in the same hospital or in a different hospital — may be an indication that the "active treatment" requirements are not met (i.e., there is no reasonable expectation of improvement) and the stay should not be covered. Accordingly, there should be documentation to establish that "readmission" to the hospital setting for alcohol rehabilitation services can reasonably be expected to result in improvement of the patient's condition. For example, the documentation should indicate what changes in the patient's medical condition, social or emotional status, or treatment plan make improvement likely, or why the patient's initial hospital treatment was not sufficient.

C. Combined Alcohol Detoxification/Rehabilitation Programs. — Fiscal intermediaries should apply the guidelines in A. and B. above to both phases of a combined inpatient hospital alcohol detoxification/rehabilitation program. Not all patients who require the inpatient hospital setting for detoxification also need the inpatient hospital setting for rehabilitation. (See §130.1 of the NCD Manual for coverage of outpatient hospital alcohol rehabilitation services.) Where the inpatient hospital setting is medically necessary for both alcohol detoxification and rehabilitation, generally a 3-week period is reasonable and necessary to bring the patient to the point where care can be continued in other than an inpatient hospital setting.Decisions regarding reasonableness and necessity of treatment, the need for an inpatient hospital level of care, and length of treatment should be made by intermediaries based on accepted medical practice with the advice of their medical consultant. (In hospitals under PSRO review, PSRO determinations of medical necessity of services and appropriateness of the level of care at which services are provided are binding on the title XVIII fiscal intermediaries for purposes of adjudicating claims for payment.)

Pub. 100-3, Section 130.2

Outpatient Hospital Services for Treatment of Alcoholism

Coverage is available for both diagnostic and therapeutic services furnished for the treatment of alcoholism by the hospital to outpatients subject to the same rules applicable to outpatient hospital services in general. While there is no coverage for day hospitalization programs, per se, individual services which meet the requirements in the Medicare Benefit Policy Manual, Chapter 6, §20 may be covered. (Meals, transportation and recreational and social activities do not fall within the scope of covered outpatient hospital services under Medicare.)

All services must be reasonable and necessary for diagnosis or treatment of the patient's condition (see the Medicare Benefit Policy Manual, chapter 16 §20). Thus, educational services and family counseling would only be covered where they are directly related to treatment of the patient's condition. The frequency of treatment and period of time over which it occurs must also be reasonable and necessary.

Pub. 100-3, Section 130.3

Chemical Aversion Therapy for Treatment of Alcoholism

Available evidence indicates that chemical aversion therapy may be an effective component of certain alcoholism treatment programs, particularly as part of multimodality treatment programs which include other behavioral techniques and therapies, such as psychotherapy. Based on this evidence, CMS's medical consultants have recommended that chemical aversion therapy be covered under Medicare. However, since chemical aversion therapy is a demanding therapy which may not be appropriate for all Medicare beneficiaries needing treatment for alcoholism, a physician should certify to the appropriateness of chemical aversion therapy in the individual case. Therefore, if chemical aversion therapy for treatment of alcoholism is determined to be reasonable and necessary for an individual patient, it is covered under Medicare.

When it is medically necessary for a patient to receive chemical aversion therapy as a hospital inpatient, coverage for care in that setting is available. (See §130.1 regarding coverage of multimodality treatment programs.) Followup treatments for chemical aversion therapy can generally be provided on an outpatient basis. Thus, where a patient is admitted as an inpatient for receipt of chemical aversion therapy, there must be documentation by the physician of the need in the individual case for the inpatient hospital admission.

Decisions regarding reasonableness and necessity of treatment and the need for an inpatient hospital level of care should be made by intermediaries based on accepted medical practice with the advice of their medical consultant. (In hospitals under QIO review, QIO determinations of medical necessity of services and appropriateness of the level of care at which services are provided are binding on the title XVIII fiscal intermediaries for purposes of adjudicating claims for payment.)

Pub. 100-3, Section 130.4

Electrical Aversion Therapy for Treatment of Alcoholism

Electrical aversion therapy has not been shown to be safe and effective and therefore is excluded from coverage.

Pub. 100-3, Section 130.5

Treatment of Alcoholism and Drug Abuse in a Freestanding Clinic

Coverage is available for alcoholism or drug abuse treatment services (such as drug therapy, psychotherapy, and patient education) that are provided incident to a physician's professional service in a freestanding clinic to patients who, for example, have been discharged from an inpatient hospital stay for the treatment of alcoholism or drug abuse or to individuals who are not in the acute stages of alcoholism or drug abuse but require treatment. The coverage available for these services is subject to the same rules generally applicable to the coverage of clinic services. Of course, the services also must be reasonable and necessary for the diagnosis or treatment of the individual's alcoholism or drug abuse. The Part B psychiatric limitation would apply to alcoholism or drug abuse treatment services furnished by physicians to individuals who are not hospital inpatients.

Pub. 100-3, Section 130.6

Treatment of Drug Abuse (Chemical Dependency)

Accordingly, when it is medically necessary for a patient to receive detoxification and/or rehabilitation for drug substance abuse as a hospital inpatient, coverage for care in that setting is available. Coverage is also available for treatment services that are provided in the outpatient department of a hospital to patients who, for example, have been discharged from an inpatient stay for the treatment of drug substance abuse or who require treatment but do not require the availability and intensity of services found only in the inpatient hospital setting. The coverage available for these services is subject to the same rules generally applicable to the coverage of outpatient hospital services. The services must also be reasonable and necessary for treatment of the individual's condition. Decisions regarding reasonableness and necessity of treatment, the need for an inpatient hospital level of care, and length of treatment should be made by intermediaries based on accepted medical practice with the advice of their medical consultant. (In hospitals under QIO review, QIO determinations of medical necessity of services and appropriateness of the level of care at which services are provided are binding on the title XVIII fiscal intermediaries for purposes of adjudicating claims for payment.)

Pub. 100-3, Section 130.7

Withdrawal Treatments for Narcotic Addictions

Withdrawal is an accepted treatment for narcotic addiction, and Part B payment can be made for these services if they are provided by the physician directly or under his personal supervision and if they are reasonable and necessary. In reviewing claims, reasonableness and necessity are determined with the aid of the contractor's medical staff.

Drugs that the physician provides in connection with this treatment are also covered if they cannot be self-administered and meet all other statutory requirements.

Pub. 100-3, Section 130.8

Hemodialysis for Treatment of Schizophrenia

Scientific evidence supporting use of hemodialysis as a safe and effective means of treatment for schizophrenia is inconclusive at this time. Accordingly, Medicare does not cover hemodialysis for treatment of schizophrenia.

Pub. 100-3, Section 140.1

Abortion

Abortions are not covered Medicare procedures except:

1. If the pregnancy is the result of an act of rape or incest; or

2. In the case where a woman suffers from a physical disorder, physical injury, or physical illness, including a life-endangering physical condition caused by or arising from the pregnancy itself, that would, as certified by a physician, place the woman in danger of death unless an abortion is performed.

Pub. 100-3, Section 140.2

Breast Reconstruction Following Mastectomy

Reconstruction of the affected and the contralateral unaffected breast following a medically necessary mastectomy is considered a relatively safe and effective noncosmetic procedure. Accordingly, program payment may be made for breast reconstruction surgery following removal of a breast for any medical reason.

Program payment may not be made for breast reconstruction for cosmetic reasons. (Cosmetic surgery is excluded from coverage under §l862(a)(l0) of the Social Security Act.)

Pub. 100-3, Section 140.3

Transsexual Surgery

Transsexual surgery for sex reassignment of transsexuals is controversial. Because of the lack of well controlled, long term studies of the safety and effectiveness of the surgical procedures and attendant therapies for transsexualism, the treatment is considered experimental. Moreover, there is a high rate of serious complications for these surgical procedures. For these reasons, transsexual surgery is not covered.

Pub. 100-3, Section 140.4

Plastic Surgery to Correct "Moon Face"

The cosmetic surgery exclusion precludes payment for any surgical procedure directed at improving appearance. The condition giving rise to the patient's preoperative appearance is generally not a consideration. The only exception to the exclusion is surgery for the prompt repair of an accidental injury or for the improvement of a malformed body member which coincidentally serves some cosmetic purpose. Since surgery to correct a condition of "moon face" which developed as a side effect of cortisone therapy does not meet the exception to the exclusion, it is not covered under Medicare (§1862(a)(10) of the Act).

Pub. 100-3, Section 140.5

Laser Procedures

Medicare recognizes the use of lasers for many medical indications. Procedures performed with lasers are sometimes used in place of more conventional techniques. In the absence of a specific noncoverage instruction, and where a laser has been approved for marketing by the Food and Drug Administration, contractor discretion may be used to determine whether a procedure performed with a laser is reasonable and necessary and, therefore, covered.

The determination of coverage for a procedure performed using a laser is made on the basis that the use of lasers to alter, revise, or destroy tissue is a surgical procedure. Therefore, coverage of laser procedures is restricted to practitioners with training in the surgical management of the disease or condition being treated.

Pub. 100-3, Section 150.1

Manipulation

A. Manipulation of the Rib Cage. — Manual manipulation of the rib cage contributes to the treatment of respiratory conditions such as bronchitis, emphysema, and asthma as part of a regimen which includes other elements of therapy, and is covered only under such circumstances.

B. Manipulation of the Head. — Manipulation of the occipitocervical or temporomandibular regions of the head when indicated for conditions affecting those portions of the head and neck is a covered service.

Pub. 100-3, Section 150.2

Osteogenic Stimulators

Electrical Osteogenic Stimulators

B. Nationally Covered Indications

1. Noninvasive Stimulator.

The noninvasive stimulator device is covered only for the following indications:

- Nonunion of long bone fractures;
- Failed fusion, where a minimum of nine months has elapsed since the last surgery;
- Congenital pseudarthroses; and
- Effective July 1, 1996, as an adjunct to spinal fusion surgery for patients at high risk of pseudarthrosis due to previously failed spinal fusion at the same site or for those undergoing multiple level fusion. A multiple level fusion involves 3 or more vertebrae (e.g., L3-L5, L4-S1, etc.).
- Effective September 15, 1980, nonunion of long bone fractures is considered to exist only after 6 or more months have elapsed without healing of the fracture.
- Effective April 1, 2000, nonunion of long bone fractures is considered to exist only when serial radiographs have confirmed that fracture healing has ceased for 3 or more months prior to starting treatment with the electrical osteogenic stimulator. Serial radiographs must include a minimum of 2 sets of radiographs, each including multiple views of the fracture site, separated by a minimum of 90 days.

2. Invasive (Implantable) Stimulator.

The invasive stimulator device is covered only for the following indications:

- Nonunion of long bone fractures
- Effective July 1, 1996, as an adjunct to spinal fusion surgery for patients at high risk of pseudarthrosis due to previously failsed spinal fusion at the same site or for those undergoing multiple level fusion. A multiple level fusion involves 3 or more vertebrae (e.g., L3-5, L4-S1, etc.)
- Effective September 15, 1980, nonunion of long bone fractures is considered to exist only after 6 or more months have elapsed without healing of the fracture.
- Effective April 1, 2000, non union of long bone fractures is considered to exist only when serial radiographs have confirmed that fracture healing has ceased for 3 or more months prior to starting treatment with the electrical osteogenic stimulator. Serial radiographs must include a minimum of 2 sets of radiographs, each including multiple views of the fracture site, separated by a minimum of 90 days.

Effective for services performed on or after January 1, 2001, ultrasonic osteogenic stimulators are covered as medically reasonable and necessary for the treatment of non-union fractures. In demonstrating nonunion of fractures, we would expect:

- A minimum of two sets of radiographs obtained prior to starting treatment with the osteogenic stimulator, separated by a minimum of 90 days. Each radiograph must include multiple views of the fracture site accompanied with a written interpretation by a physician stating that there has been no clinically significant evidence of fracture healing between the two sets of radiographs.
- Indications that the patient failed at least one surgical intervention for the treatment of the fracture.
- Effective April 27, 2005, upon the recommendation of the ultrasound stimulation for nonunion fracture healing, CMS determins that the evidence is adequate to condlude that noninvasive ultrasound stimulation for the treatment of nonunion bone fractures prior to surfical intervention is reasonable and necessary. In demonstrating non-union fracturs, CMS expects::
- A minimum of 2 sets of radiographs, obtained prior to starting treating with the osteogenic stimulator, separated by a minimum of 90 days. Each radiograph set must include multiple views of the fracture site accompanied with a written interpretation by a physician stating that there has been no clinically significant evidence of fracture healing between the 2 sets of radiographs.

C. Nationally Non-Covered Indications

Nonunion fractures of the skull, vertebrae and those that are tumor-related are excluded from coverage.

Ultrasonic osteogenic stimulators may not be used concurrently with other non-invasive osteogenic devices.

Ultrasonic osteogenic stimulators for fresh fractures and delayed unions remain non-covered.

(This NCD last reviewed June 2005)

Pub. 100-3, Section 150.3

Bone (Mineral) Density Studies

The Following Bone (Mineral) Density Studies Are Covered Under Medicare:

A. Single Photon Absorptiometry

A non-invasive radiological technique that measures absorption of a monochromatic photon beam by bone material. The device is placed directly on the patient, uses a low dose of radionuclide, and measures the mass absorption efficiency of the energy used. It provides a quantitative measurement of the bone mineral of cortical and trabecular bone, and is used in assessing an individual's treatment response at appropriate intervals.

Single photon absorptiometry is covered under Medicare when used in assessing changes in bone density of patients with osteodystrophy or osteoporosis when performed on the same individual at intervals of 6 to 12 months.

B. Bone Biopsy

A physiologic test which is a surgical, invasive procedure. A small sample of bone (usually from the ilium) is removed, generally by a biopsy needle. The biopsy sample is then examined histologically, and provides a qualitative measurement of the bone mineral of trabecular bone. This procedure is used in ascertaining a differential diagnosis of bone disorders and is used primarily to differentiate osteomalacia from osteoporosis.

Bone biopsy is covered under Medicare when used for the qualitative evaluation of bone no more than four times per patient, unless there is special justification given. When used more than four times on a patient, bone biopsy leaves a defect in the pelvis and may produce some patient discomfort.

C. Photodensitometry(radiographic absorptiometry)

A noninvasive radiological procedure that attempts to assess bone mass by measuring the optical density of extremity radiographs with a photodensitometer, usually with a reference to a standard density wedge placed on the film at the time of exposure. This procedure provides a quantitative measurement of the bone mineral of bone, and is used for monitoring gross bone change.

The Following Bone (Mineral) Density Study Is Not Covered Under Medicare:

D. Dual Photon Absorptiometry

A noninvasive radiological technique that measures absorption of a dichromatic beam by bone material. This procedure is not covered under Medicare because it is still considered to be in the investigational stage.

Pub. 100-3, Section 150.5

Diathermy Treatment

High energy pulsed wave diathermy machines have been found to produce some degree of therapeutic benefit for essentially the same conditions and to the same extent as standard diathermy. Accordingly, where the contractor's medical staff has determined that the pulsed wave diathermy apparatus used is one which is considered therapeutically effective, the treatments are considered a covered service, but only for those conditions for which standard diathermy is medically indicated and only when rendered by a physician or incident to a physician's professional services.

Pub. 100-3, Section 150.6

Vitamin B12 Injections to Strengthen Tendons, Ligaments, etc., of the Foot

Vitamin B12 injections to strengthen tendons, ligaments, etc., of the foot are not covered under Medicare because (1) there is no evidence that vitamin B12 injections are effective for the purpose of strengthening weakened tendons and ligaments, and (2) this is nonsurgical treatment under the subluxation exclusion. Accordingly, vitamin B12 injections are not considered reasonable and necessary within the meaning of §1862(a)(1) of the Act.

Pub. 100-3, Section 150.7

Prolotherapy, Joint Sclerotherapy, and Ligamentous Injections with Sclerosing Agents

The medical effectiveness of the above therapies has not been verified by scientifically controlled studies. Accordingly, reimbursement for these modalities should be denied on the ground that they are not reasonable and necessary as required by §1862(a)(1) of the Act.

Pub. 100-3, Section 160.1

Induced Lesions of Nerve Tracts

Accordingly, program payment may be made for these denervation procedures when used in selected cases (concurred in by contractor's medical staff) to treat chronic pain.

Pub. 100-3, Section 160.2

Treatment of Motor Function Disorders with Electric Nerve Stimulation

Where electric nerve stimulation is employed to treat motor function disorders, no reimbursement may be made for the stimulator or for the services related to its implantation since this treatment cannot be considered reasonable and necessary.

Note: For Medicare coverage of deep brain stimulation for essential tremor and Parkinson's disease, see §160.24 of the NCD Manual.

Pub. 100-3, Section 160.4

Stereotactic Cingulotomy as a Means of Psychosurgery

Stereotactic cingulotomy is not covered under Medicare because the procedure is considered to be investigational.

Pub. 100-3, Section 160.5

Stereotaxic Depth Electrode Implantation

Stereotaxic depth electrode implantation prior to surgical treatment of focal epilepsy for patients who are unresponsive to anticonvulsant medications has been found both safe and effective for diagnosing resectable seizure foci that may go undetected by conventional scalp electroencephalographs (EEGs).

Pub. 100-3, Section 160.7

Electrical Nerve Stimulators

Two general classifications of electrical nerve stimulators are employed to treat chronic intractable pain: peripheral nerve stimulators and central nervous system stimulators.

A-Implanted Peripheral Nerve Stimulators

Payment may be made under the prosthetic device benefit for implanted peripheral nerve stimulators. Use of this stimulator involves implantation of electrodes around a selected peripheral nerve. The stimulating electrode is connected by an insulated lead to a receiver unit which is implanted under the skin at a depth not greater than 1/2 inch. Stimulation is induced by a generator connected to an antenna unit which is attached to the skin surface over the receiver unit. Implantation of electrodes requires surgery and usually necessitates an operating room.

NOTE: Peripheral nerve stimulators may also be employed to assess a patient's suitability for continued treatment with an electric nerve stimulator. As explained in §160.7.1, such use of the stimulator is covered as part of the total diagnostic service furnished to the beneficiary rather than as a prosthesis.

B-Central Nervous System Stimulators (Dorsal Column and Depth Brain Stimulators).The implantation of central nervous system stimulators may be covered as therapies for the relief of chronic intractable pain, subject to the following conditions:

1-Types of Implantations

There are two types of implantations covered by this instruction:

- Dorsal Column (Spinal Cord) Neurostimulation. – The surgical implantation of neurostimulator electrodes within the dura mater (endodural) or the percutaneous insertion of electrodes in the epidural space is covered.

- Depth Brain Neurostimulation. – The stereotactic implantation of electrodes in the deep brain (e.g., thalamus and periaqueductal gray matter) is covered.

2-Conditions for Coverage

No payment may be made for the implantation of dorsal column or depth brain stimulators or services and supplies related to such implantation, unless all of the conditions listed below have been met:

- The implantation of the stimulator is used only as a late resort (if not a last resort) for patients with chronic intractable pain;

- With respect to item a, other treatment modalities (pharmacological, surgical, physical, or psychological therapies) have been tried and did not prove satisfactory, or are judged to be unsuitable or contraindicated for the given patient;

- Patients have undergone careful screening, evaluation and diagnosis by a multidisciplinary team prior to implantation. (Such screening must include psychological, as well as physical evaluation);

- All the facilities, equipment, and professional and support personnel required for the proper diagnosis, treatment training, and followup of the patient (including that required to satisfy item c) must be available; and

- Demonstration of pain relief with a temporarily implanted electrode precedes permanent implantation.

Contractors may find it helpful to work with QIOs to obtain the information needed to apply these conditions to claims.

Pub. 100-3, Section 160.7.1

Assessing Patient's Suitability for Electrical Nerve Stimulation Therapy

Indications and Limitations of Coverage

CIM 35-46

Electrical nerve stimulation is an accepted modality for assessing a patient's suitability for ongoing treatment with a transcutaneous or an implanted nerve stimulator.

Accordingly, program payment may be made for the following techniques when used to determine the potential therapeutic usefulness of an electrical nerve stimulator:

A. Transcutaneous Electrical Nerve Stimulation(TENS)

This technique involves attachment of a transcutaneous nerve stimulator to the surface of the skin over the peripheral nerve to be stimulated. It is used by the patient on a trial basis and its effectiveness in modulating pain is monitored by the physician, or physical therapist. Generally, the physician or physical therapist is able to determine whether the patient is likely to derive a significant therapeutic benefit from continuous use of a transcutaneous stimulator within a trial period of 1 month; in a few cases this determination may take longer to make. Document the medical necessity for such services which are furnished beyond the first month. (See §160.13 for an explanation of coverage of medically necessary supplies for the effective use of TENS.)

If TENS significantly alleviates pain, it may be considered as primary treatment; if it produces no relief or greater discomfort than the original pain electrical nerve stimulation therapy is ruled out. However, where TENS produces incomplete relief, further evaluation with percutaneous electrical nerve stimulation may be considered to determine whether an implanted peripheral nerve stimulator would provide significant relief from pain.

Usually, the physician or physical therapist providing the services will furnish the equipment necessary for assessment. Where the physician or physical therapist advises the patient to rent the TENS from a supplier during the trial period rather than supplying it himself/herself, program payment may be made for rental of the TENS as well as for the services of the physician or physical therapist who is evaluating its use. However, the combined program payment which is made for the physician's or physical therapist's services and the rental of the stimulator from a supplier should not exceed the amount which would be payable for the total service, including the stimulator, furnished by the physician or physical therapist alone.

B. Percutaneous Electrical Nerve Stimulation (PENS)

This diagnostic procedure which involves stimulation of peripheral nerves by a needle electrode inserted through the skin is performed only in a physician's office, clinic, or hospital outpatient department. Therefore, it is covered only when performed by a physician or incident to physician's service. If pain is effectively controlled by percutaneous stimulation, implantation of electrodes is warranted.

As in the case of TENS (described in subsection A), generally the physician should be able to determine whether the patient is likely to derive a significant therapeutic benefit from continuing use of an implanted nerve stimulator within a trial period of 1 month. In a few cases, this determination may take longer to make. The medical necessity for such diagnostic services which are furnished beyond the first month must be documented.

NOTE: Electrical nerve stimulators do not prevent pain but only alleviate pain as it occurs. A patient can be taught how to employ the stimulator, and once this is done, can use it safely and effectively without direct physician supervision. Consequently, it is inappropriate for a patient to visit his/her physician, physical therapist, or an outpatient clinic on a continuing basis for treatment of pain with electrical nerve stimulation. Once it is determined that electrical nerve stimulation should be continued as therapy and the patient has been trained to use the stimulator, it is expected that a stimulator will be implanted or the patient will employ the TENS on a continual basis in his/her home. Electrical nerve stimulation treatments furnished by a physician in his/her office, by a physical therapist or outpatient clinic are excluded from coverage by §1862(a)(1) of the Act. (See §160.7 for an explanation of coverage of the therapeutic use of implanted peripheral nerve stimulators under the prosthetic devices benefit. See §280.13 for an explanation of coverage of the therapeutic use of TENS under the durable medical equipment benefit.)

Pub. 100-3, Section 160.8

Electroencephalographic Monitoring During Surgical Procedures Involving the Cerebral Vasculature

Electroencephalographic (EEG) monitoring is a safe and reliable technique for the assessment of gross cerebral blood flow during general anesthesia and is covered under Medicare. Very characteristic changes in the EEG occur when cerebral perfusion is inadequate for ce rebral function. EEG monitoring as an indirect measure of cerebral perfusion requires the expertise of an electroencephalographer, a neurologist trained in EEG, or an advanced EEG technician for its proper interpretation.

The EEG monitoring may be covered routinely in carotid endarterectomies and in other neurological procedures where cerebral perfusion could be reduced. Such other procedures might include aneurysm surgery where hypotensive anesthesia is used or other cerebral vascular procedures where cerebral blood flow may be interrupted. Transmittal Number 48

Pub. 100-3, Section 160.9

Electronecephalographic (EEG) Monitoring during Open-Heart Surgery

The value of EEG monitoring during open heart surgery and in the immediate post-operative period is debatable because there are little published data based on well designed studies regarding its clinical effectiveness. The procedure is not frequently used and does not enjoy widespread acceptance of benefit.

Accordingly, Medicare does not cover EEG monitoring during open heart surgery and during the immediate post-operative period.

Pub. 100-3, Section 160.10

Evoked Response Tests

Evoked response tests, including brain stem evoked response and visual evoked response tests, are generally accepted as safe and effective diagnostic tools. Program payment may be made for these procedures.

Pub. 100-3, Section 160.13

Supplies Used in the Delivery of Transcutaneous Electrical Nerve Stimulation (TENS) and Neuromuscular Electrical Stimulation (NMES)

A form-fitting conductive garment (and medically necessary related supplies) may be covered under the program only when:

1. It has received permission or approval for marketing by the Food and Drug Administration;

2. It has been prescribed by a physician for use in delivering covered TENS or NMES treatment; and

3. One of the medical indications outlined below is met:

- The patient cannot manage without the conductive garment because there is such a large area or so many sites to be stimulated and the stimulation would have to be delivered so frequently that it is not feasible to use conventional electrodes, adhesive tapes and lead wires;

- The patient cannot manage without the conductive garment for the treatment of chronic intractable pain because the areas or sites to be stimulated are inaccessible with the use of conventional electrodes, adhesive tapes and lead wires;

- The patient has a documented medical condition such as skin problems that preclude the application of conventional electrodes, adhesive tapes and lead wires;

- The patient requires electrical stimulation beneath a cast either to treat disuse atrophy, where the nerve supply to the muscle is intact, or to treat chronic intractable pain; or:

- The patient has a medical need for rehabilitation strengthening (pursuant to a written plan of rehabilitation) following an injury where the nerve supply to the muscle is intact.

A conductive garment is not covered for use with a TENS device during the trial period specified in §35-46 unless:

4. The patient has a documented skin problem prior to the start of the trial period; and

5. The carrier's medical consultants are satisfied that use of such an item is medically necessary for the patient.

Pub. 100-3, Section 160.15

Electrotherapy for Treatment of Facial Nerve Paralysis (Bell's Palsy)

Electrotherapy for the treatment of facial nerve paralysis, commonly known as Bell's Palsy, is not covered under Medicare because its clinical effectiveness has not been established.

Pub. 100-3, Section 160.17

L-DOPA

A. Part A Payment for L-Dopa and Associated Inpatient Hospital Services. — A hospital stay and related ancillary services for the administration of L-Dopa are covered if medically required for this purpose. Whether a drug represents an allowable inpatient hospital cost during such stay depends on whether it meets the definition of a drug in §1861(t) of the Act; i.e., on its inclusion in the compendia named in the Act or approval by the hospital's pharmacy and drug therapeutics (P&DT) or equivalent committee. (Levodopa (L-Dopa) has been favorably evaluated for the treatment of Parkinsonism by A.M.A. Drug Evaluations, First Edition 1971, the replacement compendia for "New Drugs.")

Inpatient hospital services are frequently not required in many cases when L-Dopa therapy is initiated. Therefore, determine the medical need for inpatient hospital services on the basis of medical facts in the individual case. It is not necessary to hospitalize the typical, well-functioning, ambulatory Parkinsonian patient who has no concurrent disease at the start of L-Dopa treatment. It is reasonable to provide inpatient hospital services for Parkinsonian patients with concurrent diseases, particularly of the cardiovascular, gastrointestinal, and neuropsychiatric systems. Although many patients require hospitalization for a period of under 2 weeks, a 4-week period of inpatient care is not unreasonable.

Laboratory tests in connection with the administration of L-Dopa. — The tests medically warranted in connection with the achievement of optimal dosage and the control of the side effects of L-Dopa include a complete blood count, liver function tests such as SGOT, SGPT, and/or alkaline phosphatase, BUN or creatinine and urinalysis, blood sugar, and electrocardiogram.

Whether or not the patient is hospitalized, laboratory tests in certain cases are reasonable at weekly intervals although some physicians prefer to perform the tests much less frequently.

Physical therapy furnished in connection with administration of L-Dopa. — Where, following administration of the drug, the patient experiences a reduction of rigidity which permits the reestablishment of a restorative goal for him/her, physical therapy services required to enable him/her to achieve this goal are payable provided they require the skills of a qualified physical therapist and are furnished by or under the supervision of such a therapist. However, once the individual's restoration potential has been achieved, the services required to maintain him/her at this level do not generally require the skills of a qualified physical therapist. In such situations, the role of the therapist is to evaluate the patient's needs in consultation with his/her physician and design a program of exercise appropriate to the capacity and tolerance of the patient and treatment objectives of the physician, leaving to others the actual carrying out of the program. While the evaluative services rendered by a qualified physical therapist are payable as physical therapy, services furnished by others in connection with the carrying out of the maintenance program established by the therapist are not.

B. Part A Reimbursement for L-Dopa Therapy in SNFs. — Initiation of L-Dopa therapy can be appropriately carried out in the SNF setting, applying the same guidelines used for initiation of L-Dopa therapy in the hospital, including the types of patients who should be covered for inpatient services, the role of physical therapy, and the use of laboratory tests. (See subsection A.)

Where inpatient care is required and L-Dopa therapy is initiated in the SNF, limit the stay to a maximum of 4 weeks; but in many cases the need may be no longer than 1 or 2 weeks, depending upon the patient's condition. However, where L-Dopa therapy is begun in the hospital and the patient is transferred to an SNF for continuation of the therapy, a combined length of stay in hospital and SNF of no longer than 4 weeks is reasonable (i.e., 1 week hospital stay followed by 3 weeks SNF stay; or 2 weeks hospital stay followed by 2 weeks SNF stay; etc.). Medical need must be demonstrated in cases where the combined length of stay in hospital and SNF is longer than 4 weeks. The choice of hospital or SNF, and the decision regarding the relative length of time spent in each, should be left to the medical judgment of the treating physician.

C. L-Dopa Coverage Under Part B. — Part B reimbursement may not be made for the drug L-Dopa since it is a self-administrable drug. (See Intermediary Manual, §3112.4B; Carriers Manual, §2050.5B; and Hospital Manual, §230.4B.) However, physician services rendered in connection with its administration and control of its side effects are covered if determined to be reasonable and necessary. Initiation of L-Dopa therapy on an outpatient basis is possible in most cases. Visit

frequency ranging from every week to every 2 or 3 months is acceptable. However, after half a year of therapy, visits more frequent than every month would usually not be reasonable.

Pub. 100-3, Section 160.18

Vagus Nerve Stimulation for Treatment of Seizures

Clinical evidence has shown that vagus nerve stimulation is safe and effective treatment for patients with medically refractory partial onset seizures, for whom surgery is not recommended or for whom surgery has failed. Vagus nerve stimulation is not covered for patients with other types of seizure disorders which are medically refractory and for whom surgery is not recommended or for whom surgery has failed.

A partial onset seizure has a focal onset in one area of the brain and may or may not involve a loss of motor control or alteration of consciousness. Partial onset seizures may be simple, complex, or complex partial seizures, secondarily generalized.

Pub. 100-3, Section 160.20

Transfer Factor for Treatment of Multiple Sclerosis

Transfer factor is the dialysate of an extract from sensitized leukocytes which increases cellular immune activity in the recipient. It is not covered as a treatment for multiple sclerosis because its use for the purpose is still experimental.

Pub. 100-3, Section 160.21

Telephone Transmission of Electroencephalograms

Telephone transmission of electroencephalograms (EEGs) is covered as a physician's service or as incident to a physician's service when reasonable and necessary for the individual patient, under appropriate circumstances. The service is safe, and may save time and cost in sending EEGs from remote areas without special competence in neurology, neurosurgery, and electroencephalography, by avoiding the need to transport patients to large medical centers for standard EEG testing.

Pub. 100-3, Section 160.22

Ambulatory Electroencephalographic (EEG) Monitoring

Ambulatory EEG monitoring is a diagnostic procedure for patients in whom a seizure diathesis is suspected but not defined by history, physical or resting EEG. Ambulatory EEG can be utilized in the differential diagnosis of syncope and transient ischemic attacks if not elucidated by conventional studies. Ambulatory EEG should always be preceded by a resting EEG.

Ambulatory EEG monitoring is considered an established technique and covered under Medicare for the above purposes.

Pub. 100-3, Section 170.3

Speech Pathology Services for the Treatment of Dysphagia

Speech pathology services are covered under Medicare for the treatment of dysphagia, regardless of the presence of a communication disability.

Pub. 100-3, Section 180.1

Medical Nutrition Therapy

Effective October 1, 2002, basic coverage of MNT for the first year a beneficiary receives MNT with either a diagnosis of renal disease or diabetes as defined at 42 CFR §410.130 is 3 hours. Also effective October 1, 2002, basic coverage in subsequent years for renal disease or diabetes is 2 hours. The dietitian/nutritionist may choose how many units are performed per day as long as all of the other requirements in this NCD and 42 CFR §§410.130-410.134 are met. Pursuant to the exception at 42 CFR §410.132(b)(5), additional hours are considered to be medically necessary and covered if the treating physician determines that there is a change in medical condition, diagnosis, or treatment regimen that requires a change in MNT and orders additional hours during that episode of care.

Effective October 1, 2002, if the treating physician determines that receipt of both MNT and DSMT is medically necessary in the same episode of care, Medicare will cover both DSMT and MNT initial and subsequent years without decreasing either benefit as long as DSMT and MNT are not provided on the same date of service. The dietitian/nutritionist may choose how many units are performed per day as long as all of the other requirements in the NCD and 42 CFR §§410.130-410.134 are met. Pursuant to the exception at 42 CFR 410.132(b)(5), additional hours are considered to be medically necessary and covered if the treating physician determines that there is a change in medical condition, diagnosis, or treatment regimen that requires a change in MNT and orders additional hours during that episode of care.

Pub. 100-3, Section 190.1

Histocompatibility Testing

This testing is safe and effective when it is performed on patients:

A. In preparation for a kidney transplant;

B. In preparation for bone marrow transplantation;

C. In preparation for blood platelet transfusions (particularly where multiple infusions are involved); or

D. Who are suspected of having ankylosing spondylitis.

This testing is covered under Medicare when used for any of the indications listed in A, B, and C and if it is reasonable and necessary for the patient.

It is covered for ankylosing spondylitis in cases where other methods of diagnosis would not be appropriate or have yielded inconclusive results. Request documentation supporting the medical necessity of the test from the physician in all cases where ankylosing spondylitis is indicated as the reason for the test.

Pub. 100-3, Section 190.2

Diagnostic Pap Smears

A diagnostic pap smear and related medically necessary services are covered under Medicare Part B when ordered by a physician under one of the following conditions:

- Previous cancer of the cervix, uterus, or vagina that has been or is presently being treated;
- Previous abnormal pap smear;
- Any abnormal findings of the vagina, cervix, uterus, ovaries, or adnexa;
- Any significant complaint by the patient referable to the female reproductive system; or
- Any signs or symptoms that might in the physician's judgment reasonably be related to a gynecologic disorder.

Screening Pap Smears and Pelvic Examinations for Early Detection of Cervical or Vaginal Cancer. (See section 210.2.)

Pub. 100-3, Section 190.3

Cytogenetic Studies

Medicare covers these tests when they are reasonable and necessary for the diagnosis or treatment of the following conditions:

- Genetic disorders (e.g., mongolism) in a fetus (See Medicare Benefit Policy Manual, Chapter 15, "Covered medical and Other health Services," §20.1);
- Failure of sexual development;
- Chronic myelogenous leukemia;
- Acute leukemias lymphoid (FAB L1-L3), myeloid (FAB M0-M7), and unclassified; or:
- Mylodysplasia:

Pub. 100-3, Section 190.4

Electron Microscope

The electron microscope has been used in the examination of biopsies for years; its efficacy, and therefore its Medicare coverage, is not being questioned. However, there are less expensive methods for examining biopsies which are normally adequate. The additional expense for the electron microscope is normally warranted only when distinguishing different types of nephritis from renal needle biopsies or when there is an uncertain diagnosis from the pathologist. When an uncertain diagnosis from the pathologists results from a less expensive method of examination and an electron microscope examination is therefore necessary, both biopsy examinations are covered. Where the additional expense for an electron microscope examination is not warranted, payment is based upon the less costly methods of examining biopsies.

Pub. 100-3, Section 190.5

Sweat Test

The sweat test is an important diagnostic tool in cystic fibrosis and may be covered when used for that purpose. Usage of the sweat test as a predictor of efficacy of sympathectomy in peripheral vascular disease is unproven and, therefore, is not covered.

Pub. 100-3, Section 190.6

Hair Analysis

Indications and Limitations of Coverage

Hair analysis to detect mineral traces as an aid in diagnosing human disease is not a covered service under Medicare.

The correlation of hair analysis to the chemical state of the whole body is not possible at this time, and therefore this diagnostic procedure cannot be considered to be reasonable and necessary under §1862(a)(1) of the Act.

Pub. 100-3, Section 190.8

Lymphocyte Mitogen Response Assays

It is a covered test under Medicare when it is medically necessary to assess lymphocytic function in diagnosed immunodeficiency diseases and to monitor immunotherapy.

It is not covered when it is used to monitor the treatment of cancer, because its use for that purpose is experimental.

Pub. 100-3, Section 190.9

Serologic Testing for Acquired Immunodeficiency Syndrome (AIDS)

These tests may be covered when performed to help determine a diagnosis for symptomaticpatients. They are not covered when furnished as part of a screening program for asymptomatic persons.

NOTE: Two enzyme-linked immunosorbent assay (ELISA) tests that were conducted on the same specimen must both be positive before Medicare will cover the Western blot test.

Pub. 100-3, Section 190.10

Laboratory Tests - CRD Patients

A. Laboratory tests are essential to monitor the progress of CRD patients. The following list and frequencies of tests constitute the level and types of routine laboratory tests that are covered. Bills for other types of tests are considered nonroutine. Routine tests at greater frequencies must include medical justification. Nonroutine tests generally are justified by the diagnosis. The routinely covered regimen includes the following tests:

Per Dialysis

All hematocrit or hemoglobin and clotting time tests furnished incident to dialysis treatments.

Per Week

Prothrombin time for patients on anticoagulant therapy

Serum Creatinine

Per Week or Thirteen Per Quarter

BUN

Monthly

CBC	Serum Calcium
Serum Potassium	Serum Chloride
Serum Bicarbonate	Serum Phosphorous
Total ProteiSerum Albumin	
Alkaline Phospatase	AST, SGOT
LDH	

Guidelines for tests other than those routinely performed include:

Serum Aluminum - one every 3 months

Serum Ferritin - one every 3 months

The following tests for hepatitis B are covered when patients first enter a dialysis facility: hepatitis B surface antigen (HBsAg) and Anti-HBs. Coverage of future testing in these patients depends on their serologic status and on whether they have been successfully immunized against hepatitis B virus. The following table summarizes the frequency of serologic surveillance for hepatitis B. Tests furnished according to this table do not require additional documentation and are paid separately because payment for maintenance dialysis treatments does not take them into account.

	Frequency of Screening	
Vaccination andSerologic Status	HBsAg Patients	Anti-HBs Patients
UNVACCINATED		
Susceptible	Monthly	Semiannually
HBsAg Carrier	Annually	None
Anti-HBs-Positive (1)	None	Annually
VACCINATED		
Anti-HBs-Positive (1)		
Low Level or No	None	Annually
Anti-HBs	Monthly	Semiannually

(1) At least 10 sample ration units by radioimmunoassay or positive by enzyme immunoassay.

Patients who are in the process of receiving hepatitis B vaccines, but have not received the complete series, should continue to be routinely screened as susceptible. Between one and six months after the third dose, all vaccines should be tested for anti-HBs to confirm their response to the vaccine. Patients who have a level of anti-HBs of at least 10 sample ratio units (SRUs) by radioimmunoassay (RIA) or who are positive by enzyme immunoassay (EIA) are considered adequate responders to vaccine and need only be tested for anti-HBs annually to verify their immune status. If anti-HBs drops below 10 SRUs by RIA or is negative by EIA, a booster dose of hepatitis B vaccine should be given.

B. Laboratory tests are subject to the normal coverage requirements. If the laboratory services are performed by a free-standing facility, be sure it meets the conditions of coverage for independent laboratories.

Pub. 100-3, Section 190.12

Urine Culture, Bacterial

Indications

1. A patient's urinalysis is abnormal suggesting urinary tract infection, for example, abnormal microscopic (hematuria, pyuria, bacteriuria); abnormal biochemical urinalysis (positive leukocyte esterase, nitrite, protein, blood); a Gram's stain positive for microorganisms; positive bacteriuria screen by a non?culture technique; or other significant abnormality of a urinalysis. While it is not essential to evaluate a urine specimen by one of these methods before a urine culture is performed, certain clinical presentations with highly suggestive signs and symptoms may lend themselves to an antecedent urinalysis procedure where follow-up culture depends upon an initial positive or abnormal test result.

2. A patient has clinical signs and symptoms indicative of a possible urinary tract infection (UTI). Acute lower UTI may present with urgency, frequency, nocturia, dysuria, discharge or incontinence. These findings may also be noted in upper UTI with additional systemic symptoms (for example, fever, chills, lethargy); or pain in the costovertebral, abdominal, or pelvic areas. Signs and symptoms may overlap considerably with other inflammatory conditions of the genitourinary tract (for example, prostatitis, urethritis, vaginitis, or cervicitis). Elderly or immunocompromised patients, or patients with neurologic disorders may present atypically (for example, general debility, acute mental status changes, declining functional status).

3. The patient is being evaluated for suspected urosepsis, fever of unknown origin, or other systemic manifestations of infection but without a known source. Signs and symptoms used to define sepsis have been well established.

4. A test-of-cure is generally not indicated in an uncomplicated infection. However, it may be indicated if the patient is being evaluated for response to therapy and there is a complicating co-existing urinary abnormality including structural or functional abnormalities, calculi, foreign bodies, or ureteral/renal stents or there is clinical or laboratory evidence of failure to respond as described in Indications 1 and 2.

5. In surgical procedures involving major manipulations of the genitourinary tract, preoperative examination to detect occult infection may be indicated in selected cases (for example, prior to renal transplantation, manipulation or removal of kidney stones, or transurethral surgery of the bladder or prostate).

6. Urine culture may be indicated to detect occult infection in renal transplant recipients on immunosuppressive therapy.

Limitations

1. CPT 87086 may be used one time per encounter.

2. Colony count restrictions on coverage of CPT 87088 do not apply as they may be highly variable according to syndrome or other clinical circumstances (for example, antecedent therapy, collection time, degree of hydration).

3. CPT 87088, 87184, and 87186 may be used multiple times in association with or independent of 87086, as urinary tract infections may be polymicrobial.

4. Testing for asymptomatic bacteriuria as part of a prenatal evaluation may be medically appropriate but is considered screening and, therefore, not covered by Medicare. The US Preventive Services Task Force has concluded that screening for asymptomatic bacteriuria outside of the narrow indication for pregnant women is generally not indicated. There are insufficient data to recommend screening in ambulatory elderly patients including those with diabetes. Testing may be clinically indicated on other grounds including likelihood of recurrence or potential adverse effects of antibiotics, but is considered screening in the absence of clinical or laboratory evidence of infection.

Pub. 100-3, Section 190.13

Human Immunodeficiency Virus Testing (Prognosis Including Monitoring)

Indications:

1. A plasma HIV RNA baseline level may be medically necessary.in any patient with confirmed HIV infection.

2. Regular periodic measurement of plasma HIV RNA levels may be medically necessary to determine risk for disease progression in an HIV-infected individual and to determine when to initiate or modify antiretroviral treatment regimens.

3. In clinical situations where the risk of HIV infection is significant and initiation of therapy is anticipated, a baseline HIV quantification may be performed. These situations include:

a. Persistence of borderline or equivocal serologic reactivity in an at-risk individual.

b. Signs and symptoms of acute retroviral syndrome characterized by fever, malaise, lymphadenopathy and rash in an at-risk individual.

Limitations:

1. Viral quantification may be appropriate for prognostic use including baseline determination, periodic monitoring, and monitoring of response to therapy. Use as a diagnostic test method is not indicated.

2. Measurement of plasma HIV RNA levels should be performed at the time of establishment of an HIV infection diagnosis. For an accurate baseline, 2 specimens in a 2-week period are appropriate.

3. For prognosis including anti-retroviral therapy monitoring, regular, periodic measurements are appropriate. The frequency of viral load testing should be consistent with the most current Centers for Disease Control and Prevention guidelines for use of anti-retroviral agents in adults and adolescents or pediatrics.

4. Because differences in absolute HIV copy number are known to occur using different assays, plasma HIV RNA levels should be measured by the same analytical method. A change in assay method may necessitate re-establishment of a baseline.

5. Nucleic acid quantification techniques are representative of rapidly emerging and evolving new technologies. As such, users are advised to remain current on FDA-approval status.

Note: Scroll down for links to the quarterly Covered Code Lists (including narrative).

Pub. 100-3, Section 190.14

Human Immunodeficiency Virus Testing (Diagnosis)

Indications

Diagnostic testing to establish HIV infection may be indicated when there is a strong clinical suspicion supported by one or more of the following clinical findings:

1. The patient has a documented, otherwise unexplained, AIDS-defining or AIDS-associated opportunistic infection.

2. The patient has another documented sexually transmitted disease which identifies significant risk of exposure to HIV and the potential for an early or subclinical infection.

3. The patient has documented acute or chronic hepatitis B or C infection that identifies a significant risk of exposure to HIV and the potential for an early or subclinical infection.

4. The patient has a documented AIDS-defining or AIDS-associated neoplasm.

5. The patient has a documented AIDS-associated neurologic disorder or otherwise unexplained dementia.

6. The patient has another documented AIDS-defining clinical condition, or a history of other severe, recurrent, or persistent conditions which suggest an underlying immune deficiency (for example, cutaneous or mucosal disorders).

7. The patient has otherwise unexplained generalized signs and symptoms suggestive of a chronic process with an underlying immune deficiency (for example, fever, weight loss, malaise, fatigue, chronic diarrhea, failure to thrive, chronic cough, hemoptysis, shortness of breath, or lymphadenopathy).

8. The patient has otherwise unexplained laboratory evidence of a chronic disease process with an underlying immune deficiency (for example, anemia, leukopenia, pancytopenia, lymphopenia, or low CD4+ lymphocyte count).

9. The patient has signs and symptoms of acute retroviral syndrome with fever, malaise, lymphadenopathy, and skin rash.

10. The patient has documented exposure to blood or body fluids known to be capable of transmitting HIV (for example, needlesticks and other significant blood exposures) and antiviral therapy is initiated or anticipated to be initiated.

11. The patient is undergoing treatment for rape. (HIV testing is a part of the rape treatment protocol.)

Limitations

1. HIV antibody testing in the United States is usually performed using HIV-1 or HIV-2 combination tests. HIV-2 testing is indicated if clinical circumstances suggest HIV-2 is likely (that is, compatible clinical findings and HIV-1 test negative). HIV-2 testing may also be indicated in areas of the country where there is greater prevalence of HIV-2 infections.

2. The Western Blot test should be performed only after documentation that the initial EIA tests are repeatedly positive or equivocal on a single sample.

3. The HIV antigen tests currently have no defined diagnostic usage.

4. Direct viral RNA detection may be performed in those situations where serologictesting does not establish a diagnosis but strong clinical suspicion persists (for example, acute retroviral syndrome, nonspecific serologic evidence of HIV, or perinatal HIV infection).

5. If initial serologic tests confirm an HIV infection, repeat testing is not indicated.

6. If initial serologic tests are HIV EIA negative and there is no indication for confirmation of infection by viral RNA detection, the interval prior to retesting is 3-6 months.

7. Testing for evidence of HIV infection using serologic methods may be medically appropriate in situations where there is a risk of exposure to HIV. However, in the absence of a documented AIDS defining or HIV- associated disease, an HIV associated sign or symptom, or documented exposure to a known HIV-infected source, the testing is considered by Medicare to be screening and thus is not covered by Medicare (for example, history of multiple blood component transfusions, exposure to blood or body fluids not resulting in consideration of therapy, history of transplant, history of illicit drug use, multiple sexual partners, same-sex encounters, prostitution, or contact with prostitutes).

8. The CPT Editorial Panel has issued a number of codes for infectious agent detection by direct antigen or nucleic acid probe techniques that have not yet been developed or are only being used on an investigational basis. Laboratory providers are advised to remain current on FDA-approval status for these tests.

Note: Scroll down for links to the quarterly Covered Code Lists (including narrative).

Pub. 100-3, Section 190.15

Blood Counts

Indications and Limitations of Coverage

Indications

Indications for a CBC or hemogram include red cell, platelet, and white cell disorders. Examples of these indications are enumerated individually below.

1. Indications for a CBC generally include the evaluation of bone marrow dysfunction as a result of neoplasms, therapeutic agents, exposure to toxic substances, or pregnancy. The CBC is also useful in assessing peripheral destruction of blood cells, suspected bone marrow failure or bone marrow infiltrate, suspected myeloproliferative, myelodysplastic, or lymphoproliferative processes, and immune disorders.

2. Indications for hemogram or CBC related to red cell (RBC) parameters of the hemogram include signs, symptoms, test results, illness, or disease that can be associated with anemia or other red blood cell disorder (e.g., pallor, weakness, fatigue, weight loss, bleeding, acute injury associated with blood loss or suspected blood loss, abnormal menstrual bleeding, hematuria, hematemesis, hematochezia, positive fecal occult blood test, malnutrition, vitamin deficiency, malabsorption, neuropathy, known malignancy, presence of acute or chronic disease that may have associated anemia, coagulation or hemostatic disorders, postural dizziness, syncope, abdominal pain, change in bowel habits, chronic marrow hypoplasia or decreased RBC production, tachycardia, systolic heart murmur, congestive heart failure, dyspnea, angina, nailbed deformities, growth retardation, jaundice, hepatomegaly, splenomegaly, lymphadenopathy, ulcers on the lower extremities).

3. Indications for hemogram or CBC related to red cell (RBC) parameters of the hemogram include signs, symptoms, test results, illness, or disease that can be associated with polycythemia (for example, fever, chills, ruddy skin, conjunctival redness, cough, wheezing, cyanosis, clubbing of the fingers, orthopnea, heart murmur, headache, vague cognitive changes including memory changes, sleep apnea, weakness, pruritus, dizziness, excessive sweating, visual symptoms, weight loss, massive obesity, gastrointestinal bleeding, paresthesias, dyspnea, joint symptoms, epigastric distress, pain and erythema of the fingers or toes, venous or arterial thrombosis, thromboembolism, myocardial infarction, stroke, transient ischemic attacks, congenital heart disease, chronic obstructive pulmonary disease, increased erythropoietin production associated

with neoplastic, renal or hepatic disorders, androgen or diuretic use, splenomegaly, hepatomegaly, diastolic hypertension.)

4. Specific indications for CBC with differential count related to the WBC include signs, symptoms, test results, illness, or disease associated with leukemia, infections or inflammatory processes, suspected bone marrow failure or bone marrow infiltrate, suspected myeloproliferative, myelodysplastic or lymphoproliferative disorder, use of drugs that may cause leukopenia, and immune disorders (e.g., fever, chills, sweats, shock, fatigue, malaise, tachycardia, tachypnea, heart murmur, seizures, alterations of consciousness, meningismus, pain such as headache, abdominal pain, arthralgia, odynophagia, or dysuria, redness or swelling of skin, soft tissue bone, or joint, ulcers of the skin or mucous membranes, gangrene, mucous membrane discharge, bleeding, thrombosis, respiratory failure, pulmonary infiltrate, jaundice, diarrhea, vomiting, hepatomegaly, splenomegaly, lymphadenopathy, opportunistic infection such as oral candidiasis.)

5. Specific indications for CBC related to the platelet count include signs, symptoms, test results, illness, or disease associated with increased or decreased platelet production and destruction, or platelet dysfunction(e.g., gastrointestinal bleeding, genitourinary tract bleeding, bilateral epistaxis, thrombosis, ecchymosis, purpura, jaundice, petechiae, fever, heparin therapy, suspected DIC, shock, pre-eclampsia, neonate with maternal ITP, massive transfusion, recent platelet transfusion, cardiopulmonary bypass, hemolytic uremic syndrome, renal diseases, lymphadenopathy, hepatomegaly, splenomegaly, hypersplenism, neurologic abnormalities, viral or other infection, myeloproliferative, myelodysplastic, or lymphoproliferative disorder, thrombosis, exposure to toxic agents, excessive alcohol ingestion, autoimmune disorders (SLE, RA and other).

6. Indications for hemogram or CBC related to red cell (RBC) parameters of the hemogram include, in addition to those already listed, thalassemia, suspected hemoglobinopathy, lead poisoning, arsenic poisoning, and spherocytosis.

7. Specific indications for CBC with differential count related to the WBC include, in addition to those already listed, storage diseases/mucopolysaccharidoses, and use of drugs that cause leukocytosis such as G-CSF or GM-CSF.

8. Specific indications for CBC related to platelet count include, in addition to those already listed, May-Hegglin syndrome and Wiskott-Aldrich syndrome.

Limitations

1. Testing of patients who are asymptomatic, or who do not have a condition that could be expected to result in a hematological abnormality, is screening and is not a covered service.

2. In some circumstances it may be appropriate to perform only a hemoglobin or hematocrit to assess the oxygen carrying capacity of the blood. When the ordering provider requests only a hemoglobin or hematocrit, the remaining components of the CBC are not covered.

3. When a blood count is performed for an end-stage renal disease (ESRD) patient, and is billed outside the ESRD rate, documentation of the medical necessity for the blood count must be submitted with the claim.

4. In some patients presenting with certain signs, symptoms or diseases, a single CBC may be appropriate. Repeat testing may not be indicated unless abnormal results are found, or unless there is a change in clinical condition. If repeat testing is performed, a more descriptive diagnosis code (e.g., anemia) should be reported to support medical necessity. However, repeat testing may be indicated where results are normal in patients with conditions where there is a continued risk for the development of hematologic abnormality.

Note: Scroll down for links to the quarterly Covered Code Lists (including narrative).

Pub. 100-3, Section 190.16

Partial Thromboplastin Time (PTT)

Indications:

1. Ferritin (82728), iron (83540) and either iron binding capacity (83550) or transferrin (84466) are useful in the differential diagnosis of iron deficiency, anemia, and for iron overload conditions.

a. The following presentations are examples that may support the use of these studies for evaluating iron deficiency:

- Certain abnormal blood count values (i.e., decreased mean corpuscular volume (MCV), decreased hemoglobin/hematocrit when the MCV is low or normal, or increased red cell distribution width (RDW) and low or normal MCV);

- Abnormal appetite (pica);

- Acute or chronic gastrointestinal blood loss;

- Hematuria;

- Menorrhagia;

- Malabsorption;

- Status post-gastrectomy;

- Status post-gastrojejunostomy;

- Malnutrition;

- Preoperative autologous blood collection(s);

- Malignant, chronic inflammatory and infectious conditions associated with anemia which may present in a similar manner to iron deficiency anemia;

- Following a significant surgical procedure where blood loss had occurred and had not been repaired with adequate iron replacement.

b. The following presentations are examples that may support the use of these studies for evaluating iron overload:

- Chronic Hepatitis;
- Diabetes;
- Hyperpigmentation of skin;
- Arthropathy;
- Cirrhosis;
- Hypogonadism;
- Hypopituitarism;
- Impaired porphyrin metabolism;
- Heart failure;
- Multiple transfusions;
- Sideroblastic anemia;
- Thalassemia major;
- Cardiomyopathy, cardiac dysrhythmias and conduction disturbances.

2. Follow-up testing may be appropriate to monitor response to therapy, e.g., oral or parenteral iron, ascorbic acid, and erythropoietin.

3. Iron studies may be appropriate in patients after treatment for other nutritional deficiency anemias, such as folate and vitamin B12, because iron deficiency may not be revealed until such a nutritional deficiency is treated.

4. Serum ferritin may be appropriate for monitoring iron status in patients with chronic renal disease with or without dialysis.

5. Serum iron may also be indicated for evaluation of toxic effects of iron and other metals (e.g., nickel, cadmium, aluminum, lead) whether due to accidental, intentional exposure or metabolic causes.

Limitations:

1. Iron studies should be used to diagnose and manage iron deficiency or iron overload states. These tests are not to be used solely to assess acute phase reactants where disease management will be unchanged. For example, infections and malignancies are associated with elevations in acute phase reactants such as ferritin, and decreases in serum iron concentration, but iron studies would only be medically necessary if results of iron studies might alter the management of the primary diagnosis or might warrant direct treatment of an iron disorder or condition.

2. If a normal serum ferritin level is documented, repeat testing would not ordinarily be medically necessary unless there is a change in the patient's condition, and ferritin assessment is needed for the ongoing management of the patient. For example, a patient presents with new onset insulin-dependent diabetes mellitus and has a serum ferritin level performed for the suspicion of hemochromatosis. If the ferritin level is normal, the repeat ferritin for diabetes mellitus would not be medically necessary.

3. When an End Stage Renal Disease (ESRD) patient is tested for ferritin, testing more frequently than every three months (the frequency authorized by 3167.3, Fiscal Intermediary manual) requires documentation of medical necessity [e.g., other than "Chronic Renal Failure" (ICD-9-CM 585) or "Renal Failure, Unspecified" (ICD-9-CM 586)].

4. It is ordinarily not necessary to measure both transferrin and TIBC at the same time because TIBC is an indirect measure of transferrin. When transferrin is ordered as part of the nutritional assessment for evaluating malnutrition, it is not necessary to order other iron studies unless iron deficiency or iron overload is suspected as well.

5. It is not ordinarily necessary to measure both iron/TIBC (or transferrin) and ferritin in initial patient testing. If clinically indicated after evaluation of the initial iron studies, it may be appropriate to perform additional iron studies either on the initial specimen or on a subsequently obtained specimen. After a diagnosis of iron deficiency or iron overload is established, either iron/TIBC (or transferrin) or ferritin may be medically necessary for monitoring, but not both.

6. It would not ordinarily be considered medically necessary to do a ferritin as a preoperative test except in the presence of anemia or recent autologous blood collections prior to the surgery.

Pub. 100-3, Section 190.17

Prothrombin Time (PT)

Indications:

1. A PT may be used to assess patients taking warfarin. The prothrombin time is generally not useful in monitoring patients receiving heparin who are not taking warfarin.

2. A PT may be used to assess patients with signs or symptoms of abnormal bleeding or thrombosis. For example:

a. swollen extremity with or without prior trauma;

b. unexplained bruising;

c. abnormal bleeding, hemorrhage or hematoma;

d. petechiae or other signs of thrombocytopenia that could be due to Disseminated Intravascular Coagulation.

3. A PT may be useful in evaluating patients who have a history of a condition known to be associated with the risk of bleeding or thrombosis that is related to the extrinsic coagulation pathway. Such abnormalities may be genetic or acquired. For example:

a. dysfibrinogenemia;

b. afibrinogenemia (complete);

c. acute or chronic liver dysfunction or failure, including

d. Wilson's disease and Hemochromatosis;

e. disseminated intravascular coagulation (DIC);

f. congenital and acquired deficiencies of factors II, V, VII, X;

g. vitamin K deficiency;

h. lupus erythematosus;

i. hypercoagulable state;

j. paraproteinemia;

k. lymphoma;

l. amyloidosis;

m. acute and chronic leukemias;

n. plasma cell dyscrasia;

o. HIV infection;

p. malignant neoplasms;

q. hemorrhagic fever;

r. salicylate poisoning;

s. obstructive jaundice;

t. intestinal fistula;

u. malabsorption syndrome;

v. colitis;

w. chronic diarrhea;

x. presence of peripheral venous or arterial thrombosis or pulmonary emboli or myocardial infarction;

y. patients with bleeding or clotting tendencies;

z. organ transplantation;

aa. presence of circulating coagulation inhibitors.

4. A PT may be used to assess the risk of hemorrhage or thrombosis in patients who are going to have a medical intervention known to be associated with increased risk of bleeding or thrombosis. For example:

a. evaluation prior to invasive procedures or operations of patients with personal history of bleeding or a condition associated with coagulopathy

b. prior to the use of thrombolytic medication.

Limitations:

1. When an ESRD patient is tested for PT, testing more frequently than weekly (the frequency authorized by 3171.2, Fiscal Intermediary Manual, or 2231.3 Medicare Carrier Manual) requires documentation of medical necessity (e.g. other than a diagnosis of "Chronic Renal Failure" or "Renal Failure, Unspecified").

2. The need to repeat this test is determined by changes in the underlying medical condition and/or the dosing of warfarin. In a patient on stable warfarin therapy, it is ordinarily not necessary to repeat testing more than every two to three weeks. When testing is performed to evaluate a patient with signs or symptoms of abnormal bleeding or thrombosis and the initial test result is normal, it is ordinarily not necessary to repeat testing unless there is a change in the patient's medical status.

3. Since the INR is a calculation, it will not be paid in addition to the PT when expressed in seconds, and is considered part of the conventional prothrombin time.

4. Testing prior to any medical intervention associated with a risk of bleeding and thrombosis (other than thrombolytic therapy) will generally be considered medically necessary only where there are signs or symptoms of a bleeding or thrombotic abnormality or a personal history of bleeding, thrombosis or a condition associated with a coagulopathy. Hospital/clinic-specific policies, protocols, etc., in and of themselves, cannot alone justify coverage.

Note: Scroll down for links to the quarterly Covered Code Lists (including narrative).

Pub. 100-3, Section 190.18

Serum Iron Studies

Indications:

1. Ferritin (82728), iron (83540) and either iron binding capacity (83550) or transferrin (84466) are useful in the differential diagnosis of iron deficiency, anemia, and for iron overload conditions.

a. The following presentations are examples that may support the use of these studies for evaluating iron deficiency:

Certain abnormal blood count values (i.e., decreased mean corpuscular volume (MCV), decreased hemoglobin/hematocrit when the MCV is low or normal, or increased red cell distribution width (RDW) and low or normal MCV);

Abnormal appetite (pica);

Acute or chronic gastrointestinal blood loss;

Hematuria;

Menorrhagia;

Malabsorption;

Status post-gastrectomy;

Status post-gastrojejunostomy;

Malnutrition;

Preoperative autologous blood collection(s);

Malignant, chronic inflammatory and infectious conditions associated with anemia which may present in a similar manner to iron deficiency anemia;

Following a significant surgical procedure where blood loss had occurred and had not been repaired with adequate iron replacement.

b. The following presentations are examples that may support the use of these studies for evaluating iron overload:

Chronic Hepatitis;

Diabetes;

Hyperpigmentation of skin;

Arthropathy;

Cirrhosis;

Hypogonadism;

Hypopituitarism;

Impaired porphyrin metabolism;

Heart failure;

Multiple transfusions;

Sideroblastic anemia;

Thalassemia major;

Cardiomyopathy, cardiac dysrhythmias and conduction disturbances.

2. Follow-up testing may be appropriate to monitor response to therapy, e.g., oral or parenteral iron, ascorbic acid, and erythropoietin.

3. Iron studies may be appropriate in patients after treatment for other nutritional deficiency anemias, such as folate and vitamin B12, because iron deficiency may not be revealed until such a nutritional deficiency is treated.

4. Serum ferritin may be appropriate for monitoring iron status in patients with chronic renal disease with or without dialysis.

5. Serum iron may also be indicated for evaluation of toxic effects of iron and other metals (e.g., nickel, cadmium, aluminum, lead) whether due to accidental, intentional exposure or metabolic causes.

Limitations:

1. Iron studies should be used to diagnose and manage iron deficiency or iron overload states. These tests are not to be used solely to assess acute phase reactants where disease management will be unchanged. For example, infections and malignancies are associated with elevations in acute phase reactants such as ferritin, and decreases in serum iron concentration, but iron studies would only be medically necessary if results of iron studies might alter the management of the primary diagnosis or might warrant direct treatment of an iron disorder or condition.

2. If a normal serum ferritin level is documented, repeat testing would not ordinarily be medically necessary unless there is a change in the patient's condition, and ferritin assessment is needed for the ongoing management of the patient. For example, a patient presents with new onset insulin-dependent diabetes mellitus and has a serum ferritin level performed for the suspicion of hemochromatosis. If the ferritin level is normal, the repeat ferritin for diabetes mellitus would not be medically necessary.

3. When an End Stage Renal Disease (ESRD) patient is tested for ferritin, testing more frequently than every three months (the frequency authorized by 3167.3, Fiscal Intermediary manual) requires documentation of medical necessity [e.g., other than "Chronic Renal Failure" (ICD-9-CM 585) or "Renal Failure, Unspecified" (ICD-9-CM 586)].

4. It is ordinarily not necessary to measure both transferrin and TIBC at the same time because TIBC is an indirect measure of transferrin. When transferrin is ordered as part of the nutritional assessment for evaluating malnutrition, it is not necessary to order other iron studies unless iron deficiency or iron overload is suspected as well.

5. It is not ordinarily necessary to measure both iron/TIBC (or transferrin) and ferritin in initial patient testing. If clinically indicated after evaluation of the initial iron studies, it may be appropriate to perform additional iron studies either on the initial specimen or on a subsequently obtained specimen. After a diagnosis of iron deficiency or iron overload is established, either iron/TIBC (or transferrin) or ferritin may be medically necessary for monitoring, but not both.

6. It would not ordinarily be considered medically necessary to do a ferritin as a preoperative test except in the presence of anemia or recent autologous blood collections prior to the surgery.

Pub. 100-3, Section 190.19

Collagen Crosslinks, Any Method

Indications:

Generally speaking, collagen crosslink testing is useful mostly in "fast losers" of bone. The age when these bone markers can help direct therapy is often pre-Medicare. By the time a fast loser of bone reaches age 65, she will most likely have been stabilized by appropriate therapy or have lost so much bone mass that further testing is useless. Coverage for bone marker assays may be established, however, for younger Medicare beneficiaries and for those men and women who might become fast losers because of some other therapy such as glucocorticoids. Safeguards should be incorporated to prevent excessive use of tests in patients for whom they have no clinical relevance.

Collagen crosslinks testing is used to:

1. Identify individuals with elevated bone resorption, who have osteoporosis in whom response to treatment is being monitored;

2. Predict response (as assessed by bone mass measurements) to FDA approved antiresorptive therapy in postmenopausal women; and

3. Assess response to treatment of patients with osteoporosis, Paget's disease of the bone, or risk for osteoporosis where treatment may include FDA approved antiresorptive agents, anti-estrogens or selective estrogen receptor moderators.

Limitations:

Because of significant specimen to specimen collagen crosslink physiologic variability (15-20%), current recommendations for appropriate utilization include: one or two base-line assays from specified urine collections on separate days; followed by a repeat assay about three months after starting anti-resorptive therapy; followed by a repeat assay in 12 months after the three-month assay; and thereafter not more than annually, unless there is a change in therapy in which circumstance an additional test may be indicated three months after the initiation of new therapy.

Some collagen crosslink assays may not be appropriate for use in some disorders, according to FDA labeling restrictions.

Note: Scroll down for links to the quarterly Covered Code Lists (including narrative).

Pub. 100-3, Section 190.20

Blood Glucose Testing

Indications:

Blood glucose values are often necessary for the management of patients with diabetes mellitus, where hyperglycemia and hypoglycemia are often present. They are also critical in the determination of control of blood glucose levels in the patient with impaired fasting glucose (FPG 110-125 mg/dL), the patient with insulin resistance syndrome and/or carbohydrate intolerance (excessive rise in glucose following ingestion of glucose or glucose sources of food), in the patient with a hypoglycemia disorder such as nesidioblastosis or insulinoma, and in patients with a catabolic or malnutrition state. In addition to those conditions already listed, glucose testing may be medically necessary in patients with tuberculosis, unexplained chronic or recurrent infections, alcoholism, coronary artery disease (especially in women), or unexplained skin conditions (including pruritis, local skin infections, ulceration and gangrene without an established cause).

Many medical conditions may be a consequence of a sustained elevated or depressed glucose level. These include comas, seizures or epilepsy, confusion, abnormal hunger, abnormal weight loss or gain, and loss of sensation. Evaluation of glucose may also be indicated in patients on medications known to affect carbohydrate metabolism.

Effective January 1, 2005, the Medicare law expanded coverage to diabetic screening services. Some forms of blood glucode testing covered under this national coverage determination may be covered for screening purposes subject to specified frequencies. See 42 CFR 410.18 and section 90, chapter 18 of the Claims Processing Manual, for a full description of this screening benefit.

Limitations:

Frequent home blood glucose testing by diabetic patients should be encouraged. In stable, non-hospitalized patients who are unable or unwilling to do home monitoring, it may be reasonable and necessary to measure quantitative blood glucose up to four times annually.

Depending upon the age of the patient, type of diabetes, degree of control, complications of diabetes, and other co-morbid conditions, more frequent testing than four times annually may be reasonable and necessary.

In some patients presenting with nonspecific signs, symptoms, or diseases not normally associated with disturbances in glucose metabolism, a single blood glucose test may be medically necessary. Repeat testing may not be indicated unless abnormal results are found or unless there is a change in clinical condition. If repeat testing is performed, a specific diagnosis code (e.g., diabetes) should be reported to support medical necessity. However, repeat testing may be indicated where results are normal in patients with conditions where there is a confirmed continuing risk of glucose metabolism abnormality (e.g., monitoring glucocorticoid therapy).

Pub. 100-3, Section 190.21

Glycated Hemoglobin/Glycated Protein

Indications:

Glycated hemoglobin/protein testing is widely accepted as medically necessary for the management and control of diabetes. It is also valuable to assess hyperglycemia, a history of hyperglycemia or dangerous hypoglycemia. Glycated protein testing may be used in place of glycated hemoglobin in the management of diabetic patients, and is particularly useful in patients who have abnormalities of erythrocytes such as hemolytic anemia or hemoglobinopathies.

Limitations:

It is not considered reasonable and necessary to perform glycated hemoglobin tests more often than every three months on a controlled diabetic patient to determine whether the patient's metabolic control has been on average within the target range. It is not considered reasonable and necessary for these tests to be performed more frequently than once a month for diabetic pregnant women. Testing for uncontrolled type one or two diabetes mellitus may require testing more than four times a year. The above Description Section provides the clinical basis for those

situations in which testing more frequently than four times per annum is indicated, and medical necessity documentation must support such testing in excess of the above guidelines.

Many methods for the analysis of glycated hemoglobin show significant interference from elevated levels of fetal hemoglobin or by variant hemoglobin molecules. When the glycated hemoglobin assay is initially performed in these patients, the laboratory may inform the ordering physician of a possible analytical interference. Alternative testing, including glycated protein, for example, fructosamine, may be indicated for the monitoring of the degree of glycemic control in this situation. It is therefore conceivable that a patient will have both a glycated hemoglobin and glycated protein ordered on the same day. This should be limited to the initial assay of glycated hemoglobin, with subsequent exclusive use of glycated protein. These tests are not considered to be medically necessary for the diagnosis of diabetes.

Pub. 100-3, Section 190.22

Thyroid Testing

Indications:

Thyroid function tests are used to define hyper function, euthyroidism, or hypofunction of thyroid disease. Thyroid testing may be reasonable and necessary to:distinguish between primary and secondary hypothyroidism; confirm or rule out primary hypothyroidism; monitor thyroid hormone levels (for example, patients with goiter, thyroid nodules, or thyroid cancer); monitor drug therapy in patients with primary hypothyroidism; confirm or rule out primary hyperthyroidism; and monitor therapy in patients with hyperthyroidism.

Thyroid function testing may be medically necessary in patients with disease or neoplasm of the thyroid and other endocrine glands. Thyroid function testing may also be medically necessary in patients with metabolic disorders; malnutrition; hyperlipidemia; certain types of anemia; psychosis and non-psychotic personality disorders; unexplained depression; ophthalmologic disorders; various cardiac arrhythmias; disorders of menstruation; skin conditions; myalgias; and a wide array of signs and symptoms, including alterations in consciousness; malaise; hypothermia; symptoms of the nervous and musculoskeletal system; skin and integumentary system; nutrition and metabolism; cardiovascular; and gastrointestinal system.

It may be medically necessary to do follow-up thyroid testing in patients with a personal history of malignant neoplasm of the endocrine system and in patients on long-term thyroid drug therapy.

Limitations:

Testing may be covered up to two times a year in clinically stable patients; more frequent testing may be reasonable and necessary for patients whose thyroid therapy has been altered or in whom symptoms or signs of hyperthyroidism or hypothyroidism are noted.

Pub. 100-3, Section 190.23

Lipid Testing

Indications and Limitations of Coverage

Indications

The medical community recognizes lipid testing as appropriate for evaluating atherosclerotic cardiovascular disease. Conditions in which lipid testing may be indicated include:

- Assessment of patients with atherosclerotic cardiovascular disease.

- Evaluation of primary dyslipidemia.

- Any form of atherosclerotic disease, or any disease leading to the formation of atherosclerotic disease.

- Diagnostic evaluation of diseases associated with altered lipid metabolism, such as: nephrotic syndrome, pancreatitis, hepatic disease, and hypo and hyperthyroidism.

- Secondary dyslipidemia, including diabetes mellitus, disorders of gastrointestinal absorption, chronic renal failure.

- Signs or symptoms of dyslipidemias, such as skin lesions.

As follow-up to the initial screen for coronary heart disease (total cholesterol + HDL cholesterol) when total cholesterol is determined to be high (>240 mg/dL), or borderline-high (200-240 mg/dL) plus two or more coronary heart disease risk factors, or an HDL cholesterol, <35 mg/dl.

To monitor the progress of patients on anti-lipid dietary management and pharmacologic therapy for the treatment of elevated blood lipid disorders, total cholesterol, HDL cholesterol and LDL cholesterol may be used. Triglycerides may be obtained if this lipid fraction is also elevated or if the patient is put on drugs (for example, thiazide diuretics, beta blockers, estrogens, glucocorticoids, and tamoxifen) which may raise the triglyceride level.

When monitoring long term anti-lipid dietary or pharmacologic therapy and when following patients with borderline high total or LDL cholesterol levels, it may be reasonable to perform the lipid panel annually. A lipid panel at a yearly interval will usually be adequate while measurement of the serum total cholesterol or a measured LDL should suffice for interim visits if the patient does not have hypertriglyceridemia.

Any one component of the panel or a measured LDL may be reasonable and necessary up to six times the first year for monitoring dietary or pharmacologic therapy. More frequent total cholesterol HDL cholesterol, LDL cholesterol and triglyceride testing may be indicated for marked elevations or for changes to anti-lipid therapy due to inadequate initial patient response to dietary or pharmacologic therapy. The LDL cholesterol or total cholesterol may be measured three times yearly after treatment goals have been achieved.

Electrophoretic or other quantitation of lipoproteins may be indicated if the patient has a primary disorder of lipoid metabolism.

Effective January 1, 2005, the Medicare law expanded coverage to cardiovascular screening services. Several of the procedures included in this NCD may be covered for screening purposes subject to specified frequencies. See 42 CFR 410.17 and section 100, chapter 18, of the Claims Processing Manual, for a full description of this benefit.Limitations

Lipid panel and hepatic panel testing may be used for patients with severe psoriasis which has not responded to conventional therapy and for which the retinoid etretinate has been prescribed and who have developed hyperlipidemia or hepatic toxicity. Specific examples include erythrodermia and generalized pustular type and psoriasis associated with arthritis.

Routine screening and prophylactic testing for lipid disorder are not covered by Medicare. While lipid screening may be medically appropriate, Medicare by statute does not pay for it. Lipid testing in asymptomatic individuals is considered to be screening regardless of the presence of other risk factors such as family history, tobacco use, etc.

Once a diagnosis is established, one or several specific tests are usually adequate for monitoring the course of the disease. Less specific diagnoses (for example, other chest pain) alone do not support medical necessity of these tests.

When monitoring long term anti-lipid dietary or pharmacologic therapy and when following patients with borderline high total or LDL cholesterol levels, it is reasonable to perform the lipid panel annually. A lipid panel at a yearly interval will usually be adequate while measurement of the serum total cholesterol or a measured LDL should suffice for interim visits if the patient does not have hypertriglyceridemia.

Any one component of the panel or a measured LDL may be medically necessary up to six times the first year for monitoring dietary or pharmacologic therapy. More frequent total cholesterol HDL cholesterol, LDL cholesterol and triglyceride testing may be indicated for marked elevations or for changes to anti-lipid therapy due to inadequate initial patient response to dietary or pharmacologic therapy. The LDL cholesterol or total cholesterol may be measured three times yearly after treatment goals have been achieved.

If no dietary or pharmacological therapy is advised, monitoring is not necessary.

When evaluating non-specific chronic abnormalities of the liver (for example, elevations of transaminase, alkaline phosphatase, abnormal imaging studies, etc.), a lipid panel would generally not be indicated more than twice per year

Pub. 100-3, Section 190.24

Digoxin Therapeutic Drug Assay

Indications and Limitations of Coverage

Indications

Digoxin levels may be performed to monitor drug levels of individuals receiving digoxin therapy because the margin of safety between side effects and toxicity is narrow or because the blood level may not be high enough to achieve the desired clinical effect.

Clinical indications may include individuals on digoxin:

- With symptoms, signs or electrocardiogram (ECG) suggestive of digoxin toxicity.
- Taking medications that influence absorption, bioavailability, distribution, and/or elimination of digoxin.
- With impaired renal, hepatic, gastrointestinal, or thyroid function.
- With pH and/or electrolyte abnormalities.
- With unstable cardiovascular status, including myocarditis.
- Requiring monitoring of patient compliance.
- Clinical indications may include individuals:
- Suspected of accidental or intended overdose.
- Who have an acceptable cardiac diagnosis (as listed) and for whom an accurate history of use of digoxin is unobtainable.

The value of obtaining regular serum digoxin levels is uncertain, but it may be reasonable to check levels once yearly after a steady state is achieved. In addition, it may be reasonable to check the level if:

- Heart failure status worsens.
- Renal function deteriorates.
- Additional medications are added that could affect the digoxin level.
- Signs or symptoms of toxicity develop.

Steady state will be reached in approximately 1 week in patients with normal renal function, although 2?3 weeks may be needed in patients with renal impairment. After changes in dosages or the addition of a medication that could affect the digoxin level, it is reasonable to check the digoxin level one week after the change or addition. Based on the clinical situation, in cases of digoxin toxicity, testing may need to be done more than once a week.

Digoxin is indicated for the treatment of patients with heart failure due to systolic dysfunction and for reduction of the ventricular response in patients with atrial fibrillation or flutter. Digoxin may also be indicated for the treatment of other supraventricular arrhythmias, particularly in the presence of heart failure.

Limitations

This test is not appropriate for patients on digitoxin or treated with digoxin FAB (fragment antigen binding) antibody.

Pub. 100-3, Section 190.25

Alpha-Fetoprotein

Indications and Limitations of Coverage

AFP is useful for the diagnosis of hepatocellular carcinoma in high-risk patients (such as alcoholic cirrhosis, cirrhosis of viral etiology, hemochromatosis, and alpha 1-antitrypsin deficiency) and in separating patients with benign hepatocellular neoplasms or metastases from those with hepatocellular carcinoma and, as a non-specific tumor associated antigen, serves in marking germ cell neoplasms of the testis, ovary, retro peritoneum, and mediastinum.

Note: Scroll down for links to the quarterly Covered Code Lists (including narrative).

Pub. 100-3, Section 190.26

Carcinoembryonic Antigen

Indications

CEA may be medically necessary for follow-up of patients with colorectal carcinoma. It would however only be medically necessary at treatment decision?making points. In some clinical situations (e.g. adenocarcinoma of the lung, small cell carcinoma of the lung, and some gastrointestinal carcinomas) when a more specific marker is not expressed by the tumor, CEA may be a medically necessary alternative marker for monitoring. Preoperative CEA may also be helpful in determining the post?operative adequacy of surgical resection and subsequent medical management. In general, a single tumor marker will suffice in following patients with colorectal carcinoma or other malignancies that express such tumor markers.

In following patients who have had treatment for colorectal carcinoma, ASCO guideline suggests that if resection of liver metastasis would be indicated, it is recommended that post-operative CEA testing be performed every two to three months in patients with initial stage II or stage III disease for at least two years after diagnosis.

For patients with metastatic solid tumors which express CEA, CEA may be measured at the start of the treatment and with subsequent treatment cycles to assess the tumor's response to therapy.

Limitations:

Serum CEA determinations are generally not indicated more frequently than once per chemotherapy treatment cycle for patients with metastatic solid tumors which express CEA or every two months post-surgical treatment for patients who have had colorectal carcinoma. However, it may be proper to order the test more frequently in certain situations, for example, when there has been a significant change from prior CEA level or a significant change in patient status which could reflect disease progression or recurrence.

Testing with a diagnosis of an in situ carcinoma is not reasonably done more frequently than once, unless the result is abnormal, in which case the test may be repeated once.

Note: Scroll down for links to the quarterly Covered Code Lists (including narrative).

Pub. 100-3, Section 190.27

Human Chorionic Gonadotropin

Indications:

hCG is useful for monitoring and diagnosis of germ cell neoplasms of the ovary, testis, mediastinum, retroperitoneum, and central nervous system. In addition, hCG is useful for monitoring pregnant patients with vaginal bleeding, hypertension and/or suspected fetal loss.

Limitations:

Not more than once per month for diagnostic purposes. As needed for monitoring of patient progress and treatment. Qualitative hCG assays are not appropriate for medically managing patients with known or suspected germ cell neoplasms.

Pub. 100-3, Section 190.28

Tumor Antigen by Immunoassay - CA125

Indications

CA 125 is a high molecular weight serum tumor marker elevated in 80% of patients who present with epithelial ovarian carcinoma. It is also elevated in carcinomas of the fallopian tube, endometrium, and endocervix. An elevated level may also be associated with the presence of a malignant mesothelioma or primary peritoneal carcinoma.

A CA125 level may be obtained as part of the initial pre-operative work-up for women presenting with a suspicious pelvic mass to be used as a baseline for purposes of post-operative monitoring. Initial declines in CA 125 after initial surgery and/or chemotherapy for ovarian carcinoma are also measured by obtaining three serum levels during the first month post treatment to determine the patient's CA 125 half-life, which has significant prognostic implications.

The CA 125 levels are again obtained at the completion of chemotherapy as an index of residual disease. Surveillance CA125 measurements are generally obtained every 3 months for 2 years, every 6 months for the next 3 years, and yearly thereafter. CA 125 levels are also an important indicator of a patient's response to therapy in the presence of advanced or recurrent disease. In this setting, CA 125 levels may be obtained prior to each treatment cycle.

Limitations

These services are not covered for the evaluation of patients with signs or symptoms suggestive of malignancy. The service may be ordered at times necessary to assess either the presence of recurrent disease or the patient's response to treatment with subsequent treatment cycles.

The CA 125 is specifically not covered for aiding in the differential diagnosis of patients with a pelvic mass as the sensitivity and specificity of the test is not sufficient. In general, a single "tumor marker" will suffice in following a patient with one of these malignancies.

(This NCD last reviewed November 2005)

Pub. 100-3, Section 190.29

Tumor Antigen by Immunoassay CA 15-3/CA 27.29

Indications:

Multiple tumor markers are available for monitoring the response of certain malignancies to therapy and assessing whether residual tumor exists post-surgical therapy.

CA 15-3 is often medically necessary to aid in the management of patients with breast cancer. Serial testing must be used in conjunction with other clinical methods for monitoring breast cancer. For monitoring, if medically necessary, use consistently either CA 15-3 or CA 27.29, not both.

CA 27.29 is equivalent to CA 15-3 in its usage in management of patients with breast cancer.

Limitations:

These services are not covered for the evaluation of patients with signs or symptoms suggestive of malignancy. The service may be ordered at times necessary to assess either the presence of recurrent disease or the patient's response to treatment with subsequent treatment cycles.

Pub. 100-3, Section 190.30

Tumor Antigen by Immunoassay CA 19-9

Indications:

Multiple tumor markers are available for monitoring the response of certain malignancies to therapy and assessing whether residual tumor exists post-surgical therapy.

Levels are useful in following the course of patients with established diagnosis of pancreatic and biliary ductal carcinoma. The test is not indicated for diagnosing these two diseases.

Limitations:

These services are not covered for the evaluation of patients with signs or symptoms suggestive of malignancy. The service may be ordered at times necessary to assess either the presence of recurrent disease or the patient's response to treatment with subsequent treatment cycles.

Pub. 100-3, Section 190.31

Prostate Specific Antigen

Indications:

PSA is of proven value in differentiating benign from malignant disease in men with lower urinary tract signs and symptoms (e.g., hematuria, slow urine stream, hesitancy, urgency, frequency, nocturia and incontinence) as well as with patients with palpably abnormal prostate glands on physician exam, and in patients with other laboratory or imaging studies that suggest the possibility of a malignant prostate disorder. PSA is also a marker used to follow the progress of prostate cancer once a diagnosis has been established, such as in detecting metastatic or persistent disease in patients who may require additional treatment. PSA testing may also be useful in the differential diagnosis of men presenting with as yet undiagnosed disseminated metastatic disease.

Limitations:

Generally, for patients with lower urinary tract signs or symptoms, the test is performed only once per year unless there is a change in the patient's medical condition.

Testing with a diagnosis of in situ carcinoma is not reasonably done more frequently than once, unless the result is abnormal, in which case the test may be repeated once.

Note: Scroll down for links to the quarterly Covered Code Lists (including narrative).

Pub. 100-3, Section 190.32

Gamma Glutamyl Transferase

Indications and Limitations of Coverage

Indications

1. To provide information about known or suspected hepatobiliary disease, for example:

a. Following chronic alcohol or drug ingestion.

b. Following exposure to hepatotoxins.

c. When using medication known to have a potential for causing liver toxicity (e.g., following the drug manufacturer's recommendations).

d. Following infection (e.g., viral hepatitis and other specific infections such as amoebiasis, tuberculosis, psittacosis, and similar infections).

2. To assess liver injury/function following diagnosis of primary or secondary malignant neoplasms.

3. To assess liver injury/function in a wide variety of disorders and diseases known to cause liver involvement (e.g., diabetes mellitus, malnutrition, disorders of iron and mineral metabolism, sarcoidosis, amyloidosis, lupus, and hypertension).

4. To assess liver function related to gastrointestinal disease.

5. To assess liver function related to pancreatic disease.

6. To assess liver function in patients subsequent to liver transplantation.

7. To differentiate between the different sources of elevated alkaline phosphatase activity.

Limitations

When used to assess liver dysfunction secondary to existing non-hepatobiliary disease with no change in signs, symptoms, or treatment, it is generally not necessary to repeat a GGT determination after a normal result has been obtained unless new indications are present.

If the GGT is the only "liver" enzyme abnormally high, it is generally not necessary to pursue further evaluation for liver disease for this specific indication.

When used to determine if other abnormal enzyme tests reflect liver abnormality rather than other tissue, it generally is not necessary to repeat a GGT more than one time per week.

Because of the extreme sensitivity of GGT as a marker for cytochrome oxidase induction or cell membrane permeability, it is generally not useful in monitoring patients with known liver disease

Pub. 100-3, Section 190.33

Hepatitis Panel/Acute Hepatitis Panel

Indications:

1. To detect viral hepatitis infection when there are abnormal liver function test results, with or without signs or symptoms of hepatitis.

2. Prior to and subsequent to liver transplantation.

Limitations:

After a hepatitis diagnosis has been established, only individual tests, rather than the entire panel, are needed.

Pub. 100-3, Section 190.34

Fecal Occult Blood

Indications

1. To evaluate known or suspected alimentary tract conditions that might cause bleeding into the intestinal tract.

2. To evaluate unexpected anemia.

3. To evaluate abnormal signs, symptoms, or complaints that might be associated with loss of blood.

4. To evaluate patient complaints of black or red-tinged stools.

Limitations

1. The FOBT is reported once for the testing of up to three separate specimens (comprising either one or two tests per specimen).

2. In patients who are taking non-steroidal anti-inflammatory drugs and have a history of gastrointestinal bleeding but no other signs, symptoms, or complaints associated with gastrointestinal blood loss, testing for occult blood may generally be appropriate no more than once every three months.

3. When testing is done for the purpose of screening for colorectal cancer in the absence of signs, symptoms, conditions, or complaints associated with gastrointestinal blood loss, report the HCPCS code for colorectal cancer screening; fecal-occult blood test, 1-3 simultaneous determinations should be used.

Note: Scroll down for links to the quarterly Covered Code Lists (including narrative).

Pub. 100-3, Section 210.1

Prostate Cancer Screening Tests

Indications and Limitations of Coverage

CIM 50-55

Covered

A. General

Section 4103 of the Balanced Budget Act of 1997 provides for coverage of certain prostate cancer screening tests subject to certain coverage, frequency, and payment limitations. Medicare will cover prostate cancer screening tests/procedures for the early detection of prostate cancer. Coverage of prostate cancer screening tests includes the following procedures furnished to an individual for the early detection of prostate cancer:

• Screening digital rectal examination; and

• Screening prostate specific antigen blood test

B. Screening Digital Rectal Examinations

Screening digital rectal examinations are covered at a frequency of once every 12 months for men who have attained age 50 (at least 11 months have passed following the month in which the last Medicare-covered screening digital rectal examination was performed). Screening digital rectal examination means a clinical examination of an individual's prostate for nodules or other abnormalities of the prostate. This screening must be performed by a doctor of medicine or osteopathy (as defined in §1861(r)(1) of the Act), or by a physician assistant, nurse practitioner, clinical nurse specialist, or certified nurse midwife (as defined in §1861(aa) and §1861(gg) of the Act) who is authorized under State law to perform the examination, fully knowledgeable about the beneficiary's medical condition, and would be responsible for using the results of any examination performed in the overall management of the beneficiary's specific medical problem.

C. Screening Prostate Specific Antigen Tests

Screening prostate specific antigen tests are covered at a frequency of once every 12 months for men who have attained age 50 (at least 11 months have passed following the month in which the last Medicare-covered screening prostate specific antigen test was performed). Screening prostate specific antigen tests (PSA) means a test to detect the marker for adenocarcinoma of prostate. PSA is a reliable immunocytochemical marker for primary and metastatic adenocarcinoma of prostate. This screening must be ordered by the beneficiary's physician or by the beneficiary's physician assistant, nurse practitioner, clinical nurse specialist, or certified nurse midwife (the term "attending physician" is defined in §1861(r)(1) of the Act to mean a doctor of medicine or osteopathy and the terms "physician assistant, nurse practitioner, clinical nurse specialist, or certified nurse midwife" are defined in §1861(aa) and §1861(gg) of the Act) who is fully knowledgeable about the beneficiary's medical condition, and who would be responsible for using the results of any examination (test) performed in the overall management of the beneficiary's specific medical problem.

Pub. 100-3, Section 210.2

Screening Pap Smears and Pelvic Examinations for Early Detection of Cervical or Vaginal Cancer

Indications and Limitations of Coverage

CIM 50-20.1

Screening Pap Smear

A screening pap smear and related medically necessary services provided to a woman for the early detection of cervical cancer (including collection of the sample of cells and a physician's interpretation of the test results) and pelvic examination (including clinical breast examination) are covered under Medicare Part B when ordered by a physician (or authorized practitioner) under one of the following conditions:

- She has not had such a test during the preceding two years or is a woman of childbearing age (§1861(nn) of the Act).

- There is evidence (on the basis of her medical history or other findings) that she is at high risk of developing cervical cancer and her physician (or authorized practitioner) recommends that she have the test performed more frequently than every two years.

High risk factors for cervical and vaginal cancer are:

- Early onset of sexual activity (under 16 years of age).

- Multiple sexual partners (five or more in a lifetime).

- History of sexually transmitted disease (including HIV infection).

- Fewer than three negative or any pap smears within the previous 7 years.; and

- DES (diethylstilbestrol) - exposed daughters of women who took DES during pregnancy.

NOTE: Claims for pap smears must indicate the beneficiary's low or high risk status by including the appropriate ICD-9-CM on the line item (Item 24E of the Form CMS-1500).

Definitions

A woman as described in §1861(nn) of the Act is a woman who is of childbearing age and has had a pap smear test during any of the preceding three years that indicated the presence of cervical or vaginal cancer or other abnormality, or is at high risk of developing cervical or vaginal cancer.

A woman of childbearing age is one who is premenopausal and has been determined by a physician or other qualified practitioner to be of childbearing age, based upon the medical history or other findings.

Other qualified practitioner, as defined in 42 CFR 410.56(a) includes a certified nurse midwife (as defined in §1861(gg) of the Act), or a physician assistant, nurse practitioner, or clinical nurse specialist (as defined in §1861(aa) of the Act) who is authorized under State law to perform the examination.

Screening Pelvic Examination

Section 4102 of the Balanced Budget Act of 1997 provides for coverage of screening pelvic examinations (including a clinical breast examination) for all female beneficiaries, subject to certain frequency and other limitations. A screening pelvic examination (including a clinical breast examination) should include at least seven of the following eleven elements:

Inspection and palpation of breasts for masses or lumps, tenderness, symmetry, or nipple discharge.

Digital rectal examination including sphincter tone, presence of hemorrhoids, and rectal masses. Pelvic examination (with or without specimen collection for smears and cultures) including:

- External genitalia (for example, general appearance, hair distribution, or lesions).

- Urethral maetus (for example, size, location, lesions, or prolapse).

- Urethra (for example, masses, tenderness, or scarring).

- Bladder (for example, fullness, masses, or tenderness).

- Vagina (for example, general appearance, estrogen effect, discharge lesions, pelvic support, cystocele, or rectocele).

- Cervix (for example, general appearance, lesions, or discharge).

- Uterus (for example, size, contour, position, mobility, tenderness, consistency, descent, or support).

- Adnexa/parametria (for example, masses, tenderness, organomegaly, or nodularity).

- Anus and perineum.

This description is from Documentation Guidelines for Evaluation and Management Services, published in May 1997 and was developed by the Centers for Medicare and Medicaid Services and the American Medical Association.

Pub. 100-3, Section 220.1

Computerized Tomography

A. General

Diagnostic examinations of the head (head scans) and of other parts of the body (body scans) performed by computerized tomography (CT) scanners are covered if you find that the medical and scientific literature and opinion support the effective use of a scan for the condition, and the scan is: (1) reasonable and necessary for the individual patient; and (2) performed on a model of CT equipment that meets the criteria in C below.

CT scans have become the primary diagnostic tool for many conditions and symptoms. CT scanning used as the primary diagnostic tool can be cost effective because it can eliminate the need for a series of other tests, is non-invasive and thus virtually eliminates complications, and does not require hospitalization.

B. Determining Whether a CT Scan Is Reasonable and Necessary

Sufficient information must be provided with claims to differentiate CT scans from other radiology services and to make coverage determinations. Carefully review claims to insure that a scan is reasonable and necessary for the individual patient; i.e., the use must be found to be medically appropriate considering the patient's symptoms and preliminary diagnosis.

There is no general rule that requires other diagnostic tests to be tried before CT scanning is used. However, in an individual case the contractor's medical staff may determine that use of a CT scan as the initial diagnostic test was not reasonable and necessary because it was not supported by the patient's symptoms or complaints stated on the claim form; e.g., "periodic headaches."

Claims for CT scans are reviewed for evidence of abuse which might include the absence of reasonable indications for the scans, an excessive number of scans or unnecessarily expensive types of scans considering the facts in the particular cases.

C-Approved Models of CT Equipment

1. Criteria for Approval

In the absence of evidence to the contrary, you may assume that a CT scan for which payment is requested has been performed on equipment that meets the following criteria:

a. The model must be known to the Food and Drug Administration, and

b. Must be in the full market release phase of development.

Should it be necessary to confirm that those criteria are met, ask the manufacturer to submit the information in subsection C.2. If manufacturers inquire about obtaining Medicare approval for their equipment, inform them of the foregoing criteria.

2. Evidence of Approval

a. The letter sent by the Bureau of Radiological Health, Food and Drug Administration (FDA), to the manufacturer acknowledging the FDA's receipt of information on the specific CT scanner system model submitted as required under Public Law 90-602, "The Radiation Control for Health and Safety Act of 1968."

b. A letter signed by the chief executive officer or other officer acting in a similar capacity for the manufacturer which:

1. Furnishes the CT scanner system model number, all names that hospitals and physicians' offices may use to refer to the CT scanner system on claims, and the accession number assigned by FDA to the specific model;

2. Specifies whether the scanner performs head scans only, body scans only (i.e., scans of parts of the body other than the head), or head and body scans;

3. States that the company or corporation is satisfied with the results of the developmental stages that preceded the full market release phase of the equipment, that the equipment is in the full market release phase, and the date on which it was decided to put the product into the full market release phase.

D-Mobile Ct Equipment

CT scans performed on mobile units are subject to the same Medicare coverage requirements applicable to scans performed on stationary units, as well as certain health and safety requirements recommended by PHS. As with scans performed on stationary units, the scans must be determined medically necessary for the individual patient. The scans must be performed on types of CT scanning equipment that have been approved for use as stationary units (see C above), and must be in compliance with applicable State laws and regulations for control of radiation.

1. Hospital Setting

The hospital must assume responsibility for the quality of the scan furnished to inpatients and outpatients and must assure that a radiologist or other qualified physician is in charge of the procedure. The radiologist or other physician (i.e., one who is with the mobile unit) who is responsible for the procedure must be approved by the hospital for similar privileges.

2. Ambulatory Setting

If mobile CT scan services are furnished at an ambulatory health care facility other than a hospital-based facility, e.g., a freestanding physician-directed clinic, the diagnostic procedure must be performed by or under the direct personal supervision of a radiologist or other qualified physician. In addition, the facility must maintain a record of the attending physician's order for a scan performed on a mobile unit.

3. Billing for Mobile CT Scans

Hospitals, hospital-associated radiologists, ambulatory health care facilities, and physician owner/operators of mobile units may bill for mobile scans as they would for scans performed on stationary equipment.

4. Claims Review

Evidence of compliance with applicable State laws and regulations for control of radiation should be requested from owners of mobile CT scan units upon receipt of the first claims. All mobile scan claims should be reviewed very carefully in accordance with instructions applicable to scans performed on fixed units, with particular emphasis on the medical necessity for scans performed in an ambulatory setting.

E-Multi-Planar Diagnostic Imaging (MPDI)

In usual computerized tomography (CT) scanning procedures, a series of transverse or axial images are reproduced. These transverse images are routinely translated into coronal and/or sagittal views. Multiplanar diagnostic imaging (MPDI) is a process which further translates the data produced by CT scanning by providing reconstructed oblique images which can contribute to diagnostic information. MPDI, also known as planar image reconstruction or reformatted imaging, is covered under Medicare when provided as a service to an entity performing a covered CT scan.

Pub. 100-3, Section 220.2

Magnetic Resonance Imaging (MRI)

B - Nationally Covered Indications (Effective November 22, 1985)

Although several uses of MRI are still considered investigational and some uses are clearly contraindicated (see subsection D), MRI is considered medically efficacious for a number of uses. Use the following descriptions as general guidelines or examples of what may be considered covered rather than as a restrictive list of specific covered indications. Coverage is limited to MRI units that have received FDA premarket approval, and such units must be operated within the parameters specified by the approval. In addition, the services must be reasonable and necessary for the diagnosis or treatment of the specific patient involved.

The MRI is useful in examining the head, central nervous system, and spine. Multiple sclerosis can be diagnosed with MRI and the contents of the posterior fossa are visible. The inherent tissue contrast resolution of MRI makes it an appropriate standard diagnostic modality for general neuroradiology.

The MRI can assist in the differential diagnosis of mediastinal and retroperitoneal masses, including abnormalities of the large vessels such as aneurysms and dissection. When a clinical need exists to visualize the parenchyma of solid organs to detect anatomic disruption or neoplasia, this can be accomplished in the liver, urogenital system, adrenals, and pelvic organs without the use of radiological contrast materials. When MRI is considered reasonable and necessary, the use of paramagnetic contrast materials may be covered as part of the study. MRI may also be used to detect and stage pelvic and retroperitoneal neoplasms and to evaluate disorders of cancellous bone and soft tissues. It may also be used in the detection of pericardial thickening. Primary and secondary bone neoplasm and aseptic necrosis can be detected at an early stage and monitored with MRI. Patients with metallic prostheses, especially of the hip, can be imaged in order to detect the early stages of infection of the bone to which the prothesis is attached.

Disc Disease Diagnosis (Effective March 22, 1994)

The MRI may also be covered to diagnose disc disease without regard to whether radiological imaging has been tried first to diagnose the problem.

Gating Devices and Surface Coils (Effective March 4, 1991)

Gating devices that eliminate distorted images caused by cardiac and respiratory movement cycles are now considered state of the art techniques and may be covered. Surface and other specialty coils may also be covered, as they are used routinely for high resolution imaging where small limited regions of the body are studied. They produce high signal-to-noise ratios resulting in images of enhanced anatomic detail.

C - Contraindications and Nationally Noncovered Indications

1. ContraindicationsThe MRI is not covered when the following patient-specific contraindications are present. It is not covered for patients with cardiac pacemakers or with metallic clips on vascular aneurysms. MRI during a viable pregnancy is also contraindicated at this time. The danger inherent in bringing ferromagnetic materials within range of MRI units generally constrains the use of MRI on acutely ill patients requiring life support systems and monitoring devices that employ ferromagnetic materials. In addition, the long imaging time and the enclosed position of the patient may result in claustrophobia, making patients who have a history of claustrophobia unsuitable candidates for MRI procedures.

2. Nationally Noncovered Indications

The CMS has determined that blood flow measurement, imaging of cortical bone and calcifications, and procedures involving spatial resolution of bone and calcifications, are not considered reasonable and necessary indications within the meaning of section 1862(a)(1)(A) of the Social Security Act, and are therefore noncovered.

D. Other

All other uses of MRI for which CMS has not specifically indicated coverage or noncoverage continue to be eligible for coverage through individual local contractor discretion.

(This NCD last reviewed September 2004.)

Pub. 100-3, Section 220.3

Magnetic Resonance Angiography (MRA)

B. Nationally Covered Indications

1. Head and Neck

Studies have proven that MRA is effective for evaluating flow in internal carotid vessels of the head and neck. However, not all potential applications of MRA have been shown to be reasonable and necessary. All of the following criteria must apply in order for Medicare to provide coverage for MRA of the head and neck:

a. MRA is used to evaluate the carotid arteries, the circle of Willis, the anterior, middle or posterior cerebral arteries, the vertebral or basilar arteries or the venous sinuses;

b. MRA is performed on patients with conditions of the head and neck for which surgery is anticipated and may be found to be appropriate based on the MRA. These conditions include, but are not limited to, tumor, aneurysms, vascular malformations, vascular occlusion or thrombosis. Within this broad category of disorders, medical necessity is the underlying determinant of the

need for an MRA in specific diseases. The medical records should clearly justify and demonstrate the existence of medical necessity; and

c. MRA and contrast angiography (CA) are not expected to be performed on the same patient for diagnostic purposes prior to the application of anticipated therapy. Only one of these tests will be covered routinely unless the physician can demonstrate the medical need to perform both tests.

2. Peripheral Arteries of Lower Extremities

Studies have proven that MRA of peripheral arteries is useful in determining the presence and extent of peripheral vascular disease in lower extremities. This procedure is non-invasive and has been shown to find occult vessels in some patients for which those vessels were not apparent when CA was performed. Medicare will cover either MRA or CA to evaluate peripheral arteries of the lower extremities. However, both MRA and CA may be useful is some cases, such as:

a. A patient has had CA and this test was unable to identify a viable run-off vessel for bypass. When exploratory surgery is not believed to be a reasonable medical course of action for this patient, MRA may be performed to identify the viable runoff vessel; or

b. A patient has had MRA, but the results are inconclusive.

3. Abdomen and Pelvis

a. Pre-operative Evaluation of Patients Undergoing Elective Abdominal Aortic Aneurysm (AAA) Repair (Effective July 1, 1999)The MRA is covered for pre-operative evaluation of patients undergoing elective AAA repair if the scientific evidence reveals MRA is considered comparable to CA in determining the extent of AAA, as well as in evaluating aortoiliac occlusion disease and renal artery pathology that may be necessary in the surgical planning of AAA repair. These studies also reveal that MRA could provide a net benefit to the patient. If preoperative CA is avoided, then patients are not exposed to the risks associated with invasive procedures, contrast media, end-organ damage, or arterial injury.

b. Imaging the Renal Arteries and the Aortoiliac Arteries in the Absence of AAA or Aortic Dissection (Effective July 1, 2003)The MRA coverage is expanded to include imaging the renal arteries and the aortoiliac arteries in the absence of AAA or aortic dissection. MRA should be obtained in those circumstances in which using MRA is expected to avoid obtaining CA, when physician history, physical examination, and standard assessment tools provide insufficient information for patient management, and obtaining an MRA has a high probability of positively affecting patient management. However, CA may be ordered after obtaining the results of an MRA in those rare instances where medical necessity is demonstrated.

4. Chest

a. Diagnosis of Pulmonary EmbolismCurrent scientific data has shown that diagnostic pulmonary MRAs are improving due to recent developments such as faster imaging capabilities and gadolinium-enhancement. However, these advances in MRA are not significant enough to warrant replacement of pulmonary angiography in the diagnosis of pulmonary embolism for patients who have no contraindication to receiving intravenous iodinated contrast material. Patients who are allergic to iodinated contrast material face a high risk of developing complications if they undergo pulmonary angiography or computed tomography angiography. Therefore, Medicare will cover MRA of the chest for diagnosing a suspected pulmonary embolism when it is contraindicated for the patient to receive intravascular iodinated contrast material.

b. Evaluation of Thoracic Aortic Dissection and AneurysmStudies have shown that MRA of the chest has a high level of diagnostic accuracy for pre-operative and post-operative evaluation of aortic dissection of aneurysm. Depending on the clinical presentation, MRA may be used as an alternative to other non-invasive imaging technologies, such as transesophageal echocardiography and CT. Generally, Medicare will provide coverage only for MRA or for CA when used as a diagnostic test. However, if both MRA and CA of the chest are used, the physician must demonstrate the medical need for performing these tests.While the intent of this policy is to provide reimbursement for either MRA or CA, CMS is also allowing flexibility for physicians to make appropriate decisions concerning the use of these tests based on the needs of individual patients. CMS anticipates, however, low utilization of the combined use of MRA and CA. As a result, CMS encourages contractors to monitor the use of these tests and, where indicated, requires evidence of the need to perform both MRA and CA.

C. Nationally Noncovered Indications

All other uses of MRA for which CMS has not specifically indicated coverage continue to be noncovered.

D. Other

Not applicable.

(This NCD last reviewed September 2004.)

Pub. 100-3, Section 220.4

Mammograms

A diagnostic mammography is a covered service if it is ordered by a doctor of medicine or osteopathy as defined in §1861(r)(1) of the Act.

Payment may not be made for screening mammography performed on a woman under age 35. Payment may be made for only one screening mammography performed on a woman over age 34, but under age 40. For an asymptomatic woman over age 39, payment may be made for a screening mammography performed after at least 11 months have passed following the month in which the last screening mammography was performed.

A radiological mammogram is a covered diagnostic test under the following conditions:

- A patient has distinct signs and symptoms for which a mammogram is indicated;

- A patient has a history of breast cancer; or

- A patient is asymptomatic but, on the basis of the patient's history and other factors the physician considers significant, the physician's judgment is that a mammogram is appropriate.

Use of mammograms in routine screening of (1) asymptomatic women aged 50 and over, and (2) asymptomatic women aged 40 or over whose mothers or sisters have had the disease, is considered medically appropriate, but would not be covered for Medicare purposes.

Pub. 100-3, Section 220.5

Ultrasound Diagnostic Procedures

Ultrasound diagnostic procedures are listed below and are divided into two categories:

1. Medicare coverage is extended to the procedures listed in Category I. Periodic claims review by the intermediary's medical consultants should be conducted to insure that the techniques are medically appropriate and the general indications specified in these categories are met.

2. Techniques in Category II are considered experimental and should not be covered at this time.

Category I - (Clinically effective, usually part of initial patient evaluation, may be an adjunct to radiologic and nuclear medicine diagnostic technique):

Echoencephalography, (Diencephalic Midline) (A-Mode).

Echoencephalography, Complete (Diencephalic Midline and Ventricular Size).

Ocular and Orbital Echography (A-Mode).

Covered procedures include efforts to determine the suitability of aphakic patients for implantation of an artificial lens (pseudophakoi) following cataract surgery.

Ocular and Orbital Sonography (B-Mode).

Echocardiography, Pericardial Effusion (M-Mode).

Pericardiocentesis, by Ultrasonic Guidance.

Echocardiography, Cardiac Valve(s) (M-Mode).

Echocardiography, Complete (M-Mode).

Echocardiography, limited (e.g., follow-up or limited study) (M-Mode).

Pleural Effusion Echography.

Thoracentesis, by Ultrasonic Guidance.

Abdominal Sonography, complete survey study (B-Scan).

Abdominal Sonography, limited (e.g., follow-up or limited study) (B-Scan).

Abdominal sonography is not synonymous with ultrasound examination of individual organs.

Renal Cyst Aspiration, by Ultrasonic Guidance.

Renal Biopsy, by Ultrasonic Guidance.

Pancreas Sonography (B-Scan).

Pancreatic sonography has proven effective in diagnosing pseudocysts.

Spleen Sonography (B-Scan).

Abdominal Aorta Echography (A-Mode).

Abdominal Aorta Sonography (B-Scan).

Retroperitoneal Sonography (B-Scan).

Retroperitoneal sonography does not include planning of fields for radiation therapy.

Urinary Bladder Sonography (B-Scan).

Urinary bladder sonography does not include staging of bladder tumors.

Pregnancy Diagnosis sonography (B-Scan).

Fetal Age Determination (Biparietal Diameter) Sonography (B-Scan).

Fetal Growth Rate Sonography (B-Scan).

Placenta Localization Sonography (B-Scan).

Pregnancy Sonography, Complete (B-Scan).

Molar Pregnancy Diagnosis Sonography (B-Scan).

Ectopic Pregnancy Diagnosis sonography (B-Scan).

Passive Testing (Antepartum Monitoring of Fetal Heart Rate In the Resting Fetus).

Intrauterine Contraceptive Device Sonography (B-Scan).

Pelvic Mass Diagnosis Sonography (B-Scan).

Amniocentesis, by Ultrasonic Guidance.

Arterial Flow Study, Peripheral (Doppler).

Venous Flow Study, Peripheral (Doppler).

Arterial Aneurysm, Peripheral (B-Scan).

Radiation Therapy Planning Sonography (B-Scan).

Thyroid Echography (A-Mode).

Thyroid Sonography (B-Scan).

Breast Echography (A-Mode).

Breast Sonography (B-Scan).

Hepatic Sonography (B-Scan).

Gallbladder Sonography.

Renal Sonography.

Two-Dimensional Echocardiography (B-Mode).

Category II - (Clinical reliability and efficacy not proven):

B-Scan for atherosclerotic narrowing of peripheral arteries.

Monitoring of cardiac output (Doppler).

In view of the rapid changes in the field of ultrasound diagnosis, uses for ultrasound diagnostic procedures other than those listed under Categories I and II should be carefully reviewed before payment. Medical justification may be required. When appropriate, new uses for ultrasound diagnostic procedures should be forwarded to CMS so that revisions may be made in the coverage policy when appropriate.

Pub. 100-3, Section 220.6

PET Scans

The following indications may be covered for PET under certain circumstances. Details of Medicare PET coverage are discussed later in this section. Unless otherwise indicated, the clinical conditions below are covered when PET utilizes FDG as a tracer.

NOTE: This manual section 220.6 lists all Medicare-covered uses of PET scans. Except as set forth below in cancer indications listed as "Coverage with Evidence Development", a particular use of PET scans is not covered unless this manual specifically provides that such use is covered. Although this section 220.6 lists some non-covered uses of PET scans, it does not constitute an exhaustive list of all non-covered uses.

Clinical Condition	Effective Date	Coverage
Solitary Pulmonary Nodules (SPNs)	January 1, 1998	Characterization
Lung Cancer (Non Small Cell)	January 1, 1998	Initial staging
Lung Cancer (Non Small Cell)	July 1, 2001	Diagnosis, staging, restaging
Esophageal Cancer	July 1, 2001	Diagnosis, staging, restaging
Colorectal Cancer	July 1, 1999	Determining location of tumors if rising CEA level suggests recurrence
Colorectal Cancer	July 1, 2001	Diagnosis, staging, restaging
Lymphoma	July 1, 1999	Staging and restaging only when used as alternative to Gallium scan
Lymphoma	July 1, 2001	Diagnosis, staging and restaging
Melanoma	July 1, 1999	Evaluating recurrence prior to surgery as alternative to Gallium scan
Melanoma	July 1, 2001	Diagnosis, staging, restaging; Non-covered for evaluating regional node
Breast Cancer	October 1, 2002	As an adjunct to standard imaging modalities for staging patients with distant metastasis or restaging patients with loco-regional recurrence or metastasis; as an adjunct to standard imaging modalities for monitoring tumor response to treatment for women with locally advanced and metastatic breast cancer when a change in therapy is anticipated
Head and Neck Cancers (excluding CNS and thyroid)	July 1, 2001	Diagnosis, staging, restaging
Thyroid Cancer	October 1, 2003	Restaging of recurrent or residual thyroid cancers of follicular cell origin previously treated by thyroidectomy and radioiodine ablation and have a serum thyroglobulin >10ng/ml and negative I-131 whole body scan performed

Clinical Condition	Effective Date	Coverage
Myocardial Viability	July 1, 2001 to September 30, 2002	Only following inconclusive SPECT
Myocardial Viability	October 1, 2002	Primary or initial diagnosis, or following an inconclusive SPECT prior to revascularization. SPECT may not be used following an inconclusive PET scan
Refractory Seizures	July 1, 2001	Pre-surgical evaluation only
Perfusion of the heart using Rubidium 82*tracer	March 14, 1995	Noninvasive imaging of the perfusion of the heart
Perfusion of the heart using ammonia N-13*tracer	October 1, 2003	Noninvasive imaging of the perfusion of the heart

Not FDG-PET.

EFFECTIVE JANUARY 28, 2005: This manual section lists Medicare-covered uses of PET scans effective for services performed on or after January 28, 2005. Except as set forth below in cancer indications listed as "coverage with evidence development", a particular use of PET scans is not covered unless this manual specifically provides that such use is covered. Although this section 220.6 lists some non-covered uses of PET scans, it does not constitute an exhaustive list of all non-covered uses.

For cancer indications listed as "coverage with evidence development" CMS determines that the evidence is sufficient to conclude that an FDG PET scan is reasonable and necessary only when the provider is participating in, and patients are enrolled in, one of the following types of prospective clinical studies that is designed to collect additional information at the time of the scan to assist in patient management:

A clinical trial of FDG PET that meets the requirements of Food and Drug Administration (FDA) category B investigational device exemption (42 CFR 405.201);

An FDG PET clinical study that is designed to collect additional information at the time of the scan to assist in patient management. Qualifying clinical studies must ensure that specific hypotheses are addressed; appropriate data elements are collected; hospitals and providers are qualified to provide the PET scan and interpret the results; participating hospitals and providers accurately report data on all enrolled patients not included in other qualifying trials through adequate auditing mechanisms; and, all patient confidentiality, privacy, and other Federal laws must be followed.

Effective January 28, 2005: For PET services identified as "Coverage with Evidence Development. Medicare shall notify providers and beneficiaries where these services can be accessed, as they become available, via the following:

Federal Register Notice

CMS coverage Web site at: www.cms.gov/coverage

Indication	Covered [1]	Nationally Non-covered [2]	Coverage with Evidence Development [3]
Brain			X
Breast-Diagnosis-Initial staging of axillary nodes-Staging of distant metastasis-Restaging, monitoring *	XX	XX	
Cervical-Staging as adjunct to conventional imaging-Other staging-Diagnosis, restaging, monitoring *	X		XX
Colorectal-Diagnosis, staging, restaging-Monitoring *	X		X
Esophagus-Diagnosis, staging, restaging-Monitoring *	X		X
Head and Neck (non-CNS/thyroid)-Diagnosis, staging, restaging-Monitoring *	X		X

Indication	Covered [1]	Nationally Non-covered [2]	Coverage with Evidence Development [3]
Lymphoma-Diagnosis, staging, restaging-Monitoring *	X		X
Melanoma-Diagnosis, staging, restaging-Monitoring *	X		X
Non-Small Cell Lung-Diagnosis, staging, restaging-Monitoring *	X		X
Ovarian			X
Pancreatic			X
Small Cell Lung			X
Soft Tissue Sarcoma			X
Solitary Pulmonary Nodule (characterization)	X		
Thyroid-Staging of follicular cell tumors-Restaging of medullary cell tumors-Diagnosis, other staging & restaging-Monitoring *	X		XXX
Testicular			X
All other cancers not listed herein (all indications)			X

1 Covered nationally based on evidence of benefit. Refer to National Coverage Determination Manual Section 220.6 in its entirety for specific coverage language and limitations for each indication.

2 Non-covered nationally based on evidence of harm or no benefit.

3 Covered only in specific settings discussed above if certain patient safeguards are provided. Otherwise, non-covered nationally based on lack of evidence sufficient to establish either benefit or harm or no prior decision addressing this cancer. Medicare shall notify providers and beneficiaries where these services can be accessed, as they become available, via the following:

Federal Register Notice

CMS coverage Web site at: www.cms.gov/coverage

Monitoring = monitoring response to treatment when a change in therapy is anticipated.

II. General Conditions of Coverage for FDG PET

A. Allowable FDG PET Systems

1. Definitions: For purposes of this section:

a. "Any FDA-approved" means all systems approved or cleared for marketing by the Food and Drug Administration (FDA) to image radionuclides in the body.

b. "FDA-approved" means that the system indicated has been approved or cleared for marketing by the FDA to image radionuclides in the body.

c. "Certain coincidence systems" refers to the systems that have all the following features:

• Crystal at least 5/8-inch thick;

• Techniques to minimize or correct for scatter and/or randoms; and

• Digital detectors and iterative reconstruction.

Scans performed with gamma camera PET systems with crystals thinner than 5/8" will not be covered by Medicare. In addition, scans performed with systems with crystals greater than or equal to 5/8" in thickness, but that do not meet the other listed design characteristics are not covered by Medicare.

2. Allowable PET systems by covered clinical indication:

Allowable Type of FDG PET System

Covered Clinical Condition	Prior to July 1, 2001	July 1, 2001 through December 31, 2001	On or after January 1, 2002

Characterization of single pulmonary nodules	Effective 1/1/1998, any FDA-approved	Any FDA-approved	FDA-approved: Full/Partial ring, certain coincidence systems
Initial staging of lung cancer (non small cell)	Effective 1/1/1998, any FDA-approved	Any FDA-approved	FDA-approved: Full/Partial ring, certain coincidence systems
Determining location of colorectal tumors if rising CEA level suggests recurrence	Effective 7/1/1999, any FDA-approved	Any FDA-approved	FDA approved: Full/Partial ring, certain coincidence systems
Staging or restaging of lymphoma only when used as alternative to gallium scan	Effective 7/1/1999, any FDA-approved	Any FDA-approved	FDA-approved: Full/Partial ring, certain coincidence systems
Evaluating recurrence of melanoma prior to surgery as alternative to gallium scan	Effective 7/1/1999, any FDA-approved.	Any FDA-approved	FDA-approved: Full/Partial ring, certain coincidence systems
Diagnosis, staging, restaging of colorectal cancer	Not covered by Medicare	Full ring	FDA-approved: Full/Partial ring
Diagnosis, staging, restaging of esophageal cancer	Not covered by Medicare	Full ring	FDA-approved: Full/Partial ring
Diagnosis, staging, restaging of head and neck cancers (excluding CNS and thyroid)	Not covered by Medicare	Full ring	FDA-approved: Full/Partial ring
Diagnosis, staging, restaging of lung cancer (non small cell)	Not covered by Medicare	Full ring	FDA-approved: Full/Partial ring
Diagnosis, staging, restaging of lymphoma	Not covered by Medicare	Full ring	FDA-approved: Full/Partial ring
Diagnosis, staging, restaging of melanoma (non-covered for evaluating regional nodes)	Not covered by Medicare	Full ring	FDA-approved: Full/Partial ring
Determination of myocardial viability only following inconclusive SPECT	Not covered by Medicare	Full ring	FDA-approved: Full/Partial ring
Pre-surgical evaluation of refractory seizures	Not covered by Medicare	Full ring	FDA-approved: Full ring
Breast Cancer	Not covered	Not covered	Effective October 1, 2002, Full/Partial ring
Thyroid Cancer	Not covered	Not covered	Effective October 1, 2003, Full/Partial ring
Myocardial Viability Primary or initial diagnosis prior to revascularization	Not covered	Not covered	Effective October 1, 2002, Full/Partial ring
All other oncology indications not previously specified	Not covered	Not covered	Effective January 28, 2005, Full/Partial ring

B. Regardless of any other terms or conditions, all uses of FDG PET scans, in order to be covered by the Medicare program, must meet the following general conditions prior to June 30, 2001:

1. Submission of claims for payment must include any information Medicare requires to ensure the PET scans performed were: (a) medically necessary, (b) did not unnecessarily duplicate other covered diagnostic tests, and (c) did not involve investigational drugs or procedures using investigational drugs, as determined by the FDA.

2. The PET scan entity submitting claims for payment must keep such patient records as Medicare requires on file for each patient for whom a PET scan claim is made.

C. Regardless of any other terms or conditions, all uses of FDG PET scans, in order to be covered by the Medicare program, must meet the following general conditions as of July 1, 2001:

1. The provider of the PET scan should maintain on file the doctor's referral and documentation that the procedure involved only FDA-approved drugs and devices, as is normal business practice.

2. The ordering physician is responsible for documenting the medical necessity of the study and ensuring that it meets the conditions specified in the instructions. The physician should have documentation in the beneficiary's medical record to support the referral to the PET scan provider.

III. Covered Indications for PET Scans and Limitations/Requirements for Usage

For all uses of PET relating to malignancies the following conditions apply:

1. Diagnosis: PET is covered only in clinical situations in which: (1) the PET results may assist in avoiding an invasive diagnostic procedure, or in which (2) the PET results may assist in determining the optimal anatomical location to perform an invasive diagnostic procedure. In general, for most solid tumors, a tissue diagnosis is made prior to the performance of PET scanning. PET scans following a tissue diagnosis are generally performed for staging rather than diagnosis.

PET is not covered as a screening test (i.e., testing patients without specific signs and symptoms of disease).

2. Staging: PET is covered for staging in clinical situations in which: (1)(a) the stage of the cancer remains in doubt after completion of a standard diagnostic workup, including conventional imaging (computed tomography (CT), magnetic resonance imaging (MRI), or ultrasound), or (1)(b) it could potentially replace one or more conventional imaging studies when it is expected that conventional study information is insufficient for the clinical management of the patient, and 2) clinical management of the patient would differ depending on the stage of the cancer identified.

3. Restaging: PET is covered for restaging: (1) after completion of treatment for the purpose of detecting residual disease, (2) for detecting suspected recurrence or metastasis, (3) to determine the extent of a known recurrence, or (4) if it could potentially replace one or more conventional imaging studies when it is expected that conventional study information is insufficient for the clinical management of the patient. Restaging applies to testing after a course of treatment is completed, and is covered subject to the conditions above.

4. Monitoring: This refers to use of PET to monitor tumor response to treatment during the planned course of therapy (i.e., when a change in therapy is anticipated).

NOTE: In the absence of national frequency limitations, contractors, should, if necessary, develop frequency requirements on any or all of the indications covered on and after July 1, 2001.

(This NCD last reviewed December 2004.)

Pub. 100-3, Section 220.7

Xenon Scan

Program payment may be made for this diagnostic procedure which involves perfusion lung imaging with 133 xenon. However, review for evidence of abuse which might include absence of reasonable indications, inappropriate sequence, or excessive number or kinds of procedures used in the care of individual patients.

Pub. 100-3, Section 220.8

Nuclear Radiology Procedure

Nuclear radiology procedures, including nuclear examinations performed with mobile radiological equipment, are covered if reasonable and necessary for the individual patient. Although these procedures may not be widely used, they are generally accepted. Review claims for these procedures for evidence of abuse which might absence of reasonable indications, inappropriate sequence, or excessive number or kinds of procedures used in the care of individual patients.

Pub. 100-3, Section 220.9

Digital Subtraction Angiography

Contractors should be alert to possible increases in utilization of DSA over conventional angiographic procedures, as well as to the fact that ordinarily patients should not require inpatient hospitalization solely to perform the procedure.

Payment for DSA should not exceed, and may be less than, that being paid for conventional angiographic techniques.

Pub. 100-3, Section 220.11

Thermography

Thermography for any indication (including breast lesions which were excluded from Medicare coverage on July 20, 1984) is excluded from Medicare coverage because the available evidence does not support this test as a useful aid in the diagnosis or treatment of illness or injury. Therefore, it is not considered effective. This exclusion was published as a HCFA Final Notice in the Federal Register on November 20, 1992.

Pub. 100-3, Section 220.12

Single Photon Emission Tomography - Covered

Frequency limitations: Contractor discretion.

In the case of myocardial viability, FDG PET may be used following a SPECT that was found to be inconclusive. However, SPECT may not be used following an inconclusive FDG PET performed to evaluate myocardial viability.

Pub. 100-3, Section 220.13

Percutaneous Image-Guided Breast Biopsy

The Breast Imaging Reporting and Data System (or BIRADS system) employed by the American College of Radiology provides a standardized lexicon with which radiologists may report their interpretation of a mammogram. The BIRADS grading of mammograms is as follows: Grade I-Negative, Grade II-Benign finding, Grade III-Probably benign, Grade IV-Suspicious abnormality, and Grade V-Highly suggestive of malignant neoplasm.

A. Nonpalpable Breast Lesions. —

Effective January 1, 2003, Medicare covers percutaneous image-guided breast biopsy using stereotactic or ultrasound imaging for a radiographic abnormality that is nonpalpable and is graded as a BIRADS III, IV, or V.

B. Palpable Breast Lesions. —

Effective January 1, 2003, Medicare covers percutaneous image guided breast biopsy using stereotactic or ultrasound imaging for palpable lesions that are difficult to biopsy using palpation alone. Contractors have the discretion to decide what types of palpable lesions are difficult to biopsy using palpation.

Pub. 100-3, Section 230.1

Treatment of Kidney Stones

In addition to the traditional surgical/endoscopic techniques for the treatment of kidney stones, the following lithotripsy techniques are also covered for services rendered on or after March I5, I985.

A. Extracorporeal Shock Wave Lithotripsy. — Extracorporeal Shock Wave Lithotripsy (ESWL) is a non-invasive method of treating kidney stones using a device called a lithotriptor. The lithotriptor uses shock waves generated outside of the body to break up upper urinary tract stones. It focuses the shock waves specifically on stones under X-ray visualization, pulverizing them by repeated shocks. ESWL is covered under Medicare for use in the treatment of upper urinary tract kidney stones.

B. Percutaneous Lithotripsy. — Percutaneous lithotripsy (or nephrolithotomy) is an invasive method of treating kidney stones by using ultrasound, electrohydraulic or mechanical lithotripsy. A probe is inserted through an incision in the skin directly over the kidney and applied to the stone. A form of lithotripsy is then used to fragment the stone. Mechanical or electrohydraulic lithotripsy may be used as an alternative or adjunct to ultrasonic lithotripsy. Percutaneous lithotripsy of kidney stones by ultrasound or by the related techniques of electrohydraulic or mechanical lithotripsy is covered under Medicare.

The following is covered for services rendered on or after January 16, 1988.

C. Transurethral Ureteroscopic Lithotripsy. — Transurethral ureteroscopic lithotripsy is a method of fragmenting and removing ureteral and renal stones through a cystoscope. The cystoscope is inserted through the urethra into the bladder. Catheters are passed through the scope into the opening where the ureters enter the bladder. Instruments passed through this opening into the ureters are used to manipulate and ultimately disintegrate stones, using either mechanical crushing, transcystoscopic electrohydraulic shock waves, ultrasound or laser. Transurethral ureteroscopic lithotripsy for the treatment of urinary tract stones of the kidney or ureter is covered under Medicare.

Pub. 100-3, Section 230.2

Uroflowmetric Evaluations

Uroflowmetric evaluations (also referred to as urodynamic voiding or urodynamic flow studies) are covered under Medicare for diagnosing various urological dysfunctions, including bladder outlet obstructions.

Pub. 100-3, Section 230.3

Sterilization

A - Covered Conditions

Payment may be made only where sterilization is a necessary part of the treatment of an illness or injury, e.g., removal of a uterus because of a tumor, removal of diseased ovaries (bilateral oophorectomy), or bilateral orchidectomy in a case of cancer of the prostate. Deny claims when the pathological evidence of the necessity to perform any such procedures to treat an illness or injury is absent; and

Sterilization of a mentally retarded beneficiary is covered if it is a necessary part of the treatment of an illness or injury.

Monitor such surgeries closely and obtain the information needed to determine whether in fact the surgery was performed as a means of treating an illness or injury or only to achieve sterilization.

B - Noncovered Conditions

Elective hysterectomy, tubal ligation, and vasectomy, if the stated reason for these procedures is sterilization;

A sterilization that is performed because a physician believes another pregnancy would endanger the overall general health of the woman is not considered to be reasonable and necessary for the diagnosis or treatment of illness or injury within the meaning of §1862(a)(1) of the Act. The same conclusion would apply where the sterilization is performed only as a measure to prevent the possible development of, or effect on, a mental condition should the individual become pregnant; and

Sterilization of a mentally retarded person where the purpose is to prevent conception, rather than the treatment of an illness or injury.

Pub. 100-3, Section 230.4

Diagnosis and Treatment of Impotence

Program payment may be made for diagnosis and treatment of sexual impotence. Since causes and, therefore, appropriate treatment vary, if abuse is suspected it may be necessary to request documentation of appropriateness in individual cases. If treatment is furnished to patients (other than hospital inpatients) in connection with a mental condition, apply the psychiatric service limitation described in the Medicare General Information, Eligibility, and Entitlement Manual, Chapter 3.

Pub. 100-3, Section 230.6

Vabra Aspirator

Program payment cannot be made for the aspirator or the related diagnostic services when furnished in connection with the examination of an asymptomatic patient. Payment for routine physical checkups is precluded under the statute (§1862(a)(7) of the Act).

Pub. 100-3, Section 230.9

Cryosurgery of Prostate

Cryosurgery of the prostate as a salvage therapy is not covered for any services performed prior to June 30, 2001.

Salvage cryosurgery of the prostate for recurrent cancer is medically necessary and appropriate only for those patients with localized disease who:

a. Have failed a trial of radiation therapy as their primary treatment; and

b. Meet one of the following conditions: Stage T2B or below, Gleason score <9, PSA <8 ng/mL.

Cryosurgery as salvage therapy is therefore not covered under Medicare after failure of other therapies as the primary treatment. Cryosurgery as salvage is only covered after the failure of a trial of radiation therapy, under the conditions noted above.

Pub. 100-3, Section 230.10

Incontinence Control Devices

A. Mechanical/Hydraulic Incontinence Control Devices. — Mechanical/hydraulic incontinence control devices are accepted as safe and effective in the management of urinary incontinence in patients with permanent anatomic and neurologic dysfunctions of the bladder. This class of devices achieves control of urination by compression of the urethra. The materials used and the success rate may vary somewhat from device to device. Such a device is covered when its use is reasonable and necessary for the individual patient.

B. Collagen Implant. — A collagen implant, which is injected into the submucosal tissues of the urethra and/or the bladder neck and into tissues adjacent to the urethra, is a prosthetic device used in the treatment of stress urinary incontinence resulting from intrinsic sphincter deficiency (ISD). ISD is a cause of stress urinary incontinence in which the urethral sphincter is unable to contract and generate sufficient resistance in the bladder, especially during stress maneuvers.

Prior to collagen implant therapy, a skin test for collagen sensitivity must be administered and evaluated over a 4 week period.

In male patients, the evaluation must include a complete history and physical examination and a simple cystometrogram to determine that the bladder fills and stores properly. The patient then is asked to stand upright with a full bladder and to cough or otherwise exert abdominal pressure on his bladder. If the patient leaks, the diagnosis of ISD is established.

In female patients, the evaluation must include a complete history and physical examination (including a pelvic exam) and a simple cystometrogram to rule out abnormalities of bladder compliance and abnormalities of urethral support. Following that determination, an abdominal leak point pressure (ALLP) test is performed. Leak point pressure, stated in cm H2O, is defined as the intra-abdominal pressure at which leakage occurs from the bladder (around a catheter) when the bladder has been filled with a minimum of 150 cc fluid. If the patient has an ALLP of less than 100 cm H2O, the diagnosis of ISD is established.

To use a collagen implant, physicians must have urology training in the use of a cystoscope and must complete a collagen implant training program.

Coverage of a collagen implant, and the procedure to inject it, is limited to the following types of patients with stress urinary incontinence due to ISD:

Male or female patients with congenital sphincter weakness secondary to conditions such as myelomeningocele or epispadias;

Male or female patients with acquired sphincter weakness secondary to spinal cord lesions;

Male patients following trauma, including prostatectomy and/or radiation; and

Female patients without urethral hypermobility and with abdominal leak point pressures of 100 cm H2O or less.

Patients whose incontinence does not improve with 5 injection procedures (5 separate treatment sessions) are considered treatment failures, and no further treatment of urinary incontinence by collagen implant is covered. Patients who have a reoccurrence of incontinence following successful treatment with collagen implants in the past (e.g., 6-12 months previously) may benefit from additional treatment sessions. Coverage of additional sessions may be allowed but must be supported by medical justification.

C. Non-Implantable Pelvic Floor Electrical Stimulator. — (See §60-24.)

Pub. 100-3, Section 230.12

Dimethyl Sulfoxide (DMSO)

The Food and Drug Administration has determined that the only purpose for which DMSO is safe and effective for humans is in the treatment of the bladder condition, interstitial cystitis. Therefore, the use of DMSO for all other indications is not considered to be reasonable and necessary. Payment may be made for its use only when reasonable and necessary for a patient in the treatment of interstitial cystitis.

Pub. 100-3, Section 230.14

Ultrafiltration Monitor

Covered:

Ultrafiltration and ultrafiltration monitoring as a component of hemodialysis has an established and critical role in maintaining the well-being of ESRD patients and is a covered service. The Ultrafiltration Monitor is covered under the Medicare program when it is used to calculate fluid rates for those recipients who present difficult fluid management problems. Determine the medical necessity of this device on a case-by-case basis.

Not Covered:

Ultrafiltration, independent of conventional dialysis, is considered experimental, and technology exclusively designed for this purpose is not covered under Medicare.

Pub. 100-3, Section 240.3

Heat Treatment, including the Use of Diathermy and Ultrasound for Pulmonary Conditions

There is no physiological rationale or valid scientific documentation of effectiveness of diathermy or ultrasound heat treatments for asthma, bronchitis, or any other pulmonary condition and for such purpose this treatment cannot be considered reasonable and necessary within the meaning of section 1862(a)(1) of the Act.

Pub. 100-3, Section 240.6

Transvenous (Catheter) Pulmonary Embolectomy

It is not covered under Medicare because it is still experimental.

Pub. 100-3, Section 240.7

Postural Drainage Procedures and Pulmonary Exercises

In most cases, postural drainage procedures and pulmonary exercises can be carried out safely and effectively by nursing personnel. However, in some cases patients may have acute or severe pulmonary conditions involving complex situations in which these procedures or exercises require the knowledge and skills of a physical therapist or a respiratory therapist. Therefore, if the attending physician determines as part of his/her plan of treatment that for the safe and effective administration of such services the procedures or exercises in question need to be performed by a physical therapist, the services of such a therapist constitute covered physical therapy when provided as an inpatient hospital service, extended care service, home health service, or outpatient physical therapy service.

NOTE: Physical therapy furnished in the outpatient department of a hospital is covered under the outpatient physical therapy benefit.

If the attending physician determines that the services should be performed by a respiratory therapist, the services of such a therapist constitute covered respiratory therapy when provided as an inpatient hospital service, outpatient hospital service, or extended care service, assuming that such services are furnished to the skilled nursing facility by a hospital with which the facility has a transfer agreement. Since the services of a respiratory therapist are not covered under the home health benefit, payment may not be made under the home health benefit for visits by a respiratory therapist to a patient's home to provide such services. Postural drainage procedures and pulmonary exercises are also covered when furnished by a physical therapist or a respiratory therapist as incident to a physician's professional service.

Pub. 100-3, Section 250.1

Treatment of Psoriasis

Psoriasis is a chronic skin disease, for which several conventional methods of treatment have been recognized as covered. These include topical application of steroids or other drugs; ultraviolet light (actinotherapy); and coal tar alone or in combination with ultraviolet B light (Goeckerman treatment).

A newer treatment for psoriasis uses a psoralen derivative drug in combination with ultraviolet A light, known as PUVA. PUVA therapy is covered for treatment of intractable, disabling psoriasis, but only after the psoriasis has not responded to more conventional treatment. The contractor should document this before paying for PUVA therapy.

In addition, reimbursement for PUVA therapy should be limited to amounts paid for other types of photochemotherapy; ordinarily, payment should not be allowed for more than 30 days of treatment, unless improvement is documented.

Pub. 100-3, Section 250.4

Treatment of Actinic Keratosis

Medicare covers the destruction of actinic keratoses without restrictions based on lesion or patient characteristics.

Pub. 100-3, Section 260.1

Adult Liver Transplantation

A - General

Effective July 15, 1996, adult liver transplantation when performed on beneficiaries with end stage liver disease other than hepatitis B or malignancies is covered under Medicare when performed in a facility which is approved by CMS as meeting institutional coverage criteria.

Effective December 10, 1999, adult liver transplantation when performed on beneficiaries with end stage liver disease other than malignancies is covered under Medicare when performed in a facility which is approved by CMS as meeting institutional coverage criteria.

Effective September 1, 2001, Medicare covers adult liver transplantation for hepatocellular carcinoma when the following conditions are met:

The patient is not a candidate for subtotal liver resection;

The patient's tumor(s) is less than or equal to 5 cm in diameter;

There is no macrovascular involvement;

There is no identifiable extrahepatic spread of tumor to surrounding lymph nodes, lungs, abdominal organs or bone; and

The transplant is furnished in a facility which is approved by CMS as meeting institutional coverage criteria for liver transplants (See 65 FR 15006).

Adult liver transplantation for other malignancies remains excluded from coverage.

Coverage of adult liver transplantation is effective as of the date of the facility's approval, but for applications received before July 13, 1991, can be effective as early as March 8, 1990. (See [ITAL]Federal Register[ITAL] 56 FR 15006 dated April 12, 1991.)

B - Follow-up Care

Follow-up care or retransplantation (ICD-9-M 996.82, Complications of Transplanted Organ, Liver required as a result of a covered liver transplant is covered, provided such services are otherwise reasonable and necessary. Follow-up care is also covered for patients who have been discharged from a hospital after receiving noncovered liver transplant. Coverage for follow-up care is for items and services that are reasonable and necessary as determined by Medicare guidelines.

C - Immunosuppressive Drugs

See the Medicare Benefit Policy Manual, Chapter 15, "Covered Medical and Other Health Services," §50.5.1 and the Medicare Claims Processing Manual, Chapter 17, "Drugs and Biologicals," §80.3.

Pub. 100-3, Section 260.2

Pediatric Liver Transplantation

Effective for services performed on or after February 9, 1984, liver transplantation is covered for children (under age 18) with extrahepatic biliary atresia or any other form of end stage liver disease, except that coverage is not provided for children with a malignancy extending beyond the margins of the liver or those with persistent viremia.

Effective for services performed on or after April 12, 1991, liver transplantation is covered for Medicare beneficiaries when performed in a pediatric hospital that performs pediatric liver transplants if the hospital submits an application which CMS approves documenting that:

The hospital's pediatric liver transplant program is operated jointly by the hospital and another facility that has been found by CMS to meet the institutional coverage criteria in the Federal Register notice of April 12, 1991;

The unified program shares the same transplant surgeons and quality assurance program (including oversight committee, patient protocol, and patient selection criteria); and:

The hospital is able to provide the specialized facilities, services, and personnel that are required by pediatric liver transplant patients.

Pub. 100-3, Section 260.3

Pancreas Transplants

B. National Covered Indications

CMS determines that whole organ pancreas transplantation will be nationally covered by Medicare only when performed siumltaneous with or after a kidney transplant. If the pancreas transplant occurs after the kidney transplant, immunosuppressive therapy will begin with the date of discharge from the inpatient stay for the pancrease transplant.

C. Nationally Noncovered Indications

CMS determines that the following procedures are not considered reasonable and necessary within the meaning of section 1862(a)(1)(A) of the Social Security Act:

1. Pancreas transplantation for diabetic patients who have not experienced end stage renal failure secondary to diabetes.

2. Transplantation of partial pancreatic tissue or islet cells (except in the context of a clinical trial (see section 260.3.1 of the NCD Manual)).

D. Other

Not applicable

(This NCD last reviewed July 2004.)

Pub. 100-3, Section 260.7

Lymphocyte Immune Globulin, Anti-Thymocyte Globulin (Equine)

The FDA has approved one lymphocyte immune globulin preparation for marketing, lymphocyte immune globulin, anti-thymocyte globulin (equine). This drug is indicated for the management of allograft rejection episodes in renal transplantation. It is covered under Medicare when used for this purpose. Other forms of lymphocyte globulin preparation which the FDA approves for this indication in the future may be covered under Medicare.

Pub. 100-3, Section 260.9

Heart Transplants

A. General. — Cardiac transplantation is covered under Medicare when performed in a facility which is approved by Medicare as meeting institutional coverage criteria. (See HCFA Ruling 87-1.)

B. Exceptions. — In certain limited cases, exceptions to the criteria may be warranted if there is justification and if the facility ensures our objectives of safety and efficacy. Under no circumstances will exceptions be made for facilities whose transplant programs have been in existence for less than two years, and applications from consortia will not be approved.Although consortium arrangements will not be approved for payment of Medicare heart transplants, consideration will be given to applications from heart transplant facilities that consist of more than one hospital where all of the following conditions exist:

The hospitals are under the common control or have a formal affiliation arrangement with each other under the auspices of an organization such as a university or a legally-constituted medical research institute; and

The hospitals share resources by routinely using the same personnel or services in their transplant programs. The sharing of resources must be supported by the submission of operative notes or other information that documents the routine use of the same personnel and services in all of the individual hospitals. At a minimum, shared resources means:- The individual members of the transplant team, consisting of the cardiac transplant surgeons, cardiologists and pathologists, must practice in all the hospitals and it can be documented that they otherwise function as members of the transplant team; and- The same organ procurement organization, immunology, and tissue-typing services must be used by all the hospitals; and:

The hospitals submit, in the manner required (Kaplan-Meier method) their individual and pooled experience and survival data; and

The hospitals otherwise meet the remaining Medicare criteria for heart transplant facilities; that is, the criteria regarding patient selection, patient management, program commitment, etc.

C. Pediatric Hospitals. — Cardiac transplantation is covered for Medicare beneficiaries when performed in a pediatric hospital that performs pediatric heart transplants if the hospital submits an application which HCFA approves as documenting that:

The hospital's pediatric heart transplant program is operated jointly by the hospital and another facility that has been found by HCFA to meet the institutional coverage criteria in HCFA Ruling 87-1;

The unified program shares the same transplant surgeons and quality assurance program (including oversight committee, patient protocol, and patient selection criteria); and:

The hospital is able to provide the specialized facilities, services, and personnel that are required by pediatric heart transplant patients.

D. Follow-up Care. —

Follow-up care required as a result of a covered heart transplant is covered, provided such services are otherwise reasonable and necessary. Follow-up care is also covered for patients who have been discharged from a hospital after receiving a noncovered heart transplant. Coverage for follow-up care would be for items and services that are reasonable and necessary, as determined by Medicare guidelines. (See Medicare Benefit Policy Manual, chapter 16, "General Exclusions from Coverage," §180.)

E. Immunosuppressive Drugs.

See the Medicare Claims Processing Manual, Chapter 17, "Drugs and Biologicals," §80.3.1, and Chapter 8, "Outpatient ESRD Hospital, Independent Facility, and Physician/Supplier Claims," §120.1.

F. Artificial Hearts

Medicare does not cover the use of artificial hearts as a permanent replacement for a human heart or as a temporary life-support system until a human heart becomes available for transplant (often referred to as a "bridge to transplant"). Medicare does cover a ventricular assist device (VAD) when used in conjunction with specific criteria listed in §20.9 of the NCD Manual.

Pub. 100-3, Section 270.1

Electrical Stimulation (ES) and Electromagnetic Therapy for the Treatment of Wounds

A. Nationally Covered Indications

The use of ES and electromagnetic therapy for the treatment of wounds are considered adjunctive therapies, and will only be covered for chronic Stage III or Stage IV pressure ulcers, arterial ulcers, diabetic ulcers, and venous stasis ulcers. Chronic ulcers are defined as ulcers that have not healed within 30 days of occurrence. ES or electromagnetic therapy will be covered only after appropriate standard wound therapy has been tried for at least 30 days and there are no measurable signs of improved healing. This 30-day period may begin while the wound is acute.

Standard wound care includes: optimization of nutritional status, debridement by any means to remove devitalized tissue, maintenance of a clean, moist bed of granulation tissue with appropriate moist dressings, and necessary treatment to resolve any infection that may be present. Standard wound care based on the specific type of wound includes: frequent repositioning of a patient with pressure ulcers (usually every 2 hours), offloading of pressure and good glucose control for diabetic ulcers, establishment of adequate circulation for arterial ulcers, and the use of a compression system for patients with venous ulcers.

Measurable signs of improved healing include: a decrease in wound size (either surface area or volume), decrease in amount of exudates, and decrease in amount of necrotic tissue. ES or electromagnetic therapy must be discontinued when the wound demonstrates 100% epithelilized wound bed.

ES and electromagnetic therapy services can only be covered when performed by a physician, physical therapist, or incident to a physician service. Evaluation of the wound is an integral part of wound therapy. When a physician, physical therapist, or a clinician incident to a physician, performs ES or electromagnetic therapy, the practitioner must evaluate the wound and contact the treating physician if the wound worsens. If ES or electromagnetic therapy is being used, wounds must be evaluated at least monthly by the treating physician.

B. Nationally Noncovered Indications

1. ES and electromagnetic therapy will not be covered as an initial treatment modality.

2. Continued treatment with ES or electromagnetic therapy is not covered if measurable signs of healing have not been demonstrated within any 30-day period of treatment.

3. Unsupervised use of ES or electromagnetic therapy for wound therapy will not be covered, as this use has not been found to be medically reasonable and necessary.C. Other

All other uses of ES and electromagnetic therapy not otherwise specified for the treatment of wounds remain at local contractor discretion.

(This NCD last reviewed March 2004.)

Pub. 100-3, Section 270.2

Noncontact Normothermic Wound Therapy (NNWT)

There is insufficient scientific or clinical evidence to consider this device as reasonable and necessary for the treatment of wounds within the meaning of §1862(a)(1)(A) of the Social Security Act and will not be covered by Medicare.

Pub. 100-3, Section 270.4

Treatment of Decubitus Ulcers

Hydrotherapy (whirlpool) treatment for decubitus ulcers is a covered service under Medicare for patients when treatment is reasonable and necessary.

Some other methods of treating decubitus ulcers, the safety and effectiveness of which have not been established, are not covered under the Medicare program. Some examples of these types of treatments are: ultraviolet light, low intensity direct current, topical application of oxygen, and topical dressings with Balsam of Peru in castor oil.

Pub. 100-3, Section 270.5

Porcine Skin and Gradient Pressure Dressings

Porcine (pig) skin dressings are covered, if reasonable and necessary for the individual patient as an occlusive dressing for burns, donor sites of a homograft, and decubiti and other ulcers.

Gradient pressure dressings are Jobst elasticized heavy duty dressings used to reduce hypertrophic scarring and joint contractures following burn injury. They are covered when used for that purpose.

Pub. 100-3, Section 280.13

Transcutaneous Electrical Nerve Stimulators (TENS)

Payment for TENS may be made under the durable medical equipment benefit.

Pub. 100-3, Section 280.14

Infusion Pumps

B. Nationally Covered Indications

The following indications for treatment using infusion pumps are covered under Medicare:

1. External Infusion Pumps

a. Iron Poisoning (Effective for Services Performed On or After September 26, 1984)When used in the administration of deferoxamine for the treatment of acute iron poisoning and iron overload, only external infusion pumps are covered.

b. Thromboembolic Disease (Effective for Services Performed On or After September 26, 1984)When used in the administration of heparin for the treatment of thromboembolic disease and/or pulmonary embolism, only external infusion pumps used in an institutional setting are covered.

c. Chemotherapy for Liver Cancer (Effective for Services Performed On or After January 29, 1985)The external chemotherapy infusion pump is covered when used in the treatment of primary hepatocellular carcinoma or colorectal cancer where this disease is unresectable; OR, where the patient refuses surgical excision of the tumor.

d. Morphine for Intractable Cancer Pain (Effective for Services Performed On or After April 22, 1985)Morphine infusion via an external infusion pump is covered when used in the treatment of intractable pain caused by cancer (in either an inpatient or outpatient setting, including a hospice).

e. Continuous Subcutaneous Insulin Infusion (CSII) Pumps (Effective for Services Performed On or after December 17, 2004)Continuous subcutaneous insulin infusion (CSII) and related drugs/supplies are covered as medically reasonable and necessary in the home setting for the treatment of diabetic patients who: (1) either meet the updated fasting C-Peptide testing requirement, or, are beta cell autoantibody positive; and, (2) satisfy the remaining criteria for insulin pump therapy as described below. Patients must meet either Criterion A or B as follows:Criterion A: The patient has completed a comprehensive diabetes education program, and has been on a program of multiple daily injections of insulin (i.e., at least 3 injections per day), with frequent self-adjustments of insulin doses for at least 6 months prior to initiation of the insulin pump, and has documented frequency of glucose self-testing an average of at least 4 times per day during the 2 months prior to initiation of the insulin pump, and meets one or more of the following criteria while on the multiple daily injection regimen:

- Glycosylated hemoglobin level (HbAlc) > 7.0 percent;

- History of recurring hypoglycemia;

- Wide fluctuations in blood glucose before mealtime;

- Dawn phenomenon with fasting blood sugars frequently exceeding 200 mg/dl; or,

- History of severe glycemic excursions.

Criterion B: The patient with diabetes has been on a pump prior to enrollment in Medicare and has documented frequency of glucose self-testing an average of at least 4 times per day during the month prior to Medicare enrollment.

General CSII Criteria

In addition to meeting Criterion A or B above, the following general requirements must be met:

The patient with diabetes must be insulinopenic per the updated fasting C-peptide testing requirement, or, as an alternative, must be beta cell autoantibody positive.

Updated fasting C-peptide testing requirement:

- Insulinopenia is defined as a fasting C-peptide level that is less than or equal to 110% of the lower limit of normal of the laboratory's measurement method.

- For patients with renal insufficiency and creatinine clearance (actual or calculated from age, gender, weight, and serum creatinine) <50 ml/minute, insulinopenia is defined as a fasting C-peptide level that is less than or equal to 200% of the lower limit of normal of the laboratory's measurement method.

- Fasting C-peptide levels will only be considered valid with a concurrently obtained fasting glucose <225 mg/dL.

- Levels only need to be documented once in the medical records.

Continued coverage of the insulin pump would require that the patient be seen and evaluated by the treating physician at least every 3 months.

The pump must be ordered by and follow-up care of the patient must be managed by a physician who manages multiple patients with CSII and who works closely with a team including nurses, diabetes educators, and dietitians who are knowledgeable in the use of CSII.

Other Uses of CSII

The CMS will continue to allow coverage of all other uses of CSII in accordance with the Category B investigational device exemption (IDE) clinical trials regulation (42 CFR 405.201) or as a routine cost under the clinical trials policy (Medicare National Coverage Determinations (NCD) Manual 310.1).

f. Other Uses -- Other uses of external infusion pumps are covered if the contractor's medical staff verifies the appropriateness of the therapy and the prescribed pump for the individual patient.

NOTE: Payment may also be made for drugs necessary for the effective use of a covered external infusion pump as long as the drug being used with the pump is itself reasonable and necessary for the patient's treatment.

2. Implantable Infusion Pumps

a. Chemotherapy for Liver Cancer (Effective for Services Performed On or After September 26, 1984)

The implantable infusion pump is covered for intra-arterial infusion of 5-FUdR for the treatment of liver cancer for patients with primary hepatocellular carcinoma or Duke's Class D colorectal cancer, in whom the metastases are limited to the liver, and where: (1) the disease is unresectable, or (2) the patient refuses surgical excision of the tumor.

b. Anti-Spasmodic Drugs for Severe Spasticity

An implantable infusion pump is covered when used to administer anti-spasmodic drugs intrathecally (e.g., baclofen) to treat chronic intractable spasticity in patients who have proven unresponsive to less invasive medical therapy as determined by the following criteria:

- As indicated by at least a 6-week trial, the patient cannot be maintained on noninvasive methods of spasm control, such as oral anti-spasmodic drugs, either because these methods fail to control adequately the spasticity or produce intolerable side effects, and prior to pump implantation, the patient must have responded favorably to a trial intrathecal dose of the anti-spasmodic drug.

c. Opioid Drugs for Treatment of Chronic Intractable Pain

An implantable infusion pump is covered when used to administer opioid drugs (e.g., morphine) intrathecally or epidurally for treatment of severe chronic intractable pain of malignant or nonmalignant origin in patients who have a life expectancy of at least 3 months, and who have proven unresponsive to less invasive medical therapy as determined by the following criteria:

- The patient's history must indicate that he/she would not respond adequately to noninvasive methods of pain control, such as systemic opioids (including attempts to eliminate physical and behavioral abnormalities which may cause an exaggerated reaction to pain); and a preliminary trial of intraspinal opioid drug administration must be undertaken with a temporary intrathecal/epidural catheter to substantiate adequately acceptable pain relief and degree of side effects (including effects on the activities of daily living) and patient acceptance.

d. Coverage of Other Uses of Implanted Infusion Pumps

Determinations may be made on coverage of other uses of implanted infusion pumps if the contractor's medical staff verifies that:

- The drug is reasonable and necessary for the treatment of the individual patient;

- It is medically necessary that the drug be administered by an implanted infusion pump; and,

- The Food and Drug Administration (FDA)-approved labeling for the pump must specify that the drug being administered and the purpose for which it is administered is an indicated use for the pump.

e. Implantation of Infusion Pump Is ContraindicatedThe implantation of an infusion pump is contraindicated in the following patients:

- With a known allergy or hypersensitivity to the drug being used (e.g., oral baclofen, morphine, etc.);

- Who have an infection;

- Whose body size is insufficient to support the weight and bulk of the device; and,

- With other implanted programmable devices since crosstalk between devices may inadvertently change the prescription.NOTE: Payment may also be made for drugs necessary for the effective use of an implantable infusion pump as long as the drug being used with the pump is itself reasonable and necessary for the patient's treatment.

C. Nationally Noncovered Indications

The following indications for treatment using infusion pumps are not covered under Medicare:

1. External Infusion Pumps

a. Vancomycin (Effective for Services Beginning On or After September 1, 1996)

Medicare coverage of vancomycin as a durable medical equipment infusion pump benefit is not covered. There is insufficient evidence to support the necessity of using an external infusion pump, instead of a disposable elastomeric pump or the gravity drip method, to administer vancomycin in a safe and appropriate manner.

2. Implantable Infusion Pump

a. Thromboembolic Disease (Effective for Services Performed On or After September 26, 1984)

According to the Public Health Service, there is insufficient published clinical data to support the safety and effectiveness of the heparin implantable pump. Therefore, the use of an implantable infusion pump for infusion of heparin in the treatment of recurrent thromboembolic disease is not covered.

b. Diabetes

An implanted infusion pump for the infusion of insulin to treat diabetes is not covered. The data does not demonstrate that the pump provides effective administration of insulin.

D. Other

Not applicable.

(This NCD last reviewed January 2005.)

Pub. 100-3, Section 300.1

Obsolete or Unreliable Diagnostic Tests

Indications and Limitations of Coverage

CIM 50-34

A. Diagnostic Tests -- Do not routinely pay for the following diagnostic tests because they are obsolete and have been replaced by more advanced procedures. The listed tests may be paid for only if the medical need for the procedure is satisfactorily justified by the physician who performs it. When the services are subject to the Quality Improvement Organization (QIO) Review, the QIO is responsible for determining that satisfactory medical justification exists. When the services are not subject to QIO review, the intermediary or carrier is responsible for determining that satisfactory medical justification exists. This includes:

- Amylase, blood isoenzymes, electrophoretic,

- Chromium, blood,

- Guanase, blood,

- Zinc sulphate turbidity, blood,

- Skin test, cat scratch fever,

- Skin test, lymphopathia venereum,

- Circulation time, one test,

- Cephalin flocculation,

- Congo red, blood,

- Hormones, adrenocorticotropin quantitative animal tests,

- Hormones, adrenocorticotropin quantitative bioassay,

- Thymol turbidity, blood,

- Skin test, actinomycosis,

- Skin test, brucellosis,

- Skin test, psittacosis,

- Skin test, trichinosis,

- Calcium, feces, 24-hour quantitative,

- Starch, feces, screening,

- Chymotrypsin, duodenal contents,

- Gastric analysis, pepsin,

- Gastric analysis, tubeless,

- Calcium saturation clotting time,

- Capillary fragility test (Rumpel-Leede),

- Colloidal gold,

- Bendien's test for cancer and tuberculosis,

- Bolen's test for cancer,

- Rehfuss test for gastric acidity, and

- Serum seromucoid assay for cancer and other diseases.

B. Cardiovascular Tests -- Do not pay for the following phonocardiography and vectorcardiography diagnostic tests because they have been determined to be outmoded and of little clinical value. They include:

Phonocardiogram with or without ECG lead; with supervision during recording with interpretation and report (when equipment is supplied by the physician),

- Phonocardiogram; tracing only, without interpretation and report (e.g., when equipment is supplied by the hospital, clinic),

- Phonocardiogram; interpretation and report,

- Phonocardiogram with ECG lead, with indirect carotid artery and/or jugular vein tracing, and/or apex cardiogram; with interpretation and report,

- Phonocardiogram; without interpretation and report,

- Phonocardiogram; interpretation and report only, Intracardiac,

- Vectorcardiogram (VCG), with or without ECG; with interpretation and report,

- Vectorcardiogram; tracing only, without interpretation and report, and

- Vectorcardiogram; interpretation and report only.

Transmittal Number48

Transmittal Link -- http://www.cms.hhs.gov/transmittals/downloads/R48NCD.pdf

Revision History -- 04/01/1997 - Excluded coverage of 10 phonocardiography and vectorcardiography diagnostic tests. Effective 1/1/1997. (TN 96)03/2006 - Delete coding information. Effective/Implementation date: 06/19/2006. (TN 48) (CR4278)Other VersionsObsolete or Unreliable Diagnostic Tests - Version 1, Effective between 01/01/1997 - 06/19/2006

Pub. 100-4, Chapter 1, Section 30.3.5

Effect of Assignment Upon Purchase of Cataract Glasses From Participating Physician or Supplier on Claims Submitted to Carriers

B3-3045.4

A pair of cataract glasses is comprised of two distinct products: a professional product (the prescribed lenses) and a retail commercial product (the frames). The frames serve not only as a holder of lenses but also as an article of personal apparel. As such, they are usually selected on the basis of personal taste and style. Although Medicare will pay only for standard frames, most patients want deluxe frames. Participating physicians and suppliers cannot profitably furnish such deluxe frames unless they can make an extra (noncovered) charge for the frames even though they accept assignment.

Therefore, a participating physician or supplier (whether an ophthalmologist, optometrist, or optician) who accepts assignment on cataract glasses with deluxe frames may charge the Medicare patient the difference between his/her usual charge to private pay patients for glasses with standard frames and his/her usual charge to such patients for glasses with deluxe frames, in addition to the applicable deductible and coinsurance on glasses with standard frames, if all of the following requirements are met:

A. The participating physician or supplier has standard frames available, offers them for sale to the patient, and issues and ABN to the patient that explains the price and other differences between standard and deluxe frames. Refer to Chapter 30.

B. The participating physician or supplier obtains from the patient (or his/her representative) and keeps on file the following signed and dated statement:

_____

Name of Patient Medicare Claim Number

Having been informed that an extra charge is being made by the physician or supplier for deluxe frames, that this extra charge is not covered by Medicare, and that standard frames are available for purchase from the physician or supplier at no extra charge, I have chosen to purchase deluxe frames. _____ Signature Date

C. The participating physician or supplier itemizes on his/her claim his/her actual charge for the lenses, his/her actual charge for the standard frames, and his/her actual extra charge for the deluxe frames (charge differential).

Once the assigned claim for deluxe frames has been processed, the carrier will follow the ABN instructions as described in §60.

Pub. 100-4, Chapter 1, Section 60.4.5

Clarification of Liability for Preventive Screening Benefits Subject to Frequency Limits

Some Medicare preventive benefits are subject to frequency limits, and are also specifically cited at §1862 (a)(1) (F) ff. of the Act as subject to "medical necessity." There has been some confusion as to the basis of denial and how such services are adjudicated. When medical necessity is the basis for denial (i.e., §1862 (a)(1) (F) ff. of the Act), a ABN is necessary in order to shift the liability to the beneficiary, and special ABN-related billing must be used (see III. E. above). Services above frequency limits, however, had been erroneously considered noncovered services by some, and billed as such, not requiring ABNs. In these cases default liability in Medicare systems is the provider, unless specific billing methods and modifiers were used to signal beneficiary liability (see sections III A. and B. above).

Medicare FIs systems had been programmed with frequency as the primary reason for denial at one time, and Medicare carrier systems have used medical necessity. FI systems have changed so that medical necessity is the primary reason for denial.

It may be contrary to provider practices to submit services over the frequency limit as covered charges, as ABN billing requires. However, it can be pointed out that existing Common Working

File (CWF) frequency edits should still result in the denial of these services. Remittance denial reason codes and MSN messages to be used in this situation are listed below for beneficiary and provider liability should either circumstance occur:

TABLE 10:

Preventive Benefit	HCPCS Code(s)	PROVIDER LIABLE (ANSI)			
Remittance Group and Reason Code		PROVIDER LIABLE MSN			
Message		BENE. LIABLE			
ANSI) Remittance Group and Reason Code		BENE. LIABLE MSN			
Message					
Screening mammography	G0202, 76092, 76083	CO – 57 [57: Payment denied/reduced because the payer deems the information submitted does not support this level of service, this many services, this length of service, this dosage, or this day's supply.]	15. 21 The information provided does not support the need for this many services or items in this period of time but you do not have to pay this amount. [Le informacion proporcionada no justifica la necesidad do esta cantidad de servicios o articulos an este periodo de tiempo pero usted no tiene que pagar esta cantidad.]	PR – 57*[57: Payment denied/reduced because the payer deems the information submitted does not support this level of service, this many services, this length of service, this dosage, or this day's supply.]	15. 22 The information provided does not support the need for this many services or items in this period of time so Medicare will not pay for this item or service. [Le informacion proporcionada no justifica la necesidad do esta cantidad de servicios o articulos an este periodo de tiempo por lo cual Medicare no pagara por este articulo o servicio.]
Screening pap smear	G0123, G0143, G0144, G0145, G0147, G0148, P3000, Q0091	CO - 57	Ditto above	PR – 57*	Ditto above
Screening pelvic exam	G0101	CO - 57	Ditto above	PR – 57*	Ditto above
Screening glaucoma	G0117, G0118	CO - 57	Ditto above	PR – 57*	Ditto above
Prostate cancer screening test	G0102, G0103	CO - 57	Ditto above	PR – 57*	Ditto above
Colorectal cancer screening test	G0104, G0106, G0107, G0120, G0122	CO - 57	Ditto above	PR – 57*	Ditto above

- This ANSI ASC X12 reason code becomes obsolete with implementation of the 835 remittance version 4050. For the purpose of this table, use of 57 in the 835 version 4050 and subsequent versions can be crosswalked to code 151: "Payment adjusted because the payer deems the information submitted does not support this many services".

Pub. 100-4, Chapter 3, Section 10.4

Payment of Nonphysician Services for Inpatients

HO-407

All items and nonphysician services furnished to inpatients must be furnished directly by the hospital or billed through the hospital under arrangements. This provision applies to all hospitals, regardless of whether they are subject to PPS.

A. Other Medical Items, Supplies, and Services

The following medical items, supplies, and services furnished to inpatients are covered under Part A. Consequently, they are covered by the prospective payment rate or reimbursed as reasonable costs under Part A to hospitals excluded from PPS.

- Laboratory services (excluding anatomic pathology services and certain clinical pathology services);

- Pacemakers and other prosthetic devices including lenses, and artificial limbs, knees, and hips;

- Radiology services including computed tomography (CT) scans furnished to inpatients by a physician's office, other hospital, or radiology clinic;

- Total parenteral nutrition (TPN) services; and

- Transportation, including transportation by ambulance, to and from another hospital or freestanding facility to receive specialized diagnostic or therapeutic services not available at the facility where the patient is an inpatient.

The hospital must include the cost of these services in the appropriate ancillary service cost center, i.e., in the cost of the diagnostic or therapeutic service. It must not show them separately under revenue code 0540.

EXCEPTIONS:

- Pneumococcal Vaccine - is payable under Part B only and is billed by the hospital on the Form CMS-1450.

- Ambulance Service - For purposes of this section "hospital inpatient" means a beneficiary who has been formally admitted it does not include a beneficiary who is in the process of being transferred from one hospital to another. Where the patient is transferred from one hospital to another, and is admitted as an inpatient to the second, the ambulance service is payable under only Part B. If transportation is by a hospital owned and operated ambulance, the hospital bills separately on Form CMS-1450 as appropriate. Similarly, if the hospital arranges for the ambulance transportation with an ambulance operator, including paying the ambulance operator, it bills separately. However, if the hospital does not assume any financial responsibility, the billing is to the carrier by the ambulance operator or beneficiary, as appropriate, if an ambulance is used for the transportation of a hospital inpatient to another facility for diagnostic tests or special treatment

the ambulance trip is considered part of the DRG, and not separately billable, if the resident hospital is under PPS.

- Part B Inpatient Services - Where Part A benefits are not payable, payment may be made to the hospital under Part B for certain medical and other health services. See Chapter 4 for a description of Part B inpatient services

- Anesthetist Services "Incident to" Physician Services - If a physician's practice was to employ anesthetists and to bill on a reasonable charge basis for these services and that practice was in effect as of the last day of the hospital's most recent 12-month cost reporting period ending before September 30, 1983, the physician may continue that practice through cost reporting periods beginning October 1, 1984. However, if the physician chooses to continue this practice, the hospital may not add costs of the anesthetist's service to its base period costs for purposes of its transition payment rates. If it is the existing or new practice of the physician to employ certified registered nurse anesthetists (CRNAs) and other qualified anesthetists and include charges for their services in the physician bills for anesthesiology services for the hospital's cost report periods beginning on or after October 1, 1984, and before October 1, 1987, the physician may continue to do so.

B. Exceptions/Waivers

These provisions were waived before cost reporting periods beginning on or after October 1, 1986, under certain circumstances. The basic criteria for waiver was that services furnished by outside suppliers are so extensive that a sudden change in billing practices would threaten the stability of patient care. Specific criteria for waiver and processing procedures are in §2804 of the Provider Reimbursement Manual (CMS Pub. 15-1).

Pub. 100-4, Chapter 3, Section 20

Payment Under Prospective Payment System (PPS) Diagnosis Related Groups (DRGs)

A. General

The Social Security Amendments of 1983 (P.L. 98-21) provided for establishment of a prospective payment system (PPS) for Medicare payment of inpatient hospital services. (See §20.4 for corresponding information for PPS capital payments and computation of capital and operating outliers for FY 1992.) Under PPS, hospitals are paid a predetermined rate per discharge for inpatient hospital services furnished to Medicare beneficiaries. Each type of Medicare discharge is classified according to a list of DRGs. These amounts are, with certain exceptions, payment in full to the hospital for inpatient operating costs. Beneficiary cost-sharing is limited to statutory deductibles, coinsurance, and payment for noncovered items and services. Section 4003 of OBRA of 1990 (P.L. 101-508) expands the definition of inpatient operating costs to include certain preadmission services. (See §40.3.)

The statute excludes children's hospitals and cancer hospitals, hospitals located outside the 50 States. In addition to these categorical exclusions, the statute provides other special exclusions, such as hospitals that are covered under State reimbursement control systems. These excluded hospitals and units are paid on the

basis of reasonable costs subject to the target rate of increase limits.

In accordance with Section 1814 (b) (3) of the Act, services provided by hospitals in Maryland subject to the Health Services Cost Review Commission (provider numbers 21000-21099) are paid according to the terms of the waiver, that is 94% of submitted charges subject to any unmet Part B deductible and coinsurance.

For discharges occurring on or after April 1, 1988, separate standardized payment amounts are established for large urban areas and rural areas. Large urban areas are urban areas with populations of more than 1,000,000 as determined by the Secretary of HHS on the basis of the most recent census population data. In addition, any New England County Metropolitan Area (NECMA) with a population of more than 970,000 is a large urban area.

The OBRA 1987 required payment of capital costs under PPS effective with cost reporting periods that began October 1, 1991, or later. A 10-year transition period was provided to protect hospitals that had incurred capital obligations in excess of the standardized national rate from major disruption. High capital cost hospitals are known as "hold harmless" hospitals. The transition period also provides for phase-in of the national Federal capital payment rate for hospitals with capital obligations that are less than the national rate. New hospitals that open during the transition period are exempt from capital PPS payment for their first 2 years of operation. Hospitals and hospital distinct part units that are excluded from PPS for operating costs are also excluded from PPS for capital costs.

Capital payments are based on the same DRG designations and weights, outlier guidelines, geographic classifications, wage indexes, and disproportionate share percentages that apply to operating payments under PPS. The indirect teaching adjustment is based on the ratio of residents to average daily census. The hospital split bill, adjustment bill, waiver of liability and remaining guidelines that have historically been applied to operating payments also apply to capital payments under PPS.

B. Hospitals and Units Excluded

The following hospitals and distinct part hospital units (DPU) are excluded from PPS and are paid on a reasonable cost or other basis:

- Pediatric hospitals whose inpatients are predominately under the age of 18.

Hospitals located outside the 50 States.

- Hospitals participating in a CMS-approved demonstration project or State payment control system.

- Nonparticipating hospitals furnishing emergency services have not been affected by the PPS statute (P.L. 97-21). They are paid under their existing basis.

C. Situations Requiring Special Handling

1. Sole Community Hospitals are paid in accordance with the methods used to establish the operating prospective rates for the first year of the PPS transition for operating costs. The appropriate percentage of hospital-specific rate and the Federal regional rate is applied by the Pricer program in accordance with the current values for the appropriate fiscal year.

2. Hospitals have the option to continue to be reimbursed on a reasonable cost basis subject to the target ceiling rate or to be reimbursed under PPS if the following are met:

- Recognized as of April 20, 1983, by the National Cancer Institute as Comprehensive Cancer Centers or Clinical Research Centers;

- Demonstrating that the entire facility is organized primarily for treatment of, and research on, cancer; and

- Having a patient population that is at least 50 percent of the hospital's total discharges with a principal diagnosis of neoplastic disease.

The hospital makes this decision at the beginning of its fiscal year. The choice continues until the hospital requests a change. If it selects reasonable cost subject to the target ceiling, it can later request PPS. No further option is allowed.

3. Regional and national referral centers within short-term acute care hospital complexes. Rural hospitals that meet the criteria have their prospective rate determined on the basis of the urban, rather than the rural, adjusted standardized amounts, as adjusted by the applicable DRG weighting factor and the hospital's area wage index.

4. Hospitals in Alaska and Hawaii have the nonlabor related portion of the wage index adjusted by their appropriate cost-of-living factor. These calculations are made by the Pricer program and are included in the Federal portion of the rate.

5. Kidney, heart, and liver acquisition costs incurred by approved transplant centers are treated as an adjustment to the hospital's payments. These payments are adjusted in each cost reporting period to compensate for the reasonable expenses of the acquisition and are not included in determining prospective payment.

6. Religious Nonmedical Health Care Institutions are paid on the basis of a predetermined fixed amount per discharge. Payment is based on the historical inpatient operating costs per discharge and is not calculated by "Pricer."

7. Transferring hospitals with discharges assigned to DRG 385 (Neonates, Died or Transferred) or DRG 504-511 (burns, transferred to another acute care facility) have their payments calculated by the Pricer program on the same basis as those receiving the full prospective payment. They are also eligible for cost outliers.

8. Nonparticipating hospitals furnishing emergency services are not included in PPS.

9. Veterans Administration (VA) Hospitals are generally excluded from participation. Where payments are made for Medicare patients, the payments are determined in accordance with 38 U.S.C. 5053(d).

10. A hospital that loses its urban area status as a result of the Executive Office of Management and Budget redesignation occurring after April 20, 1983, may qualify for special consideration by having its rural Federal rate phased-in over a 2-year period. The hospital will receive, in addition to its rural Federal rate in the first cost reporting period, two-thirds of the difference between its rural Federal rate and the urban Federal rate that would have been paid had it retained its urban status. In the second reporting period, one-third of the difference is applied. The adjustment is applied for two successive cost reporting periods beginning with the cost-reporting period in which CMS recognizes the reclassification.

11. The payment per discharge under the PPS for hospitals in Puerto Rico is the sum of:

- 50 percent of the Puerto Rico discharge weighted urban or rural standardized rate.

- 50 percent of the national discharge weighted standardized rate.

(The special treatment of referral centers and sole community hospitals does not apply to prospective payment hospitals in Puerto Rico.)

There are special criteria that facilities must meet in order to obtain approval for payment for heart transplants and special processing procedures for these bills. (See §90.2.) Facilities that wish to obtain coverage of heart transplants for their Medicare patients must submit an application and documentation showing their initial and ongoing compliance with the criteria. For facilities that are approved, Medicare covers under Part A all medically reasonable and necessary inpatient services.

12. Hospitals with high percentage of ESRD discharges may qualify for additional payment. These payments are handled as adjustments to cost reports.

13. Exception payments are provided for hospitals with inordinately high levels of capital obligations. They will expire at the end of the 10-year transition period. Exception payments ensure that for FY 1992 and FY 1993:

- Sole community hospitals receive 90 percent of Medicare inpatient capital costs:

- Urban hospitals with 100 or more beds and a disproportionate share patient percentage of at least 20.2 percent receive 80 percent of their Medicare inpatient capital costs; and

- All other hospitals receive 70 percent of their Medicare inpatient capital costs.

A limited capital exception payment is also provided during the 10-year capital transition period for hospitals that experience extraordinary circumstances that require an unanticipated major capital expenditure. Events such as a tornado, earthquake, catastrophic fire, or a hurricane are examples of extraordinary circumstances. The capital project must cost at least $5 million to qualify for this exception.

D. DRG Classification

The DRGs are a patient classification system which provides a means of relating types of patients a hospital treats (i.e., its case mix) to the costs incurred by the hospital. Payment for inpatient hospital services is made on the basis of a rate per discharge that varies according to the DRG to which a beneficiary's stay is assigned. All inpatient transfer/discharge bills from both PPS and non-PPS facilities, including those from waiver States, long-term care facilities, and excluded units are classified by the Grouper software program into one of 489 diagnosis related groups (DRGs).

The following DRGs receive special attention:

- DRG No. 468 - Represents a discharge with valid data but where the surgical procedure is unrelated to the principal diagnosis. This DRG has a weight assigned and will be paid. The hospital must review the record on each DRG in the remittance record and where either the principle diagnosis or surgical procedure was reported incorrectly, prepare an adjustment bill. The FI may elect to avoid the adjustment bill by returning the bill to the hospital prior to adjustment. Further, Quality Improvement Organizations (QIOs) will review all DRG 468 cases.

- DRG No. 469 - Represents a discharge with a valid diagnosis in the principle diagnosis field, but one not acceptable as a principal diagnosis. Examples include a diagnosis of diabetes mellitus or an infection of the genitourinary tract during pregnancy, both unspecified as to episode of care. These diagnoses may be valid, but they are not sufficient to determine the principal diagnosis for DRG assignment purposes. FIs will return the claims. The hospital must enter the corrected principal diagnosis for proper DRG assignment and resubmit the claim.

- DRG No. 470 - Represents a discharge with invalid data. FIs return the claims for correction of data elements affecting proper DRG assignment. The hospital resubmits the corrected claim.

When the bills are processed in conjunction with the MCE (see §20.2.1) coding inconsistencies in the information and data are identified.

The MCE must be run before Grouper to identify inconsistencies before the bills are processed through the Grouper.

E. Difference in Age/Admission Versus Discharge

HO-415.4

When a beneficiary's age changes between the date of admission and date of discharge, the DRG and related payment amount are determined from the patient's age at admission.

Pub. 100-4, Chapter 3, Section 20.1.2.8

Special Outlier Payments for Burn Cases

For discharges occurring on or after April 1, 1988, the additional payment amount for the DRGs related to burn cases, which are identified in the most recent annual notice of prospective payment rates is computed using the same methodology (as stated above in section 20.1.2.3) except that the payment is made using a marginal cost factor of 90 percent instead of 80 percent.

Pub. 100-4, Chapter 3, Section 20.2.1

Medicare Code Editor (MCE)

A3-3656.1, HO-417.1

A. General

The MCE edits claims to detect incorrect billing data. In determining the appropriate DRG for a Medicare patient, the age, sex, discharge status, principal diagnosis, secondary diagnosis, and procedures performed must be reported accurately to the Grouper program. The logic of the

Grouper software assumes that this information is accurate and the Grouper does not make any attempt to edit the data for accuracy. Only where extreme inconsistencies occur in the patient information will a patient not be assigned to a DRG. Therefore, the MCE is used to improve the quality of information given to Grouper.

The MCE addresses three basic types of edits which will support the DRG assignment:

Code Edits - Examines a record for the correct use of ICD-9-CM codes that describe a patient's diagnoses and procedures. They include basic consistency checks on the interrelationship among a patient's age, sex, and diagnoses and procedures.

Coverage Edits - Examines the type of patient and procedures performed to determine if the services where covered.

Clinical Edits - Examines the clinical consistency of the diagnostic and procedural information on the medical claim to determine if they are clinically reasonable and, therefore, should be paid.

B. Implementation Requirements

The FI processes all inpatient Part A discharge/transfer bills for both PPS and non-PPS facilities (including waiver States, long-term care hospitals, and excluded units) through the MCE. It processes claims that have been reviewed by the QIO prior to billing through the MCE only for edit types 1, 2, 3, 4, 7, and 12. It does not process the following kinds of bills through the MCE include:

- Where no Medicare payment is due (amounts reported by value codes 12, 13, 14, 15, or 16 equal or exceed charges).

- Where no Medicare payment is being made. Where partial payment is made, editing is required.

- Where QIO reviewed prior to billing (code C1 or C3 in FL 24-30). It may process these exceptions through the program and ignore development codes or bypass the program.

The MCE software contains multiple versions. The version of the MCE accessed by the program depends upon the patient discharge date entered on the claim.

C. Bill System/MCE Interface

The FI installs the MCE online, if possible, so that prepayment edit requirements identified in subsection C can be directed to hospitals without clerical handling.

The MCE needs the following data elements to analyze the bill:

- Age;

- Sex;

- Discharge status;

- Diagnosis (5 maximum);

- Procedures (3 maximum); and

- Discharge date.

The MCE provides the FI an analysis of "errors" on the bill as described in subsection D. The FI develops its own interface program to provide data to MCE and receive data from it.

The MCE Installation Manual describes the installation and operation of the program, including data base formats and locations.

D. Processing Requirements

The hospital must follow the procedure described below for each error code. For bills returned to the provider, the FI considers the bill improperly completed for control and processing time purposes. (See Chapter 1.)

1. Invalid Diagnosis or Procedure Code

The MCE checks each diagnosis code, including the admitting diagnosis, and each procedure code against a table of valid ICD-9-CM codes. An admitting diagnosis, a principle diagnosis, and up to eight additional diagnoses may be reported. A principle procedure code and up to five other procedure codes may be reported on an inpatient claim. If the recorded code is not in this table, the code is invalid, and the FI returns the bill to the provider.

For a list of all valid ICD-9-CM codes see "International Classification of Diseases, 9th Revision, Clinical Modification (ICD-9-CM), January 1979, Volume I (Diseases)" and "Volume 3 (Procedures)," and the "Addendum/Errata" and new codes furnished by the FI. The hospital must review the medical record and/or face sheet and enter the correct diagnosis/procedure before returning the bill.

2. Invalid Fourth or Fifth Digit

The MCE identifies any diagnosis code, including the admitting diagnosis or any procedure that requires a fourth or fifth digit, which is either missing or not valid for the code in question.

For a list of all valid fourth and fifth digit ICD-9-CM codes see "International Classification of Diseases, 9th Revision, Clinical Modification (ICD-9-CM), January 1979, Volume 1 (Diseases)" and "Volume 3 (Procedures)," and the "Addendum/Errata" and new codes furnished by the FI. The FI returns claims edited for this reason to the hospital. The hospital must review the medical record and/or face sheet and enter the correct diagnosis/procedure before returning the bill.

3. E-Code as Principal Diagnosis

E-codes describe the circumstances that caused an injury, not the nature of the injury, and therefore are not principal diagnoses. E-codes are all ICD-9-CM diagnosis codes that begin with the letter E. For a list of all E-codes, see "International Classification of Diseases, 9th Revision, Clinical Modification (ICD-9-CM), January 1979, Volume I (Diseases)." The hospital must review the medical record and/or face sheet and enter the correct diagnosis before returning the bill.

4. Duplicate of PDX

Any secondary diagnosis that is the same code as the principal diagnosis is identified as a duplicate of the principal diagnoses, because the secondary diagnosis may cause assignment to a complication/co-morbidity DRG in error. Hospitals may not repeat a diagnosis. The FI will delete the duplicate secondary diagnosis and process the bill.

5. Age Conflict

The MCE detects inconsistencies between a patient's age and any diagnosis on the patient's record. Examples are:

- A 5-year-old patient with benign prostatic hypertrophy.

- A 78-year-old delivery.

In the above cases, the diagnosis is clinically impossible in a patient of the stated age. Therefore, either the diagnosis or age is presumed to be incorrect. Four age code categories are described below.

- A subset of diagnoses is intended only for newborns and neonates. These are "Newborn" diagnoses. For "Newborn" diagnoses, the patient's age must be 0 years.

- Certain diagnoses are considered reasonable only for children between the ages of 0 and 17. These are "Pediatric" diagnoses.

- Diagnoses identified as "Maternity" are coded only for patients between the ages of 12 and 55 years.

- A subset of diagnoses is considered valid only for patients over the age of 14. These are "Adult" diagnoses. For "Adult" diagnoses the age range is 15 through 124.

The diagnoses described in Addendum E, pages E-2-17 are acceptable only for the age categories shown. If the FI edits online, it will return such bills for a proper diagnosis or correction of age as applicable. If the FI edits in batch operations after receipt of the admission query response, it uses the age based on CMS records and returns bills that fail this edit. The hospital must review the medical record and/or face sheet and enter the proper diagnosis before returning the bill.

6. Sex Conflict

The MCE detects inconsistencies between a patient's sex and a diagnosis or procedure on the patient's record. Examples are:

- Male patient with cervical cancer (diagnosis).

- Male patient with a hysterectomy (procedure).

In both instances, the indicated diagnosis or the procedure conflicts with the stated sex of the patient. Therefore, either the patient's diagnosis, procedure or sex is incorrect.

Addendum E, pages E-18-38 contain listings of male and female related ICD-9-CM diagnosis and procedure codes and the corresponding English descriptions. The hospital should review the medical record and/or face sheet and enter the proper sex, diagnosis, and procedure before returning the bill.

7. Manifestation Code As Principal Diagnosis

A manifestation code describes the manifestation of an underlying disease, not the disease itself, and therefore, cannot be a principal diagnosis. Addendum E, pages E-39-41 contain listings of ICD-9-CM diagnoses identified as manifestation codes. The hospital should review the medical record and/or face sheet and enter the proper diagnosis before returning the bill.

8. Nonspecific Principal Diagnosis

A set of diagnosis codes, particularly those described as "not otherwise specified," are identified by the MCE as nonspecific diagnoses. While these codes are valid according to the ICD-9-CM coding scheme, more precise codes must be used for the principal diagnosis.

The edit is performed only if the patient was discharged alive. Deceased patients often do not receive a complete diagnostic workup, thus, the specification of precise principal diagnosis may not be possible.

Addendum E, pages E-42-50 contain listings of ICD-9-CM diagnosis codes identified as "nonspecific" when used as principal diagnosis.

If the hospital's coding can be processed by the Grouper program, its FI processes the bill. If not, the claim is returned for the hospital to provide a specific principal diagnoses.

If over 10 percent of a hospital's bills result in the MCE error type, its FI will contact it about improving it's coding.

9. Questionable Admission

There are some diagnoses, which are not usually sufficient justification for admission to an acute care hospital. For example, if a patient is given a principal diagnosis of:

4011 - Benign Hypertension

then this patient would have a questionable admission, since benign hypertension is not normally sufficient justification for admission.

Addendum E, page E-51 contains a listing of ICD-9-CM diagnosis codes identified as "Questionable Admission" when used as principal diagnosis.

QIOs review on a post-payment basis all questionable admission cases. Where the QIO determines the denial rate is sufficiently high to warrant, it requests the FI to refer claims for review before payment.

The FIs will not interrupt processing based upon MCE identification of questionable admission.

10. Unacceptable Principal Diagnosis

There are selected codes that describe a circumstance which influences an individual's health status but is not a current illness or injury; therefore, they are unacceptable as a principal

diagnosis. For example, VI73 (Family History of Ischemic Heart Disease) is an unacceptable principal diagnosis.

In a few cases, there are codes that are acceptable if a secondary diagnosis is coded. If no secondary diagnosis is present for them, MCE returns the message "requires secondary dx." Codes that follow this rule are indicated with an asterisk (*) in Addendum E, pages E-52-57.

The QIO reviews claims with diagnosis V571, V572, V573, V5789, and V579 and a secondary diagnosis.

If these codes are identified without a secondary diagnosis, the FI returns the bill to the hospital and requests a secondary diagnosis that describes the origin of the impairment. Also, bills containing other "unacceptable principal diagnosis" codes are returned.

The hospital reviews the medical record and/or face sheet and enters the principal diagnosis that describes the illness or injury before returning the bill.

11. Nonspecific O.R. Procedures

A set of O.R. procedure codes, particularly those described as "not otherwise specified" are identified by the MCE as nonspecific. While these codes are valid according to the ICD-9-CM coding scheme, the hospital must use more precise codes for Medicare. For example, 8020 (Arthroscopy NOS) is identified as a nonspecific O.R. procedure because the site is not specified by the code. Codes 8021-8029 specify the precise site.

MCE reports the nonspecific O.R. procedure condition only if all the O.R. procedures performed have been coded as nonspecific.

If the hospital's coding can be processed by the Grouper program, the FI processes the bill. If not, the FI returns the bill for the hospital to provide a specific O.R. procedure code.

The FI counts monthly by provider for this exception. If over 10 percent of a hospital's bills result in the MCE error type, it contacts the hospital about improving it's coding.

12. Noncovered O.R. Procedures

There are some O.R. procedures for which Medicare does not provide payment.

The FI will return the bill requesting either:

- A no pay bill, or

- A correction in the procedure code.

- A bill indicating the covered and noncovered procedures.

If the hospital indicates that there are covered and noncovered procedures, the FI refers the bill to the QIO for prepayment review. Upon receipt of the QIOs response, it either deletes the noncovered procedures and charges or requires the hospital to delete them. It does not process the noncovered procedures through Grouper or the noncovered charges through Pricer.

13. Open Biopsy Check

Biopsies can be performed as open (i.e., a body cavity is entered surgically), or percutaneously or endoscopically. The DRG definitions assign a patient to different DRGs depending upon whether or not the biopsy was open. In general, for most organ systems, open biopsies are performed infrequently.

Effective October 1, 1987, there are revised biopsy codes that distinguish between open and closed biopsies. To make sure that hospitals are using ICD-9-CM codes correctly, the FI requests O.R. reports on a sample of 10 percent of claims with open biopsy procedures for review on a postpayment basis.

If the O.R. report reveals that the biopsy was closed (performed percutaneously, endoscopically, etc.) the FI changes the procedure code on the bill to the closed biopsy code and processes an adjustment bill. Some biopsy codes (3328 and 5634) have two related closed biopsy codes, one for closed endoscopic and for closed percutaneous biopsies. The FI assigns the appropriate closed biopsy code after reviewing the medical information.

14. Medicare as Secondary Payer - MSP Alert

The MCE identifies situations that may involve automobile medical, no-fault or liability insurance. The hospital must develop other insurance coverage as provided in the Medicare Secondary Payer Manuals, before billing Medicare.

15. Bilateral Procedure

There are codes that do not accurately reflect performed procedures in one admission on two or more different bilateral joints of the lower extremities. A combination of these codes show a bilateral procedure when, in fact, they could be single joint procedures (i.e., duplicate procedures).

If two more of these procedures are coded, and the principal diagnosis is in MDC 8, the claim is flagged for post-pay development. The FI processes the bill as coded but requests an O.R. report. If the report substantiates bilateral surgery, no further action is necessary. If the O.R. report does not substantiate bilateral surgery, an adjustment bill is processed.

If the error rate for any provider is sufficiently high, the FI may develop claims prior to payment on a provider-specific basis.

16. Invalid Age

If the hospital reports an age over 124, the FI requests the hospital to determine if it made a bill preparation error. If the beneficiary's age is established at over 124, the hospital enters 123.

17. Invalid Sex

A patient's sex is sometimes necessary for appropriate DRG determination. Usually the FI can resolve the issue without hospital assistance. The sex code reported must be either 1 (male) or 2 (female).

18. Invalid Discharge Status

A patient's discharge status is sometimes necessary for appropriate DRG determination. Discharge status must be coded according to the Form CMS-1450 conventions. See Chapter 25.

19. Invalid Discharge Date

An invalid discharge date is a discharge date that does not fall into the acceptable range of numbers to represent, either the month, day or year (e.g., 13/03/01, 12/32/01). If no discharge date is entered, it is also invalid. MCE reports when an invalid discharge date is entered.

20 – Limited Coverage

Effective October 1, 2003, for certain procedures whose medical complexity and serious nature incur extraordinary associated costs, Medicare limits coverage. The edit message indicates the type of limited coverage (e.g., LVRS, heart transplant, etc). The procedures receiving limited coverage edits previously were listed as non-covered procedures, but were covered under Medicare in certain circumstances. The FIs will handle these procedures as they had previously.

Pub. 100-4, Chapter 3, Section 20.7.3

Payment for Blood Clotting Factor Administered to Hemophilia Inpatients

Section 6011 of Public Law (P.L.) 101-239 amended §1886(a)(4) of the Social Security Act (the Act) to provide that prospective payment system (PPS) hospitals receive an additional payment for the costs of administering blood clotting factor to Medicare hemophiliacs who are hospital inpatients. Section 6011(b) of P.L. 101.239 specified that the payment be based on a predetermined price per unit of clotting factor multiplied by the number of units provided. This add-on payment originally was effective for blood clotting factors furnished on or after June 19, 1990, and before December 19, 1991. Section 13505 of P. L. 103-66 amended §6011 (d) of P.L. 101-239 to extend the period covered by the add-on payment for blood clotting factors administered to Medicare inpatients with hemophilia through September 30, 1994. Section 4452 of P.L. 105-33 amended §6011(d) of P.L. 101-239 to reinstate the add-on payment for the costs of administering blood-clotting factor to Medicare beneficiaries who have hemophilia and who are hospital inpatients for discharges occurring on or after October 1, 1998.

Local carriers shall process non-institutional blood clotting factor claims.

The FIs shall process institutional blood clotting factor claims payable under either Part A or Part B.

A. Inpatient Bills

Under the Inpatient Prospective Payment System (PPS), hospitals receive a special add-on payment for the costs of furnishing blood clotting factors to Medicare beneficiaries with hemophilia, admitted as inpatients of PPS hospitals. The clotting factor add-on payment is calculated using the number of units (as defined in the HCPCS code long descriptor) billed by the provider under special instructions for units of service.

The PPS Pricer software does not calculate the payment amount. The Fiscal Intermediary Standard System (FISS) calculates the payment amount and subtracts the charges from those submitted to Pricer so that the clotting factor charges are not included in cost outlier computations.

Blood clotting factors not paid on a cost or PPS basis are priced as a drug/biological under the Medicare Part B Drug Pricing File effective for the specific date of service. As of January 1, 2005, the average sales price (ASP) plus 6 percent shall be used.

If a beneficiary is in a covered Part A stay in a PPS hospital, the clotting factors are paid in addition to the DRG/HIPPS payment (For FY 2004, this payment is based on 95 percent of average wholesale price.) For a SNF subject to SNF/PPS, the payment is bundled into the SNF/PPS rate.

For SNF inpatient Part A, there is no add-on payment for blood clotting factors.

The codes for blood-clotting factors are found on the Medicare Part B Drug Pricing File. This file is distributed on a quarterly basis.

For discharges occurring on or after October 1, 2000, and before December 31, 2005, report HCPCS Q0187 based on 1 billing unit per 1.2 mg. Effective January 1, 2006, HCPCS code J7189 replaces Q0187 and is defined as 1 billing unit per 1 microgram (mcg).

The examples below include the HCPCS code and indicate the dosage amount specified in the descriptor of that code. Facilities use the units field as a multiplier to arrive at the dosage amount.

EXAMPLE 1

HCPCS	Drug	Dosage
J7189	Factor VIIa	1 mcg

Actual dosage: 13,365 mcg

On the bill, the facility shows J7189 and 13,365 in the units field (13,365 mcg divided by 1 mcg = 13,365 units).

NOTE: The process for dealing with one international unit (IU) is the same as the process of dealing with one microgram.

EXAMPLE 2

HCPCS	Drug	Dosage
J9355	Trastuzumab	10 mg

Actual dosage: 140 mg

On the bill, the facility shows J9355 and 14 in the units field (140 mg divided by 10mg = 14 units).

When the dosage amount is greater than the amount indicated for the HCPCS code, the facility rounds up to determine units. When the dosage amount is less than the amount indicated for the HCPCS code, use 1 as the unit of measure.

EXAMPLE 3

HCPCS	Drug	Dosage
J3100	Tenecteplase	50 mg

Actual Dosage: 40 mg

The provider would bill for 1 unit, even though less than 1 full unit was furnished.

At times, the facility provides less than the amount provided in a single use vial and there is waste, i.e.; some drugs may be available only in packaged amounts that exceed the needs of an individual patient. Once the drug is reconstituted in the hospital's pharmacy, it may have a limited shelf life. Since an individual patient may receive less than the fully reconstituted amount, we encourage hospitals to schedule patients in such a way that the hospital can use the drug most efficiently. However, if the hospital must discard the remainder of a vial after administering part of it to a Medicare patient, the provider may bill for the amount of drug discarded plus the amount administered.

Example 1:

Drug X is available only in a 100-unit size. A hospital schedules three Medicare patients to receive drug X on the same day within the designated shelf life of the product. An appropriate hospital staff member administers 30 units to each patient. The remaining 10 units are billed to Medicare on the account of the last patient. Therefore, 30 units are billed on behalf of the first patient seen and 30 units are billed on behalf of the second patient seen. Forty units are billed on behalf of the last patient seen because the hospital had to discard 10 units at that point.

Example 2:

An appropriate hospital staff member must administer 30 units of drug X to a Medicare patient, and it is not practical to schedule another patient who requires the same drug. For example, the hospital has only one patient who requires drug X, or the hospital sees the patient for the first time and did not know the patient's condition. The hospital bills for 100 units on behalf of the patient, and Medicare pays for 100 units.

When the number of units of blood clotting factor administered to hemophiliac inpatients exceeds 99,999, the hospital reports the excess as a second line for revenue code 0636 and repeats the HCPCS code. One hundred thousand fifty (100,050) units are reported on one line as 99,999, and another line shows 1,051.

Revenue Code 0636 is used. It requires HCPCS. Some other inpatient drugs continue to be billed without HCPCS codes under pharmacy.

No changes in beneficiary notices are required. Coverage is applicable to hospital Part A claims only. Coverage is also applicable to inpatient Part B services in SNFs and all types of hospitals, including CAHs. Separate payment is not made to SNFs for beneficiaries in an inpatient Part A stay.

B. FI Action

The FI is responsible for the following:

- It accepts HCPCS codes for inpatient services;

- It edits to require HCPCS codes with Revenue Code 0636. Multiple iterations of the revenue code are possible with the same or different HCPCS codes. It does not edit units except to ensure a numeric value;

- It reduces charges forwarded to Pricer by the charges for hemophilia clotting factors in revenue code 0636. It retains the charges and revenue and HCPCS codes for CWF; and

- It modifies data entry screens to accept HCPCS codes for hospital (including CAH) swing bed, and SNF inpatient claims (bill types 11X, 12X, 18x, 21x and, 22x).

The September 1, 1993, IPPS final rule (58 FR 46304) states that payment will be made for the blood clotting factor only if an ICD-9-CM diagnosis code for hemophilia is included on the bill.

Since inpatient blood-clotting factors are covered only for beneficiaries with hemophilia, the FI must ensure that one of the following hemophilia diagnosis codes is listed on the bill before payment is made:

286.0	Congenital factor VIII disorder
286.1	Congenital factor IX disorder
286.2	Congenital factor IX disorder
286.3	Congenital deficiency of other clotting factor
286.4	von Willebrands' disease

Effective for discharges on or after August 1, 2001, payment may also be made if one of the following diagnosis codes is reported:

286.5	Hemorrhagic disorder due to circulating anticoagulants
286.7	Acquired coagulation factor deficiency

C. Part A Remittance Advice

1. X12.835 Ver. 003030M

For remittance reporting PIP and/or non-PIP payments, the Hemophilia Add on will be reported in a claims level 2-090-CAS segment (CAS is the element identifier) exhibiting an "OA" Group Code and adjustment reason code "97" (payment is included in the allowance for the basic service/

procedure) followed by the associated dollar amount (POSITIVE) and units of service. For this version of the 835, "OA" group coded line level CAS segments are informational and are not included in the balancing routine. The Hemophilia Add On amount will always be included in the 2-010-CLP04 Claim Payment Amount.

For remittance reporting PIP payments, the Hemophilia Add On will also be reported in the provider level adjustment (element identifier PLB) segment with the provider level adjustment reason code "CA" (Manual claims adjustment) followed by the associated dollar amount (NEGATIVE).

NOTE: A data maintenance request will be submitted to ANSI ASC X12 for a new PLB adjustment reason code specifically for PIP payment Hemophilia Add On situations for future use. However, continue to use adjustment reason code "CA" until further notice.

The FIs enter MA103 (Hemophilia Add On) in an open MIA (element identifier) remark code data element. This will alert the provider that the reason code 97 and PLB code "CA" adjustments are related to the Hemophilia Add On.

2. X12.835 Ver. 003051

For remittances reporting PIP and/or non-PIP payments, Hemophilia Add On information will be reported in the claim level 2-062-AMT and 2-064-QTY

segments. The 2-062-AMTO1 element will carry a "ZK" (Federal Medicare claim MANDATE - Category 1) qualifier code followed by the total claim level Hemophilia Add On amount (POSITIVE). The 2-064QTYO1 element will carry a "FL" (Units) qualifier code followed by the number of units approved for the Hemophilia Add On for the claim. The Hemophilia Add On amount will always be included in the 2-010-CLP04 Claim Payment Amount.

NOTE: A data maintenance request will be submitted to ANSI ASC X12 for a new AMT qualifier code specifically for the Hemophilia Add On for future use. However, continue to use adjustment reason code "ZK" until further notice.

For remittances reporting PIP payments, the Hemophilia Add On will be reported in the provider level adjustment PLB segment with the provider level adjustment reason "ZZ" followed by the associated dollar amount (NEGATIVE).

NOTE: A data maintenance request will be submitted to ANSI ASC X12 for a new PLB, adjustment reason code specifically for the Hemophilia Add On for future use. However, continue to use PLB adjustment reason code "ZZ" until further notice.

The FIs enter MA103 (Hemophilia Add On) in an open MIA remark code data element. This will alert the provider that the ZK, FL and ZZ entries are related to the Hemophilia Add On. (Effective with version 4010 of the 835, report ZK in lieu of FL in the QTY segment.)

3. Standard Hard Copy Remittance Advice

For paper remittances reporting non-PIP payments involving Hemophilia Add On, add a "Hemophilia Add On" category to the end of the "Pass Thru Amounts" listings in the "Summary" section of the paper remittance. Enter the total of the Hemophilia Add On amounts due for the claims covered by this remittance next to the Hemophilia Add On heading.

The FIs add the Remark Code "MA103" (Hemophilia Add On) to the remittance advice under the REM column for those claims that qualify for Hemophilia Add On payments.

This will be the full extent of Hemophilia Add On reporting on paper remittance notices; providers wishing more detailed information must subscribe to the Medicare Part A specifications for the ANSI ASC X12N 835, where additional information is available.

See chapter 22, for detailed instructions and definitions.

Pub. 100-4, Chapter 3, Section 40.2.2

Charges to Beneficiaries for Part A Services

The hospital submits a bill even where the patient is responsible for a deductible which covers the entire amount of the charges for non-PPS hospitals, or in PPS hospitals, where the DRG payment amount will be less than the deductible.

A beneficiary's liability for payment is governed by the limitation on liability notification rules in Chapter 30 where the admission is found not to be reasonable and necessary and no payment will be made for the stay under limitation on liability. A hospital receiving payment for a covered hospital stay (or PPS hospital that includes at least one covered day, or one treated as covered under guarantee of payment or limitation on liability) may charge the beneficiary, or other person, for items and services furnished during the stay only as described in subsections A through H.

A - Deductible and Coinsurance

The hospital may charge the beneficiary or other person for applicable deductible and coinsurance amounts. The deductible is satisfied only by charges for covered services. The FI deducts the deductible and coinsurance first from the PPS payment. Where the deductible exceeds the PPS amount, the excess will be applied to a subsequent payment to the hospital. (See Chapter 3 of the Medicare General Information, Eligibility, and Entitlement Manual for specific policies.)

B - Blood Deductible

The Part A blood deductible provision applies and reporting of the number of pints is applicable to both PPS and non-PPS hospitals. (See Chapter 3 of the Medicare General Information, Eligibility, and Entitlement Manual for specific policies.)

C - Inpatient Care No Longer Required

The hospital may charge for services that are not reasonable and necessary or that constitute custodial care, furnished on or after the third day following the date of the written notification when the following requirements are met:

- The hospital (acting directly or through its URC) determined that the beneficiary no longer required inpatient hospital care. (For this purpose, a beneficiary is considered to require

inpatient hospital care if the beneficiary needed a SNF level of care but an SNF-level bed was unavailable.) The hospital cannot issue a notice of noncoverage if a bed is not available. Medicare pays for days awaiting placement until a bed is available and it is documented in the medical record that SNF placement is actively being sought.

- The attending physician agreed with the hospital's determination in writing, i.e., by issuing a written discharge order. Or, if the physician disagreed with the hospital's determination, the hospital requested a review by the QIO and the QIO concurred with the hospitals' notice.

Prior to charging for the noncovered period, the hospital (acting directly or through the URC) notified the beneficiary (or person acting on the beneficiary's behalf) in writing that:

- In its opinion and with the concurrence of the attending physician (or of the QIO), the beneficiary no longer requires inpatient hospital care (See §§130 for coordination with a QIO); or

- Customary charges will be made for continued hospital care beginning with the third day following the date of the notice.

The beneficiary may request that the QIO make a formal determination on the validity of the hospital's finding if the beneficiary remains in the hospital after becoming liable for charges. If the beneficiary wants an immediate review by the QIO, the beneficiary must request it within 3 days of receiving the hospital's notice. Any patient during the course of a stay will receive the QIO decision within 2 workdays.

The determination of the QIO may be appealed if it is unfavorable to the beneficiary in any way and the QIO decision will be made within 30 days.

To the extent that a finding is made that the beneficiary required continued hospital care beyond the point indicated by the hospital, the charges for the continued care will be invalidated and any money paid by the beneficiary, or on the beneficiary's behalf, refunded.

The manner in which the hospital gives the notice to the beneficiary is in Chapter 30.

If a hospital furnishing covered inpatient hospital services is able to determine in advance that the beneficiary will not require inpatient hospital care as of a certain date, it may give the notice in advance of that date, but ordinarily no earlier than 3 days before that date. If a hospital determines, however, that a beneficiary needs (or by the third day thereafter, will need) only a SNF-level of care but a SNF bed is not or will not be available, it may notify the beneficiary (or the beneficiary's representative) that the beneficiary will be subject to charges beginning with the third day after the date of the notice that the SNF bed becomes available. This can be done as an advance beneficiary notice. The hospital needs to notify the beneficiary or representative the day the bed becomes available or has knowledge of the bed available.

The beneficiary has the same right to appeal the QIO's determination that the beneficiary no longer required inpatient hospital care as of a certain date as applies to QIO determinations regarding medical necessity. The hospital also has the right to appeal a QIO's determination that is unfavorable to the beneficiary.

When the hospital appeals in such cases the following entries are required on the bill:

- Occurrence code 31 (and date) to indicate the date the hospital notified the patient in accordance with the first bullet above;

- Occurrence span code 76 (and dates) to indicate the period of noncovered care for which it is charging the beneficiary;

- Occurrence span code 77 (and dates) to indicate the period of noncovered care for which the provider is liable, when it is aware of this prior to billing; and

- Value code 31 (and amount) to indicate the amount of charges it may bill the beneficiary for days for which inpatient care was no longer required. They are included as noncovered charges on the bill.

D - Change in the Beneficiary's Condition

If the beneficiary remains in the hospital after receiving notice as described in subsection C, and the hospital, the physician who concurred in the hospital's determination, or the QIO, subsequently determines that the beneficiary again requires inpatient hospital care, the hospital may not charge the beneficiary or other person for services furnished after the beneficiary again required inpatient hospital care until the conditions in subsection C. are again met. If a patient who needs only a SNF level of care remains in the hospital after the SNF bed becomes available, and the bed ceases to be available, the hospital may continue to charge the beneficiary. It need not provide the beneficiary with a subsequent notice when the patient chose not to be discharged to the SNF bed.

E - Admission Denied

If the entire hospital admission is determined to be not reasonable or necessary:

- If the beneficiary was notified in writing prior to, or upon admission, the hospital may charge for the entire period of hospitalization.

- If the beneficiary was notified in writing on the day following the admission or subsequently, the hospital may charge the beneficiary for the hospitalization beginning with the day following the day the written notice was given. In this circumstance, the provider is liable for the period between admission and the day after the beneficiary was notified.

The notice to the beneficiary must state:

- The basis of the determination that inpatient hospital care is not necessary or reasonable (e.g., coverage exclusions);

- That customary charges will be made for hospital care beginning with the day following the day on which the notice is given to either the beneficiary or to a representative on his behalf;

- The beneficiary may request that the QIO make a formal determination on the validity of the hospital's finding if the beneficiary remains in the hospital. If the beneficiary wishes immediate QIO review, it must be requested within 3 days of receiving the hospital's notice;

- The beneficiary may appeal the determination of the QIO if it is unfavorable to the beneficiary in any way. The hospital also has the right to appeal a QIO's decision; and

- If a finding is made that the beneficiary required the hospitalization, the charges for the hospital stay will be invalidated, and money paid by the beneficiary or on his behalf will be refunded.

In such cases the following entries are required on the bill:

- Occurrence code 31 (and date) to indicate the date the hospital notified the beneficiary.

- Occurrence span code 76 (and dates) to indicate the period of noncovered care for which the hospital is charging the beneficiary.

- Occurrence span code 77 (and dates) to indicate any period of noncovered care for which the provider is liable (e.g., the period between issuing the notice and the time it may charge the beneficiary) when the provider is aware of this prior to billing.

- Value code 31 (and amount) to indicate the amount of charges the hospital may bill the beneficiary for hospitalization that was not necessary or reasonable. They are included as noncovered charges on the bill.

F - Procedures, Studies and Courses of Treatment That Are Not Reasonable or Necessary

If diagnostic procedures, studies, therapeutic studies and courses of treatment are excluded from coverage as not reasonable and necessary (even though the beneficiary requires inpatient hospital care) the hospital may charge the beneficiary or other person for the services or care under the following circumstances:

- If the beneficiary was notified in writing prior to receipt of the care or services that the hospital may charge for the excluded care or services; and

- The notice to the beneficiary must state:

  — The basis of the determination that inpatient hospital care is not necessary or reasonable (i.e., coverage exclusions);

  — The determination is the hospital's opinion. (If the hospital obtained concurrence from the FI or the QIO this may be stated);

  — Customary charges will be made if the beneficiary receives the services;

  — The beneficiary may request the FI, or the QIO when medical necessity is involved, to make a formal determination on the validity of the hospital's finding if the beneficiary receives the items or services. If the beneficiary wants immediate QIO review, the beneficiary must request it within 3 days of receiving the hospital's notice;

  — The FI's determination, or the QIO's where a medical necessity determination is involved, may be appealed by the beneficiary if unfavorable to the beneficiary in any way. The hospital also has the right to appeal the FI's or the QIO's decision; and

  — The charges for the services will be invalidated and refunded if they are found to be covered.

The hospital may consult with the FI (on coverage exclusions) or the QIO (on medical necessity determinations) prior to issuing the notice to the beneficiary.

The following bill entries apply to these circumstances:

- Occurrence code 32 (and date) to indicate the date the hospital provided the notice to the beneficiary.

- Value code 31 (and amount) to indicate the amount of such charges to be billed to the beneficiary. They are included as noncovered charges on the bill.

G - Nonentitlement Days and Days after Benefits Exhausted

If a hospital stay exceeds the day outlier threshold, the hospital may charge for some, or all, of the days on which the patient is not entitled to Medicare Part A, or after the Part A benefits are exhausted (i.e., the hospital may charge its customary charges for services furnished on those days). It may charge the beneficiary for the lesser of:

- The number of days on which the patient was not entitled to benefits or after the benefits were exhausted; or

- The number of outlier days. (Day outliers were discontinued at the end of FY 1997.)

If the number of outlier days exceeds the number of days on which the patient was not entitled to benefits, or after benefits were exhausted, the hospital may charge for all days on which the patient was not entitled to benefits or after benefits were exhausted. If the number of days on which the beneficiary was not entitled to benefits, or after benefits were exhausted, exceeds the number of outlier days, the hospital determines the days for which it may charge by starting with the last day of the stay (i.e., the day before the day of discharge) and identifying and counting off in reverse order, days on which the patient was not entitled to benefits or after the benefits were exhausted, until the number of days counted off equals the number of outlier days. The days counted off are the days for which the hospital may charge.

H - Contractual Exclusions

In addition to receiving the basic prospective payment, the hospital may charge the beneficiary for any services that are excluded from coverage for reasons other than, or in addition to, absence of medical necessity, provision of custodial care, non-entitlement to Part A, or exhaustion of benefits. For example, it may charge for most cosmetic and dental surgery.

I - Private Room Care

Payment for medically necessary private room care is included in the prospective payment. Where the beneficiary requests private room accommodations, the hospital must inform the beneficiary of the additional charge. (See the Medicare Benefit Policy Manual, Chapter 1.) When the beneficiary accepts the liability, the hospital will supply the service, and bill the beneficiary directly. If the beneficiary believes the private room was medically necessary, the beneficiary has a right to a determination and may initiate a Part A appeal.

J - Deluxe Item or Service

Where a beneficiary requests a deluxe item or service, i.e., an item or service which is more expensive than is medically required for the beneficiary's condition, after the hospital informs the beneficiary of the additional charge, it may collect the additional charge. That charge is the difference between the customary charge for the item or service most commonly furnished by the hospital to private pay patients with the beneficiary's condition, and the charge for the more expensive item or service requested. If the beneficiary believes that the more expensive item or service was medically necessary, the beneficiary has a right to a determination and may initiate a Part A appeal.

K - Inpatient Acute Care Hospital Admission Followed By a Death or Discharge Prior To Room Assignment

A patient of an acute care hospital is considered an inpatient upon issuance of written doctor's orders to that effect. If a patient either dies or is discharged prior to being assigned and/or occupying a room, a hospital may enter an appropriate room and board charge on the claim. If a patient leaves of their own volition prior to being assigned and/or occupying a room, a hospital may enter an appropriate room and board charge on the claim as well as a patient status code 07 which indicates they left against medical advice. A hospital is not required to enter a room and board charge, but failure to do so may have a minimal impact on future DRG weight calculations.

Pub. 100-4, Chapter 3, Section 40.3

Outpatient Services Treated as Inpatient Services

A3-3610.3, HO-415.6, HO-400D, A-03-008, A-03-013, A-03-054

A Outpatient Services Followed by Admission Before Midnight of the Following Day (Effective For Services Furnished Before October 1, 1991)

When a beneficiary receives outpatient hospital services during the day immediately preceding the hospital admission, the outpatient hospital services are treated as inpatient services if the beneficiary has Part A coverage. Hospitals and FIs apply this provision only when the beneficiary is admitted to the hospital before midnight of the day following receipt of outpatient services. The day on which the patient is formally admitted as an inpatient is counted as the first inpatient day.

When this provision applies, services are included in the applicable PPS payment and not billed separately. When this provision applies to hospitals and units excluded from the hospital PPS, services are shown on the bill and included in the Part A payment. See Chapter 1 for FI requirements for detecting duplicate claims in such cases.

B Preadmission Diagnostic Services (Effective for Services Furnished On or After January 1, 1991)

Diagnostic services (including clinical diagnostic laboratory tests) provided to a beneficiary by the admitting hospital, or by an entity wholly owned or wholly operated by the admitting hospital (or by another entity under arrangements with the admitting hospital), within 3 days prior to and including the date of the beneficiary's admission are deemed to be inpatient services and included in the inpatient payment, unless there is no Part A coverage. For example, if a patient is admitted on a Wednesday, outpatient services provided by the hospital on Sunday, Monday, Tuesday, or Wednesday are included in the inpatient Part A payment.

This provision does not apply to ambulance services and maintenance renal dialysis services (see the Medicare Benefit Policy Manual, Chapters 10 and 11, respectively). Additionally, Part A services furnished by skilled nursing facilities, home health agencies, and hospices are excluded from the payment window provisions.

For services provided before October 31, 1994, this provision applies to both hospitals subject to the hospital inpatient prospective payment system (IPPS) as well as those hospitals and units excluded from IPPS.

For services provided on or after October 31, 1994, for hospitals and units excluded from IPPS, this provision applies only to services furnished within one day prior to and including the date of the beneficiary's admission. The hospitals and units that are excluded from IPPS are: psychiatric hospitals and units; inpatient rehabilitation facilities (IRF) and units; long-term care hospitals (LTCH); children's hospitals; and cancer hospitals.

Critical access hospitals (CAHs) are not subject to the 3-day (nor 1-day) DRG payment window.

An entity is considered to be "wholly owned or operated" by the hospital if the hospital is the sole owner or operator. A hospital need not exercise administrative control over a facility in order to operate it. A hospital is considered the sole operator of the facility if the hospital has exclusive responsibility for implementing facility policies (i.e., conducting or overseeing the facility's routine operations), regardless of whether it also has the authority to make the policies.

For this provision, diagnostic services are defined by the presence on the bill of the following revenue and/or HCPCS codes:

0254 -	Drugs incident to other diagnostic services
0255 -	Drugs incident to radiology
030X -	Laboratory
031X -	Laboratory pathological
032X -	Radiology diagnostic
0341 -	Nuclear medicine, diagnostic

035X -	CT scan
0371 -	Anesthesia incident to Radiology
0372 -	Anesthesia incident to other diagnostic services
040X -	Other imaging services
046X -	Pulmonary function
0471 -	Audiology diagnostic
048X -	Cardiology, with HCPCS codes 93015, 93307, 93308, 93320, 93501, 93503, 93505, 93510, 93526, 93541, 93542, 93543, 93544 - 93552, 93561, or 93562
053X -	Osteopathic services
061X -	MRT
062X -	Medical/surgical supplies, incident to radiology or other diagnostic services
073X -	EKG/ECG
074X -	EEG
092X -	Other diagnostic services

The CWF rejects services furnished January 1, 1991, or later when outpatient bills for diagnostic services with through dates or last date of service (occurrence span code 72) fall on the day of admission or any of the 3 days immediately prior to admission to an IPPS or IPPS-excluded hospital. This reject applies to the bill in process, regardless of whether the outpatient or inpatient bill is processed first. Hospitals must analyze the two bills and report appropriate corrections. For services on or after October 31, 1994, for hospitals and units excluded from IPPS, CWF will reject outpatient diagnostic bills that occur on the day of or one day before admission. For IPPS hospitals, CWF will continue to reject outpatient diagnostic bills for services that occur on the day of or any of the 3 days prior to admission.

Hospitals in Maryland that are under the jurisdiction of the Health Services Cost Review Commission are subject to the 3-day payment window.

C Other Preadmission Services (Effective for Services Furnished On or After October 1, 1991)

Nondiagnostic outpatient services that are related to a patient's hospital admission and that are provided by the hospital, or by an entity wholly owned or wholly operated by the admitting hospital (or by another entity under arrangements with the admitting hospital), to the patient during the 3 days immediately preceding and including the date of the patient's admission are deemed to be inpatient services and are included in the inpatient payment. Effective March 13, 1998, we defined nondiagnostic preadmission services as being related to the admission only when there is an exact match (for all digits) between the ICD-9-CM principal diagnosis code assigned for both the preadmission services and the inpatient stay. Thus, whenever Part A covers an admission, the hospital may bill nondiagnostic preadmission services to Part B as outpatient services only if they are not related to the admission. The FI shall assume, in the absence of evidence to the contrary, that such bills are not admission related and, therefore, are not deemed to be inpatient (Part A) services. If there are both diagnostic and nondiagnostic preadmission services and the nondiagnostic services are unrelated to the admission, the hospital may separately bill the nondiagnostic preadmission services to Part B. This provision applies only when the patient has Part A coverage. This provision does not apply to ambulance services and maintenance renal dialysis. Additionally, Part A services furnished by skilled nursing facilities, home health agencies, and hospices are excluded from the payment window provisions.

For services provided before October 31, 1994, this provision applies to both hospitals subject to IPPS as well as those hospitals and units excluded from IPPS (see section B above).

For services provided on or after October 31, 1994, for hospitals and units excluded from IPPS, this provision applies only to services furnished within one day prior to and including the date of the beneficiary's admission.

Critical access hospitals (CAHs) are not subject to the 3-day (nor 1-day) DRG payment window.

Hospitals in Maryland that are under the jurisdiction of the Health Services Cost Review Commission are subject to the 3-day payment window.

Pub. 100-4, Chapter 3, Section 90.1

General

A3-3612, HO-E414

A major treatment for patients with ESRD is kidney transplantation. This involves removing a kidney, usually from a living relative of the patient or from an unrelated person who has died, and surgically placing the kidney into the patient. After the beneficiary receives a kidney transplant, Medicare pays the transplant hospital for the transplant and appropriate standard acquisition charges. Special provisions apply to payment.

A transplant hospital may acquire cadaver kidneys by:

- Excising kidneys from cadavers in its own hospital; and
- Arrangements with a freestanding organ procurement organization that provides cadaver kidneys to any transplant hospital.

A transplant hospital that is also a certified organ procurement organization may acquire cadaver kidneys by:

- Having its organ procurement team excise kidneys from cadavers in other hospitals;
- Arrangements with participating community hospitals, whether they excise kidneys on a regular or irregular basis; and
- Arrangements with an organ procurement organization that services the transplant hospital as a member of a network.

When the transplant hospital also excises the cadaver kidney, the cost of the procedure is included in its kidney acquisition costs and is considered in arriving at its standard cadaver kidney acquisition charge. When the transplant hospital excises a kidney to provide another hospital, it may use its standard cadaver kidney acquisition charge or its standard detailed departmental charges to bill that hospital.

When the excising hospital is not a transplant hospital, it bills its customary charges for services used in excising the cadaver kidney to the transplant hospital or organ procurement agency.

If the transplanting hospital's organ procurement team excises the cadaver kidney at another hospital, the cost of operating such a team is included in the transplanting hospital's kidney acquisition costs, along with the reasonable charges billed by the other hospital of its services.

Pub. 100-4, Chapter 3, Section 90.1.1

The Standard Kidney Acquisition Charge

A3-3612.1, A3-3612.3, HO-E417, HO-406, HO-E408, HO-E410, HO-E412, HO-E416, HO-E418, HO-E420

There are two basic standard charges that must be developed by transplant hospitals from costs expected to be incurred in the acquisition of kidneys:

- The standard charge for acquiring a live donor kidney; and
- The standard charge for acquiring a cadaver kidney.

The standard charge is not a charge representing the acquisition cost of a specific kidney; rather, it is a charge that reflects the average cost associated with each type of kidney acquisition.

When the transplant hospital bills the program for the transplant, it shows its standard kidney acquisition charge on a separate line on the billing form.

Acquisition services are billed from the excising hospital to the transplant hospital. A billing form is not submitted from the excising hospital to the FI. The transplant hospital keeps an itemized statement that identifies the services furnished, the charges, the person receiving the service (donor/recipient), and whether this is a potential transplant donor or recipient. These charges are reflected in the transplant hospital's kidney acquisition cost center and are used in determining the hospital's standard charge for acquiring a live donor's kidney or a cadaver's kidney. The standard charge is not a charge representing the acquisition cost of a specific kidney. Rather, it is a charge that reflects the average cost associated with each type of kidney acquisition. Also, it is an all-inclusive charge for all services required in acquisition of a kidney, i.e., tissue typing, post-operative evaluation.

A. Billing For Blood And Tissue Typing of the Transplant Recipient Whether or Not Medicare Entitlement Is Established

Tissue typing and pre-transplant evaluation can be reflected only through the kidney acquisition charge of the hospital where the transplant will take place. The transplant hospital includes in its kidney acquisition cost center the reasonable charges it pays to the independent laboratory or other hospital which typed the potential transplant recipient, either before or after his entitlement. It also includes reasonable charges paid for physician tissue typing services, applicable to live donors and recipients (during the pre-entitlement period and after entitlement, but prior to hospital admission for transplantation).

B. Billing for Blood and Tissue Typing and Other Pre-Transplant Evaluation of Live Donors

The entitlement date of the beneficiary who will receive the transplant is not a consideration in reimbursing for the services to donors, since no bill is submitted directly to Medicare. All charges for services to donors prior to admission into the hospital for excision are "billed" indirectly to Medicare through the live donor acquisition charge of transplanting hospitals.

C. Billing Donor And Recipient Pre-Transplant Services (Performed by Transplant Hospitals or Other Providers) to the Kidney Acquisition Cost Center

The transplant hospital prepares an itemized statement of the services rendered for submittal to its cost accounting department. Regular Medicare billing forms are not necessary for this purpose, since no bills are submitted to the FI at this point.

The itemized statement should contain information that identifies the person receiving the service (donor/recipient), the health care insurance number, the service rendered and the charge for the service, as well as a statement as to whether this is a potential transplant donor or recipient. If it is a potential donor, the provider must identify the prospective recipient.

EXAMPLE:

    Mary Jones

    Health care insurance number

    200 Adams St.

    Anywhere, MS

Transplant donor evaluation services for recipient:

    John Jones

    Health care insurance number

    200 Adams St.

    Anywhere, MS

Services performed in a hospital other than the potential transplant hospital or by an independent laboratory are billed by that facility to the potential transplant hospital. This holds true regardless of where in the United States the service is performed. For example, if the donor services are performed in a Florida hospital and the transplant is to take place in a California hospital, the Florida hospital bills the California hospital (as described in above). The Florida hospital is paid by the California hospital which recoups the monies through the kidney acquisition cost center.

D. Billing for Cadaveric Donor Services

Normally, various tests are performed to determine the type and suitability of a cadaver kidney. Such tests may be performed by the excising hospital (which may also be a transplant hospital) or an independent laboratory. When the excising-only hospital performs the tests, it includes the related charges on its bill to the transplant hospital or to the organ procurement agency.

When the tests are performed by the transplant hospital, it uses the related costs in establishing the standard charge for acquiring the cadaver kidney. The transplant hospital includes the costs and charges in the appropriate departments for final cost settlement purposes.

When the tests are performed by an independent laboratory for the excising-only hospital or the transplant hospital, the laboratory bills the hospital that engages its services or the organ procurement agency. The excising-only hospital includes such charges in its charges to the transplant hospital, which then includes the charges in developing its standard charge for acquiring the cadaver kidney. It is the transplant hospitals' responsibility to assure that the independent laboratory does not bill both hospitals.

The cost of these services cannot be billed directly to the program, since such tests and other procedures performed on a cadaver are not identifiable to a specific patient.

E. Billing For Physicians' Services Prior to Transplantation

Physicians' services applicable to kidney excisions involving live donors and recipients (during the pre-entitlement period and after entitlement, but prior to entrance into the hospital for transplantation) as well as all physicians' services applicable to cadavers are considered Part A hospital services (kidney acquisition costs).

F. Billing for Physicians' Services After Transplantation

All physicians' services rendered to the living donor and all physicians' services rendered to the transplant recipient are billed to the Medicare program in the same manner as all Medicare Part B services are billed. All donor physicians' services must be billed to the account of the recipient (i.e., the recipient's Medicare number).

G. Billing For Physicians' Renal Transplantation Services

To ensure proper payment when submitting a Part B bill for the renal surgeon's services to the recipient, the appropriate HCPCS codes must be submitted, including HCPCS codes for concurrent surgery, as applicable.

The bill must include all living donor physicians' services, e.g., Revenue Center code 081X.

Pub. 100-4, Chapter 3, Section 90.1.2

Billing for Kidney Transplant and Acquisition Services
A3-3612.2

Applicable standard kidney acquisition charges are identified separately in FL 42 by revenue code 0811 (Living Donor Kidney Acquisition) or 0812 (Cadaver Donor Kidney Acquisition). Where interim bills are submitted, the standard acquisition charge appears on the billing form for the period during which the transplant took place. This charge is in addition to the hospital's charges for services rendered directly to the Medicare recipient.

The FI deducts kidney acquisition charges for PPS hospitals for processing through Pricer. These costs, incurred by approved kidney transplant hospitals, are not included in the prospective payment DRG 302 (kidney transplant). They are paid on a reasonable cost basis. Interim payment is paid as a "pass through" item. (See the Provider Reimbursement Manual, Part 1, §2802 B.8.) The FI includes kidney acquisition charges under the appropriate revenue code in CWF.

Pub. 100-4, Chapter 3, Section 90.2

Heart Transplants
A3-3613, HO-416

Cardiac transplantation is covered under Medicare when performed in a facility which is approved by Medicare as meeting institutional coverage criteria. On April 6, 1987, CMS Ruling 87-1, "Criteria for Medicare Coverage of Heart Transplants" was published in the "Federal Register." For Medicare coverage purposes, heart transplants are medically reasonable and necessary when performed in facilities that meet these criteria. If a hospital wishes to bill Medicare for heart transplants, it must submit an application and documentation, showing its ongoing compliance with each criterion.

The facility mails the application to the address below in a manner which provides it with documentation that it was received, e.g., return receipt requested.

    Director

    Division of Integrated Delivery Systems

    Centers for Medicare & Medicaid Services

    Mailstop C4-25-02

    7500 Security Blvd.

    Baltimore, MD 21244-1850

If an FI has any questions concerning the effective or approval dates of its hospitals, it should contact its RO.

For a complete list of transplant centers, please visit
http://www.cms.hhs.gov/providers/transplant/hartlist.asp.

A. Effective Dates

The effective date of coverage for heart transplants performed at facilities applying after July 6, 1987, is the date the facility receives approval as a heart transplant facility. Coverage is effective for discharges October 17, 1986 for facilities that would have qualified and that applied by July 6, 1987.

The CMS informs each hospital of its effective date in an approval letter.

B. Drugs

Medicare Part B covers immunosuppressive drugs following a covered transplant in an approved facility.

C. Noncovered Transplants

Medicare will not cover transplants or re-transplants in facilities that have not been approved as meeting the facility criteria. If a beneficiary is admitted for and receives a heart transplant from a hospital that is not approved, physicians' services, and inpatient services associated with the transplantation procedure are not covered.

If a beneficiary received a heart transplant from a hospital while it was not an approved facility and later requires services as a result of the noncovered transplant, the services are covered when they are reasonable and necessary in all other respects.

D. Charges for Heart Acquisition Services

The excising hospital bills the transplant (implant) hospital for applicable services. It should not submit a bill to its FI. The transplant hospital must keep an itemized statement that identifies the services rendered, the charges, the person receiving the service (donor/recipient), and whether this person is a potential transplant donor or recipient. These charges are reflected in the transplant hospital's heart acquisition cost center and are used in determining its standard charge for acquiring a donor's heart. The standard charge is not a charge representing the acquisition cost of a specific heart; rather, it reflects the average cost associated with each type of heart acquisition. Also, it is an all inclusive charge for all services required in acquisition of a heart, i.e., tissue typing, post-operative evaluation, etc.

E. Bill Review Procedures

The FI takes the following actions to process heart transplant bills. It may accomplish them manually or modify its MCE and Grouper interface programs to handle the processing.

1. Change MCE Interface

The MCE creates a Limited Coverage edit for procedure code 37.51 (heart transplant). Where this procedure code is identified by MCE, the FI checks the provider number to determine if the provider is an approved transplant center, and checks the effective approval date. If payment is appropriate (i.e., the center is approved and the service is on or after the approval date) it overrides the limited coverage edit.

2. Handling Heart Transplant Billings From Nonapproved Hospitals

Where a heart transplant and covered services are provided by a nonapproved hospital, the bill data processed through Grouper and Pricer must exclude transplant procedure codes and related charges.

Pub. 100-4, Chapter 3, Section 90.2.1

Artificial Hearts and Related Devices

Medicare does not cover the use of artificial hearts, either as a permanent replacement for a human heart or as a temporary life-support system until a human heart becomes available for transplant (often referred to a "bridge to transplant").

Medicare does cover a Ventricular Assist Device (VAD). A ventricular assist device (VAD) is used to assist a damaged or weakened heart in pumping blood. VADs are used as a bridge to a heart transplant, for support of blood circulation postcardiotomy or destination therapy. Please refer to the NCD Manual, section 20.9 for coverage criteria.

The MCE creates a Limited Coverage edit for procedure code 37.66. This procedure code has limited coverage due to the stringent conditions that must be met by hospitals. Where this procedure code is identified by MCE, the FI shall determine if coverage criteria is met and override the MCE if appropriate.

Pub. 100-4, Chapter 3, Section 90.3

Stem Cell Transplantation
A3-3614, HO-416.1

Stem cell transplantation is a process in which stem cells are harvested from either a patient's or donor's bone marrow or peripheral blood for intravenous infusion. Autologous stem cell transplants (AuSCT) must be used to effect hematopoietic reconstitution following severely myelotoxic doses of chemotherapy (HDCT) and/or radiotherapy used to treat various malignances. Allogeneic stem cell transplant may also be used to restore function in recipients having an inherited or acquired deficiency or defect.

Bone marrow and peripheral blood stem cell transplantation is a process which includes mobilization, harvesting, and transplant of bone marrow or peripheral blood stem cells and the administration of high dose chemotherapy or radiotherapy prior to the actual transplant. When bone marrow or peripheral blood stem cell transplantation is covered, all necessary steps are included in coverage. When bone marrow or peripheral blood stem cell transplantation is non-covered, none of the steps are covered.

Allogeneic and autologous stem cell transplants are covered under Medicare for specific diagnoses. Effective October 1, 1990, these cases were assigned to the DRG 481, Bone Marrow Transplant.

The FI's Medicare Code Editor (MCE) will edit stem cell transplant procedure codes against diagnosis codes to determine which cases meet specified coverage criteria. Cases with a diagnosis code for a covered condition will pass (as covered) the MCE noncovered procedure edit. When a stem cell transplant case is selected for review based on the random selection of beneficiaries, the QIO will review the case on a post-payment basis to assure proper coverage decisions

Procedure code 41.00 (bone marrow transplant, not otherwise specified) will be classified as noncovered and the claim will be returned to the hospital for a more specific procedure code.

Pub. 100-4, Chapter 3, Section 90.3.1

Allogeneic Stem Cell Transplantation

A3-3614.1, HO-416.2, A3-3614.2, HO-416.3

A. General

Allogeneic stem cell transplantation (ICD-9-CM Procedure Codes 41.02, 41.03, 41.05, and 41.08, CPT-4 Code 38240) is a procedure in which a portion of a healthy donor's stem cells are obtained and prepared for intravenous infusion to restore normal hematopoietic function in recipients having an inherited or acquired hematopoietic deficiency or defect. See the National Coverage Determinations Manual for more information.

Expenses incurred by a donor are a covered benefit to the recipient/beneficiary but, except for physician services, are not paid separately. Services to the donor include physician services, hospital care in connection with screening the stem cell, and ordinary follow-up care.

B. Covered Conditions

1. Effective for services performed on or after August 1, 1978:

- For the treatment of leukemia, leukemia in remission (ICD-9-CM codes 204.00 through 208.91), or aplastic anemia (ICD-9-CM codes 284.0 through 284.9) when it is reasonable and necessary; and

2. Effective for services performed on or after June 3, 1985:

- For the treatment of severe combined immunodeficiency disease (SCID) (ICD-9-CM code 279.2), and for the treatment of Wiskott - Aldrich syndrome (ICD-9-CM 279.12).

C. Noncovered Conditions

3. Effective for services performed on or after May 24, 1996:

- Allogeneic stem cell transplantation is not covered as treatment for multiple myeloma (ICD-9-CM codes 203.00 and 203.01).

NOTE: Coverage for conditions other than these specifically designated as covered or noncovered in this section or National Coverage Determination Manual are left to individual FI's discretion.

Pub. 100-4, Chapter 3, Section 90.3.2

Autologous Stem Cell Transplantation (AuSCT)

A. General

Autologous stem cell transplantation (AuSCT) (ICD-9-CM procedure code 41.01, 41.04, 41.07, and 41.09 and CPT-4 code 38241) is a technique for restoring stem cells using the patient's own previously stored cells. AuSCT must be used to effect hematopoietic reconstitution following severely myelotoxic doses of chemotherapy(high dose chemotherapy (HDCT)) and/or radiotherapy used to treat various malignancies.

B. Covered Conditions

1. Effective for services performed on or after April 28, 1989:

- Acute leukemia in remission (ICD-9-CM codes 204.01, lymphoid; 205.01, myeloid; 206.01, monocytic; 207.01, acute erythremia and erythroleukemia; and 208.01 unspecified cell type) patients who have a high probability of relapse and who have no human leucocyte antigens (HLA)-matched;

- Resistant non-Hodgkin's lymphomas (ICD-9-CM codes 200.00-200.08, 200.10-200.18, 200.20-200.28, 200.80-200.88, 202.00-202.08, 202.80-202.88, and 202.90-202.98) or those presenting with poor prognostic features following an initial response;

- Recurrent or refractory neuroblastoma (see ICD-9-CM Neoplasm by site, malignant); or

- Advanced Hodgkin's disease (ICD-9-CM codes 201.00-201.98) patients who have failed conventional therapy and have no HLA-matched donor.

2. Effective for services performed on or after October 1, 2000:

- Durie-Salmon Stage II or III that fit the following requirement: Newly diagnosed or responsive multiple myeloma (ICD-9-CM codes 203.00 and 238.6). This includes those patients with previously untreated disease, those with at least a partial response to prior chemotherapy (defined as a 50% decrease either in measurable paraprotein [serum and/or urine] or in bone marrow infiltration, sustained for at least 1 month), and those in responsive relapse, and adequate cardiac, renal, pulmonary, and hepatic function.

3. Effective for services performed on or after March 15, 2005, when recognized clinical risk factors are employed to select patients for transplantation, high-dose melphalan (HDM), together with AuSCT, in treating Medicare beneficiaries of any age group with primary amyloid light-chain (AL) amyloidosis who meet the following criteria:

1. Amyloid deposition in 2 or fewer organs; and,

2. Cardiac left ventricular ejection fraction (EF) of 45% or greater.

C. Noncovered Conditions

Insufficient data exist to establish definite conclusions regarding the efficacy of autologous stem cell transplantation for the following conditions:

- Acute leukemia not in remission (ICD-9-CM codes 204.00, 205.00, 206.00, 207.00 and 208.00);

- Chronic granulocytic leukemia (ICD-9-CM codes 205.10 and 205.11);

- Solid tumors (other than neuroblastoma) (ICD-9-CM codes 140.0-199.1); or

- Multiple myeloma (ICD-9-CM code 203.00 and 238.6), through September 30, 2000.

- Tandem transplantation (multiple rounds of autologous stem cell transplantation) for patients with multiple myeloma (ICD-9-CM code 203.00 and 238.6)

- Non-primary (AL) amyloidosis (ICD-9-CM code 277.3), effective October 1, 2000; or

- Primary (AL) amyloidosis (ICD-9-CM code 277.3) for Medicare beneficiaries age 64 or older, effective October 1, 2000, through March 14, 2005.

NOTE: Coverage for conditions other than these specifically designated as covered or non-covered is left to the FI's discretion.

Pub. 100-4, Chapter 3, Section 90.3.3

Billing for Stem Cell Transplantation

A. Billing for Acquisition Services

The hospital identifies stem cell acquisition charges separately in FL 42 of Form CMS-1450 by using revenue code 0819 (Other Organ Acquisition). The FI does not make separate payment for these acquisition charges, since they are included in the DRG payment.

For allogeneic stem cell transplants (procedure codes 41.02 or 41.03) where the hospital submits interim bills, the acquisition charge will appear on the billing form for the period during which the transplant took place. Since claims for stem cell transplants are paid using PPS, the hospital submits an adjustment bill whenever an interim bill has been processed. Charges will appear on the transplant bill if there are no interim bills involved.

The transplant hospital keeps an itemized statement that identifies the services furnished, the charges, the person receiving the service (donor/recipient), and whether this is a potential transplant donor or recipient. These charges will be reflected in the transplant hospital's stem cell/bone marrow acquisition cost center. Revenue code 0819 is to include all services required in acquisition of stem cell, e.g., tissue typing or post-operative evaluation.

The donor is covered for medically necessary inpatient hospital days of care in connection with the bone marrow transplant operation. Expenses incurred for complications are covered only if they are directly and immediately attributable to the stem cell donation procedure If the donor receives hospital services in connection with a stem cell transplant, they are covered under Part A. The hospital reports the charges on the billing form for the recipient. It does not charge the donor's days of care against the recipient's utilization record. For cost reporting purposes, it includes the covered donor days and charges as Medicare days and charges.

The hospital shows charges for the transplant itself in revenue center code 0362. Selection of the cost center is up to the hospital.

C. Billing for Autologous Stem Cell Transplants

Since there are no covered acquisition charges for autologous stem cell transplant, the hospital shows all charges in the usual manner. It shows charges for the transplant, procedure code 41.01, in revenue center code 0362 or other appropriate cost center.

Pub. 100-4, Chapter 3, Section 90.4

Liver Transplants

A3-3615, A3-3615.5, HO-416.5

A. Background

For Medicare coverage purposes, liver transplants are considered medically reasonable and necessary for specified conditions when performed in facilities that meet specific criteria.

To review the current list of Approved Liver Transplant Centers, see http://www.cms.hhs.gov/providers/transplant/livrlist.asp

Pub. 100-4, Chapter 3, Section 90.4.1

Standard Liver Acquisition Charge

For allogeneic stem cell transplants (procedure codes 41.02 and 41.03, 41.05, or 41.08), the hospital includes charges for acquisition and any applicable storage charges on the recipient's transplant bill.

Acquisition charges do not apply to autologous stem cell acquisitions. On the transplant bill, the hospital reports the charges, cost report days, and utilization days for the stay in which the stem cell was obtained.

B. Billing for Allogeneic Stem Cell Transplants

A3-3615.1, A3-3615.3

Each transplant facility must develop a standard charge for acquiring a cadaver liver from costs it expects to incur in the acquisition of livers.

This standard charge is not a charge that represents the acquisition cost of a specific liver. Rather, it is a charge that reflects the average cost associated with a liver acquisition.

Services associated with liver acquisition are billed from the organ procurement organization or, in some cases, the excising hospital to the transplant hospital. The excising hospital does not submit a billing form to the FI. The transplant hospital keeps an itemized statement that identifies the services furnished, the charges, the person receiving the service (donor/recipient), and the potential transplant donor. These charges are reflected in the transplant hospital's liver acquisition cost center and are used in determining the hospital's standard charge for acquiring a cadaver's liver. The standard charge is not a charge representing the acquisition cost of a specific liver. Rather, it is a charge that reflects the average cost associated with liver acquisition. Also, it is an all-inclusive charge for all services required in acquisition of a liver, e.g., tissue typing, transportation of organ, and surgeons' retrieval fees.

Pub. 100-4, Chapter 3, Section 90.4.2

Billing for Liver Transplant and Acquisition Services

A3-3615.2

Form CMS-1450 or its electronic equivalent is completed, in accordance with instructions in Chapter 25 for the beneficiary who receives a covered liver transplant. Applicable standard liver acquisition charges are identified separately in FL 42 by revenue code 0817 (Donor-Liver). Where interim bills are submitted, the standard acquisition charge appears on the billing form for the period during which the transplant took place. This charge is in addition to the hospital's charge for services furnished directly to the Medicare recipient.

The FI deducts liver acquisition charges for PPS hospitals prior to processing through Pricer. Costs of liver acquisition incurred by approved liver transplant facilities are not included in prospective payment DRG 480 (Liver Transplant). They are paid on a reasonable cost basis. This item is a "pass-through" cost for which interim payments are made. (See the Provider Reimbursement Manual, Part 1, §2802 B.8.) The FI includes liver acquisition charges under revenue code 0817 in the HUIP record that it sends to CWF and the QIO.

A. Bill Review Procedures

The FI takes the following actions to process liver transplant bills.

1. Operative Report

The FI requires the operative report with all claims for liver transplants, or sends a development request to the hospital for each liver transplant with a diagnosis code for a covered condition.

2. MCE Interface

The MCE creates an exception for procedure codes 50.51 and 50.59 (liver transplant). Where one of these procedure codes is identified by the MCE, the FI must check the provider number and effective date to determine if the provider is an approved liver transplant facility at the time of the transplant. If yes, the claim is suspended for review of the operative report to determine whether the beneficiary has at least one of the covered conditions when the diagnosis code is for a covered condition. If payment is appropriate (i.e., the facility is approved, the service is furnished on or after the approval date, and the beneficiary has a covered condition), the FI sends the claim to Grouper and Pricer.

If none of the diagnoses codes are for a covered condition, or if the provider is not an approved liver transplant facility, the FI denies the claim.

NOTE: Some non-covered conditions are included in the covered diagnostic codes. (The diagnostic codes are broader than the covered conditions. For example, primary biliary cirrhosis is a covered condition, secondary biliary cirrhosis is not a covered condition. Both primary and secondary biliary cirrhosis have the same diagnosis code ICD 9 571.6) Do not pay for noncovered conditions.

3. Grouper

If the bill shows a discharge date before March 8, 1990, the procedure is not covered. If the discharge date is March 8, 1990 or later, the FI processes the bill through Grouper and Pricer. If the discharge date is after March 7, 1990, and before October 1, 1990, Grouper assigns DRG 191 or 192. The FI sends the bill to Pricer with review code 08. Pricer overlays DRG 191 or 192 with DRG 480 and the weights and thresholds for DRG 480 to price the bill. If the discharge date is after September 30, 1990, Grouper assigns DRG 480 and Pricer is able to price without using review code 08.

4. Liver Transplant Billing From Non-approved Hospitals

Where a liver transplant and covered services are provided by a non-approved hospital, the bill data processed through Grouper and Pricer must exclude transplant procedure codes and related charges.

When CMS approves a hospital to furnish liver transplant services, it informs the hospital of the effective date in the approval letter. The FI will receive a copy of the letter.

Pub. 100-4, Chapter 3, Section 90.5

Pancreas Transplants With Kidney Transplants

A. Background

Effective July 1, 1999, Medicare will cover pancreas transplantation when it is performed simultaneously with or following a kidney transplant (ICD-9-CM procedure code 55.69). Pancreas transplantation is performed to induce an insulin independent, euglycemic state in diabetic patients. The procedure is generally limited to those patients with severe secondary complications of diabetes including kidney failure. However, pancreas transplantation is sometimes performed on patients with labile diabetes and hypoglycemic unawareness.

Medicare has had a policy of not covering pancreas transplantation. The Office of Health Technology Assessment performed an assessment on pancreas-kidney transplantation in 1994. They found reasonable graft survival outcomes for patients receiving either simultaneous pancreas-kidney (SPK) transplantation or pancreas after kidney (PAK) transplantation.

B. Billing for Pancreas Transplants

There are no special provisions related to managed care participants. Managed care plans are required to provide all Medicare covered services. Medicare does not restrict which hospitals or physicians may perform pancreas transplantation.

The transplant procedure and revenue code 0360 for the operating room are paid under these codes. Procedures must be reported using the current ICD-9-CM procedure codes for pancreas and kidney transplants. Providers must place at least one of the following transplant procedure codes on the claim:

52. 80

Transplant of pancreas

52. 82

Homotransplant of pancreas

The Medicare Code Editor (MCE) has been updated to include 52.80 and 52.82 as covered procedures. (Effective October 1, 2000, ICD-9-CM code 52.83 was moved in the MCE to non-

covered. The FI must override any deny edit on claims that came in with 52.82 prior to October 1, 2000 and adjust, as 52.82 is the correct code.)

If the discharge date is July 1, 1999, or later: the FI processes the bill through Grouper and Pricer.

Pancreas transplantation is reasonable and necessary for the following diagnosis codes. However, since this is not an all-inclusive list, the contractor is permitted to determine if any additional diagnosis codes will be covered for this procedure.

Diabetes Diagnosis Codes

250.00	Diabetes mellitus without mention of complication, type II (non-insulin dependent) (NIDDM) (adult onset) or unspecified type, not stated as uncontrolled.
250.01	Diabetes mellitus without mention of complication, type I (insulin dependent) (IDDM) (juvenile), not stated as uncontrolled.
250.02	Diabetes mellitus without mention of complication, type II (non-insulin dependent) (NIDDM) (adult onset) or unspecified type, uncontrolled.
250.03	Diabetes mellitus without mention of complication, type I (insulin dependent) (IDDM) (juvenile), uncontrolled.
250.1X	Diabetes with ketoacidosis
250.2X	Diabetes with hyperosmolarity
250.3X	Diabetes with coma
250.4X	Diabetes with renal manifestations
250.5X	Diabetes with ophthalmic manifestations
250.6X	Diabetes with neurological manifestations
250.7X	Diabetes with peripheral circulatory disorders
250.8X	Diabetes with other specified manifestations
250.9X	Diabetes with unspecified complication

NOTE: X=0-3

- Hypertensive Renal Diagnosis Codes:

403.01	Malignant hypertensive renal disease, with renal failure
403.11	Benign hypertensive renal disease, with renal failure
403.91	Unspecified hypertensive renal disease, with renal failure
404.02	Malignant hypertensive heart and renal disease, with renal failure
404.03	Malignant hypertensive heart and renal disease, with congestive heart failure or renal failure
404.12	Benign hypertensive heart and renal disease, with renal failure
404.13	Benign hypertensive heart and renal disease, with congestive heart failure or renal failure
404.92	Unspecified hypertensive heart and renal disease, with renal failure
404.93	Unspecified hypertensive heart and renal disease, with congestive heart failure or renal failure

585.1 - 585.6, 585.9 Chronic Renal Failure Code

NOTE: If a patient had a kidney transplant that was successful, the patient no longer has chronic kidney failure, therefore it would be inappropriate for the provider to bill 585.1 - 585.6, 585.9 on such a patient. In these cases one of the following V-codes should be present on the claim or in the beneficiary's history.

The provider uses the following V-codes only when a kidney transplant was performed before the pancreas transplant:

V42.0   Organ or tissue replaced by transplant kidney

V43.89   Organ tissue replaced by other means, kidney or pancreas

NOTE: If a kidney and pancreas transplants are performed simultaneously, the claim should contain a diabetes diagnosis code and a renal failure code or one of the hypertensive renal failure diagnosis codes. The claim should also contain two transplant procedure codes. If the claim is for a pancreas transplant only, the claim should contain a diabetes diagnosis code and a V-code to indicate a previous kidney transplant. If the V-code is not on the claim for the pancreas transplant, the FI will search the beneficiary's claim history for a V-code.

Pancreas Transplant HCPCS Code

Carriers shall ensure the following HCPCS code is present on the claim:

48554 - Transplantation of pancreatic allograft

C. Drugs

If the pancreas transplant occurs after the kidney transplant, immunosuppressive therapy will begin with the date of discharge from the inpatient stay for the pancreas transplant.

D. Charges for Pancreas Acquisition Services

A separate organ acquisition cost center has been established for pancreas transplantation. The Medicare cost report will include a separate line to account for pancreas transplantation costs. The 42 CFR 412.2(e)(4) was changed to include pancreas in the list of organ acquisition costs that are paid on a reasonable cost basis.

Acquisition costs for pancreas transplantation as well as kidney transplants will occur in Revenue Center 081X. The FI overrides any claims that suspend due to repetition of revenue code

081X on the same claim if the patient had a simultaneous kidney/pancreas transplant. It pays for acquisition costs for both kidney and pancreas organs if transplants are performed simultaneously. It will not pay for more than two organ acquisitions on the same claim.

E. Medicare Summary Notices (MSN) and Remittance Advice Messages

If the provider submits a claim for simultaneous pancreas kidney transplantation or pancreas transplantation following a kidney transplant, and omits one of the appropriate diagnosis/procedure codes, the FI rejects and the carrier denies the claim, using the following MSN:

- MSN 16.32, "Medicare does not pay separately for this service."

- Use the following Remittance Advice Message:

- Claim adjustment reason code B15, "Claim/service denied/reduced because this procedure or service is not paid separately."

- If a claim is denied because no evidence of a prior kidney transplant is presented, use the following MSN message:

- MSN 15.4, "The information provided does not support the need for this service or item."

The contractor uses the following Remittance Advice Message:

- Claim adjustment reason code 50, "These are non-covered services because this is not deemed a 'medical necessity' by the payer."

To further clarify the situation, the contractor should also use new claim level remark code MA 126, "Pancreas transplant not covered unless kidney transplant performed."

Pub. 100-4, Chapter 3, Section 90.6

Visceral Transplants

A3-3615.7, Transmittal R1878A3

A. Background

Effective for services on or after April 1, 2001, Medicare covers intestinal and multi-visceral transplantation for the purpose of restoring intestinal function in patients with irreversible intestinal failure. Intestinal failure is defined as the loss of absorptive capacity of the small bowel secondary to severe primary gastrointestinal disease or surgically induced short bowel syndrome. Intestinal failure prevents oral nutrition and may be associated with both mortality and profound morbidity. Multi-Visceral transplantation includes organs in the digestive system (stomach, duodenum, liver, and intestine). See §260.5 of the National Coverage Determinations Manual for further information.

B. Approved Transplant Facilities

Medicare will cover intestinal transplantation if performed in an approved facility. The approved facilities are located at: http://www.cms.hhs.gov/ApprovedTransplantCenters.

C. Billing

ICD-9-CM procedure code 46.97 is effective for discharges on or after April 1, 2001. The Medicare Code Editor (MCE) lists this code as a non-covered procedure with no exceptions. The FI is to override the MCE when this procedure code is listed and the coverage criteria are met in an approved transplant facility.

For this procedure where the provider is approved as transplant facility, and the service is performed on or after the transplant approval date, the FI must suspend the claim for clerical review of the operative report to determine whether the beneficiary has at least one of the covered conditions listed when the diagnosis code is for a covered condition.

This review is not part of the FI's medical review workload. Instead, the FI should complete this review as part of its claims processing workload.

Charges for ICD-9-CM procedure code 46.97 should be billed under revenue code 0360, Operating Room Services.

For discharge dates on or after October 1, 2001, acquisition charges are billed under revenue code 081X, Organ Acquisition. For discharge dates between April 1, 2001, and September 30, 2001, hospitals were to report the acquisition charges on the claim, but there was no interim pass-through payment made for these costs.

Bill the procedure used to obtain the donor's organ on the same claim, using appropriate ICD-9-CM procedure codes.

The 11X bill type should be used when billing for intestinal transplants.

Immunosuppressive therapy for intestinal transplantation is covered and should be billed consistent with other organ transplants under the current rules.

There is no specific ICD-9-CM diagnosis code for intestinal failure. Diagnosis codes exist to capture the causes of intestinal failure. Some examples of intestinal failure include, but are not limited to:

- Volvulus 560.2,

- Volvulus gastroschisis 756.79, other [congenital] anomalies of abdominal wall,

- Volvulus gastroschisis 569.89, other specified disorders of intestine,

- Necrotizing enterocolitis 777.5, necrotizing enterocolitis in fetus or newborn,

- Necrotizing enterocolitis 014.8, other tuberculosis of intestines, peritoneum, and mesenteric,

- Necrotizing enterocolitis and splanchnic vascular thrombosis 557.0, acute vascular insufficiency of intestine,

- Inflammatory bowel disease 569.9, unspecified disorder of intestine,

- Radiation enteritis 777.5, necrotizing enterocolitis in fetus or newborn, and

- Radiation enteritis 558.1.

D. Acquisition Costs

A separate organ acquisition cost center was established for acquisition costs incurred on or after October 1, 2001. The Medicare Cost Report will include a separate line to account for these transplantation costs. For intestinal and multi-visceral transplants performed between April 1, 2001, and October 1, 2001, the DRG payment was payment in full for all hospital services related to this procedure.

E. Medicare Summary Notices (MSN), Remittance Advice Messages, and Notice of Utilization Notices (NOU)

If an intestinal transplant is billed by an unapproved facility after April 1, 2001, the FI must deny the claim and use MSN message 21.6, "This item or service is not covered when performed, referred, or ordered by this provider;" 21.18, "This item or service is not covered when performed or ordered by this provider;" or, 16.2, "This service cannot be paid when provided in this location/facility;" and Remittance Advice Message, Claim Adjustment Reason Code 52, "The referring/prescribing/rendering provider is not eligible to refer/prescribe/order/perform the service billed."

Pub. 100-4, Chapter 3, Section 100.1

Billing for Abortion Services

A3-3652

Effective October 1, 1998, abortions are not covered under the Medicare program except for instances where the pregnancy is a result of an act of rape or incest; or the woman suffers from a physical disorder, physical injury, or physical illness, including a life endangering physical condition caused by the pregnancy itself that would, as certified by a physician, place the woman in danger of death unless an abortion is performed.

A. "G" Modifier

The "G7" modifier is defined as "the pregnancy resulted from rape or incest, or pregnancy certified by physician as life threatening."

Beginning July 1, 1999, providers should bill for abortion services using the new Modifier G7. This modifier can be used on claims with dates of services October 1, 1998, and after. CWF will be able to recognize the modifier beginning July 1, 1999.

B. FI Billing Instructions

1. Hospital Inpatient Billing

Hospitals will bill the FI on Form CMS-1450 using bill type 11X. Medicare will pay only when condition code A7 or A8 is used in FLs 24-30 of UB92 along with an appropriate ICD-9-CM principal diagnosis code that will group to DRG 380 or with an appropriate ICD-9-CM principal diagnosis code and one of the four appropriate ICD-9-CM operating room procedure codes listed below that will group to DRG 381.

69.01

69.02

69.51

74.91

Providers must use ICD-9-CM codes 69.01 and 69.02 to describe exactly the procedure or service performed.

The FI must manually review claims with the above ICD-9-CM procedure codes to verify that all of the above conditions are met.

2. Outpatient Billing

Hospitals will bill the FI on Form CMS-1450 using bill type 13X, 83X and 85X. Medicare will pay only if one of the following CPT codes is used with the "G7" modifier.

59840

59851

59856

59841

59852

59857

59850

59855

59866

C. Common Working File (CWF) Edits

For hospital outpatient claims, CWF will bypass its edits for a managed care beneficiary who is having an abortion outside their plan and the claim is submitted with the "G7" modifier and one of the above CPT codes.

For hospital inpatient claims, CWF will bypass its edits for a managed care beneficiary who is having an abortion outside their plan and the claim is submitted with one of the above ICD-9-CM procedure codes.

D. Medicare Summary Notices (MSN)/Explanation of Your Medicare Benefits Remittance Advice Message

If a claim is submitted with one of the above CPT procedure codes but no "G7" modifier, the claim is denied. The FI states on the MSN the following message:

This service was denied because Medicare covers this service only under certain circumstances." (MSN Message 21.21).

For the remittance advice the FI uses existing American National Standard Institute (ANSI) X12-835 claim adjustment reason code B5, "Claim/service denied/reduced because coverage guidelines were not met or were exceeded."

Pub. 100-4, Chapter 3, Section 100.2

Payment for CRNA or AA Services
A3-3660.9

Anesthesia services furnished on or after January 1, 1990, at a qualified rural hospital by a hospital employed or contracted CRNA or AA can be paid on a reasonable cost basis. The FI determines the hospital's qualification using the following criteria.

The hospital must be located in a rural area (as defined for PPS purposes) to be considered. A rural hospital that qualified and was paid on a reasonable cost basis

for CRNA or AA services during calendar year 1989 could continue to be paid on a reasonable cost basis for these services furnished during calendar year 1990 if it could establish before January 1, 1990, that it did not provide more than 500 surgical procedures, both inpatient and outpatient, requiring anesthesia services during 1989.

A rural hospital that was not paid on a reasonable cost basis for CRNA or AA services during calendar year 1989 could be paid on a reasonable cost basis for these services furnished during calendar year 1990 if it established before January 1, 1990, that:

- As of January 1, 1988, it employed or contracted with a CRNA or AA (but not more than one full-time equivalent CRNA or AA); and

- In both 1987 and 1989, it had a volume of 500 or fewer surgical procedures, including inpatient and outpatient procedures, requiring anesthesia services.

Each CRNA or AA employed by, or under contract with the hospital, must agree in writing not to bill on a fee schedule basis for services furnished at the hospital. A rural hospital can qualify and continue to be paid on a reasonable cost basis for qualified CRNA or AA services for a calendar year beyond 1990 if it could establish before January 1 of that year that it did not provide more than 500 surgical procedures, both inpatient and outpatient, requiring anesthesia services during the preceding year. For a calendar year beyond 1990, it must make its election after September 30, but before January 1. The FI determines the number of anesthetics by annualizing the number of surgical procedures for the 9-month period ending September 30.

A rural hospital that first elects reasonable cost payment for CRNA services for a calendar year after 1990 must demonstrate that:

- It had a volume of 500 or fewer surgical procedures, including inpatient and outpatient, requiring anesthesia services in the preceding year; and

- It meets the criteria that would have been met by a rural hospital first electing reasonable cost in calendar year 1990.

To prevent duplicate payments, the FI informs carriers of the names of CRNAs or AAs, the hospitals with which they have agreements, and the effective dates of the agreements. If the CRNA or AA bills Part B for anesthesia services furnished prior to the hospital's election of reasonable cost payments, the carrier must recover the overpayment from the CRNA or AA.

Pub. 100-4, Chapter 3, Section 100.6

Inpatient Renal Services
HO-E400

Section 405.103l of Subpart J of Regulation 5 stipulates that only approved hospitals may bill for ESRD services. Hence, to allow hospitals to bill and be reimbursed for inpatient dialysis services furnished under arrangements, both facilities participating in the arrangement must meet the conditions of 405.2120 and 405.2160 of Subpart U of Regulation 5. In order for renal dialysis facilities to have a written arrangement with each other to provide inpatient dialysis care both facilities must meet the minimum utilization rate requirement, i.e., two dialysis stations with a performance capacity of at least four dialysis treatments per week.

Dialysis may be billed by an SNF as a service if: (a) it is provided by a hospital with which the facility has a transfer agreement in effect, and that hospital is approved to provide staff-assisted dialysis for the Medicare program; or (b) it is furnished directly by an SNF meeting all nonhospital maintenance dialysis facility requirements, including minimum utilization requirements. (See §§1861(h)(6), 1861(h)(7), title XVIII.)

Pub. 100-4, Chapter 3, Section 100.7

Lung Volume Reduction Surgery

Lung Volume Reduction Surgery (LVRS) (also known as reduction pneumoplasty, lung shaving, or lung contouring) is an invasive surgical procedure to reduce the volume of a hyperinflated lung in order to allow the underlying compressed lung to expand, and thus, establish improved respiratory function.

Effective for discharges on or after January 1, 2004, Medicare will cover LVRS under certain conditions as described in §240 of Pub. 100-03, "National Coverage Determinations".

The Medicare Code Editor (MCE) creates a Limited Coverage edit for procedure code 32.22. This procedure code has limited coverage due to the stringent conditions that must be met by hospitals. Where this procedure code is identified by MCE, the FI shall determine if coverage criteria is met and override the MCE if appropriate.

The LVRS can only be performed in the facilities listed on the following Web site: www.cms.hhs.gov/coverage/lvrsfacility.pdf

Medicare previously only covered LVRS as part of the National Emphysema Treatment Trial (NETT). The study was limited to 18 hospitals, and patients were randomized into two arms, either medical management and LVRS or medical management. The study was conducted by The

National Heart, Lung, and Blood Institute of the National Institutes of Health and coordinated by Johns Hopkins University (JHU). Hospital claims for patients in the NETT were identified by the presence of Condition Code EY. The JHU instructed hospitals of the correct billing procedures for billing claims under the NETT.

Pub. 100-4, Chapter 4, Section 10.4

Packaging

Initial packaging rules for OPPS implementation are:

- Initially, only minimal packaging, i.e., payment for a procedure or medical visits does not include payment for the related ancillary services such as laboratory tests or x-rays;

- Payment for clinical diagnostic laboratory tests which are paid under the clinical diagnostic fee schedule and radiology and other diagnostic services paid under OPPS will be made in addition to the OPPS payment for a surgical procedure or medical visit performed on the same day; and

- APC payments will include certain packaged items, such as anesthesia, supplies, certain drugs and the use of recovery and observation rooms.

Under OPPS, packaged services are items and services that are considered to be an integral part of another service that is paid under the OPPS. No separate payment is made for packaged services, because the cost of these items is included in the APC payment for the service of which they are an integral part. For example, routine supplies, anesthesia, recovery room and most drugs are considered to be an integral part of a surgical procedure so payment for these items is packaged into the APC payment for the surgical procedure.

A. Claims Resulting in APC Payments

If a claim contains services that result in an APC payment but also contains packaged services, separate payment for the packaged services is not made since payment is included in the APC. However, charges related to the packaged services are used for outlier and Transitional Corridor Payments (TOPs) as well as for future rate setting.

Claims Resulting in No APC Payments

If the claim contains only services payable under cost reimbursement, such as corneal tissue, and services that would be packaged services if an APC were payable, then the packaged services are not separately payable. In addition, these charges for the packaged services are not used to calculate TOPs.

If the claim contains only services payable under a fee schedule, such as clinical diagnostic laboratory, and also contains services that would be packaged services if an APC were payable, the packaged services are not separately payable. In addition, the charges are not used to calculate TOPs.

If a claim contains services payable under cost reimbursement, services payable under a fee schedule, and services that would be package services if an APC were payable, the packaged services are not separately payable. In addition, the charges are not used to calculate TOPs payments.

During claims processing of bill types 12X and 13X cost reimbursement payments may not be made to hospital outpatient departments for any items or services except for corneal tissue and certain CRNA services, orphan drugs, and ESRD drugs and supplies not included in the composite rate. Effective 4/1/06, 14X type of bill is for non-patient laboratory specimens and is no longer applicable for cost reimbursement payment.

Pub. 100-4, Chapter 4, Section 10.5

Discounting
A-01-93

- Multiple surgical procedures furnished during the same operative session are discounted;

- The full amount is paid for the surgical procedure with the highest weight;

- Fifty percent is paid for any other surgical procedure(s) performed at the same time;

- Similar discounting occurs now under the physician fee schedule and the payment system for ASCs;

- Surgical procedures terminated after a patient is prepared for surgery but before induction of anesthesia are paid at 50 percent of the APC payment; and

- When multiple surgical procedures are performed during the same operative session, beneficiary coinsurance is discounted in proportion to the APC payment.

Pub. 100-4, Chapter 4, Section 10.10

Biweekly Interim Payments for Certain Hospital Outpatient Items and Services That Are Paid on a Cost Basis, and Direct Medical Education Payments, Not Included in the Hospital Outpatient Prospective
A-01-32

For hospitals subject to the OPPS, payment for certain items that are not paid under the OPPS, but which are reimbursable in addition to OPPS, are made through biweekly interim payments subject to retrospective adjustment based on a settled cost report. These payments include:

- Direct medical education payments;

- Costs of nursing and allied health programs;

- Costs associated with interns and residents not in an approved teaching program as described in 42 CFR 415.202;

- Teaching physicians costs attributable to Part B services for hospitals that elect cost-based reimbursement for teaching physicians under 42 CFR 415.160;

- CRNA services;

- For hospitals that meet the requirements under 42 CFR 412.113(c), the reasonable costs of anesthesia services furnished to hospital outpatients by qualified nonphysician anesthetists (i.e., certified registered nurse anesthetists and anesthesiologists' assistants) employed by the hospital or obtained under arrangements;

- Bad debts for uncollectible deductibles and coinsurance;

- Organ acquisition costs paid under Part B.

For hospitals that are paid under the OPPS, interim payments for these items attributable to both hospital outpatients, as well as inpatients whose services are paid under Part B of the Medicare program are made on a biweekly basis. The FI determines the amount of the biweekly payment by estimating a hospital's reimbursement amount for these items for the cost reporting period by using:

- Medicare principles of cost reimbursement for cost-based items; and

- Medicare rules for determining payment for graduate medical education for direct medical education, and dividing the total annual estimated amount for these items into 26 equal biweekly payments.

The estimated annual amount is based on the most current data available. Biweekly interim payments are reviewed and, if necessary, adjusted at least twice during the reporting period, with final settlement based on a submitted cost report.

Because hospitals subject to the OPPS have not received payment for these items attributable to services furnished on or after August 1, 2000, the date the OPPS was implemented, the first payment to each hospital included all the payments due to the hospital retroactive to August 1, 2000. Thereafter, FIs continue to make payment on a biweekly basis. Each payment is made two weeks after the end of a biweekly period of services. The FI was required to make retroactive payments and begin making biweekly interim payments to all hospitals that are due these payments no later than 60 days after March 8, 2001.

These biweekly payments may be combined with the inpatient biweekly payments that the FI makes under §2405.2 of the Medicare Provider Reimbursement Manual (CMS Pub.15-I). However, if a single payment is made, for purposes of final cost report settlement, they must maintain records to separately identify the amount of the hospital's combined payment that is paid out of the Part A or Part B trust fund.

Pub. 100-4, Chapter 4, Section 20.5

HCPCS/Revenue Code Chart

A-01-93, A-01-50, A-03-066

The following chart reflects HCPCS coding to be reported under OPPS by hospital outpatient departments. This chart is intended only as a guide to be used by hospitals to assist them in reporting services rendered. Hospitals that are currently utilizing different revenue/HCPCS reporting may continue to do so. They are not required to change the way they currently report their services to agree with this chart. Note that this chart does not represent all HCPCS coding subject to OPPS.

Revenue Code	HCPCS Code	Description
	10040-69990	Surgical Procedure
	92950-92961	Cardiovascular
	96570, 96571	Photodynamic Therapy
	99170, 99185, 99186	Other Services and Procedures
	99291-99292	Critical Care
	99440	Newborn Care
	90782-90799	Therapeutic or Diagnostic Injections
	D0150, D0240-D0274, D0277, D0460, D0472- D0999, D1510-D1550, D2970, D2999, D3460, D3999, D4260-D4264, D4270-D4273, D4355-D4381, D5911-D5912, D5983-D5985, D5987, D6920, D7110-D7260, D7291, D7940, D9630, D9930, D9940, D9950-D9952	Dental Services
	92502-92596, 92599	Otorhinolaryngologic Services (ENT)
0278	E0749, E0782, E0783, E0785	Implanted Durable Medical Equipment
0278	E0751, E0753, L8600, L8603, L8610, L8612, L8613, L8614, L8630, L8641, L8642, L8658, L8670, L8699	Implanted Prosthetic Devices
0302	86485-86586	Immunology
0305	85060-85102, 86077-86079	Hematology

Revenue Code	HCPCS Code	Description
031X	80500-80502	Pathology - Lab
0310	88300-88365, 88399	Surgical Pathology
0311	88104-88125, 88160-88199	Cytopathology
032X	70010-76092, 76094-76999	Diagnostic Radiology
0333	77261-77799	Radiation Oncology
034X	78000-79999	Nuclear Medicine
037X	99141-99142	Anesthesia
045X	99281-99285, 99291	Emergency
046X	94010-94799	Pulmonary Function
0480	93600-93790, 93799, G0166	Intra Electrophysiological Procedures and Other Vascular Studies
0481	93501-93572	Cardiac Catheterization
0482	93015-93024	Stress Test
0483	93303-93350	Echocardiography
051X	92002-92499	Ophthalmological Services
051X	99201-99215, 99241-99245, 99271-99275	Clinic Visit
0510, 0517, 0519	95144-95149, 95165, 95170, 95180, 95199	Allergen Immunotherapy
0519	95805-95811	Sleep Testing
0530	98925-98929	Osteopathic Manipulative Procedures
0636	A4642, A9500, A9605	Radionucleides
0636	90476-90665, 90675-90749	Vaccines, Toxoids
0636	90296-90379, 90385, 90389-90396	Immune Globulins
073X	G0004-G0006, G0015	Event Recording ECG
0730	93005-93009, 93011-93013, 93040-93224, 93278	Electrocardiograms (ECGs)
0731	93225-93272	Holter Monitor
074X	95812-95827, 95950-95962	Electroencephalogram (EEG)
0771	G0008-G0010	Vaccine Administration
088X	90935-90999	Non-ESRD Dialysis
0900	90801, 90802, 90865,90899	Behavioral Health Treatment/Services
0901	90870, 90871	Psychiatry
0903	90910, 90911, 90812-90815, 90823, 90824, 90826-90829	Psychiatry
0909	90880	Psychiatry
0914	90804-90809, 90816-90819, 90821, 90822, 90845, 90862	Psychiatry
0915	90853, 90857	Psychiatry
0916	90846,90847, 90849	Psychiatry
0917	90901-90911	Biofeedback
0918	96100-96117	Central Nervous System Assessments/Tests
092X	95829-95857, 95900-95937, 95970-95999	Miscellaneous Neurological Procedures
0920, 0929	93875-93990	Non Invasive Vascular Diagnosis Studies

Revenue Code	HCPCS Code	Description
0922	95858-95875	Electromyography (EMG)
0924	95004-95078	Allergy Test
0940	96900-96999	Special Dermatological Procedures
0940	98940-98942	Chiropractic Manipulative Treatment
0940	99195	Other Services and Procedures
0943	93797-93798	Cardiac Rehabilitation

Revenue codes have not been identified for these procedures, as they can be performed in a number of revenue centers within a hospital, such as emergency room (0450), operating room (0360), or clinic (0510). Hospitals are to report these HCPCS codes under the revenue center where they were performed.

NOTE: The listing of HCPCS codes contained in the above chart does not assure coverage on the specific service. Current coverage criteria apply. FIs are not to install additional edits for matching of revenue codes and HCPCS codes.

20. 5.1 – Appropriate Revenue Codes to Report Medical Devices That Have Been Granted Pass-Through Status

A-03-035

The FIs shall instruct their hospitals to use an appropriate HCPCS code and one of the following revenue codes:

0272, 0275, 0276, 0278, 0279, 0280, 0289 or 0624 to bill implantable devices that have been granted pass-through status under the OPPS. Devices eligible for pass-through payment, as designated by payment status indicator "H," should not be reported utilizing any other revenue code series or subcategories.

The FIs shall instruct their hospitals to report implantable orthotic and prosthetic devices and implantable durable medical equipment (DME) under another revenue code such as 0278- other implants. Hospitals are not to use revenue codes 0274 or 0290 to report implantable orthotic and prosthetic devices or implantable DME. Similar requirements apply to reporting revenue codes for non-pass-through devices.

Pub. 100-4, Chapter 4, Section 20.6

Use of Modifiers

The following is a list of all modifiers that are reported under OPPS as of April 1, 2002. Definitions may be found in the current CPT guide or the HCPCS Guide.

Modifiers Used for Outpatient Prospective Payment System

Modifiers Used for Outpatient Prospective Payment System	Level I (CPT) Modifiers	Level II (HCPCS) Modifiers
-25	-50	-73
-91	-CA	-E1
-FA	-GA	-LC
-QL	-RC	-TA
-27	-52	-74
-E2	-F1	-GG
-LD	-QM	-RT
-T1	-58	-76
-E3	-F2	-GH
-LT	-T2	-59
-77	-E4	-F3
-GY	-T3	-78
-F4	-GZ	-T4
-79	-F5	-T5
-F6	-T6	-F7
-T7	-F8	-T8
-F9	-T9	

As indicated in §20.6.2, modifier -50, while it may be used with diagnostic and radiology procedures as well as with surgical procedures, should be used to report bilateral procedures that are performed at the same operative session as a single line item. Modifiers RT and LT are not used when modifier -50 applies. A bilateral procedure is reported on one line using modifier -50. Modifier -50 applies to any bilateral procedure performed on both sides at the same session.

NOTE: Use of modifiers applies to services/procedures performed on the same calendar day.

Other valid modifiers that are used under other payment methods are still valid and should continue to be reported, e.g., those that are used to report outpatient rehabilitation and ambulance services. Modifiers may be applied to surgical, radiology, and other diagnostic procedures. Providers must use any applicable modifier where appropriate.

Providers do not use a modifier if the narrative definition of a code indicates multiple occurrences.

EXAMPLES:

The code definition indicates two to four lesions. The code indicates multiple extremities.

Providers do not use a modifier if the narrative definition of a code indicates that the procedure applies to different body parts.

EXAMPLES:

Code 11600 (Excision malignant lesion, trunks, arms, or legs; lesion diameter 0.5 cm. or less)

Code 11640 (Excision malignant lesion, face, ears, eyelids, nose, lips; lesion diameter 0.5 cm. or less)

Modifiers -GN, -GO, and -GP must be used to identify the therapist performing speech language therapy, occupational therapy, and physical therapy respectively.

Modifier 50 (bilateral) applies to diagnostic, radiological, and surgical procedures.

Modifiers -52 applies to radiological procedures.

Modifiers -73, and -74 apply only to certain diagnostic and surgical procedures that require anesthesia.

Following are some general guidelines for using modifiers. They are in the form of questions to be considered. If the answer to any of the following questions is yes, it is appropriate to use the applicable modifier.

1. Will the modifier add more information regarding the anatomic site of the procedure?

EXAMPLE: Cataract surgery on the right or left eye.

2. Will the modifier help to eliminate the appearance of duplicate billing?

EXAMPLES: Use modifier 77 to report the same procedure performed more than once on the same date of service but at different encounters.

Use modifier 25 to report significant, separately identifiable evaluation and management service by the same physician on the same day of the procedure or other service.

Use modifier 58 to report staged or related procedure or service by the same physician during the postoperative period.

Use modifier 78 to report a return to the operating room for a related procedure during the postoperative period.

Use modifier 79 to report an unrelated procedure or service by the same physician during the postoperative period.

3. Would a modifier help to eliminate the appearance of unbundling?

EXAMPLE: CPT codes 90780 (Infusion therapy, using other than chemotherapeutic drugs, per visit) and 36000 (Introduction of needle or intra catheter, vein): If procedure 36000 was performed for a reason other than as part of the IV infusion, modifier -59 would be appropriate.

Pub. 100-4, Chapter 4, Section 20.6.4

Use of Modifiers for Discontinued Services
A. General

Modifiers provide a way for hospitals to report and be paid for expenses incurred in preparing a patient for surgery and scheduling a room for performing the procedure

where the service is subsequently discontinued. This instruction is applicable to both outpatient hospital departments and to ambulatory surgical centers.

Modifier -73 is used by the facility to indicate that a surgical or diagnostic procedure requiring anesthesia was terminated due to extenuating circumstances or to circumstances that threatened the well being of the patient after the patient had been prepared for the procedure (including procedural pre-medication when provided), and been taken to the room where the procedure was to be performed, but prior to administration of anesthesia. For purposes of billing for services furnished in the hospital outpatient department, anesthesia is defined to include local, regional block(s), moderate sedation/analgesia ("conscious sedation"), deep sedation/analgesia, or general anesthesia. This modifier code was created so that the costs incurred by the hospital to prepare the patient for the procedure and the resources expended in the procedure room and recovery room (if needed) could be recognized for payment even though the procedure was discontinued. Prior to January 1, 1999, modifier -52 was used for reporting these discontinued services.

Modifier -74 is used by the facility to indicate that a surgical or diagnostic procedure requiring anesthesia was terminated after the induction of anesthesia or after the procedure was started (e.g., incision made, intubation started, scope inserted) due to extenuating circumstances or circumstances that threatened the well being of the patient. For purposes of billing for services furnished in the hospital outpatient department, anesthesia is defined to include local, regional block(s), moderate sedation/analgesia ("conscious sedation"), deep sedation/analgesia, and general anesthesia. This modifier code was created so that the costs incurred by the hospital to initiate the procedure (preparation of the patient, procedure room, recovery room) could be recognized for payment even though the procedure was discontinued prior to completion. Prior to January 1, 1999, modifier -53 was used for reporting these discontinued services.

Modifiers -52 and -53 are no longer accepted as modifiers for certain diagnostic and surgical procedures under the hospital outpatient prospective payment system. Coinciding with the addition of the modifiers -73 and -74, modifiers -52 and -53 were revised. Modifier -52 is used to indicate partial reduction or discontinuation of radiology procedures and other services that do not require anesthesia. The modifier provides a means for reporting reduced services without disturbing the identification of the basic service. Modifier -53 is used to indicate discontinuation of physician services and is not approved for use for outpatient hospital services.

The elective cancellation of a procedure should not be reported.

Modifiers -73 and -74 are used to indicate discontinued surgical and certain diagnostic procedures only. They are not used to indicate discontinued radiology procedures.

B. Effect on Payment

Surgical or certain diagnostic procedures that are discontinued after the patient has been prepared for the procedure and taken to the procedure room for which modifier -73 is coded, will be paid at 50 percent of the full OPPS payment amount.

Surgical or certain diagnostic procedures that are discontinued after the procedure has been initiated and/or the patient has received anesthesia for which modifier -74 is coded, will be paid at the full OPPS payment amount.

C. Termination Where Multiple Procedures Planned

When one or more of the procedures planned is completed, the completed procedures are reported as usual.

When one or more of the procedures planned is completed, the completed procedures are reported as usual. The other(s) that were planned, and not started, are not reported. When none of the procedures that were planned were completed, and the patient has been prepared and taken to the procedure room, the first procedure that was planned, but not completed is reported with modifier -73. If the first procedure has been started (scope inserted, intubation started, incision made, etc.) and/or the patient has received anesthesia, modifier -74 is used. The other procedures are not reported.

If the first procedure is terminated prior to the induction of anesthesia and before the patient is wheeled into the procedure room, the procedure should not be reported. The patient has to be taken to the room where the procedure is to be performed in order to report modifier -73 or -74.

Pub. 100-4, Chapter 4, Section 61.2

Edits for Claims on Which Specified Procedures are to be Reported With Device Codes

The OCE will return to the provider any claim that reports a HCPCS code for a procedure listed in the table of device edits that does not also report at least one device HCPCS code required for that procedure as listed on the CMS Web site at http://www.cms.hhs.gov/providers/hopps/. The table shows the effective date for each edit. If the claim is returned to the provider for failure to pass the edits, the hospital will need to modify the claim by either correcting the procedure code or ensuring that one of the required device codes is on the claim before resubmission. While all devices that have device HCPCS codes, and that were used in a given procedure should be reported on the

claim, where more than one device code is listed for a given procedure code, only one of the possible device codes is required to be on the claim for payment to be made, unless otherwise specified.

Device edits do not apply to the specified procedure code if the provider reports one of the following modifiers with the procedure code:

52 - Reduced Services;

73 — Discontinued outpatient procedure prior to anesthesia administration; and

74 — Discontinued outpatient procedure after anesthesia administration.

Where a procedure that normally requires a device is interrupted, either before or after the administration of anesthesia if anesthesia is required or at any point if anesthesia is not required, and the device is not used, hospitals should report modifier 52, 73 or 74 as applicable. The device edits are not applied in these cases.

Pub. 100-4, Chapter 4, Section 160

Coding for Clinic and Emergency Visits

A-01-93

The OPPS hospitals previously reported CPT code 99201 to indicate a visit of any type. Under OPPS, 31 codes are used to indicate visits, with payment differentials for more or less intense services.

Hospitals code the site of the visit and the level of intensity, using the following codes:

92002, 92004, 92012, 92014, 99201, 99202, 99203, 99204, 99205, 99211, 99212, 99213, 99214, 99215, 99241, 99242, 99243, 99244, 99245, 99271, 99272, 99273, 99274, 99275, 99281, 99282, 99283, 99284, 99285, 99291, and G0175.

Because CPT is more descriptive of practitioner than of facility services, hospitals must use CPT guidelines when applicable, or crosswalk hospital coding structures to CPT. For example, a hospital that has eight levels of emergency and trauma care, depending on nursing ratios, should crosswalk those eight levels to the CPT codes for emergency care.

Pub. 100-4, Chapter 4, Section 180.3

Unlisted Service or Procedure

This section does not apply to OPPS hospitals.

There may be services or procedures performed that are not found in HCPCS. These are typically services that are rarely provided, unusual, variable, or new. A number of specific code numbers have been designated for reporting unlisted procedures. When an unlisted procedure code is used, a report describing the service is submitted with the claim. Pertinent information includes a definition or description of the nature, extent, and need for the procedure and the time, effort, and equipment necessary to provide the service.

When an FI receives a claim with an unlisted procedure code, it reviews it to verify that there is no existing code that adequately describes the procedure. If it determines that an adequately descriptive code is contained in HCPCS, it advises the hospital of the proper code and processes the claim. If it determines that no existing code is sufficiently descriptive, it pays the claim using the unlisted procedure code. If the frequency of the procedure warrants assignment of a local code, the FI forwards a copy and the operative report to the RO HCPCS coordinator for a code determination. When it receives a determination, the FI informs the hospital of the correct code for future reporting. Local codes are not accepted under OPPS and line items for local codes are no longer paid on cost.

NOTE: If the claim is submitted via EMC or identified after the bill has been processed, an operative report, the provider number, revenue codes, and charges are sufficient.

The "Unlisted Procedures" and codes for surgery are:

HCPCS code	Unlisted Procedure
15999	Unlisted procedure, excision pressure ulcer
17999	Unlisted procedure, skin, mucous membrane and subcutaneous tissue
19499	Unlisted procedure, breast
20999	Unlisted procedure, musculoskeletal system, general
21299	Unlisted craniofacial and maxillofacial procedures
21499	Unlisted orthopedic procedure, head
21899	Unlisted procedure, neck or thorax
22899	Unlisted procedure, spine
22999	Unlisted procedure, abdomen, musculoskeletal system
23929	Unlisted procedure, shoulder
24999	Unlisted procedure, humerus or elbow
25999	Unlisted procedure, forearm or wrist
26989	Unlisted procedure, hands or fingers
27299	Unlisted procedure, pelvis or hip joint
27599	Unlisted procedure, femur or knee
27899	Unlisted procedure, leg or ankle
28899	Unlisted procedure, foot or toes
29799	Unlisted procedure, casting or strapping
29909	Unlisted procedure, arthroscopy
30999	Unlisted procedure, nose
31299	Unlisted procedure, accessory sinuses
31599	Unlisted procedure, larynx
31899	Unlisted procedure, trachea, bronchi
32999	Unlisted procedure, lungs, and pleura
33999	Unlisted procedure, cardiac surgery
36299	Unlisted procedure, vascular injection
37799	Unlisted procedure, vascular surgery
38999	Unlisted procedure, hemic or lymphatic system
39499	Unlisted procedure, mediastinum
39599	Unlisted procedure, diaphragm
40799	Unlisted procedure, lips
40899	Unlisted procedure, vestibule of mouth
41599	Unlisted procedure, tongue, floor of mouth
41899	Unlisted procedure, dentoalveolar structures

HCPCS code	Unlisted Procedure
42299	Unlisted procedure, palate, uvula
42699	Unlisted procedure, salivary glands or ducts
42999	Unlisted procedure, pharynx, adenoids, or tonsils
43499	Unlisted procedure, esophag
43999	Unlisted procedure, stomach
44799	Unlisted procedure, intestine
44899	Unlisted procedure, Meckel's diverticulum and the mesentery
45999	Unlisted procedure, rectum
46999	Unlisted procedure, anus
47399	Unlisted procedure, liver
47999	Unlisted procedure, biliary tract
48999	Unlisted procedure, pancreas
49999	Unlisted procedure, abdomen, peritoneum, and omentum
53899	Unlisted procedure, urinary system
55899	Unlisted procedure, male genital system
56399	Unlisted procedure, laparoscopy, hysteroscopy
58999	Unlisted procedure, female genital system non-obstetrical
59899	Unlisted procedure, maternity care and delivery
60699	Unlisted procedure, endocrine system
64999	Unlisted procedure, nervous system
66999	Unlisted procedure, anterior segment of eye
67299	Unlisted procedure, posterior segment
67399	Unlisted procedure, ocular muscle
67599	Unlisted procedure, orbit
67999	Unlisted procedure, eyelids
68399	Unlisted procedure, conjunctiva
68899	Unlisted procedure, lacrimal system
69399	Unlisted procedure, external ear
69799	Unlisted procedure, middle ear
69949	Unlisted procedure, inner ear
69979	Unlisted procedure, temporal bone, middle fossa approach

Pub. 100-4, Chapter 4, Section 220.1

Billing for IMRT Planning and Delivery

A-02-026

Effective for services furnished on or after April 1, 2002, codes G0174, and G0178 are no longer valid codes. Hospitals must use CPT code 77301 for IMRT planning and CPT code 77418 for IMRT delivery. Any of the CPT codes 77401 through 77416 or 77418 may be reported on the same day as long as the services are furnished at a separate treatment sessions. In these cases, modifier -59 must be appended to the appropriate codes.

Pub. 100-4, Chapter 4, Section 220.4

Additional Billing Instructions for IMRT and SR Planning

A-02-026

Payment for the services identified by CPT codes 77280 through 77295, 77300, and 77305 through 77321, 77336, and 77370 are included in the APC payment for IMRT and SR planning. These codes should not be billed in addition to 77301 and G0242.

Payment for IMRT and SR planning does not include payment for services described by CPT codes 77332 through 77334. When provided, these services should be billed in addition to the IMRT and SR planning codes 77301 and G0242.

Payment for CPT code 20660 is included in G0243; therefore, hospitals should not report 20660 separately.

Pub. 100-4, Chapter 4, Section 230.1

Coding and Payment for Drugs and Biologicals

This section provides hospitals with coding instructions and payment information for drugs paid under OPPS.

Pub. 100-4, Chapter 4, Section 230.2.1

Administration of Drugs Via Implantable or Portable Pumps

Table 2: CY 2006 OPPS Drug Administration Codes for Implantable or Portable Pumps

	2005 CPT		Final CY 2006 OPPS		
2005 CPT	2005 Descrip	Code	Descrip	SI	APC
n/a	n/a	C8957	Intravenous infusion for therapy/diagnosis; initiation of prolonged infusion (more than 8 hours), requiring use of portable or implantable pump	S	0120
96414	Chemotherapy administration, intravenous; infusion technique, initiation of prolonged infusion (more than 8 hours), requiring the use of a portable or implantable pump	96416	Chemotherapy administration, intravenous infusion technique; initiation of prolonged chemotherapy infusion (more than 8 hours), requiring use of portable or implantable pump	S	0117
96425	Chemotherapy administration, infusion technique, initiation of prolonged infusion (more than 8 hours), requiring the use of a portable or implantable pump)	96425	Chemotherapy administration, intra-arterial; infusion technique, initiation of prolonged infusion (more than 8 hours), requiring the use of a portable or implantable pump	S	0117
96520	Refilling and maintenance of portable pump	96521	Refilling and maintenance of portable pump	T	0125
96530	Refilling and maintenance of implantable pump or reservoir for drug delivery, systemic [e.g., Intravenous, intra-arterial]	96522	Refilling and maintenance of implantable pump or reservoir for drug delivery, systemic (e.g., intravenous, intra-arterial)	T	125
n/a	n/a	96523	Irrigation of implanted venous access device for drug delivery systems	N	-

Hospitals are to report HCPCS code C8957 and CPT codes 96416 and 96425 to indicate the initiation of a prolonged infusion that requires the use of an implantable or portable pump. CPT codes 96521, 92522, and 96523 should be used by hospitals to indicate refilling and maintenance of drug delivery systems or irrigation of implanted venous access devices for such systems, and may be reported for the servicing of devices used for therapeutic drugs other than chemotherapy.

Pub. 100-4, Chapter 4, Section 230.2.2

Chemotherapy Drug Administration

A. Overview

AMA chemotherapy administration instructions for CPT codes 96401-96549 additionally apply to HCPCS codes C8954, C8955 and C8953. Therefore, hospitals are to report chemotherapy drug administration HCPCS codes when providing non-radionuclide anti-neoplastic drugs to treat cancer and when administering non-radionuclide anti-neoplastic drugs, anti-neoplastic agents, monoclonal antibody agents, and biologic response modifiers for treatment of noncancer diagnoses.

Medicare's general policy regarding physician supervision within hospital outpatient departments meets the physician supervision requirements for use of CPT codes 96401-96549. (Reference: Medicare Benefit Policy Manual, Pub.100-02, Chapter 6, §20.4.1.)

B. Administration of Chemotherapy Drugs by Intravenous Infusion

Effective for services furnished on or after January 1, 2006, hospitals paid under the OPPS (12x and 13x bill types) are to report an appropriate HCPCS code for chemotherapy drug administration by intravenous infusion as listed in Table 3.

Table 3: CY 2006 OPPS Chemotherapy Drug Administration – Intravenous Infusion Technique

2005 CPT	2005 Descrip	Code	Descrip	SI	APC
			Final CY 2006 OPPS		
96410	Chemotherapy administration, intravenous; infusion technique, up to one hour	C8954	Chemotherapy administration, intravenous; infusion technique, up to one hour	S	0117
96412	Chemotherapy administration, intravenous; infusion technique, one to 8 hours, each additional hour (List separately in addition to code for primary procedure)	C8955	Chemotherapy administration, intravenous; infusion technique, each additional hour (List separately in addition to C8954)	N	-
96414	Chemotherapy administration, intravenous; infusion technique, initiation of prolonged infusion (more than 8 hours), requiring the use of a portable or implantable pump	96416	Chemotherapy administration, intravenous infusion technique; initiation of prolonged chemotherapy infusion (more than 8 hours), requiring use of portable or implantable pump	S	0117

For services furnished in hospital outpatient departments prior to January 1, 2005, chemotherapy drug infusions were reported using HCPCS alphanumeric code Q0084, Administration of Chemotherapy by Infusion only, per visit. Chemotherapy infusion services furnished in hospital outpatient departments during CY 2005 were reported using CPT codes 96410, 96412 and 96414.

Table 3 maps CY 2005 chemotherapy administration via intravenous infusion CPT codes to OPPS drug administration codes effective January 1, 2006.

HCPCS code C8955 is an add-on code. HCPCS code C8955 should be used by hospitals to report the total number of additional infusion hours after the first hour of chemotherapy infusion. Additional hours of chemotherapy infusion beyond 9 hours will no longer need to be reported on separate lines, as there is no hour limit associated with this code.

The OCE logic assumes that all services for chemotherapy infusions billed on the same date of service were provided during the same encounter. In those unusual cases where the beneficiary makes two separate visits to the hospital for chemotherapy infusions in the same day, the hospital reports modifier 59 for chemotherapy infusion codes during the second encounter that were also furnished in the first encounter. The OCE identifies modifier 59 and pays up to a maximum number of units per day, as listed in Table 1.

EXAMPLE 1

A beneficiary receives one injection of non-hormonal anti-neoplastic drugs and an infusion for 2 hours of anti-neoplastic drugs in one encounter. The patient leaves the hospital and later that same day returns to the hospital for two injections of non-hormonal anti-neoplastic drugs. To bill for the first encounter, the hospital reports one unit of 96401 (without modifier 59), one unit of C8954, and one unit of C8955 (without modifier 59). To bill for the second encounter, the hospital reports one unit of 96401 (with modifier 59) and one unit of 96401 (without modifier 59). The hospital will be paid two units of APC 0116 (once for each encounter with 96401 - one unit in the first, two units in the second)) and one unit of APC 0117 (for the one unit of C8954 and the one unit of C8955). (NOTE: See §230.1 for drug billing instructions.)

EXAMPLE 2

A beneficiary receives an infusion of anti-neoplastic drugs for 2 hours using a hydrating solution to which the anti-neoplastic drug has been added, without a specific medically necessary order for hydration. The hospital reports one unit of C8954 and one unit of C8955. The OCE will pay one unit of APC 0117 (for the one unit each of C8954 and C8955). (NOTE: See §230.1 for drug billing instructions.)

C. Administration of Chemotherapy Drugs by a Route Other Than Intravenous Infusion

Effective for services furnished on or after January 1, 2006, hospitals paid under the OPPS (12x and 13x bill types) are to report an appropriate HCPCS code for chemotherapy drug administration by route other than infusion as listed in Table 4.

Table 4: CY 2006 OPPS Chemotherapy Drug Administration – Route Other Than Intravenous Infusion

2005 CPT	2005 Descrip	Code	Descrip	SI	APC
			Final CY 2006 OPPS		
96408	Chemotherapy administration, intravenous; push technique	C8953	Chemotherapy administration, intravenous; push technique	S	0116
96400	Chemotherapy administration, subcutaneous or intramuscular, with or without local anesthesia	96401	Chemotherapy administration, subcutaneous or intramuscular; non-hormonal anti-neoplastic	S	0116
96400	Chemotherapy administration, subcutaneous or intramuscular, with or without local anesthesia	96402	Chemotherapy administration, subcutaneous or intramuscular; hormonal anti neoplastic	S	0116
96405	Chemotherapy administration, intralesional; up to and including 7 lesions	96405	Chemotherapy administration; intralesional, up to and including 7 lesions	S	0116
96406	Chemotherapy administration, intralesional; more than 7 lesions	96406	Chemotherapy administration; intralesional, more than 7 lesions	S	0116
96420	Chemotherapy administration, intra-arterial; push technique	96420	Chemotherapy administration, intra-arterial; push technique	S	0116
96422	Chemotherapy administration, infusion technique up to one hour	96422	Chemotherapy administration, intra-arterial; infusion technique, up to one hour	S	0117
96440	Chemotherapy administration into pleural cavity, requiring and including thoracentesis	96440	Chemotherapy administration into pleural cavity, requiring and including thoracentesis	S	0116
96445	Chemotherapy administration into peritoneal cavity, requiring and including peritoneocentesis	96445	Chemotherapy administration into peritoneal cavity, requiring and including peritoneocentesis	S	0116
96450	Chemotherapy administration, into CNS (e.g. Intrathecal) requiring and including spinal puncture	96450	Chemotherapy administration, into CNS (e.g., intrathecal), requiring and including spinal puncture	S	0116

2005 CPT	2005 Descrip	Code	Descrip	SI	APC
96542	Chemotherapy injection, subarachnoid or intraventricular via subcutaneous reservoir, single or multiple agents	96542	Chemotherapy injection, subarachnoid or intraventricular via subcutaneous reservoir, single or multiple agents	S	0116
96549	Unlisted chemotherapy procedure	96549	Unlisted chemotherapy procedure	S	0116
96423	Chemotherapy administration, infusion technique, one to 8 hours, each additional hour (List separately in addition to code for primary procedure)	96423	Chemotherapy administration, intra-arterial; infusion technique, each additional hour up to 8 hours (List separately in addition to code for primary procedure)	N	-

Column headers: **2005 CPT** / **Final CY 2006 OPPS**

Chemotherapy drug administration services other than intravenous infusion that were furnished in hospital outpatient departments during CY 2005 were reported using CPT codes 96420-96549.

Table 4 maps CY 2005 chemotherapy administration via routes other than intravenous infusion CPT codes to OPPS drug administration HCPCS codes effective January 1, 2006.

CPT code 96423 is an add-on code to indicate the total number of hours of intra-arterial infusion that are provided in addition to the first hour of administration. CPT code 96423 should be used by hospitals to report the total number of additional infusion hours. Additional hours of infusion beyond 8 should be reported on another separate line with CPT code 96423 and the appropriate number of hours.

OCE logic assumes that all services for chemotherapy drug administration by a route other than infusion that are billed on the same date of service were provided during the same encounter. In those unusual cases where the beneficiary makes two separate visits to the hospital for chemotherapy treatment in the same day, hospitals are instructed to report modifier 59 for chemotherapy drug administration (by a route other than infusion) codes during the second encounter that were also furnished in the first encounter. The OCE identifies modifier 59 and pays up to a maximum number of units per day, as listed in Table 1.

Pub. 100-4, Chapter 4, Section 230.2.3

Chemotherapy Drug Administration

A. Administration of Non-Chemotherapy Drugs by Intravenous Infusion

Table 5: CY 2006 OPPS Non-Chemotherapy Drug Administration – Intravenous Infusion Technique

2005 CPT	2005 Descrip	Code	Descrip	SI	APC
90780	Intravenous infusion for therapy/diagnosis, administered by physician or under direct supervision of physician; up to one hour	C8950	Intravenous infusion for therapy/diagnosis; up to 1 hour	S	0120

Column headers: **2005 CPT** / **Final CY 2006 OPPS**

2005 CPT	2005 Descrip	Code	Descrip	SI	APC
90781	Intravenous infusion for therapy/diagnosis, administered by physician or under direct supervision of physician; each additional hour, up to eight (8) hours (List separately in addition to code for primary procedure)	C8951	Intravenous infusion for therapy/diagnosis; each additional hour (List separately in addition to C8950)	N	-
n/a	n/a	C8957	Intravenous infusion for therapy/diagnosis; initiation of prolonged infusion (more than 8 hours), requiring use of portable or implantable pump	S	0120

Hospitals are to report HCPCS code C8950 to indicate an infusion of drugs other than anti-neoplastic drugs furnished on or after January 1, 2006 (except as noted at 230.2.2(A) above). HCPCS code C8951 should be used to report all additional infusion hours, with no limit on the number of hours billed per line. Medically necessary separate therapeutic or diagnostic hydration services should be reported with C8950 and C8951, as these are considered intravenous infusions for therapy/diagnosis.

HCPCS codes C8950 and C8951 should not be reported when the infusion is a necessary and integral part of a separately payable OPPS procedure.

When more than one nonchemotherapy drug is infused, hospitals are to code HCPCS codes C8950 and C8951 (if necessary) to report the total duration of an infusion, regardless of the number of substances or drugs infused. Hospitals are reminded to bill separately for each drug infused, in addition to the drug administration services.

The OCE pays one APC for each encounter reported by HCPCS code C8950, and only pays one APC for C8950 per day (unless Modifier 59 is used). Payment for additional hours of infusion reported by HCPCS code C8951 is packaged into the payment for the initial infusion. While no separate payment will be made for units of HCPCS code C8951, hospitals are instructed to report all codes that appropriately describe the services provided and the corresponding charges so that CMS may capture specific historical hospital cost data for future payment rate setting activities.

OCE logic assumes that all services for non-chemotherapy infusions billed on the same date of service were provided during the same encounter. Where a beneficiary makes two separate visits to the hospital for non-chemotherapy infusions in the same day, hospitals are to report modifier 59 for non-chemotherapy infusion codes during the second encounter that were also furnished in the first encounter. The OCE identifies modifier 59 and pays up to a maximum number of units per day, as listed in Table 1.

EXAMPLE 1

A beneficiary receives infused drugs that are not anti-neoplastic drugs (including hydrating solutions) for 2 hours. The hospital reports one unit of HCPCS code C8950 and one unit of HCPCS code C8951. The OCE will pay one unit of APC 0120. Payment for the unit of HCPCS code C8951 is packaged into the payment for one unit of APC 0120. (NOTE: See §230.1 for drug billing instructions.)

EXAMPLE 2

A beneficiary receives infused drugs that are not anti-neoplastic drugs (including hydrating solutions) for 12 hours. The hospital reports one unit of HCPCS code C8950 and eleven units of HCPCS code C8951. The OCE will pay one unit of APC 0120. Payment for the 11 units of HCPCS code C8951 is packaged into the payment for one unit of APC 0120. (NOTE: See §230.1 for drug billing instructions.)

EXAMPLE 3

A beneficiary experiences multiple attempts to initiate an intravenous infusion before a successful infusion is started 20 minutes after the first attempt. Once started, the infusion lasts one hour. The hospital reports one unit of HCPCS code C8950 to identify the 1 hour of infusion time. The 20 minutes spent prior to the infusion attempting to establish an IV line are not separately billable in the OPPS. The OCE pays one unit of APC 0120. (NOTE: See §230.1 for drug billing instructions.)

B. Administration of Non-Chemotherapy Drugs by a Route Other Than Intravenous Infusion

Table 6: CY 2006 OPPS Non-Chemotherapy Drug Administration – Route Other Than Intravenous Infusion

2005 CPT	2005 Descrip	Code	Descrip	SI	APC
			Final CY 2006 OPPS		
90784	Therapeutic, prophylactic or diagnostic injection (specify material injected); intravenous	C8952	Therapeutic, prophylactic or diagnostic injection; intravenous push	X	0359
90782	Therapeutic, prophylactic or diagnostic injection (specify material injected); subcutaneous or intramuscular	90772	Therapeutic, prophylactic or diagnostic injection (specify substance or drug); subcutaneous or intramuscular	X	0353
90783	Therapeutic, prophylactic or diagnostic injection (specify material injected); intra-arterial	90773	Therapeutic, prophylactic or diagnostic injection (specify substance or drug); intra-arterial	X	0359
90779	Unlisted therapeutic, prophylactic or diagnostic intravenous or intra-arterial, injection or infusion	90779	Unlisted therapeutic, prophylactic or diagnostic intravenous or intra-arterial injection or infusion	X	0352

Pub. 100-4, Chapter 4, Section 231.9

Billing for Pheresis and Apheresis Services

Apheresis/pheresis services are billed on a per visit basis and not on a per unit basis. OPPS providers should report the charge for an Evaluation and Management (E&M) visit only if there is a separately identifiable E&M service performed which extends beyond the evaluation and management portion of a typical apheresis/pheresis service. If the OPPS provider is billing an E&M visit code in addition to the apheresis/pheresis service, it may be appropriate to use the HCPCS modifier -25.

Pub. 100-4, Chapter 4, Section 240

Inpatient Part B Hospital Services

Inpatient Part B services which are paid under OPPS include:

- Diagnostic x-ray tests, and other diagnostic tests (excluding clinical diagnostic laboratory tests);
- X-ray, radium, and radioactive isotope therapy, including materials and services of technicians;
- Surgical dressings applied during an encounter at the hospital and splints, casts, and other devices used for reduction of fractures and dislocations (splints and casts, etc., include dental splints);
- Implantable prosthetic devices;
- Hepatitis B vaccine and its administration, and certain preventive screening services (pelvic exams, screening sigmoidoscopies, screening colonoscopies, bone mass measurements, and prostate screening.)
- Bone Mass measurements;
- Prostate screening;
- Immunosuppressive drugs;
- Oral anti-cancer drugs;
- Oral drug prescribed for use as an acute anti-emetic used as part of an anti-cancer chemotherapeutic regimen; and
- Epoetin Alfa (EPO)

NOTE: Payment for some of these services is packaged into the payment rate of other separately payable services.

Inpatient Part B services paid under other payment methods include:

- Clinical diagnostic laboratory tests, prosthetic devices other than implantable ones and other than dental which replace all or part of an internal body organ (including contiguous

tissue), or all or part of the function of a permanently inoperative or malfunctioning internal body organ, including replacement or repairs of such devices;

- Leg, arm, back and neck braces; trusses and artificial legs; arms and eyes including adjustments, repairs, and replacements required because of breakage, wear, loss, or a change in the patient's physical condition; take home surgical dressings; outpatient physical therapy; outpatient occupational therapy; and outpatient speech pathology services;
- Ambulance services;
- Screening pap smears, screening colorectal tests, and screening mammography;
- Influenza virus vaccine and its administration, pneumococcal vaccine and its administration;
- Diabetes self-management;
- Hemophilia clotting factors for hemophilia patients competent to use these factors without supervision).

See Chapter 6 of the Medicare Benefit Policy Manual for a discussion of the circumstances under which the above services may be covered as Part B Inpatient services.

Pub. 100-4, Chapter 4, Section 250.1.3

Clarification of HCPCS Code to Revenue Code Reporting

A-03-035

Generally, CMS does not instruct hospitals on the assignment of HCPCS codes to revenue codes for services provided under OPPS since hospitals' assignment of cost vary. Where explicit instructions are not provided, the contractor advises hospitals to report their charges under the revenue code that will result in the charges being assigned to the same cost center to which the cost of those services are assigned in the cost report.

Pub. 100-4, Chapter 4, Section 250.3.1

Anesthesia File

Record Layout for the Anesthesia Conversion Factor File

Data Element Name	Picture	Location	Length
Carrier Number	X (5)	1-5	5
Locality Number	X (2)	13-14	2
Locality Name	X (30)	19-48	30
Anesthesia CF 2002	99V99	74-77	4

Pub. 100-4, Chapter 4, Section 250.3.2

Physician Rendering Anesthesia in a Hospital Outpatient Setting

When a medically necessary anesthesia service is furnished within a HPSA area by a physician, a HPSA bonus is payable. In addition to using the PC/TC indicator on the CORF extract of the MPFS Summary File to identify HPSA services, pay physicians the HPSA bonus when CPT codes 00100 through 01999 are billed with the following modifiers: QY, QK, AA, or GC and "QB" or "QU" in revenue code 963. The modifiers signify that a physician performed an anesthesia service. Using the Anesthesia File (See Section above) the physician service will be 115 percent times the payment amount to be paid to a CAH on Method payment plus 10 percent HPSA bonus payment.

Anesthesiology modifiers:

AA = anesthesia services performed personally by anesthesiologist.

GC =service performed, in part, by a resident under the direction of a teaching physician.

QK = medical direction of two, three, or four concurrent anesthesia procedures involving qualified individuals.

QY = medical direction of one CRNA by an anesthesiologist.

Modifiers AA and GC result in physician payment at 80% of the allowed amount. Modifiers QK and QY result in physician payment at 50% of the allowed amount.

Data elements needed to calculate payment:

- HCPCS plus Modifier,
- Base Units,
- Time units, based on standard 15 minute intervals,
- Locality specific anesthesia Conversion factor, and
- Allowed amount minus applicable deductions and coinsurance amount.

Formula 1: Calculate payment for a physician performing anesthesia alone

HCPCS = xxxxx

Modifier = AA

Base Units = 4

Anesthesia Time is 60 minutes. Anesthesia time units = 4 (60/15)

Sum of Base Units plus Time Units = 4 + 4 = 8

Locality specific Anesthesia conversion factor = $17.00 (varies

by localities)

Coinsurance = 20%

Example 1: Physician personally performs the anesthesia case

Base Units plus time units - 4+4=8

Total units multiplied by the anesthesia conversion factor times.80

8 x $17= ($136.00 — (deductible*) x.80 = $108.80

Payment amount times 115 percent for the CAH method II payment.

$108.80 x 1.15 = $125.12 (Payment amount)

$125.12 x.10 = $12.51 (HPSA bonus payment)

Assume the Part B deductible has already been met for the calendar year

Formula 2: Calculate the payment for the physician's medical direction service when the physician directs two concurrent cases involving CRNAs. The medical direction allowance is 50% of the allowance for the anesthesia service personally performed by the physician.

HCPCS = xxxxx

Modifier = QK

Base Units = 4

Time Units 60/15=4

Sum of base units plus time units = 8

Locality specific anesthesia conversion factor = $17(varies

by localities)

Coinsurance = 20 %

(Allowed amount adjusted for applicable deductions and coinsurance and to reflect payment percentage for medical direction).

Example 2: Physician medically directs two concurrent cases involving CRNAs

Base units plus time - 4+4=8

Total units multiplied by the anesthesia conversion factor times. 50 equal allowed amount minus any remaining deductible

8 x $17 = $136 x.50 = $68.00 — (deductible*) = $68.00

Allowed amount Times 80 percent times 1.15

$68.00 x.80 = $54.40 x 1.15 = 62.56 (Payment amount)

$62.56 x.10 = $6.26 (HPSA bonus payment)

Assume the deductible has already been met for the calendar year.

Pub. 100-4, Chapter 4, Section 250.3.3

Anesthesia and CRNA Services in a Critical Access Hospital (CAH)

Pub. 100-4, Chapter 4, Section 300

Medical Nutrition Therapy (MNT) Services

Section 105 of the Medicare, Medicaid, and SCHIP Benefits Improvement and Protection Act of 2000 (BIPA) permits Medicare coverage of Medical Nutrition Therapy (MNT) services when furnished by a registered dietitian or nutrition professional meeting certain requirements. The benefit is available for beneficiaries with diabetes or renal disease, when referral is made by a physician as defined in §1861(r)(l) of the Act. It also allows registered dietitians and nutrition professionals to receive direct Medicare reimbursement for the first time. The effective date of this provision is January 1, 2002.

The benefit consists of an initial visit for an assessment; follow-up visits for interventions; and reassessments as necessary during the 12-month period beginning with the initial assessment ("episode of care") to assure compliance with the dietary plan. Effective October 1, 2002, basic coverage of MNT for the first year a beneficiary receives MNT with either a diagnosis of renal disease or diabetes as defined at 42 CFR, 410.130 is 3 hours. Also effective October 1, 2002, basic coverage in subsequent years for renal disease is 2 hours.

For the purposes of this benefit, renal disease means chronic renal insufficiency or the medical condition of a beneficiary who has been discharged from the hospital after a successful renal transplant within the last 6 months. Chronic renal insufficiency means a reduction in renal function not severe enough to require dialysis or transplantation (glomerular filtration rate (GFR) 13-50 ml/min/1.73m²s). Effective January 1, 2004, CMS updated the definition of diabetes to be as follows: Diabetes is defined as diabetes mellitus, a condition of abnormal glucose metabolism diagnosed using the following criteria: a fasting blood sugar greater than or equal to 126 mg/dL on two different occasions; a 2 hour post-glucose challenge greater than or equal to 200 mg/dL on 2 different occasions; or a random glucose test over 200 mg/dL for a person with symptoms of uncontrolled diabetes.

The MNT benefit is a completely separate benefit from the diabetes self-management training (DSMT) benefit. CMS had originally planned to limit how much of both benefits a beneficiary might receive in the same time period. However, the national coverage decision, published May 1, 2002, allows a beneficiary to receive the full amount of both benefits in the same period. Therefore, a beneficiary can receive the full 10 hours of initial DSMT and the full 3 hours of MNT. However, providers are not allowed to bill for both DSMT and MNT on the same date of service for the same beneficiary.

Pub. 100-4, Chapter 5, Section 10

General

Section 4541(a)(2) of the Balanced Budget Act (BBA) (P.L. 105-33), which added §1834(k)(5) to the Social Security Act (the Act), required that all claims for outpatient rehabilitation, certain audiology services and comprehensive outpatient rehabilitation facility (CORF) services, be reported using a uniform coding system. The CMS chose HCPCS (Healthcare Common Procedure Coding System) as the coding system to be used for the reporting of these services. This coding requirement is effective for all claims for outpatient rehabilitation services including certain audiology services and CORF services submitted on or after April 1, 1998.

The BBA also required payment under a prospective payment system for outpatient rehabilitation services including audiology and CORF services. Effective for claims with dates of service on or after January 1, 1999, the Medicare Physician Fee Schedule (MPFS) became the method of payment for outpatient physical therapy (which includes outpatient speech-language pathology) services furnished by:

- Comprehensive Outpatient Rehabilitation Facilities (CORFs);
- Outpatient Physical Therapy Providers (OPTs);
- Other Rehabilitation Facilities (ORFs);
- Hospitals (to outpatients and inpatients who are not in a covered Part A stay);
- Skilled Nursing Facilities (SNFs) (to residents not in a covered Part A stay and to nonresidents who receive outpatient rehabilitation services from the SNF); and
- Home Health Agencies (HHAs) (to individuals who are not homebound or otherwise are not receiving services under a home health plan of care (POC)).

The MPFS is used as a method of payment for outpatient rehabilitation services furnished under arrangement with any of these providers.

In addition, the MPFS is used as the payment system for audiology and CORF services identified by the HCPCS codes in §20 Assignment is mandatory.

The Medicare allowed charge for the services is the lower of the actual charge or the MPFS amount. The Medicare payment for the services is 80 percent of the allowed charge after the Part B deductible is met. Coinsurance is made at 20 percent of the lower of the actual charge or the MPFS amount. The general coinsurance rule (20 percent of the actual charges) does not apply when making payment under the MPFS. This is a final payment.

The MPFS does not apply to outpatient rehabilitation services furnished by critical access hospitals (CAHs). CAHs are to be paid on a reasonable cost basis.

Fiscal Intermediaries (FIs) process outpatient rehabilitation claims from hospitals, including CAHs, SNFs, CORFs, outpatient rehabilitation agencies, and outpatient physical therapy providers for which they have received a tie in notice from the RO. Carriers process claims from physicians, certain nonphysician practitioners (NPPs), and physical and occupational therapists in private practice (PTPPs and OTPPs). A physician-directed clinic that bills for services furnished incident to a physician's service (see Chapter 15 in Pub. 100-02, Medicare Benefit Policy Manual for a definition of "incident to") bills the carrier.

There are different fee rates for nonfacility and facility services. Chapter 23 describes the differences in these two rates. (See fields 28 and 29 of the record therein described). Facility rates apply to professional services performed in a facility other than the professional's office. Nonfacility rates apply when the service is performed in the professional's office. The nonfacility rate (that is paid when the provider performs the services in its own facility) accommodates overhead and indirect expenses the provider incurs by operating its own facility. Thus it is somewhat higher than the facility rate.

FIs pay the nonfacility rate for services performed in the provider's facility. Carriers may pay the facility or nonfacility rate depending upon where the service is performed (place of service on the claim), and the provider specialty.

Carriers pay the codes in §20 under the MPFS regardless of whether they may be considered rehabilitation services. However, FIs must use this list to determine whether to pay under outpatient rehabilitation rules or whether payment rules for other types of service may apply, e.g., OPPS for hospitals, reasonable costs for CAHs.

Note that because a service is considered an outpatient rehabilitation service does not automatically imply payment for that service. Additional criteria, including coverage, plan of care and physician certification must also be met. These criteria are described in Pub. 100-02, Medicare Benefit Policy Manual, Chapters 1 and 15.

Payment for rehabilitation services provided to Part A inpatients of hospitals or SNFs is included in the respective PPS rate. Also, for SNFs (but not hospitals), if the beneficiary has Part B, but not Part A coverage (e.g., Part A benefits are exhausted), the SNF must bill the FI for any rehabilitation service (except audiologic function tests). Independent audiologists may bill the carrier directly for services rendered to Part B Medicare entitled beneficiaries residing in a SNF, but not in a SNF Part A covered stay. Payment is made based on the MPFS, whether by the carrier or the FI. For beneficiaries not in a covered Part A SNF stay, who are sometimes referred to as beneficiaries in a Part B SNF stay, audiologic function tests are payable under Part B when billed by the SNF as type of bill 22X, or when billed directly to the carrier by the provider or supplier of the service. For tests that include both a professional component and technical component, the SNF may elect to bill the technical component to the FI, but is not required to bill the service. (The professional component of a service is the direct patient care provided by the physician or audiologist, e.g., the interpretation of a test.)

Payment for rehabilitation services provided by home health agencies under a home health plan of care is included in the home health PPS rate. HHAs may submit bill type 34X and be paid under the MPFS if there are no home health services billed under a home health plan of care at the same time, and there is a valid rehabilitation POC (e.g., the patient is not homebound).

An institutional employer (other than a SNF) of the PTPPs, OTPPs, or physician performing outpatient services, (e.g., hospital, CORF, etc.), or a clinic billing on behalf of the physician or therapist may bill the carrier on Form CMS-1500.

The MPFS is the basis of payment for outpatient rehabilitation services furnished by PTPPs and OTPPs, physicians, and certain nonphysician practitioners or for diagnostic tests provided incident to the services of such physicians or nonphysician practitioners. (See Pub. 100-02, Medicare Benefit Policy Manual, Chapter 15, for a definition of "incident to.") Such services are billed to the Part B carrier. Assignment is mandatory.

The following table identifies the provider types or physician/nonphysician and to which contractor they may submit bills.

Provider/ Service Type	Bill to	Bill Type	Comment
Inpatient hospital Part A	FI	11X	Included in PPS
Inpatient SNF Part A	FI	21X	Included in PPS
Inpatient hospital Part B	FI	12X	Hospital may obtain services under arrangements and bill, or rendering provider may bill.
Inpatient SNF Part B except for audiology function tests.	FI	22X	SNF must provide and bill, or obtain under arrangements and bill.
Inpatient SNF Part B audiology function tests only.	FI	22X	SNF may bill the FI or provider of service may bill the carrier.
Outpatient hospital	FI	13X	Hospital may provide and bill or obtain under arrangements and bill, or rendering provider may bill
Outpatient SNF	FI	23X	SNF must provide and bill or obtain under arrangements and bill
HHA billing for services rendered under a Part A or Part B home health plan of care.	FI	32X	Service is included in PPS rate. CMS determines whether payment is from Part A or Part B trust fund.
HHA billing for services not rendered under a Part A or Part B home health plan of care, but rendered under a therapy plan of care.	FI	34X	Service not under home health plan of care.
Other Rehabilitation Facility (ORF)	FI	74X	Paid MPFS for outpatient rehabilitation services effective January 1, 1999, and all other services except drugs effective July 1, 2000. Starting April 1, 2002, drugs are paid 95% of the AWP. For claims with dates of service on or after July 1, 2003, drugs and biologicals do not apply in an OPT setting. Therefore, FIs are to advise their OPTs not to bill for them.

Provider/ Service Type	Bill to	Bill Type	Comment
Comprehensive Outpatient Rehabilitation Facility (CORF)	FI	75X	Paid MPFS for outpatient rehabilitation services effective January 1, 1999, and all other services except drugs effective July 1, 2000. Starting April 1, 2002, drugs are paid 95% of the AWP.
Physician, NPPs, PTPPs, OTPPs, and, for diagnostic tests only, audiologists (service in hospital or SNF)	Carrier	See Chapter 26 for place of service, and type of service coding.	Payment may not be made for therapy services to Part A inpatients of hospitals or SNFs, or for Part B SNF residents. Otherwise, carrier billing. Note that physician/ NPP/PTPP/OTPP employee of facility may assign benefits to the facility, enabling the facility to bill for physician/therapist to carrier
Physician/NPP/PTPP/ OTPP office, independent clinic or patient's home	Carrier	See Chapter 26 for place of service, and type of service coding.	Paid via Physician fee schedule.
Practicing audiologist for services defined as diagnostic tests only	Carrier	See Chapter 26 for place of service, and type of service coding.	Some audiologists tests provided in hospitals are considered other diagnostic tests and are subject to HOPPS instead of MPFS for outpatient therapy fee schedule.
Critical Access Hospital - inpatient Part A	FI	85X	Rehabilitation services are paid cost.
Critical Access Hospital - inpatient Part B	FI	85X	Rehabilitation services are paid cost.
Critical Access Hospital – outpatient Part B	FI	85X	Rehabilitation services are paid cost.

Complete Claim form completion requirements are contained in Chapters 25 and 26.

For a list of the outpatient rehabilitation HCPCS codes see §20.

If an FI receives a claim for one of the these HCPCS codes with dates of service on or after July 1, 2003, that does not appear on the supplemental file it currently uses to pay the therapy claims, it contacts its local carrier to obtain the price in order to pay the claim. When requesting the pricing data, it advises the carrier to provide it with the nonfacility fee.

NOTE: The list of codes in §20 contains commonly utilized codes for outpatient rehabilitation services. FIs may consider other codes for payment under the MPFS as outpatient rehabilitation services to the extent that such codes are determined to be medically reasonable and necessary and those that could be performed within the scope of practice of the therapist providing the service.

Pub. 100-4, Chapter 5, Section 20

HCPCS Coding Requirement

A. Uniform Coding

Section 1834(k)(5) of the Act requires that all claims for outpatient rehabilitation therapy services and all comprehensive outpatient rehabilitation facility (CORF) services be reported using a uniform coding system. The Healthcare Common Procedure Coding System/Current Procedural Terminology, 2006 Edition (HCPCS/CPT-4) is the coding system used for the reporting of these services. The uniform coding requirement in the Act is specific to payment for all CORF services and outpatient rehabilitation therapy services - including physical therapy, occupational therapy, and speech-language pathology - that is provided and billed to carriers and fiscal intermediaries (FIs). The Medicare physician fee schedule (MPFS) is used to make payment for these therapy services at the nonfacility rate.

Effective for claims submitted on or after April 1, 1998, providers that had not previously reported HCPCS/CPT for outpatient rehabilitation and CORF services began using HCPCS to report these services. This requirement does not apply to outpatient rehabilitation services provided by:

Critical access hospitals, which are paid on a cost basis, not MPFS;

RHCs, and FQHCs for which therapy is included in the all-inclusive rate; or

Providers that do not furnish therapy services.

The following "providers of services" must bill the FI for outpatient rehabilitation services using HCPCS codes:

Hospitals (to outpatients and inpatients who are not in a covered Part A1 stay);

Skilled nursing facilities (SNFs) (to residents not in a covered Part A1 stay and to nonresidents who receive outpatient rehabilitation services from the SNF);

Home health agencies (HHAs) (to individuals who are not homebound or otherwise are not receiving services under a home health plan of care2 (POC);

Comprehensive outpatient rehabilitation facilities (CORFs); and

Providers of outpatient physical therapy and speech-language pathology services (OPTs), also known as rehabilitation agencies (previously termed outpatient physical therapy facilities in this instruction).

Note 1. The requirements for hospitals and SNFs apply to inpatient Part B and outpatient services only. Inpatient Part A services are bundled into the respective prospective payment system payment; no separate payment is made.

Note 2. For HHAs, HCPCS/CPT coding for outpatient rehabilitation services is required only when the HHA provides such service to individuals that are not homebound and, therefore, not under a Home Health plan of care.

The following practitioners must bill the carriers for outpatient rehabilitation therapy services using HCPCS/CPT codes:

Physical therapists in private practice (PTPPs),

Occupational therapists in private practice (OTPPs),

Physicians, including MDs, DOs, podiatrists and optometrists, and

Certain nonphysician practitioners (NPPs), acting within their State scope of practice, e.g., nurse practitioners and clinical nurse specialists.

Providers billing to intermediaries shall report:

The date the therapy plan of care was either established or last reviewed (see §220.1.3B) in Occurrence Code 17, 29, or 30.

The first day of treatment in Occurrence Code 35, 44, or 45.

B. Applicable Outpatient Rehabilitation HCPCS Codes

The CMS identifies the following codes as therapy services, regardless of the presence of a financial limitation. Therapy services include only physical therapy, occupational therapy and speech-language pathology services. Therapist means only a physical therapist, occupational therapist or speech-language pathologist. Therapy modifiers are GP for physical therapy, GO for occupational therapy, and GN for speech-language pathology. Check the notes below the chart for details about each code.

When in effect, any financial limitation will also apply to services represented by the following codes, except as noted below.

NOTE: Listing of the following codes does not imply that services are covered or applicable to all provider settings.

64550+	90901+	92506	92507	92508	92526
92597	92605****	92606****	92607	92608	92609
92610+	92611+	92612+	92614+	92616+	95831+
95832+	95833+	95834+	95851+	95852+	96105+
96110+✓	96111+✓	96115+	97001	97002	97003
97004	97010****	97012	97016	97018	97020
97022	97024	97026	97028	97032	97033
97034	97035	97036	97039*◆	97110	97112
97113	97116	97124	97139*◆	97140	97150
97530	97532+	97533	97535	97537	97542
97597+✗	97598+✗	97602+✗****	97605+✗	97606+✗	97750
97755	97760**▲	97761	97762	97799*	G0281
G0283	G0329	0019T+***	0029T+***		

* The physician fee schedule abstract file does not contain a price for CPT codes 97039, 97139, or 97799, since the carrier prices them. Therefore, the FI must contact the carrier to obtain the appropriate fee schedule amount in order to make proper payment for these codes.

◆ Effective January 1, 2006, these codes will no longer be valued under the MPFS. They will be priced by the carriers.

▲ Effective January 1, 2006, the code descriptors for these services have been changed.

CPT code 97760 should not be reported with CPT code 97116 for the same extremity.

The physician fee schedule abstract file does not contain a price for CPT codes 0019T or 0029T since they are priced by the carrier. In addition, the carrier determines coverage for these codes. Therefore, the FI contacts the carrier to obtain the appropriate fee schedule amount.

****These HCPCS/CPT codes are bundled under the MPFS. They are bundled with any therapy codes. Regardless of whether they are billed alone or in conjunction with another therapy code, never make payment separately for these codes. If billed alone, HCPCS/CPT codes marked as "****" shall be denied using the existing MSN language. For remittance advice notices, use group code CO and claim adjustment reason code 97 that says: "Payment is included in the allowance for another service/procedure." Use reason code 97 to deny a procedure code that should have been bundled. Alternatively, reason code B15, which has the same intent, may also be used.

✓ If billed by an outpatient hospital department, these HCPCS codes are paid using the Outpatient Prospective Payment System (OPPS).

Underlined codes are "always therapy" services, regardless of who performs them. These codes always require therapy modifiers (GP, GO, GN).

✗ If billed by a hospital subject to OPPS for an outpatient service, these HCPCS codes – also indicated as "sometimes therapy" services - will be paid under the OPPS when the service is not performed by a qualified therapist and it is inappropriate to bill the service under a therapy plan of care. The requirements for other "sometimes therapy" codes, described below, apply.

+ These HCPCS/CPT codes sometimes represent therapy services. However, these codes always represent therapy services and require the use of a therapy modifier when performed by therapists.

There are some circumstances when these codes will not be considered representative of therapy services and therapy limits (when they are in effect) will not apply. Codes marked + are not therapy services when:

- It is not appropriate to bill the service under a therapy plan of care, and

- They are billed by practitioners/providers of services who are not therapists, i.e., physicians, clinical nurse specialists, nurse practitioners and psychologists; or they are billed to fiscal intermediaries by hospitals for outpatient services which are performed by non-therapists as noted in Note ¿"" above.

While the "+" designates that a particular HCPCS/CPT code will not of itself always indicate that a therapy service was rendered, these codes always represent therapy services when rendered by therapists or by practitioners who are not therapists in situations where the service provided is integral to an outpatient rehabilitation therapy plan of care. For these situations, these codes must always have a therapy modifier. For example, when the service is rendered by either a doctor of medicine or a nurse practitioner (acting within the scope of his or her license when performing such service), with the goal of rehabilitation, a modifier is required. When there is doubt about whether a service should be part of a therapy plan of care, the contractor shall make that determination.

"Outpatient rehabilitation therapy" refers to skilled therapy services, requiring the skills of qualified therapists, performed for restorative purposes and generally involving ongoing treatments as part of a therapy plan of care. In contrast, a non-therapy service is a service performed by non-therapist practitioners, without an appropriate rehabilitative plan or goals, e.g., application of a surface (transcutaneous) neurostimulator – CPT code 64550, and biofeedback training by any modality – CPT code 90901. When performed by therapists, these are "always" therapy services. Contractors have discretion to determine whether circumstances describe a therapy service or require a rehabilitation plan of care.

The underlined HCPCS codes on the above list do not have a + sign because they are considered "always therapy" codes and always require a therapy modifier. Therapy services, whether represented by "always therapy" codes, or + codes in the above list performed as outpatient rehabilitation therapy services, must follow all the policies for therapy services (e.g., Pub. 100-04, chapter 5; Pub. 100-02, chapters 12 and 15).

C. Additional HCPCS Codes

Some HCPCS/CPT codes that are not on the list of therapy services should not be billed with a modifier. For example, outpatient non-rehabilitation HCPCS codes G0237, G0238, and G0239 should be billed without therapy modifiers. These HCPCS codes describe services for the improvement of respiratory function and may represent either "incident to" services or respiratory therapy services that may be appropriately billed in the CORF setting. When the services described by these G-codes are provided by physical therapists (PTs) or occupational therapists (OTs) treating respiratory conditions, they are considered therapy services and must meet the other conditions for physical and occupational therapy. The PT or OT would use the appropriate HCPCS/CPT code(s) in the 97000 – 97799 series and the corresponding therapy modifier, GP or GO, must be used.

Another example of codes that are not on the list of therapy services and should not be billed with a therapy modifier includes the following HCPCS codes: 95860, 95861, 95863, 95864, 95867, 95869, 95870, 95900, 95903, 95904, and 95934. These services represent diagnostic services - not therapy services; they must be appropriately billed and shall not include therapy modifiers.

Other codes not on the above list, and not paid under another fee schedule, are appropriately billed with therapy modifiers when the services are furnished by therapists or provided under a therapy plan of care and where the services are covered and appropriately delivered (e.g., the therapist is qualified to provide the service). One example of non-listed codes where a therapy modifier is indicated, regards the provision of services described in the CPT code series, 29000 through 29590, for the application of casts and strapping. Some of these previously appeared on the above list, but were deleted because we determined that they represented services that are most often performed outside a therapy plan of care. However, when these services are provided by therapists or as an integral part of a therapy plan of care, the CPT code must be accompanied with the appropriate therapy modifier.

NOTE: The above lists of HCPCS/CPT codes are intended to facilitate the contractor's ability to pay claims under the MPFS. It is not intended to be an exhaustive list of covered services, imply applicability to provider settings, and does not assure coverage of these services.

Pub. 100-4, Chapter 5, Section 100.10

Group Therapy Services (Code 97150)

CR 2225, A3-1872 Dated 1-24-03, A3-3653, B3-15302-15304

Carriers pay for outpatient physical therapy services (which includes outpatient speech-language pathology services) and outpatient occupational therapy services provided simultaneously to two or more individuals by a practitioner as group therapy services. The individuals can be, but need not be performing the same activity. The physician or therapist involved in group therapy services must be in constant attendance, but one-on-one patient contact is not required.

Pub. 100-4, Chapter 11, Section 10

Overview

Medicare beneficiaries entitled to hospital insurance (Part A) who have terminal illnesses and a life expectancy of six months or less have the option of electing hospice benefits in lieu of standard Medicare coverage for treatment and management of their terminal condition. Only care provided by a Medicare certified hospice is covered under the hospice benefit provisions.

Hospice care is available for two 90-day periods and an unlimited number of 60-day periods during the remainder of the hospice patient's lifetime. However, a beneficiary may voluntarily terminate his hospice election period. Election/termination dates are retained on CWF.

When hospice coverage is elected, the beneficiary waives all rights to Medicare Part B payments for services that are related to the treatment and management of his/her terminal illness during any period his/her hospice benefit election is in force, except for professional services of an attending physician, which may include a nurse practitioner. If the attending physician, who may be a nurse practitioner, is an employee of the designated hospice, he or she may not receive compensation from the hospice for those services under Part B. These physician professional services are billed to Medicare Part A by the hospice.

To be covered, hospice services must be reasonable and necessary for the palliation or management of the terminal illness and related conditions. The individual must elect hospice care and a certification that the individual is terminally ill must be completed by the patient's attending physician (if there is one), and the Medical Director (or the physician member of the Interdisciplinary Group (IDG)). Nurse practitioners serving as the attending physician may not certify or re-certify the terminal illness. A plan of care must be established before services are provided. To be covered, services must be consistent with the plan of care. Certification of terminal illness is based on the physician's or medical director's clinical judgment regarding the normal course of an individual's illness. It should be noted that predicting life expectancy is not always exact.

See the Medicare Benefit Policy Manual, Chapter 9, for additional general information about the Hospice benefit.

See Chapter 29 of this manual for information on the appeals process that should be followed when an entity is dissatisfied with the determination made on a claim.

See Chapter 9 of the Medicare Benefit Policy Manual for hospice eligibility requirements and election of hospice care.

Pub. 100-4, Chapter 11, Section 40.1.3

Attending Physician Services

When hospice coverage is elected, the beneficiary waives all rights to Medicare Part B payments for professional services that are related to the treatment and management of his/her terminal illness during any period his/her hospice benefit election is in force, except for professional services of an "attending physician," who is not an employee of the designated hospice nor receives compensation from the hospice for those services. For purposes of administering the hospice benefit provisions, an "attending physician" means an individual who:

- Is a doctor of medicine or osteopathy or

- A nurse practitioner (for professional services related to the terminal illness that are furnished on or after December 8, 2003); and

- Is identified by the individual, at the time he/she elects hospice coverage, as having the most significant role in the determination and delivery of their medical care.

Even though a beneficiary elects hospice coverage, he/she may designate and use an attending physician, who is not employed by nor receives compensation from the hospice for professional services furnished, in addition to the services of hospice-employed physicians. The professional services of an attending physician, who may be a nurse practitioner as defined in Chapter 9, that are reasonable and necessary for the treatment and management of a hospice patient's terminal illness are not considered hospice services.

Where the service is considered a hospice service (i.e., a service related to the hospice patient's terminal illness that was furnished by someone other than the designated "attending physician" [or a physician substituting for the attending physician]) the physician or other provider must look to the hospice for payment.

Professional services related to the hospice patient's terminal condition that were furnished by the "attending physician", who may be a nurse practitioner, are billed to carriers. When the attending physician furnishes a terminal illness related service that includes both a professional and technical component (e.g., x-rays), he/she bills the professional component of such services

to the carrier and looks to the hospice for payment for the technical component. Likewise, the attending physician, who may be a

nurse practitioner, would look to the hospice for payment for terminal illness related services furnished that have no professional component (e.g., clinical lab tests). The remainder of this section explains this in greater detail.

When a Medicare beneficiary elects hospice coverage he/she may designate an attending physician, who may be a nurse practitioner, not employed by the hospice, in addition to receiving care from hospice-employed physicians. The professional services of a non-hospice affiliated attending physician for the treatment and management of his/her terminal illness are not considered "hospice services." These attending physician services are billed to the carrier, provided they were not furnished under a payment arrangement with the hospice. The attending physician codes services with the GV modifier "Attending physician not employed or paid under agreement by the patient's hospice provider" when billing his/her professional services furnished for the treatment and management of a hospice patient's terminal condition. Carriers make payment to the attending physician or beneficiary, as appropriate, based on the payment and deductible rules applicable to each covered service.

Payments for the services of attending physician are not counted in determining whether the hospice cap amount has been exceeded because services provided by an independent attending physician are not part of the hospice's care.

Services provided by an independent attending physician who may be a nurse practitioner must be coordinated with any direct care services provided by hospice physicians.

Only the direct professional services of an independent attending physician, who may be a nurse practitioner, to a patient may be billed; the costs for services such as lab or x-rays are not to be included in the bill.

If another physician covers for a hospice patient's designated attending physician, the services of the substituting physician are billed by the designated attending physician under the reciprocal or locum tenens billing instructions. In such instances, the attending physician bills using the GV modifier in conjunction with either the Q5 or Q6 modifier.

When services related to a hospice patient's terminal condition are furnished under a payment arrangement with the hospice by the designated attending physician who may be a nurse practitioner, the physician must look to the hospice for payment. In this situation the physicians' services are hospice services and are billed by the hospice to its FI.

Carriers must process and pay for covered, medically necessary Part B services that physicians furnish to patients after their hospice benefits are revoked even if the patient remains under the care of the hospice. Such services are billed without the GV or GW modifiers. Make payment based on applicable Medicare payment and deductible rules for each covered service even if the beneficiary continues to be treated by the hospice after hospice benefits are revoked.

The CWF response contains the period of hospice entitlement. This information is a permanent part of the notice and is furnished on all CWF replies and automatic notices.

Carriers use the CWF reply for validating dates of hospice coverage and to research, examine and adjudicate services coded with the GV or GW modifiers.

Pub. 100-4, Chapter 12, Section 10

General

B3-2020

This chapter provides claims processing instructions for physician and nonphysician practitioner services.

Most physician services are paid according to the Medicare Physician Fee Schedule. Section 20 below offers additional information on the fee schedule application. Chapter 23 includes the fee schedule format and payment localities, and identifies services that are paid at reasonable charge rather than based on the fee schedule. In addition:

- Chapter 13 describes billing and payment for radiology services.

- Chapter 16 outlines billing and payment under the laboratory fee schedule.

- Chapter 17 provides a description of billing and payment for drugs.

- Chapter 18 describes billing and payment for preventive services and screening tests.

The Medicare Manual Pub 100-1, Medicare General Information, Eligibility, and Entitlement Manual, Chapter 5, provides definitions for the following:

- Physician;

- Doctors of Medicine and Osteopathy;

- Dentists;

- Doctors of Podiatric Medicine;

- Optometrists;

- Chiropractors (but only for spinal manipulation); and

- Interns and Residents.

- The Medicare Benefit Policy Manual, Chapter 15, provides coverage policy for the following services.

- Telephone services;

- Consultations;

- Patient initiated second opinions; and

- Concurrent care.

- Chapter 26 provides guidance on completing and submitting Medicare claims.

Pub. 100-4, Chapter 12, Section 30.1

49999)

B3-15100

A. Upper Gastrointestinal Endoscopy Including Endoscopic Ultrasound (EUS) (Code 43259)

If the person performing the original diagnostic endoscopy has access to the EUS and the clinical situation requires an EUS, the EUS may be done at the same time. The procedure, diagnostic and EUS, is reported under the same code, CPT 43259. This code conforms to CPT guidelines for the indented codes. The service represented by the indented code, in this case code 43259 for EUS, includes the service represented by the unintended code preceding the list of indented codes. Therefore, when a diagnostic examination of the upper gastrointestinal tract "including esophagus, stomach, and either the duodenum or jejunum as appropriate," includes the use of endoscopic ultrasonography, the service is reported by a single code, namely 43259.

Interpretation, whether by a radiologist or endoscopist, is reported under CPT code 76975-26. These codes may both be reported on the same day.

B. Incomplete Colonoscopies (Codes 45330 and 45378)

An incomplete colonoscopy, e.g., the inability to extend beyond the splenic flexure, is billed and paid using colonoscopy code 45378 with modifier "-53." The Medicare physician fee schedule database has specific values for code 45378-53. These values are the same as for code 45330, sigmoidoscopy, as failure to extend beyond the splenic flexure means that a sigmoidoscopy rather than a colonoscopy has been performed. However, code 45378-53 should be used when an incomplete colonoscopy has been done because other MPFSDB indicators are different for codes 45378 and 45330.

Pub. 100-4, Chapter 12, Section 30.2

55899)

B3-15200

A. Cystourethroscopy With Ureteral Catheterization (Code 52005)

Code 52005 has a zero in the bilateral field (payment adjustment for bilateral procedure does not apply) because the basic procedure is an examination of the bladder and urethra (cystourethroscopy), which are not paired organs. The work RVUs assigned take into account that it may be necessary to examine and catheterize one or both ureters. No additional payment is made when the procedure is billed with bilateral modifier "-50." Neither is any additional payment made when both ureters are examined and code 52005 is billed with multiple surgery modifier "-51." It is inappropriate to bill code 52005 twice, once by itself and once with modifier "-51," when both ureters are examined.

B. Cystourethroscopy With Fulgration and/or Resection of Tumors (Codes 52234, 52235, and 52240)

The descriptors for codes 52234 through 52240 include the language "tumor(s)."

This means that regardless of the number of tumors removed, only one unit of a single code can be billed on a given date of service. It is inconsistent to allow payment for removal of a small (code 52234) and a large (code 52240) tumor using two codes when only one code is allowed for the removal of more than one large tumor. For these three codes only one unit may be billed for any of these codes, only one of the codes may be billed, and the billed code reflects the size of the largest tumor removed.

Pub. 100-4, Chapter 12, Section 30.4

93799)

A. Echocardiography Contrast Agents

Effective October 1, 2000, physicians may separately bill for contrast agents used in echocardiography. Physicians should use HCPCS Code A9700 (Supply of Injectable Contrast Material for Use in Echocardiography, per study). The type of service code is 9. This code will be carrier-priced.

B. Electronic Analyses of Implantable Cardioverter-defibrillators and Pacemakers

The CPT codes 93731, 93734, 93741 and 93743 are used to report electronic analyses of single or dual chamber pacemakers and single or dual chamber implantable cardioverter-defibrillators. In the office, a physician uses a device called a programmer to obtain information about the status and performance of the device and to evaluate the patient's cardiac rhythm and response to the implanted device.

Advances in information technology now enable physicians to evaluate patients with implanted cardiac devices without requiring the patient to be present in the physician's office. Using a manufacturer's specific monitor/transmitter, a patient can send complete device data and specific cardiac data to a distant receiving station or secure Internet server. The electronic analysis of cardiac device data that is remotely obtained provides immediate and long-term data on the device and clinical data on the patient's cardiac functioning equivalent to that obtained during an in-office evaluation. Physicians should report the electronic analysis of an implanted cardiac device using remotely obtained data as described above with CPT code 93731, 93734, 93741 or 93743, depending on the type of cardiac device implanted in the patient.

Pub. 100-4, Chapter 12, Section 30.5

Payment for Codes for Chemotherapy Administration and Nonchemotherapy Injections and Infusions

A. General

Codes for Chemotherapy administration and nonchemotherapy injections and infusions include the following three categories of codes in the American Medical Association's Current Procedural Terminology (CPT):

1. Hydration;

2. Therapeutic, prophylactic, and diagnostic injections and infusions (excluding chemotherapy); and

3. Chemotherapy administration.

Physician work related to hydration, injection, and infusion services involves the affirmation of the treatment plan and the supervision (pursuant to incident to requirements) of nonphysician clinical staff.

B. Hydration

The hydration codes are used to report a hydration IV infusion which consists of a pre-packaged fluid and /or electrolytes (e.g. normal saline, D5-1/2 normal saline +30 mg EqKC1/liter) but are not used to report infusion of drugs or other substances.

C. Therapeutic, prophylactic, and diagnostic injections and infusions (excluding chemotherapy)

A therapeutic, prophylactic, or diagnostic IV infusion or injection, other than hydration, is for the administration of substances/drugs. The fluid used to administer the drug (s) is incidental hydration and is not separately payable.

If performed to facilitate the infusion or injection or hydration, the following services and items are included and are not separately billable:

1. Use of local anesthesia;

2. IV start;

3. Access to indwelling IV, subcutaneous catheter or port;

4. Flush at conclusion of infusion; and

5. Standard tubing, syringes and supplies.

Payment for the above is included in the payment for the chemotherapy administration or nonchemotherapy injection and infusion service.

If a significant separately identifiable evaluation and management service is performed, the appropriate E & M code should be reported utilizing modifier 25 in addition to the chemotherapy administration or nonchemotherapy injection and infusion service. For an evaluation and management service provided on the same day, a different diagnosis is not required.

The CPT 2006 includes a parenthetical remark immediately following CPT code 90772 (Therapeutic, prophylactic or diagnostic injection; (specify substance or drug); subcutaneous or intramuscular.) It states, "Do not report 90772 for injections given without direct supervision. To report, use 99211."

This coding guideline does not apply to Medicare patients. If the RN, LPN or other auxiliary personnel furnishes the injection in the office and the physician is not present in the office to meet the supervision requirement, which is one of the requirements for coverage of an incident to service, then the injection is not covered. The physician would also not report 99211 as this would not be covered as an incident to service.

D. Chemotherapy Administration

Chemotherapy administration codes apply to parenteral administration of non-radionuclide anti-neoplastic drugs; and also to anti-neoplastic agents provided for treatment of noncancer diagnoses (e.g., cyclophosphamide for auto-immune conditions) or to substances such as monoclonal antibody agents, and other biologic response modifiers. The following drugs are commonly considered to fall under the category of monoclonal antibodies: infliximab, rituximab, alemtuzumb, gemtuzumab, and trastuzumab. Drugs commonly considered to fall under the category of hormonal antineoplastics include leuprolide acetate and goserelin acetate. The drugs cited are not intended to be a complete list of drugs that may be administered using the chemotherapy administration codes. Local carriers may provide additional guidance as to which drugs may be considered to be chemotherapy drugs under Medicare.

The administration of anti-anemia drugs and anti-emetic drugs by injection or infusion for cancer patients is not considered chemotherapy administration.

If performed to facilitate the chemotherapy infusion or injection, the following services and items are included and are not separately billable:

1. Use of local anesthesia;

2. IV access;

3. Access to indwelling IV, subcutaneous catheter or port;

4. Flush at conclusion of infusion;

5. Standard tubing, syringes and supplies; and

6. Preparation of chemotherapy agent(s).

Payment for the above is included in the payment for the chemotherapy administration service.

If a significant separately identifiable evaluation and management service is performed, the appropriate E & M code should be reported utilizing modifier 25 in addition to the chemotherapy code. For an evaluation and management service provided on the same day, a different diagnosis is not required.

E. Coding Rules for Chemotherapy Administration and Nonchemotherapy Injections and Infusion Services

Instruct physicians to follow the CPT coding instructions to report chemotherapy administration and nonchemotherapy injections and infusion services with the exception listed in subsection C for CPT code 90772. The physician should be aware of the following specific rules.

When administering multiple infusions, injections or combinations, the physician should report only one "initial" service code unless protocol requires that two separate IV sites must be used. The initial code is the code that best describes the key or primary reason for the encounter and should always be reported irrespective of the order in which the infusions or injections occur. If an injection or infusion is of a subsequent or concurrent nature, even if it is the first such service within that group of services, then a subsequent or concurrent code should be reported. For example, the first IV push given subsequent to an initial one-hour infusion is reported using a subsequent IV push code.

If more than one "initial" service code is billed per day, the carrier shall deny the second initial service code unless the patient has to come back for a separately identifiable service on the same day or has two IV lines per protocol. For these separately identifiable services, instruct the physician to report with modifier 59.

The CPT includes a code for a concurrent infusion in addition to an intravenous infusion for therapy, prophylaxis or diagnosis. Allow only one concurrent infusion per patient per encounter. Do not allow payment for the concurrent infusion billed with modifier 59 unless it is provided during a second encounter on the same day with the patient and is documented in the medical record.

For chemotherapy administration and therapeutic, prophylactic and diagnostic injections and infusions, an intravenous or intra-arterial push is defined as: 1.) an injection in which the healthcare professional is continuously present to administer the substance/drug and observe the patient; or 2.) an infusion of 15 minutes or less.

The physician may report the infusion code for "each additional hour" only if the infusion interval is greater than 30 minutes beyond the 1 hour increment. For example if the patient receives an infusion of a single drug that lasts 1 hour and 45 minutes, the physician would report the "initial" code up to 1 hour and the add-on code for the additional 45 minutes.

Several chemotherapy administration and nonchemotherapy injection and infusion service codes have the following parenthetical descriptor included as a part of the CPT code, "List separately in addition to code for primary procedure." Each of these codes has a physician fee schedule indicator of "ZZZ" meaning this service is allowed if billed with another chemotherapy administration or nonchemotherapy injection and infusion service code.

Do not interpret this parenthetical descriptor to mean that the add-on code can be billed only if it is listed with another drug administration primary code. For example, code 90761 will be ordinarily billed with code 90760. However, there may be instances when only the add-on code, 90761, is billed because an "initial" code from another section in the drug administration codes, instead of 90760, is billed as the primary code.

Pay for code 96523, "Irrigation of implanted venous access device for drug delivery systems," if it is the only service provided that day. If there is a visit or other chemotherapy administration or nonchemotherapy injection or infusion service provided on the same day, payment for 96523 is included in the payment for the other service.

F. Chemotherapy Administration (or Nonchemotherapy Injection and Infusion) and Evaluation and Management Services Furnished on the Same Day

For services furnished on or after January 1, 2004, do not allow payment for CPT code 99211, with or without modifier 25, if it is billed with a nonchemotherapy drug infusion code or a chemotherapy administration code. Apply this policy to code 99211 when it is billed with a diagnostic or therapeutic injection code on or after January 1, 2005.

Physicians providing a chemotherapy administration service or a nonchemotherapy drug infusion service and evaluation and management services, other than CPT code 99211, on the same day must bill in accordance with §30.6.6 using modifier 25. The carriers pay for evaluation and management services provided on the same day as the chemotherapy

administration services or a nonchemotherapy injection or infusion service if the evaluation and management service meets the requirements of section §30.6.6 even though the underlying codes do not have global periods. If a chemotherapy service and a significant separately identifiable evaluation and management service are provided on the same day, a different diagnosis is not required.

In 2005, the Medicare physician fee schedule status database indicators for therapeutic and diagnostic injections were changed from T to A. Thus, beginning in 2005, the policy on evaluation and management services, other than 99211, that is applicable to a chemotherapy or a nonchemotherapy injection or infusion service applies equally to these codes.

Pub. 100-4, Chapter 12, Section 30.6

General (Codes 99201 - 99499)

B3-15501-15501.1

Pub. 100-4, Chapter 12, Section 30.6.2

Billing for Medically Necessary Visit on Same Occasion as Preventive Medicine Service

See Chapter 18 for payment for covered preventive services.

When a physician furnishes a Medicare beneficiary a covered visit at the same place and on the same occasion as a noncovered preventive medicine service (CPT codes 99381-99397), consider the covered visit to be provided in lieu of a part of the preventive medicine service of equal value to the visit. A preventive medicine service (CPT codes 99381-99397) is a noncovered service. The physician may charge the beneficiary, as a

charge for the noncovered remainder of the service, the amount by which the physician's current established charge for the preventive medicine service exceeds his/her current established charge for the covered visit. Pay for the covered visit based on the lesser of the fee schedule amount or the physician's actual charge for the visit. The physician is not required to give the beneficiary written advance notice of noncoverage of the part of the visit that constitutes a routine preventive visit. However, the physician is responsible for notifying the patient in advance of his/her liability for the charges for services that are not medically necessary to treat the illness or injury.

There could be covered and noncovered procedures performed during this encounter (e.g., screening x-ray, EKG, lab tests.). These are considered individually. Those procedures which are

for screening for asymptomatic conditions are considered noncovered and, therefore, no payment is made. Those procedures ordered to diagnose or monitor a symptom, medical condition, or treatment are evaluated for medical necessity and, if covered, are paid.

Pub. 100-4, Chapter 12, Section 30.6.7

99215)

A Definition of New Patient for Selection of E/M Visit Code

Interpret the phrase "new patient" to mean a patient who has not received any professional services, i.e., E/M service or other face-to-face service (e.g., surgical procedure) from the physician or physician group practice (same physician specialty) within the previous 3 years. For example, if a professional component of a previous procedure is billed in a 3 year time period, e.g., a lab interpretation is billed and no E/M

service or other face-to-face service with the patient is performed, then this patient remains a new patient for the initial visit. An interpretation of a diagnostic test, reading an x-ray or EKG etc., in the absence of an E/M service or other face-to-face service with the patient does not affect the designation of a new patient.

B Office/Outpatient E/M Visits Provided on Same Day for Unrelated Problems

As for all other E/M services except where specifically noted, carriers may not pay two E/M office visits billed by a physician (or physician of the same specialty from the same group practice) for the same beneficiary on the same day unless the physician documents that the visits were for unrelated problems in the office or outpatient setting which could not be provided during the same encounter (e.g., office visit for blood pressure medication evaluation, followed five hours later by a visit for evaluation of leg pain following an accident).

C Office/Outpatient or Emergency Department E/M Visit on Day of Admission to Nursing Facility

Carriers may not pay a physician for an emergency department visit or an office visit and a comprehensive nursing facility assessment on the same day. Bundle E/M visits on the same date provided in sites other than the nursing facility into the initial nursing facility care code when performed on the same date as the nursing facility admission by the same physician.

D Drug Administration Services and E/M Visits Billed on Same Day of Service

Carriers must advise physicians that CPT code 99211 cannot be paid if it is billed with a drug administration service such as a chemotherapy or nonchemotherapy drug infusion code (effective January 1, 2004). This drug administration policy was expanded in the Physician Fee Schedule Final Rule, November 15, 2004, to also include a therapeutic or diagnostic injection code (effective January 1, 2005). Therefore, when a medically necessary, significant and separately identifiable E/M service (which meets a higher complexity level than CPT code 99211) is performed, in addition to one of these drug administration services, the appropriate E/M CPT code should be reported with modifier -25. Documentation should support the level of E/M service billed. For an E/M service provided on the same day, a different diagnosis is not required.

Pub. 100-4, Chapter 12, Section 30.6.8

99220)

B3-15504

A. Who May Bill Initial Observation Care

Carriers pay for initial observation care billed by only the physician who admitted the patient to hospital observation and was responsible for the patient during his/her stay in observation. A physician who does not have inpatient admitting privileges but who is authorized to admit a patient to observation status may bill these codes.

For a physician to bill the initial observation care codes, there must be a medical observation record for the patient which contains dated and timed physician's admitting

orders regarding the care the patient is to receive while in observation, nursing notes, and progress notes prepared by the physician while the patient was in observation status. This record must be in addition to any record prepared as a result of an emergency department or outpatient clinic encounter.

Payment for an initial observation care code is for all the care rendered by the admitting physician on the date the patient was admitted to observation. All other physicians who see the patient while he or she is in observation must bill the office and other outpatient service codes or outpatient consultation codes as appropriate when they provide services to the patient.

For example, if an internist admits a patient to observation and asks an allergist for a consultation on the patient's condition, only the internist may bill the initial observation care code. The allergist must bill using the outpatient consultation code that best represents the services he or she provided. The allergist cannot bill an inpatient consultation since the patient was not a hospital inpatient.

B. Physician Billing for Observation Care Following Admission to Observation

If the patient is discharged on the same date as admission to observation, pay only the initial observation care code because that code represents a full day of care.

If the patient remains in observation after the first date following the admission to observation, it is expected that the patient would be discharged on that second calendar date. The physician bills CPT code 99217 for observation care discharge services provided on the second date.

In the rare circumstance when a patient is held in observation status for more than two calendar dates, the physician must bill subsequent services furnished before the date of discharge using the outpatient/office visit codes. The physician may not use the subsequent hospital care codes since the patient is not an inpatient of the hospital.

C. Admission to Inpatient Status from Observation

If the same physician who admitted a patient to observation status also admits the patient to inpatient status from observation before the end of the date on which the patient was admitted to observation, pay only an initial hospital visit for the evaluation and management services provided on that date. Medicare payment for the initial hospital visit includes all services provided to the patient on the date of admission by that physician, regardless of the site of service. The physician may not bill an initial observation care code for services on the date that he or she admits the patient to inpatient status. If the patient is admitted to inpatient status from observation subsequent to the date of admission to observation, the physician must bill an initial hospital visit for the services provided on that date. The physician may not bill the hospital observation discharge management code (code 99217) or an outpatient/office visit for the care provided in observation on the date of admission to inpatient status.

D. Hospital Observation During Global Surgical Period

The global surgical fee includes payment for hospital observation (codes 99217, 99218, 99219, and 99220, 99234, 99235, 99236) services unless the criteria for use of CPT modifiers "-24," "-25," or "-57" are met. Carriers must pay for these services in addition to the global surgical fee only if both of the following requirements are met:

- The hospital observation service meets the criteria needed to justify billing it with CPT modifiers "-24," "-25," or "-57" (decision for major surgery); and

- The hospital observation service furnished by the surgeon meets all of the criteria for the hospital observation code billed.

Examples of the decision for surgery during a hospital observation period are:

- A patient is admitted by an emergency department physician to an observation unit for observation of a head injury. A neurosurgeon is called in to do a consultation on the need for surgery while the patient is in the observation unit and decides that the patient requires surgery. The surgeon would bill an outpatient consultation with the "-57" modifier to indicate that the decision for surgery was made during the consultation. The surgeon must bill an outpatient consultation because the patient in an observation unit is not an inpatient of the hospital. Only the physician who admitted the patient to hospital observation may bill for initial observation care.

- A patient is admitted by a neurosurgeon to a hospital observation unit for observation of a head injury. During the observation period, the surgeon makes the decision for surgery. The surgeon would bill the appropriate level of hospital observation code with the "-57" modifier to indicate that the decision for surgery was made while the surgeon was providing hospital observation care.

Examples of hospital observation services during the postoperative period of a surgery are:

- A patient at the 80th day following a TURP is admitted to observation by the surgeon who performed the procedure with abdominal pain from a kidney stone. The surgeon decides that the patient does not require surgery. The surgeon would bill the observation code with CPT modifier "-24" and documentation to support that the observation services are unrelated to the surgery.

- A patient at the 80th day following a TURP is admitted to observation with abdominal pain by the surgeon who performed the procedure. While the patient is in hospital observation, the surgeon decides that the patient requires kidney surgery. The surgeon would bill the observation code with HCPCS modifier "-57" to indicate that the decision for surgery was made while the patient was in hospital observation. The subsequent surgical procedure would be reported with modifier "-79."

- A patient at the 20th day following a resection of the colon is admitted to observation for abdominal pain by the surgeon who performed the surgery. The surgeon determines that the patient requires no further colon surgery and discharges the patient. The surgeon may not bill for the observation services furnished during the global period because they were related to the previous surgery.

An example of a billable hospital observation service on the same day as a procedure is a patient is admitted to the hospital observation unit for observation of a head injury by a physician who repaired a laceration of the scalp in the emergency department. The physician would bill the observation code with a CPT modifier 25 and the procedure code.

Pub. 100-4, Chapter 12, Section 30.6.9

General (Codes 99221 - 99239)

B3-15505-15505.2

A. Hospital Visit and Critical Care on Same Day

See §30.6.12.E for billing of critical care on the day of another evaluation and management service.

B. Two Hospital Visits Same Day

Carriers pay a physician for only one hospital visit per day for the same patient, whether the problems seen during the encounters are related or not. The inpatient hospital visit descriptors contain the phrase "per day" which means that the code and the payment established for the code represent all services provided on that date. The physician should select a code that reflects all services provided during the date of the service.

C. Hospital Visits Same Day But by Different Physicians

In a hospital inpatient situation involving one physician covering for another, if physician A sees the patient in the morning and physician B, who is covering for A, sees the same patient in the evening, carriers do not pay physician B for the second visit. The hospital visit descriptors include the phrase "per day" meaning care for the day.

If the physicians are each responsible for a different aspect of the patient's care, pay both visits if the physicians are in different specialties and the visits are billed with different diagnoses. There are circumstances where concurrent care may be billed by physicians of the same specialty.

D. Visits to Patients in Swing Beds

If the inpatient care is being billed by the hospital as inpatient hospital care, the hospital care codes apply. If the inpatient care is being billed by the hospital as nursing facility care, then the nursing facility codes apply.

Pub. 100-4, Chapter 12, Section 30.6.10

99255)

A. Consultation Services versus Other Evaluation and Management (E/M) Visits

Carriers pay for a reasonable and medically necessary consultation service when all of the following criteria for the use of a consultation code are met:

- Specifically, a consultation service is distinguished from other evaluation and management (E/M) visits because it is provided by a physician or qualified nonphysician practitioner (NPP) whose opinion or advice regarding evaluation and/or management of a specific problem is requested by another physician or other appropriate source. The qualified NPP may perform consultation services within the scope of practice and licensure requirements for NPPs in the State in which he/she practices. Applicable collaboration and general supervision rules apply as well as billing rules;

- A request for a consultation from an appropriate source and the need for consultation (i.e., the reason for a consultation service) shall be documented by the consultant in the patient's medical record and included in the requesting physician or qualified NPP's plan of care in the patient's medical record; and

- After the consultation is provided, the consultant shall prepare a written report of his/her findings and recommendations, which shall be provided to the referring physician.

The intent of a consultation service is that a physician or qualified NPP or other appropriate source is asking another physician or qualified NPP for advice, opinion, a recommendation, suggestion, direction, or counsel, etc. in evaluating or treating a patient because that individual has expertise in a specific medical area beyond the requesting professional's knowledge. Consultations may be billed based on time if the counseling/coordination of care constitutes more than 50 percent of the face-to-face encounter between the physician or qualified NPP and the patient. The preceding requirements (request, evaluation (or counseling/coordination) and written report) shall also be met when the consultation is based on time for counseling/coordination.

A consultation shall not be performed as a split/shared E/M visit.

B. Consultation Followed by Treatment

A physician or qualified NPP consultant may initiate diagnostic services and treatment at the initial consultation service or subsequent visit. Ongoing management, following the initial consultation service by the consultant physician, shall not be reported with consultation service codes. These services shall be reported as subsequent visits for the appropriate place of service and level of service. Payment for a consultation service shall be made regardless of treatment initiation unless a transfer of care occurs.

Transfer of Care

A transfer of care occurs when a physician or qualified NPP requests that another physician or qualified NPP take over the responsibility for managing the patients' complete care for the condition and does not expect to continue treating or caring for the patient for that condition.

When this transfer is arranged, the requesting physician or qualified NPP is not asking for an opinion or advice to personally treat this patient and is not expecting to continue treating the patient for the condition. The receiving physician or qualified NPP shall document this transfer of the patient's care, to his/her service, in the patient's medical record or plan of care.

In a transfer of care the receiving physician or qualified NPP would report the appropriate new or established patient visit code according to the place of service and level of service performed and shall not report a consultation service.

C. Initial and Follow-Up Consultation Services

Initial Consultation Service

In the hospital setting, the consulting physician or qualified NPP shall use the appropriate Initial Inpatient Consultation codes (99251 – 99255) for the initial consultation service.

In the nursing facility setting, the consulting physician or qualified NPP shall use the appropriate Initial Inpatient Consultation codes (99251 – 99255) for the initial consultation service.

The Initial Inpatient Consultation may be reported only once per consultant per patient per facility admission.

In the office or other outpatient setting, the consulting physician or qualified NPP shall use the appropriate Office or Other Outpatient Consultation (new or established patient) codes (99241 – 99245) for the initial consultation service.

If an additional request for an opinion or advice, regarding the same or a new problem with the same patient, is received from the same or another physician or qualified NPP and documented in the medical record, the Office or Other Outpatient Consultation (new or established patient) codes (99241 – 99245) may be used again. However, if the consultant continues to care for the patient for the original condition following his/her initial consultation, repeat consultation services shall not be reported by this physician or qualified NPP during his/her ongoing management of this condition.

Follow-Up Consultation Service

Effective January 1, 2006, the follow-up inpatient consultation codes (99261 – 99263) are deleted.

In the hospital setting, following the initial consultation service, the Subsequent Hospital Care codes (99231 – 99233) shall be reported for additional follow-up visits.

In the nursing facility setting, following the initial consultation service, the Subsequent Nursing Facility (NF) Care codes (new CPT codes 99307 – 99310) shall be reported for additional follow-up visits. Effective January 1, 2006, CPT codes 99311 – 99313 are deleted and not valid for Subsequent NF visits.

In the office or other outpatient setting, following the initial consultation service, the Office or Other Outpatient Established Patient codes (99212 – 99215) shall be reported for additional follow-up visits. The CPT code 99211 shall not be reported as a consultation service. The CPT code 99211 is not included by Medicare for a consultation service since this service typically does not require the presence of a physician or qualified NPP and would not meet the consultation service criteria.

D. Second Opinion E/M Service Requests

Effective January 1, 2006, the Confirmatory Consultation codes (99271 – 99275) are deleted.

A second opinion E/M service is a request by the patient and/or family or mandated (e.g., by a third-party payer) and is not requested by a physician or qualified NPP. A consultation service requested by a physician, qualified NPP or other appropriate source that meets the requirements stated in Section A shall be reported using the initial consultation service codes as discussed in Section C. A written report is not required by Medicare to be sent to a physician when an evaluation for a second opinion has been requested by the patient and/or family.

A second opinion, for Medicare purposes, is generally performed as a request for a second or third opinion of a previously recommended medical treatment or surgical procedure. A second opinion E/M service initiated by a patient and/or family is not reported using the consultation codes.

In both the inpatient hospital setting and the NF setting, a request for a second opinion would be made through the attending physician or physician of record. If an initial consultation is requested of another physician or qualified NPP by the attending physician and meets the requirements for a consultation service (as identified in Section A) then the appropriate Initial Inpatient Consultation code shall be reported by the consultant. If the service does not meet the consultation requirements, then the E/M service shall be reported using the Subsequent Hospital Care codes (99231 – 99233) in the inpatient hospital setting and the Subsequent NF Care codes (99307 – 99310) in the NF setting.

A second opinion E/M service performed in the office or other outpatient setting shall be reported using the Office or Other Outpatient new patient codes (99201 – 99205) for a new patient and established patient codes (99212 – 99215) for an established patient, as appropriate. The 3 year rule regarding "new patient" status applies. Any medically necessary follow-up visits shall be reported using the appropriate subsequent visit/established patient E/M visit codes.

The CPT modifier -32 (Mandated Services) is not recognized as a payment modifier in Medicare. A second opinion evaluation service to satisfy a requirement for a third party payer is not a covered service in Medicare.

E. Consultations Requested by Members of Same Group

Carriers pay for a consultation if one physician or qualified NPP in a group practice requests a consultation from another physician in the same group practice when the consulting physician or qualified NPP has expertise in a specific medical area beyond the requesting professional's knowledge. A consultation service shall not be reported on

every patient as a routine practice between physicians and qualified NPPs within a group practice setting.

F. Documentation for Consultation Services

Consultation Request

A written request for a consultation from an appropriate source and the need for a consultation must be documented in the patient's medical record. The initial request may be a verbal interaction between the requesting physician and the consulting physician; however, the verbal conversation shall be documented in the patient's medical record, indicating a request for a consultation service was made by the requesting physician or qualified NPP.

The reason for the consultation service shall be documented by the consultant (physician or qualified NPP) in the patient's medical record and included in the requesting physician or qualified NPP's plan of care. The consultation service request may be written on a physician order form by the requestor in a shared medical record.

Consultation Report

A written report shall be furnished to the requesting physician or qualified NPP.

In an emergency department or an inpatient or outpatient setting in which the medical record is shared between the referring physician or qualified NPP and the consultant, the request may be documented as part of a plan written in the requesting physician or qualified NPP's progress note, an order in the medical record, or a specific written request for the consultation. In these settings, the report may consist of an appropriate entry in the common medical record.

In an office setting, the documentation requirement may be met by a specific written request for the consultation from the requesting physician or qualified NPP or if the consultant's records show a specific reference to the request. In this setting, the consultation report is a separate document communicated to the requesting physician or qualified NPP.

In a large group practice, e.g., an academic department or a large multi-specialty group, in which there is often a shared medical record, it is acceptable to include the consultant's report in the medical record documentation and not require a separate letter from the consulting physician or qualified NPP to the requesting physician or qualified NPP. The written request and the consultation evaluation, findings and recommendations shall be available in the consultation report.

G. Consultation for Preoperative Clearance

Preoperative consultations are payable for new or established patients performed by any physician or qualified NPP at the request of a surgeon, as long as all of the requirements for performing and reporting the consultation codes are met and the service is medically necessary and not routine screening.

H. Postoperative Care by Physician Who Did Preoperative Clearance Consultation

If subsequent to the completion of a preoperative consultation in the office or hospital, the consultant assumes responsibility for the management of a portion or all of the patient's condition(s) during the postoperative period, the consultation codes should not be used postoperatively. In the hospital setting, the physician or qualified NPP who has performed a preoperative consultation and assumes responsibility for the management of a portion or all of the patient's condition(s) during the postoperative period should use the appropriate subsequent hospital care codes to bill for the concurrent care he or she is providing. In the office setting, the appropriate established patient visit codes should be used during the postoperative period.

A physician (primary care or specialist) or qualified NPP who performs a postoperative evaluation of a new or established patient at the request of the surgeon may bill the appropriate consultation code for evaluation and management services furnished during the postoperative period following surgery when all of the criteria for the use of the consultation codes are met and that same physician has not already performed a preoperative consultation.

I. Surgeon's Request That Another Physician Participate In Postoperative Care

If the surgeon asks a physician or qualified NPP who had been treating the patient preoperatively or who had not seen the patient for a preoperative consultation to take responsibility for the management of an aspect of the patient's condition during the postoperative period, the physician or qualified NPP may not bill a consultation because the surgeon is not asking the physician or qualified NPP's opinion or advice for the surgeon's use in treating the patient. The physician or qualified NPP's services would constitute concurrent care and should be billed using the appropriate subsequent hospital care codes in the hospital inpatient setting, subsequent NF care codes in the SNF/NF setting or the appropriate office or other outpatient visit codes in the office or outpatient settings.

J. Examples That Meet the Criteria for Consultation Services

For brevity, the consultation request and the consultation written report is not repeated in each of these examples. Criteria for consultation services shall always include a request and a written report in the medical record as described above.

EXAMPLE 1:

An internist sees a patient that he has followed for 20 years for mild hypertension and diabetes mellitus. He identifies a questionable skin lesion and asks a dermatologist to evaluate the lesion. The dermatologist examines the patient and decides the lesion is probably malignant and needs to be removed. He removes the lesion which is determined to be an early melanoma. The dermatologist dictates and forwards a report to the internist regarding his evaluation and treatment of the patient. Modifier -25 shall be used with the consultation service code in addition to the procedure code. Modifier -25 is required to identify the consultation service as a significant, separately identifiable E/M service in addition to the procedure code reported for the incision/removal of lesion. The internist resumes care of the patient and continues surveillance of the skin on the advice of the dermatologist.

EXAMPLE 2:

A rural family practice physician examines a patient who has been under his care for 20 years and diagnoses a new onset of atrial fibrillation. The family practitioner sends the patient to a cardiologist at an urban cardiology center for advice on his care and management. The cardiologist examines the patient, suggests a cardiac catheterization and other diagnostic tests which he schedules and then sends a written report to the requesting physician. The cardiologist subsequently periodically sees the patient once a year as follow-up. Subsequent visits provided by the cardiologist should be billed as an established patient visit in the office or other outpatient setting, as appropriate. Following the advice and intervention by the cardiologist the family practice physician resumes the general medical care of the patient.

EXAMPLE 3:

A family practice physician examines a female patient who has been under his care for some time and diagnoses a breast mass. The family practitioner sends the patient to a general surgeon for advice and management of the mass and related patient care. The general surgeon examines the patient and recommends a breast biopsy, which he schedules, and then sends a written report to the requesting physician. The general surgeon subsequently performs a biopsy and then periodically sees the patient once a year as follow-up. Subsequent visits provided by the surgeon should be billed as an established patient visit in the office or other outpatient setting, as appropriate. Following the advice and intervention by the surgeon the family practice physician resumes the general medical care of the patient.

I. Examples That Do Not Meet the Criteria for Consultation Services

EXAMPLE 1: Standing orders in the medical record for consultations.

EXAMPLE 2: No order for a consultation.

EXAMPLE 3: No written report of a consultation.

EXAMPLE 4: The emergency room physician treats the patient for a sprained ankle. The patient is discharged and instructed to visit the orthopedic clinic for follow-up. The physician in the orthopedic clinic shall not report a consultation service because advice or opinion is not required by the emergency room physician. The orthopedic physician shall report the appropriate office or other outpatient visit code.

Pub. 100-4, Chapter 12, Section 30.6.11

99288)

B3-15507

A. Use of Emergency Department Codes by Physicians Not Assigned to Emergency Department

Any physician seeing a patient registered in the emergency department may use emergency department visit codes (for services matching the code description). It is not required that the physician be assigned to the emergency department.

B. Use of Emergency Department Codes In Office

Emergency department coding is not appropriate if the site of service is an office or outpatient setting or any sight of service other than an emergency department. The emergency department codes should only be used if the patient is seen in the emergency

department and the services described by the HCPCS code definition are provided. The emergency department is defined as an organized hospital-based facility for the provision of unscheduled or episodic services to patients who present for immediate medical attention.

C. Use of Emergency Department Codes to Bill Nonemergency Services

Services in the emergency department may not be emergencies. However the codes (99281 - 99288) are payable if the described services are provided.

However, if the physician asks the patient to meet him or her in the emergency department as an alternative to the physician's office and the patient is not registered as a patient in the emergency department, the physician should bill the appropriate office/outpatient visit codes. Normally a lower level emergency department code would be reported for a nonemergency condition.

D. Emergency Department or Office/Outpatient Visits on Same Day As Nursing Facility Admission

Emergency department visit provided on the same day as a comprehensive nursing facility assessment are not paid. Payment for evaluation and management services on the same date provided in sites other than the nursing facility are included in the payment for initial nursing facility care when performed on the same date as the nursing facility admission.

E. Physician Billing for Emergency Department Services Provided to Patient by Both Patient's Personal Physician and Emergency Department Physician

If a physician advises his/her own patient to go to an emergency department (ED) of a hospital for care and the physician subsequently is asked by the ED physician to come to the hospital to evaluate the patient and to advise the ED physician as to whether the patient should be admitted to the hospital or be sent home, the physicians should bill as follows:

- If the patient is admitted to the hospital by the patient's personal physician, then the patient's regular physician should bill only the appropriate level of the initial hospital care (codes 99221 - 99223) because all evaluation and management services provided by that physician in conjunction with that admission are considered part of the initial hospital care when performed on the same date as the admission. The ED physician who saw the patient in the emergency department should bill the appropriate level of the ED codes.

- If the ED physician, based on the advice of the patient's personal physician who came to the emergency department to see the patient, sends the patient home, then the ED physician should bill the appropriate level of emergency department service. The patient's personal physician should also bill the level of emergency department code that describes the service he or she provided in the emergency department. The patient's personal physician would not bill a consultation because he or she is not providing information to the emergency department physician for his or her use in treating the patient. If the patient's personal physician does not come to the hospital to see the patient, but only advises the emergency department physician by telephone, then the patient's personal physician may not bill.

F. Emergency Department Physician Requests Another Physician to See the Patient in Emergency Department or Office/Outpatient Setting

If the emergency department physician requests that another physician evaluate a given patient, the other physician should bill a consultation if the criteria for consultation are met. If the criteria for a consultation are not met and the patient is discharged from the Emergency Department or admitted to the hospital by another physician, the physician contacted by the Emergency Department physician should bill an emergency department visit. If the consulted physician admits the patient to the hospital and the criteria for a consultation are not met, he/she should bill an initial hospital care code.

Pub. 100-4, Chapter 12, Section 30.6.12

99292)

B3-15508

A. Use of Critical Care (Code 99292) in Cases Which are Not Medical Emergencies

Critical care includes the care of critically ill and unstable patients who require constant physician attention, whether the patient is in the course of a medical emergency or not. It involves decision making of high complexity to assess, manipulate, and support circulatory, respiratory, central nervous, metabolic, or other vital system function to prevent or treat single or multiple vital organ system failure. It often also requires extensive interpretation of multiple databases and the application of advanced technology to manage the critically ill patient.

Critical care is usually, but not always, given in a critical care area such is the coronary care unit, intensive care unit, respiratory care unit, or the emergency department. However, payment may be made for critical care services provided in any location as long as the care provided meets the definition of critical care. Services for a patient who is not critically ill and unstable but who happens to be in a critical care, intensive care, or other specialized care unit are reported using subsequent hospital care codes (99231-99233) or hospital consultation codes (99251 - 99263). Critical care may include neonatal intensive care.

B. Constant Attendance or Constant Attention as Prerequisite for Use of Critical Care Codes

The duration of critical care time to be reported is the time the physician spent working on the critical care patient's case, whether that time was spent at the immediate bedside or elsewhere on the floor, but immediately available to the patient.

For example, time spent reviewing laboratory test results or discussing the critically ill patient's care with other medical staff in the unit or at the nursing station on the floor would be reported as critical care, even if it does not occur at the bedside.

Time spent in activities that occur outside of the unit or off the floor (e.g., telephone calls, whether taken at home, in the office, or elsewhere in the hospital) may not be reported as critical

care since the physician is not immediately available to the patient. This work is the typical pre and post-service work that accompanies any evaluation and management service. Time spent in activities that do not directly contribute to the treatment of the patient may not be reported as critical care, even if they are performed in the critical care unit at a patient's bedside (e.g., telephone calls to discuss other patients, reviewing literature).

For critical care to be billed, the physician must devote his or her full attention to the patient and, therefore, cannot render evaluation and management services to any other patient during the same period of time.

The time spent with the individual patient and the service rendered should be recorded in the patient's record to support the claim for critical care services.

C. Hours and Days of Critical Care

Payment for critical care is not restricted to a fixed number of days. As long as the critical care criteria are met and the services are reasonable and necessary to treat illness or injury, payment for critical care services is appropriate. However, claims for seemingly improbable amounts of critical care on the same date are subjected to review to determine if the physician has filed a false claim.

D. Counting of Units of Critical Care Services

Code 99291 (critical care, first hour) is used to report the services of a physician providing constant attention to a critically ill patient for a total of 30 to 74 minutes on a given day. Only one unit of code 99291 may be billed by a physician for a patient on a given date.

If the total duration of critical care provided by the physician on a given day is less than 30 minutes, the appropriate evaluation and management code should be used. In the hospital setting, it is expected that the Level 3 subsequent hospital care code 99233 would most often be used.

Code 99292 (critical care, each additional 30 minutes) is used to report the services of a physician providing constant attention to the critically ill patient for 15 to 30 minutes beyond the first 74 minutes of critical care on a given day.

The following illustrates the correct reporting of critical care services:

Total Duration of Critical Care	*Code(s)*
Less than 30 minutes	99232 or 99233
30-74 minutes	99291 x 1
75-104 minutes	99291 x 1 and 99292 x 1
105-134 minutes	99291 x 1 and 99292 x 2
135-164 minutes	99291 x 1 and 99292 x 3
165-194 minutes	99291 x 1 and 99292 x 4

E. Critical Care Service and other Evaluation and Management Services Provided on Same Day

If critical care is required upon the patient's presentation to the emergency department, only critical care codes 99291-99292 may be reported. Emergency department codes will not be paid for the same day. If there is a hospital or office/outpatient evaluation and management service furnished early in the day and at that time the patient does not require critical care, but the patient requires critical care later in the day, both critical care and the evaluation and management service may be paid.

Physicians must submit supporting documentation when critical care is billed on the same day as other evaluation and management services.

F. Critical Care Services Provided During Preoperative Portion of Global Period of Procedure With 90 Day Global Period in Trauma and Burn Cases

Preoperative critical care may be paid in addition to a global fee if the patient is critically ill and requires the constant attendance of the physician, and the critical care is unrelated to the specific anatomic injury or general surgical procedure performed. Such patients are potentially unstable or have conditions that could pose a significant threat to life or risk of prolonged impairment.

In order for these services to be paid, two reporting requirements must be met. Codes 99291/99292 and modifier "-25" (significant, separately identifiable evaluation and management services by the same physician on the day of the procedure) must be used, and documentation that the critical care was unrelated to the specific anatomic injury or general surgical procedure performed must be submitted. An ICD-9-CM code in the range 800.0 through 959.9 (except 930-939), which clearly indicates that the critical care was unrelated to the surgery, is acceptable documentation.

G. Critical Care Services Provided During Postoperative Period of Procedure With Global Period in Trauma and Burn Cases

Postoperative critical care may be paid in addition to a global fee if the patient is critically ill and requires the constant attendance of the physician, and the critical care is unrelated to the specific anatomic injury or general surgical procedure performed. Such patients are potentially unstable or have conditions that could pose a significant threat to life or risk of prolonged impairment.

In order for these services to be paid, two reporting requirements must be met. Codes 99291/99292 and modifier "-24" (Unrelated evaluation and management service by the same physician during a postoperative period) must be used, and documentation that the critical care was unrelated to the specific anatomic injury or general surgical procedure performed must be submitted. An ICD-9-CM code in the range 800.0 through 959.9 (except 930-939), which clearly indicates that the critical care was unrelated to the surgery, is acceptable documentation.

Pub. 100-4, Chapter 12, Section 30.6.13

99318)

A. Visits to Perform the Initial Comprehensive Assessment and Annual Assessments

The distinction made between the delegation of physician visits and tasks in a skilled nursing facility (SNF) and in a nursing facility (NF) is based on the Medicare Statute. Section 1819 (b) (6) (A) of the Social Security Act (the Act) governs SNFs while section 1919 (b) (6) (A) of the Act governs NFs. For further information refer to Medlearn Matters article number SE0418 at www.cms.hhs.gov/medlearn/matters

The initial visit in a SNF and NF must be performed by the physician except as otherwise permitted (42 CFR 483.40 (c) (4)). The initial visit is defined in S&C-04-08 (see www.cms.hhs.gov/medlearn/matters) as the initial comprehensive assessment visit during which the physician completes a thorough assessment, develops a plan of care and writes or verifies admitting orders for the nursing facility resident. For Survey and Certification requirements, a visit must occur no later than 30 days after admission.

Further, per the Long Term Care regulations at 42 CFR 483.40 (c)(4) and (e) (2), the physician may not delegate a task that the physician must personally perform. Therefore, as stated in S&C-04-08 the physician may not delegate the initial visit in a SNF. This also applies to the NF with one exception.

The only exception, as to who performs the initial visit, relates to the NF setting. In the NF setting, a qualified NPP (i.e., a nurse practitioner (NP), physician assistant (PA), or a clinical nurse specialist (CNS), who is not employed by the facility, may perform the initial visit when the State law permits this. The evaluation and management (E/M) visit shall be within the State scope of practice and licensure requirements where the E/M visit is performed and the requirements for physician collaboration and physician supervision shall be met.

Under Medicare Part B payment policy, other medically necessary E/M visits may be performed and reported prior to and after the initial visit, if the medical needs of the patient require an E/M visit. A qualified NPP may perform medically necessary E/M visits prior to and after the initial visit if all the requirements for collaboration, general physician supervision, licensure and billing are met.

The CPT Nursing Facility Services codes shall be used with place of service (POS) 31 (SNF) if the patient is in a Part A SNF stay. They shall be used with POS 32 (nursing facility) if the patient does not have Part A SNF benefits or if the patient is in a NF or in a non-covered SNF stay (e.g., there was no preceding 3-day hospital stay). The CPT Nursing Facility code definition also includes POS 54 (Intermediate Care Facility/Mentally Retarded) and POS 56 (Psychiatric Residential Treatment Center). For further guidance on POS codes and associated CPT codes refer to §30.6.14.

Effective January 1, 2006, the Initial Nursing Facility Care codes 99301 – 99303 are deleted.

Beginning January 1, 2006, the new CPT codes, Initial Nursing Facility Care, per day, (99304 – 99306) shall be used to report the initial visit. Only a physician may report these codes for an initial visit performed in a SNF or NF (with the exception of the qualified NPP in the NF setting who is not employed by the facility and when State law permits, as explained above).

A readmission to a SNF or NF shall have the same payment policy requirements as an initial admission in both the SNF and NF settings.

A physician who is employed by the SNF/NF may perform the E/M visits and bill independently to Medicare Part B for payment. An NPP who is employed by the SNF or NF may perform and bill Medicare Part B directly for those services where it is permitted as discussed above. The employer of the PA shall always report the visits performed by the PA. A physician, NP or CNS has the option to bill Medicare directly or to reassign payment for his/her professional service to the facility.

As with all E/M visits for Medicare Part B payment policy, the E/M documentation guidelines apply.

B. Visits to Comply With Federal Regulations (42 CFR 483.40 (c) (1)) in the SNF and NF

Payment is made under the physician fee schedule by Medicare Part B for federally mandated visits. Following the initial visit by the physician, payment shall be made for federally mandated visits that monitor and evaluate residents at least once every 30 days for the first 90 days after admission and at least once every 60 days thereafter.

Effective January 1, 2006, the Subsequent Nursing Facility Care, per day, codes 99311 – 99313 are deleted.

Beginning January 1, 2006, the new CPT codes, Subsequent Nursing Facility Care, per day, (99307 – 99310) shall be used to report federally mandated physician E/M visits and medically necessary E/M visits.

Carriers shall not pay for more than one E/M visit performed by the physician or qualified NPP for the same patient on the same date of service. The Nursing Facility Services codes represent a "per day" service.

The federally mandated E/M visit may serve also as a medically necessary E/M visit if the situation arises (i.e., the patient has health problems that need attention on the day the scheduled mandated physician E/M visit occurs). The physician/qualified NPP shall bill only one E/M visit.

Beginning January 1, 2006, the new CPT code, Other Nursing Facility Service (99318), may be used to report an annual nursing facility assessment visit on the required schedule of visits on an annual basis. For Medicare Part B payment policy, an annual nursing facility assessment visit code may substitute as meeting one of the federally mandated physician visits if the code requirements for CPT code 99318 are fully met and in lieu of reporting a Subsequent Nursing Facility Care, per day, service (codes 99307 – 99310). It shall not be performed in addition to the

required number of federally mandated physician visits. The new CPT annual assessment code does not represent a new benefit service for Medicare Part B physician services.

Qualified NPPs, whether employed or not by the SNF, may perform alternating federally mandated physician visits, at the option of the physician, after the initial visit by the physician in a SNF.

Qualified NPPs in the NF setting, who are not employed by the NF, may perform federally mandated physician visits, at the option of the State, after the initial visit by the physician.

Medicare Part B payment policy does not pay for additional E/M visits that may be required by State law for a facility admission or for other additional visits to satisfy facility or other administrative purposes. E/M visits, prior to and after the initial physician visit, that are reasonable and medically necessary to meet the medical needs of the individual patient (unrelated to any State requirement or administrative purpose) are payable under Medicare Part B.

C. Visits by Qualified Nonphysician Practitioners

All E/M visits shall be within the State scope of practice and licensure requirements where the visit is performed and all the requirements for physician collaboration and physician supervision shall be met when performed and reported by qualified NPPs. General physician supervision and employer billing requirements shall be met for PA services in addition to the PA meeting the State scope of practice and licensure requirements where the E/M visit is performed.

Medically Necessary Visits

Qualified NPPs may perform medically necessary E/M visits prior to and after the physician's initial visit in both the SNF and NF. Medically necessary E/M visits for the diagnosis or treatment of an illness or injury or to improve the functioning of a malformed body member are payable under the physician fee schedule under Medicare Part B. CPT codes, Subsequent Nursing Facility Care, per day (99307 - 99310), shall be reported for these E/M visits even if the visits are provided prior to the initial visit by the physician.

SNF Setting – Place of Service Code 31

Following the initial visit by the physician, the physician may delegate alternate federally mandated physician visits to a qualified NPP who meets collaboration and physician supervision requirements and is licensed as such by the State and performing within the scope of practice in that State.

NF Setting – Place of Service Code 32

Per the regulations at 42 CFR 483.40 (f), a qualified NPP, who meets the collaboration and physician supervision requirements, the State scope of practice and licensure requirements, and who is not employed by the NF, may at the option of the State, perform the initial visit in a NF, and may perform any other federally mandated physician visit in a NF in addition to performing other medically necessary E/M visits.

Questions pertaining to writing orders or certification and recertification issues in the SNF and NF settings shall be addressed to the appropriate State Survey and Certification Agency departments for clarification.

D Medically Complex Care

Payment is made for E/M visits to patients in a SNF who are receiving services for medically complex care upon discharge from an acute care facility when the visits are reasonable and medically necessary and documented in the medical record. Physicians and qualified NPPs shall report E/M visits using the Subsequent Nursing Facility Care, per day (codes 99307 - 99310) for these E/M visits even if the visits are provided prior to the initial visit by the physician.

E Incident to Services

Where a physician establishes an office in a SNF/NF, the "incident to" services and requirements are confined to this discrete part of the facility designated as his/her office. "Incident to" E/M visits, provided in a facility setting, are not payable under the Physician Fee Schedule for Medicare Part B. Thus, visits performed outside the designated "office" area in the SNF/NF would be subject to the coverage and payment rules applicable to SNF/NF setting and shall not be reported using the CPT codes for office or other outpatient visits or use place of service code 11.

F Use of the Prolonged Services Codes and Other Time-Related Services

Beginning January 1, 2006, typical/average time units for the new CPT codes for E/M visits in the SNF/NF settings have not yet been determined by the American Medical Association (AMA) and therefore, typical/average time units cannot be associated with prolonged services for E/M visits until typical/average time units are determined by the AMA. Effective January 1, 2006, the Prolonged Services (codes 99354 – 99357) may not be billed with the Nursing Facility Services (codes 99304-99306, 99307-99310 and 99318).

Counseling and Coordination of Care Visits

Until typical/average time units are determined by the AMA, E/M visits for counseling/coordination of care, for the Nursing Facility Services, that are time-based must be billed based on the key components of an E/M service (history, exam and medical decision making).

G Gang Visits

The complexity level of an E/M visit and the CPT code billed must be a covered and medically necessary visit for each patient (refer to §§1862 (a)(1)(A) of the Act). Claims for an unreasonable number of daily E/M visits by the same physician to multiple patients at a facility within a 24-hour period may result in medical review to determine medical necessity for the visits. The E/M visit (Nursing Facility Services) represents a "per day" service per patient as defined by the CPT code. The medical record must be personally documented by the physician or qualified NPP who performed the E/M visit and the documentation shall support the specific level of E/M visit to each individual patient.

H Split/Shared E/M Visit

A split/shared E/M visit cannot be reported in the SNF/NF setting. A split/shared E/M visit is defined by Medicare Part B payment policy as a medically necessary encounter with a patient where the physician and a qualified NPP each personally perform a substantive portion of an E/M visit face-to-face with the same patient on the same date of

service. A substantive portion of an E/M visit involves all or some portion of the history, exam or medical decision making key components of an E/M service. The physician and the qualified NPP must be in the same group practice or be employed by the same employer. The split/shared E/M visit applies only to selected E/M visits and settings (i.e., hospital inpatient, hospital outpatient, hospital observation, emergency department, hospital discharge, office and non facility clinic visits, and prolonged visits associated with these E/M visit codes). The split/shared E/M policy does not apply to consultation services, critical care services or procedures.

I SNF/NF Discharge Day Management Service

Medicare Part B payment policy requires a face-to-face visit with the patient provided by the physician or the qualified NPP to meet the SNF/NF discharge day management service as defined by the CPT code. The E/M discharge day management visit shall be reported for the date of the actual visit by the physician or qualified NPP even if the patient is discharged from the facility on a different calendar date. The CPT codes 99315 – 99316 shall be reported for this visit. The Discharge Day Management Service may be reported using CPT code 99315 or 99316, depending on the code requirement, for a patient who has expired, but only if the physician or qualified NPP personally performed the death pronouncement.

Pub. 100-4, Chapter 12, Section 30.6.14

99350)

Physician Visits to Patients Residing in Various Places of Service

The American Medical Association's Current Procedural Terminology (CPT) 2006 new patient codes 99324 — 99328 and established patient codes 99334 - 99337(new codes beginning January 2006), for Domiciliary, Rest Home (e.g., Boarding Home), or Custodial Care Services, are used to report evaluation and management (E/M) services to residents residing in a facility which provides room, board, and other personal assistance services, generally on a long-term basis. These CPT codes are used to report E/M services in facilities assigned places of service (POS) codes 13 (Assisted Living Facility), 14 (Group Home), 33 (Custodial Care Facility) and 55 (Residential Substance Abuse Facility). Assisted living facilities may also be known as adult living facilities.

Physicians and qualified nonphysician practitioners (NPPs) furnishing E/M services to residents in a living arrangement described by one of the POS listed above must use the level of service code in the CPT code range 99324 — 99337 to report the service they provide. The CPT codes 99321 — 99333 for Domiciliary, Rest Home (e.g., Boarding Home), or Custodial Care Services are deleted beginning January, 2006.

Beginning in 2006, reasonable and medically necessary, face-to-face, prolonged services, represented by CPT codes 99354 — 99355, may be reported with the appropriate companion E/M codes when a physician or qualified NPP, provides a prolonged service involving direct (face-to-face) patient contact that is beyond the usual E/M visit service for a Domiciliary, Rest Home (e.g., Boarding Home) or Custodial Care Service. All the requirements for prolonged services at §30.6.15.1 must be met.

The CPT codes 99341 through 99350, Home Services codes, are used to report E/M services furnished to a patient residing in his or her own private residence (e.g., private home, apartment, town home) and not residing in any type of congregate/shared facility living arrangement including assisted living facilities and group homes. The Home Services codes apply only to the specific 2-digit POS 12 (Home). Home Services codes may not be used for billing E/M services provided in settings other than in the private residence of an individual as described above.

Beginning in 2006, E/M services provided to patients residing in a Skilled Nursing Facility (SNF) or a Nursing Facility (NF) must be reported using the appropriate CPT level of service code within the range identified for Initial Nursing Facility Care (new CPT codes 99304 — 99306) and Subsequent Nursing Facility Care (new CPT codes 99307 — 99310). Use the CPT code, Other Nursing Facility Services (new CPT code 99318), for an annual nursing facility assessment. Use CPT codes 99315 — 99316 for SNF/NF discharge services. The CPT codes 99301 — 99303 and 99311 — 99313 are deleted beginning January, 2006. The Home Services codes should not be used for these places of service.

The CPT SNF/NF code definition includes intermediate care facilities (ICFs) and long term care facilities (LTCFs). These codes are limited to the specific 2-digit POS 31 (SNF), 32 (Nursing Facility), 54 (Intermediate Care Facility/Mentally Retarded) and 56 (Psychiatric Residential Treatment Center).

The CPT nursing facility codes should be used with POS 31 (SNF) if the patient is in a Part A SNF stay and POS 32 (nursing facility) if the patient does not have Part A SNF benefits. There is no longer a standard payment amount for a Part A or Part B benefit period in these POS settings.

Pub. 100-4, Chapter 12, Section 30.6.15

99360)

B3-15511-15511.3

Pub. 100-4, Chapter 12, Section 30.6.16

99373)

B3-15512

A. Team Conferences

Team conferences (codes 99361-99362) may not be paid separately. Payment for these services is included in the payment for the services to which they relate.

B. Telephone Calls

Telephone calls (codes 99371-99373) may not be paid separately. Payment for telephone calls is included in payment for billable services (e.g., visit, surgery, diagnostic procedure results).

Pub. 100-4, Chapter 12, Section 40.6

Claims for Multiple Surgeries

B3-4826, B3-15038, B3-15056

A. General

Multiple surgeries are separate procedures performed by a single physician or physicians in the same group practice on the same patient at the same operative session or on the same day for which separate payment may be allowed. Co-surgeons, surgical teams, or assistants-at-surgery may participate in performing multiple surgeries on the same patient on the same day.

Multiple surgeries are distinguished from procedures that are components of or incidental to a primary procedure. These intra-operative services, incidental surgeries, or components of more major surgeries are not separately billable. See Chapter 23 for a description of mandatory edits to prevent separate payment for those procedures. Major surgical procedures are determined based on the MFSDB approved amount and not on the submitted amount from the providers. The major surgery, as based on the MFSDB, may or may not be the one with the larger submitted amount.

Also, see subsection D below for a description of the standard payment policy on multiple surgeries. However, these standard payment rules are not appropriate for certain procedures. Field 21 of the MFSDB indicates whether the standard payment policy rules apply to a multiple surgery, or whether special payment rules apply. Site of service payment adjustments (codes with an indicator of "1" in Field 27 of the MFSDB) should be applied before multiple surgery payment adjustments.

B. Billing Instructions

The following procedures apply when billing for multiple surgeries by the same physician on the same day.

- Report the more major surgical procedure without the multiple procedures modifier "-51."

- Report additional surgical procedures performed by the surgeon on the same day with modifier "-51."

There may be instances in which two or more physicians each perform distinctly different, unrelated surgeries on the same patient on the same day (e.g., in some multiple trauma cases). When this occurs, the payment adjustment rules for multiple surgeries may not be appropriate. In such cases, the physician does not use modifier "-51" unless one of the surgeons individually performs multiple surgeries.

C. Carrier Claims Processing System Requirements

Carriers must be able to:

1. Identify multiple surgeries by both of the following methods:

- The presence on the claim form or electronic submission of the "-51" modifier; and

- The billing of more than one separately payable surgical procedure by the same physician performed on the same patient on the same day, whether on different lines or with a number greater than 1 in the units column on the claim form or inappropriately billed with modifier "-78" (i.e., after the global period has expired);

2. Access Field 34 of the MFSDB to determine the Medicare fee schedule payment amount for each surgery;

3. Access Field 21 for each procedure of the MFSDB to determine if the payment rules for multiple surgeries apply to any of the multiple surgeries billed on the same day;

4. If Field 21 for any of the multiple procedures contains an indicator of "0," the multiple surgery rules do not apply to that procedure. Base payment on the lower of the billed amount or the fee schedule amount (Field 34 or 35) for each code unless other payment adjustment rules apply;

5. For dates of service prior to January 1, 1995, if Field 21 contains an indicator of "1," the standard rules for pricing multiple surgeries apply (see items 6-8 below);

6. Rank the surgeries subject to the standard multiple surgery rules (indicator "1") in descending order by the Medicare fee schedule amount;

7. Base payment for each ranked procedure on the lower of the billed amount, or:

- 100 percent of the fee schedule amount (Field 34 or 35) for the highest valued procedure;

- 50 percent of the fee schedule amount for the second highest valued procedure; and

- 25 percent of the fee schedule amount for the third through the fifth highest valued procedures;

8. If more than five procedures are billed, pay for the first five according to the rules listed in 5, 6, and 7 above and suspend the sixth and subsequent procedures for manual review and payment, if appropriate, "by report." Payment determined on a "by report" basis for these codes should never be lower than 25 percent of the full payment amount;

9. For dates of service on or after January 1, 1995, new standard rules for pricing multiple surgeries apply. If Field 21 contains an indicator of "2," these new standard rules apply (see items 10-12 below);

10. Rank the surgeries subject to the multiple surgery rules (indicator "2") in descending order by the Medicare fee schedule amount;

11. Base payment for each ranked procedure (indicator "2") on the lower of the billed amount:

- 100 percent of the fee schedule amount (Field 34 or 35) for the highest valued procedure; and

- 50 percent of the fee schedule amount for the second through the fifth highest valued procedures; or

12. If more than five procedures with an indicator of "2" are billed, pay for the first five according to the rules listed in 9, 10, and 11 above and suspend the sixth and subsequent procedures for manual review and payment, if appropriate, "by report." Payment determined on a "by report" basis for these codes should never be lower than 50 percent of the full payment amount. Pay by the unit for services that are already reduced (e.g., 17003). Pay for 17340 only once per session, regardless of how many lesions were destroyed;

NOTE: For dates of service prior to January 1, 1995, the multiple surgery indicator of "2" indicated that special dermatology rules applied. The payment rules for these codes have not changed. The rules were expanded, however, to all codes that previously had a multiple surgery indicator of "1." For dates of service prior to January 1, 1995, if a dermatological procedure with an indicator of "2" was billed with the "-51" modifier with other procedures that are not dermatological procedures (procedures with an indicator of "1" in Field 21), the standard multiple surgery rules applied. Pay no less than 50 percent for the dermatological procedures with an indicator of "2." See §§40.6.C.6-8 for required actions.

13. If Field 21 contains an indicator of "3," and multiple endoscopies are billed, the special rules for multiple endoscopic procedures apply. Pay the full value of the highest valued endoscopy, plus the difference between the next highest and the base endoscopy. Access Field 31A of the MFSDB to determine the base endoscopy.

EXAMPLE

In the course of performing a fiber optic colonoscopy (CPT code 45378) a physician performs a biopsy on a lesion (code 45380) and removes a polyp (code 45385) from a different part of the colon. The physician bills for codes 45380 and 45385. The value of codes 45380 and 45385 have the value of the diagnostic colonoscopy (45378) built in. Rather than paying 100 percent for the highest valued procedure (45385) and 50 percent for the next (45380), pay the full value of the higher valued endoscopy (45385), plus the difference between the next highest endoscopy (45380) and the base endoscopy (45378).

Carriers assume the following fee schedule amounts for these codes:

45378 - $255.40

45380 - $285.98

45385 - $374.56

Pay the full value of 45385 ($374.56), plus the difference between 45380 and 45378 ($30.58), for a total of $405.14.

NOTE: If an endoscopic procedure with an indicator of "3" is billed with the "-51" modifier with other procedures that are not endoscopies (procedures with an indicator of "1" in Field 21), the standard multiple surgery rules apply. See §§40.6.C.6-8 for required actions.

14. Apply the following rules where endoscopies are performed on the same day as unrelated endoscopies or other surgical procedures:

- Two unrelated endoscopies (e.g., 46606 and 43217): Apply the usual multiple surgery rules;

- Two sets of unrelated endoscopies (e.g., 43202 and 43217; 46606 and 46608): Apply the special endoscopy rules to each series and then apply the multiple surgery rules. Consider the total payment for each set of endoscopies as one service;

- Two related endoscopies and a third, unrelated procedure: Apply the special endoscopic rules to the related endoscopies, and, then apply the multiple surgery rules. Consider the total payment for the related endoscopies as one service and the unrelated endoscopy as another service.

15. If two or more multiple surgeries are of equal value, rank them in descending dollar order billed and base payment on the percentages listed above (i.e., 100 percent for the first billed procedure, 50 percent for the second, etc.);

16. If any of the multiple surgeries are bilateral surgeries, consider the bilateral procedure at 150 percent as one payment amount, rank this with the remaining procedures, and apply the appropriate multiple surgery reductions. See §40.7 for bilateral surgery payment instructions.);

17. Round all adjusted payment amounts to the nearest cent;

18. If some of the surgeries are subject to special rules while others are subject to the standard rules, automate pricing to the extent possible. If necessary, price manually;

19. In cases of multiple interventional radiological procedures, both the radiology code and the primary surgical code are paid at 100 percent of the fee schedule amount. The subsequent surgical procedures are paid at the standard multiple surgical percentages (50 percent, 50 percent, 50 percent and 50 percent);

20. Apply the requirements in §§40 on global surgeries to multiple surgeries;

21. Retain the "-51" modifier in history for any multiple surgeries paid at less than the full global amount; and

22. Follow the instructions on adjudicating surgery claims submitted with the "-22" modifier. Review documentation to determine if full payment should be made for those distinctly different, unrelated surgeries performed by different physicians on the same day.

D. Ranking of Same Day Multiple Surgeries When One Surgery Has a "-22" Modifier and Additional Payment is Allowed

B3-4826

If the patient returns to the operating room after the initial operative session on the same day as a result of complications from the original surgery, the complications rules apply to each procedure required to treat the complications from the original surgery. The multiple surgery rules would not apply.

However, if the patient is returned to the operating room during the postoperative period of the original surgery, not on the same day of the original surgery, for multiple procedures that are required as a result of complications from the original surgery, the complications rules would apply. The multiple surgery rules would also not apply.

Multiple surgeries are defined as separate procedures performed by a single physician or physicians in the same group practice on the same patient at the same operative session or on the same day for which separate payment may be allowed. Co-surgeons, surgical teams, or assistants-at-surgery may participate in performing multiple surgeries on the same patient on the same day.

Multiple surgeries are distinguished from procedures that are components of or incidental to a primary procedure. These intra-operative services, incidental surgeries, or components of more major surgeries are not separately billable. See Chapter 23 for a description of mandatory edits to prevent separate payment for those procedures.

Pub. 100-4, Chapter 12, Section 40.7

Claims for Bilateral Surgeries

B3-4827, B3-15040

A. General

Bilateral surgeries are procedures performed on both sides of the body during the same operative session or on the same day.

The terminology for some procedure codes includes the terms "bilateral" (e.g., code 27395; Lengthening of the hamstring tendon; multiple, bilateral.) or "unilateral or bilateral" (e.g., code 52290; cystourethroscopy; with ureteral meatotomy, unilateral or bilateral). The payment adjustment rules for bilateral surgeries do not apply to procedures identified by CPT as "bilateral" or "unilateral or bilateral" since the fee schedule reflects any additional work required for bilateral surgeries.

Field 22 of the MFSDB indicates whether the payment adjustment rules apply to a surgical procedure.

B. Billing Instructions for Bilateral Surgeries

If a procedure is not identified by its terminology as a bilateral procedure (or unilateral or bilateral), physicians must report the procedure with modifier "-50." They report such procedures as a single line item. (NOTE: This differs from the CPT coding guidelines which indicate that bilateral procedures should be billed as two line items.)

If a procedure is identified by the terminology as bilateral (or unilateral or bilateral), as in codes 27395 and 52290, physicians do not report the procedure with modifier "-50."

C. Claims Processing System Requirements

Carriers must be able to:

1. Identify bilateral surgeries by the presence on the claim form or electronic submission of the "-50" modifier or of the same code on separate lines reported once with modifier "-LT" and once with modifier "-RT";

2. Access Field 34 or 35 of the MFSDB to determine the Medicare payment amount;

3. Access Field 22 of the MFSDB:

- If Field 22 contains an indicator of "0," "2," or "3," the payment adjustment rules for bilateral surgeries do not apply. Base payment on the lower of the billed amount or 100 percent of the fee schedule amount (Field 34 or 35) unless other payment adjustment rules apply.

NOTE: Some codes which have a bilateral indicator of "0" in the MFSDB may be performed more than once on a given day. These are services that would never be considered bilateral and thus should not be billed with modifier "-50." Where such a code is billed on multiple line items or with more than 1 in the units field and carriers have determined that the code may be reported more than once, bypass the "0" bilateral indicator and refer to the multiple surgery field for pricing;

- If Field 22 contains an indicator of "1," the standard adjustment rules apply. Base payment on the lower of the billed amount or 150 percent of the fee schedule amount (Field 34 or 35). (Multiply the payment amount in Field 34 or 35 for the surgery by 150 percent and round to the nearest cent.)

4. Apply the requirements §§40 - 40.4 on global surgeries to bilateral surgeries; and

5. Retain the "-50" modifier in history for any bilateral surgeries paid at the adjusted amount.

(NOTE: The "-50" modifier is not retained for surgeries which are bilateral by definition such as code 27395.)

Pub. 100-4, Chapter 12, Section 50

Payment for Anesthesiology Services

B3-15018

A. General Payment Rule

The fee schedule amount for physician anesthesia services furnished on or after January 1, 1992 is, with the exceptions noted, based on allowable base and time units multiplied by an anesthesia conversion factor specific to that locality. The base unit for each anesthesia procedure is listed in §50.K, Exhibit 1. The way in which time units are calculated is described in §50.G. CMS releases the conversion factor annually. Carriers may not allow separate payment for the anesthesia service performed by the physician who also furnishes the medical or surgical service. In that case, payment for the anesthesia service is made through the payment for the medical or surgical service. For example, carriers may not allow separate payment for the surgeon's performance of a local or surgical anesthesia if the surgeon also performs the surgical procedure. Similarly, separate payment is not allowed for the psychiatrist's performance of the anesthesia service associated with the electroconvulsive therapy if the psychiatrist performs the electroconvulsive therapy.

B. Payment at Personally Performed Rate

Carriers must determine the fee schedule payment, recognizing the base unit for the anesthesia code and one time unit per 15 minutes of anesthesia time if:

- The physician personally performed the entire anesthesia service alone;

- The physician is involved with one anesthesia case with a resident, the physician is a teaching physician as defined in §100, and the service is furnished on or after January 1, 1996;

The physician is continuously involved in a single case involving a student nurse anesthetist;

- The physician is continuously involved in one anesthesia case involving a CRNA (or AA) and the service was furnished prior to January 1, 1998. If the physician is involved with a single case with a CRNA (or AA) and the service was furnished on or after January 1, 1998, carriers may pay the physician service and the CRNA (or AA) service in accordance with the medical direction payment policy; or

- The physician and the CRNA (or AA) are involved in one anesthesia case and the services of each are found to be medically necessary. Documentation must be submitted by both the CRNA and the physician to support payment of the full fee for each of the two providers. The physician reports the "AA" modifier and the CRNA reports the "QZ" modifier for a nonmedically directed case.

C. Payment at the Medically Directed Rate

Carriers determine payment for the physician's medical direction service furnished on or after January 1, 1998 on the basis of 50 percent of the allowance for the service performed by the physician alone. Medical direction occurs if the physician medically directs qualified individuals in two, three, or four concurrent cases and the physician performs the following activities.

- Performs a pre-anesthetic examination and evaluation;

- Prescribes the anesthesia plan;

- Personally participates in the most demanding procedures in the anesthesia plan, including induction and emergence;

- Ensures that any procedures in the anesthesia plan that he or she does not perform are performed by a qualified anesthetist;

- Monitors the course of anesthesia administration at frequent intervals;

- Remains physically present and available for immediate diagnosis and treatment of emergencies; and

- Provides indicated-post-anesthesia care.

Prior to January 1, 1999 the physician was required to participate in the most demanding procedures of the anesthesia plan, including induction and emergence.

For medical direction services furnished on or after January 1, 1999, the physician must participate only in the most demanding procedures of the anesthesia plan, including, if applicable, induction and emergence. Also for medical direction services furnished on or after January 1, 1999, the physician must document in the medical record that he or she performed the pre-anesthetic examination and evaluation. Physicians must also document that they provided indicated post-anesthesia care, were present during some portion of the anesthesia monitoring, and were present during the most demanding procedures, including induction and emergence, where indicated.

For services furnished on or after January 1, 1994, the physician can medically direct two, three, or four concurrent procedures involving qualified individuals, all of whom could be CRNAs, AAs, interns, residents or combinations of these individuals. The medical direction rules apply to cases involving student nurse anesthetists if the physician directs two concurrent cases, each of which involves a student nurse anesthetist, or the physician directs one case involving a student nurse anesthetist and another involving a CRNA, AA, intern or resident.

If anesthesiologists are in a group practice, one physician member may provide the pre-anesthesia examination and evaluation while another fulfills the other criteria. Similarly, one physician member of the group may provide post-anesthesia care while another member of the group furnishes the other component parts of the anesthesia service. However, the medical record must indicate that the services were furnished by physicians and identify the physicians who furnished them.

A physician who is concurrently directing the administration of anesthesia to not more than four surgical patients cannot ordinarily be involved in furnishing additional services to other patients. However, addressing an emergency of short duration in the immediate area, administering an epidural or caudal anesthetic to ease labor pain, or periodic, rather than continuous, monitoring of an obstetrical patient does not substantially diminish the scope of control exercised by the physician in directing the administration of anesthesia to surgical patients. It does not constitute a separate service for the purpose of determining whether the medical direction criteria are met. Further, while directing concurrent anesthesia procedures, a physician may receive patients entering the operating suite for the next surgery, check or discharge patients in the recovery room, or handle scheduling matters without affecting fee schedule payment.

However, if the physician leaves the immediate area of the operating suite for other than short durations or devotes extensive time to an emergency case or is otherwise not available to respond to the immediate needs of the surgical patients, the physician's services to the surgical patients are supervisory in nature. Carriers may not make payment under the fee schedule.

See §50.J for a definition of concurrent anesthesia procedures.

D. Payment at Medically Supervised Rate

Carriers may allow only three base units per procedure when the anesthesiologist is involved in furnishing more than four procedures concurrently or is performing other services while directing the concurrent procedures. An additional time unit may be recognized if the physician can document he or she was present at induction.

E. Billing and Payment for Multiple Anesthesia Procedures

B3-4830.C and D

Physicians bill for the anesthesia services associated with multiple bilateral surgeries by reporting the anesthesia procedure with the highest base unit value with the multiple procedure modifier "-51." They report the total time for all procedures in the line item with the highest base unit value.

If the same anesthesia CPT code applies to two or more of the surgical procedures, billers enter the anesthesia code with the "-51" modifier and the number of surgeries to which the modified CPT code applies.

Payment can be made under the fee schedule for anesthesia services associated with multiple surgical procedures or multiple bilateral procedures. Payment is determined based on the base unit of the anesthesia procedure with the highest base unit value and time units based on the actual anesthesia time of the multiple procedures. See §§40.6-40.7 for a definition and appropriate billing and claims processing instructions for multiple and bilateral surgeries.

F. Payment for Medical and Surgical Services Furnished in Addition to Anesthesia Procedure

Payment may be made under the fee schedule for specific medical and surgical services furnished by the anesthesiologist as long as these services are reasonable and medically necessary or provided that other rebundling provisions (see §30 and Chapter 23) do not preclude separate payment. These services may be furnished in conjunction with the anesthesia procedure to the patient or may be furnished as single services, e.g., during the day of the day before the anesthesia service. These services include the insertion of a Swan Ganz catheter, the insertion of central venous pressure lines, emergency intubation, and critical care visits.

G. Anesthesia Time and Calculation of Anesthesia Time Units

Anesthesia time is defined as the period during which an anesthesia practitioner is present with the patient. It starts when the anesthesia practitioner begins to prepare the patient for anesthesia services in the operating room or an equivalent area and ends when the anesthesia practitioner is no longer furnishing anesthesia services to the patient, that is, when the patient may be placed safely under postoperative care. Anesthesia time is a continuous time period from the start of anesthesia to the end of an anesthesia service. In counting anesthesia time for services furnished on or after January 1, 2000, the anesthesia practitioner can add blocks of time around an interruption in anesthesia time as long as the anesthesia practitioner is furnishing continuous anesthesia care within the time periods around the interruption.

Actual anesthesia time in minutes is reported on the claim. For anesthesia services furnished on or after January 1, 1994, carriers compute time units by dividing reported

anesthesia time by 15 minutes. Round the time unit to one decimal place. Carriers do not recognize time units for CPT codes 01995 or 01996.

For purposes of this section, anesthesia practitioner means a physician who performs the anesthesia service alone, a CRNA who is not medically directed, or a CRNA or AA, who is medically directed. The physician who medically directs the CRNA or AA would ordinarily report the same time as the CRNA or AA reports for the CRNA service.

H. Base Unit Reduction for Concurrent Medically Directed Procedures

If the physician medically directs concurrent medically directed procedures prior to January 1, 1994, reduce the number of base units for each concurrent procedure as follows.

- For two concurrent procedures, the base unit on each procedure is reduced 10 percent.

- For three concurrent procedures, the base unit on each procedure is reduced 25 percent.

- For four concurrent procedures, the base on each concurrent procedure is reduced 40 percent.

- If the physician medically directs concurrent procedures prior to January 1, 1994, and any of the concurrent procedures are cataract or iridectomy anesthesia, reduce the base units for each cataract or iridectomy procedure by 10 percent.

I. Monitored Anesthesia Care

Carriers pay for reasonable and medically necessary monitored anesthesia care services on the same basis as other anesthesia services. Anesthesiologists use modifier QS to report monitored anesthesia care cases. Monitored anesthesia care involves the intra-operative monitoring by a physician or qualified individual under the medical direction of a physician or of the patient's vital physiological signs in anticipation of the need for administration of general anesthesia or of the development of adverse physiological patient reaction to the surgical procedure. It also includes the performance of a pre-anesthetic examination and evaluation, prescription of the anesthesia care required, administration of any necessary oral or parenteral medications (e.g., etropine, demerol, valium) and provision of indicated postoperative anesthesia care.

Payment is made under the fee schedule using the payment rules in subsection B if the physician personally performs the monitored anesthesia care case or under the rules in subsection C if the physician medically directs four or fewer concurrent cases and monitored anesthesia care represents one or more of these concurrent cases.

J. Definition of Concurrent Medically Directed Anesthesia Procedures

Concurrency is defined with regard to the maximum number of procedures that the physician is medically directing within the context of a single procedure and whether these other procedures overlap each other. Concurrency is not dependent on each of the cases involving a Medicare patient. For example, if an anesthesiologist directs three concurrent procedures, two of which involve non-Medicare patients and the remaining a Medicare patient, this represents three concurrent cases. The following example illustrates this concept and guides physicians in determining how many procedures they are directing.

EXAMPLE

Procedures A through E are medically directed procedures involving CRNAs and furnished between January 1, 1992 and December 31, 1997 (1998 concurrent instructions can be found in subsection C.) The starting and ending times for each procedure represent the periods during which anesthesia time is counted. Assume that none of the procedures were cataract or iridectomy anesthesia.

Procedure A begins at 8:00 a.m. and lasts until 8:20 a.m.

Procedure B begins at 8:10 a.m. and lasts until 8:45 a.m.

Procedure C begins at 8:30 a.m. and lasts until 9:15 a.m.

Procedure D begins at 9:00 a.m. and lasts until 12:00 noon.

Procedure E begins at 9:10 a.m. and lasts until 9:55 a.m.

Procedure	Number of Concurrent Medically Directed Procedures	Base Unit Reduction Percentage
A	2	10%
B	2	10%
C	3	25%
D	3	25%
E	3	25%

From 8:00 a.m. to 8:20 a.m., the length of procedure A, the anesthesiologist medically directed two concurrent procedures, A and B.

From 8:10 a.m. to 8:45 a.m., the length of procedure B, the anesthesiologist medically directed two concurrent procedures. From 8:10 to 8:20 a.m., the anesthesiologist medically directed procedures A and B. From 8:20 to 8:30 a.m., the anesthesiologist medically directed only procedure B. From 8:30 to 8:45 a.m., the anesthesiologist medically directed procedures B and C. Thus, during procedure B, the anesthesiologist medically directed, at most, two concurrent procedures.

From 8:30 a.m. to 9:15 a.m., the length of procedure C, the anesthesiologist medically directed three concurrent procedures. From 8:30 to 8:45 a.m., the anesthesiologist medically directed procedures B and C. From 8:45 to 9:00 a.m., the anesthesiologist medically directed procedure C. From 9:00 to 9:10 a.m., the anesthesiologist medically directed procedures C and D. From 9:10 to 9:15 a.m., the anesthesiologist medically

directed procedures C, D and E. Thus, during procedure C, the anesthesiologist medically directed, at most, three concurrent procedures.

The same analysis shows that during procedure D or E, the anesthesiologist medically directed, at most, three concurrent procedures.

K. Anesthesia Claims Modifiers

B3-4830, B3-15018.K

Physicians report the appropriate anesthesia modifier to denote whether the service was personally performed, medically directed, or medically supervised.

Specific anesthesia modifiers include:

AA - Anesthesia Services performed personally by the anesthesiologist

AD - Medical Supervision by a physician; more than 4 concurrent anesthesia procedures;

G8 - Monitored anesthesia care (MAC) for deep complex complicated, or markedly invasive surgical procedures;

G9 - Monitored anesthesia care for patient who has a history of severe cardio-pulmonary condition

QK - Medical direction of two, three or four concurrent anesthesia procedures involving qualified individuals

QS - Monitored anesthesia care service

QX - CRNA service; with medical direction by a physician

QY - Medical direction of one certified registered nurse anesthetist by an anesthesiologist

QZ - CRNA service: Without medical direction by a physician.

The QS modifier is for informational purposes. Providers must report actual anesthesia time on the claim.

Carriers must determine payment for anesthesia in accordance with these instructions. They must be able to determine the uniform base unit that is assigned to the anesthesia code and apply the appropriate reduction where the anesthesia procedures is medically directed. They must also be able to determine the number of anesthesia time units from actual anesthesia time reported on the claim, differentiating 15 minute time unit intervals for personally performed anesthesia procedures and 30 minute time unit intervals for medically directed procedures. Carriers must multiply allowable units by the anesthesia-specific conversion factor used to determine fee schedule payment for the payment area.

Exhibit 1: Base Unit for Each Anesthesia Procedure

HEAD

Anesthesia Code	Anesthesia Procedure	Base Units
00100	Anesthesia for procedures on Integumentary system of head and/or salivary glands, including biopsy; not otherwise specified	5
00102	Plastic repair of cleft lip	6
00103	Anesthesia for procedures in eye, blepharoplasty	5
00104	Anesthesia for electroconvulsive therapy	4
00120	Anesthesia for procedures on external, middle, and inner ear, including biopsy; not otherwise specified	5
00124	Otoscopy	4
00126	Tympanotomy	4
00140	Anesthesia for procedures on eye; not otherwise specified	5
00142	Lens surgery	4
00144	Corneal transplant	6
00145	Vitrectomy	6
00147	Iridectomy	4
00148	Ophthalmoscopy	4
00160	Anesthesia for procedures on nose and accessory sinuses; not otherwise specified	5
00162	Radical surgery	7
00164	Biopsy, soft tissue	4
00170	Anesthesia for intraoral procedures, including biopsy; not otherwise specified	5
00172	Repair of cleft palate	6
00174	Excision of retropharyngeal tumor	6
00176	Radical surgery	7
00190	Anesthesia for procedures on facial bones; not otherwise	5
00192	Radical surgery (including prognathism)	7
00210	Anesthesia for intracranial procedures; not otherwise specified	11
00212	Subdural taps	5
00214	Burr holes (For burr holes for ventriculography, see 01902.)	9
00215	Anesthesia for intracranial procedures; elevation of depressed skull fracture, extradural (simple or compound)	9
00216	Vascular procedures	15
00218	Procedures in sitting position	13
00220	Spinal fluid shunting procedures	10

Anesthesia Code	Anesthesia Procedure	Base Units
00222	Electrocoagulation of intracranial nerve	6

NECK

Anesthesia Code	Anesthesia Procedure	Base Units
00300	Anesthesia for all procedures on integumentary system of neck, including subcutaneous tissue	5
00320	Anesthesia for all procedures on esophagus, thyroid, larynx, trachea and lymphatic system of neck; not otherwise specified	6
00322	Needle biopsy of thyroid (For procedures on cervical spine and cord see 00600, 00604, 00670)	3
00350	Anesthesia for procedures on major vessels of neck; not otherwise specified	10
00352	Simple ligation (For arteriography; see radiologic procedure 01916)	5

THORAX (CHEST WALL AND SHOULDER GIRDLE)

Anesthesia Code	Anesthesia Procedure	Base Units
00400	Anesthesia for procedures on anterior integumentary system of chest, including subcutaneous tissue; not otherwise specified	3
00402	Reconstructive procedures on breast (e.g.,reduction or augmentation mammoplasty, muscle flaps)	5
00404	Radical or modified radical procedures on breast	5
00406	Radical or modified radical procedures on breast with internal mammary node dissection	
00410	Electrical conversion of arrhythmias	4
00420	Anesthesia for procedures on posterior integumentary system of chest, including subcutaneous tissue	5
00450	Anesthesia for procedures on clavicle and scapula; not otherwise specified	5
00452	Radical surgery	6
00454	Biopsy of clavicle	3
00470	Anesthesia for partial rib resection; not otherwise specified	6
00472	Thoracoplasty (any type)	10
00474	Radical procedures, (e.g., pectus excavatum)	13

INTRATHORACIC

Anesthesia Code	Anesthesia Procedure	Base Units
00500	Anesthesia for all procedures on esophagus	15
00520	Anesthesia for closed chest procedures (including esophagoscopy, bronchoscopy, thoracoscopy); not otherwise specified	6
00522	Needle biopsy of pleura	4
00524	Pneumocentesis	4
00528	Mediastinoscopy	8
00530	Anesthesia for transvenous pacemaker insertion	4
00532	Anesthesia for vascular access to central venous circulation	4
00534	Anesthesia for thoracotomy procedures involving lungs, pleura, diaphragm, and mediastinum; not otherwise specified	7
00537	Anesthesia for cardiac electrophys	7
00540	Anesthesia for thoracotomy procedures involving lungs, pleura, diaphragm, and mediastinum; not otherwise specified	13
00542	Decortication	15
00544	Pleurectomy	15
00546	Pulmonary resection with thoracoplasty	15
00548	Intrathoracic repair of trauma to trachea and bronchi	15
00550	Anesthesia for sternal debridement	-
00560	Anesthesia for procedures on heart, pericardium, and great vessels of chest; without pump oxygenator	15
00562	With pump oxygenator	20
00563	Anesthesia for heart proc with pump	25
00566	Anesthesia for cabg without pump	25
00580	Anesthesia for heart or heart/lung transplant	20

SPINE AND SPINAL CORD

Anesthesia Code	Anesthesia Procedure	Base Units
00600	Anesthesia for procedures on cervical spine and cord; not otherwise specified (For myelography and discography, see radiological procedures 01906-01914.)	10
00604	Posterior cervical laminectomy in sitting position	

Anesthesia Code	Anesthesia Procedure	Base Units
00620	Anesthesia for procedures on thoracic spine and cord; not otherwise specified	10
00622	Thoracolumbar sympathectomy	13
00630	Anesthesia for procedures in lumbar region; not otherwise specified	8
00632	Lumbar sympathectomy	7
00634	Chemonucleolysis	10
00635	Anesthesia for lumbar puncture	4
00670	Anesthesia for extensive spine and spinal cord procedures (e.g., Harrington rod technique)	13

UPPER ABDOMEN

Anesthesia Code	Anesthesia Procedure	Base Units
00700	Anesthesia for procedures on upper anterior abdominal wall; not otherwise specified	3
00702	Percutaneous liver biopsy	4
00730	Anesthesia for procedures on upper posterior abdominal wall	5
00740	Anesthesia for upper gastrointestinal endoscopic procedures	5
00750	Anesthesia for hernia repairs in upper abdomen; not otherwise specified	4
00752	Lumbar and ventral (incisional) hernias and/or wound dehiscence	6
00754	Omphalocele	7
00756	Transabdominal repair of diaphragmatic hernia	7
00770	Anesthesia for all procedures on major abdominal blood vessels	15
00790	Anesthesia for intraperitoneal procedures in upper abdomen including laparoscopy; not otherwise specified	7
00792	Partial hepatectomy (excluding liver biopsy)	13
00794	Pancreatectomy, partial or total (e.g., Whipple procedure)	8
00796	Liver transplant (recipient)	30
00797	Anesthesia, surgery for obesity	8

LOWER ABDOMEN

Anesthesia Code	Anesthesia Procedure	Base Units
00800	Anesthesia for procedures on lower anterior abdominal wall; not otherwise specified	3

Anesthesia Code	Anesthesia Procedure	Base Units
00802	Panniculectomy	5
00810	Anesthesia for intestinal endoscopic procedures	6
00820	Anesthesia for procedures on lower posterior abdominal wall	5
00830	Anesthesia for hernia repairs in lower abdomen; not otherwise specified	4
00832	Ventral and incisional hernias	
00840	Anesthesia for intraperitoneal procedures in lower abdomen including laparoscopy; not otherwise specified	6
00842	Amniocentesis	4
00844	Abdominoperineal resection	7
00846	Radical hysterectomy	8
00848	Pelvic exenteration	8
00851	Anestheisa, tubal ligation	6
00860	Anesthesia for extraperitoneal procedures in lower abdomen, including urinary tract; not otherwise specified	6
00862	Renal procedures, including upper 1/3 of ureter or donor nephrectomy	7
00864	Total cystectomy	8
00865	Anesthesia for removal of prostate	7
00866	Adrenalectomy	
00868	Renal transplant (recipient) (For donor nephrectomy, use 00862.) (For harvesting kidney from brain-dead patient, use 01990.)	10
00869	Anesthesia for vasectomy	3
00870	Cystolithotomy	5
00872	Anesthesia for lithotripsy, extracorporeal shock wave; with water bath	7
00873	Without water bath	5
00880	Anesthesia for procedures on major lower abdominal vessels; not otherwise specified	15
00882	Inferior vena cava ligation	10
00884	Transvenous umbrella insertion	5

PERINEUM

Anesthesia Code	Anesthesia Procedure	Base Units
00902	Anorectal procedure (including endoscopy and/or biopsy)	4
00904	Radical perineal procedure	7
00906	Vulvectomy	4
00908	Perineal prostatectomy	6

Anesthesia Code	Anesthesia Procedure	Base Units
00910	Anesthesia for transurethral procedures (including urethrocystoscopy); not otherwise specified	3
00912	Transurethral resection of bladder tumor(s)	5
00914	Transurethral resection of prostate	5
00916	Post-transurethral resection bleeding	5
00918	With fragmentation and/or fragmentation removal of ureteral calculus	5
00920	Anesthesia for procedures on male external genitalia; not otherwise specified	3
00922	Seminal vesicles	6
00924	Undescended testis, unilateral or bilateral	4
00926	Radical orchiectomy, inguinal	4
00928	Radical orchiectomy, abdominal	6
00930	Orchiopexy, unilateral and bilateral	4
00932	Complete amputation of penis	4
00934	Radical amputation of penis with bilateral inguinal lymphadenectomy	6
00936	Radical amputation of penis with bilateral inguinal and iliac lymphadenectomy	8
00938	Insertion of penile prosthesis (perineal approach)	4
00940	Anesthesia for vaginal procedures (including biopsy of labia, vagina, cervix or endometrium); not otherwise specified	3
00942	Colpotomy, colpectomy, colporrhaphy	4
00944	Vaginal hysterectomy	6
00948	Cervical cerlage	4
00950	Culdoscopy	5
00952	Hysteroscopy	4
00955	Continuous epidural and analgesic for labor and vaginal delivery	5

PELVIS (EXCEPT HIP)

Anesthesia Code	Anesthesia Procedure	Base Units
01000	Anesthesia for procedures on anterior integumentary system of pelvis (anterior to iliac crest), except external genitalia	3
01110	Anesthesia for procedures on posterior integumentary system of pelvis (posterior to iliac crest), except perineum	5

Anesthesia Code	Anesthesia Procedure	Base Units
01112	Anesthesia for bone aspirate/bx	5
01120	Anesthesia for procedures on bony pelvis	6
01130	Anesthesia for body cast application or revision	3
01140	Anesthesia for interpelviabdominal (hind quarter) amputation	15
01150	Anesthesia for radical procedures for tumor of pelvis, except hind quarter amputation	8
01160	Anesthesia for closed procedures involving symphysis pubis or sacroiliac joint	4
01170	Anesthesia for open procedures involving symphysis pubis or sacroiliac joint	8
01180	Anesthesia for obturator neurectomy; extrapelvic	3
01190	Intrapelvic	4

UPPER LEG (EXCEPT KNEE)

Anesthesia Code	Anesthesia Procedure	Base Units
01200	Anesthesia for all closed procedures involving hip joint	4
01202	Anesthesia for arthroscopic procedures of hip joint	4
01210	Anesthesia for open procedures involving hip joint; not otherwise specified	6
01212	Hip disarticulation	10
01214	Total hip replacement or revision	10
01215	Anesthesia for revise hip repair	10
01220	Anesthesia for all closed procedures involving upper 2/3 of femur	4
01230	Anesthesia for open procedures involving upper 2/3 of femur; not otherwise specified	6
01232	Amputation	5
01234	Radical resection	8
01240	Anesthesia for all procedures on integumentary system of upper leg	3
01250	Anesthesia for all procedures on nerves, muscles, tendons, fascia, and bursae of upper leg	4
01260	Anesthesia for all procedures involving veins of upper leg, including exploration	3

Anesthesia Code	Anesthesia Procedure	Base Units
01270	Anesthesia for procedures involving arteries of upper leg, including bypass graft; not otherwise specified	8
01272	Femoral artery ligation	4
01274	Femoral artery embolectomy	6

KNEE AND POPLITEAL AREA

Anesthesia Code	Anesthesia Procedure	Base Units
01320	Anesthesia for all procedures on nerves, muscles, tendons, fascia and bursae of knee and/or popliteal area	4
01340	Anesthesia for all closed procedures on lower 1/3 of femur	4
01360	Anesthesia for all open procedures on lower 1/3 of femur	5
01380	Anesthesia for all closed procedures on knee joint	3
01382	Anesthesia for arthroscopic procedures of knee joint	3
01390	Anesthesia for all closed procedures on upper ends of tibia and fibula, and/or patella	3
01392	Anesthesia for all open procedures on upper ends of tibia and fibula and/or patella	4
01400	Anesthesia for open procedures on knee joint; not otherwise specified	4
01402	Total knee replacement	7
01404	Disarticulation at knee	5
01420	Anesthesia for all cast applications, removal, or repair involving knee joint	3
01430	Anesthesia for procedures on veins of knee and popliteal area; not otherwise specified	3
01432	Arteriovenous fistula	5
01440	Anesthesia for procedures on arteries of knee and Popliteal area; not otherwise specified	5
01442	Popliteal thromboendarterectomy, with or without patch graft	8
01444	Popliteal excision and graft or repair for occlusion or aneurysm	8

LOWER LEG (Below knee - includes ankle and foot)

Anesthesia Code	Anesthesia Procedure	Base Units
01462	Anesthesia for all closed procedures on lower leg, ankle, and foot	3
01464	Anesthesia for arthroscopic procedures of ankle joint	3

Anesthesia Code	Anesthesia Procedure	Base Units
01470	Anesthesia for procedures on nerves, muscles, tendons, and fascia of lower leg, ankle, and foot; not otherwise specified	3
01472	Repair of ruptured Achilles tendon, with or without graft	5
01474	Gastrocnemius recession (e.g., Strayer procedure)	5
01480	Anesthesia for open procedures on bones of lower leg, ankle, and foot; not otherwise specified	3
01482	Radical resection	4
01484	Osteotomy or osteoplasty of tibia and/or fibula	4
01486	Total ankle replacement	7
01490	Anesthesia for lower leg cast application, removal, or repair	3
01500	Anesthesia for procedures on arteries of lower leg, including bypass graft; not otherwise specified	8
01502	Embolectomy, direct or catheter	6
01520	Anesthesia for procedures on veins of lower leg; not otherwise specified	3
01522	Venous thrombectomy, direct or catheter	5

SHOULDER AND AXILLA

(Includes humeral head and neck, sternoclavicular joint, acromioclavicular joint, and shoulder joint)

Anesthesia Code	Anesthesia Procedure	Base Units
01610	Anesthesia for all procedures on nerves, muscles, tendons, fascia, and bursae of shoulder and axilla	5
	(Includes humeral head and neck, sternoclavicular joint, acromioclavicular joint, and shoulder joint)	
01620	Anesthesia for all closed procedures on humeral head and neck, sternoclavicular joint, and shoulder joint	4
01622	Anesthesia for arthroscopic procedures of shoulder joint	4
01630	Anesthesia for open procedures on humeral head and neck, sternoclavicular joint, acromioclavicular oint, and shoulder joint; not otherwise specified	5
01632	Radical resection	6
01634	Shoulder disarticulation	9
01636	Interthoracoscapular (forequarter) amputation	15
01638	Total shoulder replacement	10

Anesthesia Code	Anesthesia Procedure	Base Units
01650	Anesthesia for procedures on arteries of shoulder and axilla; not otherwise specified	6
01652	Axillary-brachial aneurysm	10
01654	Bypass graft	8
01656	Axillary-femoral bypass graft	10
01670	Anesthesia for all procedures on veins of shoulder and axilla	4
01680	Anesthesia for shoulder cast application, removal or repair; not otherwise specified	3
01682	Shoulder spica	4

UPPER ARM AND ELBOW

Anesthesia Code	Anesthesia Procedure	Base Units
01710	Anesthesia for procedures on nerves, muscles, tendons, fascia, bursae of upper arm and elbow; not otherwise specified	3
01712	Tenotomy, elbow to shoulder, open	5
01714	Tenoplasty, elbow to shoulder	5
01716	Tenodesis, rupture of long tendon of biceps	5
01730	Anesthesia for all closed procedures on humerus and elbow	3
01732	Anesthesia for arthroscopic procedures of elbow joint	3
01740	Anesthesia for open procedures on humerus and elbow; not otherwise specified	4
01742	Osteotomy of humerus	5
01744	Repair of nonunion or malunion of humerus	5
01756	Radical procedures	6
01758	Excision of cyst or tumor of humerus	5
01760	Total elbow replacement	7
01770	Anesthesia for procedures on arteries of upper arm; not otherwise specified	8
01772	Embolectomy	6
01780	Anesthesia for procedures on veins of upper arm and elbow; not otherwise specified	3
01782	Phleborrhaphy	4

FOREARM, WRIST AND HAND

Anesthesia Code	Anesthesia Procedure	Base Units
01810	Anesthesia for all procedures on nerves, muscles, tendons, fascia, bursae of forearm, wrist, and hand	3

Anesthesia Code	Anesthesia Procedure	Base Units
01820	Anesthesia for all closed procedures on radius, ulna, wrist, or hand bones	3
01830	Anesthesia for open procedures on radius, ulna, wrist, or hand bones; not otherwise specified	3
01832	Total wrist replacement	6
01840	Anesthesia for procedures on arteries of forearm, wrist, and hand; not otherwise specified	6
01842	Embolectomy	6
01844	Anesthesia for vascular shunt, or shunt revision, any type (e.g., dialysis)	6
01850	Anesthesia for procedures on veins of forearm, wrist, and hand; not otherwise specified	3
01852	Phleborrhaphy	4
01860	Anesthesia for forearm, wrist, or hand cast application, removal or repair	3

RADIOLOGICAL PROCEDURES

Anesthesia Code	Anesthesia Procedure	Base Units
01905		5
01916	Anesthesia for arteriograms, needle; carotid, or vertebral	5
01920	Anesthesia for cardiac catheterization including coronary arteriography and ventriculography (not to include Swan-Ganz catheter)	7
01922	Anesthesia for noninvasive imaging or radiation therapy	7
01924	Anesthesia, ther intervene rad, art	5
01925	Anesthesia, ther intervene rad, car	7
01926	Anesthesia, tx interv rad hrt/cran	8

MISCELLANEOUS PROCEDURE(S)

Anesthesia Code	Anesthesia Procedure	Base Units
01930	Anesthesia, ther intervene rad, vein	5
01931	Anesthesia, ther intervene rad, tip	7
01932	Anesthesia, tx interv rad, th vein	6
01952	Anesthesia, burn, less 4 percent	5
01953	Anesthesia, burn 4-9 percent	5
01960	Anesthesia, vaginal delivery	5
01961	Anesthesia, caesarean delivery	7

Anesthesia Code	Anesthesia Procedure	Base Units
01962	Anesthesia, emergency hysterectomy	8
01963	Anesthesia, caesarean hysterectomy	8
01964	Anesthesia, abortion procedures	4
01967	Anesthesia/analg, vaginal delivery	5
01968	Anesthesia/analg caesarean delivery add-on	2
01969	Anesthesia/analg caesarean hysterectomy add-on	5
01990	Physiological support for harvesting of organ(s) from brain-dead patient	7
01995	Region IV administration of local anesthetic agent (upper or lower extremity)	5
01996	Daily management of epidural or subarachnoid drug administration	3
01999	Unlisted anesthesia procedure(s)	I. C.* Individual Consideration

Pub. 100-4, Chapter 12, Section 60

Payment for Pathology Services

B3-15020, AB-01-47 (CR1499)

A. General Payment Rule

Payment may be made under the fee schedule for the professional component of physician laboratory or physician pathology services furnished to hospital inpatients or outpatients by hospital physicians or by independent laboratories, if they qualify as the reassignee for the physician service. Payment may be made under the fee schedule, as noted below, for the technical component (TC) of pathology services furnished by an independent laboratory to hospital inpatients or outpatients. Payment may be made under the fee schedule for the technical component of physician pathology services furnished by an independent laboratory, or a hospital if it is acting as an independent laboratory, to non-hospital patients. The Medicare physician fee schedule identifies those physician laboratory or physician pathology services that have a technical component service.

CMS published a final regulation in 1999 that would no longer allow independent laboratories to bill under the physician fee schedule for the TC of physician pathology services. The implementation of this regulation was delayed by Section 542 of the Benefits and Improvement and Protection Act of 2000 (BIPA). Section 542 allows the Medicare carrier to continue to pay for the TC of physician pathology services when an independent laboratory furnishes this service to an inpatient or outpatient of a covered hospital. This provision is applicable to TC services furnished in 2001, 2002, 2003, 2004, 2005 or 2006.

For this provision, a covered hospital is a hospital that had an arrangement with an independent laboratory that was in effect as of July 22, 1999, under which a laboratory furnished the TC of physician pathology services to fee-for-service Medicare beneficiaries who were hospital inpatients or outpatients, and submitted claims for payment for the TC to a carrier. The TC could have been submitted separately or combined with the professional component and reported as a combined service.

The term, fee-for-service Medicare beneficiary, means an individual who:

Is entitled to benefits under Part A or enrolled under Part B of title XVIII or both; and

Is not enrolled in any of the following: A Medicare + Choice plan under Part C of such title; a plan offered by an eligible organization under §1876 of the Social Security Act; a program of all-inclusive care for the elderly under §1894; or a social health maintenance organization demonstration project established under Section 4108 of the Omnibus Budget Reconciliation Act of 1987.

In implementing Section 542, the carriers should consider as independent laboratories those entities that it has previously recognized as independent laboratories.

An independent laboratory that has acquired another independent laboratory that had an arrangement of July 22, 1999, with a covered hospital, can bill the TC of physician pathology services for that hospital's inpatients and outpatients under the physician fee schedule.

An independent laboratory that furnishes the TC of physician pathology services to inpatients or outpatients of a hospital that is not a covered hospital may not bill the carrier for the TC of physician pathology services during the time §542 is in effect.

If the arrangement between the independent laboratory and the covered hospital limited the provision of TC physician pathology services to certain situations or at particular times, then the independent laboratory can bill the carrier only for these limited services.

The carrier shall require independent laboratories that had an arrangement, on or prior to July 22, 1999 with a covered hospital, to bill for the technical component of physician pathology services to provide a copy of this agreement, or other documentation substantiating that an arrangement was in effect between the hospital and the independent laboratory as of this date. The independent laboratory must submit this documentation for each covered hospital that the independent laboratory services.

See Chapter 16 for additional instruction on laboratory services including clinical diagnostic laboratory services.

Physician laboratory and pathology services are limited to:

- Surgical pathology services;

- Specific cytopathology, hematology and blood banking services that have been identified to require performance by a physician and are listed below;

- Clinical consultation services that meet the requirements in subsection D below; and

- Clinical laboratory interpretation services that meet the requirements and which are specifically listed in subsection E below.

B. Surgical Pathology Services

Surgical pathology services include the gross and microscopic examination of organ tissue performed by a physician, except for autopsies, which are not covered by Medicare. Surgical pathology services paid under the physician fee schedule are reported under the following CPT codes:

88300, 88302, 88304, 88305, 88307, 88309, 88311, 88312, 88313, 88314, 88318, 88319, 88321, 88323, 88325, 88329, 88331, 88332, 88342, 88346, 88347, 88348, 88349, 88355, 88356, 88358, 88361, 88362, 88365, 88380.

Depending upon circumstances and the billing entity, the carriers may pay professional component, technical component or both.

C. Specific Hematology, Cytopathology and Blood Banking Services

Cytopathology services include the examination of cells from fluids, washings, brushings or smears, but generally excluding hematology. Examining cervical and vaginal smears are the most common service in cytopathology. Cervical and vaginal smears do not require interpretation by a physician unless the results are or appear to be abnormal. In such cases, a physician personally conducts a separate microscopic evaluation to determine the nature of an abnormality. This microscopic evaluation ordinarily does require performance by a physician. When medically necessary and when furnished by a physician, it is paid under the fee schedule.

These codes include 88104, 88106, 88107, 88108, 88112, 88125, 88141, 88160, 88161, 88162, 88172, 88173, 88180, 88182.

For services furnished prior to January 1, 1999, carriers pay separately under the physician fee schedule for the interpretation of an abnormal pap smear furnished to a hospital inpatient by a physician. They must pay under the clinical laboratory fee

schedule for pap smears furnished in all other situations. This policy also applies to screening pap smears requiring a physician interpretation. For services furnished on or after January 1, 1999, carriers allow separate payment for a physician's interpretation of a pap smear to any patient (i.e., hospital or non-hospital) as long as: (1) the laboratory's screening personnel suspect an abnormality; and (2) the physician reviews and interprets the pap smear.

This policy also applies to screening pap smears requiring a physician interpretation and described in the National Coverage Determination Manual and Chapter 18. These services are reported under codes P3000 or P3001.

Physician hematology services include microscopic evaluation of bone marrow aspirations and biopsies. It also includes those limited number of peripheral blood smears which need to be referred to a physician to evaluate the nature of an apparent abnormality identified by the technologist. These codes include 85060, 38220, 85097, and 38221.

Carriers pay the professional component for the interpretation of an abnormal blood smear (code 85060) furnished to a hospital inpatient by a hospital physician or an independent laboratory.

For the other listed hematology codes, payment may be made for the professional component if the service is furnished to a patient by a hospital physician or independent laboratory. In addition, payment may be made for these services furnished to patients by an independent laboratory.

Codes 38220 and 85097 represent professional-only component services and have no technical component values.

Blood banking services of hematologists and pathologists are paid under the physician fee schedule when analyses are performed on donor and/or patient blood to determine compatible donor units for transfusion where cross matching is difficult or where contamination with transmissible disease of donor is suspected.

The blood banking codes are 86077, 86078, and 86079 and represent professional component only services. These codes do not have a technical component.

D. Clinical Consultation Services

Clinical consultations are paid under the physician fee schedule only if they:

Are requested by the patient's attending physician;

Relate to a test result that lies outside the clinically significant normal or expected range in view of the condition of the patient;

Result in a written narrative report included in the patient's medical record; and

Require the exercise of medical judgment by the consultant physician.

Clinical consultations are professional component services only. There is no technical component. The clinical consultation codes are 80500 and 80502.

Routine conversations held between a laboratory director and an attending physician about test orders or results do not qualify as consultations unless all four requirements are

met. Laboratory personnel, including the director, may from time to time contact attending physicians to report test results or to suggest additional testing or be contacted by attending physicians on similar matters. These contacts do not constitute clinical consultations. However, if in the course of such a contact, the attending physician requests a consultation from the pathologist, and if that consultation meets the other criteria and is properly documented, it is paid under the fee schedule.

EXAMPLE: A pathologist telephones a surgeon about a patient's suitability for surgery based on the results of clinical laboratory test results. During the course of their conversation, the surgeon ask the pathologist whether, based on test results, patient history and medical records, the patient is a candidate for surgery. The surgeon's request requires the pathologist to render a medical judgment and provide a consultation. The pathologist follows up his/her oral advice with a written report and the surgeon notes in the patient's medical record that he/she requested a consultation. This consultation is paid under the fee schedule.

In any case, if the information could ordinarily be furnished by a nonphysician laboratory specialist, the service of the physician is not a consultation payable under the fee schedule.

See the Program Integrity Manual for guidelines for related data analysis to identify inappropriate patterns of billing for consultations.

E. Clinical Laboratory Interpretation Services

Only clinical laboratory interpretation services listed below and which meet the criteria in subsections D.1, D.3, and D.4 for clinical consultations and, as a result, are billable under the fee schedule. These services are reported under the clinical laboratory code with modifier 26. These services can be paid under the physician fee schedule if they are furnished to a patient by a hospital pathologist or an independent laboratory. Note that a hospital's standing order policy can be used as a substitute for the individual request by the patient's attending physician. Carriers are not allowed to revise CMS's list to accommodate local medical practice. The CMS periodically reviews this list and adds or deletes clinical laboratory codes as warranted.

Clinical Laboratory Interpretation Services

Code	Definition
83020	Hemoglobin; electrophoresis
83912	Nucleic acid probe, with electrophoresis, with examination and report
84165	Protein, total, serum; electrophoretic fractionation and quantitation
84181	Protein; Western Blot with interpretation and report, blood or other body fluid
84182	Protein; Western Blot, with interpretation and report, blood or other body fluid, immunological probe for band identification; each
85390	Fibrinolysin; screening
85576	Platelet; aggregation (in vitro), any agent
86255	Fluorescent antibody; screen
86256	Fluorescent antibody; titer
86320	Immunoelectrophoresis; serum, each specimen
86325	Immunoelectrophoresis; other fluids (e.g.urine) with concentration, each specimen
86327	Immunoelectrophoresis; crossed (2 dimensional assay)
86334	Immunofixation electrophoresis
87164	Dark field examination, any source (e.g. penile, vaginal, oral, skin); includes specimen collection
87207	Smear, primary source, with interpretation; special stain for inclusion bodies or intracellular parasites (e.g. malaria, kala azar, herpes)
88371	Protein analysis of tissue by Western Blot, with interpretation and report.
88372	Protein analysis of tissue by Western Blot, immunological probe for band identification, each
89060	Crystal identification by light microscopy with or without polarizing lens analysis, any body fluid (except urine)

Pub. 100-4, Chapter 12, Section 70

Payment Conditions for Radiology Services
B3-15022

See chapter 13, for claims processing instructions for radiology.

Pub. 100-4, Chapter 12, Section 80.3

Unusual Travel (CPT Code 99082)
B3-15026

In general, travel has been incorporated in the MPFSDB individual fees and is thus not separately payable. Carriers must pay separately for unusual travel (CPT code 99082) only when the physician submits documentation to demonstrate that the travel was very unusual.

Pub. 100-4, Chapter 12, Section 90.3

Physicians' Services Performed in Ambulatory Surgical Centers (ASC)
B3-2265, B3-2265.4

See Chapter 14, for a description of services that may be billed by an ASC and services separately billed by physicians.

The ASC payment does not include the professional services of the physician. These are billed separately by the physician. Physicians' services include the services of anesthesiologists administering or supervising the administration of anesthesia to ASC patients and the patients' recovery from the anesthesia. The term physicians' services also includes any routine pre- or postoperative services, such as office visits, consultations, diagnostic tests, removal of stitches, changing of dressings, and other services which the individual physician usually performs.

The physician must enter the place of service code (POS) 24 on the claim to show that the procedure was performed in an ASC.

The carrier pays the "facility" fee from the MPFSDB to the physician. The facility fee is for services done in a facility other than the physician's office and is less then the nonfacility fee for services performed in the physician's office.

Pub. 100-4, Chapter 12, Section 100

Teaching Physician Services
Definitions

For purposes of this section, the following definitions apply.

Resident - An individual who participates in an approved graduate medical education (GME) program or a physician who is not in an approved GME program but who is authorized to practice only in a hospital setting. The term includes interns and fellows in GME programs recognized as approved for purposes of direct GME payments made by the FI. Receiving a staff or faculty appointment or participating in a fellowship does not by itself alter the status of "resident". Additionally, this status remains unaffected regardless of whether a hospital includes the physician in its full time equivalency count of residents.

Student - An individual who participates in an accredited educational program (e.g., a medical school) that is not an approved GME program. A student is never considered to be an intern or a resident. Medicare does not pay for any service furnished by a student. See §100.1.1B for a discussion concerning E/M service documentation performed by students.

Teaching Physician - A physician (other than another resident) who involves residents in the care of his or her patients.

Direct Medical and Surgical Services - Services to individual beneficiaries that are either personally furnished by a physician or furnished by a resident under the supervision of a physician in a teaching hospital making the reasonable cost election for physician services furnished in teaching hospitals. All payments for such services are made by the FI for the hospital.

Teaching Hospital - A hospital engaged in an approved GME residency program in medicine, osteopathy, dentistry, or podiatry.

Teaching Setting - Any provider, hospital-based provider, or nonprovider setting in which Medicare payment for the services of residents is made by the FI under the direct graduate medical education payment methodology or freestanding SNF or HHA in which such payments are made on a reasonable cost basis.

Critical or Key Portion - That part (or parts) of a service that the teaching physician determines is (are) a critical or key portion(s). For purposes of this section, these terms are interchangeable.

Documentation - Notes recorded in the patient's medical records by a resident, and/or teaching physician or others as outlined in the specific situations below regarding the service furnished. Documentation may be dictated and typed or hand-written, or computer-generated and typed or handwritten. Documentation must be dated and include a legible signature or identity. Pursuant to 42 CFR 415.172 (b), documentation must identify, at a minimum, the service furnished, the participation of the teaching physician in providing the service, and whether the teaching physician was physically present.

In the context of an electronic medical record, the term 'macro' means a command in a computer or dictation application that automatically generates predetermined text that is not edited by the user.

When using an electronic medical record, it is acceptable for the teaching physician to use a macro as the required personal documentation if the teaching physician adds it personally in a secured (password protected) system. In addition to the teaching physician's macro, either the resident or the teaching physician must provide customized information that is sufficient to support a medical necessity determination. The note in the electronic medical record must sufficiently describe the specific services furnished to the specific patient on the specific date. It is insufficient documentation if both the resident and the teaching physician use macros only.

Physically Present - The teaching physician is located in the same room (or partitioned or curtained area, if the room is subdivided to accommodate multiple patients) as the patient and/or performs a face-to-face service.

Pub. 100-4, Chapter 12, Section 100.1.7

Assistants at Surgery in Teaching Hospitals

A. General

Carriers do not pay for the services of assistants at surgery furnished in a teaching hospital which has a training program related to the medical specialty required for the surgical procedure and has a qualified resident available to perform the service unless the requirements of one of subsections C, D, or E are met. Each teaching hospital has a different situation concerning numbers of residents, qualifications of residents, duties of residents, and types of surgeries performed.

Contact those affected by these instructions to learn the circumstances in individual teaching hospitals. There may be some teaching hospitals in which carriers can apply a presumption about the availability of a qualified resident in a training program related to the medical specialty required for the surgical procedures, but there are other teaching hospitals in which there are often no qualified residents available. This may be due to their involvement in other activities, complexity of the surgery, numbers of residents in the program, or other valid reasons. Carriers process assistant at surgery claims for services furnished in teaching hospitals on the basis of the following certification by the assistant, or through the use of modifier -82 which indicates that a qualified resident surgeon was not available. This certification is for use only when the basis for payment is the unavailability of qualified residents.

I understand that §1842(b)(7)(D) of the Act generally prohibits Medicare physician fee schedule payment for the services of assistants at surgery in teaching hospitals when qualified residents are available to furnish such services. I certify that the services for which payment is claimed were medically necessary and that no qualified resident was available to perform the services. I further understand that these services are subject to post-payment review by the Medicare carrier.

Carriers retain the claim and certification for four years and conduct post-payment reviews as necessary. For example, carriers investigate situations in which it is always certified that there are no qualified residents available, and undertake recovery if warranted.

Assistant at surgery claims denied based on these instructions do not qualify for payment under the limitation on liability provision.

B. Definition

An assistant at surgery is a physician who actively assists the physician in charge of a case in performing a surgical procedure. (Note that a nurse practitioner, physician assistant or clinical nurse specialist who is authorized to provide such services under State law can also serve as an assistant at surgery). The conditions for coverage of such services in teaching hospitals are more restrictive than those in other settings because of the availability of residents who are qualified to perform this type of service.

C. Exceptional Circumstances

Payment may be made for the services of assistants at surgery in teaching hospitals, subject to the special limitation in §20.4.3 notwithstanding the availability of a qualified resident to furnish the services. There may be exceptional medical circumstances (e.g.,

emergency, life-threatening situations such as multiple traumatic injuries) which require immediate treatment. There may be other situations in which the medical staff may find that exceptional medical circumstances justify the services of a physician assistant at surgery even though a qualified resident is available.

D. Physicians Who Do Not Involve Residents in Patient Care

Payment may be made for the services of assistants at surgery in teaching hospitals, subject to the limitations in §20.4.3, above, if the primary surgeon has an across-the-board policy of never involving residents in the preoperative, operative, or postoperative care of his or her patients. Generally, this exception is applied to community physicians who have no involvement in the hospital's GME program. In such situations, payment may be made for reasonable and necessary services on the same basis as would be the case in a nonteaching hospital. However, if the assistant is not a physician primarily engaged in the field of surgery, no payment be made unless either of the criteria of subsection E is met.

E. Multiple Physician Specialties Involved in Surgery

Complex medical procedures, including multistage transplant surgery and coronary bypass, may require a team of physicians. In these situations, each of the physicians performs a unique, discrete function requiring special skills integral to the total procedure. Each physician is engaged in a level of activity different from assisting the surgeon in charge of the case. The special payment limitation in §20.4.3 is not applied. If payment is made on the basis of a single team fee, additional claims are denied. The carrier will determine which procedures performed in the service area require a team approach to surgery. Team surgery is paid for on a "By Report" basis.

The services of physicians of different specialties may be necessary during surgery when each specialist is required to play an active role in the patient's treatment because of the existence of more than one medical condition requiring diverse, specialized medical services. For example, a patient's cardiac condition may require a cardiologist be present to monitor the patient's condition during abdominal surgery. In this type of situation, the physician furnishing the concurrent care is functioning at a different level than that of an assistant at surgery, and payment is made on a regular fee schedule basis.

Pub. 100-4, Chapter 12, Section 100.1.8

Physician Billing in the Teaching Setting

B3-8204, B3-15016

A. Reimbursement to the Hospital

When a hospital is billing the carrier, as opposed to the physician billing the carrier, for covered services, it must bill the carrier on the Form CMS-1500 or equivalent electronic format. It no longer has the option to establish any other type of agreement with the carrier.

B. Carrier Claims

The method by which services performed in a teaching setting must be billed is determined by the manner in which reimbursement is made for such services. For carriers, the shared system suspends claims submitted by a teaching physician, for review.

Pub. 100-4, Chapter 12, Section 110.2

Outpatient Mental Health Limitation

B3-4112, B3-2472.4

The carrier must apply the outpatient mental health limitation to all covered mental health therapeutic services furnished by PAs. The reduction is 62.5 percent applied after the 85 percent.

Refer to §210 below for a complete discussion of the outpatient mental health limitation.

Pub. 100-4, Chapter 12, Section 140

Certified Registered Nurse Anesthetist (CRNA) Services

B3-16003, B3-16003 A, B3-3040.4, B3-4172

Section 9320 of OBRA 1986 provides for payment under a fee schedule to certified registered nurse anesthetists (CRNAs) and anesthesia assistants (AAs). CRNAs and AAs may bill Medicare directly for their services or have payment made to an employer or an entity under which they have a contract. This could be a hospital, physician or ASC. This provision is effective for services rendered on or after January 1, 1989.

Anesthesia services are subject to the usual Part B coinsurance and deductible and when furnished on or after January 1, 1992 by a qualified nurse anesthetist and are paid at the lesser of the actual charge, the physician fee schedule, or the CRNA fee schedule. Payment for CRNA services is made only on an assignment basis.

Pub. 100-4, Chapter 12, Section 140.2

Entity or Individual to Whom CRNA Fee Schedule is Payable

B3-16003.C, B3-4830.A

Payment for the services of a CRNA may be made to the CRNA who furnished the anesthesia services or to a hospital, physician, group practice, or ASC with which the CRNA has an employment or contractual relationship.

Pub. 100-4, Chapter 12, Section 140.3.2

Anesthesia Time and Calculation of Anesthesia Time Units

B3-15018.G

Anesthesia time means the time during which a CRNA is present with the patient. It starts when the CRNA begins to prepare the patient for anesthesia services in the operating room or an equivalent area and ends when the CRNA is no longer furnishing anesthesia services to the patient, that is, when the patient may be placed safely under postoperative care. Anesthesia time is a continuous time period from the start of anesthesia to the end of an anesthesia service. In counting anesthesia time for services furnished on or after January 1, 2000, the CRNA can add blocks of time around an interruption in anesthesia time as long as the CRNA is furnishing continuous anesthesia care within the time periods around the interruption.

Pub. 100-4, Chapter 12, Section 150

Clinical Social Worker (CSW) Services

B3-2152, B3-17000

See Medicare Benefit Policy Manual, Chapter 15, for coverage requirements.

Assignment of benefits is required.

Payment is at 75 percent of the physician fee schedule.

CSWs are identified on the provider file by specialty code 80 and provider type 56.

Medicare applies the outpatient mental health limitation to all covered therapeutic services furnished by qualified CSWs. Refer to §210, below, for a discussion of the outpatient mental health limitation. The modifier "AJ" must be applied on CSN services.

Pub. 100-4, Chapter 12, Section 160

Independent Psychologist Services

B3-2150, B3-2070.2

See the Medicare Benefit Policy Manual, Chapter 15, for coverage requirements.

There are a number of types of psychologists. Educational psychologists engage in identifying and treating education-related issues. In contrast, counseling psychologists provide services that include a broader realm including phobias, familial issues, etc. Psychometrists are psychologists who have been trained to administer and interpret tests. However, clinical psychologists are defined as a provider of diagnostic and therapeutic services. Because of the differences in services provided, services provided by psychologists who do not provide clinical services are subject to different billing guidelines. One service often provided by nonclinical psychologist is diagnostic testing.

NOTE: Diagnostic psychological testing services performed by persons who meet these requirements are covered as other diagnostic tests. When, however, the psychologist is not practicing independently, but is on the staff of an institution, agency, or clinic, that entity bills for the diagnostic services.

Expenses for such testing are not subject to the payment limitation on treatment for mental, psychoneurotic, and personality disorders. Independent psychologists are not required by law to accept assignment when performing psychological tests. However, regardless of whether the psychologist accepts assignment, he or she must report on the claim form the name and address of the physician who ordered the test.

Pub. 100-4, Chapter 12, Section 160.1

Payment

Diagnostic testing services are not subject to the outpatient mental health limitation. Refer to §210, below, for a discussion of the outpatient mental health limitation.

The diagnostic testing services performed by a psychologist (who is not a clinical psychologist) practicing independently of an institution, agency, or physician's office are covered as other diagnostic tests if a physician orders such testing. Medicare covers this type of testing as an outpatient service if furnished by any psychologist who is licensed or certified to practice psychology in the State or jurisdiction where he or she is furnishing services or, if the jurisdiction does not issue licenses, if provided by any practicing psychologist. (It is CMS' understanding that all States, the District of Columbia, and Puerto Rico license psychologists, but that some trust territories do not. Examples of psychologists, other than clinical psychologists, whose services are covered under this provision include, but are not limited to, educational psychologists and counseling psychologists.)

To determine whether the diagnostic psychological testing services of a particular independent psychologist are covered under Part B in States which have statutory licensure or certification, carriers must secure from the appropriate State agency a current listing of psychologists holding the required credentials. In States or territories which lack statutory licensing and certification, carriers must check individual qualifications as claims are submitted. Possible reference sources are the national directory of membership of the American Psychological Association, which provides data about the educational background of individuals and indicates which members are board-certified, and records and directories of the State or territorial psychological association. If qualification is dependent on a doctoral degree from a currently accredited program, carriers must verify the date of accreditation of the school involved, since such accreditation is not retroactive. If the reference sources listed above do not provide enough information (e.g., the psychologist is not a member of the association), carriers must contact the psychologist personally for the required information. Carriers may wish to maintain a continuing list of psychologists whose qualifications have been verified.

Medicare excludes expenses for diagnostic testing from the payment limitation on treatment for mental/psychoneurotic/personality disorders.

Carriers must identify the independent psychologist's choice whether or not to accept assignment when performing psychological tests.

Carriers must accept an independent psychologist claim only if the psychologist reports the name/UPIN of the physician who ordered a test.

Carriers pay nonparticipating independent psychologists at 95 percent of the physician fee schedule allowed amount. Carriers pay participating independent psychologists at 100 percent of the physician fee schedule allowed amount.

Independent psychologists are identified on the provider file by specialty code 62 and provider type 35.

Pub. 100-4, Chapter 12, Section 170

Clinical Psychologist Services

B3-2150

See Medicare Benefit Policy Manual, Chapter 15, for general coverage requirements.

Direct payment may be made under Part B for professional services. However, services furnished incident to the professional services of CPs to hospital patients remain bundled. Therefore, payment must continue to be made to the hospital (by the FI) for such "incident to" services.

Pub. 100-4, Chapter 12, Section 170.1

Payment

B3-2150, B3-17001.1

All covered therapeutic services furnished by qualified CPs are subject to the outpatient mental health services limitation (i.e., only 62 1/2 percent of expenses for these services are considered incurred expenses for Medicare purposes). The limitation does not apply to diagnostic services. Refer to §210 below for a discussion of the outpatient mental health limitation.

Payment for the services of CPs is made on the basis of a fee schedule or the actual charge, whichever is less, and only on the basis of assignment.

CPs are identified by specialty code 68 and provider type 27. Modifier "AH" is required on CP services.

Pub. 100-4, Chapter 12, Section 190

Medicare Payment for Telehealth Services

A3-3497, A3-3660.2, B3-4159, B3-15516

Pub. 100-4, Chapter 12, Section 190.7

Contractor Editing of Telehealth Claims

Medicare telehealth services (as listed in section 190.3) are billed with either the "GT" or "GQ" modifier. The contractor shall approve covered telehealth services if the physician or practitioner is licensed under State law to provide the service. Contractors must familiarize themselves with licensure provisions of States for which they process claims and disallow telehealth services furnished by physicians or practitioners who are not authorized to furnish the applicable telehealth service under State law. For example, if a nurse practitioner is not licensed to provide individual psychotherapy under State law, he or she would not be permitted to receive payment for individual psychotherapy under Medicare. The contractor shall install edits to ensure that only properly licensed physicians and practitioners are paid for covered telehealth services.

If a contractor receives claims for professional telehealth services coded with the "GQ" modifier (representing "via asynchronous telecommunications system"), it shall approve/pay for these services only if the physician or practitioner is affiliated with a Federal telemedicine demonstration conducted in Alaska or Hawaii. The contractor may require the physician or practitioner at the distant site to document his or her participation in a Federal telemedicine demonstration program conducted in Alaska or Hawaii prior to paying for telehealth services provided via asynchronous, store and forward technologies.

If a contractor denies telehealth services because the physician or practitioner may not bill for them, the contractor uses MSN message 21.18: "This item or service is not covered when performed or ordered by this practitioner." The contractor uses remittance advice message 52 when denying the claim based upon MSN message 21.18.

If a service is billed with one of the telehealth modifiers and the procedure code is not designated as a covered telehealth service, the contractor denies the service using MSN message 9.4: "This item or service was denied because information required to make payment was incorrect." The remittance advice message depends on what is incorrect, e.g., B18 if procedure code or modifier is incorrect, 125 for submission billing errors, 4-12 for difference inconsistencies. The contractor uses B18 as the explanation for the denial of the claim.

The only claims from institutional facilities that FIs shall pay for telehealth services at the distant site, except for MNT services, are for physician or practitioner services when the distant site is located in a CAH that has elected Method II, and the physician or practitioner has reassigned his/her benefits to the CAH. The CAH bills its regular FI for the professional services provided at the distant site via a telecommunications system, in

any of the revenue codes 096x, 097x or 098x. All requirements for billing distant site telehealth services apply.

Claims from hospitals or CAHs for MNT services are submitted to the hospital's or CAH's regular FI. Payment is based on the non-facility amount on the Medicare Physician Fee Schedule for the particular HCPCS codes.

Pub. 100-4, Chapter 12, Section 200

Allergy Testing and Immunotherapy

B3-15050

A. Allergy Testing

The MPFSDB fee amounts for allergy testing services billed under codes 95004-95078 are established for single tests. Therefore, the number of tests must be shown on the claim.

EXAMPLE: If a physician performs 25 percutaneous tests (scratch, puncture, or prick) with allergenic extract, the physician must bill code 95004 and specify 25 in the units field of Form CMS-1500 (paper claims or electronic format). To compute payment, the Medicare carrier multiplies the payment for one test (i.e., the payment listed in the fee schedule) by the quantity listed in the units field.

B. Allergy Immunotherapy

For services rendered on or after January 1, 1995, all antigen/allergy immunotherapy services are paid for under the Medicare physician fee schedule. Prior to that date, only the antigen injection services, i.e., only codes 95115 and 95117, were paid for under the fee schedule. Codes representing antigens and their preparation and single codes representing both the antigens and their injection were paid for under the Medicare reasonable charge system. A legislative change brought all of these services under the fee schedule at the beginning of 1995 and the following policies are effective as of January 1, 1995:

1. CPT codes 95120 through 95134 are not valid for Medicare. Codes 95120 through 95134 represent complete services, i.e., services that include both the injection service as well as the antigen and its preparation.

2. Separate coding for injection only codes (i.e., codes 95115 and 95117) and/or the codes representing antigens and their preparation (i.e., codes 95144 through 95170) must be used.

If both services are provided both codes are billed.

This includes allergists who provide both services through the use of treatment boards.

3. If a physician bills both an injection code plus either codes 95165 or 95144, carriers pay the appropriate injection code (i.e., code 95115 or code 95117) plus the code 95165 rate. When a provider bills for codes 95115 or 95117 plus code 95144, carriers change 95144 to 95165 and pay accordingly. Code 95144 (single dose vials of antigen) should be billed only if the physician providing the antigen is providing it to be injected by some other entity. Single dose vials, which

should be used only as a means of insuring proper dosage amounts for injections, are more costly than multiple dose vials (i.e., code 95165) and therefore their payment rate is higher. Allergists who prepare antigens are assumed to be able to administer proper doses from the less costly multiple dose vials. Thus, regardless of whether they use or bill for single or multiple dose vials at the same time that they are billing for an injection service, they are paid at the multiple dose vial rate.

4. The fee schedule amounts for the antigen codes (95144 through 95170) are for a single dose. When billing those codes, physicians are to specify the number of doses provided. When making payment, carriers multiply the fee schedule amount by the number of doses specified in the units field.

5. If a patient's doses are adjusted, e.g., because of patient reaction, and the antigen provided is actually more or fewer doses than originally anticipated, the physician is to make no change in the number of doses for which he or she bills. The number of doses anticipated at the time of the antigen preparation is the number of doses to be billed. This is consistent with the notes on page 30 of the Spring 1994 issue of the American Medical Association's CPT Assistant. Those notes indicate that the antigen codes mean that the physician is to identify the number of doses "prospectively planned to be provided." The physician is to "identify the number of doses scheduled when the vial is provided." This means that in cases where the patient actually gets more doses than originally anticipated (because dose amounts were decreased during treatment)

and in cases where the patient gets fewer doses (because dose amounts were increased), no change is to be made in the billing. In the first case, carriers are not to pay more because the number of doses provided in the original vial(s) increased. In the second case, carriers are not to seek recoupment (if carriers have already made payment) because the number of doses is less than originally planned. This is the case for both venom and nonvenom antigen codes.

6. Venom Doses and Catch-Up Billing - Venom doses are prepared in separate vials and not mixed together - except in the case of the three vespid mix (white and yellow hornets and yellow jackets). A dose of code 95146 (the two-venom code) means getting some of two venoms. Similarly, a dose of code 95147 means getting some of three venoms; a dose of code 95148 means getting some of four venoms; and a dose of code 95149 means getting some of five venoms. Some amount of each of the venoms must be provided. Questions arise when the administration of these venoms does not remain synchronized because of dosage adjustments due to patient reaction. For example, a physician prepares ten doses of code 95148 (the four venom code) in two vials - one containing 10 doses of three vespid mix and another containing 10 doses of wasp venom. Because of dose adjustment, the three vespid mix doses last longer, i.e., they last for 15 doses. Consequently, questions arise regarding the amount of "replacement" wasp venom antigen that should be prepared and how it should be billed. Medicare pricing amounts have savings built into the use of the higher venom codes. Therefore, if a patient is in two venom, three venom, four venom or five venom therapy, the carrier objective is to pay at the highest venom level possible. This means that, to the greatest

extent possible, code 95146 is to be billed for a patient in two venom therapy, code 95147 is to be billed for a patient in three venom therapy, code 95148 is to be billed for a patient in four venom therapy, and code 95149 is to be billed for a patient in five venom therapy. Thus, physicians are to be instructed that the venom antigen preparation, after dose adjustment, must be done in a manner that, as soon as possible, synchronizes the preparation back to the highest venom code possible. In the above example, the physician should prepare and bill for only 5 doses of "replacement" wasp venom - billing five doses of code 95145 (the one venom code). This will permit the physician to get back to preparing the four venoms at one time and therefore billing the doses of the "cheaper" four venom code. Use of a code below the venom treatment number for the particular patient should occur only for the purpose of "catching up."

7. Code 95165 Doses. - Code 95165 represents preparation of vials of non-venom antigens. As in the case of venoms, some non-venom antigens cannot be mixed together, i.e., they must be prepared in separate vials. An example of this is mold and pollen. Therefore, some patients will be injected at one time from one vial — containing in one mixture all of the appropriate antigens — while other patients will be injected at one time from more than one vial. In establishing the practice expense component for mixing a multidose vial of antigens, we observed that the most common practice was to prepare a 10 cc vial; we also observed that the most common use was to remove aliquots with a volume of 1 cc. Our PE computations were based on those facts. Therefore, a physician's removing 10 1cc aliquot doses captures the entire PE component for the service.

This does not mean that the physician must remove 1 cc aliquot doses from a multidose. It means that the practice expenses payable for the preparation of a 10cc vial remain the same irrespective of the size or number of aliquots removed from the vial. Therefore, a physician may not bill this vial preparation code for more than 10 doses per vial; paying more than 10 doses per multidose vial would significantly overpay the practice expense component attributable to this service. (Note that this code does not include the injection of antigen(s); injection of antigen(s) is separately billable.)

When a multidose vial contains less than 10cc, physicians should bill Medicare for the number of 1 cc aliquots that may be removed from the vial. That is, a physician may bill Medicare up to a maximum of 10 doses per multidose vial, but should bill Medicare for fewer than 10 doses per vial when there is less than 10cc in the vial.

If it is medically necessary, physicians may bill Medicare for preparation of more than one multidose vial.

EXAMPLES:

(1) If a 10cc multidose vial is filled to 6cc with antigen, the physician may bill Medicare for 6 doses since six 1cc aliquots may be removed from the vial.

If a 5cc multidose vial is filled completely, the physician may bill Medicare for 5 doses for this vial.

(3) If a physician removes 2 cc aliquots from a 10cc multidose vial for a total of 20 doses from one vial, he/she may only bill Medicare for 10 doses. Billing for more

than 10 doses would mean that Medicare is overpaying for the practice expense of making the vial.

(4) If a physician prepares two 10cc multidose vials, he/she may bill Medicare for 20 doses. However, he/she may remove aliquots of any amount from those vials. For example, the physician may remove 2 aliquots from one vial, and 1cc aliquots from the other vial, but may bill no more than a total of 20 doses.

(5) If a physician prepares a 20cc multidose vial, he/she may bill Medicare for 20 doses, since the practice expense is calculated based on the physician's removing 1cc aliquots from a vial. If a physician removes 2cc aliquots from this vial, thus getting only 10 doses, he/she may nonetheless bill Medicare for 20 doses because the PE for 20 doses reflects the actual practice expense of preparing the vial.

(6) If a physician prepares a 5cc multidose vial, he may bill Medicare for 5 doses, based on the way that the practice expense component is calculated. However, if the physician removes ten 2 cc aliquots from the vial, he/she may still bill only 5 doses because the practice expense of preparing the vial is the same, without regard to the number of additional doses that are removed from the vial.

C. Allergy Shots and Visit Services on the Same Day

At the outset of the physician fee schedule, the question was posed as to whether visits should be billed on the same day as an allergy injection (CPT codes 95115-95117), since these codes

have status indicators of A rather than T. Visits should not be billed with allergy injection services 95115 or 95117 unless the visit represents another separately identifiable service. This language parallels CPT editorial language that accompanies the allergen immunotherapy codes, which include codes 9515 and 95117. Prior to January 1, 1995, you appeared to be enforcing this policy through three (3) different means:

- Advising physician to use modifier 25 with the visit service;

- Denying payment for the visit unless documentation has been provided; and

- Paying for both the visit and the allergy shot if both are billed for.

For services rendered on or after January 1, 1995, you are to enforce the requirement that visits not be billed and paid for on the same day as an allergy injection through the following means. Effective for services rendered on or after that date, the global surgery policies will apply to all codes in the allergen immunotherapy series, including the allergy shot codes 95115 and 95117. To accomplish this, CMS changed the global surgery indicator for allergen immunotherapy codes from XXX, which meant that the global surgery concept did not apply to those codes, to 000, which means that the global surgery concept applies, but that there are no days in the postoperative global period. Now that the global surgery policies apply to these services, you are to rely on the use of modifier 25 as the only means through which you can make payment for visit services provided on the same day as allergen immunotherapy services. In order for a physician to receive payment for a visit service provided on the same day that the physician also provides a service in the allergen immunotherapy series (i.e., any service in the series from 95115 through 95199), the physician is to bill a modifier 25 with the visit code,

indicating that the patient's condition required a significant, separately identifiable visit service above and beyond the allergen immunotherapy service provided.

D. Reasonable Supply of Antigens

See CMS Manual System, Internet Only Manual, Medicare Benefits Policy Manual, CMS Pub. 100-02 Chapter 15, section 50.4.4, regarding the coverage of antigens, including what constitutes a reasonable supply of antigens.

Pub. 100-4, Chapter 12, Section 210

Outpatient Mental Health Limitation
B3-2470

Regardless of the actual expenses a beneficiary incurs for treatment of mental, psychoneurotic, and personality disorders while the beneficiary is not an inpatient of a hospital at the time such expenses are incurred, the amount of those expenses that may be recognized for Part B deductible and payment purposes is limited to 62.5 percent of the Medicare allowed amount for those services. This limitation is called the outpatient mental health treatment limitation. Expenses for diagnostic services (e.g., psychiatric testing and evaluation to diagnose the patient's illness) are not subject to this limitation. This limitation applies only to therapeutic services and to services performed to evaluate the progress of a course of treatment for a diagnosed condition.

Pub. 100-4, Chapter 13, Section 10

9-CM Coding for Diagnostic Tests
B3-15021.1

The ICD-9-CM Coding Guidelines for Outpatient Services (hospital-based and physician office) have instructed physicians to report diagnoses based on test results. Instructions and examples for coding specialists, contractors, physicians, hospitals, and other health care providers to use in determining the use of ICD-9-CM codes for coding diagnostic test results is found in Chapter 23.

Pub. 100-4, Chapter 13, Section 20

Payment Conditions for Radiology Services
B3-15022

Pub. 100-4, Chapter 13, Section 30

Computerized Axial Tomography (CT) Procedures
Carriers do not reduce or deny payment for medically necessary multiple CT scans of different areas of the body that are performed on the same day.

The TC RVUs for CT procedures that specify "with contrast" include payment for high osmolar contrast media. When separate payment is made for low osmolar contrast media under the conditions set forth in §30.1.1, reduce payment for the contrast media as set forth in §30.1.2.

Pub. 100-4, Chapter 13, Section 40

Magnetic Resonance Imaging (MRI) Procedures
Carriers do not make additional payments for three or more MRI sequences. The RVUs reflect payment levels for two sequences.

The TC RVUs for MRI procedures that specify "with contrast" include payment for paramagnetic contrast media. Carriers do not make separate payment under code A4647.

A diagnostic technique has been developed under which an MRI of the brain or spine is first performed without contrast material, then another MRI is performed with a standard (0.1mmol/kg) dose of contrast material, and, based on the need to achieve a better image, a third MRI is performed with an additional double dosage (0.2mmol/kg) of contrast material. When the high-dose contrast technique is utilized, carriers:

- Do not pay separately for the contrast material used in the second MRI procedure;

- Pay for the contrast material given for the third MRI procedure through supply code A4643 when billed with CPT codes 70553, 72156, 72157, and 72158;

- Do not pay for the third MRI procedure. For example, in the case of an MRI of the brain, if CPT code 70553 (without contrast material, followed by with contrast material(s) and further sequences) is billed, make no payment for CPT code 70551 (without contrast material(s)), the additional procedure given for the purpose of administering the double dosage, furnished during the same session. Medicare does not pay for the third procedure (as distinguished from the contrast material) because the CPT definition of code 70553 includes all further sequences; and

- Do not apply the payment criteria for low osmolar contrast media in §30.1.2 to billings for code A4643.

Pub. 100-4, Chapter 13, Section 40.1

Magnetic Resonance Angiography

R1 795B3, B3-4602, R1 883A3, A3-3665

Pub. 100-4, Chapter 13, Section 40.1.1

Magnetic Resonance Angiography Coverage Summary

Section 1861(s)(2)(C) of the Act provides for coverage of diagnostic testing. Coverage of magnetic resonance angiography (MRA) of the head and neck, and MRA of the peripheral vessels of the lower extremities is limited as described in the Medicare National Coverage Determinations Manual. This instruction has been revised as of July 1, 2003, based on a determination that coverage is reasonable and necessary in additional circumstances. Under that instruction, MRA is generally covered only to the extent that it is used as a substitute for contrast angiography, except to the extent that there are documented circumstances consistent with that instruction that demonstrate the medical necessity of both tests. There is no coverage of MRA outside of the indications and circumstances described in that instruction.

Because the status codes for HCPCS codes 71555, 71555-TC, 71555-26, 74185, 74185-TC, and 74185-26 were changed in the MPFSDB from N to R on April 1, 1998, any MRA claims with those HCPCS codes with dates of service between April 1, 1998, and June 30, 1999, are to be processed according to the contractor's discretionary authority to determine payment in the absence of national policy.

Pub. 100-4, Chapter 13, Section 60

General Information

Positron emission tomography (PET) is a noninvasive imaging procedure that assesses perfusion and the level of metabolic activity in various organ systems of the human body. A positron camera (tomograph) is used to produce cross-sectional tomographic images which are obtained by detecting radioactivity from a radioactive tracer substance (radiopharmaceutical) that emits a radioactive tracer substance (radiopharmaceutical FDG) such as 2 — [F-18] flouro-D-glucose FDG, that is administered intravenously to the patient.

The Medicare National Coverage Determinations (NCD) Manual, Chapter 1, §220.6, contains additional coverage instructions to indicate the conditions under which a PET scan is performed.

A. Definitions

For all uses of PET, excluding Rubidium 82 for perfusion of the heart, myocardial viability and refractory seizures, the following definitions apply:

- Diagnosis: PET is covered only in clinical situations in which the PET results may assist in avoiding an invasive diagnostic procedure, or in which the PET results may assist in determining the optimal anatomical location to perform an invasive diagnostic procedure. In general, for most solid tumors, a tissue diagnosis is made prior to the performance of PET scanning. PET scans following a tissue diagnosis are generally performed for the purpose of staging, rather than diagnosis. Therefore, the use of PET in the diagnosis of lymphoma, esophageal and colorectal cancers, as well as in melanoma, should be rare. PET is not covered for other diagnostic uses, and is not covered for screening (testing of patients without specific signs and symptoms of disease).

- Staging: PET is covered in clinical situations in which (1) (a) the stage of the cancer remains in doubt after completion of a standard diagnostic workup, including conventional imaging (computed tomography, magnetic resonance imaging, or ultrasound) or, (b) the use of PET would also be considered reasonable and necessary if it could potentially replace one or more conventional imaging studies when it is expected that conventional study information is insufficient for the clinical management of the patient and, (2) clinical management of the patient would differ depending on the stage of the cancer identified.

- Restaging: PET will be covered for restaging: (1) after the completion of treatment for the purpose of detecting residual disease, (2) for detecting suspected recurrence or metastasis, (3) to determine the extent of a known recurrence, or (4) if it could potentially replace one or more conventional imaging studies when it is expected that conventional study information is to determine the extent of a known recurrence, or if study information is insufficient for the clinical management of the patient. Restaging applies to testing after a course of treatment is completed and is covered subject to the conditions above.

- Monitoring: Use of PET to monitor tumor response to treatment during the planned course of therapy (i.e., when a change in therapy is anticipated).

B. Limitations

For staging and restaging: PET is covered in either/or both of the following circumstances:

- The stage of the cancer remains in doubt after completion of a standard diagnostic workup, including conventional imaging (computed tomography, magnetic resonance imaging, or ultrasound); and/or

- The clinical management of the patient would differ depending on the stage of the cancer identified. PET will be covered for restaging after the completion of treatment for the purpose of detecting residual disease, for detecting suspected recurrence, or to determine the extent of a known recurrence. Use of PET would also be considered reasonable and necessary if it could potentially replace one or more conventional imaging

studies when it is expected that conventional study information is insufficient for the clinical management of the patient.

The PET is not covered for other diagnostic uses, and is not covered for screening (testing of patients without specific symptoms). Use of PET to monitor tumor response during the planned course of therapy (i.e. when no change in therapy is being contemplated) is not covered.

Pub. 100-4, Chapter 13, Section 60.1

Billing Instructions

A. Billing and Payment Instructions or Responsibilities for Carriers

Claims for PET scan services must be billed on Form-CMS 1500 or the electronic equivalent with the appropriate HCPCS or CPT code and diagnosis codes to the local carrier. Effective for claims received on or after July 1, 2001, PET modifiers were discontinued and are no longer a claims processing requirement for PET scan claims. Therefore, July 1, 2001, and after the MSN messages regarding the use of PET modifiers can be discontinued. The type of service (TOS) for the new PET scan procedure codes is TOS 4, Diagnostic Radiology. Payment is based on the Medicare Physician Fee Schedule.

B. Billing and Payment Instructions or Responsibilities for FIs

Claims for PET scan procedures must be billed to the FI on Form CMS-1450 (UB-92) or the electronic equivalent with the appropriate diagnosis and HCPCS "G" code or CPT code to indicate the conditions under which a PET scan was done. These codes represent the technical component costs associated with these procedures when furnished to hospital and SNF outpatients. They are paid as follows:

- under OPPS for hospitals subject to OPPS

- under current payment methodologies for hospitals not subject to OPPS

- on a reasonable cost basis for critical access hospitals.

- on a reasonable cost basis for skilled nursing facilities.

Institutional providers bill these codes under Revenue Code 0404 (PET Scan).

Medicare contractors shall pay claims submitted for services provided by a critical access hospital (CAH) as follows: Method I technical services are paid at 101% of reasonable cost; Method II technical services are paid at 101% of reasonable cost, and professional services are paid at 115% of the Medicare Physician Fee Schedule Data Base.

C. Frequency

In the absence of national frequency limitations, for all indications covered on and after July 1, 2001, contractors can, if necessary, develop frequency limitations on any or all covered PET scan services.

D. Post-Payment Review for PET Scans

As with any claim, but particularly in view of the limitations on this coverage, Medicare may decide to conduct post-payment reviews to determine that the use of PET scans is consistent with coverage instructions. Pet scanning facilities must keep patient record information on file for each Medicare patient for whom a PET scan claim is made. These medical records can be used in any post-payment reviews and must include the information necessary to substantiate the need for the PET scan. These records must include standard information (e.g., age, sex, and height) along with sufficient patient histories to allow determination that the steps required in the coverage instructions were followed. Such information must include, but is not limited to, the date, place and results of previous diagnostic tests (e.g., cytopathology and surgical pathology reports, CT), as well as the results and reports of the PET scan(s) performed at the center. If available, such records should include the prognosis derived from the PET scan, together with information regarding the physician or institution to which the patient proceeded following the scan for treatment or evaluation. The ordering physician is responsible for forwarding appropriate clinical data to the PET scan facility.

Effective for claims received on or after July 1, 2001, CMS no longer requires paper documentation to be submitted up front with PET scan claims. Contractors shall be aware and advise providers of the specific documentation requirements for PET scans for dementia and neurodegenerative diseases. This information is outlined in section 60.12. Documentation requirements such as physician referral and medical necessity determination are to be maintained by the provider as part of the beneficiary's medical record. This information must be made available to the carrier or FI upon request of additional documentation to determine appropriate payment of an individual claim.

Pub. 100-4, Chapter 13, Section 60.2

Use of Gamma Cameras and Full Ring and Partial Ring PET Scanners for PET Scans

See the Medicare NCD Manual, Section 220.6, concerning 2-[F-18] Fluoro-D-Glucose (FDG) PET scanners and details about coverage.

On July 1, 2001, HCPCS codes G0210 - G0230 were added to allow billing for all currently covered indications for FDG PET. Although the codes do not indicate the type

of PET scanner, these codes were used until January 1, 2002, by providers to bill for services in a manner consistent with the coverage policy.

Effective January 1, 2002, HCPCS codes G0210 — G0230 were updated with new descriptors to properly reflect the type of PET scanner used. In addition, four new HCPCS codes became effective for dates of service on and after January 1, 2002, (G0231, G0232, G0233, G0234) for covered conditions that may be billed if a gamma camera is used for the PET scan. For services performed from January 1, 2002, through January 27, 2005, providers should bill using the revised HCPCS codes G0210 - G0234. Beginning January 28, 2005 providers should bill using the appropriate CPT code.

Pub. 100-4, Chapter 13, Section 60.3

PET Scan Qualifying Conditions and HCPCS Code Chart

Below is a summary of all covered PET scan conditions, with effective dates.

NOTE: The G codes below except those a # can be used to bill for PET Scan services through January 27, 2005. Effective for dates of service on or after January 28, 2005, providers must bill for PET Scan services using the appropriate CPT codes. See section 60.3.1. The G codes with a # can continue to be used for billing after January 28, 2005 and these remain non-covered by Medicare. (NOTE: PET Scanners must be FDA-approved.)

Conditions	Coverage Effective Date	HCPCS/CPT
Myocardial perfusion imaging (following previous PET G0030-G0047) single study, rest or stress (exercise and/or pharmacologic)	3/14/95	G0030
Myocardial perfusion imaging (following previous PET G0030-G0047) multiple studies, rest or stress (exercise and/or pharmacologic)	3/14/95	G0031
Myocardial perfusion imaging (following rest SPECT, 78464); single study, rest or stress (exercise and/or pharmacologic)	3/14/95	G0032
Myocardial perfusion imaging (following rest SPECT 78464); multiple studies, rest or stress (exercise and/or pharmacologic)	3/14/95	G0033
Myocardial perfusion (following stress SPECT 78465); single study, rest or stress (exercise and/or pharmacologic)	3/14/95	G0034
Myocardial Perfusion Imaging (following stress SPECT 78465); multiple studies, rest or stress (exercise and/or pharmacologic)	3/14/95	G0035
Myocardial Perfusion Imaging (following coronary angiography 93510-93529); single study, rest or stress (exercise and/or pharmacologic)	3/14/95	G0036
Myocardial Perfusion Imaging, (following coronary angiography), 93510-93529); multiple studies, rest or stress (exercise and/or pharmacologic)	3/14/95	G0037
Myocardial Perfusion Imaging (following stress planar myocardial perfusion, 78460); single study, rest or stress (exercise and/or pharmacologic)	3/14/95	G0038
Myocardial Perfusion Imaging (following stress planar myocardial perfusion, 78460); multiple studies, rest or stress (exercise and/or pharmacologic)	3/14/95	G0039
Myocardial Perfusion Imaging (following stress echocardiogram 93350); single study, rest or stress (exercise and/or pharmacologic)	3/14/95	G0040
Myocardial Perfusion Imaging (following stress echocardiogram, 93350); multiple studies, rest or stress (exercise and/or pharmacologic)	3/14/95	G0041
Myocardial Perfusion Imaging (following stress nuclear ventriculogram 78481 or 78483); single study, rest or stress (exercise and/or pharmacologic)	3/14/95	G0042
Myocardial Perfusion Imaging (following stress nuclear ventriculogram 78481 or 78483); multiple studies, rest or stress (exercise and/or pharmacologic)	3/14/95	G0043
Myocardial Perfusion Imaging (following stress ECG, 93000); single study, rest or stress (exercise and/or pharmacologic)	3/14/95	G0044
Myocardial perfusion (following stress ECG, 93000), multiple studies; rest or stress (exercise and/or pharmacologic)	3/14/95	G0045
Myocardial perfusion (following stress ECG, 93015), single study; rest or stress (exercise and/or pharmacologic)	3/14/95	G0046
Myocardial perfusion (following stress ECG, 93015); multiple studies, rest or stress (exercise and/or pharmacologic)	3/14/95	G0047

Conditions	Coverage Effective Date	HCPCS/CPT
PET imaging regional or whole body; single pulmonary nodule	1/1/98	G0125
Lung cancer, non-small cell (PET imaging whole body) Diagnosis, Initial Staging, Restaging	7/1/01	G0210, G0211, G0212
Colorectal cancer (PET imaging whole body) Diagnosis, Initial Staging, Restaging	7/1/01	G0213, G0214, G0215
Melanoma (PET imaging whole body) Diagnosis, Initial Staging, Restaging	7/1/01	G0216, G0217, G0218
Melanoma for non-covered indications	7/1/01	#G0219
Lymphoma (PET imaging whole body) Diagnosis, Initial Staging, Restaging	7/1/01	G0220, G0221, G0222
Head and neck cancer; excluding thyroid and CNS cancers (PET imaging whole body or regional) Diagnosis, Initial Staging, Restaging	7/1/01	G0223, G0224, G0225
Esophageal cancer (PET imaging whole body) Diagnosis, Initial Staging, Restaging	7/1/01	G0226, G0227, G0228
Metabolic brain imaging for pre-surgical evaluation of refractory seizures	7/1/01	G0229
Metabolic assessment for myocardial viability following inconclusive SPECT study	7/1/01	G0230
Recurrence of colorectal or colorectal metastatic cancer (PET whole body, gamma cameras only)	1/1/02	G0231
Staging and characterization of lymphoma (PET whole body, gamma cameras only)	1/1/02	G0232
Recurrence of melanoma or melanoma metastatic cancer (PET whole body, gamma cameras only)	1/1/02	G0233
Regional or whole body, for solitary pulmonary nodule following CT, or for initial staging of non-small cell lung cancer (gamma cameras only)	1/1/02	G0234
Non-Covered Service PET imaging, any site not otherwise specified	1/28/05	#G0235
Non-Covered Service Initial diagnosis of breast cancer and/or surgical planning for breast cancer (e.g., initial staging of axillary lymph nodes), not covered (full- and partial-ring PET scanners only)	10/1/02	#G0252
Breast cancer, staging/restaging of local regional recurrence or distant metastases, i.e., staging/restaging after or prior to course of treatment (full- and partial-ring PET scanners only)	10/1/02	G0253
Breast cancer, evaluation of responses to treatment, performed during course of treatment (full- and partial-ring PET scanners only)	10/1/02	G0254
Myocardial imaging, positron emission tomography (PET), metabolic evaluation)	10/1/02	78459
Restaging or previously treated thyroid cancer of follicular cell origin following negative I-131 whole body scan (full- and partial-ring PET scanner only)	10/1/03	G0296
Tracer Rubidium**82 (Supply of Radiopharmaceutical Diagnostic Imaging Agent) (This is only billed through Outpatient Perspective Payment System, OPPS.) (Carriers must use HCPCS Code A4641).	10/1/03	Q3000
Supply of Radiopharmaceutical Diagnostic Imaging Agent, Ammonia N-13***	01/1/04	A9526
PET imaging, brain imaging for the differential diagnosis of Alzheimer's disease with aberrant features vs. fronto-temporal dementia	09/15/04	Appropriate CPT Code from section 60.3.1
PET Cervical Cancer Staging as adjunct to conventional imaging, other staging, diagnosis, restaging, monitoring	1/28/05	Appropriate CPT Code from section 60.3.1

NOTE: Carriers must report A4641 for the tracer Rubidium 82 when used with PET scan codes G0030 through G0047 for services performed on or before January 27, 2005

NOTE: Not FDG PET

NOTE: For dates of service October 1, 2003, through December 31, 2003, use temporary code Q4078 for billing this radiopharmaceutical.

Pub. 100-4, Chapter 13, Section 60.3.1

Appropriate CPT Codes Effective for PET Scans for Services Performed on or After January 28, 2005

NOTE: All PET scan services require the use of a radiopharmaceutical diagnostic imaging agent (tracer). The applicable tracer code should be billed when billing for a PET scan service. See section 60.3.2 below for applicable tracer codes.

CPT Code	Description
78459	Myocardial imaging, positron emission tomography (PET), metabolic evaluation
78491	Myocardial imaging, positron emission tomography (PET), perfusion, single study at rest or stress
78492	Myocardial imaging, positron emission tomography (PET), perfusion, multiple studies at rest and/or stress
78608	Brain imaging, positron emission tomography (PET); metabolic evaluation
78609	Brain imaging, positron emission tomography (PET); perfusion evaluation
78811	Tumor imaging, positron emission tomography (PET); limited area (e.g., chest, head/neck)
78812	Tumor imaging, positron emission tomography (PET); skull base to mid thigh
78813	Tumor imaging, positron emission tomography (PET); whole body
78814	Tumor imaging, positron emission tomography (PET) with concurrently acquired computed tomography (CT) for attenuation correction and anatomical localization; limited area (e.g., chest, head/neck)
78815	Tumor imaging, positron emission tomography (PET) with concurrently acquired computed tomography (CT) for attenuation correction and anatomical localization; skull base to mid thigh
78816	Tumor imaging, positron emission tomography (PET) with concurrently acquired computed tomography (CT) for attenuation correction and anatomical localization; whole body

Pub. 100-4, Chapter 13, Section 60.4

PET Scans for Imaging of the Perfusion of the Heart Using Rubidium 82 (Rb 82)

For dates of service on or after March 14, 1995, Medicare covers one PET scan for imaging of the perfusion of the heart using Rubidium 82 (Rb 82), provided that the following conditions are met:

- The PET is done at a PET imaging center with a PET scanner that has been approved by the FDA;

- The PET scan is a rest alone or rest with pharmacologic stress PET scan, used for noninvasive imaging of the perfusion of the heart for the diagnosis and management of patients with known or suspected coronary artery disease, using Rb 82; and

- Either the PET scan is used in place of, but not in addition to, a single photon emission computed tomography (SPECT) or the PET scan is used following a SPECT that was found inconclusive.

Pub. 100-4, Chapter 13, Section 60.9

Coverage of PET Scans for Myocardial Viability

FDG PET is covered for the determination of myocardial viability following an inconclusive single photon computed tomography test (SPECT) from July 1, 2001, through September 30, 2002. Only full ring scanners are covered as the scanning medium for this service from July 1, 2001, through December 31, 2001. However, as of January 1, 2002, full and partial ring scanners are covered for myocardial viability following an inconclusive SPECT.

Beginning October 1, 2002, Medicare will cover FDG PET for the determination of myocardial viability as a primary or initial diagnostic study prior to revascularization, and will continue to cover FDG PET when used as a follow-up to an inconclusive SPECT. However, if a patient received a FDG PET study with inconclusive results, a follow-up SPECT is not covered. FDA full and partial ring PET scanners are covered. In the event that a patient receives a SPECT with inconclusive results, a PET scan may be performed and covered by Medicare. However, a SPECT is not covered following a FDG PET with inconclusive results. See the Medicare National Coverage Determinations Manual, Section 220.6 for specific frequency limitations for Myocardial Viability following an inconclusive SPECT.

Documentation that these conditions are met should be maintained by the referring provider as part of the beneficiary's medical record.

HCPCS Code for PET Scan for Myocardial Viability

78459 - Myocardial imaging, positron emission tomography (PET), metabolic evaluation

Pub. 100-4, Chapter 13, Section 60.11

13

Effective for service performed on or after October 1, 2003, PET scans performed at rest or with pharmacological stress used for noninvasive imaging of the perfusion of the heart for the diagnosis and management of patients with known or suspected coronary artery disease using the FDA-approved radiopharmaceutical ammonia N-13 are covered, provided the following requirements are met.

Pub. 100-4, Chapter 13, Section 60.12

Coverage for PET Scans for Dementia and Neurodegenerative Diseases

Effective for dates of service on or after September 15, 2004, Medicare will cover FDG PET scans for a differential diagnosis of fronto-temporal dementia (FTD) and Alzheimer's disease OR; its use in a CMS-approved practical clinical trial focused on the utility of FDG-PET in the diagnosis or treatment of dementing neurodegenerative diseases. Refer to Pub. 100-03, NCD Manual, section 220.6.13, for complete coverage conditions and clinical trial requirements and section 60.15 of this manual for claims processing information.

A. Carrier and FI Billing Requirements for PET Scan Claims for FDG-PET for the Differential Diagnosis of Fronto-temporal Dementia and Alzheimer's Disease:

- CPT Code for PET Scans for Dementia and Neurodegenerative Diseases

Contractors shall advise providers to use the appropriate CPT code from section 60.3.1 for dementia and neurodegenerative diseases for services performed on or after January 28, 2005.

- Diagnosis Codes for PET Scans for Dementia and Neurodegenerative Diseases

The contractor shall ensure one of the following appropriate diagnosis codes is present on claims for PET Scans for AD:

- 290.0, 290.10 - 290.13, 290.20 - 290, 21, 290.3, 331.0, 331.11, 331.19, 331.2, 331.9, 780.93

Medicare contractors shall use an appropriate Medicare Summary Notice (MSN) message such as 16.48, "Medicare does not pay for this item or service for this condition" to deny claims when submitted with an appropriate CPT code from section 60.3.1 and with a diagnosis code other than the range of codes listed above. Also, contractors shall use an appropriate Remittance Advice (RA) such as 11, "The diagnosis is inconsistent with the procedure."

Medicare contractors shall instruct providers to issue an Advanced Beneficiary Notice to beneficiaries advising them of potential financial liability prior to delivering the service if one of the appropriate diagnosis codes will not be present on the claim.

- Provider Documentation Required with the PET Scan Claim

Medicare contractors shall inform providers to ensure the conditions mentioned in the NCD Manual, section 220.6.13, have been met. The information must also be maintained in the beneficiary's medical record.

- Date of onset of symptoms;

- Diagnosis of clinical syndrome (normal aging, mild cognitive impairment or MCI: mild, moderate, or severe dementia);

- Mini mental status exam (MMSE) or similar test score;

- Presumptive cause (possible, probably, uncertain AD);

- Any neuropsychological testing performed;

- Results of any structural imaging (MRI, CT) performed;

- Relevant laboratory tests (B12, thyroid hormone); and,

Number and name of prescribed medications.

Pub. 100-4, Chapter 13, Section 70.3

77417)

Carriers pay for these TC services on a daily basis under CPT codes 77401-77416 for radiation treatment delivery. They do not use local codes and RVUs in paying for the TC of radiation oncology services. Multiple treatment sessions on the same day are payable as long as there has been a distinct break in therapy services, and the individual sessions are of the character usually furnished on different days. Carriers pay for CPT code 77417 (Therapeutic radiology port film(s)) on a weekly (five fractions) basis.

Pub. 100-4, Chapter 13, Section 70.4

77799)

Carriers must apply the bundled services policy to procedures in this family of codes other than CPT code 77776. For procedures furnished in settings in which TC payments are made, carriers must pay separately for the expendable source associated with these procedures under CPT code 79900 except in the case of remote after-loading high intensity brachytherapy procedures (CPT codes 77781-77784). In the four codes cited, the expendable source is included in the RVUs for the TC of the procedures.

Pub. 100-4, Chapter 13, Section 90

Ray Suppliers

B3-2070.4, B3-15022.G, B3-4131, B3-4831

Services furnished by portable x-ray suppliers may have as many as four components. Carriers must follow the following rules.

Pub. 100-4, Chapter 13, Section 100

Interpretation of Diagnostic Tests
B3-15023

Pub. 100-4, Chapter 13, Section 140.2

Frequency Standard
SNF-533.5.B, B3-4181.2, A3-3631.n

Medicare pays for a bone mass measurement meeting the criteria as stated above once every 2 years (at least 23 months have passed since the month the last bone mass measurement was performed). However, if it is medically necessary, Medicare may pay for a bone mass measurement for a beneficiary more frequently than every two years. Examples of situations where more frequent bone mass measurement procedures may be medically necessary include, but are not limited to, the following medical circumstances:

- Monitoring beneficiaries on long-term glucocorticoid (steroid) therapy of more than 3 months; and

- Allowing for a confirmatory baseline bone mass measurement (either central or peripheral) to permit monitoring of beneficiaries in the future if the initial test was performed with a technique that is different from the proposed monitoring method (for example, if the initial test was performed using bone sonometry and monitoring is anticipated using bone densitometry, cover the baseline measurement using bone densitometry).

Pub. 100-4, Chapter 13, Section 140.3

Payment Methodology and HCPCS Coding
Carriers pay for bone mass measurement procedures based on the Medicare physician fee schedule. Claims from physicians, other practitioners, or suppliers where assignment was not taken are subject to the Medicare limiting charge.

The FIs pay for bone mass measurement procedures under the current payment methodologies for radiology services according to the type of provider.

Deductible and coinsurance apply.

Any of the following codes may be used when billing for bone mass measurements. All of these codes are bone densitometry measurements except code 76977 which is bone sonometry measurements. Codes are applicable to billing FIs and carriers.

76070 76071 76075 76076 76078 76977 78350 G0130

The FIs are billed using the ANSI X12N 837 I or hardcopy Form CMS-1450 (UB-92). The appropriate bill types are: 12X, 13X, 22X, 23X, 34X, 71X (Provider-based and independent), 72X, 73X (Provider-based and freestanding), 83X, and 85X. Effective 4/1/06, type of bill 14X is for non-patient laboratory specimens and is no longer applicable for bone mass measurements.

Providers who use the hard copy UB-92 (Form CMS-1450) report the applicable bill type in Form Locator (FL) 4, Type of Bill.

Providers must report HCPCS codes for bone mass measurements under revenue code 320 with number of units and line item dates of service per revenue code line for each bone mass measurement reported.

Carriers are billed for bone mass measurement procedures using the ANSI X12N 837 P or hardcopy Form CMS-1500.

Pub. 100-4, Chapter 14, Section 10

General
B3-2265

Payment is made under Part B for certain surgical procedures that are furnished in ASCs and are approved for being furnished in an ASC. These procedures are those that generally do not exceed 90 minutes in length and do not require more than four hours recovery or convalescent time.

To be paid under this provision, a facility must be certified as meeting the requirements for an ASC and must enter into a written agreement with the Centers for Medicare & Medicaid Services (CMS). The certification process is described in the State Operations Manual.

Medicare will not pay an ASC for those procedures that require more than an ASC level of care, or for minor procedures that are normally performed in a physician's office.

The CMS publishes updates to the list of procedures for which an ASC may be paid each year. The complete list of procedures is available through the Public Use files (PUF) at http://www.cms.hhs.gov/researchers/. This includes applicable codes, payment groups, and payment amounts for each ASC group before adjustments for regional wage variations. Applicable wage indices are also published via program memorandum.

ASCs must accept Medicare's payment for such procedures as payment in full for the facility service with respect to those services defined as ASC facility services. The physician and anesthesiologist may bill and be paid for the professional component of the service also.

Certain other services may be performed in an ASC facility, billed by the appropriate certified provider/supplier, or in certain cases by the ASC facility itself, and paid outside of the facility rate.

Pub. 100-4, Chapter 16, Section 10

Background
B3-2070, B3-2070.1, B3-4110.3, B3-5114

Diagnostic X-ray, laboratory, and other diagnostic tests, including materials and the services of technicians, are covered under the Medicare program. Some clinical laboratory procedures or tests require Food and Drug Administration (FDA) approval before coverage is provided.

A diagnostic laboratory test is considered a laboratory service for billing purposes, regardless of whether it is performed in:

- A physician's office, by an independent laboratory;

- By a hospital laboratory for its outpatients or nonpatients;

- In a rural health clinic; or

- In an HMO or Health Care Prepayment Plan (HCPP) for a patient who is not a member.

When a hospital laboratory performs laboratory tests for nonhospital patients, the laboratory is functioning as an independent laboratory, and still bills the fiscal intermediary (FI). Also, when physicians and laboratories perform the same test, whether manually or with automated equipment, the services are deemed similar.

Laboratory services furnished by an independent laboratory are covered under SMI if the laboratory is an approved Independent Clinical Laboratory. However, as is the case of all diagnostic services, in order to be covered these services must be related to a patient's illness or injury (or symptom or complaint) and ordered by a physician. A small number of laboratory tests can be covered as a preventive screening service.

See the Medicare Benefit Policy Manual, Chapter 15, for detailed coverage requirements.

See the Medicare Program Integrity Manual, Chapter 10, for laboratory/supplier enrollment guidelines.

See the Medicare State Operations Manual for laboratory/supplier certification requirements.

Pub. 100-4, Chapter 16, Section 10.1

Definitions
B3-2070.1, B3-2070.1.B, RHC-406.4

"Independent Laboratory" - An independent laboratory is one that is independent both of an attending or consulting physician's office and of a hospital that meets at least the requirements to qualify as an emergency hospital as defined in §1861(e) of the Social Security Act (the Act.) (See the Medicare Benefits Policy Manual, Chapter 15, for detailed discussion.)

"Physician Office Laboratory" — A physician office laboratory is a laboratory maintained by a physician or group of physicians for performing diagnostic tests in connection with the physician practice.

"Clinical Laboratory" - See the Medicare Benefits Policy Manual, Chapter 15.

"Qualified Hospital Laboratory" - A qualified hospital laboratory is one that provides some clinical laboratory tests 24 hours a day, 7 days a week, to serve a hospital's emergency room that is also available to provide services 24 hours a day, 7 days a week. For the qualified hospital laboratory to meet this requirement, the hospital must have physicians physically present or available within 30 minutes through a medical staff call roster to handle emergencies 24 hours a day, 7 days a week; and hospital laboratory technologists must be on duty or on call at all times to provide testing for the emergency room.

"Hospital Outpatient" - See the Medicare Benefit Policy Manual, Chapter 2.

"Referring laboratory" - A Medicare-approved laboratory that receives a specimen to be tested and that refers the specimen to another laboratory for performance of the laboratory test.

"Reference laboratory" - A Medicare-enrolled laboratory that receives a specimen from another, referring laboratory for testing and that actually performs the test.

"Billing laboratory" - The laboratory that submits a bill or claim to Medicare.

"Service" - A clinical diagnostic laboratory test. Service and test are synonymous.

"Test" - A clinical diagnostic laboratory service. Service and test are synonymous.

"CLIA" - The Clinical Laboratory Improvement Act and CMS implementing regulations and processes.

"Certification" - A laboratory that has met the standards specified in the CLIA.

"Draw Station' - A place where a specimen is collected but no Medicare-covered clinical laboratory testing is performed on the drawn specimen.

"Medicare-approved laboratory - A laboratory that meets all of the enrollment standards as a Medicare provider including the certification by a CLIA certifying authority.

Pub. 100-4, Chapter 16, Section 110.4

Carrier Contacts With Independent Clinical Laboratories
B3-2070.1.F

An important role of the carrier is as a communicant of necessary information to independent clinical laboratories. Failure to inform independent laboratories of Medicare regulations and claims processing procedures may have an adverse effect on prosecution of laboratories suspected of fraudulent activities with respect to tests performed by, or billed on behalf of, independent laboratories. United States Attorneys often must prosecute under a handicap or may refuse to prosecute cases where there is no evidence that a laboratory has been specifically informed of Medicare regulations and claims processing procedures.

To assure that laboratories are aware of Medicare regulations and carrier's policy, notification must be sent to independent laboratories when any changes are made in coverage policy or claims processing procedures. Additionally, to completely document efforts to fully inform independent laboratories of Medicare policy and the laboratory's responsibilities, previously issued newsletters should be periodically re-issued to remind laboratories of existing requirements.

Some items which should be discussed are the requirements to have the same charges for Medicare and private patients, to document fully the medical necessity for collection of specimens from a skilled nursing facility or a beneficiary's home, and, in cases when a laboratory service is referred from one independent laboratory to another independent laboratory, to identify the laboratory actually performing the test.

Additionally, when carrier professional relations representatives make personal contacts with particular laboratories, they should prepare and retain reports of contact indicating dates, persons present, and issues discussed.

Pub. 100-4, Chapter 18, Section 60.1

Payment

Payment (carrier and FI) is under the MPFS except as follows:

Fecal occult blood tests (82270*(G0107*and G0328) are paid under the clinical diagnostic lab fee schedule except reasonable cost is paid to CAHs when submitted on TOB 85X. See section A below for payment to Maryland waiver on TOB 13X. Payment from all hospitals for non-patient laboratory specimens on TOB 14X will be based on the clinical diagnostic fee schedule, including CAHs and Maryland waiver hospitals.

Flexible sigmoidoscopy (code G0104) is paid under OPPS for hospital outpatient departments and on a reasonable cost basis for CAHs; or current payment methodologies for hospitals not subject to OPPS.

Colonoscopy (G0105) and barium enemas (G0106 and G0120) are paid under OPPS for hospital outpatient departments and on a reasonable costs basis for CAHs or current payment methodologies for hospitals not subject to OPPS. Also colonoscopies may be done in an Ambulatory Surgical Center (ASC) and when done in an ASC the ASC rate applies. The ASC rate is the same for diagnostic and screening colonoscopies.

The following screening codes must be paid at rates consistent with the diagnostic codes indicated.

A. Special Payment Instructions for TOB 13X Maryland Waiver Hospitals

For hospitals in Maryland under the jurisdiction of the Health Services Cost Review Commission, screening colorectal services HCPCS codes G0104, G0105, G0106, 82270*(G0107*) G0120, G0121 and G0328 are paid according to the terms of the waiver, that is 94% of submitted charges minus any unmet existing deductible, co-insurance and non-covered charges. Maryland Hospitals bill TOB 13X for outpatient colorectal cancer screenings.

B. Special Payment Instructions for Non-Patient Laboratory Specimen (TOB 14X) for all hospitals

Payment for colorectal cancer screenings (82270*(G0107*) and G0328) to a hospital for a non-patient laboratory specimen (TOB 14X), is the lesser of the actual charge, the fee schedule amount, or the National Limitation Amount (NLA), (including CAHs and Maryland Waiver hospitals). Part B deductible and coinsurance do not apply.

NOTE: For claims with dates of service prior to January 1, 2007, physicians, suppliers, and providers report HCPCS code G0107. Effective January 1, 2007, code G0107 is discontinued and replaced with CPT code 82270.

Pub. 100-4, Chapter 18, Section 60.2

HCPCS Codes, Frequency Requirements, and Age Requirements (If Applicable)

B3-4180.2, A3-3660.17.A, AB-03-114

Effective for services furnished on or after January 1, 1998, the following codes are used for colorectal cancer screening services:

82270*(G0107*) - Colorectal cancer screening; fecal-occult blood tests, 1-3 simultaneous determinations;

G0104 - Colorectal cancer screening; flexible sigmoidoscopy;

G0105 - Colorectal cancer screening; colonoscopy on individual at high risk;

G0106 - Colorectal cancer screening; barium enema; as an alternative to G0104, screening sigmoidoscopy;

G0120 - Colorectal cancer screening; barium enema; as an alternative to G0105, screening colonoscopy.

Effective for services furnished on or after July 1, 2001 the following codes are used for colorectal cancer screening services:

G0121 - Colorectal cancer screening; colonoscopy on individual not meeting criteria for high risk. Note that the description for this code has been revised to remove the term "noncovered."

G0122 - Colorectal cancer screening; barium enema (noncovered).

Effective for services furnished on or after January 1, 2004, the following code is used for colorectal cancer screening services as an alternative to 82270*(G0107*):

G0328 - Colorectal cancer screening; immunoassay, fecal-occult blood test, 1-3 simultaneous determinations

NOTE: For claims with dates of service prior to January 1, 2007, physicians, suppliers, and providers report HCPCS code G0107. Effective January 1, 2007, code G0107 is discontinued and replaced with CPT code 82270.

G0104 - Colorectal Cancer Screening; Flexible Sigmoidoscopy

Screening flexible sigmoidoscopies (code G0104) may be paid for beneficiaries who have attained age 50, when performed by a doctor of medicine or osteopathy at the frequencies noted below.

For claims with dates of service on or after January 1, 2002, contractors pay for screening flexible sigmoidoscopies (code G0104) for beneficiaries who have attained age 50 when these services were performed by a doctor of medicine or osteopathy, or by a physician assistant, nurse practitioner, or clinical nurse specialist (as defined in §1861(aa)(5) of the Act and in the

Code of Federal Regulations at 42 CFR 410.74, 410.75, and 410.76) at the frequencies noted above. For claims with dates of service prior to January 1, 2002, contractors pay for these services under the conditions noted only when a doctor of medicine or osteopathy performs them.

For services furnished from January 1, 1998, through June 30, 2001, inclusive:

Once every 48 months (i.e., at least 47 months have passed following the month in which the last covered screening flexible sigmoidoscopy was done).

For services furnished on or after July 1, 2001:

Once every 48 months as calculated above unless the beneficiary does not meet the criteria for high risk of developing colorectal cancer (refer to §60.3 of this chapter) and he/she has had a screening colonoscopy (code G0121) within the preceding 10 years. If such a beneficiary has had a screening colonoscopy within the preceding 10 years, then he or she can have covered a screening flexible sigmoidoscopy only after at least 119 months have passed following the month that he/she received the screening colonoscopy (code G0121).

NOTE: If during the course of a screening flexible sigmoidoscopy a lesion or growth is detected which results in a biopsy or removal of the growth; the appropriate diagnostic procedure classified as a flexible sigmoidoscopy with biopsy or removal should be billed and paid rather than code G0104.

G0105 - Colorectal Cancer Screening; Colonoscopy on Individual at High Risk

Ref: AB-03-114

Screening colonoscopies (code G0105) may be paid when performed by a doctor of medicine or osteopathy at a frequency of once every 24 months for beneficiaries at high risk for developing colorectal cancer (i.e., at least 23 months have passed following the month in which the last covered G0105 screening colonoscopy was performed). Refer to §60.3 of this chapter for the criteria to use in determining whether or not an individual is at high risk for developing colorectal cancer.

NOTE: If during the course of the screening colonoscopy, a lesion or growth is detected which results in a biopsy or removal of the growth, the appropriate diagnostic procedure classified as a colonoscopy with biopsy or removal should be billed and paid rather than code G0105.

A. Colonoscopy Cannot be Completed Because of Extenuating Circumstances

1. FIs

When a covered colonoscopy is attempted but cannot be completed because of extenuating circumstances, Medicare will pay for the interrupted colonoscopy as long as the coverage conditions are met for the incomplete procedure. However, the frequency standards associated with screening colonoscopies will not be applied by CWF. When a covered colonoscopy is next attempted and completed, Medicare will pay for that colonoscopy according to its payment methodology for this procedure as long as coverage conditions are met, and the frequency standards will be applied by CWF. This policy is applied to both screening and diagnostic colonoscopies. When submitting a facility claim for the interrupted colonoscopy, providers are to suffix the colonoscopy HCPCS codes with a modifier of " – 73" or" – 74" as appropriate to indicate that the procedure was interrupted. Payment for covered incomplete screening colonoscopies shall be consistent with payment methodologies currently in place for complete screening colonoscopies, including those contained in 42 CFR 419.44(b). In situations where a critical access hospital (CAH) has elected payment Method II for CAH patients, payment shall be consistent with payment methodologies currently in place as outlined in Chapter 3. As such, instruct CAHs that elect Method II payment to use modifier " – 53" to identify an incomplete screening colonoscopy (physician professional service(s) billed in revenue code 096X, 097X, and/or 098X). Such CAHs will also bill the technical or facility component of the interrupted colonoscopy in revenue code 075X (or other appropriate revenue code) using the "-73" or "-74" modifier as appropriate.

Note that Medicare would expect the provider to maintain adequate information in the patient's medical record in case it is needed by the contractor to document the incomplete procedure.

2. Carriers

When a covered colonoscopy is attempted but cannot be completed because of extenuating circumstances (see Chapter 12), Medicare will pay for the interrupted colonoscopy at a rate consistent with that of a flexible sigmoidoscopy as long as coverage conditions are met for the incomplete procedure. When a covered colonoscopy is next attempted and completed, Medicare will pay for that colonoscopy according to its payment methodology for this procedure as long as coverage conditions are met. This policy is applied to both screening and diagnostic colonoscopies. When submitting a claim for the interrupted colonoscopy, professional providers are to suffix the colonoscopy code with a modifier of " – 53" to indicate that the procedure was interrupted. When submitting a claim for the facility fee associated with this procedure, Ambulatory Surgical Centers (ASCs) are to suffix the colonoscopy code with " – 73" or " – 74" as appropriate. Payment for covered screening colonoscopies, including that for the associated ASC facility fee when applicable, shall be consistent with payment for diagnostic colonoscopies, whether the procedure is complete or incomplete.

Note that Medicare would expect the provider to maintain adequate information in the patient's medical record in case it is needed by the contractor to document the incomplete procedure.

G0106 - Colorectal Cancer Screening; Barium Enema; as an Alternative to G0104, Screening Sigmoidoscopy

Screening barium enema examinations may be paid as an alternative to a screening sigmoidoscopy (code G0104). The same frequency parameters for screening sigmoidoscopies (see those codes above) apply.

In the case of an individual aged 50 or over, payment may be made for a screening barium enema examination (code G0106) performed after at least 47 months have passed following the month in which the last screening barium enema or screening flexible sigmoidoscopy was performed. For example, the beneficiary received a screening barium enema examination as an alternative to a screening flexible sigmoidoscopy in January 1999. Start counts beginning February 1999. The beneficiary is eligible for another screening barium enema in January 2003.

The screening barium enema must be ordered in writing after a determination that the test is the appropriate screening test. Generally, it is expected that this will be a screening double contrast enema unless the individual is unable to withstand such an exam. This means that in the case of a particular individual, the attending physician must determine that the estimated screening potential for the barium enema is equal to or greater than the screening potential that has been estimated for a screening flexible sigmoidoscopy for the same individual. The screening single contrast barium enema also requires a written order from the beneficiary's attending physician in the same manner as described above for the screening double contrast barium enema examination.

82270*(G0107*) - Colorectal Cancer Screening; Fecal-Occult Blood Test, 1-3 Simultaneous Determinations

Effective for services furnished on or after January 1, 1998, screening FOBT 82270*(G0107*) may be paid for beneficiaries who have attained age 50, and at a frequency of once every 12 months (i.e., at least 11 months have passed following the month in which the last covered screening FOBT was performed). This screening FOBT means a guaiac-based test for peroxidase activity, in which the beneficiary completes it by taking samples from two different sites of three consecutive stools. This screening requires a written order from the beneficiary's attending physician. (The term "attending physician" is defined to mean a doctor of medicine or osteopathy (as defined in §1861(r)(1) of the Act) who is fully knowledgeable about the beneficiary's medical condition, and who would be responsible for using the results of any examination performed in the overall management of the beneficiary's specific medical problem.)

Effective for services furnished on or after January 1, 2004, payment may be made for a immunoassay-based FOBT (G0328, described below) as an alternative to the guaiac-based FOBT, 82270*(G0107*).

Medicare will pay for only one covered FOBT per year, either82270*(G0107*)or G0328, but not both. *NOTE: For claims with dates of service prior to January 1, 2007, physicians, suppliers, and providers report HCPCS code G0107. Effective January 1, 2007, code G0107 is discontinued and replaced with CPT code 82270.

G0328 - Colorectal Cancer Screening; Immunoassay, Fecal-Occult Blood Test, 1-3 Simultaneous Determinations

Effective for services furnished on or after January 1, 2004, screening FOBT, (code G0328) may be paid as an alternative to 82270*(G0107*) for beneficiaries who have attained age 50. Medicare will pay for a covered FOBT (either82270*(G0107*) or G0328, but not both) at a frequency of once every 12 months (i.e., at least 11 months have passed following the month in which the last covered screening FOBT was performed). Screening FOBT, immunoassay, includes the use of a spatula to collect the appropriate number of samples or the use of a special brush for the collection of samples, as determined by the individual manufacturer's instructions. This screening requires a written order from the beneficiary's attending physician. (The term "attending physician" is defined to mean a doctor of medicine or osteopathy (as defined in §1861(r)(1) of the Act) who is fully knowledgeable about the beneficiary's medical condition, and who would be responsible for using the results of any examination performed in the overall management of the beneficiary's specific medical problem.)

G0120 - Colorectal Cancer Screening; Barium Enema; as an Alternative to or G0105, Screening Colonoscopy

Screening barium enema examinations may be paid as an alternative to a screening colonoscopy (code G0105) examination. The same frequency parameters for screening colonoscopies (see those codes above) apply.

In the case of an individual who is at high risk for colorectal cancer, payment may be made for a screening barium enema examination (code G0120) performed after at least 23 months have passed following the month in which the last screening barium enema or the last screening colonoscopy was performed. For example, a beneficiary at high risk for developing colorectal cancer received a screening barium enema examination (code G0120) as an alternative to a screening colonoscopy (code G0105) in January 2000. Start counts beginning February 2000. The beneficiary is eligible for another screening barium enema examination (code G0120) in January 2002.

The screening barium enema must be ordered in writing after a determination that the test is the appropriate screening test. Generally, it is expected that this will be a screening double contrast enema unless the individual is unable to withstand such an exam. This means that in the case of a particular individual, the attending physician must determine that the estimated screening potential for the barium enema is equal to or greater than the screening potential that has been estimated for a screening colonoscopy, for the same individual. The screening single contrast barium enema also requires a written order from the beneficiary's attending physician in the same manner as described above for the screening double contrast barium enema examination.

G0121 - Colorectal Screening; Colonoscopy on Individual Not Meeting Criteria for High Risk - Applicable On and After July 1, 2001

Effective for services furnished on or after July 1, 2001, screening colonoscopies (code G0121) performed on individuals not meeting the criteria for being at high risk for developing colorectal cancer (refer to §60.2 of this chapter) may be paid under the following conditions:

At a frequency of once every 10 years (i.e., at least 119 months have passed following the month in which the last covered G0121 screening colonoscopy was performed).

If the individual would otherwise qualify to have covered a G0121 screening colonoscopy based on the above but has had a covered screening flexible sigmoidoscopy (code G0104), then he or she may have covered a G0121 screening colonoscopy only after at least 47 months have passed following the month in which the last covered G0104 flexible sigmoidoscopy was performed.

NOTE: If during the course of the screening colonoscopy, a lesion or growth is detected which results in a biopsy or removal of the growth, the appropriate diagnostic procedure classified as a colonoscopy with biopsy or removal should be billed and paid rather than code G0121.

G0122 - Colorectal Cancer Screening; Barium Enema

The code is not covered by Medicare.

Pub. 100-4, Chapter 18, Section 60.2.1

Common Working Files (CWF) Edits

Effective for dates of service January 1, 1998, and later, CWF will edit all colorectal screening claims for age and frequency standards. The CWF will also edit FI claims for valid procedure codes (G0104, G0105, G0106, 82270*(G0107*), G0120, G0121, G0122, and G0328) and for valid bill types. The CWF currently edits for valid HCPCS codes for carriers. (See §60.6 of this chapter for bill types.)

NOTE: For claims with dates of service prior to January 1, 2007, physicians, suppliers, and providers report HCPCS code G0107. Effective January 1, 2007, code G0107 is discontinued and replaced with CPT code 82270.

Pub. 100-4, Chapter 18, Section 60.6

Billing Requirements for Claims Submitted to FIs

Follow the general bill review instructions in Chapter 25. Hospitals use the ANSI X12N 837I to bill the FI or on the hardcopy Form CMS-1450. Hospitals bill revenue codes and HCPCS codes as follows:

82270***

(G0107)***

G0328

The appropriate revenue code when reporting any other surgical procedure.

14X is only applicable for non-patient laboratory specimens

For claims with dates of service prior to January 1, 2007, physicians, suppliers, and providers report HCPCS code G0107. Effective January 1, 2007, code G0107, is discontinued and replaced with CPT code 82270.

CAHs that elect Method II bill revenue code 096X, 097X, and/or 098X for professional services and 075X (or other appropriate revenue code) for the technical or facility component.

A - Special Billing Instructions for Hospital Inpatients

When these tests/procedures are provided to inpatients of a hospital, they are covered under this benefit. However, the provider bills on bill type 13X using the discharge date of the hospital stay to avoid editing in the Common Working File (CWF) as a result of the hospital bundling rules.

Pub. 100-4, Chapter 20, Section 50.3

Payment for Replacement of Parenteral and Enteral Pumps

B3-3324

Payment for replacement of PEN pumps purchased more than eight years prior to the current date may be considered, with documentation that indicates proof of purchase date. Medicare will consider payment for either a replacement by purchase or 15 months of rental.

Pub. 100-4, Chapter 20, Section 100.2.2

Evidence of Medical Necessity for Parenteral and Enteral Nutrition (PEN) Therapy

B3-3324, B3-4450

The PEN coverage is determined by information provided by the treating physician and the PEN supplier. A completed certification of medical necessity (CMN) must accompany and support initial claims for PEN to establish whether coverage criteria are met and to ensure that the PEN therapy provided is consistent with the attending or ordering physician's prescription. Contractors ensure that the CMN contains pertinent information from the treating physician. Uniform specific medical data facilitate the review and promote consistency in coverage determinations and timelier claims processing.

The medical and prescription information on a PEN CMN can be most appropriately completed by the treating physician or from information in the patient's records by an employee of the physician for the physician's review and signature. Although PEN suppliers sometimes may assist in providing the PEN services, they cannot complete the CMN since they do not have the same access to patient information needed to properly enter medical or prescription information. Contractors use appropriate professional relations issuances, training sessions, and meetings to ensure that all persons and PEN suppliers are aware of this limitation of their role.

When properly completed, the PEN CMN includes the elements of a prescription as well as other data needed to determine whether Medicare coverage is possible. This practice will facilitate prompt delivery of PEN services and timely submittal of the related claim.

Pub. 100-4, Chapter 20, Section 160.1

Billing for Total Parenteral Nutrition and Enteral Nutrition Furnished to Part B Inpatients

A3-3660.6, SNF-544, SNF-559, SNF-260.4, SNF-261, HHA-403, HO-438, HO-229

Inpatient Part A hospital or SNF care includes total parenteral nutrition (TPN) systems and enteral nutrition (EN).

For inpatients for whom Part A benefits are not payable (e.g., benefits are exhausted or the beneficiary is entitled to Part B only), total parenteral nutrition (TPN) systems and enteral nutrition (EN) delivery systems are covered by Medicare as prosthetic devices when the coverage criteria are met. When these criteria are met, the medical equipment and medical supplies (together with nutrients) being used comprise covered prosthetic devices for coverage purposes rather than durable medical equipment. However, reimbursement rules relating to DME continue to apply to such items.

When a facility supplies TPN or EN systems that meet the criteria for coverage as a prosthetic device to an inpatient whose care is not covered under Part A, the facility must bill one of the DMERCs. Additionally, HHAs, SNFs, and hospitals that provide PEN supplies, equipment and nutrients as a prosthetic device under Part B must use the CMS-1500 or the related NSF or ANSI ASC X12N 837 format to bill the appropriate DMERC. The DMERC is determined according to the residence of the beneficiary. Refer to §10 for jurisdiction descriptions.

FIs return claims containing PEN charges for Part B services where the bill type is 12x, 13x, 22x, 23x, 32x, 33x, or 34x with instructions to the provider to bill the DMERC.

Pub. 100-4, Chapter 32, Section 10.1

Ambulatory Blood Pressure Monitoring (ABPM) Billing Requirements

A. Coding Applicable to Local Carriers & Fiscal Intermediaries (FIs)

Effective April 1, 2002, a National Coverage Decision was made to allow for Medicare coverage of ABPM for those beneficiaries with suspected "white coat hypertension" (WCH). ABPM involves the use of a non-invasive device, which is used to measure blood pressure in 24-hour cycles. These 24-hour measurements are stored in the device and are later interpreted by a physician. Suspected "WCH" is defined as: (1) Clinic/office blood pressure >140/90 mm Hg on at least three separate clinic/office visits with two separate measurements made at each visit; (2) At least two documented separate blood pressure measurements taken outside the clinic/office which are <140/90 mm Hg; and (3) No evidence of end-organ damage. ABPM is not covered for any other uses. Coverage policy can be found in Medicare National Coverage Determinations Manual, Chapter 1, Section 20.19. (www.cms.hhs.gov/masnuals/103 cov determ/ncd103index.asp).

The ABPM must be performed for at least 24 hours to meet coverage criteria. Payment is not allowed for institutionalized beneficiaries, such as those receiving Medicare covered skilled nursing in a facility. In the rare circumstance that ABPM needs to be performed more than once for a beneficiary, the qualifying criteria described above must be met for each subsequent ABPM test.

Effective dates for applicable Common Procedure Coding System (HCPCS) codes for ABPM for suspected WCH and their covered effective dates are as follows:

HCPCS	Definition	Effective Date
93784	ABPM, utilizing a system such as magnetic tape and/or computer disk, for 24 hours or longer; including recording, scanning analysis, interpretation and report.	04/01/2002
93786	ABPM, utilizing a system such as magnetic tape and/or computer disk, for 24 hours or longer; recording only.	04/01/2002
93788	ABPM, utilizing a system such as magnetic tape and/or computer disk, for 24 hours or longer; scanning analysis with report.	01/01/2004
93790	ABPM, utilizing a system such as magnetic tape and/or computer disk, for 24 hours or longer; physician review with interpretation and report.	04/01/2002

In addition, the following diagnosis code must be present:

796.2   Elevated blood pressure reading without diagnosis of hypertension.

B. FI Billing Instructions

The applicable types of bills acceptable when billing for ABPM services are 13X, 23X, 71X, 73X, 75X, and 85X. Chapter 25 of this manual provides general billing instructions that must be followed for bills submitted to FIs. The FIs pay for hospital outpatient ABPM services billed on a 13X type of bill with HCPCS 93786 and/or 93788 as follows: (1) Outpatient Prospective Payment System (OPPS) hospitals pay based on the Ambulatory Payment Classification (APC); (2) non-OPPS hospitals (Indian Health Services Hospitals, Hospitals that provide Part B services only, and hospitals located in American Samoa, Guam, Saipan and the Virgin Islands) pay based on reasonable cost, except for Maryland Hospitals which are paid based on a percentage of cost. Effective 4/1/06, type of bill 14X is for non-patient laboratory specimens and is no longer applicable for ABPM.

The FIs pay for comprehensive outpatient rehabilitation facility (CORF) ABPM services billed on a 75x type of bill with HCPCS code 93786 and/or 93788 based on the Medicare Physician Fee Schedule (MPFS) amount for that HCPCS code.

The FIs pay for ABPM services for critical access hospitals (CAHs) billed on a 85x type of bill as follows: (1) for CAHs that elected the Standard Method and billed HCPCS code 93786 and/or 93788, pay based on reasonable cost for that HCPCS code; and (2) for CAHs that elected the Optional Method and billed any combination of HCPCS codes 93786, 93788 and 93790 pay based on reasonable cost for HCPCS 93786 and 93788 and pay 115% of the MPFS amount for HCPCS 93790.

The FIs pay for ABPM services for skilled nursing facility (SNF) outpatients billed on a 23x type of bill with HCPCS code 93786 and/or 93788, based on the MPFS.

The FIs accept independent and provider-based rural health clinic (RHC) bills for visits under the all-inclusive rate when the RHC bills on a 71x type of bill with revenue code 052x for providing the professional component of ABPM services. The FIs should not make a separate payment to a RHC for the professional component of ABPM services in addition to the all-inclusive rate. RHCs

are not required to use ABPM HCPCS codes for professional services covered under the all-inclusive rate.

The FIs accept free-standing and provider-based federally qualified health center (FQHC) bills for visits under the all-inclusive rate when the FQHC bills on a 73x type of bill with revenue code 052x for providing the professional component of ABPM services.

The FIs should not make a separate payment to a FQHC for the professional component of ABPM services in addition to the all-inclusive rate. FQHCs are not required to use ABPM HCPCS codes for professional services covered under the all-inclusive rate.

The FIs pay provider-based RHCs/FQHCs for the technical component of ABPM services when billed under the base provider's number using the above requirements for that particular base provider type, i.e., a OPPS hospital based RHC would be paid for the ABPM technical component services under the OPPS using the APC for code 93786 and/or 93788 when billed on a 13x type of bill.

Independent and free-standing RHC/FQHC practitioners are only paid for providing the technical component of ABPM services when billed to the carrier following the carrier instructions.

C. Carrier Claims

Local carriers pay for ABPM services billed with diagnosis code 796.2 and HCPCS codes 93784 or for any combination of 93786, 93788 and 93790, based on the MPFS for the specific HCPCS code billed.

D. Coinsurance and Deductible

The FIs and local carriers shall apply coinsurance and deductible to payments for ABPM services except for services billed to the FI by FQHCs. For FQHCs only co-insurance applies.

11 - Wound Treatments

(Rev 124a, 03-19-04)

Pub. 100-4, Chapter 32, Section 12.1

HCPCS and Diagnosis Coding

The following HCPCS codes should be reported when billing for smoking and tobacco- use cessation counseling services:

G0375 - Smoking and tobacco-use cessation counseling visit; intermediate, greater than 3 minutes up to 10 minutes

Short Descriptor: Smoke/Tobacco counseling 3-10

G0376 - Smoking and tobacco-use cessation counseling visit; intensive, greater than 10 minutes

Short Descriptor: Smoke/Tobacco counseling greater than 10

NOTE: The above G codes will NOT be active in contractors' systems until July 5, 2005. Therefore, contractors shall advise providers to use unlisted code 99199 to bill for smoking and tobacco- use cessation counseling services during the interim period of March 22, 2005, through July 4, 2005, and received prior to July 5, 2005.

On July 5, 2005, contractors' systems will accept the new G codes for services performed on and after March 22, 2005.

Contractors shall allow payment for a medically necessary E/M service on the same day as the smoking and tobacco-use cessation counseling service when it is clinically appropriate. Physicians and qualified non-physician practitioners shall use an appropriate HCPCS code, such as HCPCS 99201 — 99215, to report an E/M service with modifier 25 to indicate that the E/M service is a separately identifiable service from G0375 or G0376.

Contractors shall only pay for 8 Smoking and Tobacco-Use Cessation Counseling sessions in a 12-month period. The beneficiary may receive another 8 sessions during a second or subsequent year after 11 full months have passed since the first Medicare covered cessation session was performed. To start the count for the second or subsequent 12-month period, begin with the month after the month in which the first Medicare covered cessation session was performed and count until 11 full months have elapsed.

Claims for smoking and tobacco use cessation counseling services shall be submitted with an appropriate diagnosis code. Diagnosis codes should reflect: the condition the patient has that is adversely affected by tobacco use or the condition the patient is being treated for with a therapeutic agent whose metabolism or dosing is affected by tobacco use.

NOTE: This decision does not modify existing coverage for minimal cessation counseling (defined as 3 minutes or less in duration) which is already considered to be covered as part of each Evaluation and Management (E/M) visit and is not separately billable.

Pub. 100-4, Chapter 32, Section 30

Hyperbaric Oxygen (HBO) Therapy

Pub. 100-4, Chapter 32, Section 40

Sacral Nerve Stimulation

A sacral nerve stimulator is a pulse generator that transmits electrical impulses to the sacral nerves through an implanted wire. These impulses cause the bladder muscles to contract, which gives the patient ability to void more properly.

Pub. 100-4, Chapter 32, Section 50

Deep Brain Stimulation for Essential Tremor and Parkinson's Disease

Deep brain stimulation (DBS) refers to high-frequency electrical stimulation of anatomic regions deep within the brain utilizing neurosurgically implanted electrodes. These DBS electrodes are stereotactically placed within targeted nuclei on one (unilateral) or both (bilateral) sides of the brain. There are currently three targets for DBS — the thalamic ventralis intermedius nucleus (VIM), subthalamic nucleus (STN) and globus pallidus interna (GPi).

Essential tremor (ET) is a progressive, disabling tremor most often affecting the hands. ET may also affect the head, voice and legs. The precise pathogenesis of ET is unknown. While it may start at any age, ET usually peaks within the second and sixth decades. Beta-adrenergic blockers and anticonvulsant medications are usually the first line treatments for reducing the severity of tremor. Many patients, however, do not adequately respond or cannot tolerate these medications. In these medically refractory ET patients, thalamic VIM DBS may be helpful for symptomatic relief of tremor.

Parkinson's disease (PD) is an age-related progressive neurodegenerative disorder involving the loss of dopaminergic cells in the substantia nigra of the midbrain. The disease is characterized by tremor, rigidity, bradykinesia and progressive postural instability. Dopaminergic medication is typically used as a first line treatment for reducing the primary symptoms of PD. However, after prolonged use, medication can become less effective and can produce significant adverse events such as dyskinesias and other motor function complications. For patients who become unresponsive to medical treatments and/or have intolerable side effects from medications, DBS for symptom relief may be considered.

Pub. 100-4, Chapter 32, Section 90

Stem Cell Transplantation

Stem cell transplantation is a process in which stem cells are harvested from either a patient's or donor's bone marrow or peripheral blood for intravenous infusion. Autologous stem cell transplantation (AuSCT) must be used to effect hematopoietic reconstitution following severely myelotoxic doses of chemotherapy (HDCT) and/or radiotherapy used to treat various malignancies. Allogeneic stem cell transplant may also be used to restore function in recipients having an inherited or acquired deficiency or defect.

Bone marrow and peripheral blood stem cell transplantation is a process which includes mobilization, harvesting, and transplant of bone marrow or peripheral blood stem cells and the administration of high dose chemotherapy or radiotherapy prior to the actual transplant. When bone marrow or peripheral blood stem cell transplantation is covered, all necessary steps are included in coverage. When bone marrow or peripheral blood stem cell transplantation is non-covered, none of the steps are covered.

Allogeneic and autologous stem cell transplants are covered under Medicare for specific diagnoses. See Pub. 100-03, National Coverage Determinations Manual, section 110.8.1, for a complete description of covered and noncovered conditions. The following sections contain claims processing instructions for carrier claims. For institutional claims processing instructions, please refer to Pub. 100-04, chapter 3, section 90.3.

Pub. 100-4, Chapter 32, Section 100

Billing Requirements for Expanded Coverage of Cochlear Implantation

Effective for dates of services on and after April 4, 2005, the Centers for Medicare & Medicaid Services (CMS) has expanded the coverage for cochlear implantation to cover moderate-to-profound hearing loss in individuals with hearing test scores equal to or less than 40% correct in the best aided listening condition on tape-recorded tests of open-set sentence recognition and who demonstrate limited benefit from amplification. (See Publication 100-03, chapter 1, section 50.3, for specific coverage criteria).

In addition CMS is covering cochlear implantation for individuals with open-set sentence recognition test scores of greater than 40% to less than or equal to 60% correct but only when the provider is participating in, and patients are enrolled in, either:

- A Food and Drug Administration(FDA)-approved category B investigational device exemption (IDE) clinical trial; or

- A trial under the CMS clinical trial policy (see Pub. 100-03, section 310.1); or

A prospective, controlled comparative trial approved by CMS as consistent with the evidentiary requirements for national coverage analyses and meeting specific quality standards.

APPENDIX E — GLOSSARY

Abdominal lymphadenectomy — Cutting out (removing) the lymph node grouping, with or without para-aortic and vena caval nodes, and dissecting away from the surrounding tissue, nerves, and blood vessels.

Absorbable sutures — Strands prepared from collagen or a synthetic polymer and capable of being absorbed by tissue over time. Examples include surgical gut, collagen sutures, or synthetics like polydioxanone (PDS), polyglactin 910 (Vicryl), polylecapron 25 (Monocryl), polyglyconate (Maxon), and polyglycolic acid (Dexon).

Acetabuloplasty — Plastic repair/reconstruction of the acetabulum. The acetabulum is the rounded cavity on the external surface of the innominate bone that receives the head of the femur.

Air conduction — The transportation of sound from the air, through the external auditory canal, to the tympanic membrane, and ossicular chain, ending at, but not including the cochlea. Testing air conduction establishes the patency or nonpatency of these mechanisms.

Air puff device — Measures intraocular pressure by evaluating the force of a reflected amount of air blown against the cornea. A valuable screening tool, but less precise than other methods.

Allograft — Tissue obtained from a nonidentical individual of the same species. Other terms used to identify allografts include: allogenic graft, homologous graft, homoplastic graft.

Amniocentesis — Amniocentesis provides an accurate source of chromosomal information about the fetus. It is usually performed between 16 and 20 weeks gestation.

Anastomosis — Surgically created connection between ducts, blood vessels, or bowel segments to allow flow from one to the other.

Angioplasty — Reconstruction or repair of a diseased or damaged blood vessel.

Annuloplasty — The annuli are thick, fibrous rings and one is found surrounding each of the cardiac chambers. The atrial and ventricular muscle fibers attach to the annuli. In annuloplasty, weakened annuli may be surgically plicated, or tucked, to improve muscular functions.

Anorectal anometry — Measurement of pressure generated by anal sphincter to help treat incontinence.

Anterior chamber lenses — These are inserted in conjunction with intracapsular cataract extraction and posterior chamber lenses are inserted in conjunction with extracapsular cataract extraction. Anterior chamber lenses are commonly used for secondary insertion.

Applanation tomometer — Measures intraocular pressure by recording the force required to flatten an area of the cornea. It is attached to a slit lamp and is considered the most accurate methodology.

Aspirate — Physician uses a syringe or a suction device to withdraw fluid or air from a cavity.

Atrial septal defect — An atrial septal defect allows oxygenated blood to return to the lungs instead of circulating throughout the rest of the body. This can increase pulmonary blood flow, causing pulmonary hypertension if the defect is not closed.

Auricle — The external ear, or auricle, is a single elastic cartilage covered in skin and normal adnexal features (hair follicles, sweat glands, and sebaceous glands). The ridged nature of the auricle is to channel sounds into the acoustic meatus. The semicircular depression leading into the ear is named the concha, Latin for shell. The lining of the acoustic meatus is skin with ceruminous glands that secrete ear wax.

Autogenous transplant — Transplanted from one part of the patient's body to another. Autogenous bone may be freshly harvested, or preserved and stored in a bone bank for later grafting. Most commonly, the bone is cryogenically preserved. Other terms for autograft include: autogenic graft, autologous graft, autotransplant.

Bankart procedure — This procedure is also referred to as a capsulolabral reconstruction. The procedure is used to treat recurrent dislocation of the shoulder requiring reconstruction of the avulsed capsule and labrum at the glenoid lip.

Bartholin's gland — Gland on either side of vaginal opening. Also called vestibular glands.

Bartholin's gland abscess — An abscess of the Bartholin's gland is a pocket of pus and surrounding cellulitis caused by infection of the Bartholin's gland. Symptoms include localized swelling and pain in the posterior labia majora. The pain may extend into the lower vagina.

Basic value or base uUnit (anesthesia services) — The basic value, also referred to as the base unit or relative value, has two components. One component reflects all usual services included in the anesthesia service, including pre-operative and post-operative visits, administration of fluids and/or blood products incident to the procedure, and interpretation of non-invasive monitoring (ECG, temperature, blood pressure, oximetry, capnography, and mass spectrometry). The second component reflects the relative work or cost of the specific anesthesia service. Cost in this context refers to the physician's cost of doing business. For anesthesiologists, the majority of the cost goes to malpractice insurance.

Berman locator — Small, sensitive tool for detecting location of a metallic foreign body.

Bifurcated — Having two branches or divisions, such as the left pulmonary veins that split off from the left atrium to carry oxygenated blood away from the heart.

Biopsy — Tissue or fluid removed for diagnosis. A pathologist confirms a diagnosis through analysis of the cells in the biopsy material.

Blalock-Hanlon procedure — A segment of the right atrium is excised, creating an atrial septal defect. This is a palliative procedure for transposition of great vessels.

Blalock-Taussig procedure — An end-to-side anastomosis of right subclavian artery to right pulmonary artery allows arterial and venous blood to mix and flow through the shunt to the pulmonary artery and into the lungs for oxygenation.

Blepharorrhaphy — Synonym of tarsorrhaphy. See tarsorrhaphy.

Blue baby — A term commonly used for infants that are cyanotic due to oxygen deprivation.

Body positions — There are several body positions for patients during surgical procedures. These include:

- Fowler's position. Position assumed by patient when the head of the bed is raised 18 or 20 inches and the individual's knees are elevated.

- Prone. Lying horizontally when lying face downward.

- Supine. Lying horizontally on the back (also called dorsal decubitus position).

- Trendelenburg position. Position by the patient when the patient's head is lower in relation to the inclined plane of the body and legs.

Bone conduction — The transportation of sound through bone. The source of sound is placed on the skull or teeth, and the vibration stimulates the cochlea, bypassing normal air conduction routes. Bone conduction requires operational sensorineural hearing mechanisms.

Bone mass measurement — The term means a radiologic or radioisotopic procedure or other procedure approved by the FDA for identifying bone mass, detecting bone loss. or determining bone quality. The procedure includes a physician's interpretation of the results. Qualifying individuals must be an estrogen-deficient woman at clinical risk for osteoporosis with vertebral abnormalities.

Bristow procedure — This procedure transfers the tip of the coracoid process with its muscle attachments across the anteroinferior glenohumeral joint creating a musculotendinous sling.

Buccal mucosa — The mucous membrane on the inside of the cheek.

Caldwell-Luc — A large nasoantral window is created above the canine tooth in this intraoral approach to surgery. This antrostomy is usually limited to adults because of the unerupted teeth in children.

Cardiopulmonary bypass — Venous blood is diverted to a heart-lung machine, which mechanically pumps and oxygenates the blood temporarily so that the heart can be bypassed while an open procedure on the heart or coronary arteries is performed. During bypass, the lungs are deflated and immobile.

Cardioverter-defibrillator — A cardioverter-defibrillator device uses both low energy cardioversion or defibrillating shocks and antitachycardia pacing to treat ventricular tachycardia or ventricular fibrillation. It may be either a single or dual chamber device. Cardioverter-defibrillators may require the placement of multiple leads even for single chamber devices.

Care plan oversight services — The term describes the services of a physician providing ongoing review and revision of a patient's care plan involving complex or multidisciplinary care modalities. Care plan oversight services are reported separately from any necessary office/outpatient, hospital, home, nursing facility, or domiciliary services.

Case management services — Physician case management is a process of involving direct patient care as well as coordinating and controlling access to the patient or initiating and/or supervising other necessary health care services.

Cataract extraction — The most common surgical procedure performed on adults. Most ophthalmologists perform cataract surgery in an ambulatory surgical setting. Anterior chamber lenses are inserted in conjunction with intracapsular cataract extraction and posterior chamber lenses are inserted in conjunction with extracapsular cataract extraction.

Certified nurse midwife — The term means a registered nurse who has successfully completed a program of study and clinical experience or has been certified by a recognized organization.

Cervical cap — Cervical cap is similar in form and function to the diaphragm, however, it can be left in place for up to 48 hours.

Cervical intraepithelial neoplasia — This classification system is used to report abnormalities in the epithelial cell:

* CIN I. Cervical intraepithelial neoplasia I; low-grade abnormality; mild dysplasia

* CIN II. Cervical intraepithelial neoplasia II; high-grade abnormality; moderate dysplasia

* CIN III. Cervical intraepithelial neoplasia III; carcinoma in situ; severe dysplasia

Choanal atresia — A potentially dangerous congenital defect. Infants unable to breathe through their noses cannot feed properly and have difficulty keeping their air passages clear.

Cholecystectomy — The removal of the gallbladder and its contents is the most common major operation in the United States, and performed as the definitive treatment for gallstones.

Chorionic villi sampling — Chorionic villi sampling provides a rich source of fetal genetic information. Obtained between the eighth week and the twelfth week of gestation, it can provide information to diagnose some enzymatic defects.

Chronic pain management services — The term describes distinct services frequently performed by anesthesiologists who have additional training in pain management procedures. Pain management services include initial and subsequent evaluation and management (E/M) services, trigger point injections, spine and spinal cord injections, and nerve blocks.

Cineplastic amputation — This type of amputation may also be referred to as a cinematic amputation or a kineplasty procedure. In this type of amputation, the muscles and tendons of the remaining portion of the extremity are arranged so that they may be utilized for motor functions. Following this type of amputation, a specially constructed prosthetic device allows the individual to execute more complex movements because the muscles and tendons are able to communicate independent movements to the device.

Circadian — Refers to the 24 hour period.

Classification of surgical wound — Surgical wounds fall into four categories that determine methods of treatment and outcomes:

* Clean wound. No inflammation and procedure performed under sterile operating room conditions with no break in sterile technique. No alimentary, respiratory, oropharyngeal, or genitourinary tracts are involved in the surgery. Infection rate: up to 5 percent.

* Clean-contaminated wound. No inflammation and procedure performed with minor break in surgical technique. No unusual contamination found in alimentary, respiratory, genitourinary, or oropharyngeal cavity entered. Infection rate: up to 11 percent.

* Contaminated wound. Acute nonpurulent inflammation noted and procedure performed with major break in surgical technique. Open wound less than four hours old. Gross contamination from gastrointestinal tract. Infection rate: up to 20 percent.

* Dirty and infected wound. Existing infection and inflammation prior to surgery in a dirty traumatic wound more than four hours old, or an old abscess and/or existing surgical infection. In either case abscess, and nonsterile conditions were present. Wound older than four hours. Perforated viscus, fecal contamination, necrotic tissue, or foreign body may be present. Infection rate: up to 40 percent.

Clinical social worker — The term means an individual who possesses a master's or doctor's degree in social work and, after obtaining the degree, has performed at least two years of supervised clinical social work. A clinical social worker must be licensed by the state or, in the case of states without licensure, must completed at least two years or 3,000 hours of post-master's

degree supervised clinical social work practice under the supervision of a master's level social worker.

CO2 laser — A carbon dioxide laser that emits an invisible beam and vaporizes water-rich tissue. The vapor is suctioned from the site.

Colorectal cancer screening tests — The term means any of the following procedures furnished to an individual for the purpose of early detection of colorectal cancer:

* Screening fecal-occult blood test

* Screening flexible sigmoidoscopy

* In the case of an individual at high risk for colorectal cancer, screening colonoscopy

* Other tests or procedures, and modifications to tests and procedures, with such frequency and payment limits

* Individuals are considered at high risk for colorectal cancer because of family history, prior experience of cancer or precursor neoplastic polyps, history of chronic digestive disease condition (i.e., inflammatory bowel disease, Crohn's Disease, or ulcerative colitis), or the presence of any appropriate recognized gene markers for colorectal cancer.

Colostomy — Artificial surgical opening anywhere along the length of the colon to the skin surface for the diversion of feces.

Colpocleisis — Vaginal canal closure.

Commissurotomy — Surgical division or opening of a band of fibrous tissue.

Community mental health center, partial hospitalization services — The term means the services prescribed and supervised by a physician pursuant to an individualized, written plan of treatment that sets forth the diagnosis and the type, amount, frequency, and duration of care for a patient in a community mental health center. Services must be reasonable and necessary for the diagnosis or active treatment of the individual's condition and to prevent relapse or hospitalization. The items and services include the following:

* Individual and group therapy with physicians, psychologists, or other mental health professionals

* Occupational therapy requiring the skills of a qualified occupational therapist

* Services of social workers, trained psychiatric nurses, and other staff trained to work with psychiatric patients

* Drugs and biologicals for therapeutic purposes that cannot be self-administered)

* Individualized activity therapies that are not primarily recreational or diversionary

* Family counseling

* Patient training and education

* Diagnostic services, and

* Other items and services, excluding meals and transportation

Comprehensive outpatient rehabilitation facility (CORF) — The term describes a facility that provides (by or under the supervision of physicians) diagnostic, therapeutic, and restorative services to outpatients. Patients must be under the supervision of a physician and the facility must maintain the medical record of each patient. The following items and services provided by a physician or other qualified professional to an outpatient of a comprehensive outpatient rehabilitation facility under a plan established and periodically reviewed by a physician:

* Physicians' services

* Physical therapy, occupational therapy, speech-language pathology services, and respiratory therapy

* Prosthetic and orthotic devices, including testing, fitting, or training in the use of prosthetic and orthotic devices

* Social and psychological services

* Nursing care provided by or under the supervision of a registered professional nurse

* Drugs and biologicals that cannot be self-administered

* Supplies and durable medical equipment

- Other supplies and services necessary for the rehabilitation of the patient that are ordinarily available through the CORF

A CORF must provide a surety bond in an amount that is not less than $50,000 to ensure the efficiency and effectiveness of its programs.

Conjunctivodacryocystostomy — Surgical connection of the lacrimal sac directly to the conjunctival sac.

Computerized corneal topography — Digital imaging and analysis by computer of the shape of the corneal.

Conjunctivorhinostomy — Correction of an obstruction of the lacrimal canal

Consultations — The term describes consulting services provided at the request of another physician or other appropriate source for the purpose of rendering an opinion or advice regarding the evaluation and management of a specific problem. Consultations in CPT fall under four subcategories: office or other outpatient consultations, initial inpatient consultations, follow-up inpatient consultations, and confirmatory consultations.

Costochondral — Pertains to the ribs and the scapula.

Covered osteoporosis drug — The term means an injectable drug approved for the treatment of post-menopausal osteoporosis provided to an individual by a home health agency if the individual's attending physician certifies that the individual has suffered a bone fracture related to post-menopausal osteoporosis. The individual must be unable to learn the skills needed to self-administer such drug or is otherwise physically or mentally incapable of self-administering the drug and be confined to home.

Core needle biopsy — A large-bore biopsy needle is inserted into a mass and a core of tissue is removed for diagnostic study.

Craterization — Excision of a portion of bone to create a crater-like depression to facilitate drainage from infected areas of bone.

Cricoid — The circular cartilage around the trachea.

Cryolathe — Tool for reshaping a button of corneal tissue.

Cryosurgery — Local freezing of diseased tissue without causing harm to adjacent tissue. The cold causes tissue necrosis. Frozen tissue may be removed without significant bleeding during the surgical procedure, even in highly vascular tissue. Liquid nitrogen is the most commonly used source for the cold.

Cutdown — The technique of creating a small, incised opening for venipuncture.

Cytogenetic studies — The term refers to the procedures in CPT 2001 that are related to the branch of genetics that studies cellular (cyto) structure and function as it relates to heredity (genetics). White blood cells, specifically T-lymphocytes, are the most commonly used specimen for chromosome analysis.

Dacryocystorhinostomy — Performed by suturing the posterior flaps while the lacrimal obstruction is removed, preserving the conjunctiva.

Dacryocystotome — Instrument for incising lacrimal duct strictures, also spelled dacryocystitome.

Dacryorhinocystostomy — Synonym to dacryocystorhinostomy.

Debride — Procedure involves the removal of all foreign objects and damaged tissue from a burn or a wound to prevent infection and promote healing.

Dermis graft — Skin graft that has been separated from the epidermal tissue and the underlying subcutaneous fat. Used primarily as a substitute for fascia grafts in plastic surgery.

Desensitization — Administration of extracts of allergens periodically to build immunity in the patient.

Destruction — The term describes the ablation of benign, premalignant, or malignant tissue by any of the following methods used alone or in combination: electrosurgery, cryosurgery, laser, and chemical treatment.

Diabetes outpatient self-management training services — The term means educational and training services furnished by a certified provider in an outpatient setting. The physician managing the individual's diabetic condition must certify that the services are needed under a comprehensive plan of care provide the patient with the skills and knowledge necessary for therapeutic program compliance (including skills related to the self-administration of injectable drugs). The provider must meet applicable standards established by the National Diabetes Advisory or be recognized by an organization that represents individuals with diabetes as meeting standards for furnishing the services.

Diagnostic procedures — Terms describes the procedures performed to evaluate the patient's complaints or symptoms. These procedures help the physician establish the nature of the patient's disease or condition so that definitive care can be provided. Diagnostic procedures include endoscopy, arthroscopy, injection procedures, and biopsies.

Diaphragm — Flexible, dome-shaped rubber cap that fits over the cervix and acts as a barrier to sperm. It must be used in conjunction with spermicidal cream or jelly. It is generally left in place for eight hours after coitus.

Diaphysectomy — Partial removal of a portion of bone, usually a portion of the shaft of a long bone, to facilitate drainage from infected bone.

Diathermy — Heating of tissue using microwave radiation, ultrasound, or electric currents.

Dilation — Artificial increase in the diameter of an opening made by medication or by instrumentation.

Discharge planning process — The term defines a plan applicable to services furnished by the hospital to individuals entitled to medical benefits. Upon the request of a patient's physician, the hospital must arrange for the development and initial implementation of a discharge plan for the patient. The discharge planning evaluation must be included in the patient's medical record for use in establishing an appropriate discharge plan and the results of the evaluation must be discussed with the patient or the patient's representative). Plan guidelines and standards should address the following:

- Patients who are likely to suffer adverse health consequences upon discharge in the absence of adequate discharge planning and patients, their physicians, and their representatives requesting a discharge plan

- Appropriate arrangements for post-hospital care made before discharge and to avoid unnecessary delays in discharge

- An evaluation of a patient's likely need for appropriate post-hospital services, including hospice services and the availability of those services, including the availability of home health services

Dissect — A scalpel, a probe, or scissors is used to cut apart tissues for visual or microscopic study.

Dorsal — Pertaining to the back or posterior aspect.

Drugs and biologicals — The term covers drugs and biologicals included - or approved for inclusion - in the United States Pharmacopoeia, the National Formulary, the United States Homeopathic Pharmacopoeia, in New Drugs or Accepted Dental Remedies, or approved by the pharmacy and drug therapeutics committee of the medical staff of the hospital. Drugs also include those used in an anticancer chemotherapeutic regimen for a medically accepted approved by the FDA. The carrier determines medical acceptance based on supportive clinical evidence.

Durable medical equipment (DME) — The term includes iron lungs, oxygen tents, hospital beds, and wheelchairs used in the patient's home, including an institution considered the patient's home. DME also blood-testing strips and blood glucose monitors for individuals with diabetes without regard to Type I or Type II diabetes or use of insulin.

DuToit staple capsulorrhaphy — Reattachment of the capsule and glenoid labrum to the glenoid lip using staples to anchor the avulsed capsule and glenoid labrum.

Eden-Hybinette — This anterior repair utilizes an anterior bone block to augment the bony anterior glenoid lip.

EDTA — Drug used to inhibit damage to the cornea by collagenase. EDTA is especially effective in alkali burns as it neutralizes soluable alkali, including lye.

Effusion — Escape of fluid from within a body cavity.

Electrocautery — Destruction of tissue using high-frequency electrical current. The current produces heat, which destroys cells.

Emergency — A serious medical condition or symptom (including severe pain) resulting from injury, sickness, or mental illness that arises suddenly and requires immediate care and treatment, generally received within 24 hours of onset, to avoid jeopardy to the life, limb, or health of a covered person.

Endarterectomy — Removal of the endothelial lining of a diseased or damaged artery.

Epiphysiodesis — Surgical fusion of an epiphysis performed to prematurely stop further bone growth.

Escharotomy — Removal of the scab caused by the burn, which is constricting blood flow. The procedure allows the edges to separate and restore blood flow to the unburned tissues.

Established patient — Evaluation and Management guidelines define an established patient as one who has received professional services from the physician, or another physician of the same specialty who belongs to the same group practice, within the past three years.

Exenteration — Radical excision of the contents of a body cavity (e.g., orbit).

Extended care services — The term defines the items and services provided to an inpatient of a skilled nursing facility, including nursing care, physical or occupational therapy, speech pathology, drugs and supplies, and medical social services.

External electrical capacitor device — External electrical stimulation device designed to promote bone healing. This device may also promote neural regeneration, revascularization, epiphyseal growth, and ligament maturation.

External pulsating electromagnetic field — External stimulation device designed to promote bone healing. This device may also promote neural regeneration, revascularization, epiphyseal growth, and ligament maturation.

Evaluation and management (E/M) codes — E/M codes encompass services that are part of the 99000 series of CPT codes and represent the services most frequently performed by physicians (e.g., office, emergency department, inpatient visits).

Evaluation and management service components — The components of history, examination, and medical decision making are keys to selecting the correct E/M codes. In most cases, all three components must be addressed in the documentation. However, in established, subsequent, and follow-up categories, only two of the three must be met or exceeded for a given code.

Eyre-Brook capsulorrhaphy — Reattachment of the capsule and glenoid labrum to the glenoid lip.

Fascia — The fibrous tissue that envelopes the muscle.

Fasciectomy — Surgical incision through the fascia.

Fasciotomy — Excision of the fascia or strips of fascial tissue.

Fat graft — A graft composed of fatty tissue completely freed from surrounding tissue. Used primarily to fill in depressions.

Fine needle aspiration (FNA) — A 22- or through 25-gauge needle attached to a syringe is inserted into a lesion/tissue and a few cells are aspirated for diagnostic study. Aspiration is also used to remove fluid from a benign cyst.

Fluoroscopy — Radiology technique that allows visual examination of part of the body or a function of an organ using a device that projects an x-ray image on a fluorescent screen.

Focal length — Distance between the object in focus and the lens.

Free flap — Tissue that is completely detached from the donor site and reattached to the recipient site. It receives its blood supply from capillary ingrowth at the recipient site.

Free microvascular flap — Tissue that is completely detached from the donor site following careful dissection and preservation of the blood vessels. The tissue is attached to the recipient site and the transfered blood vessels are anastomosed to vessels in the recipient site.

Fulguration — Destruction of living tissue by sparks from electric current.

Gas tamponade — Absorbable gas may be injected to force the retina against the choroid. Common gases include room air, short-acting sulfahexafluoride, intermediate-acting perfluoroethane, or long-acting perfluorooctane.

Hemilaminectomy — Excision of the right or left lamina.

Hemoperitoneum — The effusion of blood into the peritoneal cavity.

Heterologous transplant — Nonhuman biotissue transplanted into the patient.

Heterotopic transplant — Tissue transplanted from a different anatomical site for usage as is natural for that tissue, for example, buccal mucosa to a conjunctival site.

Home health agency — The term means a public agency or private organization providing skilled nursing services and other therapeutic services. Home health agencies receiving federal funds must have policies governing it services and the medical services of a physician or registered professional nurse. According to law, home health agencies must maintain clinical reports of all patients. Provisions of the Balanced Budget Act of 1997, home health agencies must provide, on a continuing basis, surety bonds of $50,000 to guarantee the efficient and effective operation of the agency. The term home health agency does not include any agency or organization that is primarily for the care and treatment of mental diseases.

Home health services — The term encompasses the items and services a home health agency provides to an individual, according to a plan developed and reviewed by the patient's physician. Services may include:

- Part-time or intermittent nursing care provided by or under the supervision of a registered professional nurse
- Physical or occupational therapy or speech-language pathology services
- Medical social services under the direction of a physician
- Part-time or intermittent services of a home health aide who has successfully completed a training program
- Medical supplies (including catheters, catheter supplies, ostomy bags, and supplies related to ostomy care, and a covered osteoporosis drug and durable medical equipment
- Medical services provided by an intern or resident-in-training of a hospital affiliated with the home health agency

Homogenous transplant (homograft) — Tissue from another human transplanted to the patient. For bone transplants, the tissue is usually obtained from a cadaver.

Hospice care — The term specifies the following items and services provided to a terminally ill individual by a hospice program under a written plan established and periodically reviewed by the individual's attending physician and by the medical director:

- Nursing care provided by or under the supervision of a registered professional nurse
- Physical or occupational therapy or speech-language pathology services
- Medical social services under the direction of a physician
- Services of a home health aide who has successfully completed a training program
- Medical supplies (including drugs and biologicals) and the use of medical appliances
- Physicians' services
- Short-term inpatient care (including both respite care and procedures necessary for pain control and acute and chronic symptom management) in an inpatient facility on an intermittent basis and not consecutively over longer than five days
- Counseling (including dietary counseling) with respect to care of the terminally ill individual and adjustment to his death
- Any item or service which is specified in the plan and for which payment may be made

Hospice program — An Hospice program establishes the care and service plan and ensures that the services are available (as needed) on a 24-hour basis and also provides bereavement counseling for the immediate family of terminally ill individuals. The services may be delivered in an individual's home, on an outpatient basis, and on a short-term inpatient basis, directly or under arrangements made by the agency or organization. The Hospice agency is responsible for all services in an aggregate number of days of inpatient care provided in any 12-month period, as overseen by an interdisciplinary group of personnel that includes at least one physician, one registered professional nurse, and one social worker. A central clinical record must be maintained for each patient.

According to federal law, an Hospice cannot discontinue its services with respect to a patient because of the inability of the patient to pay for care. Volunteers may provide care and services as long as the program maintains records on the cost savings and expansion of care and services achieved through volunteers.

Hospital — The term means an institution that provides, under the supervision of physicians, diagnostic, therapeutic, and rehabilitation services for medical diagnosis, treatment, and care of patients. Hospitals receiving federal funds must maintain clinical records on all patients, provides 24-hour nursing services, and have a discharge planning process in place. The term "hospital" also includes religious nonmedical health care institutions and facilities of 50 beds or less located in rural areas.

Ileostomy — Proximal end of transected ileum is brought out through the peritoneum and muscle of the abdominal wall to the skin. Liquid or semisolid discharge is collected in a bag over the stoma.

Infundibulectomy — Excision of the anterosuperior portion of the right ventricle of the heart.

Institutional planning — The terms describes the overall plan and budget of a hospital, skilled nursing facility, comprehensive outpatient rehabilitation facility, or home health agency. Plans must be prepared by a governing and submitted to the state health agency. Plans must include:

• An annual operating budget

• A capital expenditures plan for at least a three-year period

Internal direct current stimulator — Electrostimulation device designed to promote bone regeneration by encouraging cellular response in bone and ligaments. It is placed directly into the surgical site.

Intramedullary implants — An intramedullary nail, rod, or pin is placed into the intramedullary canal at the fracture site. Intramedullary implants not only provide a method of aligning the fracture, they also act as a splint and may reduce fracture pain. Implants may be rigid or flexible. Rigid implants are preferred for prophylactic treatment of diseased bone, while flexible implants are preferred for traumatic injuries.

Irrigation — To wash out or cleanse a body cavity wound with water or other fluid.

Jatene procedure — This corrective measure for transposition of the great vessels is used when subaortic stenosis and narrowing of the left aortic ventricular junction are present requiring reconstruction of these sites as well as surgical correction of the transposed aortic and pulmonary arteries. This technique may be used in cases where the transposition is accompanied by a ventricular septal defect or a large patent ductus arteriosus.

Krypton laser — Because the krypton spectrum (red-yellow) is poorly absorbed by hemoglobin, it can be used effectively to treat retinal bleeding, macular lesions, and vessel aberrations of the choroid.

Lacrimal punctum — The opening of the lacrimal papilla of the eyelid through which tears flow to the canaliculi to the lacrimal sac.

Lacrimotome — Knife for cutting the lacrimal sac or duct.

Lacrimotomy — Incision of the lacrimal sac or duct.

Larynx — The larynx is the air passage of the neck area, serving as the voice mechanism as well as the valve to prevent food and other particles from entering the respiratory tract. The larynx is composed of three single cartilages: cricoid, epiglottis, and thyroid; and three paired cartilages: arytenoid, corniculate, and cuneiform.

Laser surgery — Laser beams deliver a sharply defined burn, and the color and wavelength of the laser determines which tissues it can best treat. The argon laser is effective in coagulating blood-rich tissue with heat. CO2 lasers are used to vaporize tissue. Potassium titanyl phosphate (KTP) lasers coagulate tissues. Nd:YAG lasers cut and cauterize.

LEEP — Loop electrosurgical excision prcedure. This uses a stainless steel or tungsten loop electrode to excise a central core of cervical tissue. This is a therapeutic technique for treatment of premalignant lesions in women of child-bearing age, since future childbearing is unaffected.

Levonorgestrel — Drug inhibiting ovulation and preventing sperm from penetrating cervical mucus. It is delivered subcutaneously in polysiloxone capsules. The capsules can be effective for up to five years, and provide a cumulative pregnancy rate of less than 2 percent. The capsules are not biodegradable, and therefore must be removed. Removal is more difficult than insertion of levonorgestrel capsules because fibrosis develops around the capsules. Normal hormonal activity and a return to fertility begins immediately upon removal.

Ligation — This procedure involves tying off a blood vessel or duct with a suture or a soft, thin wire (ligature wire).

Magnuson-Stack procedure — Recurrent anterior dislocation is treated by tightening and realigning the subscapularis tendon.

Marsupialization — Suturing of cyst walls to the edge of a wound, following evacuation of the wound, so cavity may close by granulation.

Mastectomy — The surgical removal of one or both breasts and is most often performed to remove a malignant tumor. The types of mastectomy include:

• Radical. The breast, all lymph nodes in the axilla, and some muscles of the chest wall are removed.

• Modified radical. The large muscles of the chest that move the arm are preserved.

• Simple. Only breast tissue, nipple, and a small portion of overlying skin are removed.

McDonald procedure — Polyester tape is placed around the cervix with a running stitch to assist in the prevention of pre-term delivery. Tape is removed at term for vaginal delivery.

Mitral valve — The mitral valve is located between the left atrium and left ventricle of the heart. It has two cusps and is, therefore, frequently referred to as the bicuspid valve.

Mohs micrographic surgery — This is a special technique used to treat complex or ill-defined skin cancer and requires a single physician to provide two distinct services. The first service is surgical and involves the destruction of the lesion by a combination of chemosurgery and excision. The second service is that of a pathologist and includes mapping, color coding of specimens, microscopic examination of specimens, and complete histopathologic preparation.

Mustard procedure — This corrective measure for transposition of great vessels involves an intra-atrial baffle made of pericardial tissue or synthetic material. The baffle is secured between pulmonary veins and mitral valve and between mitral and tricuspid valves. The baffle directs systemic venous flow into the left ventricle and lungs and pulmonary venous flow into the right ventricle and aorta.

Myasthenia gravis — Neuromuscular disorder with symptoms of fatigue and exhaustion with fluctuating severity.

Myotomy — Cutting of a muscle to gain access to underlying tissues or to relieve constriction in a sphincter.

Nasal polyps — Polyps usually are bilateral, but they can be unilateral. Polyps, soft, edematous growths, project from nasal or sinus mucosa and may obstruct the posterior choanae. In addition to obstructing ventilation, they may affect the sense of smell if the olfactory epithelium is blocked. The KTP laser or the CO2 laser is sometimes used in reducing or eliminating polyps.

Nasal sinus — The nasal sinuses are air-filled cavities in the crainal bones that earn their names; all are lined with mucous membrane continuous with the nasal cavity and all drain fluids into the nasal cavity. The ethmoid cells vary in size and number and feature very thin septa, or walls. The maxillary sinuses are the largest and are the most frequently infected.

Nasopharynx — The nasopharynx is the membranous passage above the level of the soft palate; the oropharynx is the region between the soft palate and the edge of the epiglottis; the hypopharynx is the region of the epiglottis to the juncture of the larynx and esophagus; the three regions collectively are called the pharynx.

Nd:YAG laser — Invisible pulsed neodyminum is used for cataract extraction and lysis of vitreous strands. The light used by the Nd:YAG laser does not require the tissues that are being treated to be pigmented.

Neurectomy — The removal of part of a nerve.

New patient — Evaluation and Management guidelines define a new patient as one who has not received any professional services from the physician, or another physician of the same specialty who belongs to the same group practice, within the past three years.

Nissen fundoplasty — Fundus of the stomach is wrapped around the lower end of the esophagus to treat reflux esophagitis.

Nonabsorbable sutures — Strands of natural or synthetic material that resist absorption into living tissue. Skin is usually closed with nonabsorbable sutures. Examples include surgical silk, surgical cotton, linen, stainless steel, surgical nylon, polyester fiber, polybutester (Novafil), polyethylene (Dermalene), and polypropylene (Prolene, Surilene).

Nystagmus — Uncontrolled rapid movement of the eye.

Oophorectomy — Removal of ovary.

Outpatient physical therapy services — The term means the physical therapy services provided to an outpatient of a clinic, rehabilitation agency, or public health agency. The attending physician must establish a plan of physical therapy or periodically review a plan developed by a qualified physical therapist. A group of professional personnel, including one or more physicians (associated with the clinic or rehabilitation agency) and one or more qualified physical therapists must govern services and maintain clinical records of all patients. Outpatient clinics must provide a surety bond of $50,000 to guarantee the efficiency and effectiveness of programs. The term outpatient physical therapy services also includes physical therapy services provided by a physical therapist in office or at the patient's home and speech-language pathology services.

Pacemaker — A pacemaker device is used to artificially stimulate the heart muscle by the use of electric impulses that aid in maintaining normal sinus rhythm.

Paratenon graft — A graft composed of the fatty tissue found between a tendon and its sheath.

Pedicle flap — Tissue that remains partially attached to the donor site by a pedicle or stem. The blood supply is provided by vessels that remain intact in the pedicle or stem of the flap.

Percutaneous intradiscal electrothermal annuloplasty — This procedure corrects tears in the vertebral annulus by applying heat to the collagen disc walls percutaneously through a catheter. The heat contracts and thickens the wall which may contract and close any annular tears.

Percutaneous skeletal fixation — Treatment that is neither open nor closed. In this procedure, the injury site is not directly visualized. Instead fixation devices (pins, screws) are placed to stabilize the dislocation using x-ray guidance.

Percutaneous transluminal coronary angioplasty (PTCA) — The term describes the procedure used to treat coronary artery obstruction. A balloon catheter is placed in the affected artery and the balloon is inflated to flatten the plaque against the wall of the artery and open the obstruction.

Pericardium — The pericardium is the thin and slippery case in which the heart lies. It is lined with fluid so that the heart is free to pulse and move as it beats.

Physical status modifiers (anesthesia services) — Physical status modifiers reflect the patient's state of health. Individuals undergoing surgery may be healthy or may have varying degrees of systemic disease. A patient's health status affects the work related to providing the anesthesia service.

Pleurodesis — The production of adhesions between the parietal and visceral pleura.

Plication — Operation involving folding, shortening, or decreasing the size of a muscle or hollow organ by taking in tucks.

Potts-Smith-Gibson procedure — A side-to-side anastomosis of the aorta and left pulmonary artery creating a shunt that enlarges as the child grows.

Profunda — Denotes a part of a structure that is deeper from the surface of the body than the rest of the structure.

Prolonged physician services — Extended pre- or post-operative care provided to a patient whose condition requires services beyond the usual.

Prostate cancer screening tests — The term means a test that consists of any (or all) of the procedures provided for the early detection of prostate cancer to a man over 50 years of age who has not had a test during the preceding year. The procedures are as follows:

- A digital rectal examination
- A prostate-specific antigen blood test

After 2002, the list of procedures may be expanded as appropriate for the early detection of prostate cancer, taking into account changes in technology and standards of medical practice, availability, effectiveness, costs, and other factors.

Provider of services — The term means a hospital, critical access hospital, skilled nursing facility, comprehensive outpatient rehabilitation facility, home health agency, hospice program.

Psychiatric hospital — The term means an institution that provides, under the supervision of physicians, services for the diagnosis and treatment of mentally ill persons. Psychiatric hospitals receiving federal funds must maintain clinical records sufficient to determine the type of treatment provided to patients.

Pulmonary artery banding — In this palliative procedure for transposition of great vessels, the pulmonary artery is surgically constricted to prevent irreversible pulmonary vascular obstructive changes. Banding is often performed when a large ventricular septal defect is present.

Putti-Platt procedure — This procedure treats recurrent anterior dislocation by tightening and realigning the subscapularis tendon, thereby partially eliminating external rotation. The anterior capsule is also tightened and reinforced.

Pyloroplasty — Enlargement of the opening between the stomach and duodenum that may be performed in patients with an obstructing pyloric ulcer in combination with a vagotomy to treat bleeding duodenal ulcers.

Radiological examination — The term in CPT refers to plain films of specific sites. Other terms used to describe plain films include standard or conventional films. Services employing other modalities and additional techniques include the following:

- Computerized Axial Tomography (CT or CAT scan) is a type of imaging that employs basic tomographic technique enhanced by computer imaging. Computer enhancement synthesizes the images obtained from different directions in a given plane, effectively reconstructing a cross-sectional plane of the body.

- Computerized Tomography Angiography (CTA) provides multiple rapid thin section CT scans, a series of x-ray beams taken from different angles to create cross-sectional images of organs, bones, and tissues.

- Magnetic Resonance Imaging (MRI) involves the application of an external magnetic field that forces a uniform alignment of hydrogen atom nuclei in the soft tissue. The nuclei emit radiofrequency signals that are converted into sets of tomographic images and displayed on a computer screen for three-dimensional visualization of the soft tissue structure.

Rashkind procedure — A balloon catheter is inserted into the left atrium, inflated, and pulled across the septum to enlarge the foramen ovale, thus creating an atrial septal defect. This is a palliative procedure for transposition of great vessels.

Repair — Repair is the surgical closure of a wound. The wound may be a result of injury/trauma or it may be a surgically created defect. Repairs are divided into three categories: simple, intermediate, and complex. Simple repair is performed when the wound is superficial and only requires simple, one layer, primary suturing. Intermediate repair is performed for wounds and lacerations in which one or more of the deeper layers of subcutaneous tissue and non-muscle fascia are repaired in addition to the skin and subcutaneous tissue. Complex repair includes repair of wounds requiring more than layered closure. See also Wound repair.

Rhinophototherapy — The application of ultraviolet and visible light to the nasal cavity. The procedure is used as a treatment for allergic rhinitis as the light inhibits histamine release and induces apoptosis in the nasal cells.

Rural health clinic — The term defines a clinic in an area where there is a shortage of health services. The clinic must provide routine diagnostic services, including clinical laboratory services and have prompt access to additional diagnostic services from facilities meeting requirements (i.e., agreements with one or more hospitals for the referral and admission of patients requiring inpatient, diagnostic, or other specialized services not available at the clinic). In addition, the clinic must be able to administer drugs and biologicals as necessary for the treatment of emergency cases and have appropriate procedures or arrangements for storing, administering, and dispensing any drugs and biologicals. Staff must include a nurse practitioner, a physician assistant, or a certified nurse-midwife available for patient care not less than 50 percent of the time the clinic operates. In the case of a facility that is not a physician-directed clinic, there must be an arrangement with one or more physicians for the periodic review of covered services furnished by physician assistants and nurse practitioners.

Saucerization — Creation of a shallow, saucer-like depression in the bone to facilitate drainage from infected areas of bone.

Schiotz tonometer — Measures intraocular pressure by recording the depth of an indentation on the cornea by a plunger of known weight. The degree of indentation is calibrated on the tonometer to correspond to the intraocular pressure.

Screening mammography — The term means a radiologic procedure provided to a woman for the purpose of early detection of breast cancer and includes a physician's interpretation of the results of the procedure.

Screening pap smear; screening pelvic exam — The term means a diagnostic laboratory test consisting of a routine exfoliative cytology test (Papanicolaou test) provided to a woman for the purpose of early detection of cervical or vaginal cancer. The exam includes a clinical breast examination and a physician's interpretation of the results. Coverage depends on several factors, including the results of an exam during the preceding three years that indicated the presence of cervical or vaginal cancer or other abnormality or is at high risk of developing cervical or vaginal cancer.

Senning procedure — Flaps of intra-atrial septum and right atrial wall are used to create two interatrial channels to divert the systemic and pulmonary venous circulation.

Sensitivity Tests — Describes a number of methods of applying selective suspected allergens to the skin or mucous.

Sensorineural conduction — The transportation of sound from the cochlea to the acoustic nerve and central auditory pathway to the brain.

Separate procedures — Term in CPT describes services that are commonly carried out as an integral part of a larger service, and as such do not warrant separate identification. These services are noted in CPT with the parenthetical phrase (separate procedure). When this phrase appears before the semicolon, all indented descriptions that follow are covered by it.

Shirodkar procedure — Mersilene tape is drawn around the internal os and tied. This requires a small incision in the vaginal mucosa and usually predicates cesarean section.

Sinus of valsalva — Small cavity in the aorta just superior to the aortic valve. It is the origin of the coronary arteries. This area may also be referred to as the aortic sinus.

Speech-language pathology services; audiology services — The term means such speech, language, and related function assessment and rehabilitation services furnished by a qualified speech-language pathologist. Audiology services include hearing and balance assessment services furnished by a qualified audiologist. A qualified speech pathologist and audiologist must have a master's or doctoral degree in their respective fields and be licensed to serve in the state. Speech pathologists and audiologists practicing in states without licensure must complete 350 hours of supervised clinical work and perform at least nine months of supervised full-time service after earning their degrees.

Speech prosthetics — Electronic speech aids are covered by Medicare under Part B as prosthetic devices when the patient has had a laryngectomy. One operates by placing a vibrating head against the throat; the other amplifies sound waves through a tube which is inserted into the user's mouth.

Sphinteroplasty — Plastic surgery done to correct, augment, or improve the function of the muscular sphincter fibers founds in organs such as the anus or intestines.

Spirometry — Measurement of the lungs' breathing capacity.

Staghorn calculus — A concretion of the renal pelvis that often fills several calices.

Surgical package — The majority of the CPT surgical codes are "package" services; they include the actual surgical procedure, local infiltration, metacarpal and digital block or topical anesthesia (when used), and the normal, uncomplicated postoperative care.

Suture — There are numerous suturing techniques employed in wound closure. Among these are:

- Buried suture. A suture placed under the skin for a layered closure. It may be continuous or interrupted.

- Continuous suture. A running stitch with tension evenly distributed across the single strand so that it provides a leak proof suture line.

- Interrupted suture. A series of single stitches with tension isolated at each stitch. If one stitch loosens, the others may not be affected, and in the presence of infection, the isolated sutures cannot act as a wick to transport the infection.

- Purse-string suture. A continuous suture placed around a lumen and tightened to reduce or close the lumen.

- Retention suture. A secondary suture bridging the primary suture. Functionally, it provides support to the primary repair. A plastic or rubber bolster may be placed over the primary repair and under the retention sutures.

Tarsocheiloplasty — Plastic operation upon the edge of the eyelid for the treatment of trichiasis.

Tarsorrhaphy — Suture of a portion or all of the opposing eyelids for the purpose of shortening the palpebral fissure, or closing it entirely. External tarsorrhaphy involves the suture of the outer edges of the eyelid margins; median tarsorraphy involves the middle eyelid margins; and internal tarsorrhaphy involves the inner eyelid margins.

Tendon allograft — Allografts are tissues obtained from another individual of the same species. Tendon allografts are usually obtained from cadavers and frozen or freeze dried for later use in soft tissue repairs where the physician elects not to obtain an autogenous graft (a graft obtained from the individual on whom the surgery is being performed).

Tendon suture material — Tendons are composed of fibrous tissue consisting primarily of collagen and containing few cells or blood vessels. This tissue heals more slowly than tissues with more vascularization. Because of this, tendons are usually repaired with nonabsorbable suture material. Examples include surgical silk, surgical cotton, linen, stainless steel, surgical nylon, polyester fiber, polybutester (Novafil), polyethylene (Dermalene), and polypropylene (Prolene, Surilene).

Tenon's capsule — Connective tissue that forms the capsule enclosing the posterior eyeball, extending from the conjunctival fornix and continuous with the muscular fascia of the eye, also called the bulbar fascia, capusula bulbi, bulbar sheath, Bonnet's ocular, or sheath of eyeball.

Tensilon — Edrophonium chloride. An agent used for evaluation and treatment of myasthenia gravis.

Terminally Ill — An individual is considered to be "terminally ill" if the medical prognosis for life expectancy is six months or less.

Tetralogy of Fallot — A combination of congenital cardiac defects that include interventricular defect, pulmonary stenosis, right ventricular hypertrophy, and malpositioning of the aorta so that it receives venous as well as arterial blood.

Therapeutic Services — Term describes the procedures performed for treatment of a specific diagnosis. These services include performance of the procedure, various incidental elements, and normal, related follow-up care.

Thoracentesis — Using a needle to perforate the chest wall and pleural space for the aspiration of fluid for diagnostic or therapeutic purposes, or for biopsy.

Thoracic lymphadenectomy — Procedure to cut out the lymph nodes near the lungs, around the heart, and behind the trachea.

Thoracostomy — Making an incision into the chest wall to provide an opening for drainage.

Thyroglossal duct — An embryonic duct through which the thyroid gland descends during fetal development. The duct may form a cyst or sinus in adulthood. It is found at the front of the neck, within the hyoid bone.

Total disc arthroplasty with artificial disc — This procedure consists of the removal of an intravertebral disc and its replacement with an implant. The implant is an artificial disc consisting of two metal plates with a weight-bearing surface of polyethylene between the plates. The plates are anchored to the vertebral immediately above and below the affected disc.

Total shoulder replacement — Prosthetic replacement of the entire shoulder joint, including the humeral head and the glenoid fossa.

Trabeculae carneae cordis — Bands of muscular tissue that line the walls of the ventricles in the heart.

Tracheostomy — Formation of a tracheal opening to create a path for respiration. This is performed to relieve obstruction or improve patency of an airway. This is generally a more long-term measure.

Tracheotomy — Incision into the trachea below the larynx. This may be a controlled procedure or an emergency procedure, but is generally considered a temporary measure.

Transcranial magnetic stimulation — This procedure is the application of electromagnetic energy to the brain through a coil placed on the scalp. The procedure stimulates cortical neurons and is intended to activate and normalize their processes.

Trephine — A saw for removing a circular disk of bone used on the skull.

Tricuspid atresia — Tricuspid atresia is the congenital absence of the valve and it may occur with other defects, such as atrial septal defect, pulmonary atresia, and transposition of great vessels.

Tympanic membrane — The tympanic membrane is a thin, sensitive tissue and is the gateway to the middle ear. The membrane vibrates in response to sound waves and the movement is transmitted via the ossicular chain to the internal ear. The tympanic membrane may be punctured and tympanum penetrated by objects placed in the ear canal or entering the canal accidentally.

Urodynamics — The term describes a diagnostic service performed to evaluate the storage of urine and urine flow through the urinary tract.

Vagotomy — Division of the vagus nerves in the treatment of chronic gastric, pyloric, and duodenal ulcers that can cause severe pain and difficulties in eating and sleeping. Procedure interrupts nerve impulses to lower gastric acid production and hastens gastric emptying.

Vasectomy — Male sterilization achieved through removal of a portion of the vas deferens (route spermatozoa must take).

VBAC — (Vaginal Birth After Cesarean) Denotes a successful vaginal delivery after a previous cesarean delivery.

Ventricular septal defect — In a large ventricular septal defect, oxygenated blood flows back into the lungs, causing pulmonary hypertension. Small defects may be asymptomatic, and treatment may be unnecessary.

Vertebral interspace — The non-bony space between two vertebral bodies containing the intervertebral disk. It includes the nucleus pulposus, annulus, fibrosus, and the two cartilagenous endplates.

Volar — Pertaining to the palm of the hand or sole of the foot. Also may refer to the flexor surface of the forearm, wrist, or hand.

Waterston procedure — Anastomosis of aorta and right pulmonary artery placed on the posterior aspect of the aorta.

Wharton's ducts — The salivary ducts below the mandible.

Wick catheter — A device used to monitor interstitial fluid pressure. It provides continuous measurement of interstitial fluid pressure. It may also be used intraoperatively during fasciotomy procedures to evaluate the effectiveness of the decompression.

Wound repair — Repairs in CPT are divided into three categories: simple, intermediate, and complex. They are further described by anatomic site and wound size.

- Simple repair is performed when the wound is superficial, e.g., involving partial or full-thickness damage to the skin and/or subcutaneous tissues. No deeper structures are involved and only simple, one layer, primary suturing is required. This procedure includes local anesthetic and chemical or electrocauterization of wounds not closed.

- Intermediate repair is performed for wounds and lacerations in which one or more of the deeper layers of subcutaneous tissue and non-muscle fascia are repaired in addition to the skin and subcutaneous tissue. Single-layer closure can also be coded as an intermediate repair if the wound is heavily contaminated and requires extensive cleaning or removal of particulate matter.

- Complex repair includes repair of wounds requiring more than layered closure. Wounds coded from this category include those requiring revision, debridement, extensive undermining, and placement of stents or retention sutures. Complex repairs also include those requiring creation of a defect (e.g., extending excision) and special preparation of the site.

Xenograft — Tissue obtained from an animal of another species. Other terms for xenograft include heterograft, heterologous graft, xenogeneic graft.

Z-plasty — A plastic surgery technique used primarily to release tension or elongate contracted scar tissue. A Z-shaped incision is made with the middle line of the Z crossing the area of greatest tension. The triangular flaps are then rotated so that they cross the incision line in the opposite direction creating a reversed Z.

APPENDIX F — ELECTRODIAGNOSTIC MEDICINE LISTING OF SENSORY, MOTOR, AND MIXED NERVES

This summary assigns each sensory, motor, and mixed nerve with its appropriate nerve conduction study code in order to enhance accurate reporting of codes 95900, 95903, and 95904. Each nerve constitutes one unit of service.

Motor Nerves Assigned to Codes 95900 and 95903.

I.   Upper extremity, cervical plexus, and brachial plexus motor nerves

   A.   Axillary motor nerve to the deltoid

   B.   Long thoracic motor nerve to the serratus anterior

   C.   Median nerve

      1.   Median motor nerve to the abductor pollicis brevis

      2.   Median motor nerve, anterior interosseous branch, to the flexor pollicis longus

      3.   Median motor nerve, anterior interosseous branch, to the pronator quadratus

      4.   Median motor nerve to the first lumbrical

      5.   Median motor nerve to the second lumbrical

   D.   Musculocutaneous motor nerve to the biceps brachii

   E.   Radial nerve

      1.   Radial motor nerve to the extensor carpi ulnaris

      2.   Radial motor nerve to the extensor digitorum communis

      3.   Radial motor nerve to the extensor indicis proprius

      4.   Radial motor nerve to the brachioradialis

   F.   Suprascapular nerve

      1.   Suprascapular motor nerve to the supraspinatus

      2.   Suprascapular motor nerve to the infraspinatus

   G.   Thoracodorsal motor nerve to the latissimus dorsi

   H.   Ulnar nerve

      1.   Ulnar motor nerve to the abductor digiti minimi

      2.   Ulnar motor nerve to the palmar interosseous

      3.   Ulnar motor nerve to the first dorsal interosseous

      4.   Ulnar motor nerve to the flexor carpi ulnaris

   I.   Other

II.   Lower extremity motor nerves

   A.   Femoral motor nerve to the quadriceps

      1.   Femoral motor nerve to the vastus medialis

      2.   Femoral motor nerve to vastus lateralis

      3.   Femoral motor nerve to vastus intermedialis

      4.   Femoral motor nerve to rectus femoris

   B.   Ilioinguinal motor nerve

   C.   Peroneal (fibular) nerve

      1.   Peroneal motor nerve to the extensor digitorum brevis

      2.   Peroneal motor nerve to the peroneus brevis

      3.   Peroneal motor nerve to the peroneus longus

      4.   Peroneal motor nerve to the tibialis anterior

   D.   Plantar motor nerve

   E.   Sciatic nerve

   F.   Tibial nerve

      1.   Tibial motor nerve, inferior calcaneal branch, to the abductor digiti minimi

      2.   Tibial motor nerve, medial plantar branch, to the abductor hallucis

      3.   Tibial motor nerve, lateral plantar branch, to the flexor digiti minimi brevis

   G.   Other

III.   Cranial nerves and trunk

   A.   Cranial nerve VII (facial motor nerve)

      1.   Facial nerve to the frontalis

      2.   Facial nerve to the nasalis

      3.   Facial nerve to the orbicularis oculi

      4.   Facial nerve to the orbicularis oris

   B.   Cranial nerve XI (spinal accessory motor nerve)

   C.   Cranial nerve XII (hypoglossal motor nerve)

   D.   Intercostal motor nerve

   E.   Phrenic motor nerve to the diaphragm

   F.   Recurrent laryngeal nerve

   G.   Other

IV.   Nerve Roots

   A.   Cervical nerve root stimulation

      1.   Cervical level 5 (CT)

      2.   Cervical level 6 (C6)

      3.   Cervical level 7 (C7)

      4.   Cervical level 8 (C8)

   B.   Thoracic nerve root stimulation

      1.   Thoracic level 1 (T1)

      2.   Thoracic level 2 (T2)

      3.   Thoracic level 3 (T3)

      4.   Thoracic level 4 (T4)

      5.   Thoracic level 5 (T5)

      6.   Thoracic level 6 (T6)

      7.   Thoracic level 7 (T7)

      8.   Thoracic level 8 (T8)

      9.   Thoracic level 9 (T9)

      10.   Thoracic level 10 (T10)

      11.   Thoracic level 11 (T11)

      12.   Thoracic level 12 (T12)

   C.   Lumbar nerve root stimulation

      1.   Lumbar level 1 (L1)

      2.   Lumbar level 2 (L2)

      3.   Lumbar level 3 (L3)

      4.   Lumbar level 4 (L4)

      5.   Lumbar level 5 (L5)

   D.   Sacral nerve root stimulation

      1.   Sacral level 1 (S1)

      2.   Sacral level 2 (S2)

      3.   Sacral level 3 (S3)

      4.   Sacral level 4 (S4)

SENSORY AND MIXED NERVES ASSIGNED TO CODE 95904

I.   Upper extremity sensory and mixed nerves

   A.   Lateral antebrachial cutaneous sensory nerve

B. Medial antebrachial cutaneous sensory nerve

C. Medial brachial cutaneous sensory nerve

D. Median nerve

    1. Median sensory nerve to the first digit

    2. Median sensory nerve to the second digit

    3. Median sensory nerve to the third digit

    4. Median sensory nerve to the fourth digit

    5. Median palmar cutaneous sensory nerve

    6. Median palmar mixed nerve

E. Posterior antebrachial cutaneous sensory nerve

F. Radial sensory nerve

    1. Radial sensory nerve to the base of the thumb

    2. Radial sensory nerve to digit 1

G. Ulnar nerve

    1. Ulnar dorsal cutaneous sensory nerve

    2. Ulnar sensory nerve to the fourth digit

    3. Ulnar sensory nerve to the fifth digit

    4. Ulnar palmar mixed nerve

H. Intercostal sensory nerve

I. Other

II. Lower extremity sensory and mixed nerves

A. Lateral femoral cutaneous sensory nerve

B. Medical calcaneal sensory nerve

C. Medial femoral cutaneous sensory nerve

D. Peroneal nerve

    1. Deep peroneal sensory nerve

    2. Superficial peroneal sensory nerve, medial dorsal cutaneous branch

    3. Superficial peroneal sensory nerve, intermediate dorsal cutaneous branch

E. Posterior femoral cutaneous sensory nerve

F. Saphenous nerve

    1. Saphenous sensory nerve (distal technique)

    2. Saphenous sensory nerve (proximal technique)

G. Sural nerve

    1. Sural sensory nerve, lateral dorsal cutaneous branch

    2. Sural sensory nerve

H. Tibial sensory nerve (digital nerve to toe 1)

I. Tibial sensory nerve (medial plantar nerve)

J. Tibial sensory nerve (lateral plantar nerve)

K. Other

III. Head and trunk sensory nerves

A. Dorsal nerve of the penis

B. Greater auricular nerve

C. Ophthalmic branch of the trigeminal nerve

D. Pudendal sensory nerve

E. Suprascapular sensory nerves

F. Other

The following table provides a reasonable maximum number of studies performed per diagnostic category necessary for a physician to arrive at a diagnosis in 90% of patients with that final diagnosis. The numbers in each column represent the number of studies recommended. The appropriate number of studies to be performed is based upon the physician's discretion.

| Indication | | Type of Study/Maximum Number of Studies | | | |
| | Needle EMG (95860-95864, 95867-95870) | Nerve Conduction Studies (95900, 95903, 95904) | | Other EMG Studies (95934, 95936, 95937) | |
		Motor NCS With and/or Without F wave	Sensory NCS	H-Reflex	Neuromuscular Junction Testing (Repetitive Stimulation)
Carpal Tunnel (Unilateral)	1	3	4	—	—
Carpal Tunnel (Bilateral)	2	4	6	—	—
Radiculopathy	2	3	2	2	—
Mononeuropathy	1	3	3	2	—
Polyneuropathy/Mononeuropathy Multiplex	3	4	4	2	—
Myopathy	2	2	2	—	2
Motor Neuronopathy (e.g., ALS)	4	4	2	—	2
Plexopathy	2	4	6	2	·
Neuromuscular Junction	2	2	2	—	3
Tarsal Tunnel Syndrome (Unilateral)	1	4	4	—	—
Tarsal Tunnel Syndrome (Bilateral)	2	5	6	—	—
Weakness, Fatigue, Cramps, or Twitching (Focal)	2	3	4	—	2
Weakness, Fatigue, Cramps, or Twitching (General)	4	4	4	—	2
Pain, Numbness, or Tingling (Unilateral)	1	3	4	2	—
Pain, Numbness, or Tingling (Bilateral)	2	4	6	2	—

APPENDIX G — VASCULAR FAMILIES

This table assumes that the starting point is catheterization of the aorta. This categorization would not be accurate, for instance, if a femoral or carotid artery were catheterized with the blood's flow.

First Order	Second Order Branch	Third Order Branch	Beyond Third Order Branches
Innominate	**Right Common Carotid**	**Right internal Carotid**	Right Ophthalmic Right Posterior Communicating Right Middle Cerebral Right Anterior Cerebral
		Right External Carotid	Right Superior Thyroid Right Ascending Pharyngeal Right Facial Right Lingual Right Occipital Right Posterior Auricular Right Superficial Temporal Right Internal Maxillary Right Middle Meningeal
	Right Subclavian and Axillary	**Right Vertebral** ———— Basilar	
		Right Internal Thoracic (Internal Mammary)	
		Right Thyrocervical Trunk	Right Inferior Thyroid Right Surascapular Right Transverse Cervical
		Right Costocervical Trunk	Right Highest Intercostal Right Deep Cervical
		Right Lateral Thoracic Right Thoracromial Right Humeral Circumflex (A/P)	
		Right Subcapular ———— Right Circumflex Scapular	
		Right Brachial	
		Right Deep Brachial	Right Ulnar Right Radial Right Interosseous Right Deep Palmar Arch Right Superficial Palmar Arch Right Metacarpals and Digitals
Left Common Carotid	**Left Internal Carotid**	Left Ophthalmic Left Posterior Communicating Left Middle Cerebral Left Anterior Cerebral	
	Left External Carotid	Left Superior Thyroid Left Ascending Pharyngeal Left Facial Left Lingual Left Occipital Left Posterior Auricular Left Superficial Temporal	
		Left Internal Maxillary ———— Left Middle Meningeal	

First Order	Second Order Branch	Third Order Branch	Beyond Third Order Branches

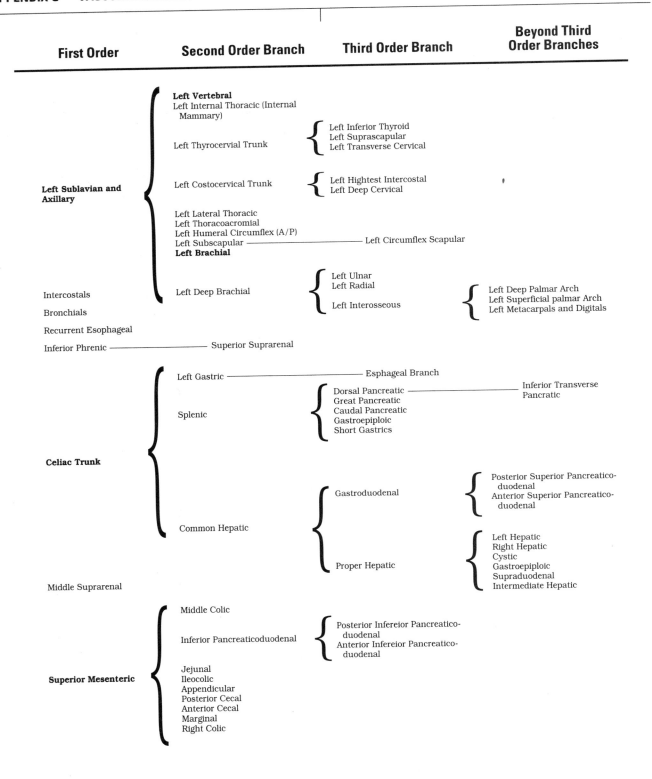

Left Sublavian and Axillary

Left Vertebral
Left Internal Thoracic (Internal Mammary)

Left Thyrocervial Trunk
{ Left Inferior Thyroid
Left Suprascapular
Left Transverse Cervical }

Left Costocervical Trunk
{ Left Hightest Intercostal
Left Deep Cervical }

Left Lateral Thoracic
Left Thoracoacromial
Left Humeral Circumflex (A/P)
Left Subscapular ——— Left Circumflex Scapular
Left Brachial

Intercostals

Bronchials

Recurrent Esophageal

Inferior Phrenic ——— Superior Suprarenal

Left Deep Brachial
{ Left Ulnar
Left Radial

Left Interosseous }
{ Left Deep Palmar Arch
Left Superficial palmar Arch
Left Metacarpals and Digitals }

Celiac Trunk

Left Gastric ——— Esphageal Branch

Splenic
{ Dorsal Pancreatic ——— Inferior Transverse Pancratic
Great Pancreatic
Caudal Pancreatic
Gastroepiploic
Short Gastrics }

Common Hepatic
{ Gastroduodenal
{ Posterior Superior Pancreatico-duodenal
Anterior Superior Pancreatico-duodenal }

Proper Hepatic
{ Left Hepatic
Right Hepatic
Cystic
Gastroepiploic
Supraduodenal
Intermediate Hepatic } }

Middle Suprarenal

Superior Mesenteric

Middle Colic

Inferior Pancreaticoduodenal
{ Posterior Infereior Pancreatico-duodenal
Anterior Infereior Pancreatico-duodenal }

Jejunal
Ileocolic
Appendicular
Posterior Cecal
Anterior Cecal
Marginal
Right Colic

First Order	Second Order Branch	Third Order Branch	Beyond Third Order Branches

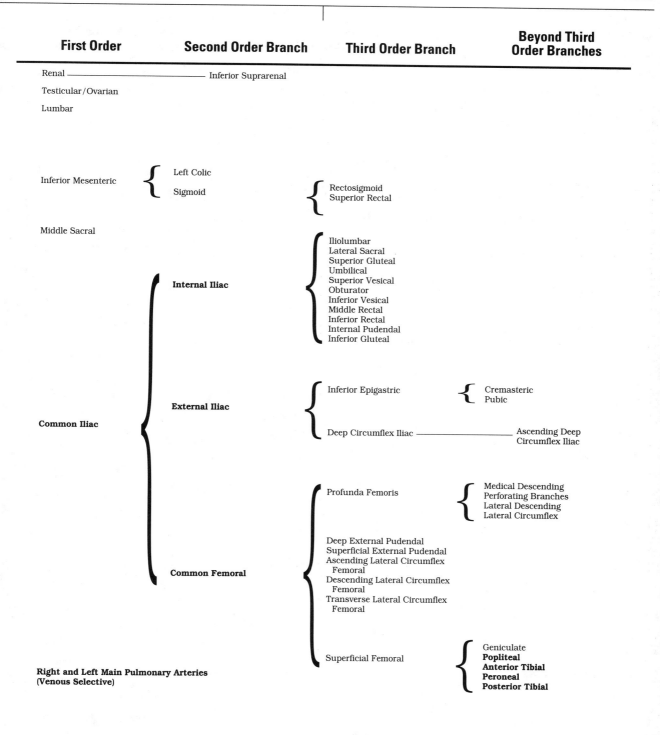

Renal —————————————— Inferior Suprarenal

Testicular/Ovarian

Lumbar

Inferior Mesenteric
{ Left Colic
  Sigmoid

Rectosigmoid
Superior Rectal

Middle Sacral

Internal Iliac
{ Iliolumbar
  Lateral Sacral
  Superior Gluteal
  Umbilical
  Superior Vesical
  Obturator
  Inferior Vesical
  Middle Rectal
  Inferior Rectal
  Internal Pudendal
  Inferior Gluteal

External Iliac
{ Inferior Epigastric
  { Cremasteric
    Pubic
  Deep Circumflex Iliac —————— Ascending Deep Circumflex Iliac

Common Iliac

Common Femoral
{ Profunda Femoris
  { Medical Descending
    Perforating Branches
    Lateral Descending
    Lateral Circumflex

  Deep External Pudendal
  Superficial External Pudendal
  Ascending Lateral Circumflex Femoral
  Descending Lateral Circumflex Femoral
  Transverse Lateral Circumflex Femoral

  Superficial Femoral
  { Geniculate
    Popliteal
    Anterior Tibial
    Peroneal
    Posterior Tibial

Right and Left Main Pulmonary Arteries (Venous Selective)

Reference: Kadir S. *Atlas of Normal and Variant Angiographic Anatomy.* Philadelphia, Pa: WB Saunders Co; 1991

APPENDIX H — CROSSWALK OF RENUMBERED CODES

This listing is a summary of the CPT 2006 codes and descriptors that have been renumbered to CPT 2007 codes.

Deleted CPT 2006 Code	CPT 2007 Code
15000	15002
15000	15004
15001	15003
15001	15005
15831	15830
15831	15847
15831	17999
17304	17311
17305	17312
17305	17314
17306	17312
17306	17314
17307	17312
17307	17314
17310	17315
19140	19300
19160	19301
19162	19302
19180	19303
19182	19304
19200	19305
19220	19306
19240	19307
25611	25606
25620	25607
25620	25608
25620	25609
26504	26390
27315	27325
27320	27326
28030	28055
33253	33254
33253	33255
33253	33256
35381	35302
35381	35303
35381	35304
35381	35305
35381	35306

Deleted CPT 2006 Code	CPT 2007 Code
35507	35506
35541	35537
35541	35538
35546	35539
35546	35540
35641	35637
35641	35638
44152	44799
44153	44799
47716	47719
48005	48105
48180	48548
49085	49402
54152	54150
54820	54865
55859	55875
56720	56442
57820	57558
67350	57346
75998	77001
76003	77002
76005	77003
76006	77071
76012	72291
76013	72292
76020	77072
76040	77073
76061	77074
76062	77075
76065	77076
76066	77077
76070	77078
76071	77079
76075	77080
76076	77081
76077	77082
76078	77083
76082	77051
76083	77052
76086	77053
76088	77054
76090	77055
76091	77056

Deleted CPT 2006 Code	CPT 2007 Code
76092	77057
76093	77058
76094	77059
76095	77031
76096	77032
76355	77011
76360	77012
76362	77013
76370	77014
76393	77021
76394	77022
76400	77084
76778	76775
76778	76776
76986	76998
78704	78707
78704	78708
78704	78709
78715	78701
78715	78707
78715	78708
78715	78709
78760	78761
92573	92700
94656	94002
94656	94004
94657	94003
94657	94004
0018T	0160T
0018T	0161T
0044T	96904
0045T	96904
0082T	77371
0082T	77372
0082T	77373
0083T	77371
0083T	77372
0083T	77373
0091T	22857
0094T	22865
0097T	22862
0120T	19105